WA 1221171 0

D1766213

ONE WEEK LOAN

REGULATION OF BREATHING

LUNG BIOLOGY IN HEALTH AND DISEASE

Executive Editor

Claude Lenfant
Director, National Heart, Lung and Blood Institute
National Institutes of Health
Bethesda, Maryland

ADDITIONAL VOLUMES IN PREPARATION

The opinions expressed in these volumes do not necessarily represent the views of the National Institutes of Health.

REGULATION OF BREATHING

SECOND EDITION
REVISED AND EXPANDED

Edited by

Jerome A. Dempsey

University of Wisconsin
Madison, Wisconsin

Allan I. Pack

University of Pennsylvania Medical Center
Philadelphia, Pennsylvania

Marcel Dekker, Inc.　　　**New York • Basel • Hong Kong**

Learning Resources
Centre
ı Z-Zı ı ᄀ ı O

Library of Congress Cataloging-in-Publication Data

Regulation of breathing / edited by Jerome A. Dempsey, Allan I. Pack.
— 2nd ed., rev. and expanded.
   p.   cm. — (Lung biology in health and disease ; 79)
   Includes bibliographical references and index.
   ISBN 0-8247-9227-0 (alk. paper)
   1. Respiration—Regulation.   I. Dempsey, Jerome A.
II. Pack, Allan I.   III. Series: Lung biology in health
and disease ; v. 79.
   [DNLM: 1. Respiration.   W1 LU62 v. 79 1994 / WF 102 R343 1994]
QP123.R425   1994
612.2—dc20
DNLM/DLC
for Library of Congress   94-3562
                                                                        CIP

The publisher offers discounts on this book when ordered in bulk quantities. For more information, write to Special Sales/Professional Marketing at the address below.

This book is printed on acid-free paper.

Copyright © 1995 by MARCEL DEKKER, INC.   All Rights Reserved.

Neither this book nor any part may be reproduced or transmitted in any form or by any means, electronic or mechanical, including photocopying, micro-filming, and recording, or by any information storage and retrieval system, without permission in writing from the publisher.

MARCEL DEKKER, INC.
270 Madison Avenue, New York, New York 10016

Current printing (last digit):
10 9 8 7 6 5 4 3 2 1

PRINTED IN THE UNITED STATES OF AMERICA

INTRODUCTION

> Since the time of Hippocrates the growth of scientific medicine has in reality been based on the study of the manner in which what we called the "nature" of the living body expresses itself in response to changes in environment, and reasserts itself in face of disturbance and injury.
>
> —J. S. Haldane, Oxford, 1920

No statement could be more correct than this, as one considers the regulation of breathing. The ancients, i.e., those who came before Galen, viewed respiration as a means to exchange heat. Galen is said to have been the first to show that the brain controls breathing. Since then, the study of the control of breathing has been an immensely fertile field of research with which some of the most respected names are associated. It is therefore not surprising that an extensive bibliography has resulted.

Now, one may ask why it is that the field has attracted so much attention and effort. Haldane gave us the answer: it is our desire to understand how we respond to changes in our environment . . . or why we do not respond! Exercise or sleep, increased or lowered barometric pressure, "pure" air or contaminated air—all constitute the environment to which we must respond through the interplay of numerous physiological mechanisms.

Over the years, the series of monographs Lung Biology in Health and Disease has included volumes concerned with the regulation of breathing, either exclusively or in part, as in the monographs on sleep and sleep disorders. But our knowledge continues to increase unabatedly as new discoveries enable us to unravel the processes that regulate breathing. Because of this, the Table of Contents of the current volume is new, and it includes topics not presented previously.

In the first edition of *Regulation of Breathing*, the editor, Dr. Thomas Hornbein, wrote in his Preface, "This monograph is filled with some science (that is, how things really work), some philosophy, and an anticipation that the best is yet to come." This new volume, edited by Drs. Jerome Dempsey and Allan Pack, will not disappoint the readership as it fulfills Dr. Hornbein's expectation.

We are grateful to Drs. Dempsey and Pack for assembling an authorship of distinction and for their effort to produce this new volume

Claude Lenfant, M.D.
Bethesda, Maryland

PREFACE

It is now 13 years since the first edition of this volume (edited by Thomas Hornbein, M.D.) was published. This extensive treatment of the subject was followed quickly by the expanded American Physiological Society Handbook series on respiration, which devoted two full volumes to the regulation of breathing. The review of the field in our current volume, some 10 years later, represents a substantial change from its predecessors, primarily because it emphasizes the striking advances made in neurobiology and its applications to the mechanisms of ventilatory control. Indeed, 14 of the 24 chapters in this second edition are predominantly devoted to neurological mechanisms, and most of the other chapters have a significant neurophysiological slant. The brain's "black boxes" of a decade ago are gradually being illuminated. For example, the current volume includes detailed outlines of the central neural pathways carrying many types of sensory input, descriptions of the basic properties of respiratory motoneurons and their efferent pathways, and even proposals for the site and model for rhythm generation in the brainstem.

Several problems discussed in the current volume were not even addressed a decade ago. These include topics such as hypothalamic contributions to respiratory motor output, the role of phrenic afferents in ventilatory control, neurotransmitter regulation of the activity of medullary respiratory neurons, and reflex regulation of upper airway patency. Even the time-honored topic of chemoreception has gained new emphasis. Mechanisms of chemosensing and transduction are detailed for the peripheral chemoreceptors, and a refreshingly new perspective and novel experimental findings are offered on "central" chemoreception—a problem that has remained relatively untouched for over a decade. The hormonal control of breathing in animal models and humans also receives extensive treatment in this volume.

Two areas of research concerned with the regulation of breathing—namely, developmental biology and sleep-disordered breathing—have expanded during the 1980s to such an extent that each now commands its own volume in the Lung Biology series. We have included three chapters in our volume devoted to current and very specific research questions within each of these research topics.

A wide variety of experimental models are currently used to study the regulation of respiration. Thus, in this book considerable emphasis is placed on the use of the isolated brainstem–spinal cord preparation, brain slice preparations from the hypothalamus and medulla, and the use of microdialysis and iontophoresis to study neurotransmitter regulatory mechanisms. Innovative techniques at the whole-animal level have been applied in the unanesthetized state, including anatomical separation of the circulation to the carotid chemoreceptors from the systemic and cerebral circulations and in vivo recording from brainstem medullary neurons. Additional models have been developed to provide further understanding of human ventilatory control, including the use of evoked potentials to study the role of the higher central nervous system (CNS) in receiving sensory input and the use of patients with specific neurological lesions in the CNS to study central mechanisms of load compensation or those with lung and/or heart transplantation to determine the effects of cardiopulmonary reflexes on ventilatory control in the human. Studies during REM sleep reveal the powerful effects of a changing CNS "state" on ventilatory control in animals and humans.

Some classic and still controversial problems in the regulation of breathing are also revisited in this volume. These classic topics include causes of respiratory failure, mechanisms of exercise hyperpnea and the sensations of dyspnea, and the inextricable coupling of alveolar ventilation to metabolism. Many important new findings and perspectives have been added to these difficult questions; however, the definitive evidence pointing to the underlying major mechanism(s) remains elusive.

We are especially fortunate and proud to have Dr. Stephen Marsh Tenney provide the introductory background for this second edition as he did for the first. Dr. Tenney has been a major contributor to our field for four decades and has directly influenced the careers of many of the authors in this second edition.

We are grateful to Mr. Daniel Barrett and Ms. Gundula Birong for their organizational expertise and efforts in compiling this volume. We are especially indebted to the outside reviewers who very generously provided peer evaluation of the manuscripts. Finally, we thank Dr. Claude Lenfant for his patience and his encouragement throughout this past year.

Jerome A. Dempsey
Allan I. Pack

CONTRIBUTORS

Dorothy M. Ainsworth, D.V.M., Ph.D. Assistant Professor of Medicine, Department of Clinical Sciences–NYSCVM, Cornell University, Ithaca, New York

Robert B. Banzett, Ph.D. Associate Professor, Physiology Program, Harvard School of Public Health, Boston, Massachusetts

Alia R. Bazzy-Asaad, M.D. Associate Professor of Pediatrics, Department of Pediatrics, Section of Respiratory Medicine, Yale University School of Medicine, New Haven, Connecticut

Mark C. Bellingham, Ph.D. Senior Research Fellow, Department of Physiology and Biophysics, University of Washington School of Medicine, Seattle, Washington

Albert J. Berger, Ph.D. Professor, Department of Physiology and Biophysics, University of Washington School of Medicine, Seattle, Washington

Gerald E. Bisgard, D.V.M., Ph.D. Professor, Department of Comparative Biosciences, University of Wisconsin, Madison, Wisconsin

Eugene N. Bruce, Ph.D.   Professor, Center for Biomedical Engineering, University of Kentucky, Lexington, Kentucky

J. Andrew Daubenspeck, Ph.D.   Professor, Department of Physiology, Dartmouth Medical School, Lebanon, New Hampshire

Paul W. Davenport, Ph.D.   Associate Professor, Department of Physiological Sciences, University of Florida, Gainesville, Florida

Richard O. Davies, D.V.M., Ph.D.   Professor of Physiology, Department of Animal Biology, School of Veterinary Medicine, University of Pennsylvania, Philadelphia, Pennsylvania

Michael S. Dekin, Ph.D.   Assistant Professor, Department of Medicine, UMDNJ–Robert Wood Johnson Medical School, New Brunswick, New Jersey

Jerome A. Dempsey, Ph.D.   Professor, Department of Preventive Medicine, University of Wisconsin, Madison, Wisconsin

Bruce G. Dinger, Ph.D.   Research Associate, Department of Physiology, University of Utah School of Medicine, Salt Lake City, Utah

David F. Donnelly, Ph.D.   Research Scientist, Department of Pediatrics, Section of Respiratory Medicine, Yale University School of Medicine, New Haven, Connecticut

Dwain L. Eckberg, M.D.   Professor, Departments of Medicine and Physiology, Hunter Holmes McGuire Department of Veterans Affairs Medical Center, and Medical College of Virginia, Richmond, Virginia

Sandra J. England, Ph.D.   Associate Professor, Department of Pediatrics, UMDNJ–Robert Wood Johnson Medical School, New Brunswick, New Jersey

Jack L. Feldman, Ph.D.   Professor of Neurosciences, Department of Physiological Science, University of California at Los Angeles, Los Angeles, California

Salvatore J. Fidone, Ph.D.   Professor and Acting Chairman, Department of Physiology, University of Utah School of Medicine, Salt Lake City, Utah

Hubert V. Forster, Ph.D.   Professor, Department of Physiology, Medical College of Wisconsin, Milwaukee, Wisconsin

Henry Gautier   Professor, Department of Physiology, Faculty of Medicine St. Antoine, Paris, France

Tapan K. Ghosh, Ph.D.   Research Associate, Department of Pediatrics, East Carolina University School of Medicine, Greenville, North Carolina

Constancio Gonzalez, M.D., Ph.D.   Professor, Department of Physiology and Biochemistry, University of Valladolid, Valladolid, Spain

Gabriel G. Haddad, M.D. Professor of Pediatrics and Cellular and Molecular Physiology, Department of Pediatrics, and Director, Section of Respiratory Medicine, Yale University School of Medicine, New Haven, Connecticut

Bernard Hannhart, M.D. Unité 14 de Recherche de Physiopathologie Respiratoire, Laboratoire INSERM, Vandoeuvre-les-Nancy, France

Rolf D. Hubmayr, M.D., F.C.C.P. Professor of Medicine and Director of Thoracic Diseases Research Unit, Division of Pulmonary and Critical Care Medicine, Mayo Clinic and Mayo Medical School, Rochester, Minnesota

Yves Jammes Professor of Physiology and Head of Laboratory, URA 1630 CNRS "Physiopathologie Respiratoire," Jean Roche Institute Faculty of Medicine, Marseilles, France

Marc P. Kaufman, Ph.D. Professor, Departments of Internal Medicine and Human Physiology, University of California—Davis, Davis, California

Leszek Kubin, Ph.D. Research Assistant Professor, Department of Animal Biology, School of Veterinary Medicine, University of Pennsylvania, Philadelphia, Pennsylvania

Robert W. Lansing, Ph.D. Professor, Department of Psychology, University of Arizona, Tucson, Arizona

J. C. Leiter, M.D. Associate Professor, Departments of Physiology and Medicine, Dartmouth Medical School, Lebanon, New Hampshire

Richard J. Martin, M.D. Professor, Department of Pediatrics, Case Western Reserve University, Cleveland, Ohio

Oommen P. Mathew, M.B.B.S., F.A.A.P. Professor, Department of Pediatrics-Neonatology, East Carolina University School of Medicine, Greenville, North Carolina

Donald R. McCrimmon, Ph.D. Associate Professor, Departments of Physiology and Anesthesia, Northwestern University Medical School, Chicago, Illinois

Martha J. Miller, M.D., Ph.D. Associate Professor of Neonatology, Department of Pediatrics, Case Western Reserve University, Cleveland, Ohio

Gordon S. Mitchell, Ph.D. Professor of Comparative Bioscience and Neuroscience, University of Wisconsin, Madison, Wisconsin

Lorna G. Moore, Ph.D. Professor, Departments of Anthropology and Medicine, University of Colorado Health Sciences Center and University of Colorado at Denver, Denver, Colorado

Jacopo P. Mortola, M.D.   Professor, Department of Physiology, McGill University, Montreal, Quebec, Canada

Eugene E. Nattie, M.D.   Professor, Department of Physiology, Dartmouth Medical School, Lebanon, New Hampshire

Judith A. Neubauer, Ph.D.   Associate Professor of Medicine, UMDNJ–Robert Wood Johnson Medical School, New Brunswick, New Jersey

Allan I. Pack, M.B., Ch.B., Ph.D.   Professor of Medicine and Director, Center for Sleep and Respiratory Neurobiology, University of Pennsylvania Medical Center, Philadelphia, Pennsylvania

James P. Porter, Ph.D.   Associate Professor, Department of Physiology, University of Louisville School of Medicine, Louisville, Kentucky

Roger L. Reep, Ph.D.   Associate Professor, Department of Physiological Sciences, University of Florida, Gainesville, Florida

Steven A. Shea, B.Sc., Ph.D.   Assistant Professor, Physiology Program, Harvard School of Public Health, Boston, Massachusetts

Gary C. Sieck, Ph.D.   Professor, Departments of Anesthesiology, Physiology, and Biophysics, Mayo Clinic and Mayo Medical School, Rochester, Minnesota

Jeffrey C. Smith, Ph.D.   Associate Professor, Department of Physiological Science, University of California at Los Angeles, Los Angeles, California

Dexter F. Speck, Ph.D.   Associate Professor, Department of Physiology, University of Kentucky, Lexington, Kentucky

Koichiro Tatsumi, M.D., Ph.D.   Department of Chest Medicine, School of Medicine, Chiba University, Chiba, Japan

S. Marsh Tenney, M.D.   Nathan Smith Professor of Physiology, Emeritus, Department of Physiology, Dartmouth Medical School, Lebanon, New Hampshire

Tony G. Waldrop, Ph.D.   Professor, Departments of Physiology and Biophysics, University of Illinois College of Medicine, Urbana, Illinois

Magdy Younes, M.D., F.R.C.P.(C), Ph.D.   Professor, Head of Respiratory Diseases, Department of Internal Medicine, University of Manitoba, Winnipeg, Manitoba, Canada

CONTENTS

Part II: CENTRAL NERVOUS CONTROL

Jack L. Feldman and Jeffrey C. Smith

Albert J. Berger and Mark C. Bellingham

Donald R. McCrimmon, Michael S. Dekin,
and Gordon S. Mitchell

Part One

OVERVIEW

1

The Control of Breathing: An Uninhibited Survey from the Perspective of Comparative Physiology

S. MARSH TENNEY and J. C. LEITER

Dartmouth Medical School
Lebanon, New Hampshire

I. Introduction

Textbooks of comparative physiology, even monographs on comparative respiratory physiology, are, with few exceptions, neglectful of the control of breathing. That omission cannot be said to come about because there is no information, although it cannot be denied that most of our current understanding of mechanisms that operate in the control system is based on experiments with common laboratory mammals. The literature on the control of breathing in submammalian vertebrates, and in invertebrates, has tended to be more descriptive than analytical or explanatory. In large measure, however, the task of surveying the relevant body of knowledge is still limited to identifying interspecific differences in behavior and response of receptors and reflexes and pathways and, above all else, in speculating about the evolution of the system and its components. That is, the strategy of comparative physiology is to examine features of organisms of different kinds, responsive to short-term changes of condition (stimulus-response characteristics), but also to long-term changes of adaptive significance when the changed condition (usually environmental) is prolonged.

In the past decade, a number of reviews of the comparative control of breathing have appeared, and taken altogether, the literature of the field can be regarded as having been thoroughly covered (1–11). Careful reading of these reviews reveals a frequent occurrence throughout of expressions such as "the location and functional significance remains far from clear," or "the reasons for this are not clear," or "the exact stimulus has yet to be determined," and so forth. In short, few fundamental mechanisms emerge to establish a foundation of comparative principles, but at a more superficial level of understanding, a continuum of some of the operational features can be glimpsed, or postulated. Even for this trivial synthesis, however, the wide variability of responses found in similar animals demands caution in interpretation. Given the existence of so many readily available, comprehensive reviews, our approach in this overview will be to set forth speculations, hypotheses, questions, and, rarely, conclusions that strike us as useful guidelines in thinking about the comparative control of breathing. Our aim has been to emphasize similarities to a greater extent than differences, the intent being to try to discern a thread of continuity in the ways a problem may be solved—sometimes by innovation, more often by modification of an underlying mechanism. The list is not exhaustive, but it is representative. The organization of what follows is traditional by stages of evolutionary progress, but a seesaw strategy has been adopted for discussion of phenomena, anticipatory of a later reappearance when a mechanism is introduced, reflective, later, of its origin and history. The references have been confined to a few, to document a point, or, if the topic has not been elaborated in existing reviews, the citations may be more extensive. The sources for our remarks can generally be found in the extensive bibliographies of the aforementioned reviews.

II. Primitive Precursors of Chemoreception

Among the variety of chemotropisms, oxygen is one that appears to attract certain invertebrate organisms (12). A similar effect is achieved in young tadpoles (13) and embryo fish whose tail muscles are excited to twitch in response to hypoxia (14), setting them into heightened motion. This leads to an apparent attractiveness of a region of high oxygen concentration, but more accurately, it is because the region of low oxygen concentration stimulates a motor activity that causes an excited random movement. This raises the probability that the organism will enter a region of higher oxygen concentration—if one exists—where the stimulus to move about is reduced, and the appearance is that of being attracted by the oxygen. This is the first, and most primitive, example of a connection between a somatomotor and respiratory response—a theme that will recur repeatedly.

       An example more specifically oriented toward a respiratory purpose can be found in those crustaceans in which the swimmerets, appendages for propelling the animal, are importantly employed to fan water over the respiratory surface (15), and in *Limulus*, the legs irrigate the respiratory surface, the central nervous system serving to coordinate locomotor and respiratory motions (16). Their beat frequency is quickened in hypoxic water. The waving and beating motions of the hind end of certain marine invertebrates (17) also fulfill a function akin to ventilation. At any respiratory surface, especially in an aqueous medium, there will be an unstirred layer that acts to increase the distance through which a respiratory molecule must travel by diffusion and thus reduces its conductance. The waving and fanning motions stir the medium and thereby reduce the partial pressure gradient (say, for oxygen).

The resemblance of oxygen tropism, and of the action of hypoxia on specialized movements that favor oxygen supply by diffusion, to chemoreceptor-mediated ventilatory drive in higher organisms invites speculation regarding analogy. However, nothing can be said about specific receptor or transducer mechanisms in these primitive organisms—only that, at the lowest levels of the animal kingdom, if oxygen is important to their survival, regulatory responses to environmental deficiency have evolved. They constitute a first step in the long path leading to the ventilatory control system of birds and mammals.

III. Primitive Ventilation and Opportunistic Employment

Size quickly becomes a limiting factor for organisms that depend solely on diffusion for their oxygen supply. The addition of convection becomes necessary, and among marine invertebrates the case of the sea cucumber is instructive (18), because the primitive "water lung" of these creatures is an example of a minor structural adaptation in an organ system primarily designed for one function that allows it to take on another. The surface of the cloaca has been modified by the introduction of "respiratory trees," which make a specialized respiratory surface that accounts for about 60% of the total oxygen uptake; the remainder is absorbed through the body surface. Convective flow is produced by a kind of peristaltic motion. A succession of cloacal contractions drives water into the animal, and this is then followed by a bodily contraction that ejects the accumulated water. If the water is hypoxic, it is pumped into the animal in the normal manner, but then, instead of being expelled, there follows a series of rapid influxes and effluxes on top of the accumulated volume. In this condition, the animal has increased in volume [equivalent to the effect of hypoxia to increase lung volume in snakes (19) and functional residual capacity in mammals?], and the pumping rate is increased. When the P_{O_2} of the water falls below 90 torr, the pumping rate decreases, or may stop, at which point the animal, inflated with a volume of stored oxygenated water, moves to a new location. Clearly, some sort of chemoreceptor mechanism is at work, and probably, a mechanism that coordinates the motor phenomena and sphincter control, but whether this requires a neural system or is simply a property of the smooth muscle is not known. Although, there is no basic information on either the chemodetection or manner of effector response, the oxygen-mediated responses depend on where the hypoxic stimulus is applied. Contact at the anterior end only increases the pumping rate but does not influence expulsion, whereas if the respiratory trees alone are made hypoxic, the rhythm becomes variable, and the expulsion rate becomes gradual.

Primitive though this organism is, its crude ventilatory system and elementary respiratory surface manifest some surprising features characteristic of a controlled system that even displays optimization of response. It can also be argued that respiratory function in the holothurians has evolved "opportunistically"; i.e., it has been grafted onto another system (it should not pass without notice that the "other" system is the alimentary tract, the same organ system out of which, further along in evolution, some primitive fish created a lung out of a diverticulum) whose apparatus fulfills the basic requirements that would otherwise have to be created de novo. In various ways, such opportunism may be regarded as a minor principle of the evolution of the respiratory apparatus and its control.

Although mechanical ventilation of the respiratory apparatus of aquatic, pulmonate snails resembles that of the holothurians—tidal ventilation of a cavity in which gas exchange occurs by diffusion across a specialized respiratory surface—snails also demonstrate more complex respiratory behaviors that are subject to control by oxygen. Gas exchange in the freshwater, pond snail, *Lymnaea stagnalis*, can occur through the skin, but the major organ of gas exchange is the mantle cavity. Access to the mantle cavity is controlled by opener and closer muscles in the pneumostome. The respiratory cycle consists of a series of stereotypical behaviors: the animal migrates to the surface, protrudes the mantle margin above the water surface, opens the pneumostome, muscles surrounding the mantle cavity compress the cavity, the cavity expands passively, the pneumostome closes, and the snail descends into the water. The cycle of pneumostome opening, mantle compression, and pneumostome closure may be repeated more than once during each visit to the surface of the water (20,21). If the Po_2 of the water is reduced or the inspiratory gas is made hypoxic, the snail returns to the surface with greater frequency and ventilates the mantle cavity for longer times. Experiments in which the Po_2 of the water and the Po_2 of the gas in the mantle were varied independently, or the atmospheric pressure was varied, demonstrated that the snails responded to the mantle cavity and skin Po_2 and the volume in the mantle cavity, but not to the hemolymph Po_2 (20,22). These findings demonstrate the presence of "peripheral" O_2 receptors and mechanoreceptors that sense the loss in buoyancy associated with reduced lung volume or the actual change in lung volume as oxygen is removed from the mantle cavity during a dive. The location of the cell bodies of the oxygen chemoreceptors has not been identified, but the neuronal effects of hypoxic chemoreceptor stimulation ramify throughout the nervous system of the snail, modifying respiratory muscle function, locomotion, and other reflexes. For example, when snails have a higher mantle Po_2, they are positively geotactic: they head toward the bottom of the pond; when hypoxic, they are negatively geotactic: they head for the surface (23). Orientation of the snails in a gravitational field depends on the function of statocysts located in the ganglia of these snails, and the variation in orientation and movement of the snails as a function of Po_2 in the mantle resembles the oxygen tropism of unicellular organisms, embryonic fish, and amphibian larvae discussed above. The most striking feature of the hypoxic response is the coordination, by reciprocal neuronal inhibition of motor neurons (24), of a number of motor behaviors all aimed, directly or indirectly, at enhancing oxygen availability.

The respiratory behavior of *L. stagnalis* follows a sequential pattern of motor behaviors, and only one behavior is present at a time: locomotion, for example, is inhibited during pneumostomal movements (21). In contrast, locusts demonstrate coordinated, parallel respiratory and locomotor activities. The respiratory rhythm is generated by a central pattern generator found primarily within the third thoracic ganglion, although there may be other subsidiary central pattern generators in the abdominal ganglia of the locust (25). The central pattern generator can function without afferent information, but afferent information does modify the frequency and some aspects of the coordination of the output of the central pattern generator. The central pattern generator controls the pattern of active abdominal compression during expiration (inspiration is passive), and the central pattern generator coordinates spiracular function to create unidirectional tracheolar ventilation (26). The coordination of flight and ventilation is strikingly similar in flying insects and vertebrates. Ventilatory-locomotor interactions in vertebrates are discussed subsequently.

Flight in insects is, like ventilation, sustained by a flight central pattern generator located primarily in the third thoracic ganglion of the locust; here as well, there may be subsidiary central pattern generators demonstrable in experiments in which the connectives between adjacent ganglia are severed (27,28). In intact animals, the central pattern generator functions like a single, dispersed polyganglionic neural network consisting of segmentally homologous interneurons (29). During flight two things occur: the rhythm of the flight central pattern generator is manifest in the motoneurons of ventilatory muscles (30), and the rhythm of the respiratory central pattern generator is manifest in the motor neurons of the flight muscle (31). Miller (32) found that spiracles 2 and 3, which control access to the tracheolar system in the region of the wings, were open during established flight and fluttered at the wing beat frequency, whereas the abdominal spiracles opened and closed without manifesting the wing beat frequency, even though the wing beat frequency is apparent in the electrical activity of abdominal, ventilatory motor neurons (30). It is tempting to view this coordination of flight and respiratory rhythms as an adaptation that optimizes the function of two independent central pattern generators to enhance gas exchange. However, we are not aware of any quantitative demonstration that ventilation is optimized by the superimposition of the wing beat rhythm on spiracular opening and closing, and intermittent inhibition of thoracic spiracular opening in phase with the wing beat during expiration, when the thoracic spiracles should be open, does not seem functionally appropriate (30). Based on a review of the fossil record and wing morphology, Kukalova-Peck concluded that insect wings evolved from a segment of the upper leg that may have functioned as a tracheal gill in primitive aquatic insects (33). These "pro-wings" may also have had other ventilatory and loco-motor functions, perhaps like swimmerets in Crustacea (34). Does this imply that the flight and respiratory central pattern generators in insects had a common, ancestral central pattern generator? It is interesting that the dominant interneurons in the central pattern generators of flight and respiration reside in the same ganglia. If true, the coordination of respiration and flight in insects, in which the muscles of locomotion derived from respiratory muscles, is the inverse of the coordination of respiration and flight in vertebrates, in which the muscles of ventilation probably derived from muscles of locomotion and posture. In any event, this extended speculation suggests that the coordination between ventilation and locomotion ought not be interpreted too quickly as evidence of optimization and adaptation: the coordination may indicate more about evolutionary history than about adaptive optimization (35).

IV. Gill Ventilation

External gills are merely bathed in the aqueous medium and are not the object of any specific control mechanism, but when the gills are internalized, an elaborate flow-through system is established with requirements for sophisticated control. Sessile organisms do not have high demands for oxygen supply, but fish are, for the most part, active swimmers with high oxygen requirements, and, therefore, the pumping mechanism that ventilates the gills must operate to produce high flow rates. The burden imposed by water as the respiratory medium is substantial, because its viscosity and density are high, and its oxygen capacity is low. The mechanical design must be refined if the respiratory purpose is to be well served (36), but there must also be a control system capable of coordinating the movements of the component parts and of regulating pump performance to match changing load, which may be introduced as either increased oxygen demand or diminished oxygen supply in the medium.

To these ends, a motor mechanism driven from the central nervous system by a rhythm generator ensures a regular breathing pattern that does not depend for its activation on a stimulating afferent input. Autorhythmic discharge persists in fish after deafferentation of the respiratory centers of the medulla, as was first demonstrated in goldfish (37), thus establishing the intrinsic character of the pacemaker. However, many factors may modulate its rhythm: chemical and mechanical afferent inputs from the periphery; descending influences on the respiratory center from more rostral regions of the brain; chemical environment of the central neurons (38).

Mechanoreceptors in the gills sense pressure, and by this means, flow can be monitored. The sensory input from the receptors travels over cranial nerves IX and X and is inhibitory on the rhythm generator and can exert an important influence on the economy of energy expenditure best illustrated in the phenomenon of ram ventilation. A fast-swimming fish has only to hold its mouth open to maintain an effective flow of water over the gill surface. The process of shifting from active to ram ventilation may proceed gradually, but the net effect is to reduce the amount of energy consumed by the gill muscles with a net gain of that available for the swimming muscles. More subtle effects on the breathing pattern can be found in many fish, but there is a wide variation in the potency of proprioceptive feedback, and there is an unexplained difference between elasmobranchs and teleosts in this regard (8). Further, if the gills of elasmobranchs are deafferented by cutting cranial nerves IX and X, the frequency of gill movements increases, but in teleosts, there is no effect. In mammals, vagotomy slows the respiratory rhythm, but it quickens if the brainstem is cut subsequently at the pontomedullary junction. The same procedure in elasmobranchs is without effect. The mammalian experiments suggest the presence of descending influences on the rhythm generator, a possibility also in teleosts, but in elasmobranchs, the inference is that such influences do not exist. How these findings fit into the evolution of proprioceptive feedback in ventilatory control is not clear, but the growing complexity of the brain inevitably complicates the phenomenology of reflex responses.

The essential fact is that in aquatic breathers, the central rhythm generator activates a regular breathing pattern, but it still cannot be said whether the mechanism originates in pacemaker cells or whether it is based on a neural network the components of which interact to produce a stable output.

V. Air Breathing Appears

With the advent of air breathing, a radical change occurred in the breathing pattern. Regular breathing disappeared, and the pattern became irregular. Evolution of air breathing appeared very early, and lungs are found in most primitive fish. Gills also were adapted to hold pockets of air that could provide a source for oxygen supply if the waters became hypoxic; diverticula of the buccal or opercular cavities became either lungs or swim bladder, structures that can be regarded as homologous with the lungs of tetrapods. Ventilation of these air-containing organs was achieved by positive-pressure filling that utilized the same muscles as in the old gill ventilation mechanism. Therefore, the origin of the significant change in rhythm is not to be found in the periphery, but in the central nervous system. Since these fish are bimodal breathers, and the gill mechanism is regular, but the lung mechanism is irregular, the evidence seems to point to two central pattern generators, one branchial, the other pulmonary. The latter appears to function as an "on demand" mechanism. It is activated when the water ceases to be an adequate source of oxygen. With the stimulus to breathe air, the gill mechanism may be inhibited in some, but not all, air-breathing fish—a response, when it occurs, that is opposite to the stimulating effect of hypoxia on gill movement in purely aquatic breathers. It is possible that the generator for air breathing existed originally, but in a dormant state; however, in those fish that encountered increasingly hypoxic waters, or were subject to environments with periodic drought, increased afferent traffic from the peripheral chemoreceptors brought the dormant cells above their threshold for excitation and thereby activated a quiescent neuronal population. In present-day lung fish, air breathing is initiated only with chemoafferent drive.

A single generator to pace gill movement that produces a nearly continuous flow of water can be of simpler design than what may be required for a tidal pattern of inspiration:expiration, but the introduction of the air mode increases the likelihood of connections between the two generators, although evidence for reciprocal inhibition is lacking. Lung inflation, via stretch receptors, affects pulmonary ventilation but not gill ventilation. Hypoxia has a more pronounced effect on the air-breathing pattern generator than on the gill generator, and it further dominates the control by a descending inhibition (39). There is no evidence for an inhibitory connection of the gill generator on the lung generator.

In air-breathing fish, the lungs relay proprioceptive information over the vagus, but determining the influence on breathing pattern is complicated by the fact that the normal rhythm is irregular. It is generally accepted that lung inflation inhibits air breathing, but whether lung inflation also inhibits gill breathing depends on the species studied. Lung deflation stimulates air breathing. Both slowly and rapidly adapting mechanoreceptors have been identified in the lungs, but their individual and combined roles remain unspecified. The control of expiratory and inspiratory timing to regulate frequency and tidal volume is an important role of pulmonary proprioceptors in mammals, but although the effects can be found in air-breathing fish and teleosts, it is difficult to see their significance in a force-pump mechanism, which requires a number of strokes to fill the lung and which operates with long times for filling, followed by a period of arrested breathing and emptying when the fish surfaces. The control over volume without reference to timing and breathing pattern is important for the respiratory function of the lung, but it may be even more so for nonrespiratory functions such as buoyancy. Proprioceptive information as lung volume shrinks during breath-holding undoubtedly contributes, along with chemoreceptor activity, to send an excitatory signal indicating that it is time to take a new breath.

Although the muscular mechanism in fish for air and water breathing is basically the same, the operation of the former "on demand" suggests a close analogy with feeding, which also is activated only when necessary and is, therefore, irregular. In fact, the force-pump ventilatory mechanism may have evolved from the swallowing mechanism. The close association of feeding and respiration in the structural and functional apparatus of both leads naturally to some common properties. It is noteworthy that internal gills may have evolved from the gills of protovertebrate filter feeders and were really a part of the alimentary tract but took on respiratory function as they were increasingly vascularized, and, as already noted, the lungs developed as outgrowths from the esophagus. So, the neuroreflex control system governing the muscles of force-pump breathing has an ancient lineage, which undoubtedly carries over features of the old as it evolves to perform new functions. Archaic remnants persist throughout evolutionary progression and are often regarded as inexplicable if seen only in a contemporary scheme of things.

VI. Invasion of the Land

Terrestrial vertebrates probably evolved from Crossopterygian fish, and it has been said that adaptation to life on land is a story of limbs and lungs. The central pattern generator in amphibians controls buccal and glottal movements and adds control of the nostrils, which must be closed when the floor of the mouth rises to force air into the lungs. The lung inflation mechanism is similar to that of air-breathing fish, and the rhythm is, likewise, irregular. For the same reason as in fish, two central pattern generators can be inferred in amphibians. The buccal movements (whose ancestor is the branchial apparatus) are driven by the primordial rhythm generator, but air breathing is dependent on a well-developed pattern generator that is responsive to chemoreceptor activation. The muscular mechanism is the same in both instances, but the rhythmic flushing of air in and out of the mouth (sniffing?) is replaced, in coordination with proper valving, by lung inflation. The African clawed frog (*Xenopus laevis*) is wholly aquatic but surfaces frequently to breathe when the water is hypoxic; the frogs of Lake Titicaca (*Telmatobius*) are also wholly aquatic, but they have only rudimentary lungs, which are of no use. *Telmatobius* depends wholly on cutaneous gas exchange and has evolved with oversize skin that hangs baggily on its body and flaps when the frog swims, slightly stirring the adjacent water layer. When hypoxic, these frogs settle on some surface under the water and execute "pushups" with the effect of stirring more vigorously the water next to their skin (40). This peculiar behavioral trait is probably another primitive example of the close relationship of postural and locomotor muscles to breathing. Somatic muscles seem to be activated by hypoxia in the examples mentioned earlier of "oxygen tropism" in embryo fish and tadpoles, and now, in an adult amphibian, of a more directly applicable respiratory response. It will be seen subsequently, further along the evolutionary path, that these skeletal muscles play more specific ventilatory roles when they can be utilized directly in an opportunistic way or modified appropriately. The linkage of limb muscles with respiratory drive is initially seen in the context of available means to implement a ventilatory act, but when that function can be performed more efficiently by other mechanisms (birds and mammals) evidence for the old linkage can still be found, and its significance in the complex of factors controlling breathing in exercise is especially apparent (41).

Weak and variable ventilatory responses to CO_2 are found in amphibians. Bimodal breathers, in contrast with purely aquatic breathers, carry a higher P_{CO_2} in their blood as a consequence of its equilibrium status with residual air in the lungs. Although this introduces the possibility of utilizing CO_2 as a controller signal, the fact that CO_2 exchange is almost entirely mediated through the skin makes it largely irrelevant as a guide for pulmonary ventilation to regulate CO_2 homeostasis. Hypoxia is a more significant stimulus to breathe, and there are peripheral chemoreceptors in the carotid labyrinth. In the case of oxygen uptake, the lungs play a predominant role, but if the inspired air is low in oxygen, and ventilation is somewhat stimulated, the more important effect is to elicit vaso-constriction in the pulmonary circulation and to shunt blood to the skin (42). It is this useful response in amphibians that carries over in mammals, where hypoxic pulmonary vasoconstriction not only serves no useful purpose, but is properly regarded as pathophysiological. Control over the site of gas exchange is thus mediated through control of perfusion to a greater extent than by ventilation in this instance, but if the ambient water is hypoxic, the effect is to stimulate pulmonary ventilation.

Amphibian lungs are innervated by the vagus, and there are, as in air-breathing fish, both slowly and rapidly adapting proprioceptors responsive to volume (pressure and tension), which, when stretched, send inhibitory signals to the brainstem. This mechanism limits the degree of inflation (if vagotomized, the lungs are pumped up to large volumes) and must be regarded as a Hering-Breuer reflex, but it is different in the sense that it works in a system that does not operate with an in-out, tidal regime, but, instead, fills over a considerable period of time before emptying. This carries implications for the adaptive characteristics of the receptors (it would be disastrous if they completely adapted within the normal filling time), and in amphibians, close control over the timing of expiration is of little consequence. The "patterning" of a respiratory cycle, a mechanism impor-tant in the control of tidal breathers, probably exists in the unrefined central pattern generator of amphibians, but its operation is largely restricted to nothing more than turning on and turning off the pulmonary force pump. End-inspiratory volume, therefore, is surely regulated, although it is probable that the duration of the end-inspiratory pause is, as well. Further refinements, like timing the duration of each inspiration, are less likely.

VII. Reptiles and Aspiration Breathing

The reptilian central nervous organization for the control of breathing is similar to that of amphibians, but the buccal mechanism is less important, and inflation of the lungs by aspiration is introduced. Regulation of the size of tidal volume is more readily achieved than is possible with the force-pump mechanism alone, but the rhythm remains irregular, as in amphibians. It is a curious fact that the rhythm becomes regular in turtles and alligators if they are decerebrated, suggesting that higher mechanisms operating to exercise a command function normally dominate the more caudal, autorhythmic centers. (Could this represent severing the connection between the two pattern generators postulated to exist in air-breathing fish? If so, the old gill motor mechanism would have been replaced, or at least, new central nervous arrangements in proximity to the gill pattern generator—possibly those for limb movements in terrestrial locomotion—would have occurred.) In the evolution of control, a developing hierarchical structure is apparent, in which each new level in the process of gradual cephalization introduces a mechanism capable of suppressing the activity at the next lower level, which, in turn, may itself have superseded (by inhibiting) the level below it. In mammals, for example, there exist in the spinal cord neurons capable of generating a respiratory rhythm (especially apparent in newborn animals), but they are suppressed by the medullary respiratory rhythmicity (which has an inherent rate higher than that in the cord) especially with maturation, and higher yet, voluntary effort can either arrest or increase breathing. It is a moot point whether volition is analogous with whatever it is in the turtle brain, situated rostral to the medulla, that accounts for decerebrate changes of breathing pattern, but breath holding at the start of submergence if not willed, is at least a conditioned response.

Seals, naturally, have an irregular pattern, because much of their time is spent in a breath-hold dive, but when they are on land, the pattern is also irregular, possibly revealing an always active command mechanism.

The main characteristic of hierarchical schemes is the introduction of successive inhibitory mechanisms, but when excitatory stimuli are introduced, the change in breathing pattern is to regularity, a phenomenon found in amphibians and reptiles under strong chemical drive. It is curious that ventilation in reptiles is decreased when hyperoxic air is breathed, but in general, hypoxia is a weak stimulus. The threshold for hypoxic response, when it does occur, varies inversely with the individual's anaerobic capacity, which says something about the relationship of response to need, but nothing at all about the chemoreceptor mechanism that sets the threshold to conform.

The reptilian ventilatory mechanism is complex and involves limb movements and contraction of pectoral and abdominal muscles; in those with ribs, the intercostals are an efficient power source. These contractions are all closely coordinated, as are the glottis opener and closer muscles. The ventilatory mechanism and the sequence of events in a ventilatory cycle vary a great deal among the reptiles, but in none is the neuroreflex control fully understood.

The respiratory rhythm in amphibians and reptiles can be regularized by raising body temperature, and it can be made irregular in mammals if they are cooled or in hibernation. Can this possibly mean that the difference in respiratory rhythm between mammals and air-breathing ectotherms is only a consequence of different body temperatures? If so, it must be a property of the second pattern generator, since the one that serves water-breathing fish is regular when cool. It is possible that a rising temperature leads to a regular rhythm, because the pacemaker (?) cells in the rhythm generator are primarily affected and dominate the system by this means. Alternatively, the hypothesized, more rostral generator, which commands the air-breathing mode, could be considered to have its neurons intermingled with those that become involved in the temperature-regulating mechanism of homeotherms. Hyperpnea in hyperthermic mammals and birds is dependent on descending excitatory influences acting on the medullary respiratory centers. Many ectotherms can manifest some crude temperature regulation (mostly behavioral), and they do become febrile when infected. Therefore, the effect of heat to regularize breathing in amphibians and reptiles could, in fact, reflect increased activity in a facilitatory neuronal pool comparable to that located in the hypothalamus of endotherms. The molding and folding of the evolving brain rearranges the location of fibers and centers to establish new relationships that lead to new functional patterns. The fact that "centers" are never discrete entities means that a region having a particular name is really made up of a heterogeneous population, but their respective functions may exhibit complementarity. Consider an elevation of body temperature, and the fact that it leads to an increase of metabolism. A ventilatory response would follow from chemoreceptor stimulation, but the fact is that the ventilatory response in endotherms is far greater because of descending facilitatory influences from the hypothalamic region for temperature control onto the medullary respiratory center. The response to hypoxia has features in common with this. Chemoreceptor afferents in hypoxia terminate not only on the respiratory center, but also in the hypothalamus where a descending facilitatory influence is initiated (43). The polypnea of hyperthermia and of hypoxia in chemodenervated cats is inhibited by CO_2 (44). These phenomena in mammals may have their roots in the organization of the premammalian brain, prior to mechanisms for controlling body temperature, but important in stimulating ventilation when body temperature is elevated.

VIII. Central Chemoreceptors

As noted above, once animals invaded the land, they entered an environment with abundant oxygen, where high levels of ventilation are no longer necessary to obtain adequate oxygen. Furthermore, CO_2 removal becomes significantly more difficult. Once air breathing is established as the dominant mechanism of gas exchange, there is a quasireciprocal relationship between P_{CO_2} and P_{O_2}. The particular value of P_{CO_2} is probably unimportant so long as adequate oxygenation is maintained, but whatever the particular P_{CO_2} value, it must be well defended because of the effect of CO_2 on acid-base balance. Defending acid-base balance presents significant problems for ectotherms. Effective protein function depends on maintaining protein conformation and relative charge state, and this requires a stable ionic and pH environment. But the pK' of proteins, nonprotein buffers and water changes as a function of temperature (45,46). Rahn et al. (46), Reeves (47), and many others have observed that active, terrestrial animals [vertebrates and invertebrates (48)] modify ventilation to keep the total CO_2 constant, and as a consequence, the $\Delta pH/\Delta T$ is appropriate to maintain the relative charge state of proteins constant. Reeves pointed out that the imidazole group of histidine is the only residue with the appropriate pK and $\Delta pK/\Delta T$ to match the $\Delta pH/\Delta T$ of blood or any other tissue: the particular pK of each imidazole group depends on the surrounding protein structure (49), and there is significant variation among imidazole groups in terms of pK. The key element is that the $\Delta pK/\Delta T$ of the dominant buffer system must be matched to the $\Delta pK/\Delta T$ of the important proteins in that tissue if protein function is to be maintained. Reeves went on to suggest that an imidazole-containing protein was ideally suited to modify ventilation so as to maintain a stable environment for protein function (47). As a consequence, the "CO_2" chemoreceptor may actually respond to the relative charge state or fractional dissociation (α) of the receptor mechanism. Hence, CO_2 may have less to do with ventilatory control and gas exchange than with protein function and acid-base balance.

In some animals (50,51), the relative change in P_{CO_2}, as a consequence of the effect of temperature on the physicochemical characteristics of blood, is the same as the relative change in $\dot{V}_{CO_2}$, and the ratio of $\dot{V}_{CO_2}/P_{CO_2}$ remains constant. In these animals, ventilation remains constant and independent of temperature. This need not be true (52), but in all ectotherms, there will be relative hypoventilation to some extent as temperature rises. For the purpose of discussion, animals in which ventilation is independent of temperature raise interesting questions. In these animals, the respiratory response to temperature has a Q_{10} of zero. In terms of the chemoreceptor, this is easy to explain, although the logic is circular: chemoreceptor activity is unchanged because the relative charge state of the sensor is unchanged. But it is more difficult to explain how the remainder of the respiratory control system remains immune to the effects of temperature. It seems unlikely that the respiratory system output is totally determined by central chemoreceptor activity. Does this imply that the central pattern generator and/or central rhythm generator also has a Q_{10} of zero? Is the activity of these processes also determined by imidazole-dependent mechanisms? Following this line of reasoning to its logical, but unrealistic, conclusion, one could argue that no function should be affected by temperature; yet this is clearly not the case (53, 54). The paradox remains: how does the respiratory controller hold respiratory system output constant and resist the effect of inputs other than the central chemoreceptor that ought to have a Q_{10} effect greater than that expected for the chemoreceptor?

IX. The Diaphragm

The reptilian mechanism for reducing intrapulmonary pressure to subatmospheric levels that aspirate air into the lungs is effective but not designed to move large minute volumes. In those reptiles with ribs, the intercostals can bring the ventilatory act into a fairly high level of performance, but the turtles and tortoises are destined to operate at a lower level. The necessary structure for pumping large volumes at high rates of flow is the muscular diaphragm. Membranous diaphragms are found in some reptiles and in birds, but the mammal is unique in its possession of a muscular diaphragm, and its evolution remains a puzzle. The hopeful anticipation of discovering a homolog in amphibians or reptiles has been frustrating, although some tantalizing proposals have been made. Some features of the ribs of some extinct reptiles suggest sites for diaphragmatic attachment, but nothing beyond speculation is possible. On the other hand, late in the last century (55) certain muscles found in the amphibian family Pipidae were referred to as the "amphibian diaphragm," and a decade alter, Keith expressed his opinion that these muscles were homologous with the mammalian diaphragm (56). The first functional study of these muscles was not made until 1974 (57), and their action was found to be mainly expiratory. Keith had called attention to the fact that their nervous innervation originated in the same brachial roots as the phrenic nerve in mammals, but if contraction of the muscle is strictly expiratory in timing, there would have to be a radical change in phase of "phrenic" discharge as evolution occurred. The two frogs *Xenopus laevis* and *Pipa pipa* are strictly aquatic and characteristically begin a respiratory cycle by emptying their lungs upon surfacing, so in that sense, the timing of their "phrenic" discharge is not different from that of mammals that inspire first, but that may be an overextended attempt to claim similarity. On a firmer base is the fact that the respiratory cycle in these frogs begins with associated body movements, the most prominent being an arching of the back, not unlike what has been described in the air-breathing fish (Arapaima) (58). The first report on that remarkable fish noted that air was aspirated into the lungs, but subsequent study failed to find any phase of subatmospheric pressure in the lung (59). A better comparison, therefore, is with events in the Pipidae, and the important fact is that the air-breathing fish and aquatic frogs provide yet another example of the use of postural muscles to assist in powering ventilation. The inspiratory/expiratory phases of the respiratory cycle in mammals can be likened to extension/flexion of the torso, and in many running quadrupeds, arching of the back is entrained with breathing. Indeed, a good case can be made for the argument that the muscular diaphragm is the old membranous diaphragm that has been invaded by postural muscles (60).

X. Mammals

The mammals offer an unexcelled opportunity for comparative study, because the range of size is so great—a few grams to several metric tons. Allometric exponents are more reliable for this class than for any other (birds are a close second), and the range of habits and habitats is extensive and varied. When it comes to quantifying the control of breathing, the vexing problem of knowing for certain what are the appropriate measures of stimulus and response arises. Because anesthesia introduces a complication, the extent of which can never be known, we elect to use ventilatory response of conscious animals as the output of choice. In addition, more data are available for analysis than would be the case, say, for phrenic discharge, but a problem still remains. Clearly, minute volume of ventilation, as measured, will not do. Absolute values would lead to the false conclusion that large animals had a higher "sensitivity" ($\Delta V/\Delta stimulus$) than small animals. It is required that ventilation be normalized. The majority of studies report weight-specific values, but we feel that this is inherently erroneous. The ventilatory control mechanism is part of a homeostatic system that maintains, within bounds, alveolar partial pressures of oxygen and carbon dioxide, and these values are subject to perturbation by metabolic rate, which is well known not to be proportional to body size or, in fact, to any other dimensional requirement of geometrical similarity. (This enigma vanishes when the problem is seen to be one for which fractal geometry is the appropriate tool.) Therefore, like Dejours (61) and others, we choose to express the output as ventilation/metabolic rate, or ventilation/BW$^{0.75}$.

If a wide range of mammals with similar habitats are examined, alveolar P_{CO_2} seems to hover about 40 ± 5 torr. There is no clearly defined relationship with size, although the highest values tend to be found in large animals, and the lowest in small (62), but this is by no means a consistent finding (63). Given the relatively narrow range of alveolar (arterial) gas values and the wide range of animal size, it is a defensible conclusion that alveolar P_{CO_2} is an interspecific "constant." From a regulatory viewpoint it can be asked, why is the P_{CO_2} "set point" 40 torr? That value can be deduced by estimating alveolar ventilation, which, in addition to measured expired ventilatory values and respiratory frequency, requires knowledge of the dead space as a function of animal size. When this calculation is made (64), the value for alveolar P_{CO_2} is found to be about 40 torr, but the residual mass exponent does indeed indicate a trend to slightly higher values in large animals.

The argument for a regulatory set point of 40 torr for P_{CO_2} can be developed along two lines: (1) if general structural design of the body and its mechanical characteristics follow a set of uniform principles, then the volumetric rate and pattern of breathing will follow predictable rules, and the result, when coupled with the size-determined metabolic rate, leads to the observed partial pressure of alveolar gases; (2) chemical reaction rates in the cells are dependent on the local pH, and, given normal mammalian body temperature and an established system of acid/base balance, a P_{CO_2} of 40 torr is best. Both the structural and chemical propositions carry the assumption that their functions have evolved to be optimal. The emphasis on CO_2 in these remarks is not meant to suggest that O_2 can be neglected; in fact, a control system oriented toward preserving tissue O_2 pressure above some "critical" value is undoubtedly the essential consideration, but CO_2 is a more easily discussed controlled variable, in part because in mammals it is the dominant controlling chemical stimulus, and any conclusion about alveolar CO_2 leads to a comparable conclusion about O_2 (so long as the exchange ratio is known).

XI. Hering-Breuer Reflexes

The lungs of mammals contain fast and slowly adapting receptors responsive to wall tension. Proprioceptive information is transmitted over the vagus and regulates tidal volume by means of its influence on inspiratory time and on frequency by influencing the duration of expiration. The extent to which the Hering-Breuer reflex is an important factor determining the pattern of normal breathing varies widely among mammalian species (65). In general, the reflex is more potent in the newborn than in the adult of any species, but this difference, and the interspecific variability have not been explained satisfactorily.

Given the well-known dependence of respiratory frequency on body size in mammals, it would be anticipated that there would be a difference in the rate of receptor adaptation among species if flow-related information is to have the same significance in all animals (66). However, contrary to expectation, it turned out that receptor adaptive characteristics were independent of body size. The information they convey must, therefore, vary and have different significance for the control of breathing in large and small animals.

The pressoreceptor in gills of fish cannot be regarded as a precursor of pulmonary stretch receptors, but the appearance of stretch receptors in the lung and swim bladder of fish probably does mark the beginning of a mechanism that progressed all the way to mammals. The essential control function in fish and amphibians was on static lung volume, but in mammals, it appears to be more important in determining pattern.

XII. Metabolic Rate and "Chemosensitivity"

There is a simple, intuitive attraction to the idea that responsiveness of the ventilatory control system ought to depend on metabolic rate. If the "load" (blood flow rate $\times$ Pv_{CO_2}) on the lungs of venous CO_2 and unsaturated hemoglobin is high, and the ventilatory response is set for a lower "load," arterial blood will leave the lungs with an elevated PCO_2 and depressed PO_2. These abnormalities will be detected by arterial chemoreceptors as an error signal, there will be an augmented stimulus to ventilate, and the blood gases will return toward normal, at which point the chemoreceptor response subsides. But then, the cycle repeats, and what is observed is an oscillation of arterial gas composition and ventilation. However, this simple analysis assumes a constant respiratory frequency. Given that condition, whether or not the mean arterial values change will depend on the sensitivity of ventilatory response, i.e., whether it is large enough to drive the PCO_2 below normal on the downswing. If that effect is small, the result would be an elevation of mean PCO_2, a prediction contrary to the evidence ($PaCO_2$ is not appreciably elevated in exercise; $PaCO_2$ is not high in small animals). A solution to the problem would lie in adjusting the "gain" of the ventilatory control system in proportion to the metabolic rate in the animal (manifest as "load" on the lung), a change that would maintain blood gas partial pressures constant interspecifically. Hypoxic ventilatory response was found (67) to vary inversely with body size (thus, directly with specific metabolic rate), although a group of mammals at the lower end of the distribution of size were uniform in their responses (68). There is no evidence for a size-dependent CO_2 ventilatory response. Sloths have an unusually low metabolic rate, a decreased hypoxic ventilatory response, but a normal CO_2 response (69). These differences bring to mind the character of ventilatory response in exercise, a state that may be compared with that of a high-metabolic-rate animal. Hypoxic ventilatory response is increased during exercise (70), but the CO_2 response is not. Is the explanation of the change of hypoxic sensitivity, but not of CO_2 sensitivity, in these examples, that the peripheral chemoreceptors (primarily responsive to hypoxia) increase their gain in relation to metabolic rate but central chemosensitive regions (primarily responsive to CO_2/H^+) do not? Whatever the mechanism, the conclusion that oxygen is of greater concern for the organism than is CO_2 seems warranted, and the higher priority is therefore assigned to "tuning" the hypoxic ventilatory control system to meet a changing need. The risk of hypoxia in the tissues can be ill afforded in contrast to that of some accumulation of CO_2 and H^+, which are minimally damaging and generally well handled by effective buffer mechanisms.

A further note of interest is raised by returning to the magnitude of oscillation in blood-borne chemical signals and this time putting aside the assumed constancy of respiratory frequency. The well-known inverse relation of respiratory frequency and body size has the effect, when its allometric mass exponent and those of metabolic rate and lung volume are all taken into consideration (71), of canceling any effect of body size on the magnitude of oscillations in arterial blood of P_{CO_2} and P_{O_2}. So, like mean blood gas values, oscillatory amplitude of arterial O_2 and CO_2 is also an interspecific constant due to the interspecific variation of respiratory frequency. Postulating a variation in magnitude of oscillation of arterial blood gases as an explanation of interspecific differences in ventilatory control must be rejected.

XIII. Hemoglobin Oxygen Affinity and Hypoxic Ventilatory Response

There is a clear-cut relationship between P_{50} (P_{O_2} at half-saturation) and body size: it is high (low O_2 affinity) in small animals; it is low in large animals (high O_2 affinity) (72). A high P_{50} is detrimental to loading but favorable for unloading; with a low P_{50}, the opposite is true. Peripheral chemoreceptor responses to hypoxia are believed to sense the partial pressure, not the content, of oxygen (at least, this is true for the carotid body), which would mean that two animals with different P_{50} ought not to have the same hypoxic threshold in their chemoreceptors if the ventilatory response that follows is appropriate for relief of the sensed hypoxia. That is because a relatively high P_{O_2} threshold, in an animal with a high hemoglobin oxygen affinity, would result in an increase of ventilation, but no consequent increase of arterial oxyhemoglobin saturation, and in an animal with a low oxygen affinity, a low hypoxic threshold would be hazardous, because too great a decrease in oxyhemoglobin saturation might exist before excitation of the chemoreceptor occurred. Experimental results in both birds and mammals (73,74) confirmed the prediction that hypoxic threshold for increasing ventilation was correlated with P_{50}. This trait in birds and mammals is consistent with the finding that "critical" P_{O_2} varies interspecifically with the hemoglobin affinity for oxygen (75) and with the fact that, in reptiles, the hypoxic ventilatory threshold varies with individual variation in anaerobic capacity. In fish, the hypoxic threshold for accelerating gill ventilation correlates with the natural activity of the species (76). The general pattern fits neatly into the class of phenomena that confirm the wisdom of the body, but it leaves unanswered the mechanism that lies behind it. Does it mean that more importance should be given to a role of detector mechanisms that sense oxygen content or saturation (like the aortic body)? Or, since a wide variability in hypoxic responses is apparent among individuals in any species (much more so than for CO_2 responses), has the process of natural selection sorted out those with the "right" threshold for the P_{50} of the species and eliminated those with the "wrong" threshold? It appears that experimental alteration of P_{50} does not influence the hypoxic threshold (77), thus indicating that the effect is not something akin to acclimitization, but may be locked into the genetic code for the species.

Based on the faintness of staining for cytochrome oxidase in carotid bodies in cattle, Lee and Mattenheimer first suggested that carotid chemoreceptor sensitivity might be related to reduced cytochrome oxidase activity (78). Subsequently, Mills and Jöbsis (79) studied the spectrophotometric characteristics of the isolated carotid body of the cat superfused with hemoglobin-free solutions equilibrated with different oxygen concentrations. They detected two cytochrome a_3 components, one of which had a low oxygen affinity. Chemoreceptor impulse activity was correlated with the redox state of the low-affinity cytochrome a_3. Hypoxic sensitivity is associated with reduced carotid body oxygen consumption (80), and an unusually low-affinity cytochrome a_3 could explain the reduction in carotid body $\dot{V}o_2$ at oxygen partial pressures well above the critical Po_2 of other tissues. Based on changes in fluorescence of NADH during carotid sinus nerve stimulation, Mills and Jöbsis thought that the low-affinity cytochrome a_3 was in the type II cell. More recently, investigators have determined that the type I cell is the oxygen sensor, but a low-affinity cytochrome continues to play a role in theories of chemotransduction (80). Biscoe and Duchen (81) have suggested that the redox state of mitochondria controls the mitochondrial membrane potential. Hypoxia modifies the redox state of mitochondria in type I cells, permitting depolarization of the mitochondrial membrane: this is the essential element in chemotransduction. Efflux of calcium from the mitochondria (where calcium is concentrated by virtue of the electrochemical gradient between mitochondria and the intracellular space) or some other intracellular pool increases the intracellular calcium concentration, promotes neurotransmitter release, and increases carotid nerve activity. The only evidence of a low-affinity cytochrome is the original spectrophotometric evidence from Mills and Jöbsis and the inference that the carotid body behaves as if it had a low-affinity cytochrome (80): such a cytochrome has not been isolated so far as we know. In view of the allometric relationships among body weight, P_{50}, critical Po_2, and the threshold of the hypoxic response, one might wonder if an allometric relationship similar to that for the P_{50} might also exist for the affinity of cytochrome a_3, but we know of no data on the subject. Furthermore, we do not know whether the affinity of cytochrome a_3 or any of the other cytochromes in mitochondria changes as a function of body weight so that the affinity of hemoglobin may be tuned to the oxygen affinity of mitochondria within the carotid body. Mitochondrial cytochromes are phylogenetically ancient and chemically quite distinct from the phylogenetically more recent hemoglobins; therefore, structural elements of the carotid body may tune a constant, but reduced, cytochrome oxidase affinity to the varying affinities of hemoglobin among different animals.

The phenomenon of hypoxic "blunting" at high altitude can be produced in cats and shown to be, not a failure of hypoxic response, but, rather, a lowering of threshold (82). What aspect of the process of ventilatory acclimitization is responsible for resetting the hypoxic chemoreceptor is not known, but it is reasonable to assume that increases in blood oxygen capacity and changes at tissue level permit a lower blood Po_2 without creating hypoxic damage and thereby permit reduction in the early hyperventilation that was maintained at a higher Po_2. The appearance is that of a system that operates with a fixed margin of safety, and if circumstances (such as acclimitization) permit reduction of Po_2 at the lower end of the oxygen cascade, there is a relaxation on regulatory demand at the upper end. Certainly, the change of hypoxic threshold in acclimatized cats is not related to any significant reduction of P_{50}, but it is possible that the condition in the tissues at sea level with a low P_{50} is not unlike that at high altitude with a higher P_{50}. In llamas (83) and yaks (84), species native to high altitudes, "blunting" is not observed. These species have a low blood P_{50}. Their hypoxic threshold is low at sea level, as well as at high altitude (73,83), and it is unaltered after acclimatization to high altitude. The fact is that all of the Camellidae have blood with a low P_{50} (85) and, therefore, are favorably equipped for oxygen uptake in a hypoxic environment; they are, in that sense, "preadapted" for life at high altitude.

XIV. Burrowing and Diving

Animals that inhabit subterranean tunnels and pockets are chronically exposed to an environment high in CO_2 and low in oxygen (74,86), a feature shared with diving animals, because their breathing pattern must include periods of prolonged breath holding. In both groups the question naturally arises whether the various homeostatic components of acclimitization to asphyxic air and, possibly, adaptive changes in the species lead to changes in the control of breathing. Burrowing and diving animals have long been known to have an elevated threshold and a depressed responsiveness to CO_2 (87,88), but there is considerable variability among species. The problem of identifying the mechanism remains unsolved. Likely candidates are a change inherent in central and/or peripheral chemoreceptor excitability and a change in buffering capacity of blood and other tissues. Basic, comparative differences in chemoreceptor characteristics have not been demonstrated, and although there is generally an increased buffering capacity in the blood of diving and fossorial animals, this is not a uniform finding, and no good correlation exists between interspecific variations of buffering and CO_2 ventilatory sensitivity. Exposure to CO_2 in the perinatal period does not affect the ventilatory response in the adult stage (89). Nothing is known in regard to possible difference in the important process governing hydrogen ion equilibria between brain and cerebrospinal fluid. Those fossorial rodents with the greatest hemoglobin oxygen affinity have the lowest hypoxic threshold, thus contributing one more factor to that pattern, as discussed earlier.

Hypoxic responsiveness has been examined in only a few species and the variability appears to be greater than for the CO_2 response, but the impression is that it is not much affected. On the one hand, this is consistent with the conclusion that guarding against hypoxia is the paramount consideration in respiratory control design and hypoxic regulatory mechanisms should be preserved under all circumstances, but, on the other hand, diving animals must tolerate high levels of chemical drive in prolonged breath holding. Too long a time and too low a Po_2 could be fatal, so, even with an attenuated CO_2 responsiveness, there must be a signal for surfacing and breaking the apnea before hypoxic damage would occur. Of course, while the animal is submerged, the lung air is compressed, and the Po_2 will remain high, but the rise to the surface and attendant fall of alveolar Po_2 as lung air is decompressed may be the most hazardous period. Presumably the signal intensity and critical time have all been worked out by natural selection.

XV. Harmony of Design

The fact that inspiratory flow velocity scales with body size (exponent is 0.74) indicates lower values in large animals (67,90) and could be interpreted to mean a body size dependence of "central drive" (91). However, experiments conducted with supramaximal phrenic stimulation, designed to control drive to the diaphragm, produced the same results as obtained in spontaneously breathing animals, which led to the conclusion that the interspecific variation of inspiratory flow velocity was attributable to mechanical properties of the lungs and chest wall and contractile properties of the respiratory muscles (90). Although that conclusion places the explanation outside of the class of phenomena normally considered under the subject of the control of breathing, it does illustrate the necessity of matching all characteristics of the components in an integrated system design, if smooth and efficient performance is to be realized.

XVI. Comparative Aspects of Upper Airway Control

As mentioned above, the upper airway force pump generates each inspiration in amphibians and air-breathing fish, but in reptiles, aspiration becomes the mechanism of inspiration, and the upper airway participates to the extent that upper airway patency must be maintained to avoid limiting inspiratory flow. It seems that animals have not had great difficulty maintaining upper airway patency during aspiratory inspiration, even though this created negative transmural pressure in the extrathoracic airway. Defense of upper airway patency has two facts, one functional and the other anatomical. Many muscles of the upper airway are activated slightly before the onset of inspiration and remain active throughout inspiration. These muscles seem to stiffen and dilate the airway (although quantitative estimates of the contribution of upper airway muscles to the size and stiffness of the airway are actually hard to find). A variety of reflexes activate these muscles in circumstances when upper airway patency may be compromised. Perhaps most interesting in this respect is the Hering-Breuer reflex. Although the reflex contributes to the timing of inspiration and expiration and limits the tidal volume by modifying diaphragmatic activation, it is striking that when tidal volume is limited and the Hering-Breuer reflex is activated, activation of upper airway muscles far exceeds activation of the diaphragm (92,93). It may be that the Hering-Breuer reflex ultimately came to have greater significance in maintaining and improving inspiratory effort during partial upper airway obstruction than as a mechanism to limit tidal volume. The anatomical feature of the upper airway that prevents airway collapse is that the upper airway is generally rigid, and those parts of the airway that are not rigid are short. The larynx sits just distal to the soft palate, and there is little if any oropharyngeal airway in animals other than humans (94).

Phylogenetic reviews often focus on the primitive precursors and early manifestations of adaptations that subsequently play an important role in mammals. But it is also true that instructive examples can be found in animals in which some adaptation has been taken to an extreme. In humans, the larynx descended and the oropharynx is elongated, probably to create a space in which to shape and enhance vocalization. It is interesting that the larynx has a more "primitive" position in newborns (the larynx is high and the oropharynx short), but the larynx descends and reaches a more adult position in babies at about the age infants begin to acquire speech (95). In a series of studies of upper airway anatomy, Lieberman et al. (96) and Laitman et al. (97) extended this analysis to the paleological record. Based on the inferred placement of the hyoid, larynx, and soft tissues and the bony features of the basicranium, these investigators deduced that Neanderthals were capable of only a limited vocal repertoire. It would be a mistake to attribute evolutionary success to a single adaptation; however, it may be significant that Neanderthals and Cro-Magnon man were contemporaries, but Cro-Magnon man superseded the Neanderthals. Cro-Magnon man had a more elongated, a more modern oropharynx capable, presumably, of more sophisticated vocalization.

Elongation of the upper airway carries a price. The airway is no longer surrounded by rigid tissues. The glottis is less well protected, and the upper airway becomes more vulnerable to collapse during inspiration. Humans are more prone than other species to choking while eating, and any factor, such as sleep, that reduces upper airway muscle activity may lead to airway collapse in susceptible individuals. The occurrence of upper airway collapse during sleep is called obstructive sleep apnea. Obstructive sleep apnea is unique to humans [dogs that manifest the illness do so only because of selective breeding programs guided by humans (98)]. Hence, obstructive sleep apnea may be viewed as part of the price humans have paid for a sophisticated "sound system" capable of speech.

XVII. Optimality

In almost all bodily functions, a case can be made for optimal performance, and its definition is most often expressed as minimum of work (mechanical or chemical) required, but other properties, like force or some sensory modality, may be introduced. Curves of ventilatory work (99) or force (100) show a minimum (a fairly broad one) at the normal respiratory frequency in humans, but little quantitative information is available for other species, except the guinea pig (100), which also appears to satisfy the criterion of minimal force. It is probably useful to note that over a 1000-fold range of animal size, passive pulmonary emptying time and the breathing frequency are in a proportional relationship (101), indicating harmony in matching the frequency demands of the central rhythm generator and the mechanical characteristics of the lung and chest wall. It is futile to ask which of the matched pair is the independent and which the dependent function. Surely, they must have evolved in parallel, but if efficiency is a driving feature, instances of poor structural design would be weeded out.

Further, more than one process may be in operation at the same time, and it may not be possible to optimize both; therefore, the issue of priority arises, and a choice will rest more on which is important for the welfare of the organism than on a matter of economy. This problem arises in muscular exercise when change of gait can be necessary to protect the limbs from rupture of tendons or fracture of bones, even though the cost in energy rises. Control of breathing can be discussed in comparable terms at the point when the oxygen consumed in maintaining a high level of ventilation approaches the net gain in oxygen introduced for use by the rest of the body. At that point the indirect cost has become excessive; it is preferable to allow blood CO_2 to rise and oxygen to fall rather than to continue expending energy driving the ventilatory muscles with no net gain for the body as a whole. There is also during exercise, particularly at high levels, the question whether entrainment of the respiratory and stepping rhythms carries any advantage in reducing the oxygen cost of breathing. The problem of indirect cost load has not been evaluated comparatively, but two facts are significant: in premammalian vertebrates, the ventilatory mechanism demands a high portion of the total metabolism of the body, but when energetic needs are high, anaerobic metabolism becomes an important part of the whole; in humans—and there is no way of being sure that their responses are representative of all mammals—the evidence indicates that ventilatory work never does reach a level at which its demands become a drain on whole-body oxygen consumption. However, ventilation at high workloads rarely goes much beyond about 65% of maximum voluntary ventilatory capacity, and it is at that value that oxygen consumption of the respiratory muscles begins to rise steeply. There is apparently an inhibitory mechanism that supervenes in the complex factors at play—a governor on the system. It is not clear whether it is reflex in nature or whether it may be sensory, possibly of effort, whatever that is.

The entrainment problem is controversial. In many birds and flying mammals, it is the rule to find a synchronous relationship between breathing and limb movements, probably related to the role of the pectoral muscles and their attachment to the chest wall, but there is no reason to conclude that the flight muscle contractions actually contribute to generating the tidal volume (102). It is more reasonable to imagine that a breath out of synchrony with wing movement would put forces in conflict and lead to an inefficient operation. When running, a quadruped experiences a forward motion of the abdominal viscera at the time the front feet strike the ground. This piston-like movement impacts the diaphragm, creating an expiratory effect on the lungs, which would be an awkward time for the animal to generate an inspiration. The metabolic cost would be excessive, and merely shifting the timing so that breathing and locomotor motions take advantage of joined, rather than opposing forces is a simple solution. In bipeds, the vector orientation of visceral movements during running does not result in a significant impact on the diaphragm and chest wall, but entrainment is sometimes seen, particularly in trained athletes. A decreased oxygen uptake has been found in runners when there is increased coupling (103), and a neurogenic mechanism based on interaction between respiratory and locomotor pattern generators has been postulated (104). Certainly, no mechanical explanation exists (105). In mammals, generally, a distinction has to be drawn between those whose gait is bipedal and those that are quadrupedal, because the mechanical influence on the thorax is different. Nonetheless, entrainment is frequently encountered in both groups and a plausible case can be made for a mechanical advantage, but nothing convincing in regard to limb motions actually assisting in powering the tidal volume has been found.

XVIII. Birds

Two things stand out in respiratory control in birds: their extraordinary tolerance to hypoxia and the presence of intrapulmonary chemoreceptors.

The unusual hypoxic tolerance in birds derives from the cross-current arrangement of pulmonary ventilation and perfusion and from the insensitivity of the cerebral vessels of birds to the vasoconstricting effects of hypocapnia. The unique structural features of the avian lung permit enhanced oxygen uptake, and the ability to sustain oxygen uptake during prolonged migratory flights over the

Himalayas perhaps demonstrates this phenomenal capacity best. Coupled with enhanced oxygen uptake in the lung, birds are able to maintain cerebral blood flow and oxygen delivery as well. Hypocapnia constricts the cerebral circulation of mammals, but this effect is absent or at least attenuated in birds (106). Hence, hypocapnia accompanying the ventilatory response to hypoxia does not limit cerebral blood flow in birds. The P_{50} of hemoglobin in birds adapted to hypoxic environments is low, as it is in similarly adapted mammals, but there is no evidence of any reduction in the Bohr effect (107).

Whereas the adaptations that enhance hypoxic tolerance in birds are reasonably clear, it is not at all clear what adaptive function intrapulmonary chemoreceptors serve. Intrapulmonary chemoreceptors are found in reptiles (except apparently in the freshwater turtle *Chrysemys picta*) and birds, but not amphibians or mammals. On the other hand, all pulmonate vertebrates possess pulmonary stretch receptors, although the evidence for a Hering-Breuer reflex in birds is not completely clear (6). The activity of intrapulmonary chemoreceptors increases when CO_2 is low or absent and decreases as the CO_2 rises. Mammalian pulmonary stretch receptors are slightly more sensitive during hypocapnia, and some intrapulmonary chemoreceptors are slightly stretch sensitive (108). It is possible that some intrapulmonary chemoreceptors are derived from pulmonary stretch receptors or from a common "primordial" receptor with equal sensitivity to stretch and CO_2, but such intermediate receptors have never been identified in any species. How one interprets the function of intrapulmonary chemoreceptors depends on how one tests them. CO_2 can be added to the inspired air, or venous blood can be loaded with CO_2. In the latter case, it seems clear in reptiles that increased venous CO_2 is associated with increased ventilation. The arterial CO_2 may remain isocapnic during venous CO_2 loading, and the response is abolished by vagotomy (109,110). If intrapulmonary chemoreceptors play a role here, it must be that reduced intrapulmonary chemoreceptor activity permits or disinhibits a ventilatory response. This is consistent with early work by Peterson and Fedde (111), in which apnea developed in unidirectionally ventilated birds when CO_2 was removed from the inspired gas (presumably, without CO_2 present, intrapulmonary chemoreceptor activity was elevated and ventilation was inhibited). However, more recently, Furilla and Bartlett have suggested that reduced inspiratory CO_2 early in inspiration leads to augmented breaths in garter snakes (112). This finding is not consistent with the suggestion that intrapulmonary chemoreceptors serve as a chemical analog of the Hering-Breuer reflex (113). In other studies, increased inspiratory CO_2 increased ventilation (114,115), and the effect seems to depend on intrapulmonary chemoreceptors. The analysis is further complicated in snakes and lizards by the presence of additional CO_2-sensitive receptors in the nose that inhibit inspiration when CO_2 is elevated (116). Suffice it to say that both intrapulmonary chemoreceptors and pulmonary stretch receptors exist in birds and reptiles, but the exact role of these receptors in controlling and shaping ventilatory output remains uncertain.

XIX. The Uniqueness of Marsupials

The special feature of marsupials that attracts interest is their state of immaturity at birth. The North American opossum, after only 13 days of gestation, must begin a life breathing air—a newborn weighing only a few milligrams, with undeveloped lungs and only the rudiments of a central nervous system, yet in its primitive way able to cope, and even to respond in ways that suggest the elements of a ventilatory control system already at work. The observation of note is the resemblance of breathing pattern in the newborn opossum to that of an amphibian. The opossum aspirates air so inflation of the lungs is different from a frog, but the respiratory rhythm is irregular in both and so too is the end-inspiratory breath-holding characteristic (117). The old dictum that ontogeny recapitulates phylogeny is notoriously inapplicable to the respiratory organ (lungs did not evolve from gills), but it does seem likely that the stages of maturation of the mammalian ventilatory control system reveal progression from archaic to contemporary mammalian design. Further, during the first few weeks of extrauterine life, the opossum illustrates the appearance of hierarchial dominance as the brain develops, and the forebrain begins to exercise a modulating influence on chemical control of breathing (118). This developmental manifestation of a progressively hierarchical system, which is complete only at maturity, can be revealed in the adult cat by employing ablation techniques to remove functional regions, proceeding in stages caudally: the classic decorticate and decerebrate preparations (43).

XX. Summary

When the unique strategy of comparative physiology is examined, its strengths and its weaknesses appear simultaneously. The search for exceptions to prove a rule may be a satisfying tactic in argument, but it can also blind an investigator to the fact that an entirely different reason underlies the operative situation of a special case. Critical thinking should suffice to circumvent that hazard, but the more difficult problem originates with the realization that evolution frequently hits on different solutions for the same question. If, for example, it is only a matter of choice of neurotransmitter say, no difficulty need arise with a description of the general behavior of a system over a range of species, but if there are fundamental differences in the neural organization of a control system, then a general principle of mechanism may have to be modified, depending, in part, on how basic the principle is. The possibility exists that, when all the types of solutions are considered, the only remaining generality will be so broad that it contains little useful information, for example, that all control systems are found to contain excitatory and inhibitory components.

Despite these hazards, we are strong advocates for intensified research on the control of breathing in primitive systems even though this approach has its own pitfalls. True, the word "primitive" is inevitably deceptive, and a search for elementary processes may only reveal an unanticipated complexity; nonetheless, there is near certainty that mechanisms and interactions in an organized control system stand a better chance of being elucidated in simple than in highly developed brains. In short, if models have a role in scientific discovery, living examples complement abstract construction. There are many promising examples in the world of invertebrates and, more difficult, but still accessible, in embryos of submammalian vertebrates, even vertebrates, when the well-organized air-breathing mechanism of newborn opossums is considered. The temptation is to think that these preparations will provide definitive models, which they sometimes may, but if they can explain how at least one elementary system works, that may help in constructing the framework of an hypothesis for how the next level of complexity may be designed.

Finally, and in homage to the dictum of August Krogh that "for many problems there is an animal on which it can be most conveniently studied," comparative physiologists should always be on the hunt for animals that manifest, by nature, special traits that offer unusual opportunities, e.g., sleep apnea in seals, or the tendency for boxer dogs to develop chemodectomas of the carotid body, or for vestigial centers in the brains of lungless salamanders. The range for exploration is limitless, and the adventure can lead to rewarding discoveries.

These remarks have been cast as a preface; they are not to be construed as a review, but rather as a biased "overview" with the aim of examining the "underview"—threads that bind together some of the important features found in a comparative survey of the control of breathing. An appreciation of identifiable threads aids in understanding the continuity of process and mechanism in evolutionary progress, but it must be admitted that there are many instances for which the pattern is a fragmented one. The following distillate lists the key discernible elements:

Protection from hypoxia defines a role of highest priority for the respiratory control system, and effects ranging from primitive behavioral responses to receptor-mediated, chemoreflex, ventilatory responses participating in a complex control system in higher animals all serve a common purpose.

Carbon dioxide as a key ventilatory stimulant appeared relatively late in evolution, and its mechanism of action (for the most part not distinguishable from the associated acidity) is ambiguous: in different orders it may be directly excitatory; it may excite by inhibiting inhibitory afferents; it may inhibit by exciting inhibitory afferents. Arterial partial pressure of CO_2 is very low in fish, somewhat higher in ectothermic, air-breathing tetrapods, and higher still in endotherms, but close control of the normal value in none appears essential.

Muscles to power ventilation have been adopted and adapted from muscle groups whose original function served some other purpose: the muscles of feeding and swallowing for gill ventilation and force-pump breathing; postural and locomotor muscles for early types of aspiration; invasion of the membranous diaphragm by somatic muscle to produce the muscular diaphragm to drive the most highly developed aspiration mechanism. As these systems evolve, their central nervous connections reveal responses indicative of their ancestral origin. The interrelationship of limb motion and ventilation, and its relevance to ventilatory control in exercise, is a case in point.

The mechanism of the inherent rhythm of a central generator has the properties of a pacemaker in invertebrates, but in vertebrates, there is no clear evidence to identify a pacemaker as distinguishable from a reverberating neural network. In fish, a population of neurons in the central nervous system acts as an intrinsically rhythmic generator to produce a regular gill motion, even though afferent signals can influence its amplitude and rate; when air breathing becomes an option in the bimodal systems of lung fish and amphibians, the rhythm becomes irregular, apparently due to a second central generator, which responds "on command" when water becomes a poor source of oxygen. At the stage reached by birds and mammals, as air breathers exclusively, the rhythm becomes regular again, but the pool of neurons in the central pattern generator in response to afferent signals from mechano- and chemoreceptors refines the timing of the phases of a breath.

The Hering-Breuer reflex in early air-breathing animals served mainly to limit tidal volume, but proprioceptive information from the lung assumes a more important role when aspiration becomes the mechanism of inspiration. In mammals, the Hering-Breuer reflex not only modifies the depth and timing of breathing, but also serves as integrate and coordinate the diaphragm and muscles of the upper airway so that inspiratory flow is not impeded.

In the construction of the complete neuromuscular and mechanical system responsive to neural signals and controlling ventilation in mammals, there is a matching of resistance, compliance, muscle properties and ventilatory requirements with velocity characteristics, respiratory frequency, and whole-body oxygen uptake rate. Controller demands and effector organ design are in harmony.

Control system design criteria throughout follow principles of optimality, most often in terms of metabolic cost.

References

1. Boggs DF. Comparative control of respiration. In: Parent RA, ed. Comparative Biology of the Normal Lung. Boca Raton, FL: CRC Press, 1992:309–350.
2. Burggren W, Johansen K, McMahon B. Respiration in phyletically ancient fishes. In: Foreman RE et al, eds. Evolutionary Biology of Primitive Fishes. New York: Plenum Press, 1985:217–252.

3. Hughes GM. Respiration of Amphibian Vertebrates. New York: Academic Press, 1976:402.

4. Hughes GM, Shelton G. Respiratory mechanism and their nervous control in fish. Adv Comp Physiol Biochem 1962; 1:275–364.

5. Milsom WK. Mechanoreceptor modulation of endogenous respiratory rhythms in vertebrates. Am J Physiol 1990; 259:R898–R910.

6. Scheid P, Piiper J. Control of breathing in birds. In: Cherniak NS, Widdicombe JG, eds. Handbook of Physiology. Section 3: The Respiratory System. Vol II. Control of Breathing. Part 2. Bethesda, MD: American Physiological Society, 1986:815–832.

7. Shelton G. The regulation of breathing. In: Hoar WS, Randall DJ, eds. Fish Physiology. London: Academic Press, 1970:293–359.

8. Shelton G, Jones DR, Milsom WK. Control of breathing in ectothermic vertebrates. In: Cherniack NS, Widdicombe JG, eds. Handbook of Physiology. Section 3: The Respiratory System. Vol II. Control of Breathing, Part 2. Bethesda, MD: American Physiological Society, 1986:851–909.

9. Smatresk NJ: Chemoreceptor modulation of endogenous respiratory rhythms in vertebrates. Am J Physiol 1990; 259:R887–R897.

10. Tenney SM, Bartlett D Jr. Some comparative aspects of the control of breathing. In: Hornbein TF, ed. Regulation of Breathing. New York: Marcel Dekker, 1981:67–104.

11. Tenney SM, Boggs DF. Comparative mammalian respiratory control. In: Cherniack NS, Widdicombe JG, eds. Handbook of Physiology: Section 3. The Respiratory System. Vol II. The Control of Breathing. Bethesda, MD: American Physiological Society, 1986:833–855.

12. Fox JM, Taylor AER. The tolerance of oxygen by aquatic invertebrates. Proc Roy Soc (Lond) Ser B. 1955; 143:214–225.

13. Savage RM. The ecology of young tadpoles, with special reference to some adaptations to the habitat of mass spawning in *Rana temporia* Linn. Proc Zool Soc (Lond) 1935; 605–610.

14. Babak E. Über provisorische Atemmechanismen bei Fischen. Zentralbl Physiol 1911; 25:370–374.

15. Fox HM, Johnson ML. The control of respiratory movements in Crustacea by oxygen and carbon dioxide. J Exp Biol 1934; 11:1–10.

16. Waterman TH, Travis DF. Respiratory reflexes and flabellum of *Limulus*. J Cell Comp Physiol 1953; 41:261–290.

17. Dausend K. Über die Atmung der Tubificiden. Z wiss Biol Z Vergleich Physiol 1931; C14:557–608.

18. Newell RC, Courtney WAM. Respiratory movements in Holothuria: *Foskali delle chiaje*. J Exp Biol 1965; 42:45–57.

19. Bartlett D Jr., Birchard GF. Effects of hypoxia on the lung volume in the garter snake. Respir Physiol 1983; 53:63–70.

20. Jones JD. Aspects of respiration in *Planorbis coneus* L. and *Lymnaea stagnalis* L. (Gastropoda: Pulmonata). Comp Biochem Physiol 1961; 4:1–29.

21. Syed NI, Harrison D, Winlow W. Respiratory behavior in the pond snail *Lymnaea stagnalis*. I. Behavioral analysis and the identification of motor neurons. J Comp Physiol A 1991; 169:541–555.

22. Janse C, van der Wilt J, van der Plas J, van der Roest M. Central and peripheral neurones involves in oxygen perception in the pulmonate snail *Lymnaea stagnalis* (Mollusca, Gastropoda). Biochem Physiol 1985; 82A:459–469.

23. Janse C. The effect of oxygen on gravity orientation in the pulmonate snail *Lymnaea stagnalis*. J Comp Physiol 1981; 142:51–59.

24. Syed NI, Winlow W. Respiratory behavior in the pond snail *Lymnaea stagnalis*. II. Neural elements of the central pattern generator (CPG). J Comp Physiol 1991; 169: 557–568.

25. Miller PI. Respiration in the desert locust. I. The control of ventilation. J Exp Biol 1960; 37:224–236.

26. Miller PL. Respiration in the desert locust. II. The control of the spiracles. J Exp Biol 1960; 37:237–263.

27. Wilson DM. The central nervous control of flight in a locust. J Exp Biol 1961; 38: 471–490.

28. Stevenson PA, Kutsch W. A reconsideration of the central pattern generator concept for locust flight. J Comp Physiol A 1987; 161:115–129.

29. Robertson RM, Pearson KG. Interneurons in the flight system of the locust: distribution, connections, and resetting properties. J Comp Neurol 1983; 215: 33–50.

30. Burrows M. Co-ordinating interneurones of the locust which convey two patterns of motor commands: their connexions with ventilatory motoneurones. J Exp Biol 1975; 63:735–753.

31. Burrows M. Co-ordinating interneurones of the locust which convey two patterns of motor commands: their connexions with flight motoneurones. J Exp Biol 1975; 63: 713–733.

32. Miller PL. Respiration in the desert locust. III. Ventilation and the spiracles during flight. J Exp Biol 1960; 37:246–278.

33. Kukalova-Peck J. Origin of the insect wing and wing articulation from the arthropodan leg. Can J Zool 1983; 61:1618–1669.

34. Kukalova-Peck J. Origin and evolution of insect wings and their relation to metamorphosis, as documented by the fossil record. J Morphol 1978; 156:53–126.

35. Dumont JPC, Robertson RM. Neuronal circuits: an evolutionary perspective. Science 1986; 233:849–852.

36. Piiper J., Scheid P. Model analysis of gas transport in fish gills. In: Hoar WS, Randall DJ, eds. Orlando, FL: Academic Press, 1984:229–262.

37. Adrian ED, Buytendijk FJJ. Potential changes in the isolated brainstem of the goldfish. J Physiol 1931; 71:121–135.

38. Ballantijn CM. Neural control of respiration in fishes and mammals. In: Proc Congr Eur Soc Comp Physiol Biochem, 3rd Noordwijkerhout, The Netherlands, 1981. Oxford, UK: Pergamon Press, 1982:127–140.

39. Fishman AP, Galante RJ, Pack AI. Diving physiology: lungfish. In: Wood SC, eds. Comparative Pulmonary Physiology. New York: Marcel Dekker, 1989:645–676.

40. Hutchinson VH, Haines HB, Engbretson G. Aquatic life at high altitude: respiratory adaptation in the Lake Titicaca frog, *Telmatobius culeus*. Respir Physiol 1976; 27:115–129.

41. Eldridge FL, Milhorn DE, Kiley JP, Waldrop TG. Stimulation by central command of locomotion, respiration and circulation during exercise. Respir Physiol 1985; 59:313–337.

42. Tenney SM. A phylogenetic perspective of control of the pulmonary circulation. In: Weir EK, Reeves JT, eds. Pulmonary Vascular Physiology and Pathophysiology. New York: Marcel Dekker, 1989:3–31.

43. Tenney SM, Ou LC. Hypoxic ventilatory response of cats at high altitude: an interpretation of "blunting." Respir Physiol 1977; 30:185–199.

44. Miller MJ, Tenney SM. Hypoxia-induced tachypnea in carotid-deafferented cats. Respir Physiol 1975; 23:31–39.

45. Somero GN. Protons, osmolytes, and fitness of internal milieu for protein function. Am J Physiol 1986; 251:R197–R213.

46. Rahn H, Reeves RB, Howell BJ. Hydrogen ion regulation, temperature, and evolution. Am Rev Respir Dis 1975; 112:165–172.

47. Reeves RB. An imidazole alphastat hypothesis for vertebrate acid-base regulation: tissue carbon dioxide content and body temperature in bullfrogs. Respir Physiol 1972; 14:219–236.

48. Barnhart MC. Control of acid-base status in active and dormant land snails, *Otala lactea* (Pulmonata, Helicidae). J Comp Physiol B 1986; 156:347–354.

49. Cameron JN. Acid-base homeostasis: past and present perspectives. Physiol Zool 1989; 62:845–865.

50. Hitzig BM. Temperature-induced changes in turtle CSF pH and central control of ventilation. Respir Physiol 1982; 49:205–222.

51. Jackson DC, Palmer SE, Meadow WL. The effects of temperature and carbon dioxide breathing on ventilation and acid-base status in turtles. Respir Physiol 1974; 20:131–146.

52. Davies DG. The effect of temperature on ventilation and gas exchange in the American alligator. Fed Proc 1975; 34:431 (abstract).

53. Douse MA, Mitchell GS. Temperature effects on CO_2-sensitive intrapulmonary chemoreceptors in the lizard, *Tupinambis nigropunctatus*. Respir Physiol 1988; 72:327–342.

54. Gallego R, Eyzaguirre C, Monit-Bloch L. Thermal and osmotic responses of arterial receptors. J Neurophysiol 1979; 42:665–680.

55. Beddard FE. On the diaphragm and on the muscular anatomy of *Xenopus*, with remarks on its affinities. Proc Zool Soc 1895; 54:841–846.

56. Keith A. The nature of the mammalian diaphragm and pleural cavities. J Anat Physiol 1905; 39:243–284.

57. Snapper JR, Tenney SM, McCann FV. Observations on the amphibian "diaphragm." Comp Biochem Physiol 1974; 49A:223–230.

58. Farrell AP, Randall DJ. Air-breathing mechanics in two Amazonian teleosts, *Arapaima gigas* and *Hoplerythrinus unitaeniatus*. Can J Zool 1978; 56:939–945.

59. Greenwood PH, Liem KF. Aspiratory inspiration in *Arapaima gigas* (*Teleostei Osteoglossomorpha*). J Zool (Lond) 1984; 203:411–425.

60. Perry SF. Evolution of the mammalian chest wall. In: Roussos C, Macklem PT, eds. The Thorax. New York: Marcel Dekker, 1985:187–198.

61. Dejours P. Respiration in Water and Air. Amsterdam: Elsevier, 1988:179.
62. Lahiri S. Blood oxygen affinity and alveolar ventilation in relation to body weight in mammals. Am J Physiol 1975; 229:529–536.
63. Tenney SM, Morrison DH. Tissue gas tensions in small wild animals. Respir Physiol 1967; 3:160–165.
64. Tenney SM, Bartlett D Jr. Comparative quantitative morphology of the mammalian lung: trachea. Respir Physiol 1967; 3:130–135.
65. Widdicombe JG. Respiratory reflexes. In: Fenn WO, Rahn H, eds. Handbook of Physiology. Respiration. Washington, DC: American Physiological Society, 1964: 585–630.
66. Bartlett D Jr, St John WM. Adaptation of pulmonary stretch receptors in different mammalian species. Respir Physiol 1979; 37:303–312.
67. Boggs DF, Tenney SM. Scaling respiratory pattern and respiratory "drive." Respir Physiol 1984; 58:245–251.
68. Frappell P, Lantheir C, Baudinette RV, Mortola JP. Metabolism and ventilation in acute hypoxia: a comparative analysis in small mammalian species. Am J Physiol 1992; 262:R1040–R1046.
69. Hill N, Tenney SM. Ventilatory responses to CO_2 and hypoxia in the two-toed sloth (*Choloepus hoffmanni*). Respir Physiol 1974; 22:311–323.
70. Asmussen R. Exercise and the regulation of ventilation. Circ Res 1967; 20:I-132–I-145.
71. Black AMS, Torrance RW. Respiratory oscillations in chemoreceptor discharge and the control of breathing. Respir Physiol 1971; 13:221–237.
72. Schmidt-Nielsen K, Larimer JL. Oxygen dissociation curves of mammalian blood in relation to body size. Am J Physiol 1958; 195:424–428.
73. Van Nice P, Black CP, Tenney SM. A comparative study of ventilatory responses to hypoxia with reference to hemoglobin O_2 affinity in llama, cat, rat, duck and goose. Comp Biochem Physiol 1980; 66A:347–350.
74. Boggs DF, Kilgore DL Jr., Birchard GF. Respiratory physiology of burrowing mammals and birds. Comp Biochem Physiol 1984; 77A:1–7.
75. Hall FG. Minimal utilizable oxygen and the oxygen dissociation curve of blood of rodents. J Appl Physiol 1966; 21:375–378.
76. Jones JRE. The reactions of fish to water of low oxygen concentration. J Exp Biol 1952; 29:403–415.
77. Birchard GF, Tenney SM. The hypoxic ventilatory response of rats with increased blood oxygen affinity. Respir Physiol 1986; 66:225–233.
78. Lee KD, Mattenheimer H. The biochemistry of the carotid body. Enzymol Biol Clin 1964; 4:199–216.
79. Mills E, Jöbsis FF. Mitochondrial respiratory chain of carotid body and chemoreceptor response to changes in oxygen tension. J Neurophysiol 1972; 35:405–428.
80. Buerk DG, Nair PK, Whalen WJ. Two-cytochrome metabolic model for carotid body Pti_{O_2} and chemosensitivity changes after hemorrhage. J Appl Physiol 1989; 67:60–68.
81. Biscoe TJ, Duchen MR. Monitoring P_{O_2} by the carotid chemoreceptor. NIPS 1990; 5:229–233.

82. Tenney SM, Ou LC. Ventilatory responses of decorticate and decerebrate cats to hypoxia and CO_2. Respir Physiol 1977; 29:81–92.
83. Brooks JG III, Tenney SM. Ventilatory response of llama to hypoxia at sea level and high altitude. Respir Physiol 1968; 5:269–278.
84. Lahiri S. Unattenuated ventilatory hypoxic drive in ovine and bovine species native to high altitude. J Appl Physiol 1972; 32:95–102.
85. Bartels H. Comparative physiology of oxygen transport in mammals. Lancet 1964; 599–604.
86. Boggs DF, Colby C, Williams BR Jr, Kilgore DL. Chemosensitivity and breathing pattern regulation of the coatimundi and woodchuck. Respir Physiol 1992; 89: 157–167.
87. Scholander PF. Experimental investigations on respiration and diving mammals and birds. Hvalradets Skr 1940; 22:1–120.
88. Irving L. The insensitivity of diving animals to CO_2. Am J Physiol 1938; 124: 729–734.
89. Birchard G, Boggs DF, Tenney SM. Effects of perinatal CO_2 exposure on adult ventilatory responses. Respir Physiol 1984; 57:341–347.
90. Leiter JC, Mortola JP, Tenney SM. A comparative analysis of contractile characteristics of the diaphragm and of respiratory system mechanics. Respir Physiol 1986; 64:267–276.
91. Milic-Emili J, Grunstein MM. Drive and timing components of ventilation. Chest 1976; 70:S131–S133.
92. Kuna ST. Inhibition of inspiratory upper airway motoneuron activity by phasic volume feedback. J Appl Physiol 1986; 60:1373–1379.
93. Bartlett D Jr, St John WM. Influence of lung volume on phrenic, hypoglossal and mylohyoid nerve activities. Respir Physiol 1988; 73:97–110.
94. Negus VE. The Comparative Anatomy and Physiology of the Larynx. London: W. Heinemann Medical Books, 1949.
95. Laitman JT, Heimbuch RC, Crelin ES. Developmental change in a basicranial line and its relationship to the upper respiratory system in living primates. Am J Anat 1978; 152:467–482.
96. Lieberman P, Crelin ES, Klatt DH. Phonetic ability and related anatomy of the newborn and adult human, Neanderthal man, and the chimpanzee. Am Anthropol 1972; 74:287–307.
97. Laitman JT, Heimbuch RC, Crelin ES. The basicranium of fossil hominids as an indicator of their upper respiratory systems. Am J Phys Anthropol 1979; 51: 15–33.
98. Hendricks JC, Kline LR, Kovalski RJ, O'Brien JA, Morrison AR, Pack AI. The English bulldog: a natural model of sleep-disordered breathing. J Appl Physiol 1987; 63:1344–1350.
99. Otis AB, Fenn WO, Rahn H. Mechanics of breathing in man. J Appl Physiol 1950; 2:592–608.
100. Mead J. Control of respiratory frequency. J Appl Physiol 1960; 15:325–336.
101. Bennett FM, Tenney SM. Comparative mechanics of mammalian respiratory system. Respir Physiol 1982; 49:131–140.

102. Banzett RB, Nations CS, Wang N, Butler JP, Lehr JL. Mechanical independence of wingbeat and breathing in starlings. Respir Physiol 1992; 89:27–36.

103. Garlando F, Kohl J, Koller EA, Pietsch P. Effect of coupling the breathing rhythms and cycling rhythms on oxygen uptake during bicycle ergometry. Eur J Appl Physiol Occup Physiol 1985; 54:497–501.

104. Perségol L, Jordan M, Viala D. Evidence for the entrainment of breathing by locomotor pattern in human. J Physiol (Paris) 1991; 85:38–43.

105. Banzett RB, Mead J, Reid MB, Topulos GP. Locomotion in men has no appreciable effect on ventilation. J Appl Physiol 1992; 72:1922–1926.

106. Grubb B, Jones JH, Schmidt-Nielsen K. Avian cerebral blood flow: influence of the Bohr effect on oxygen supply. Am J Physiol 1979; 236:H744–H749.

107. Black CP, Tenney SM. Oxygen transport during progressive hypoxia in high-altitude and sea-level waterfowl. Respir Physiol 1980; 39:217–239.

108. Powell FL, Milsom WK, Mitchell GS. Effects of intrapulmonary CO_2 and airway pressure on pulmonary vagal afferent activity in the alligator. Respir Physiol 1988; 74:285–298.

109. Furilla RA, Coates EL, Bartlett D Jr. The influence of venous CO_2 on ventilation in garter snakes. Respir Physiol 1991; 83:47–60.

110. Ballam GO, Donaldson LA. Effect of venous (gut) CO_2 loading on intrapulmonary gas fractions and ventilation in the tegu lizard. J Comp Physiol B. 1988; 158: 591–600.

111. Peterson DF, Fedde RM. Receptors sensitive to carbon dioxide in lungs of chicken. Science 1968; 162:1499–1501.

112. Furilla RA, Bartlett D Jr. Intrapulmonary CO_2 inhibits inspiration in garter snakes. Respir Physiol 1989; 78:207–218.

113. Banzett RB, Burger RE. Response of avian intrapulmonary chemoreceptors to venous CO_2 and ventilatory gas flow. Respir Physiol 1977; 29:63–72.

114. Powell FL, Fedde MR, Gratz RK, Scheid P. Ventilatory response to CO_2 in birds. I. Measurements in the unanesthetized duck. Respir Physiol 1978; 35:349–359.

115. Gratz RK. Effect of bilateral vagotomy on the ventilatory responses of the water snake *Nerodia sipedon*. Am J Physiol 1984; 246:R221–R227.

116. Coates EL, Furilla RA, Ballam GO, Bartlett D Jr. A decrease in nasal CO_2 stimulates breathing in the tegu lizard. Respir Physiol 1991; 86:65–75.

117. Farber JP. Development of pulmonary reflexes and pattern of breathing in the Virginia opossum. Respir Physiol 1972; 14:278–286.

118. Farber JP, Hultgren HN, Tenney SM. Development and the control of breathing in the Virginia opossum. Respir Physiol 1972; 14:267–277.

Part Two

CENTRAL NERVOUS CONTROL

2

Neural Control of Respiratory Pattern in Mammals: An Overview

JACK L. FELDMAN and JEFFREY C. SMITH

University of California at Los Angeles
Los Angeles, California

I. Introduction

The brain is vigilant in control of breathing. It is responsible for the regulation of blood oxygen and carbon dioxide adaptable over an order of magnitude range in metabolic demand, wide ranges of posture and body movements, compromises in muscle or cardiopulmonary function, from birth to death without lapses beyond a few minutes. It must make efficient use of the respiratory musculature, for the metabolic cost of inefficiency, integrated over time, is considerable. Moreover, serious respiratory muscle fatigue must be avoided to prevent insufficiencies, especially during and following extreme exertion or with disease.

Our current understanding of how the brain controls breathing is limited, but the future appears bright. In the past decade, a solid foundation has been established that may serve as the basis for resolution of basic mechanisms. In this chapter, we will discuss generation and control of respiratory rhythm and pattern. In order to focus on issues, we will present only a brief overview. We refer the reader to several more comprehensive reviews (1–5).

II. Overview

The apparently simple act of moving air into and out of the (mammalian) lung is the product of a complex and mutable system of many distinct components (Fig. 1). An intact brainstem and spinal cord, in situ, can generate respiratory motor nerve output, in the absence of rostral brain or sensory afferents. Mammals anesthetized or with severe rostral brain damage, including decerebration, will continue to breathe, with ventilation appropriate for blood gases and pH homeostasis. Following paralysis, provided blood gas homeostasis is maintained, rhythmic motor output in nerves innervating respiratory muscles continues. Finally, in neonatal and fetal rats (6–8), respiratory-related patterns of motor nerve activity continue following careful removal of the brainstem (and spinal cord) to an in vitro chamber; an isolated slice of a particular region of the medulla (9) will even generate respiratory-related rhythm. Taken together, this suggests that the kernel of control (10) is an intrinsic oscillator, located in the brainstem.

Rhythm generation is the first step in producing a patterned motor output, which must result in appropriate profiles of contraction in each muscle and coordination of contraction and relaxation among synergists and between antagonists. Premotor circuits transform their incoming rhythmic drive in accordance

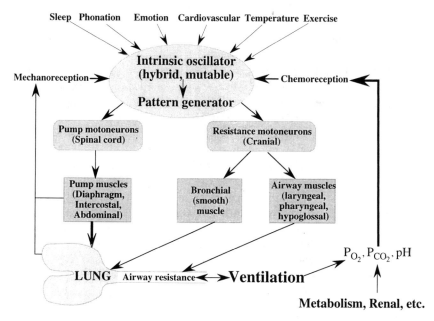

Figure 1 Cartoon of neural control of ventilation in mammals. See text for details.

with their intrinsic properties and afferent inputs into patterns of activity that drive and coordinate motoneurons. Motoneurons, which receive many inputs that can affect their excitability, are important elements in transforming the rhythm into a motor output pattern and can be categorized into two groups: spinal motoneurons innervating muscles of the respiratory pump, e.g., phrenic, intercostal, abdominal; and cranial motoneurons, innervating muscles modulating airway resistance, e.g., laryngeal and pharyngeal (skeletal) muscles, and bronchial (smooth) muscles. Contraction/relaxation of the pump muscles produces changes in intrapleural pressure resulting in inflation/deflation that depend on lung mechanics and airway resistance. The resultant alveolar ventilation, along with other factors such as metabolic load and renal function, affects blood gases and pH.

The brain mechanisms controlling breathing in intact mammals are subject to many influences, including blood and brain gas and pH values and behavioral state—emotive, cognitive, or movement-related. Signals related to these sources profoundly affect and alter the performance of the intrinsic brainstem and spinal cord neurons, and perhaps even cause reorganization of the underlying neuronal circuits. This latter possibility is important if we are to compare and contrast data obtained under different experimental conditions, at different stages of development, or from different species or even strains of mammals (see below).

There are two principal regulatory loops for breathing in mammals*:

A. Chemoreceptors

The raison d'être of breathing is to exchange O_2 and CO_2 between lung and environmental air, regulating alveolar ventilation appropriate for homeostasis. Given the markedly different natures of O_2 and CO_2 carriage in the blood and an alternative (but slower) pathway for blood CO_2 regulation via the kidney, the pathways and mechanisms for their regulation are distinct.

The principal O_2 sensors are in the carotid bodies, which signal the brain via afferent pathways in the glossopharyngeal nerve that synapse in the dorsomedial medulla in the region of the nucleus of the solitary tract. The sensors increase their discharge as O_2 levels are decreased, with steep increases below $\sim$50 mmHg; the increased discharge stimulates breathing. Under normal conditions, O_2 sensors account for only a small part of the chemical drive to breathe. Removal of carotid body chemosensory input by breathing pure O_2 reduces minute ventilation by about 15% in awake mammals.

Although the phenomenology for CO_2 responses is established in exquisite detail, the sites and mechanisms for CO_2 reception remain obscure. Peripherally chemodenervated decerebrate mammals maintain a robust CO_2 response, suggesting that CO_2 or related variables (pH, HCO_3^-) have intracranial sensors. Although

---

*In nonprimate mammals, ventilation also plays an important role in thermoregulation.

other sites have been proposed (11,12), sites in the ventral medulla have received the most attention. Recently, Nattie and colleagues suggest that the retrotrapezoid nucleus and surrounding neuronal structures (13) are critical for CO_2 regulation in decerebrate cats (14). However, identification of neurons that act as sensors has proven elusive.

B. Mechanoreceptors

There are many patterns of muscle activity that could produce alveolar ventilation appropriate for a given metabolic load; the chosen pattern depends on numerous conditions. Some patterns of respiratory muscle activity will necessarily be more efficient, depending on such factors as posture and lung and chest wall mechanics (e.g., a fibrotic lung is harder to inflate to a given tidal volume than a normal lung, and thus rapid, shallow breathing may be more efficient).

The precise regulation of muscle contraction requires feedback from muscle and joint receptors, and the influence of somatosensory receptors should also be recognized. Mechanoreceptors in the lungs and airways are critical, especially since the resultant action of respiratory muscle activity is to change lung volume (and airway resistance). Furthermore, these and other, such as irritant, receptors are required for detection of circumstances that require special respiratory reflexes, such as coughing, sneezing, sighing, gasping, and so forth.

Mechanosensory signals are critical in adapting, adjusting, and integrating breathing with other acts of brain and body. Many movements impact directly on breathing, either by utilizing the same muscles (e.g., phonation, posture, defecation, or emesis) or through mechanical disturbances, such as locomotion. These influences extend well beyond the ability to accelerate or brake ventilation. They may exert effects by reconfiguring the circuits controlling breathing (for example, the profound differences in ventilatory control between REM and slow wave sleep may be due to dynamic rewiring of the underlying neural circuits) (10); this possibility poses a serious challenge for interpretation of experimental data, especially from reduced preparations (see below).

The rest of this chapter will explore several issues related to the production of rhythm and pattern and only at the most basic level. We will first consider the fact that there is no standard experimental model for data acquisition.

III. Experimental Models

In studying brain mechanisms, the questions we ask, the data we obtain, and the interpretations we make are constrained, often severely, by the experimental models available. During this century, we have gone from using blunt spatulas, gross lesions, and macrostimulation in largely intact animals to whole-cell patch-clamp recording, molecular analysis, (micro)pharmacological manipulation, and microstimulation often in highly reduced preparations, and magnetic brain stimulation, and imaging in awake humans. We have certainly gathered a lot of facts; their relevance is not always transparent.

If our goal is to understand the neural control of breathing in humans, then ideally we should perform the necessary experiments in humans; with limited exceptions, this is impossible. Until technology provides us with the means to resolve neuronal activity noninvasively in the spatiotemporal domain of microns/ milli seconds, we are limited in human experimentation to phenomenological measures of gross variables (ventilation, regional brain metabolism/activity, etc.), and even then, we will have limited ability to clamp variables. So, we perform experiments in other species, often in reduced states that allow invasive studies.

We have argued that the circuits generating and controlling respiratory pattern can reconfigure (10), possibly transform between different brain states. Mechanisms may also differ among different species, which constrains our ability to extrapolate among experimental models. Even if restricted to mammals, the identity of mechanisms cannot be stipulated. A comparative approach can be illuminating in searching for common mechanisms (15–17), but such studies require a deep understanding of the ventilatory function in each species studied. There are certainly differences in respiratory pattern and control between related species, and there are even differences between strains in a given species (e.g., 18). Furthermore, breathing in different states in any given species (e.g., REM sleep vs. slow wave sleep vs. wakefulness; anesthetized vs. decerebrate or vagotomized vs. nonvagotomized experimental preparations) may rely on related, but not identical mechanisms and circuits. Of course, there is hardly any behavioral act or state that does not influence breathing, from sleep-wake state to menstrual cycle to locomotion to anxiety. Moreover, since breathing is homeostatically regulated, there are considerable interactions with other physiological systems.

As an example of the issues inherent in the use of any reduced preparation, we briefly examine the barbiturate-anesthetized cat, which has served as the gold standard for electrophysiologists, in large part because the suppression of non-respiratory function might reveal the most basic respiratory mechanisms. Clearly, barbiturate anesthetics suppress cognitive and volitional behaviors, as well as many homeostatic functions and reflexes. At the behavioral level, marked differences in breathing are seen between barbiturate-anesthetized and unanesthetized mammals (compare, e.g., 4,19 with 20,21). Many neurons with respiratory-related discharge patterns show remarkable plasticity in their discharge patterns in awake/sleeping (nonanesthetized) mammals (20–22) that is not seen in anesthetized animals. Are these variable firing patterns relevant or even critical to pattern generation in intact animals, or are they simply noise eliminated by anesthesia?

Reductionism and the simple fact that air either moves into or out of the lung long supported the view that respiratory rhythm had two phases: inspiration and expiration. In a thorough evaluation across various vertebrate species, Milsom (15) suggests that there are up to five distinct phases of respiratory motor pattern in vertebrates: inspiration; end-inspiratory pause; passive expiration; active expiration; and end-expiratory pause. In the past decade, postinspiration, originally described as an initial epoch of braked expiratory airflow when the diaphragm is still active and the larynx is adducted (23) and more recently as a central component of rhythm generation (24–26), has been widely accepted as a separate phase of respiratory rhythm in mammals. This hypothesis is based largely on data from barbiturate-anesthetized cats and rats (19,25,27–29). The fundamental notion that breathing rhythm involves a necessary three-phase sequence of neuronal activity (see below) needs to be considered in light of data from decerebrate unanesthetized cats (3,24,26,30,31) or rats (32,33) or from intact guinea pigs or cats during sleep or wakefulness (20,21). In contrast to anesthetized animals, the necessary class of postinspiratory neurons that are required to underlie this phase are not prevalent in the ventrolateral medulla (their reported location in the anesthetized cat); one related subclass of neurons in decerebrates has a rapid onset of bursting at the end of inspiration, but unlike postinspiratory neurons, continues to fire until the onset of the next inspiratory burst (early expiratory neurons) (34). Recently, Orem and Trotter (22) compared results from intact unanesthetized cats with conclusions drawn mostly from results in barbiturate-anesthetized cats and concluded that for five medullary cell types

> Certain features of their behavior were inconsistent with . . . their proposed role in rhythmogenesis. . . . For example, decrementing inspiratory cells switched to an augmenting pattern during the second part of the augmented breath. This behavior is inconsistent with mechanisms proposed to account for their decrementing pattern and with their postulated inhibitory actions on augmenting inspiratory neurons. . . .

Of course, whenever differences are seen among different preparations, one must recognize the possibility of recording biases; however, the differences may nonetheless be real and substantial. Several questions follow:

> How many phases of neural activity are necessary for rhythm generation?

> Is postinspiration a necessary component of rhythmogenesis or rather a component of a motor pattern (e.g., the initial component of the motor pattern underlying expiratory airflow) that is produced under barbiturate anesthesia?

> Could postinspiratory neurons be early expiratory neurons transformed by anesthesia? Whereas postinspiratory neurons are proposed to be critical in rhythmogenesis and the irreversible phase of inspiratory termination, early expiratory neurons have been proposed to play a role in terminating expiration (34,35).

At the cellular level, barbiturates, even at sedative doses, alter several important intrinsic neuronal properties, including (36–39): potentiation of voltage-dependent K^+ channels, inhibition of voltage-dependent Na^+ and Ca^{2+} channels, and inhibition of glutamate- and ACh-regulated cation channels. Of particular importance to experimental studies of the neural control of breathing is that barbiturates greatly enhance $GABA_A$-regulated Cl^--dependent inhibitory currents, which can double at sedative levels of barbiturate. At anesthetic levels, Cl^--dependent inhibitory currents are considerably higher, owing in part to the direct action on the Cl^- channel (36–39). These actions on critical neural functions must alter neuronal behavior at the membrane, synaptic, and single-neuron level; given the complexity and nonlinearity of network function, alterations in network function would also likely result. [Volatile anesthetics are no better; they can potentiate currents through $GABA_A$ Cl^--channels severalfold (40).]

Consider now that the most elaborate picture of synaptic behavior of respiratory neurons is based on observations of Cl^--dependent inhibitory currents in barbiturate anesthetized animals (see below). One might argue that these currents are best studied under conditions where they are enhanced. However, without a baseline for comparison, these currents could be sufficiently enhanced to obscure even more critical currents; they could also play a less critical role, if any, in the unanesthetized state. The relevance of inhibitory currents to respiratory rhythm and pattern generation in anesthetized cats compared to other experimental preparations, especially in the intact animal, remains to be fully established. A systematic protocol of measurements in unanesthetized i.e., decerebrate, preparations may help clarify this issue. Recognizing the limitations of a preparation should not, however, obscure its usefulness, and certainly the barbiturate-anesthetized cat has been of enormous importance.

Recently, spurred by advances in other areas of neurobiology, highly reduced in vitro preparations have been exploited to study neural control of breathing. Like the barbiturate-anesthetized cat, these preparations have led to useful observations. Since homeostatically regulated ventilation is a complex integrative process of intact animals, we need to address the relevance and, of course, the obvious limitations of in vitro preparations so far removed from this context.

A. In Vitro Preparations

Preparations with Endogenous Rhythmical Activity

We wish to consider another preparation, a decade old (8), the isolated en bloc in vitro brainstem–spinal cord from neonatal (or fetal) rat. We have reviewed the utility of this preparation, especially when compared to in vivo preparations (7,10). Its advantages include: (1) neuronal circuitry is maintained; (2) rhythmic neural activity on respiratory motor nerves is present; (3) manipulation of the extracellular environment is feasible owing to the absence of a blood-brain barrier and its relative compactness; (4) whole-cell patch-clamp and sharp electrode recording are extremely stable, in part owing to the absence of cardiopulmonary pumping. This preparation has assumed an important role in the study of basic mechanisms in the neonatal nervous system, and it is worth considering criticisms of its utility as a model system (see also 41). The criticisms fall into several categories:

"The preparation is immature." Understanding the developmental sequelae leading from zygote to adult is a fundamental question in biology; late fetal and neonatal mammals present a critical juncture for regulatory functions. This is especially true for breathing, which, unlike many systems (e.g., vision, cognition), must be functional from birth and, despite profound changes in early life especially within the brain, must remain appropriate for homeostasis and growth. Moreover, very serious dysfunctions of breathing, possibly including sudden infant death syndrome (SIDS), occur in neonatal humans, so understanding the underlying mechanisms in neonates and their ultimate transformation in adults is of obvious importance.

There is a distinct possibility that results from this neonatal preparation are relevant only to this particular stage of development. One must therefore be cautious extrapolating to mechanisms in adults (or vice versa), where virtually the entire database of respiratory neurobiology resides.

"The preparation is not breathing." In his original description, Suzue (8) suggested that the rhythmic pattern may be gasping. This view is reinforced by the criticism that the in vitro brainstem "is anoxic" (see below), since anoxia in an *adult* brainstem in situ would lead to gasping. Certainly, the pattern of motor nerve activity in vitro is different from that in the intact neonatal rat, but such differences exist for every experimental preparation when compared to the intact, undrugged mammal (and even in the intact mammal, there are differences between states, e.g., sleep-wake).

Is then the pattern in vitro so different as to be irrelevant to "normal" breathing? We think not. We have demonstrated that the pattern observed in vitro is similar to that of the anesthetized in vivo neonatal rat, following vagotomy (7). The transformation in pattern in vivo is immediate following vagotomy, too short a time for blood gas imbalance, especially hypoxia, to develop. This suggests that the neural mechanisms in vitro contain elements relevant to more intact preparations (10).

"The preparation is anoxic and/or severely acidotic." An unperfused piece of neonatal brain in vitro with any dimension ≥ 500 μm will become hypoxic, and for thicker tissue, there is the likelihood of an anoxic core. This could alter intrinsic and synaptic neuronal function, either directly or via consequential release of neuroactive chemicals. Yet, careful measurements of oxygen partial

pressure and pH in en bloc preparations in regions critical to respiratory function are consistent with aerobic metabolism and conventional neuronal function (42). At the (sub)cellular level, the intrinsic properties of individual neurons as well as synaptic properties are also consistent with normal function. At the network level: (1) the en bloc preparation produces a complex rhythmic pattern of motor nerve activity similar to that of the vagotomized neonate, which is stable for hours under control conditions; furthermore, this pattern is severely affected (eventually abolished) by removal of oxygen from the bathing medium; (2) the "oscillating" slice preparation, which is considerably thinner than the en bloc brainstem and is therefore better oxygenated, generates the same pattern of rhythmic respiratory motor activity as the en bloc brainstem (9). The robustness of the en bloc and slice preparations, perhaps surprising to those mostly familiar with adult mammals, is likely due to the special metabolic properties and resistance of neonatal (brain) tissue to the deleterious effects of low oxygen (e.g., 43, 44).

"The temperature is too low." The viability of en bloc and thick slice preparations is enhanced at lower temperature. Numerous parameters of neuronal function, including the kinetics of membrane currents (45), are temperature-dependent. In the en bloc preparation, temperature reduction from 35°C to 27°C has graded and continuous effects on respiratory phase timing but not on motor burst pattern (7) and certainly does not result in catastrophic changes. The lowered temperature of this preparation is in the mainstream of many neurobiological studies that have effectively used slice preparations of mammalian brain at reduced temperatures to illuminate neuronal properties and synaptic function (45,46).

Our position is that the en bloc in vitro preparation is useful for studying basic neural mechanisms underlying the control of breathing in mammals. In full recognition of the particular limitations of these en bloc in vitro preparations, we assert that they provide an essential bridge between more reduced systems, where many cellular and synaptic mechanisms have been illuminated in great detail (albeit in the absence of endogenous behavior), and in vivo preparations, such as more intact mammals, where current technology and experimental protocols (especially anesthesia) limit the ability to determine the role of many potentially important synaptic, cellular, and network properties in generating breathing rhythm. Given the technical advantages and reduced nature of these in vitro preparations, one may expect to make critical measurements essential to understanding rhythm generation and pattern formation. This still would leave a challenging problem: how do mechanisms generating rhythm and pattern in vitro precisely relate to those in the fully intact nervous system in vivo?

Preparations Without Endogenous Rhythmic Activity

An increasing number of studies are performed in brain slices or cultures where there is no ongoing behavior to allow identification of neurons as respiratory-related (see also discussions in 47). Consider a neuron in a brainstem region that in an intact mammal would contain neurons with respiratory-modulated activity. In a typical slice, even if this cell is demarcated by anatomical or other criteria, there is no respiratory activity; therefore, one does not know whether this particular cell received respiratory inputs when it was in the intact brain.

Although we can get exquisite measures of neuronal behavior in slices, neuronal activation is typically restricted to electrical stimulation or exogenous application of chemicals. These experimental procedures are likely to activate cells in ways different from normal (e.g., see 48). Electrical stimulation will synchronously activate inputs that may normally not be synchronous or even coactive. Exogenous application of neurotransmitter agonists will activate both synaptic and extrasynaptic receptors, with a time course that may be inappropriate [e.g., if the synaptic receptors rapidly desensitize (49)]. Some normally present neurochemicals may be absent. Furthermore, presynaptic modulation of rhythmically active neurons (see below) may be difficult to observe in the absence of endogenous activity.

Even if a cell can be inferred to be respiratory-related, there remains the question of the relevance of any particular measure. Any individual neuron can express distinctly different characteristics depending on its cellular environment, and especially its inputs. Circuits of neurons are pluripotent ensembles (50). From how a neural ensemble performs one task we may not conclude how another action is performed. (From how an acting ensemble plays Beckett, we can only guess how it will play Shakespeare, or which actor will play which role.) Respiratory-related neurons, certainly at the premotor and motoneuronal level, participate in many acts besides breathing itself (e.g., phonation, defecation, coughing, gagging, sneezing, vomiting). Most of these acts can transiently suppress breathing (anyone who has gagged can testify to the powerful transient suppression of rhythmic breathing), so at some level each act must have a stronger influence on some critical neurons than respiratory drive. If measurements of single neuron behavior are made outside the context of behavior, how can one be sure that any deduced property subserves breathing? Are the strongest features related to breath-by-breath actions, or rather to rare events that must dominate, such as gasping?

Short of noninvasive recording in intact humans (or other species of choice), and pending demonstration that observations obtained under other conditions are operational in intact humans or chosen species, all preparations are "unphysiological." A rational approach for evaluating the usefulness of experimental preparations would recognize that: (1) investigators choose a given experimental preparation because it has particular utility for making important measurements or performing critical tests; (2) preparations that differ in species [15, even strain (18)], age, state, sex, or experimental protocol are different; (3) hypotheses based on information obtained under one set of conditions can and should be tested under other conditions.

IV. Several Fundamental Questions for Control of Breathing

Regardless of the preparation, the goal of experimentation is to understand the mechanisms underlying the control of breathing. What are the questions that must be addressed?

Although the grand problem can be simply stated: "In (name your species of choice), how is respiratory rhythm generated and respiratory pattern produced and modulated?" the solution is not simple. The brain is not a black box. Regardless of how detailed or clever phenomenological descriptions are of neural control mechanisms, e.g., ventilatory responses to hypercapnea or hypoxia, we cannot deduce central mechanisms without specific reference to identified neurons and their properties. Only rarely, if ever, will behavioral descriptions sufficiently constrain the possible mechanisms to be useful for guiding contemporary neurobiological studies. Any systematic approach would seek to address the following issues:

A. What Sites Are Critically Involved?

A rough description of the critical brainstem and spinal cord regions has been available since the late 1970s (reviewed in 1,2,4; see also 13,51,52). Several brainstem regions are considered to play a direct role in the production of respiratory rhythm/pattern. In brief (Fig. 2):

Ventral Respiratory Group (VRG)

This long ventrolateral medullary cell column spans from the spinomedullary junction to the retrofacial nucleus. The location of these cells is homologous to that of ventral horn interneurons of the spinal cord. This region contains most of the premotor neurons projecting to the spinal cord (bulbospinal neurons) to provide respiratory drive to muscles of the respiratory pump. Along the rostrocaudal axis, interconnected subregions are differentiated on the basis of discharge patterns and projections of constituent neurons:

Caudal VRG (cVRG; spinomedullary junction to near obex)—contains mostly neurons with expiratory discharge patterns. Many cells project to the spinal cord (bulbospinal neurons) to provide excitatory drive to motoneurons innervating expiratory muscles, e.g., internal intercostal, abdominal.

Rostral VRG (rVRG; obex to caudal of retrofacial nucleus)—contains mostly neurons with inspiratory discharge patterns. Contains many excitatory bulbospinal neurons that provide inspiratory drive to motoneurons innervating inspiratory muscles, e.g., diaphragm, external intercostal.

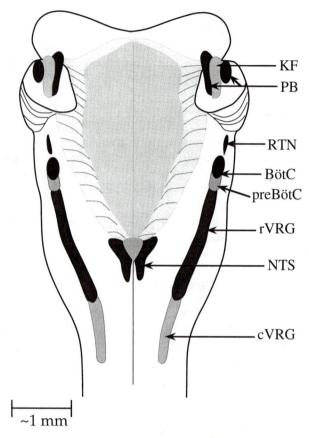

KF
PB

RTN
BötC
preBötC
rVRG
NTS
cVRG

~1 mm

Figure 2 Dorsal view of brainstem (without cerebellum) showing brainstem regions involved in control of breathing. Refer to text and reviews (1,2,4); see also Refs. 13, 51, 52. preBötC, preBötzinger complex; VRG, ventral respiratory group; PB, parabrachial nuclei; KF, Kölliker-Fuse nucleus (PB/KF comprise the pontine respiratory group); NTS, regions of nuclei of solitary tract; RTN, retrotrapezoid nucleus.

Bötzinger complex (BötC; level of retrofacial nucleus)—contains inhibitory neurons with expiratory discharge patterns. These neurons have extensive projections and act to prevent spurious discharge of inspiratory neurons during expiration (reciprocal inhibition, see below).

preBötzinger complex—This most recently identified subregion, sandwiched between the rVRG and BötC, has been hypothesized as a brainstem site generating respiratory rhythm (9). The preBötC was initially identified as the critical region required to maintain oscillations in the in vitro brainstem (9). Slices of the medulla that contain the preBötC continue to generate respiratory-related rhythms (9), and perturbation of neuronal excitability in the preBötC, both in vivo and in vitro (53), result in perturbations of rhythm. Compared to the immediately adjacent BötC and VRG, the preBötC contains a different spectrum of neuron types (3,54,55), including very few bulbospinal neurons (52). We have proposed that the preBötC is the medullary source of respiratory rhythm and that neurons in this region with bursting pacemaker properties are the kernel for rhythm generation (9; see below).

Other brainstem sites with an apparent role include: various subnuclei of the solitary tract (e.g., 56), the retrotrapezoid nucleus (13,14,57), raphe nuclei (58), and the pontine respiratory group (Kölliker-Fuse and parabrachial nuclei (4,59,60).

B. What Mechanisms Underlie Rhythmogenesis?

At present, this is a severely underconstrained problem. That is, with our limited knowledge of the intrinsic properties of neurons with *identified function* (i.e., an unequivocal demonstration of the precise role a neuron is playing in rhythmogenesis is required, which is not to be confused with descriptive properties), and with little known about their specific interconnections, a model based on contemporary experimental observations can readily be tailored to simulate respiratory rhythm. Models (Fig. 3) range from pacemaker neurons capable of generating the basic respiratory pattern (e.g., 61) to networks of platonic (46) cells (25,61,62); in between are hybrid networks of cells with active/pacemaker properties (24,26,63–65). These different classes of models are distinguished by several characteristics, including the role of complex intrinsic neuronal properties and the necessary role of postsynaptic inhibition in rhythm generation.

Role of Inhibition

In terms of timing and function, inhibition, which is any decrease in neuronal excitability, is one of at least three types (Fig. 4): recurrent, reciprocal, or phase transition.

Recurrent inhibition, present during the bursting phase of a neuron, helps to shape that burst (even to delay its onset) and may be very important in determining the precise pattern of neuronal activity.

Reciprocal inhibition, active during the normally silent phase of a neuron, acts to prevent spurious activation.

Phase transition inhibition contributes to terminating a phase.

Pacemaker   # Network

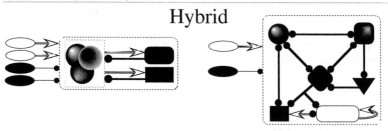

Intrinsic currents: I_{HH}, $I_{K(Ca)}$, I_Q,   Intrinsic currents: I_{HH}
$I_{Ca, LVA}$, $I_{Ca, HVA}$, $I_{Na, K}$, etc.

Hybrid

Intrinsic currents: I_{HH}, $I_{K(Ca)}$, I_Q,   Intrinsic currents: I_{HH}, $I_{K(Ca)}$, I_Q,
$I_{Ca, LVA}$, $I_{Ca, HVA}$, $I_{Na, K}$, etc. $I_{Ca, LVA}$, $I_{Ca, HVA}$, $I_{Na, K}$, etc.

Figure 3 Models of respiratory rhythm generation range from purely pacemaker driven (upper left; e.g., 61), where the rhythm is due to intrinsic currents, with interconnections serving to coordinate activity to pure network models (upper right, 1,62) of mundane cells (cells that integrate and fire, behaving much like squid axons with HH type currents) interacting with excitatory (arrow) and inhibitory (black circle) connections. More recently, hybrid models derived from a pacemaker premise (bottom left, 10,65) or from a network premise (bottom right, 24,46) have been proposed. These hybrid models postulate both active currents and ordinary excitatory and inhibitory interactions. In the hybrid pacemaker-network type model (left), synaptically coupled pacemaker neurons are embedded in a network where both tonic and phasic synaptic inputs regulate voltage-dependent oscillations of pacemaker neurons. All neurons have voltage- and time-dependent conductances, the most complex set of which is exhibited by pacemaker neurons required to generate intrinsic oscillations. In the hybrid network type models (right), neuronal behavior also results from interactions of synaptic and voltage-dependent conductances, although inhibitory interactions are still required to produce network oscillations.

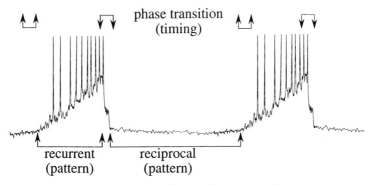

Figure 4 Role of inhibition. Hypothetical burst of an augmenting inspiratory neuron, with three different periods of synaptic inhibition (recurrent, reciprocal, and phase transition), is indicated.

In addition to these phasic inhibitory interactions, neurons may receive tonic inhibitory inputs, which can regulate membrane potential and excitability. Reduction of neuronal excitability can be produced in several distinct ways, and either post- or presynaptically:

Postsynaptic inhibition: The study of postsynaptic inhibition in respiratory neurons, pioneered by Richter and colleagues (19,25), has been informative in illuminating the events shaping neuronal behavior. In principle, synaptic inhibition results from binding of an amino acid neurotransmitter such as GABA or glycine to its postsynaptic receptor, which leads to opening of Cl^- or K^+ channels, producing, under normal conditions, an outward current that will hyperpolarize most cells. As mentioned above, Cl^- inhibition is enhanced by barbiturate anesthesia, which has been used in experiments from which most information on synaptic inhibition has been obtained.

Ion-gated hyperpolarization: The accumulation of intracellular Ca^{2+} by the entry of Ca^{2+} via ligand- (e.g., NMDA) or voltage-gated Ca^{2+} channels can open certain K^+ channels, leading to hyperpolarization, usually referred to as afterhyperpolarization (AHP), since both the Ca^{2+} inflow and the K^+-current activation requires a preceding period of depolarization. There are several different types of AHP, acting on time scales from milliseconds to seconds. AHP is seen in many different types of respiratory neurons (66–68).

Another general mechanism to reduce excitability is to decrease the depolarizing drive, either at its source (disfacilitation), before it reaches the soma (presynaptic), or by altering the somatodendritic membrane properties (shunting; voltage- (or time-) gated decreased excitability):

Disfacilitation occurs when excitatory (depolarizing) inputs are withdrawn. Disfacilitation can occur concurrently with synaptic inhibition.

Presynaptic inhibition occurs by a number of mechanisms that cause the transient reduction of excitatory neurotransmitter release from the presynaptic terminal, reducing postsynaptic excitation (see below).

Shunting inhibition occurs when the localized opening of channels on a patch of membrane serves not only as a current source, but if strategically located, as a significant sink (shunt) of more distal currents. Activation of such synapses can effectively block propagation of distal excitatory (or inhibitory) currents to the cell soma.

Voltage- (or time-) gated decreased excitability can occur when any of a variety of depolarizing conductances inactivate or hyperpolarizing currents activate simply as a result of the immediate history of neuronal potential.

Postsynaptic phase transition inhibition is a necessary component of all network models for rhythm generation. There is controversy as to whether such inhibition is a necessary component of rhythm generation, especially in highly reduced preparations. Synaptic inhibition is not essential in a purely pacemaker-driven network, for which each phase could terminate by disfacilitation, due to (a) time-dependent conductance(s) that would decrease excitability (e.g., see discussions in 61,69,70). Therefore, one *might* be able to distinguish between a network and a pacemaker-driven oscillator by examining the effects of blocking postsynaptic inhibition.

Pacemakers and Inhibition

Speculations on the possible role of pacemaker neurons in generating respiratory rhythm must certainly date from the identification of the first pacemaker neurons in *Aplysia* (71), or perhaps even before to the identification of cardiac pacemakers. The resurgence of interest in pacemaker cells originated in experiments where block of inhibition in brainstem respiratory circuits was attempted (69,70,72). When synaptic inhibition is reduced in the in vitro neonatal brainstem, respiratory-related rhythm generation is not disrupted. These results sparked an effort to identify a site for rhythmogenesis to directly test for the presence of pacemakers. The hypothesis that the preBötC is the site for rhythm generation with a pacemaker kernel requires (as a necessary but not sufficient condition) that neurons with pacemaker properties be found there; such cells are found there in vitro (9) [determination of their presence in vivo requires elaborate, carefully controlled protocols (see discussion in 61) that remain difficult to implement]. The crux of evaluating the pacemaker hypothesis is determining the causal role, if any, of pacemaker cells in rhythm generation.

The results from perturbing inhibition in vivo are even more equivocal than those obtained in vitro. Using an aortic perfused decerebrate adult guinea pig preparation, Hayashi and Lipski (73) were able to markedly alter the circulatory perfusate to presumptively reduce inhibitory activity in the brainstem *and* spinal cord (and cerebellum). In contrast to in vitro experiments in neonates, where perturbations of inhibitory transmission are restricted to the brainstem, they observed marked alterations in respiratory motor outflow, including eventual abolition. There are several possibilities:

> Blockade of inhibition extending to spinal circuits could initiate seizure-type discharge, leading to activation of ascending inputs that can modulate respiratory rhythm (originating in the brainstem) regardless of the underlying kernel for rhythm generation.
>
> Blockade of inhibition could affect inputs to or receptors on pacemaker cells and force their membrane potentials outside the range necessary for activation of the conductances underlying oscillation: too depolarized they fire tonically, too hyperpolarized they cease to oscillate (Fig. 5; see below). In either case, rhythm can be abolished.
>
> Alteration of modulatory inputs could perturb conditional pacemaker conductances (50) and block rhythm (Fig. 5).
>
> The role of inhibition is different in adult and neonatal brains.
>
> In situ brains are different than in vitro brains.

Regardless, one should not conclude that if a perturbation of inhibition (or any given conductance) (in vivo or in vitro) significantly alters respiratory pattern that inhibition (or that conductance) is *required* for normal rhythm generation. The present results do not disprove the pacemaker hypothesis, nor do they suggest a pure network model is more likely.

Network Models for Rhythmogenesis

Contemporary network models for rhythmogenesis have evolved largely from the work of Cohen (62). Based on the catalog of extracellular firing patterns of brainstem respiratory neurons, he proposed a conceptual model that accounted for the basic features of normal breathing. The model consisted of two symmetrical and reciprocally inhibitory components underlying inspiration and expiration (Fig. 3). Premotor neurons generating the burst pattern in each phase were tonically excited and reciprocally inhibited by their counterparts in the companion phase. As their discharge augmented, they excited high-threshold inhibitory neurons with recurrent connections ("off-switch neurons"). When these neurons

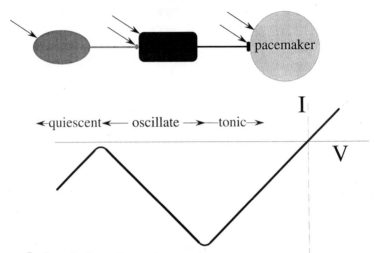

Figure 5 Perturbations of synaptic currents, including inhibitory currents, can act at many different sites that can influence respiratory rhythm generation. (Top) Cartoon of a pacemaker neuron with modulatory/tonic inputs, with arrows indicating several different sites of action, any of which could lead to abolition of oscillatory activity. (Bottom) Hypothetical steady-state current-voltage (IV) relationship of a pacemaker neuron. In contrast to most cells, these cells have a region of negative slope conductance in the subthreshold range of membrane potential, and it is in this range that the cell will oscillate. Changes in polarization level, either by effects directly on the cell or indirectly by effects on presynaptic elements, can force the pacemaker cell out of this region, causing tonic (or no) discharge.

began to fire, they quickly terminated the phase, resulting in disinhibition of premotor neurons of the reciprocal phase and initiation of the next phase. This model has been given mathematical formulation and been modified to reflect new data and changing views.

The most generally accepted and sophisticated contemporary network model has been proposed by Richter and colleagues (24,26) and represents a significant advance, since it is based on synaptic potentials and impulse discharge patterns of a now larger catalog of brainstem neurons. The initial observations of postinspiratory phrenic nerve discharge by Gesell (31) and the preferential postinspiratory firing of upper airway motoneurons have been consolidated into an hypothesis of a necessary three-phase sequence of synaptic activity in brainstem respiratory neurons. This model depends on the existence of inhibitory post-inspiratory interneurons. The basic thesis of the model is that reciprocal inhibitory interactions between postinspiratory and early inspiratory neurons underlie rhythmogenesis. Thus, as proposed in various forms (24,26,31), following the rapid decline in inspiratory activity, inhibitory postinspiratory neurons are released from inhibition from early inspiratory neurons to fire a rapid, often short-lasting burst of impulses that prevent reinitiation of inspiration, and that also delay the onset of augmenting expiratory activity. Initiation of the inspiratory phase occurs with rebound depolarization of early inspiratory neurons upon release from inhibitory inputs from postinspiratory and augmenting expiratory neurons. The sequence of burst timings has been modeled to be rather precise (24), with the limiting (but typical) case of no overlap of firing among inspiratory, postinspiratory, and late (stage 2, expiratory II) neural activity. However, such overlap appears to be the case in unanesthetized decerebrate mammals, and if so, these models will likely need to be modified.

Until recently, neurons in most models had very simple properties, at most two conductances that underlie action potential generation [Hodgkin-Huxley (HH) conductances]. Newer models (10,26,65) incorporate many different time- and voltage-dependent conductances (Fig. 3, bottom); such conductances are necessary for pacemaker activity and provide a straightforward means to account for (other) well-known phenomenology. For example, the rebound depolarization of early inspiratory and postinspiratory neurons that precedes their declining discharge can be described by endowing them with a low-voltage activated Ca^{2+} conductance to provide a postinhibitory rebound from hyperpolarized levels of membrane potential (26). The candidate pacemaker neurons in the in vitro neonatal rat medulla exhibit complex, voltage-dependent behavior, with different states ranging from quiescence to bursting oscillatory behavior to tonic modes of action potential generation (65; see Fig. 5). Models of these cells (65) suggest that a number of interacting subthreshold Na^+, K^+, and possibly Ca^{2+} conductances, in addition to HH conductances, would be required to produce this behavior. Yet, there are tens of active conductances (45,46), several of which have been tested for and observed in respiratory-related neurons (66–68). Since we do not know which neurons are generating respiratory rhythm, none of these conductances have been directly demonstrated to participate in rhythm generation; hence, one must cautiously interpret models that may imply otherwise.

Limitations of Models

Most models are based on inference from phenomenological description of neuronal behavior (e.g., firing patterns or membrane potential) and serve the useful purpose of demonstrating plausibility; i.e., neurons with a given set of properties and with postulaled connections can be organized with reasonable parameters to mimic certain experimental observations. Unfortunately, most models are retrodictive; i.e., they account for (some) known data and have yet to be usefully predictive, i.e., predict new or unusual phenomena. Moreover, they are formulated so that they are rarely falsifiable; the parameter space is so large that discrepancies usually can be remedied by modest manipulations.

Modeling should strive to generate falsifiable predictions, and even when these are not obtainable, the shortcomings of models should be acknowledged if only to better understand what they can and cannot tell us. We have discussed the limitations of current models and have proposed several conditions that models should (eventually) meet (10). Of particular importance is that: *The neuronal populations and/or associated properties that serve as the basis for the model must be shown to be critical for breathing.* This problem is often avoided by assumption, stipulation, or implication; however, there is no substitute for experimental demonstration. Unfortunately, no neuron(al population) *in any model* has been shown to participate in rhythm generation. When models describe particular connectivities, this means that under some conditions, some neurons with certain firing patterns have been shown to have an excitatory or inhibitory interaction (3,30,58,74). In no case have these neurons been definitively shown to participate in rhythm generation; such stipulated interactions among these neurons could also underlie sensory processing or pattern formation.

C. How Is the Basic Rhythm Translated into a Precise Pattern of Motoneuronal Activity to Move the Respiratory Muscles Efficiently?

At the output level, this can be broken into two problems: (1) How is the activity coordinated among motoneuron pools? (2) What factors control the activity within a motoneuron pool? (Models must also be able to account for this process.) We will focus on the second issue.

Neurons receive inputs and produce action potentials as output. This input-output relationship is determined by the cell's excitability, which is a dynamic property. For each neuron type, excitability is the convolution of intrinsic and synaptic properties. Understanding the control and modulation of respiratory (moto)neuronal excitability is essential. This is proving to be an elusive goal, confounded by the current census of 50+ distinct channels (46) and 50+ neuromessengers (75), each with up to several distinct receptors. The intrinsic properties of neurons that are presently under intense scrutiny include (76):

Type and distribution of non-ligand-gated voltage- and time-dependent ion channels.

Neuronal morphology and its relevance to function.

Electrotonic properties and the associated transfer function for ionic currents at synaptic sites throughout the somatodendritic membrane.

Second-messenger systems and their actions, intracellularly via G proteins and protein phosphatases, and intercellularly via such molecules as nitric oxide, carbon monoxide, or arachadonic acid.

Modulation of these properties by membrane voltage, second messengers, and multiple sources of current.

Synaptic properties must also be established:

Type and distribution of ligand-gated ion channels and ligand-activated second messengers, both pre- and postsynaptic.

The associated endogenous neurotransmitters and their location on the somatodendritic membrane.

The factors controlling the pattern of transmitter release in synapses containing multiple transmitters.

The interactions, including modulation, among these ligand-gated channels and messengers and between them and membrane voltage or intracellular ion concentration.

The interaction of synaptic and cellular properties, e.g., how a given pattern of synaptic input is transformed into a sequence of action potentials or the expression of certain genes.

The specific role (and interaction of) amino acid, amine, and peptide neurotransmitters.

At present, we cannot be certain which of these factors represent the most critical issues. As an example of the diversity and complexity of the problem, we consider the synaptic pharmacology affecting phrenic motoneuronal excitability, which has recently been studied in some detail.

Synaptic Pharmacology Affecting Phrenic Motoneuronal Excitability

Phrenic motoneurons have the straightforward task of controlling the diaphragm, mainly for ventilation, but also for other purposes, including protective reflexes, vocalization, and defecation. These neurons are not simple relays, especially for respiratory drive, and their synaptic control is quite complex. We have evidence for postsynaptic receptors for GABA, serotonin (5-HT), norepinephrine, substance P, neuropeptide Y, galanin, metenkephalin, CCK, and TRH (77) and presynaptic receptors for 5-HT (78), GABA$_B$ (Liu and Feldman, unpublished observations), glutamate (via AP4) (79), and adenosine (80). Given the relatively simple functional role of the phrenic nucleus, why are so many neurotransmitters required in addition to glutamate [which is the stipulated transmitter of inspiratory drive (79)] and GABA [which is the most likely transmitter of inhibition during expiration (81)]? We propose several hypotheses as to the role of these other transmitters (Figs. 6, 7):

Time Scales (10)

Fast synaptic events (~msec) are mediated in the CNS largely by amino acid transmitters; amines and peptides mostly cause actions on a slower time scale (75). The synaptic action of amino acids released onto phrenic motoneurons most likely shapes events within a single respiratory cycle; i.e., glutamate depolarizes during the bursting period, GABA and glycine provide recurrent and reciprocal inhibition. Amine and peptide actions on phrenic motoneurons could encompass a much

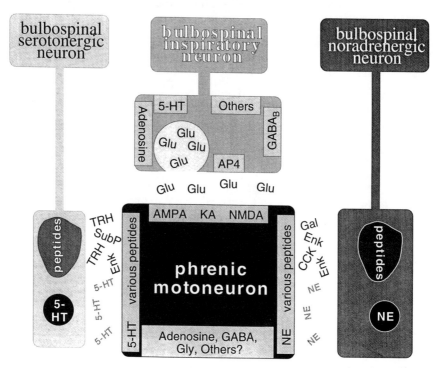

Figure 6 Descending synaptic control of phrenic motoneuronal excitability is complex, with an important component of presynaptic modulation on bulbospinal inspiratory neuronal terminals (e.g., via 5-HT, AP4, GABA$_B$, and adenosine receptors). The output of motoneuron action potentials depends critically on these elements, their sites and mode of action, and their interactions, all convolved with intrinsic neuronal properties. Some of the transmitters thought to be present in synaptic terminals at phrenic motoneurons are indicated.

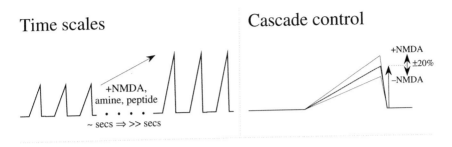

Differential control

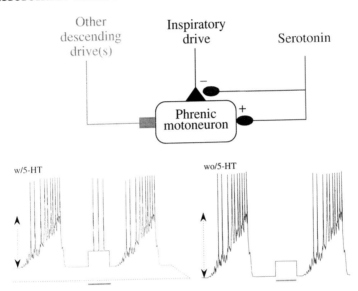

Figure 7 The host of neurotransmitters (NTs) may have several roles in regulating neuronal excitability. (Upper left). Some NTs such as amines or peptides may act slowly, and for long duration, to affect discharge. (Upper right) Some NTs (e.g., 5-HT) may only act to produce small changes in ongoing activity. Such fine tuning may be critical for efficiency. (Bottom) Some NTs, by a combination of pre- and postsynaptic action, may act to differentially alter the excitability of neurons to certain inputs, but not others.

wider range of time scales; from tens of milliseconds to tens of seconds, a range in which at most a few respiratory cycles are altered, up to months to years, in which phrenic motoneuron function undergoes long-lasting or permanent changes as during development/aging or in disease. Peptides may have a role in adaptation to physiological, state, developmental, environmental, pathological, and mechanical changes that require a sustained change in phrenic motoneuron function. Each of these adaptive challenges would produce different demands on the respiratory control system and would require different optimization strategies in an attempt to maintain homeostasis. Peptide and amine neuromessengers may have an important role in producing these adaptive changes in breathing both at the level of the phrenic nucleus and in the antecedent circuitry.

Cascade Control

To achieve precise regulation of diaphragmatic action requires tight control of phrenic motoneuronal excitability. This precise control may be mediated solely by the bulbospinal inspiratory pathway and fast EAA actions. However, for a complex system, it is difficult to achieve the degree of required regulation with only a single controlled variable, even with feedback. An alternative, called *cascade control* (Fig. 7), would allow for the principal transmitter to provide a rough degree of control (e.g., target value ±20%) and a cascade of transmitters with more limited actions (e.g., ±10%, ±5%, ±1% of the mean target value) that fine-tunes the output. It is like having amino acids to get you to the theater, and peptides and amines to help you find your seat. Testing these hypotheses is a formidable challenge (at least for the neurophysiologist), as we need to look for small changes that may take place over long time scales.

Differential Control of Excitability

Respiratory-related neurons receive multiple inputs and participate in many different motor behaviors. Could the efficacy of one (class of) input(s) to a neuron be modulated, leaving the efficacy of another input unaffected? For example, during sleep, the excitability of most motoneurons is reduced, but respiratory motor outflow is normally maintained. We propose a simple scheme, by which, through a combination of pre- and postsynaptic effects, a single neurotransmitter could do this.

Consider the effect of 5-HT on phrenic motoneurons (Fig. 6, bottom; 78). In spinal cord slices, phrenic motoneurons, like most motoneurons, depolarize in response to exogenously applied 5-HT (82). This effect is mediated postsynaptically, probably by the reduction of a K^+ current. In en bloc brainstem–spinal cord preparations, this effect is also seen. However, there is an additional effect, a specific reduction in the inspiratory drive of bulbospinal origin, which we postulate is of presynaptic origin. The combination of these two effects means that 5-HT increases the excitability of phrenic motoneurons to all inputs, but decreases inspiratory inputs, resulting in minimal change in inspiratory output from phrenic motoneurons. We propose that during sleep, when there is a dramatic drop in 5-HT release, the inspiratory throughput of phrenic motoneurons to diaphragm is maintained while their excitability to other inputs is reduced. That is, removal of 5-HT reduces excitability by increasing a K^+ current, while releasing inspiratory bulbospinal presynaptic terminals on phrenic motoneurons from their inhibition, resulting in greater synaptic activity (see also 83).

Amines may also have highly specific postsynaptic effects, differentially modulating responses of glutamate receptors (e.g., 84). Such modulation can fine-tune the postsynaptic response.

The complexity of control of phrenic motoneuronal excitability is even apparent in the synaptic processes underlying the bulbospinal transmission of inspiratory drive. During inspiration, phrenic motoneurons receive excitatory drive and during expiration are actively inhibited. Inspiratory drive is mediated by the release of glutamate acting on several postsynaptic receptors including AMPA, kainate, and NMDA receptors (79,85). Intrinsic and synaptic properties lead to a marked voltage-dependent response to inspiratory drive (Fig. 8). Thus, a small shift in background excitability of phrenic motoneurons may result in a disproportionate shift in their output; the voltage dependence itself may be affected by modulatory inputs to the motoneurons. There also appears to be a presynaptic (AP4) autoreceptor for glutamate that regulates neurotransmitter release. We propose that high levels of inspiratory drive will cause a sufficient elevation of glutamate in the synaptic cleft that acts, via this autoreceptor, to reduce further release. This would act as a governor on maximal phrenic motoneuronal activity, serving perhaps to limit the likelihood of diaphragmatic fatigue during sustained

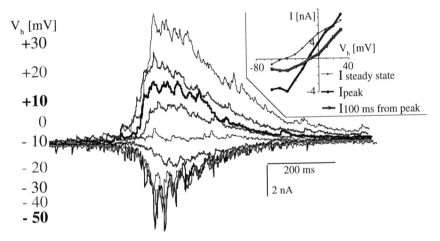

Figure 8 Voltage dependence of inspiratory drive currents in a phrenic motoneuron in a neonatal rat brainstem–spinal cord preparation in vitro. Numbers next to traces represent holding potentials for voltage-clamp recordings. (Inset) IV relationship. Note that below −40 mV, the range for subthreshold inputs, the IV relationship is relatively flat. (Redrawn from Ref. 88.)

epochs of high ventilatory demands. In addition, receptors for several other neurotransmitters appear to be present on the bulbospinal inspiratory neuronal terminal (Fig. 6), allowing for many mechanisms for presynaptic modulation of this drive.

There is undoubtedly further complexity in control of motoneuronal excitability that will be revealed with further experimentation. For example, novel gaseous neurotransmitters (86,87) remain to be fully explored.

V. Summary

Until recently, a connectionist view of the brain prevailed. Simple networks of neurons with mundane intrinsic properties and only fast excitatory or inhibitory postsynaptic inputs that added linearly were all that needed to be considered. This view is not sustainable in recognition of new data following on the extraordinary advancements in molecular neurobiology, synaptic physiology, pharmacology, and membrane biophysics. We may not need to know everything about every cell, but we have yet to figure out what we need to know and what we can safely ignore. The comfort of only a few choices for appropriate experiments has been replaced by the difficulty of choosing from a very large palette. With a close eye on function and a cautious view of reductionism, we may gain an essential understanding of the neural mechanisms controlling breathing. Finally, to fellow experimentalists, we agree that skepticism is useful, especially when it comes to (y)our own experimental preparation.

Acknowledgments

We are grateful for the generous support of our research program by the National Institutes of Health (HL 37941, NS24742, HL02204, HL40959) and the Parker B. Francis Foundation. We thank Dr. Elizabeth Dobbins for providing Figure 2, which is based on drawings made by Dr. Howard Ellenberger. We also thank our colleagues in the Systems Neurobiology Laboratory for their critical comments on this manuscript, especially Drs. Greg Funk and Steve Johnson, and Marianne R. Otto-Smith for assistance with the manuscript.

References

1.   Cohen MI. Neurogenesis of respiratory rhythm in the mammal. Physiol Rev 1979; 59: 1105–1173.
2.   Euler C von. Brain stem mechanisms for generation and control of breathing pattern. In: Cherniack NS, Widdicombe JG, eds. Handbook of Physiology. Bethesda, MD: American Physiological Society, 1986:1–68.

3. Ezure, K. Synaptic connections between medullary respiratory neurons and considerations on the genesis of respiratory rhythm. Prog Neurobiol 1990; 35:429–450.
4. Feldman JL. Neurophysiology of breathing in mammals. In Bloom FE, ed. Handbook of Physiology, Section 1: The Nervous System, Vol 4, Intrinsic Regulatory Systems of the Brain. Bethesda, MD: American Physiology Society, 1986:463–524.
5. Long SE, Duffin J. The medullary respiratory neurons: a review. Can J Physiol Pharm 1984; 62:161–182.
6. Greer JJ, Smith JC, Feldman JL. Role of excitatory amino acids in the generation and transmission of respiratory drive in neonatal rat. J Physiol 1991; 437:727–749.
7. Smith JC, Greer JJ, Liu G, Feldman JL. Neural mechanisms generating respiratory pattern in mammalian brainstem-spinal cord in vitro. I. Spatiotemporal patterns of motor and medullary neuron activity. J Neurophysiol 1990; 64:1149–1169.
8. Suzue T. Respiratory rhythm generation in the in vitro brain stem–spinal cord preparation of the neonatal rat. J Physiol 1984; 354:173–183.
9. Smith JC, Ellenberger HH, Ballanyi K, Richter DW, Feldman JL, Pre-Bötzinger complex—a brainstem region that may generate respiratory rhythm in mammals. Science 1991; 254:726–729.
10. Feldman JL, Smith JC, Ellenberger HH, Connelly CA, Liu G, Greer JJ, Lindsay AD, Otto MR. Neurogenesis of respiratory rhythm and pattern—emerging concepts. Am J Physiol 1990; 259:R879–R886.
11. Dean JB, Bayliss DA, Erickson JT, Lawing WL, Millhorn DE. Depolarization and stimulation of neurons in nucleus tractus solitarii by carbon dioxide does not require chemical synaptic input. Neuroscience 1990; 36:207–216.
12. Nattie EE, Li A, Coates EL. The centrally mediated ventilatory response to CO_2: medullary mechanisms. In: Proc XXXII Cong IUPS, 1993. Session 43:25.
13. Smith JC, Morrison DE, Ellenberger HH, Otto MR, Feldman JL. Brainstem projections to the major respiratory neuron populations in the medulla of the cat. J Comp Neurol 1989; 281:69–96.
14. Nattie EE, Li AH, St. John WM. Lesions in retrotrapezoid nucleus decrease ventilatory output in anesthetized or decerebrate cats. J Appl Physiol 1991; 71:1364–1375.
15. Milsom WK. Mechanoreceptor modulation of endogenous respiratory rhythms in vertebrates. Am J Physiol 1990; 259:R898–R910.
16. Milsom WK. Intermittent breathing in vertebrates. Annu Rev Physiol 1991; 53:87–105
17. Mitchell GS, Douse MA, Foley KI. Receptor interactions in modulating ventilatory activity. Am J Physiol 1990; 259:R911–R920.
18. Connelly CA, Otto-Smith MR, Feldman JL. Blockade of NMDA receptor-channels by MK-801 alters breathing in adult rats. Brain Res 1992; 596:99–110.
19. Ballantyne D, Richter DW. Post-synaptic inhibition of bulbar inspiratory neurones in the cat. J Physiol 1984; 348:67–87.
20. Chang FC. Modification of medullary respiratory-related discharge patterns by behaviors and states of arousal. Brain Res 1992; 571:281–292.
21. Orem J, Trotter RH. Postinspiratory neuronal activities during behavioral control, sleep, and wakefulness. J Appl Physiol 1992; 72:2369–2377.
22. Orem J, Trotter RH. Medullary respiratory neuronal activity during augmented breaths in intact unanesthetized cats. J Appl Physiol 1993; 74:761–769.

23. Bartlett DJ, Remmers JE, Gautier H. Laryngeal regulation of respiratory airflow. Respir Physiol 1973; 18:194–204.

24. Ogilvie MD, Gottschalk A, Anders K, Richter DW, Pack AI. A network model of respiratory rhythmogenesis. Am J Physiol 1992; 263:R962–R975.

25. Richter DW. Generation and maintenance of the respiratory rhythm. J Exp Biol 1982; 100:93–107.

26. Richter DW, Ballanyi K, Schwarzacher S. Mechanisms of respiratory rhythm generation. Curr Opin Neurol 1992; 2:788–793.

27. Feldman JL, Windhorst U, Anders K, Richter DW. Synaptic interaction between medullary respiratory neurones during apneusis induced by NMDA-receptor blockade in cat. J Physiol 1992; 450:303–323.

28. Richter DW, Bischoff A, Anders K, Bellingham M, Windhorst U. Response of the medullary respiratory network of the cat to hypoxia. J Physiol 1991; 443:231–256.

29. Schwarzacher SW, Willhelm Z, Anders K, Richter DW. The medullary respiratory network in the rat. J Physiol 1991; 435:631–644.

30. Ezure K, Manabe M, Otake K. Excitation and inhibition of medullary inspiratory neurons by two types of burst inspiratory neurons in the cat. Neurosci Lett 1989; 104:303–308.

31. Gesell RA. Neurophysiological interpretation of the respiratory act. Ergeb Physiol Biol Chem Exp Pharmakol 1940; 43:477–639.

32. Zheng Y, Barillot JC, Bianchi AL. Are the post-inspiratory neurons in the decerebrate rat cranial motoneurons or interneurons? Brain Res 1991; 551:256–266.

33. Zheng Y, Barillot JC, Bianchi AL. Medullary expiratory neurons in the decerebrate rat: an intracellular study. Brain Res 1992; 576:245–253.

34. Feldman JL, Cohen MI. Relation between expiratory duration and rostral medullary expiratory neuronal discharge. Brain Res 1978; 141:172–178.

35. Cohen MI, Feldman JL. Central mechanisms controlling expiratory duration. Adv Exp Med Biol 1978; 99:369–382.

36. Macdonald RL, Olsen RW. GABAA receptor channels. Annu Rev Neurosci 1994 (in press).

37. Olsen RW. Barbiturates. Int Anesth Clin 1988; 26:254–261.

38. Saunders PA, Ho IK. Barbiturates and the GABAA receptor complex. Prog Drug Res 1990; 34:261–286.

39. Tiku M. Drug modulation of $GABA_A$ mediated transmission. Semin Neurosci 1991; 3:211–218.

40. Jones MV, Harrison NL. Effects of volatile anesthetics on the kinetic of inhibitory postsynaptic currents in cultured rat hippocampal neurons. J Neurophysiol 1993; 70:1340–1349.

41. Mitchell GS. In vitro studies of respiratory control: an overview. In: Speck DF, Dekin MS, Revelette WR, Frazier DT, eds. Respiratory Control: Central and Peripheral Mechanisms. Lexington: University of Kentucky Press 1992:30–33.

42. Brochhaus J, Ballanyi K, Smith JC, Richter DW. Microenvironment of respiratory neurons in the in vitro brainstem-spinal cord of neonatal rats. J Physiol 1993; 462:421–445.

43. Hochachka PW. Defense strategies against hypoxia and hypothermia. Science 1986; 231:234–241.

44. Mortola JP, Rezzonico R, Lanthier C. Ventilation and oxygen consumption during acute hypoxia in newborn mammals: a comparative analysis. Respir Physiol 1989; 78: 31–43.

45. Hille B. Ionic Channels of Excitable Membranes. Sunderland, MA: Sinauer Associates, 1992:607.

46. Llinás, RR. The intrinsic electrophysiological properties of mammalian neurons: insights into central nervous system function. Science 1988; 242:1654–1664.

47. Berger AJ. Recent advances in respiratory neurobiology using in vitro methods. Am J Physiol 1990; 259:L24–L29.

48. Hirst GDS, Edwards FR, Bramich NJ, Klemm MF. Neural control of cardiac pacemaker potentials. NIPS 1991; 6:185–190.

49. Patneau DK, Vylicky Jr. L, Mayer ML. Hippocampal neurons exhibit cyclothiazide-sensitive rapidly desensitizing responses to kainate. J Neurosci 1993 (in press).

50. Harris-Warrick RM, Marder E. Modulation of neural networks for behavior. Annu Rev Neurosci 1991; 14:39–57.

51. Ellenberger HH, Feldman JL. Brainstem connections of the rostral ventral respiratory group of the rat. Brain Res 1990; 513:35–42.

52. Ellenberger HH, Feldman JL. Subnuclear organization of the lateral tegmental field of the rat. I. Nucleus ambiguous and ventral respiratory group. J Comp Neurol 1990; 294:202–211.

53. Funk GD, Smith JC, Feldman JL. Generation and transmission of respiratory oscillations in medullary slices: role of excitatory amino acids. J Neurophysiol 1993; 70:1497–1515.

54. Connelly CA, Dobbins EG, Feldman JL. Pre-Bötzinger complex in cats: respiratory neuronal discharge patterns. Brain Res 1992; 590:337–340.

55. Schwarzacher SW, Smith JC, Richter DW. Respiratory neurons in the pre-Bötzinger region of cats. Pflügers Arch 1991; 418:R17.

56. Bonham AC, McCrimmon DR. Neurones in a discrete region of the nucleus tractus solitarius are required for the Breuer-Hering reflex in rat. J Physiol 1990; 427:261–280.

57. Connelly CA, Ellenberger HH, Feldman JL. Respiratory activity in the retrotrapezoid nucleus in cat. Am J Physiol Lung Cell Mol Physiol 1990; 258:L33–L44.

58. Lindsey BG, Hernandez YM, Morris KF, Shannon R. Functional connectivity between brain stem midline neurons with respiratory-modulated firing rates. J Neurophysiol 1992; 67:890–904.

59. Ling L, Karius DR, Speck DF. Pontine-evoked inspiratory inhibitions after antagonism of NMDA, GABAA, or glycine receptor, J Appl Physiol 1993; 74:1265–1273.

60. Oku Y, Dick TE. Phase resetting of the respiratory cycle before and after unilateral pontine lesion in cat. J Appl Physiol 1992; 72:721–730.

61. Feldman JL, Cleland CL. Possible roles of pacemaker neurons in mammalian respiratory rhythmogenesis. In: Carpenter DO, ed. Cellular Pacemakers. New York: Wiley, 1982: 101–119.

62. Cohen MI. How respiratory rhythm originates: evidence from discharge patterns of brainstem respiratory neurones. In: Porter R, ed. Ciba Foundation Hering-Breuer Centenary Symposium; Breathing. London: J. & A. Churchill, 1970.

63. Botros SM, Bruce EN. Neural network implementation of a three-phase model of respiratory rhythm generation. Biol Cyber 1990; 63:143–153.

64. Duffin J. A model of respiratory rhythm generation. Neuroreport 1991; 2:623–626.
65. Smith JC, Funk GD, Johnson SM, Feldman JL. A hybrid pacemaker-network model for the respiratory oscillator in mammals. Soc Neurosci Abstr 1992; 18:1279.
66. Dekin MS, Getting PA, Johnson SM. In vitro characterization of neurons in the ventral part of the nucleus tractus solitarius. I. Identification of neuronal types and repetitive firing properties. J Neurophysiol 1987; 58:195–214.
67. Johnson SM, Getting PA. Electrophysiological properties of neurons within the nucleus ambiguus of adult guinea pigs. J Neurophysiol 1991; 66:744–761.
68. Viana F, Bayliss DA, Berger A. Multiple potassium conductances and their role in action potential repolarization and repetitive firing behavior of neonatal rat hypoglossal motoneurons. J Neurophysiol 1993; 69:2150–2163.
69. Feldman JL, Smith JC. Cellular mechanisms underlying modulation of breathing pattern in mammals. Ann NY Acad Sci 1989; 563:114–130.
70. Smith JC, Feldman JL. Central respiratory pattern generation studied in an in vitro mammalian brainstem-spinal cord preparation. In: Sieck GC, Cameron W, Gandivia SH, eds. Respiratory Muscles and Their Neural Control. New York: Alan R. Liss, 1987:27–36.
71. Alving B. Spontaneous activity in isolated somata of *Aplysia* pacemaker neurons. J Gen Physiol 1968; 51:29–45.
72. Onimaru H, Arata A, Homma I. Inhibitory synaptic inputs to the respiratory rhythm generator in the medulla isolated from newborn rats. Pflügers Arch 1990; 417: 425–432.
73. Hayashi F, Lipski J. The role of inhibitory amino acids in control of respiratory motor output in an arterially perfused rat. Respir Physiol 1992; 89:47–63.
74. Lindsey BG, Segers LS, Shannon R. Discharge patterns of rostrolateral medullary expiratory neurons in the cat: regulation by concurrent network processes. J Neurophysiol 1989; 61:1185–1196.
75. Siggins GR, Gruol DL. Mechanisms of transmitter action in the vertebrate central nervous system. In: Bloom FE, ed. Handbook of Physiology. The Nervous System. Bethesda, MD: American Physiological Society, 1986:1–114.
76. Jessel TM, Kandel ER, Lewin B, Reid L. Signaling at the synapse. Neuron 1993; 10(Suppl):1–149.
77. Ellenberger HH, Vera PL, Feldman JL, Holets VR. Multiple putative neuromessengers inputs to phrenic motoneurons in rat. J Chem Neuroanat 1992; 5: 375–382.
78. Lindsay AD, Feldman JL. Modulation of respiratory activity of neonatal rat phrenic motoneurones by serotonin. J Physiol 1993; 461:213–233.
79. Liu G, Feldman JL, Smith JC. Excitatory amino acid-mediated transmission of inspiratory drive to phrenic motoneurons. J Neurophysiol 1990; 64:423–436.
80. Dong X-W, Liu G, Feldman JL. Adenosine receptors modulate inspiratory drive to phrenic motoneurons. Soc Neurosci Abstr 1993; 19:1524.
81. Fedorko L, Connelly CA, Remmers JE. Neurotransmitters mediating synaptic inhibition of phrenic motoneurons. In: Sieck GC, Gandevia SC, Cameron WE, eds. Respiratory Muscles and Their Neuromotor Control. New York: Alan R. Liss, 1987: 167–173.

82. Berger AJ, Takahashi T. Serotonin enhances a low-voltage-activated calcium current in rat spinal motoneurons. J Neurosci 1990; 10:1922–1928.
83. Ziskind-Conhaim L, Seebach BS, Gao B-X. Changes in serotonin-induced potentials during spinal cord development. J Neurophysiol 1993; 69:1338–1349.
84. Cepeda C, Radisavljevic Z, Peacock W, Levine MS, Buchwald NA. Differential modulation by dopamine of responses evoked by excitatory amino acids in human cortex. Synapse 1992; 11:330–341.
85. McCrimmon DR, Smith JC, Feldman JL. Involvement of excitatory amino acids in neurotransmission of inspiratory drive to spinal respiratory motoneurons. J Neurosci 1989; 9:1910–1921.
86. Ling L, Karius DR, Fiscus RR, Speck DF. Endogenous nitric oxide required for an integrative respiratory function in the cat brain. J Neurophysiol 1992; 68:1910–1912.
87. Madison DV. Pass the nitric oxide. Proc Natl Acad Sci USA 1993; 90:4329–4331.
88. Liu G, Feldman JL. Bulbospinal transmission of respiratory drive to phrenic motoneurons. In: Speck DF, Dekin MS, Revelette WR, Frazier DT, eds. Respiratory Control: Central and Peripheral Mechanisms. Lexington: University of Kentucky Press, 1992:75–81.

3

Mechanisms of Respiratory Motor Output

ALBERT J. BERGER and MARK C. BELLINGHAM

University of Washington School of Medicine
Seattle, Washington

I. Introduction

Respiration involves spatially and temporally coordinated contraction and relaxation of various muscle groups. These muscles must function to provide the necessary pressure driving forces and airway stability that enable inspired gas to flow into and expired gas to flow out of the lungs. In addition to the act of rhythmic respiration, respiratory muscles are involved in other motor functions, such as: speaking, coughing, sneezing, and expulsive events such as childbirth, defecation, and micturition. Clearly such a repertoire of movements requires a motor control system with considerable diversity and precision. Since an obligatory synapse exists between the motoneuron and the muscle fibers it innervates, understanding the motoneuron will also enable us to understand the neural basis for contraction and relaxation of respiratory muscles. The central focus of this chapter is the respiratory motoneuron and the mechanisms both pre- and postsynaptic that govern the behavior of this important class of neuron. Two recent reviews have appeared that also focus on respiratory motoneurons (1,2). The neuropharmacology of respiratory motoneurons is discussed in Chapters 2 and 4.

What do we mean by a respiratory motoneuron? A motoneuron is a neuron whose cell body is located in the central nervous system (brainstem or spinal cord) and whose axon innervates skeletal muscle fibers. Motoneurons are further separated into two classes, α- and γ-motoneurons, depending on the type of muscle fiber innervated. The α-motoneuron innervates extrafusal and the γ-motoneuron intrafusal muscle fibers. Most of the research conducted to date has been focused on α-motoneurons, since the primary respiratory muscle, the diaphragm, has a paucity of muscle spindles and therefore γ-phrenic motoneurons are thought to be few in number and of little functional consequence (3). This characteristic is not true for the intercostal system (3), which has an important role in postural adjustments (4,5). Therefore, in this chapter when the term *motoneuron* is encountered, it can be assumed that it refers to an α-motoneuron. Finally, a motoneuron will be considered to be respiratory if the innervated muscle has a respiratory function. This function will be broadly considered to be either associated with the pump action of the thorax, related to stabilizing the airways, or involve the valve action of the upper airways. Our definition of a motoneuron as being respiratory is broad and not limited to the phrenic motoneuron, which has been regarded as the prototypic respiratory motoneuron. As a consequence, such diverse motoneurons as hypoglossal, pharyngeal, laryngeal, trigeminal, facial, phrenic, intercostal, triangularis sterni, intercartilagenous, levator costae, and abdominal muscle motoneurons will all be considered as respiratory motoneurons.

Sherrington described the motor unit as consisting of a motoneuron, its axon, and the muscle fibers it innervates (6). The motor unit is thus the smallest functional unit in a motor system. There is a matching of properties of the motoneuron with its muscle fibers. Muscle fibers exist in two broad classes that have been defined on the basis of a number of criteria. One of the most common is that determined by the contractile properties of the muscle fiber (7). Based on contraction time, separations have been made into slow-twitch (type S) and fast-twitch (type F) muscle fibers. The type F muscle fibers have been further separated on the basis of their fatigability. The motoneuron has firing properties and axonal conduction velocities that are matched to the properties of the innervated muscle fibers. For example, type S muscle fibers are innervated by motoneurons having longer-duration afterhyperpolarizations and therefore fire at slower rates and also have lower axonal conduction velocities than type F muscle fibers. The physical size of the motoneuron is also related to motor unit type. Thus type S motoneurons are smaller and their dendritic trees are less elaborate than those of type F. There are corresponding important functional implications that are at least in part related to size. For example, input resistance (R_N) of type S motoneurons is higher than that of type F. As a consequence, equal excitatory or inhibitory synaptic currents applied to both types of motoneurons (assuming these types of motoneurons have similar properties exclusive of differences in R_N) will result in different voltage responses depending on the cell's R_N. The larger the R_N, the greater will be the change in membrane potential; the depolarizing response of type S will be greater than that of type F motoneurons. These features have important functional consequences in relation to recruitment and excitability of different types of respiratory motoneurons.

II. Functional Anatomy

An important aspect in understanding the way in which a motoneuron converts synaptic input into an output is the anatomy of the motoneuron. The anatomy is relevant because of the distribution of presynaptic boutons on the soma and dendritic tree of the cell, the somatotopic relationship between the location of motoneurons in a motor nucleus and the target muscle, and possible interactions between motoneurons.

A. Spinal Motoneurons

Phrenic Motoneurons

The target muscle of phrenic motoneurons, the diaphragm, is a complex muscle having three major parts, the sternal region, with insertions into the xiphoid process, the broad costal region, with insertions along the lateral margin of the rib cage, and the crural region, with insertions into the vertebral column. The various regions are linked together through a central tendon. There is a somatotopic organization between the motoneurons in the long phrenic motor column and regions of the diaphragm (8,9). Phrenic motoneurons projecting to the sternal region are located at the rostral end of the motor column, those to the costal region are in the middle of the column, and those to the crural region are located most caudally.

The phrenic motor column is within lamina IX, which is located in the most ventral part of the ventral horn. It is a longitudinally oriented column of densely packed cells that extends over several caudal cervical spinal cord segments (10–14). In humans, this column is located from C-3 to C-5 (10), in cats from C-4 to C-6 (11), and in rats from C-3 to C-5 (13). Almost all the myelinated efferent fibers in the phrenic nerve innervate α-motoneurons in the diaphragm. Thus there are few fusimotor fibers in the phrenic nerve, which is in agreement with the paucity of muscle spindles in this muscle (3). An interesting anatomical feature of the phrenic motor nucleus is the presence, at least in some species including humans, of clustering of phrenic motoneuron cell bodies (10,11,14). The functional implications of such clustering are not clear, but it may be related to a compartmental organization in the target muscle, local motoneuronal interactions, organization of afferent inputs including segmental and supraspinal, or simply may be a consequence of maturational or metabolic factors. Another impressive structural feature is the presence of dendritic bundling, which is the close apposition of dendrites of these motoneurons. Bundling is a more prominent feature of axial motoneuron pools (15). Again, the functional relevance of bundling is unknown, but it is conceivable that it may have an important function in synchronization of activity.

The anatomy of phrenic motoneurons has been investigated in considerable detail using intracellular injection of various tracers (16–20). These studies have shown that the cell bodies are ellipsoid in shape with their major axis running parallel to the longitudinal axis of the spinal cord (17). In the cat, the largest average somal diameter oriented in the rostrocaudal direction is about 80–85 μm, while in the other planes of section the average diameter is about 25–50 μm (17) (Table 1). The vast majority of axons emerge from the cell body (17,18) and, after a short trajectory within the ventral horn, descend through the ventrolateral white matter to emerge in the cervical ventral roots. A small proportion (approx. 10%) of phrenic motoneuron axons possess axon collaterals (18,21), and these may be involved in a recurrent inhibitory pathway (18,22). At this point the functional importance of this pathway is unknown, but this pathway will be discussed below.

The dendrites of phrenic motoneurons project to different regions around and within the phrenic motor nucleus (17,20). Figure 1 shows a reconstruction of two phrenic motoneurons that were filled intracellularly with horseradish peroxidase (HRP) in the same animal. It is evident that the densest dendritic projection lies in the rostrocaudal direction and is therefore within the phrenic motor column itself. The dendritic trees extend for considerable distances; for example, an axially directed dendrite indicated by the asterisk in Figure 1 ended at a distance in excess of 2000 μm from the originating cell body. It has also been estimated that dendrites of phrenic motoneurons contain more than 97% of the total motoneuronal surface area (20). Thus phrenic motoneurons have very elaborate and extensive dendritic trees. An important functional question is to what extent synaptic inputs that are spatially remote from the cell body, owing to their location on distal dendrites, influence the behavior of these motoneurons.

The ultrastructural characteristics of adult rat phrenic motoneurons have been studied (21). In general, these characteristics were found to be similar to those of other spinal motoneurons. Direct dendrodendritic appositions were only rarely seen, and gap junctions were not observed. Thus the possibility of direct communication between neighboring dendrites, particularly within the characteristic dendritic bundles, seems unlikely. In keeping with this position, but in a different species, are the negative electrophysiological results indicating that direct electrical interactions between adult cat phrenic motoneurons could not be demonstrated (23).

Motoneurons Innervating the Muscles of the Thoracic Wall

The bony wall of the thorax has several respiratory muscles whose motoneurons lie predominantly within the ventral horn of the thoracic spinal cord. The functional

Table 1 Anatomical Properties of Adult Cat Motoneurons

Property	Phrenic			Hypoglossal			Intercostal				
							Internal		External		
	Mean	SD	Ref	Mean	SD	Ref	Mean	SD	Mean	SD	Ref
Somal diameter, μm											
Sagittal plane											
Major	84	15	17	ND	ND	54	100.3	32.0	64.2	7.4	25
Minor	32	9	17	ND	ND	54	35.5	7.8	41.2	1.9	25
Transverse plane											
Major	48	15	17	62.7	16.2	54	47.8	4.7	51.5	16.5	25
Minor	26	6	17	31.9	9.7	54	41.8	4.8	30.6	3.6	25
Number of primary dendrites	9.7	1.5	20	6.1	0.9	54	6–10[a]	ND			25

[a]Range of data from mixed population of internal and external intercostal motoneurons.
ND = no data available.

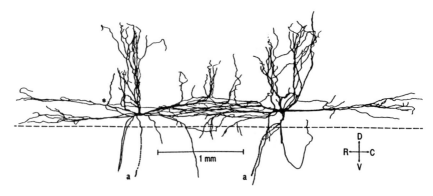

Figure 1 Reconstruction of two adult cat phrenic motoneurons filled with horseradish peroxidase in the same experiment. Note in this sagittal view the extent of overlapping dendrites. The asterisk (*) marks the site where one dendrite extended over 2000 μm from the cell body of the phrenic motoneuron on the right. Dashed line is the ventral border of the ventral horn. a, axon; C, caudal; D, dorsal; R, rostral; V, ventral. (From Ref. 17.)

anatomy of these muscles has recently been summarized by Monteau and Hilaire (1). Figure 2, adapted from their review, shows the location of the various muscle groups of the thorax. This figure shows the location of five different sets of muscles.

Between the bony portion of the ribs are the superficial external and deeper internal intercostal muscles. Traditionally, intercostal motoneurons innervating the external intercostal muscles have been deemed to be inspiratory phased, while those innervating the internal intercostal muscles have been defined as expiratory phased (24). However, this division is not true for all spinal segments, particularly for the internal intercostal motoneurons. Intracellular recordings of motoneuron activity have shown that approximately 58% of motoneurons antidromically activated from the internal intercostal nerves of the T-2 to T-5 segments showed inspiratory rather than expiratory depolarization (25), confirming previous reports of inspiratory internal intercostal motoneurons (26,27). Recordings from intercostal nerve branches have also suggested that both external and internal intercostal muscles are active during inspiration in the 1st–5th rib spaces and during expiration in the 9th–13th rib spaces, only being inspiratory and expiratory, respectively, in the 5th–9th rib spaces (28).

The more medially placed intercartilagenous (this muscle group is also known as the parasternal intercostals) and triangularis sterni muscles, which insert, at least in part, into the cartilagenous portion of the ribs, have inspiratory and expiratory actions, respectively. The levator costae (paravertebral) muscles insert into transverse processes of the thoracic vertebrae, and the opposite end of each muscle attaches to the cranial edge of the rib immediately caudal to this

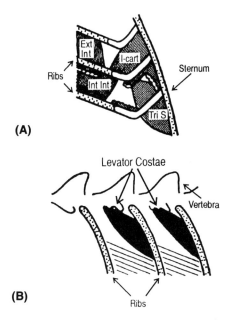

Figure 2 Schematic drawing of the location of the various muscles of the thoracic wall. (A) Location of the external intercostal (Ext Int), internal intercostal (Int Int), intercartilagenous (I-cart), and triangularis sterni (Tri S) muscles. (B) Location of the levator costae muscles. (Redrawn from Ref. 1.)

transverse process (29). Inspiratory-phase electromyographic activity has been recorded in this muscle (30). Contraction of the levator costae causes elevation of the ribs and thereby contributes to the increase in thoracic volume with each inspiration.

The neuronal anatomy of the various motor pools that excite muscles of the thoracic wall has been studied to a limited degree. The various thoracic respiratory motoneurons have cell bodies located in the most ventral portion of the thoracic ventral horn (31). For internal and external intercostals as well as triangularis sterni and intercartilagenous motoneurons, most, but not all, are located in the spinal cord segment that corresponds to the intercostal space in which the muscle is located (31). In the transverse plane, levator costae motoneurons are located in the ventromedial region of the ventral horn (30), while the intercartilagenous and trangularis sterni motoneurons are located primarily along the lateral edge of the ventral horn; finally, internal and external intercostal motoneurons are located between these motoneuron groups. External intercostal motoneurons are found more medial than internal intercostal motoneurons. There is spatial overlap of the internal and external intercostal motor pools in any given spinal cord segment (31).

Intracellular labeling of intercostal motoneurons has revealed that in the transverse plane the cell bodies are similar in size to those of phrenic motoneurons, but they are not as elongate in the direction of the spinal cord's longitudinal axis (25). Table 1 summarizes some of these data for internal and external intercostal motoneurons. Individual intercostal motoneurons have elaborate dendritic trees that extend over much of the ventral horn, and also their dendrites project over considerable distances along the longitudinal axis of the spinal cord (25). While only a small proportion of phrenic motoneurons possess axon collaterals, axon collaterals have been found in 78% of intercostal motoneurons filled intracellularly with HRP. Such axon collaterals in the intercostal motor pool may have an important function in the recurrent inhibition that has been demonstrated in intercostal motoneurons (32).

Abdominal Motoneurons

Muscles of the abdominal wall have respiratory function in addition to important functions in posture and movement as well as expulsive acts. Four different abdominal muscles comprise this group of muscles, these are: external and internal oblique, transverse abdominus, and rectus abdominus. These muscles are composed of large muscle sheets that make up the wall of the abdomen (29). Abdominal muscle contraction causes an increase in intra-abdominal pressure, and in the presence of a relaxed diaphragm, this causes a reduction in lung volume. During enhanced respiration, as during rebreathing, the abdominal muscles are rhythmically excited with each expiration (33).

The motor innervation of the abdominal muscles is derived from motoneurons located primarily in the lower thoracic and upper lumbar spinal cord. In the cat, external oblique motoneurons are in segments T-6 to L-3, internal oblique T-13 to L-3, transverse abdominus T-9 to L-3, and rectus abdominus T-4 to L-3 (34). The various motor nuclei overlap considerably in any one transverse section of the cord and are primarily located in the ventrolateral region of the ventral horn. The exception to this occurs at the lower end of the abdominal muscle motor column, where rectus abdominus motoneurons tend to be located more medially than the others (34,35). Other than studies employing retrograde labeling of abdominal motoneurons, there have been no studies utilizing intracellular labeling methods. Thus there is a lack of information on the detailed cellular morphology of this group of respiratory motoneurons.

Upper Cervical Motoneurons

Muscles in the neck and shoulder region have primary functions in head, neck, and upper limb movement, but can also contribute to respiration. These muscles include: the scaleni, sternocleidomastoid, and trapezius. Recent evidence has indicated that in humans the scaleni contribute to inspiration at rest by helping to lift and expand the upper rib cage (36). In contrast, the sternocleidomastoid and trapezius are considered accessory muscles of breathing since they are not rhythmically active at rest (36). The motoneurons innervating these neck and shoulder muscles are located in the upper cervical spinal cord. It has been reported that most neck and shoulder motoneurons have somal shape and size similar to those of phrenic motoneurons (37).

Intracellular HRP fills of trapezius motoneurons have revealed that these cervical motoneurons possess extensive dendritic arbors that extend over much of cervical ventral horn at the level of the soma. In addition, the dendrites of these motoneurons extend many hundreds of microns parallel to the longitudinal axis of the spinal cord (38), which is similar to the dendritic trees of phrenic motoneurons. Information regarding the respiratory-related behavior of upper cervical motoneurons is lacking. This may in part reflect species differences of the role of the innervated muscles when comparing bipeds, such as humans versus quadrupeds, where the action of these muscles may not be as efficient in altering lung volume (39).

B. Orofacial Motoneurons

Virtually all muscles involved in orofacial movements can show respiratory cycle-related rhythmic activity. Several orofacial motoneuron pools may thus be deemed to be respiratory in nature, such as the hypoglossal (XII), laryngeal, pharyngeal, facial (VII), and trigeminal (V) motoneuron pools. However, it is well to bear in mind that such respiratory activity may be only a secondary function of many of these muscles, as the orofacial motoneuron pools are involved in a number of other intricate behaviors, such as chewing, swallowing, and vocalization.

Hypoglossal Motoneurons

Hypoglossal motoneurons are located in paired nuclei on either side of the midline. The nuclei extend over much of the longitudinal length of the medulla. Caudal to the obex, the nuclei are immediately ventral to the dorsal motor nucleus of the vagus, while at more rostral levels, they are situated immediately below the floor of the fourth ventricle. Their axons travel in the hypoglossal nerve, which innervates the intrinsic and extrinsic muscles of the tongue.

Approximate numbers of hypoglossal motoneurons in each hypoglossal nucleus are about 3500 in the rat, based on soma and axon counts (40). Figure 3 shows that there is a somatotopic organization of the hypoglossal nucleus, in that motoneurons supplying particular muscles of the tongue are concentrated in different parts of the nucleus. Axons of motoneurons located in the ventral and medial parts of the hypoglossal nucleus travel in the medial branch of the hypo-

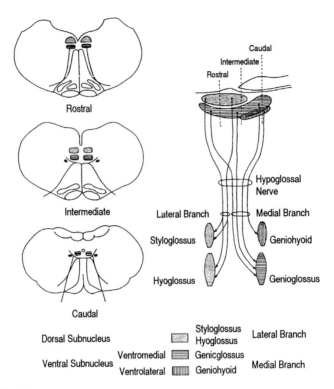

Figure 3 Somatotopic organization of the hypoglossal nucleus. (Left) Transverse section at three levels of the nucleus showing the various subnuclei. (Right) Schematic representation of the hypoglossal nucleus, the hypoglossal nerve branches, and the respective extrinsic tongue muscles innervated by those branches as well as the respective relationship between the various subnuclei and the innervated muscle. (Redrawn from Ref. 41.)

glossal nerve and supply the genioglossus or geniohyoid muscles, whose primary function is to protrude the tongue. Hypoglossal motoneurons located in the dorsal and lateral parts of the hypoglossal nucleus send their axons in the lateral nerve branch to innervate the hypoglossus and styloglossus muscles, which primarily retract the tongue (41–43).

The hypoglossal nucleus also contains interneurons that can be distinguished from hypoglossal motoneurons both morphologically and electrophysiologically. In Golgi sections from rat and monkey, these interneurons are distributed toward the lateral quarter and the ventral margin of the nucleus, appearing as smaller fusiform or ovoid somata with a few dendrites that show little branching (44–48). Electrophysiological recordings have also described interneurons that cannot be antidromically activated in vivo (49,50) and show faster maximal discharge rate (up to 250 Hz vs. 90 Hz) than hypoglossal motoneurons in vitro (51,52). Immunohistochemical staining for GABA suggests that these interneurons are GABAergic (53).

Hypoglossal motoneurons are large multipolar neurons. Intracellular staining of cat respiratory-modulated hypoglossal motoneurons with HRP revealed that soma size was 45–90 μm (major axis) and 25–50 μm (minor axis), with five to seven primary dendrites. The dendrites typically spread beyond the boundaries of the nucleus, up to 2 mm medially and laterally and up to 1–1.5 mm dorsolaterally and rostrocaudally (54,55). Dendrites course profusely through the lateral reticular formation.

Intracellular labeling of hypoglossal motoneurons in vitro has produced similar findings for soma size and number of dendrites (51,52). Recurrent collaterals have not been found to date (47,51,52,54).

Laryngeal and Pharyngeal Motoneurons

The motor innervation of the laryngeal muscles is via two branches of the vagus nerve, the recurrent and superior laryngeal nerves (56). Adduction of the vocal cords is brought about by contraction of the thyroarytenoid, interarytenoid, and lateral cricothyroid muscles, while abduction is due to contraction of the posterior cricoarytenoid and cricothyroid muscles (57). In general, abduction occurs during inspiration, beginning slightly before contraction of the diaphragm, and adduction occurs during expiration (58–62). The cricoarytenoid muscle is innervated by a branch of the superior laryngeal nerve, while all the other muscles are supplied by the recurrent laryngeal nerve. These vagal motoneurons will be referred to as laryngeal motoneurons in the rest of this chapter.

The innervation of the pharyngeal muscles is complex, as the pharyngeal branches of the vagus and glossopharyngeal nerves merge shortly after their exit from the skull, into a pharyngeal plexus that is the principal source of innervation for muscles of the oropharynx. Identification of motoneurons as being vagal or glossopharyngeal may therefore be ambiguous, depending on the site of nerve stimulation, and we suggest that it may be better to simply refer to these motoneurons as pharyngeal. Electromyographic (EMG) recordings have revealed phasic activity of pharyngeal constrictor muscles, innervated by the pharyngeal plexus, during expiration (63,64), while intracellular recordings show that motoneurons that can be antidromically activated from the pharyngeal branches of these nerves discharge during either inspiration or expiration in the cat (65,66).

Laryngeal motoneurons involved in control of upper airway diameter and pharyngeal motoneurons controlling the muscles of the oropharynx are located in the nucleus ambiguus (56,67–74).

Retrograde labeling of laryngeal motoneurons in the cat and rat shows two distinct populations. One consists of large multipolar cells in the ventral part of the nucleus ambiguus, the other of smaller neurons in the dorsal part of the nucleus ambiguus (67,69,75). Motoneurons controlling specific laryngeal muscles are somatotopically organized. Cells innervating the cricothyroid muscle are located in the rostral part of the nucleus ambiguus, while those innervating the posterior and lateral cricoarytenoid and thyroarytenoid muscles are located more caudally (67,69,74).

Retrograde labeling of motoneurons following HRP application to the pharyngeal branches of the vagus and glossopharyngeal nerves in the cat revealed two populations of cells (68). Neurons labeled from the pharyngeal branches of the vagus were found in a column in the nucleus ambiguus, extending from 1.5 to 4.1 mm rostral to the obex. Somal diameters ranged from 15 to 40 μm. Motoneurons labeled from the whole glossopharyngeal nerve were located in the retrofacial nucleus, rostral to, and partially overlapping, the neurons labeled from the vagus. Somal diameters of these glossopharyngeal motoneurons were also 15–40 μm. Distribution of the vagal pharyngeal motoneurons is similar in the rat (76).

Inspiratory and expiratory motoneurons activated from the recurrent laryngeal nerve have nearly spherical somas with 5–10 dendrites, which show profuse branching in the ventrolateral and dorsomedial directions and extending in the latter direction some 500–800 μm into the lateral tegmental field (77,78). No axon collaterals have been observed in laryngeal motoneurons (77).

Bianchi et al. (65) have described the morphology of two pharyngeal motoneurons with an augmenting inspiratory membrane potential pattern, located in the region of the retrofacial nucleus. These pharyngeal motoneurons had stellate somas with a diameter of 30–40 μm and seven to eight dendrites radiating up to 700 μm in all directions. Axons ran dorsomedially and showed no collaterals over the first 2 mm.

Trigeminal Motoneurons

On first consideration, one might dismiss trigeminal motoneurons as nonrespiratory, as their principal motor function is mastication. During quiet breathing, this is probably the case. However, under conditions of increased ventilation, such as in exercise or panting, breathing changes from being mainly nasal to oronasal, with mouth opening during inspiration (57), and many masticatory muscles show respiratory activity. Further, EMG recordings from the tensor veli palatini muscle of the nasopharynx show definite inspiratory activity during quiet breathing in humans (79), and St. John and Bledsoe (80) have reported expiratory activity in the mylohyoid branch of the trigeminal nerve of decerebrate cats.

The trigeminal motor nucleus is located in the pons, extending from the caudal pons to the middle cerebellar peduncle, and it is located medial to the principal sensory trigeminal nucleus (81–83). In the rat, each nucleus contains approximately 2500 motoneurons (84). It is composed of a large dorsolateral division, containing motoneurons innervating jaw-closing muscles (the masseter, temporalis, and medial pterygoid), and a smaller ventromedial division, present only in the caudal half of the nucleus, containing the motoneurons innervating jaw-opening muscles (the anterior digastric and mylohyoid) and those controlling the tensor veli palatini muscle (84,85). The mylohyoid branch of the trigeminal nerve innervates the jaw-opening muscles, whereas the jaw-closing muscles are supplied by the buccal, masseteric, and deep temporal nerves, which originate as a common trunk (86).

The ventromedial division of the trigeminal nucleus contains small neurons (16–20 μm diameter), likely to be intrinsic interneurons, and larger cells (24–34 μm diameter), which are the trigeminal motoneurons. Intracellular injection of HRP into jaw-closing trigeminal motoneurons of adult rat shows that they have a somal diameter ranging from 15 to 35 μm and six to eight primary dendrites, which mostly extend in a longitudinal direction, extending no more than 400 μm mediolaterally (87). In the cat, the anatomy of single trigeminal motoneurons has been studied in considerable detail (88).

Facial Motoneurons

The facial nerve controls muscles of facial expression. Of these, the small muscles controlling the diameter of the nasal openings, and the branches of the facial nerve that supply them, show definite phasic inspiratory activity in several species (89–94). Intracellular recordings from rat facial motoneurons have also revealed respiratory modulation of membrane potential, with a variety of phasic patterns (95).

The facial motor nucleus is located in the rostrovental portion of the medulla oblongata and contains approximately 5000–6000 neurons in the rat (84). The nucleus has a complex organization, with somatotopic grouping of motoneurons controlling different groups of facial muscle. Facial motoneurons innervating muscles controlling nasal diameter are located laterally in the nucleus (96–99).

Friauf (99) has described the morphology of rat facial motoneurons intracellularly injected with HRP. These motoneurons have multipolar or oval somata, with somal diameters ranging from 22 to 51 μm in their long axis and 14 to 26 μm in their short axis. Five to 11 primary dendrites are seen, which are primarily oriented rostrocaudally, and they extend beyond the border of the nucleus into the reticular formation by as much as 600 μm. Occasionally, ventral dendrites extend down to the border of the brainstem. Few dendritic spines are present, and axon collaterals are absent.

III. Intrinsic Electrical Properties of Respiratory Motoneurons

The output of a motoneuron, characterized by its spike-firing behavior, is determined by both its intrinsic properties and synaptic inputs. Ion channels in the cell membrane are important in determining a number of intrinsic properties. In recent years it has become apparent that there is considerable diversity in voltage- and time-dependent conductances present in the membranes of motoneurons (100–106). These ion channels can markedly influence both the sub- and suprathreshold behavior of the motoneuron.

In this section we will begin by discussing what is known about the passive membrane properties of respiratory motoneurons; then we will discuss the various ionic currents present and how these might affect motoneuron behavior. This section focuses on the motoneuron in the absence of synaptic inputs; in the next section we will discuss synaptic inputs.

A. Membrane Electrical Properties

A simple model of the motoneuron membrane treats it as a linear system consisting of a resistance and capacitance in parallel. In this model, the dendritic tree is collapsed so that any current injected into the somal membrane is seen by an isopotential motoneuronal membrane. Although this model is convenient, the extensive dendritic trees of respiratory motoneurons described above make this uniform model simplistic.

Perhaps the most useful passive membrane property is R_N. This is because injected or synaptic current will result in a steady-state membrane potential change that is simply proportional to R_N. For a uniform membrane, R_N is equal to the specific membrane resistivity (r_m) divided by the total membrane surface area. Thus the larger the surface area, the smaller is R_N. In phrenic motoneurons it has been observed that cell surface area is correlated with axonal conduction velocity (16), and that, as expected, there is a negative linear correlation between R_N and axonal conduction velocity (107,108). Thus larger phrenic motoneurons have higher axonal conduction velocities and lower R_N than smaller phrenic motoneurons. Table 2 summarizes the values of R_N, and axonal conduction velocities that have been observed for three different groups of respiratory motoneurons.

For the most part, the R_N values in Table 2 are derived from in vivo experiments. These values may be falsely low due to possible impalement injury with the sharp intracellular microelectrodes used in this type of experiment compared with measurements made with patch-type electrodes (109). Recordings in neonatal rat hypoglossal motoneurons in vitro have shown that R_N is approximately 25 MΩ with sharp microelectrodes (110) versus approximately 300 MΩ with patch-type microelectrodes (AJ Berger, DA Bayliss, and F Viana, unpublished observations). Thus values of R_N need to be considered with some caution since these may be dependent on the measurement technique.

The data in Table 2 reveal that R_N in both intercostal and phrenic motoneurons are similar but lower than that of hypoglossal motoneurons. This may reflect, at least in part, an apparently smaller membrane surface area of hypo-

Table 2 Electrical Properties of Adult Cat Motoneurons

Property	Phrenic				Hypoglossal				Intercostal			
	Mean	Min	Max	Ref	Mean	Min	Max	Ref	Mean	Min	Max	Ref
R_N, MΩ	2.0	1.0	4.5	107	4.3	2.0	7.9	39	2.3[b]	0.6	5.0	133
	3.3	2.0	4.2	368	13.5[a]	7.9	22.7	41	3.1[c]	1.1	5.0	133
	1.3	0.6	2.4	384	20.8[a]	ND	ND	43				
AHP_{dur}, msec	83	46	133	368	75[a]	56	95	41	ND	65[d]	110	162
	69	37	141	384								
	75	45	138	108								
AHP_{amp}, mV	3.1	1.0	8.5	384	6.1[a]	4.2	8.2	41	2.5[d]	ND	ND	162
	3.1	ND	ND	108	6.4[a]	ND	ND	43				
CV, m/sec	59	30	90	107	ND	20	41	40				
	64	35	95	368								
	73	37	94	16								
	46	22	75	386								
τ, msec	1.8	ND	ND	368	2.5	1.0	4.5	39				
					2.9[a]	1.6	4.2	385				
I_{rh}, nA	1.7	ND	ND	368	1.5	0.2	2.7	39	12.4[b]	4.5	22	133
	9.7	2	20	384	1.3[a]	0.6	2.7	41	8.1[c]	6	10	133
					2.1[a]	ND	ND	43				

[a] Data from 3-week-old motoneurons studied in slices in vitro.
[b] Data from internal intercostal motoneurons in vivo.
[c] Data from external intercostal motoneurons in vivo.
[d] Data from mixed population of internal and external intercostal motoneurons in vivo.

AHP_{amp} = afterhyperpolarization amplitude; AHP_{dur} = afterhyperpolarization duration; CV = axonal conduction velocity; I_{rh} = rheobasic current; ND = no data available; R_N = input resistance; τ = cell time constant.

glossal motoneurons compared with surface area of phrenic and intercostal motoneurons (see Table 1). This latter conclusion is based on the fewer number of primary dendrites of adult hypoglossal motoneurons compared with phrenic or intercostal motoneurons (see also Ref. 111).

Table 2 also presents additional passive membrane properties that have been measured in these motoneurons. These include the cell time constant (τ), and the rheobase current (I_{rh}). The time constant provides an estimate of the time course of response of the membrane potential to a step of injected or synaptic current. The I_{rh} is that value of depolarizing injected current that is just capable of evoking spikes in 50% of trials. Table 2 also includes some data regarding the afterpotentials following the depolarizing phase of the action potential. The afterhyperpolarization (AHP) is important in determining repetitive firing.

B. Ion Currents in Respiratory Motoneurons

In recent years in vitro methods have enabled new information to be obtained regarding the types and function of various ion channels in respiratory motoneurons (99). To date, almost all data have been obtained from studies of neonatal and adult hypoglossal motoneurons. Data regarding ion currents in spinal respiratory motoneurons, in particular phrenic motoneurons, have been very limited because spinal motoneuron in vitro preparations are viable only in the immediate postnatal period, and the focus of these studies has generally not been on identifying individual ionic currents (112).

In hypoglossal motoneurons, a number of ionic currents are activated by depolarization from resting membrane potential. It has been demonstrated that hypoglossal motoneurons possess a tetrodotoxin-sensitive, voltage-dependent transient sodium current that is responsible for the depolarizing phase of the action potential (51,100,103). A delayed rectifier K^+ current, sensitive to tetraethylammonium and responsible for the repolarizing phase of the action potential, is also present (51,100,102).

Calcium currents, both low-voltage-activated (the so-called T-type channel) and high-voltage-activated, have been demonstrated in these neurons (103). The high-voltage-activated calcium currents have recently been separated further based on their sensitivity to various calcium channel blockers (113). These results have shown that there is a diversity of high-voltage-activated calcium channels in hypoglossal motoneurons, including: large contributions from ω-conotoxin-sensitive N-type and ω-agatoxin-sensitive P-type calcium channels, and a smaller contribution from dihydropyridine-sensitive L-type channel. The various calcium channels can contribute to both the subthreshold and suprathreshold behavior of hypoglossal motoneurons. For example, following a hyperpolarizing prepulse, a rebound depolarization occurs in neonatal hypoglossal motoneurons (103). This rebound depolarization is due to activation of the low-voltage-activated calcium current, the hyperpolarizing prepulse being necessary to remove inactivation of this current. Another example of the effects of calcium currents is observed during the repolarizing phase of the action potential where an afterdepolarization is observed. This afterdepolarization is dependent on calcium influx and apparently is brought about by a contribution from both low- and high-voltage-activated calcium currents (103).

Following the action potential, there is both an early short-duration (fast) AHP, termed the fAHP, and this is followed by a later AHP of longer duration, termed the mAHP, for medium-duration AHP (51,102). Figure 4 shows these characteristic AHPs from a neonatal hypoglossal motoneuron as well as the afterdepolarization. The fAHP is blocked by extracellular application of tetra-ethylammonium ion but not by calcium channel blockers (51,102), and based on a variety of additional observations, it is thought to arise from activation of a voltage-dependent, calcium-independent K^+ conductance (102). The mAHP, on the other hand, has been shown to be due to a calcium-activated K^+ conductance. This is based on the observations that it requires influx of extracellular calcium, is blocked by the bee venom apamin, and its amplitude is dependent on membrane potential and extracellular K^+ concentration (102). This particular conductance has a considerable influence on the repetitive firing properties of hypoglossal motoneurons, as shown in Figure 5.

Adult rat hypoglossal motoneurons exhibit a slowly activating inward current during prolonged hyperpolarization (Fig. 6B) (114). In current clamp conditions this is seen as a depolarizing sag in the membrane potential during the response to hyperpolarizing current injection (Fig. 6A) (51,100,114,115). The function of this response would be to help stabilize the membrane potential of a hypoglossal motoneuron in response to inhibitory synaptic currents. Also, since this current deactivates when the hyperpolarization is removed, the current would transiently increase the excitability of the neuron, leading to a transient depolarizing overshoot in the membrane potential (Fig. 6A). Detailed analysis of this current has shown that it is the hyperpolarization-activated mixed cationic current (I_h) that has been seen in other neurons, including spinal motoneurons (106). Activation of this current in hypoglossal motoneurons has been reported to begin at about -65 to -70 mV and half activation occurs at -80 mV. Thus much of this current is on only at potentials below rest potential, which is about -70 mV (115). Another interesting feature of this current is that it is in low density in neonatal hypoglossal motoneurons and is in much higher density in adult hypoglossal motoneurons (100,114).

The interaction of the intrinsic properties described above with synaptic inputs, described in the next section, is ultimately responsible for the output of respiratory motoneurons. This output has both a subthreshold component, i.e., the membrane potential response in the absence of spike firing, and a suprathreshold component, when action potentials are generated.

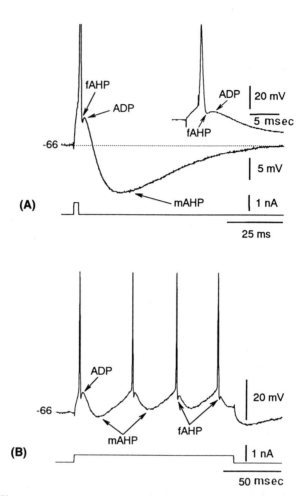

Figure 4 Characteristics of spike afterpotentials in neonatal hypoglossal motoneurons in vitro. (A) Three types of afterpotentials (arrows) following a single action potential generated by a brief (2 msec) intracellular current pulse. (Inset) Action potential on a faster time scale. (B) Presence of the three types of afterpotentials observed in the same motoneuron during slow repetitive firing. Abbreviations, see text. (Redrawn from Ref. 102.)

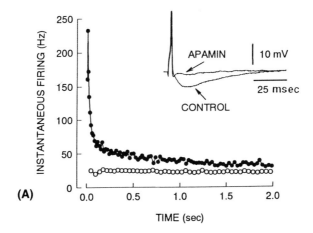

(A)

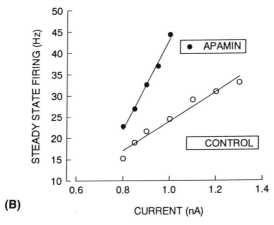

(B)

Figure 5 Importance of the mAHP in repetitive firing of neonatal hypoglossal moto-neurons in vitro. (A) Plot of the instantaneous firing frequency during a 20-sec, 0.9-nA current pulse (f-t), before (open circles) and after (filled circles) a 20-μM apamin microdroplet was applied to the slice. (Inset) Effect of apamin on the mAHP. Note that apamin abolished the mAHP and markedly altered the f-t relationship. (B) Plot of the steady-state firing frequency as a function of injected current (f-I) in control and after apamin application. Note that apamin caused a marked increase in the slope (gain) of the f-I relationship. (Redrawn from Ref. 102.)

Current Clamp

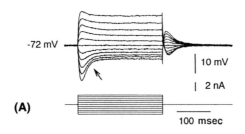

-72 mV

| 10 mV

| 2 nA

(A)

100 msec

Voltage Clamp

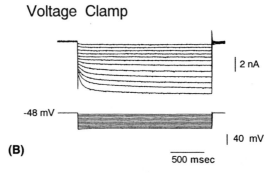

| 2 nA

-48 mV

| 40 mV

(B)

500 msec

Figure 6 Properties of the hyperpolarization activated inward current (I_h) in adult hypoglossal motoneurons in vitro. (A) Current clamp recordings showing membrane potential responses (upper traces) to hyperpolarizing and depolarizing current pulses (lower traces). Note the strong depolarizing sag in the membrane potential (arrow), which reflects activation of I_h. (B) Voltage clamp recordings showing membrane current responses (upper traces) to hyperpolarizing voltage pulses when applied from a depolarized holding potential. Note the slowly activated inward current (I_h) activated at the more hyperpolarized command voltages. A and B from different motoneurons. (Redrawn from Ref. 114.)

Figure 7 illustrates the importance of intrinsic properties on the firing behavior of phrenic motoneurons (116). This figure, obtained in vivo from cat phrenic motoneurons impaled with intracellular electrodes, illustrates the role that membrane potential history has on motoneuron behavior. This membrane potential history may, for example, remove inactivation or it could cause activation of currents that slowly deactivate at other membrane potentials. The upper four panels of Figure 7 (A_1, A_2, B_1, B_2) are taken from two phrenic motoneurons recorded during hypocapnic apnea. The upper row of traces shows the intracellular recorded (AC-coupled recording) firing response to a ramp of injected current.

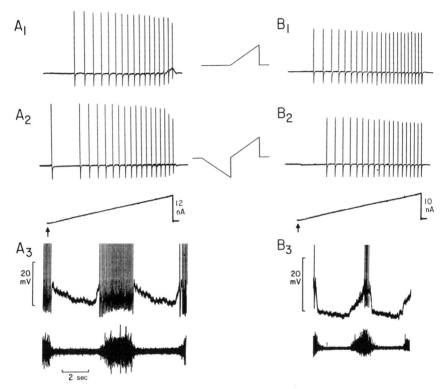

Figure 7 Potential influence of intrinsic membrane current on the excitability of two different types of cat phrenic motoneurons in vivo. (A₁ and B₁) Intracellular recording (AC-coupled) during 1-sec positive-current ramp (ramp shown schematically in insert between A₁ and B₁. (A₂ and B₂) Upper traces: Similar recording during identical positive ramps immediately preceded by mirror-image negative-current ramps (see inset between A₂ and B₂). Lower traces: Trajectories of the injected depolarizing current ramps. Arrows point to the onsets of the positive ramp current injections. (A₃ and B₃) Spontaneous inspiratory activity in the same cells as above. Upper traces: Intracellular recording (DC-coupled). Spikes truncated. Lower traces: Whole phrenic nerve activity. Time scale the same in A₃ and B₃. A and B are intracellular recordings from two different phrenic motoneurons (From Ref. 116.)

Both motoneurons fire a burst of action potentials with increase in firing frequency as the ramp progresses. Such a ramp of depolarizing injected current was chosen to roughly mimic the inspiratory-phase excitatory synaptic drive that phrenic motoneurons might experience under normocapnic or hypercapnic conditions. In addition, the first spike in each burst is somewhat delayed from the start of the ramp. In the second row of traces the firing response to the same injected current ramp is again generated, but this time the depolarizing ramp is immediately preceded by a hyperpolarizing ramp. The hyperpolarizing ramp was chosen to roughly mimic the expiratory-phase inhibitory synaptic drive these cells might experience under normocapnic or hypercapnic conditions. Now the firing pattern has changed for the phrenic motoneuron illustrated in the left-hand traces: the initial spike of the burst is advanced to the beginning or the depolarizing ramp, while for the motoneuron illustrated in the right-hand traces, the initial spike of the burst occurs later during the depolarizing current ramp. Clearly, the conditioning hyperpolarizing ramp has changed the firing pattern differently for each of these motoneurons. Next, in these experiments, apnea was replaced by rhythmic respiratory neural activity by elevating the carbon dioxide while recording intracellularly from the same phrenic motoneurons. The lower set of traces, Figure $7A_3$ and $7B_3$, show that under these conditions the motoneuron on the left with advancement of its initial spike is a phrenic motoneuron that normally fires early in the inspiratory phase and shows a progressive and large, slow expiratory-phase hyperpolarization indicative of strong active inhibition during expiration (107). In contrast, the motoneuron on the right, which had a delay in its initial spike following the hyperpolarizing ramp, fired much later during expiration. This experiment does not define the intrinsic membrane currents in these cells that may be responsible for the differences in behavior, but suggests that such properties may be an important factor in the different firing pattern that can be observed in respiratory motoneurons.

IV. Synaptic Mechanisms

A. Synaptic Inputs

Much work has been done, using both electrophysiological and neuroanatomical techniques, to elucidate the synaptic inputs to respiratory motoneurons, particularly those to the phrenic and intercostal motoneurons. The cat has been the preferred animal for such studies in the past, but the rat has also been increasingly used, particularly for neuroanatomical studies and, since the advent of in vitro preparations, for electrophysiology. Accordingly, the findings discussed below are predominantly from studies using the cat; findings in other species will be discussed specifically where they offer additional or contrasting data.

Methodologies: Cross-Correlation and Spike-
Triggered Averaging—Caveat Emptor

The methods commonly used to reveal functional (as opposed to anatomical) synaptic connections between a pre- and postsynaptic pair of neurons are cross-correlation (117,118) and spike-triggered averaging (STA) (119,120). Both techniques have advantages and disadvantages, which we will briefly discuss, as almost all of our knowledge of synaptic connectivity to respiratory neurons has been derived using these approaches. Cross-correlation histograms measure the probability of firing of a neuron relative to the occurrence of an action potential in another neuron, assuming a statistical independence of the spike trains as a null hypothesis. Thus periods of increased or decreased firing probability in the postsynaptic neuron indicate functional excitatory or inhibitory connections, respectively, once secondary effects related to internal periodicity in the correlated spike trains are removed (121). Cross-correlation studies are relatively simple, since they require only paired extracellular recordings of spike activities (often neuron and nerve fiber, but also neuron and neuron). However, the use of cross-correlation in studies of central connections have two chief problems: sensitivity and synchronization.

First, regarding the issue of sensitivity, single presynaptic fiber activity often evokes a unitary postsynaptic potential (PSP) in motoneurons having an amplitude of 100 μV or less (119,120,122–125). Such a unitary PSP will have only a relatively minor effect on firing probability of the postsynaptic neuron, necessitating the recording of a large number of firing events in order to become apparent and statistically significant. Cope et al. (126) have directly compared cross-correlation histograms and spike-triggered averages of hindlimb motoneurons, generated using the same single group Ia afferent, and shown that EPSPs of less than 86 μV did not produce positive cross-correlation histograms. In their study, the mean percentage increase in firing was significantly related to EPSP amplitude by a linear factor of 0.30–0.45%/μV. This relationship is potentially useful in estimating the amplitude of EPSPs underlying positive cross-correlation histograms, *provided* the correlation is between single pre- and postsynaptic spike trains. However, the chief point is that cross-correlation does not readily reveal smaller-amplitude synaptic inputs.

Second, the problem of synchronization of presynaptic inputs is common to both cross-correlation and spike-triggered averaging, as its presence invalidates the underlying assumption of statistical independence of random inputs to the postsynaptic neuron. In general, when peripheral afferents, such as muscle spindles, are used as trigger events, synchronization is obviated by simply removing the remaining afferents by cutting the other dorsal roots. Such a maneuver is not possible when the input is a central neuron. This is an especially relevant problem in investigating connections between respiratory neurons, as synaptic coupling of brainstem respiratory neurons is likely to produce such presynaptic synchronization (127,128). There is seemingly little that one can do to guard against this. One possibility would be to attempt to make the trigger neuron fire by other than synaptic means, e.g., by iontophoresis of an excitatory amino acid, so that its activity is at least partially desynchronized from the network. Another approach is that of Davies et al. (127,128), who excluded positive cross-correlation histograms with half-widths greater than 1.1 msec. Such short-duration peaks were mostly influenced by the rising phase of the underlying EPSP, since cross-correlation is very sensitive to the rate of change of membrane potential (121,127).

The analog averaging of whole nerve activity (129–132) or multiunit spike trains (127,128), rather than individual discriminated spike events, while having been used to assess connectivity, creates a number of potential problems in assessing the significance of cross-correlation histogram peaks. As pointed out by Merrill and Lipski (133), it is impossible to determine the relative contribution of individual fibers to either the peak height or the mean baseline count, thus precluding any estimate of the strength of synaptic coupling. These methods are also much more susceptible to presynaptic synchronization, as one is "sampling" the responses of all of (or a large part of) the motoneuron pool, which *must* be presumed to be receiving other synchronized presynaptic inputs, thus violating the assumption of independence.

STA of synaptic events is a much more sensitive measure of synaptic connectivity and can recover PSPs with amplitudes as low as 3 μV (122). Indeed, this enhanced sensitivity may become a problem, as STA can "recover" di- or trisynaptic PSPs (122). The problem thus becomes how to determine which recovered events are monosynaptically evoked and which are not. Generally, the PSPs recorded in the studies discussed here were thought to be monosynaptic because they had relatively fast rise times and had little or no variation in latency. Neither of these criteria alone is absolutely indicative of monosynaptic transmission. The longer rise time of oligosynaptically evoked PSPs is presumed to be due to the variation in latencies of individual PSPs when averaged together (122), but an often neglected factor is the slowing of PSP rise time with increasing electrotonic distance of the synapse from the soma (134–136). Watt et al. (122) have shown, using STA of mono- and disynaptic PSPs recorded from cat lumbar motoneurons, that while the mean rise time of disynaptic PSPs is longer than that of monosynaptic PSPs, individual disynaptic PSPs can have rise times well within the monosynaptic range (39% had rise times < 1.1 msec). The converse of this is that monosynaptic connections may have rise times of up to 2.5 msec (122).

A problem of sampling also occurs with STA in that, because of the technical difficulties of simultaneous extra- and intracellular recordings, it is rare to be able to test a large number of pairs, to examine whether presynaptic neurons connect to many postsynaptic neurons or see if one postsynaptic neuron receives many presynaptic inputs. Thus, unless one has a good indication of the projection site of the presynaptic neuron, STA can become a frustrating search. A second inherent problem is that sampling may be biased, as successful intracellular recording is probably biased toward larger neurons. One means of partly circumventing these difficulties is the technique of STA of small-amplitude extracellular fields due to synaptic activation (137,138). This STA technique involves extracellular recording and results in a negative-going potential when an EPSP is generated in the nearby target cell and a positive-going potential when an IPSP is generated. Generally, these so-called focal synaptic potentials are preceded by what is termed a biphasic terminal potential that is generated by the action potential entering the presynaptic terminal region (139). This technique has recently been applied successfully to map the projections of thoracic respiratory interneurons (140,141).

Inputs From Respiratory Muscle Nerve Sensory Afferents

Phrenic Motoneurons

Approximately 25% of the myelinated fibers in phrenic nerve are sensory, of which 70% have a diameter greater than 6 μm (3). In the rat, HRP-labeled phrenic afferents terminate mainly in laminae I–IV (142), although an ultrastructural study of synaptic profiles contacting rat phrenic motoneurons has also described M-type terminal boutons (21), which are thought to arise from primary afferent neurons (143). However, as described above, the numbers of muscle spindles and tendon organs in the cat diaphragm are low, with tendon organs being more numerous (144). Monosynaptic or disynaptic inputs to phrenic motoneurons from Ia or Ib afferents have not been reported. The number of these receptors in the diaphragm makes it likely that connectivity to the phrenic motor pool, if it exists, is either low or produces insignificant effects.

Electrical stimulation of the phrenic nerve at intensity levels exciting group II/III afferents causes a transient inhibition of phrenic nerve motor discharge (145–147). A part of this response seems to require supraspinal structures, presumably (but not necessarily) brainstem respiratory neurons, as phrenic stimulation has various effects on their discharge (148–150). Phrenic afferents have also been shown to project to the external cuneate nuclei (151), the cerebellar cortex (152), and the pericruciate sensorimotor cortex (153). Whether responses are due to disfacilitation of, or inhibitory synaptic inputs to, phrenic motoneurons remains to be determined by intracellular recordings.

Gill and Kuno (154) described IPSPs in phrenic motoneurons evoked by stimulation of the contralateral phrenic nerve, which appeared to be dependent on segmental mechanisms, as spinalization at C-1 did not affect their time course or magnitude. These IPSPs were present in 40% of phrenic motoneurons tested, with latencies of 5.8–9.1 msec (mean 7 msec) and duration of 15–20 msec, were dependent on the integrity of the contralateral dorsal roots, and could be reversed in polarity by injection of hyperpolarizing current. The spinal mechanism underlying this response is unknown, but it may be relevant that transection of the contralateral phrenic nerve or cutting the contralateral dorsal roots can restore activity to a diaphragm hemiparalyzed by rostral spinal hemisection, the so-called "crossed phrenic reflex" (155,156).

Stimulation of the intercostal or splanchnic nerves evokes excitation and/or inhibition of phrenic nerve discharge, depending on the site stimulated (157–161). Electrical stimulation of the intercostal nerves at middle intercostal levels causes bilateral inhibition of phrenic nerve discharge; at lower intercostal levels, this is preceded by a short burst of excitation, the so-called "intercostal-to-phrenic" reflex (160,161). The latency of phrenic nerve inhibition following middle intercostal nerve stimulation is 13–20 msec (161), while the latency of inhibition from lower intercostal nerve stimulation is 3–5 msec longer (160,161).

Selective electrical stimulation of afferent fibers in the intercostal nerves is difficult, as some cutaneous afferent fibers have conduction velocities and electrical thresholds similar to those of higher-threshold group Ia and Ib afferents (162). However, selective stimulation of Ia and Ib afferents by rib vibration has shown that these reflexes are principally due to activation of Ib and low-threshold group II afferents (163). As similar mechanical or electrical stimuli have been shown to inhibit both inspiratory and expiratory medullary respiratory neurons (164–169), it has been suggested that intercostal nerve-evoked suppression of phrenic nerve discharge is due to disfacilitation of descending excitatory drive (170).

A number of observations, however, suggest that spinal circuits may produce intercostal nerve-evoked effects on phrenic motoneurons. Stimulation of the caudal (T-9 to T-13) internal or external intercostal nerves can cause excitation of the ipsi- and contralateral phrenic nerve in intact or high spinal preparations (157,160,161,171). Intracellular recordings from phrenic motoneurons also show that membrane hyperpolarization evoked by stimulation of the 6th or 7th internal intercostal nerve is at least partly due to synaptic inhibition (172).

Intercostal Motoneurons

In contrast to diaphragm, the intercostal muscles are richly supplied with muscle spindles and tendon organs (3), and intercostal motoneurons receive an array of inputs from these muscle afferents. Shannon (170) provides an excellent review of the spinal and supraspinal effects of intercostal muscle afferent stimulation. The following section will deal with the connections of muscle afferents to the intercostal motoneuron pools.

Work in this area was pioneered by Sears and his colleagues, who recorded respiration-phased rhythmic afferent activities of muscle spindle afferents (173,174) and changes in intercostal motoneuron membrane potential (24,162, 175). Sears (162) showed that a compound EPSP, analogous to that evoked by group Ia afferents in hindlimb motoneurons, could also be elicited in homonymous intercostal motoneurons of the same and adjacent segments, while electrical stimulation at levels supramaximal for this EPSP resulted in a decrease in EPSP amplitude. This latter phenomenon may be interpreted as being due to the onset of an IPSP evoked by tendon organ afferents (170). Sears (162) also demonstrated that "reciprocal Ia inhibition," as exists between antagonistic limb motoneuron pools, did not exist between the expiratory- and inspiratory-phase intercostal motoneuron pools; i.e., stimulation of Ia afferents in the nerve to an intercostal muscle active in one respiratory phase did not produce short-latency inhibition in intercostal motoneurons active during the opposite phase.

Subsequently, Kirkwood and Sears (176), using the STA technique, recorded the unitary EPSP elicited in inspiratory intercostal motoneurons by a single primary afferent and found that the mean amplitude was 171 μV, with a mean rise time of 0.75 msec and mean half-width of 4.23 msec. Figure 8 shows an example of such an STA. In contrast to the near-universal connectivity of such afferents to hindlimb motoneuron pools (120), single intercostal primary afferents made connections with only 42–48% of tested intercostal motoneurons. Kirkwood and Sears (177) then estimated the connectivity of single primary afferents to the inspiratory motoneuron pools as a whole, by cross-correlation of the afferent and motoneuron discharges, and determined that single afferents strongly excited motoneurons of the same segment and usually also weakly excited motoneurons of adjacent segments.

Kirkwood and Sears (123) have also demonstrated that secondary muscle spindle afferents (groups II and III) make monosynaptic excitatory connections to expiratory intercostal motoneurons. The EPSPs recorded had low amplitudes (approximately 10 μV) and long latencies (1.2–2 msec).

Hypoglossal Motoneurons

Lowe (178) has reviewed the muscle nerve afferent systems to hypoglossal motoneurons. The hypoglossal nerve of cat and rat contains a number of afferent fibers, whose cell bodies have a variety of locations in the trigeminal sensory nuclei, the trigeminal ganglion, nodose ganglion, and upper two cervical ganglia (Fig. 9) (179,180). However, the proximal part of the hypoglossal nerve appears to be devoid of afferent fibers (179,181). The types of receptive organelles represented by these afferent fibers remain relatively mysterious, as muscle spindles, although present in humans and primates (182), appear to be very sparse in rat

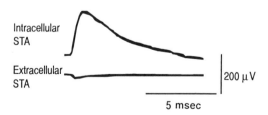

Figure 8 Spike-triggered average unitary EPSP recorded in an inspiratory intercostal motoneuron using activity in a single primary-like afferent as a trigger signal. (Upper trace) Intracellularly recorded average. (Lower trace) Extracellularly recorded average. Averages acquired only during inspiration. (Redrawn from Ref. 176.)

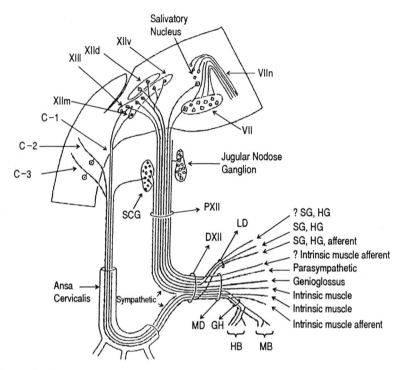

Figure 9 Summary of the hypoglossal nerve fiber composition in the rat. Hypoglossal nuclear divisions—XIId, dorsal nucleus; XIIv, ventral nucleus; XIII, lateral nucleus; XIIm, medial nucleus; C-1, C-2, C-3, ventral rami of first three cervical nerves; DXII, distal XII trunk; GH, geniohyoid branch; HB, hyoid belly of geniohyoid; HG, hyoglossus; LD, lateral division of XII; MB, mandibular belly of geniohyoid; MD, medial division of XII; PXII, proximal XII trunk; SCG, superior cervical ganglion; SG, styloglossus; VII, facial nucleus; VIIn, facial nerve. (Redrawn from Ref. 179.)

tongue muscles (179) and absent in cat (182). Less sophisticated mechanosensitive afferent nerve endings are abundant in tongue muscles of subprimate species (183).

In the cat, electrical stimulation of the hypoglossal nerve evokes changes in breathing pattern, inhibition of contralateral hypoglossal nerve discharge, and excitation of ipsilateral hypoglossal nerve branches other than the stimulated one, via afferent fibers that are directed to the nodose ganglion and enter the brainstem via ipsilateral vagal rootlets (184). In the cat, a few studies (54,185) have reported the occurrence of an IPSP following antidromic stimulation of both respiratory and nonrespiratory hypoglossal motoneurons. The latency of this response ranges from 11 to 14 msec, and it is due to GABAergic inputs, as it is chloride-dependent and sensitive to picrotoxin (185). These authors also noted that the response did not occur at stimulus frequencies higher than 6 Hz. This inhibitory response is likely to be due to excitation of high-threshold lingual afferents in the hypoglossal nerve.

Although stimulation of the hypoglossal nerve in the rat also elicits a decrease in its discharge, intracellular recordings have failed to reveal an inhibitory response (181). This finding may be in some doubt, as the stimulus frequency used was close to or above 6 Hz (185), and the proximal portion of the hypoglossal nerve, containing few afferents, was stimulated.

Inputs from Superior Laryngeal Nerve and Other Cranial Nerves

Phrenic Motoneurons

Stimulation of the superior laryngeal nerve (SLN) causes a suppression of phrenic nerve discharge (186–191). Intracellular responses of phrenic motoneurons to SLN stimulation were recorded by Biscoe and Sampson (187), who observed hyperpolarization of phrenic motoneuron membrane potential evoked by SLN stimulation during inspiration, but rarely saw hyperpolarization during expiration. They were unable to reverse this hyperpolarization by injection by hyperpolarizing current and could not detect consistent evidence of conductance changes using brief current pulses during this response. Accordingly, they ascribed the responses to disfacilitation of descending excitatory drive to phrenic motoneurons. In contrast, Bellingham et al. (191) found that SLN stimulation produced phrenic motoneuron membrane hyperpolarization in the cat during both inspiration and expiration, and that this response could be reversed by injection of hyperpolarizing current or chloride ions, indicating that at least part of the hyperpolarization was due to chloride-dependent inhibition (Fig. 10B and C). The latency of inhibition ranged from 4 to 10 msec in this study, indicating a polysynaptic input pathway.

It appears unlikely that this synaptic inhibition occurs as a result of SLN-evoked excitation of brainstem respiratory neurons, which then inhibit phrenic motoneurons. Stimulation of the SLN inhibits the great majority of brainstem respiratory neurons, both inspiratory and expiratory (192), with the exception of inspiratory bulbospinal neurons of the dorsal respiratory group (DRG), which are involved in a short-latency excitatory pathway to phrenic motoneurons described below, some propriobulbar decrementing expiratory neurons of the ventral respiratory group (VRG), and laryngeal motoneurons. In particular, augmenting expiratory bulbospinal neurons of the Bötzinger complex, which are known to inhibit phrenic motoneurons (see below), are usually inhibited by SLN stimulation (192), although SLN-evoked EPSPs, with a latency ranging from 5 to 8 msec, have been demonstrated in some of this neuron type in another study (65). Inhibition of

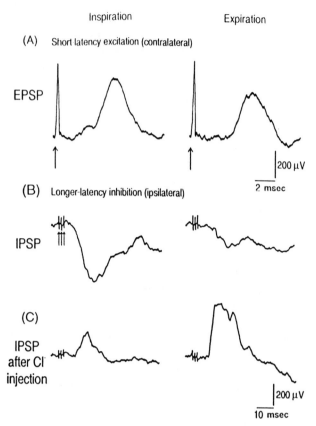

Figure 10   Evoked phrenic motoneuron responses to electrical stimulation of the superior laryngeal nerve as a function of the phase of the respiratory cycle. (A) Averaged intracellularly recorded response in an adult cat phrenic motoneuron to 50 stimuli of the contralateral superior laryngeal nerve applied in each phase of the respiratory cycle. Note the presence of an excitatory postsynaptic response during both phases of the cycle. Stimuli delivered at the arrows. (B) Averaged intracellular response in an adult cat phrenic motoneuron to 100 stimuli of the ipsilateral superior laryngeal nerve applied in each phase of the respiratory cycle. Note the presence of a hyperpolarizing response in both phases and the marked reduction of the response in expiration. (C) Averaged intracellular response of the same motoneuron as in B to 100 stimuli during constant passage of -25 nA current through the KCl-filled recording electrode. Note the reversal of the hyperpolarizing response to superior laryngeal nerve stimulation during both phases and the much larger response during expiration. Calibration is the same for B and C. (A redrawn from Ref. 190; B and C redrawn from Ref. 191.)

phrenic motoneurons by this latter subgroup may account for some longer latency IPSPs, but the other source(s) of inhibition remain unknown. One possibility is that nonrespiratory medullary neurons, which are monosynaptically activated by SLN stimulation and which have spinal axons, may directly or indirectly inhibit phrenic motoneurons (193).

Stimulation of the contralateral SLN also evokes short-latency EPSPs in phrenic motoneurons (190). The amplitude of these EPSPs in inspiration is between 0.5 and 2 mV and is reduced by some 24% in expiration (Fig. 10A). These EPSPs underlie the short-latency excitation seen in phrenic nerve records following contralateral (and sometimes ipsilateral) SLN stimulation during inspiration and are probably due to monosynaptic inputs to phrenic motoneurons from bulbospinal DRG inspiratory neurons that are excited by SLN afferents (192,194–196). In support of this proposed pathway, McCrimmon et al. (197) found that short-latency contralateral excitation of the phrenic nerve was abolished following electrolytic destruction of areas of inspiratory activity in the region of the DRG.

Hypoglossal Motoneurons

Stimulation of superior laryngeal nerve afferents by electrical shocks, pressure changes in the larynx, or chemical stimulation of the laryngeal mucosa often results in synaptic inhibition of both nonrespiratory and respiratory hypoglossal motoneurons (54,198). Evoked IPSPs have latencies ranging from 7 to 18 msec. Complex responses of EPSPs followed by IPSPs, and EPSPs alone, have also been recorded in response to SLN stimulation (54,198); latencies of the excitatory responses range from 3 to 8 msec. Neither excitatory nor inhibitory responses are likely to be due to direct inputs from laryngeal afferents, which do not project to the hypoglossal nerve (70). As electrical stimulation of the SLN can evoke both inhibition of respiration and swallowing (188), the varied responses are probably related to differences in the motor function of the particular hypoglossal motoneuron and the level of SLN stimulation.

Hypoglossal motoneurons are also affected by inputs from the pharyngeal and trigeminal afferents. The glossopharyngeal nerve is the principal sensory nerve of the pharyngeal region (178). Electrical stimulation of the glossopharyngeal nerve elicits strychnine-sensitive IPSPs in hypoglossal motoneurons of rat (181) and cat (199,200). Most rat hypoglossal motoneurons responded with hyperpolarizing potentials of 3–6 msec latency (201), which were sometimes preceded by small depolarizing potentials, while cat hypoglossal motoneurons were activated by glossopharyngeal nerve stimulation, via polysynaptic pathways (199). Glossopharyngeal nerve stimulation also exerts marked depressive effects on hypoglossal nerve reflexes evoked by stimulation of other cranial nerves, indicating that one or more sites of convergence occur in these reflex pathways (178). Stimulation of several different motor and sensory branches of the trigeminal nerve produces responses in the hypoglossal nerve and motoneurons [see Lowe (178) for a comprehensive survey of this literature]. As Kerr (202) observed no direct projections of semilunar ganglion neurons to the hypoglossal nucleus, these responses are probably mediated by one or more interneurons. The most intensively studied effect is that evoked by stimulation of the lingual branch of the trigeminal nerve, which transmits general tactile sensations, including those of mechanosensitive afferents, from the tongue (203,204). These afferents project to the sensory trigeminal nucleus. Electrical stimulation of the lingual nerve in cats elicits a reflex discharge in the hypoglossal nerve, with a latency of about 7 msec (205,206). This response is probably related to normal sensations, as Yamamoto (204) could evoke a similar reflex in rats using mechanical, thermal, and taste stimuli.

Several studies have reported the intracellular responses of hypoglossal motoneurons to lingual nerve stimulation. Depolarization and firing or hyperpolarization could be produced by mechanical stimulation (207), while electrical stimulation produces EPSPs, IPSPs, and more complex synaptic responses (185,199,207–210). Morimoto et al. (210) noted that hypoglossal motoneurons of protrusor muscles usually responded to lingual nerve stimulation with chloride-dependent IPSPs at a latency of about 6 msec, while hypoglossal motoneurons of retractor muscles responded with an EPSP/IPSP at a latency of about 4 msec. Porter (207) gives the minimal latency of EPSPs as 2 msec and that of IPSPs as 4 msec. On the basis of response latency and waveform, Porter (207) estimated that two synapses were present in this reflex pathway and proposed that units in the sensory part of the spinal trigeminal nucleus were internuncial units in this reflex pathway, as they could be synaptically activated by lingual nerve stimulation at a latency of 2 msec [see also Morimoto et al. (210)]. Alternatively, Sumino and Nakamura (209) proposed that a group of interneurons located in the nucleus of Roller just ventral to the hypoglossal nucleus might play a functional role as inhibitory interneurons, as they could be activated by a number of peripheral stimuli, with reflexogenic effects on hypoglossal motoneurons, including the lingual nerve.

The spinal trigeminal nucleus contains a large number of neurons projecting to the hypoglossal nucleus, as demonstrated by degeneration (211,212), retrograde labeling (213,214), and retrograde transsynaptic infection studies (215, 216), which may correspond in part to the internuncial neurons proposed by Porter (207) to participate in the reflex pathway from lingual nerve to hypoglossal motoneurons. Based on transsynaptic infection with pseudorabies virus, neurons in the spinal V nucleus may preferentially project to more dorsally located hypoglossal motoneurons responsible for tongue retraction (E. Dobbins, personal communication). The motor trigeminal nucleus has also been proposed as a source of afferent inputs to the hypoglossal (217), following retrograde labeling of interneurons in the motor trigeminal nucleus.

Inputs from Medullary Respiratory Neurons

The inputs to respiratory motoneurons from respiratory neurons of the medulla have been the subject of intensive inquiry for many years. Much remains to be done, however. We currently have very little knowledge of functional inputs from medullary respiratory neurons to the following motoneuron pools: pharyngeal, facial, trigeminal, abdominal, and the minor rib cage muscle motoneurons, such as triangularis sterni.

Although respiratory modulation of hypoglossal nerve discharge (218,219) and hypoglossal motoneuron membrane potential (50,54) have been described for some time, few studies have described the projections from brainstem areas containing respiratory neurons. Surprisingly, to our knowledge, no studies have directly examined synaptic inputs to hypoglossal motoneurons from identified respiratory neurons, using electrophysiological techniques. As almost 50% of cat hypoglossal motoneurons show respiratory modulation of membrane potential and also display variation in their respiratory phase of maximum depolarization, receiving both excitatory and inhibitory synaptic inputs related to respiratory phases (54), these data would be of considerable interest.

The known inputs to laryngeal motoneurons also remain relatively sparse. Therefore, the following sections concentrate heavily on inputs to the phrenic and intercostal motoneurons.

Inspiratory Neurons of the Dorsal Respiratory Group

The majority of inspiratory neurons of the DRG are bulbospinal neurons. However, antidromic mapping studies, and intracellular labeling with HRP, has shown that some also have medullary collaterals, which project principally ipsilaterally to the rostral VRG (r-VRG) (220,221). As the bulbospinal axons are excitatory (see references below), these medullary collaterals may also provide a source of excitatory drive to inspiratory laryngeal and pharyngeal motoneurons; however, no electrophysiological study of this connection has been done.

Phrenic Motoneurons. Inspiratory neurons of the DRG are thought to be the main source of excitatory input to phrenic motoneurons during inspiration (222,223). A concentration of inspiratory-phased neurons was first identified in the area of the ventrolateral nucleus of the solitary tract (functionally termed the DRG) by Baumgarten et al. (224), and they have been well characterized as bulbospinal neurons with peak depolarization and discharge in late inspiration (194,225,226). The majority of DRG inspiratory cells have axons that descend in the contralateral ventrolateral funiculus, but only a small proportion of the cells could be antidromically activated from single stimulation points in the region of the phrenic nucleus with low currents (227).

Several studies of the connectivity between DRG inspiratory neurons and phrenic motoneurons have been made, using electrophysiological techniques such as cross-correlation (127–129) or STA of phrenic motoneuron membrane potential (227–229). Figure 11 shows examples of STAs that revealed EPSPs with monosynaptic characteristics in phrenic motoneurons (227,228). These EPSPs had amplitudes ranging from 8 to 186 μV (mean = 65 μV) (228). Connectivity in these studies was relatively high, with 80% of tested DRG inspiratory neurons producing an EPSP in at least one phrenic motoneuron, and 66% of tested phrenic motoneurons showing a monosynaptic input (227,228). This was perhaps to be expected as only DRG inspiratory neurons that had axon collaterals in the region of the phrenic nucleus were tested for connectivity. Monteau et al. (229) performed STA in 80 phrenic motoneurons using a sample of DRG inspiratory neurons that were not tested for axonal arborization in the region of the phrenic nucleus; they found monosynaptic EPSPs in 39% of phrenic motoneurons, with amplitudes and rise times similar to those reported by Fedorko et al. (228) and Lipski et al. (227).

Fedorko et al. (228) measured the antidromic latency of a subset of DRG inspiratory neurons that produced EPSPs in phrenic motoneurons and found that the antidromic latency was generally within 0.5 msec of the EPSP latency, although some EPSPs occurred with a shorter latency than the antidromic latency, suggesting that they have been generated by presynaptically synchronized neurons (see also Ref. 227).

Davies et al. (127,128) cross-correlated extracellular spikes of DRG inspiratory neurons and contralateral phrenic nerve discharge and found short-latency, narrow-width peaks indicative of monosynaptic connections in 50% of cases, after careful exclusion of neurons with inappropriate antidromic latency or broader cross-correlation histogram peaks showing signs of presynaptic synchronization.

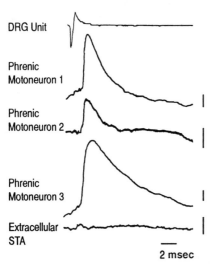

Figure 11   Spike-triggered averages of unitary EPSPs recorded intracellularly in three different adult cat phrenic motoneurons using activity from the same DRG inspiratory neuron (upper trace) as a trigger signal. (Lowest trace) Extracellularly recorded average. Vertical calibration bars are 50 μV. (Redrawn from Ref. 227.)

The conclusion to be reached from these studies is that, in the cat, DRG inspiratory neurons do make monosynaptic connections to phrenic motoneurons, with a probable frequency of 40–50%. To provide the necessary level of excitatory input to phrenic motoneurons, there must therefore be either considerable divergence in the connectivity between a relatively small number of DRG neurons (230) and the phrenic motoneuron pool or amplification of this input by interneuronal links. Divergence of monosynaptic inputs to phrenic motoneurons from single DRG inspiratory neurons does occur in some cases (227,228), but it remains doubtful whether this is sufficient, particularly when the relatively low level of monosynaptic excitatory input from VRG inspiratory neurons (228,231) and the disproportion between the numbers of DRG neurons projecting to the phrenic nucleus (232) and the much larger number of phrenic motoneurons are considered.

Brief consideration also needs to be given here to an apparent species difference between cat and rat in bulbospinal organization. The presence of a significant number of respiratory neurons in the DRG of rat remains uncertain, despite several studies that mapped activity in this area (233–237). Neuroanatomical tracing of bulbospinal projections to retrogradely labeled phrenic motoneurons in the rat has shown that relatively few neurons in the region of the DRG project to the phrenic nucleus, compared to a much larger projection originating from the region of the nucleus ambiguus, which made apparent monosynaptic contact with phrenic motoneurons (233,238). The presence of synaptic contacts between bulbospinal terminals of nucleus ambiguus neurons and phrenic motoneurons in the rat has been confirmed by electron microscopy (239). Electrophysiological studies of their synaptic pathway remain to be done.

Intercostal Motoneurons. Considerably less is known about the connections of DRG inspiratory neurons to the intercostal motoneuron pools. Retrograde labeling of neurons in the region of the DRG has been demonstrated, following injection of HRP into the regions of the contralateral intercostal motoneuron pools (240). While the discharge patterns of these labeled bulbospinal neurons remain unknown, they show a similar morphology to DRG inspiratory bulbospinal neurons intracellularly labeled with HRP (230). Duffin and Lipski (241) found that the majority (77%) of DRG inspiratory neurons had a spinal axon projecting to the contralateral T-3 to T-5 spinal segment. In this study, antidromic mapping showed that 68% of examined neurons had an axon collateral in the T-4 spinal segment, and that multiple collaterals to adjacent segments were common.

Cross-correlation of DRG inspiratory neuron discharge and intercostal nerve activity has been used to investigate inputs to intercostal motoneurons (128,132, 241). Hilaire and Monteau (132) did not find any evidence for axonal projections of DRG inspiratory neurons to the T-4 to T-10 spinal segments, or for connections to intercostal motoneurons. In contrast, the studies by Davies et al. (128) and Duffin and Lipski (241) found that short-latency cross-correlation histogram peaks were present in 9% (T-2 to T-9) and 39% (T-3 to T-5) of histograms. However, when DRG neurons with identified axon collaterals in the spinal segment whose nerve discharge was correlated were used as triggers, 70% of cross-correlation histograms were positive (241). The discrepancy in the percentage of positive cross-correlation peaks found in these two studies probably reflects the stringent criteria applied by Davies et al. (128) (see comments above) in accepting a peak as indicative of a monosynaptic connection.

Duffin and Lipski (241), using STA, demonstrated the presence of EPSPs in inspiratory intercostal motoneurons for five of 19 (28%) of DRG inspiratory neurons used as trigger spikes. Connectivity of individual trigger neurons seemed to be wide, as at least two neurons were shown to produce EPSPs in more than one motoneuron. The averaged EPSPs were small (mean amplitude 95 μV) and had relatively fast rise times (mean 0.61 msec) and short half-widths (3.9 msec). Interestingly, the trigger neurons had spinal axons with a relatively fast conduction velocity (40–60 m/sec), suggesting that monosynaptic connections might be preferentially made by a subgroup of DRG cells.

Inspiratory Neurons of the Nucleus Retroambigualis

Another group of inspiratory neurons exist in a bilateral longitudinal column within the ventrolateral medulla between 3 and 5 mm below the dorsal surface and 3 and 5 mm lateral to the midline (242–244). A large number of these neurons, a part of the so-called VRG, is commonly referred to as rostral nucleus retroambiguus (r-NRA) inspiratory neurons. The neurons have contralateral bulbospinal projections, demonstrated electrophysiologically (228,245) or neuroanatomically (246,247), with a small percentage (5–10%) also projecting ipsilaterally. Antidromic mapping studies (228,242) found that approximately 25% of r-NRA inspiratory axons in the C-5/C-6 white matter have arborizations near the phrenic nucleus, which may be quite extensive in some cases, occasionally crossing the midline [but see Fedorko et al. (231) and below]. Virtually all r-NRA inspiratory axons, including those with cervical arborizations, also descend to thoracic segments and show extensive arborization over several segments (133,242). Injection of tritiated amino acids in areas of inspiratory activity in the r-NRA resulted in anterograde labeling of axons and terminals bilaterally in the ventral horn of C-5/C-6 segments in regions in and around the phrenic nucleus and the contralateral ventral horn of segments T-1 to T-12 (247).

Phrenic Motoneurons. Cross-correlation between r-NRA inspiratory cell extracellular spike activity and phrenic nerve discharge (128,130,132,228) has estimated connectivity ranging between 27 and 61% of tested pairs. However, STA of 58 phrenic motoneurons found evidence of monosynaptic EPSPs in only one case and oligosynaptic EPSPs in three others, all triggered from the same r-NRA inspiratory cell (228). Cross-correlation in the same series of experiments resulted in positive peaks in 27% of pairs, leading these authors to conclude that such peaks must be due to scarce (and probably nondivergent) monosynaptic connections or to di- and oligosynaptic connections. A recent reexamination of this pathway by Fedorko et al. (231) found that 88% of r-NRA inspiratory neurons had axons in the contralateral C-5 segment, most of which were located in the lateral white matter. Axon collaterals within the region of the phrenic nucleus were found for 65% of r-NRA inspiratory neurons in this study, and STA of phrenic motoneurons found that 35% of the latter neurons generated monosynaptic EPSPs. Overall, however, this represents rather low (23%) connectivity for the r-NRA inspiratory population as a whole. These findings must be contrasted with those of Davies et al. (128), where positive cross-correlation peaks consistent with monosynaptic connections were seen in 50% of r-NRA inspiratory/phrenic motoneuron pairs.

Intercostal Motoneurons. Hilaire and Monteau (132) averaged the gross discharges of inspiratory intercostal nerves from T-4 to T-10, using r-NRA inspiratory units as triggers and found excitatory waves in 83% of averages. Because of the problems inherent in this method (see above), this information is questionable and contrasts with that of Davies et al. (127,128), who observed narrow-width peaks in 50% of cross-correlation histograms between r-NRA inspiratory neurons and multiunit inspiratory intercostal nerve recordings. Their study also found that single r-NRA inspiratory units often made extensive connections over several thoracic segments and that all segments received comparable amounts of monosynaptic drive. In marked contrast, STA of inspiratory intercostal motoneurons of the rostral thoracic segments failed to reveal any EPSPs consistent with monosynaptic connections (133) and found a relatively low (12%) incidence of positive cross-correlation histograms. The apparent conflict between these results and those of Davies et al. (128) may be due to the different levels of the thoracic cord tested; there is a need for this to be resolved by further investigations.

Hypoglossal Motoneurons. Intracellular HRP injection of augmenting inspiratory neurons of the r-NRA has revealed that some of these neurons have projections to the hypoglossal nucleus via axon collaterals (248), possibly providing one source of inspiratory depolarization. A study in cats by Ono (249) has also demonstrated, using retrograde double labeling, that neurons located in the DRG and in the dorsomedial aspect of the NRA project to both the hypoglossal nucleus and the phrenic nucleus. These labeled neurons are presumably respiratory, as extracellular recordings were also made from respiratory neurons in the same areas, which responded antidromically to stimulation in the hypoglossal nucleus and phrenic nucleus. Averaging of hypoglossal nerve discharge using the spontaneous spikes of these neurons revealed facilitation of nerve discharge, indicating that such neurons were excitatory.

Transsynaptic tracing of synaptic circuits from these areas to the hypoglossal motoneurons, following injections of pseudorabies virus into the tongues of neonatal and adult rats, has shown that premotor neurons are labeled in the areas of the nucleus of the solitary tract, Böt and pre-Böt complexes, and the NRA and extending caudal from this (250) (also E. Dobbins, personal communication).

While it remains to be proven that these labeled neurons are respiratory, the concentration of respiratory neurons in these areas of the rat makes it likely that this is indeed the case.

Laryngeal Motoneurons. STA has shown that inspiratory laryngeal motoneurons receive monosynaptic excitatory inputs from the medullary collaterals of augmenting inspiratory neurons of the r-VRG (251,252) and from other inspiratory propriobulbar neurons of the r-VRG and Böt complex (253).

Expiratory Neurons of the Nucleus Retroambigualis

One group of medullary expiratory neurons are located in a longitudinal column extending caudally from, and partially overlapping, the previously described rostral NRA inspiratory neurons. This column of expiratory NRA neurons (c-NRA expiratory neurons) extends from approximately the level of the obex to the C-1 rootlets (243,244). The axons of these cells descend in the contralateral ventrolateral funiculus to lumbosacral levels (133,242,244,254) and seem to have a purely premotor bulbospinal function, as electrophysiological (242,243,255) and neuroanatomical (256) experiments have failed to reveal any medullary collaterals.

Phrenic Motoneurons. No axon collaterals of these neurons at the level of the phrenic nucleus have been demonstrated electrophysiologically (242,255), in contrast with the extensive arborization seen in thoracic segments (133,242,255). STA between c-NRA expiratory units and phrenic motoneurons failed to reveal any IPSPs in a sample of 19 pairs (257). In contrast, Feldman et al. (247) found extensive bilateral anterograde labeling in the C-5/C-6 ventral horn following injection of tritiated amino acids into areas of expiratory activity in the c-NRA. It is possible that this labeling resulted from transport in nonrespiratory neurons located near the injection site, or alternatively, that anterograde transport was by inspiratory neurons, which may overlap the c-NRA expiratory neurons in their distribution (244). In other respects, however, the pattern of anterograde labeling seen by Feldman et al. (247) conforms with the results from antidromic mapping studies (242,255) and leaves open the question of whether any (presumably inhibitory) connections from c-NRA expiratory neurons to phrenic motoneurons exist. Reexamination of this connection, especially in the case of the rat, which may have a higher proportion of monosynaptic bulbospinal drive (see comments above), is warranted.

Intercostal Motoneurons. Retrograde labeling of neurons in the region of the c-NRA following injection of HRP into the region of intercostal motoneuron pools (240) and anterograde labeling in the ventral horn of intercostal segments following injection of tritiated amino acid in areas of expiratory activity in the c-NRA (247) suggests the projection of expiratory bulbospinal neurons to the region of the intercostal motoneuron pools. These results are not necessarily indicative of monosynaptic inputs to motoneurons (247), particularly given the frequent recording of respiratory interneurons in the regions of the intercostal motoneuron pools (133,258). Cohen et al. (131) averaged the whole nerve discharge of the T-8 and T-9 internal intercostal nerves using c-NRA expiratory spikes as triggers and observed excitatory peaks for 17 of 42 trigger neurons. More than half of the trigger neurons produced peaks in ipsilateral nerve averages. Since considerable evidence suggests that the thoracic projection of c-NRA neurons is overwhelmingly contralateral (133,242,247), these peaks may be due to presynaptic synchronization or disynaptic inputs via thoracic interneurons that recross the midline (140,258). Kirkwood and Sears (259) showed one EPSP revealed after averaging of an expiratory intercostal motoneuron using spike activity from a c-NRA expiratory unit; they provided no estimate of the frequency of this connection. These results have been challenged by Merrill and Lipski (133), who found little evidence for monosynaptic connections from c-NRA expiratory neurons to expiratory or inspiratory intercostal motoneurons, using both cross-correlation and STA techniques. Only two of 57 c-NRA expiratory/expiratory motoneuron pairs showed evidence of a monosynaptic connection, indicating a very low level of connectivity.

Expiratory Neurons of the Bötzinger Complex

Expiratory neurons have also been found in an area rostral to r-NRA inspiratory neurons. This group of expiratory neurons, commonly called the Bötzinger complex (Böt) has been extensively studied (65,66,257,260–267). A large proportion of Böt neurons with an augmenting expiratory-phase discharge pattern project to the spinal cord, mainly in the dorsolateral and lateral funiculi on either or both sides (261,263,268). Fedorko and Merrill (263) found that 72% of Böt neurons projected to the C-5 segment, while 29% showed evidence of arborization in the phrenic nucleus, as tested by microstimulation in the phrenic nucleus. Other studies have generally reported that fewer Böt neurons project to the cervical spinal cord; estimates range from 12% to 54% (65,261,268,269). Fedorko and Merrill (263) failed to find thoracic projections for any Böt axons, and therefore no study has tested intercostal motoneurons for inputs from these bulbospinal neurons.

Phrenic Motoneurons. It appears that the majority of the Böt expiratory axons present in the C-5/C-6 white matter do not have appropriate arborization patterns for monosynaptic connections to phrenic motoneurons (263) but may make connections via interneurons in these segments. In the only study to date, Merrill and Fedorko (257) observed IPSPs in 12 of 37 pairs, using STA. These IPSPs had latencies of 1.6–3.2 msec (mean 2.2 msec), amplitudes of 20 to 100 μV (mean = 50 μV), and 10–90% rise times of 0.54–1.4 msec (mean = 0.71 msec), and were interpreted as being due to monosynaptic connections (but see the reservations set out above). Only one attempt was made to determine the antidromic latency of a Böt expiratory neuron trigger spike that produced an IPSP.

Interestingly, antidromic latency from several points in the contralateral cord (the side of the recorded phrenic motoneuron) was always *longer* than the IPSP latency, and antidromic latency from the ipsilateral cord was only 0.2 msec longer than the IPSP latency, scarcely allowing time for synaptic delay. Given these deficiencies, further appraisal of the connectivity between Böt expiratory neurons and phrenic motoneurons is warranted.

Laryngeal Motoneurons. Expiratory laryngeal motoneurons receive monosynaptic inhibitory inputs from decrementing expiratory propriobulbar neurons (265) and from augmenting expiratory neurons (251,269) of the Böt as shown by the STA in Figure 12.

Inputs from Pontine Respiratory Group Neurons

Phrenic Motoneurons

Electrophysiological studies on respiratory neurons in the pontine respiratory group (PRG) have shown the occasional presence of spinal axons by means of antidromic activation (270). Electrical stimulation of the PRG produces respira-

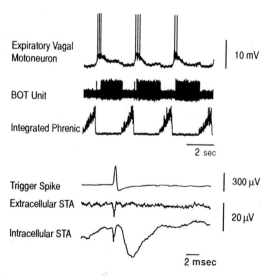

Figure 12. Spike-triggered average of unitary IPSP recorded intracellularly in an expiratory vagal (likely laryngeal) motoneuron using activity from an augmenting expiratory neuron of the Bötzinger complex. (Upper three traces) Slow time-scale recording of membrane potential in a vagal expiratory motoneuron, Bötzinger complex expiratory unit extracellularly recorded spike activity, and integrated phrenic nerve activity. (Lower three traces) Fast time-scale average records of the Bötzinger complex expiratory unit trigger spike, extracellularly recorded average, and the intracellular spike-triggered average revealing a unitary IPSP. (Redrawn from Ref. 251.)

tory phase switching (271), which is thought to be due to effects of the PRG on medullary respiratory neurons. However, Cohen (271) noted that the effect of pontine stimulation on phrenic nerve activity often preceded its effect on medullary neuron activity, opening up the possibility of a more direct projection. Considerable anatomical evidence also exists for a spinal projection of neurons in this area (272–274). Whether these projecting neurons also show respiratory activity is unknown; given the possibility of current spread during electrical stimulation, it may be stimulation of nonrespiratory neurons or axons that produces effects in motoneuron pools. Interestingly, injections of tritiated leucine in the dorsolateral pontine tegmentum produce labeling in the phrenic nucleus only when the injection site includes the lateral part of parabrachial nucleus and the Kölliker-Fuse nucleus, while injection in the lateral and medial parts of the parabrachial nucleus produce label in the ventral horn of the T-1 to T-3 segments (272).

Propriospinal/Segmental Spinal Inputs

Thus far we have examined the evidence for descending monosynaptic inputs to spinal respiratory motoneurons. Although much evidence exists for such input drive, one should realize that polysynaptic inputs to spinal motoneuron pools are by far more prevalent than monosynaptic inputs and include propriospinal systems with cell bodies located in segments away from those containing the relevant motor nuclei and segmental interneuronal systems with cell bodies located closer to the motor nuclei (275). These premotor elements receive converging inputs from various supraspinal centers and afferents, allowing both integration and amplification of these inputs. In the following section, evidence suggesting that both propriospinal and segmental respiratory spinal interneurons exist is presented.

Upper Cervical Propriospinal Neurons

One set of propriospinal respiratory interneurons, first described by Aoki et al. (276) and subsequently extensively studied, are the upper cervical interneurons. These neurons are located in the immediate zone of the gray matter near the lateral border of lamina VII and show an augmenting firing pattern during inspiration (27). They project ipsilaterally or contralaterally in the lateral funiculus to cervical, thoracic, and lumbar segments (27,277,278). Virtually all (94%) project at least as far as the T-9 segment (277). Upper cervical interneurons receive excitatory input from both DRG and r-NRA inspiratory neurons (279,280). They also receive inhibitory synaptic input during expiration (281), but the principal source of this inhibition is not the Böt expiratory neurons (268) and remains unknown.

    Using cross-correlation and STA techniques, Lipski and Duffin (27) reported that upper cervical interneurons did not make monosynaptic connections to ipsilateral phrenic motoneurons or inspiratory intercostal motoneurons of the T-3 to T-5 segments and only rarely produced disynaptic EPSPs in inspiratory intercostal motoneurons. This was despite the presence of axon collaterals in the vicinity of the motoneuron pools for 20% (phrenic) and 66% (intercostal) of tested axons. Similarly, STA of expiratory intercostal motoneurons of the T-9 to T-10 segments did not reveal any monosynaptic inputs from upper cervical interneurons, despite the presence of axon collaterals in these segments for 49% of upper cervical interneurons (277). Many of the axon collaterals of upper cervical interneurons cross the midline (27,277). Dowse et al. (278) cross-correlated upper cervical interneuron spike trains with whole nerve discharge from the ipsi- or contralateral phrenic and inspiratory intercostal nerves and with the extracellular discharges of inspiratory neurons within thoracic segments. No peaks consistent with monosynaptic inputs were seen. The function and output targets of the upper cervical interneurons remain unknown, but the collateralization of their axons at the levels of phrenic and intercostal nuclei, without the presence of direct synaptic connections, suggests that segmental interneurons may act as an intervening link between upper cervical interneurons and respiratory motoneurons.

Lower Cervical Respiratory Interneurons

Evidence for the existence of respiratory interneurons in the C-5/C-6 segments is more scarce. Anatomical evidence consists of the presence of smaller nucleolated neurons in the phrenic nucleus found intermingled with phrenic motoneurons identified by chromatolysis (282) or retrograde labeling with HRP (12). Vascik et al. (283) have also found GABA immunoreactivity in small neurons located among phrenic motoneurons retrogradely labeled with HRP. Until recently, electrophysiological evidence has also been scattered. Extracellular recordings from inspiratory and expiratory phased neurons in the ventral horn of segments containing phrenic motoneurons and intracellular records of inspiratory neurons in the region of the phrenic nucleus have been reported by Von Baumgarten et al. (284). Phrenic nerve stimulation did not antidromically activate these neurons. Dick et al. (285) recorded from the axon of an expiratory interneuron located dorsal to the phrenic nucleus and labeled the cell body and axon with HRP. The axon of this cell projected to the ventral funiculus, bifurcated, and displayed extensive collateralization into the phrenic nucleus.

More recently, further evidence has emerged for a population of respiratory interneurons in lower cervical segments. Extracellular recordings have been made from interneurons with respiratory-phased discharges in the cat (286), rabbit (287), and guinea pig (288). In these studies, classification as interneurons was assumed on the basis of location (dorsal to phrenic motor nucleus) and lack of antidromic activation by phrenic nerve stimulation. It seems unlikely that these recordings come from motoneurons innervating accessory respiratory muscles, as, in these spinal segments, they are closely associated with phrenic motoneurons (289) and are not active under conditions of anesthesia and normocapnia (90). Firing patterns of these neurons showed considerable variety, being inspiratory, expiratory, and occasionally postinspiratory. Figure 13A shows examples of

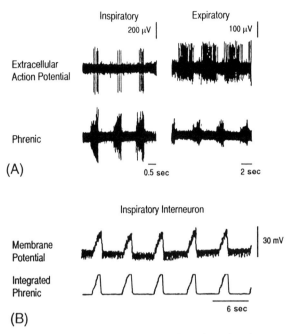

Figure 13. (A) Examples of extracellular recordings from inspiratory and expiratory interneurons in the C-5 segment of the anesthetized cat. (Upper traces) Interneuron unit activity. (Lower traces) Phrenic nerve activity. (B) Example of an intracellularly recorded membrane potential of an inspiratory cervical (C-5) interneuron recorded in the adult cat spinal cord. (Upper trace) Membrane potential of the interneuron. (Lower trace) Integrated phrenic nerve activity. (A redrawn from Ref. 286; B redrawn from Ref. 290.)

inspiratory and expiratory interneurons recorded extracellularly in the cat. SLN stimulation suppressed the firing of 36% of inspiratory interneurons and increased the firing of 15% of expiratory neurons (286).

Intracellular recordings from an area located dorsal to and within the phrenic nucleus have revealed similar neurons with rhythmic depolarizing shifts in membrane potential during inspiration, postinspiration, and expiration (290,291). Stimulation of the SLN, the pericruciate sensorimotor cortex, or the 7th internal intercostal nerve, at intensities that inhibited phrenic nerve discharge, evoked excitatory or inhibitory responses in many of these interneurons (290,291). Figure 13B shows an example of an intracellular recording from a C-5 segment inspiratory interneuron. This indicated that these interneurons may be involved in processing these inputs to phrenic motoneurons. Further evidence for such a nodal role emerged from the intracellularly recorded responses of phrenic motoneurons to combinations of test and conditioning stimuli from these sites, which indicated that these reflex pathways may converge on common interneurons at the segmental level (290).

Evidence also exists for interneurons that respond to stimulation of phrenic afferents. These interneurons are usually more dorsally located and fire bursts of action potentials after phrenic nerve stimulation at variable latencies of 5–15 msec (187,284,288). A few intracellular recordings have been made from respiratory interneurons that responded at long latency to ipsilateral stimulation of the phrenic nerve (290).

While these results establish the presence of respiratory interneurons in lower cervical spinal segments, more limited information exists regarding the target of these interneurons. The expiratory interneuron filled with HRP by Dick et al. (285) showed extensive collateralization within the ipsilateral phrenic nucleus. Partial labeling of other respiratory interneurons with HRP has shown that the initial portions of their axons are directed to the central commissure, presumably projecting to the contralateral half of the segment (290) similar to the projections of thoracic respiratory interneurons (140). Recently, STA of C-6 phrenic motoneurons using the activity of C-5 expiratory-phased interneurons has shown that these interneurons produce monosynaptic IPSPs in phrenic motoneurons (292). This provides the first evidence that these segmental interneurons directly synapse onto phrenic motoneurons.

Thoracic Respiratory Interneurons

Aminoff and Sears (293) first proposed a segmental interneuronal network transmitting mutual reciprocal inhibition between expiratory and inspiratory intercostal motoneurons to account for spinal integration of cortical, segmental, and medullary inputs. Respiratory-phased interneurons have been shown to exist in thoracic segments in several electrophysiological studies (133,258,294–296), and the presence of a large number of intercostal interneurons has been postulated on neuroanatomical grounds (297,298). In extracellular surveys of respiratory activity, respiratory interneurons were found to outnumber intercostal motoneurons from approximately 10 to 1 (295,296) to 3 to 1 (258). Cohen (296) also identified nonphasic interneurons that responded to supraspinal stimulation which produced either expiratory or inspiratory responses.

Kirkwood and his colleagues (140,141,258) have made extracellular recordings from respiratory phased interneurons in the thoracic segments of the spinal cord (Fig. 14A). These neurons were identified as interneurons, either directly by lack of antidromic activation combined with activation from other spinal cord segments or indirectly by their position and higher firing rates compared to intercostal motoneurons. Sixty-four percent fired in inspiration and 25% in expiration; the others were either postinspiratory or uncategorized (258). Interneurons were concentrated in the medial part of the ventral horn and dorsal to, but

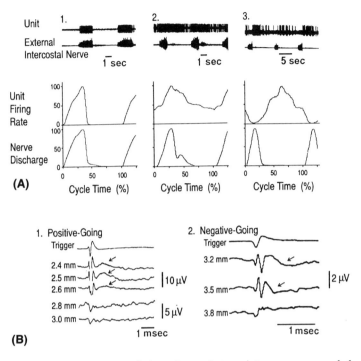

Figure 14 (A) Firing patterns of thoracic respiratory interneurons recorded extracellularly in adult cat. Panels 1, 2, and 3 are from three different interneurons with different firing patterns. (Upper trace) Unit activity. (Lower trace) External intercostal nerve recording. Lowest two panels are cycle-triggered histograms for the corresponding units above. (B) Examples of spike-triggered averaged focal synaptic potentials recorded in the thoracic ventral horn. Triggers were from respiratory interneurons recorded in the contralateral ventral horn of the same spinal cord segment. Positive-going focal synaptic potentials (on the left indicated by arrows) indicative of inhibitory effects produced by the triggering interneuron. Negative-going focal synaptic potentials (on the right indicated by arrows) indicative of excitatory effects produced by the triggering interneuron. Depths along the electrode track are indicated in each averaged record. (Redrawn from Refs. 140,141.)

overlapping, the motor nuclei (133,258). Antidromic activation showed that most of the interneurons had axons that projected contralaterally and caudally as far as five spinal segments (258). Some units responded to stimulation of peripheral nerves, but responses were generally at high thresholds (5–10 times threshold for group Ia afferents) with long latencies (10–20 msec) and consisted of bursts of spikes (133,258). More recently, extracellular STA of focal synaptic potentials (138) or retrograde labeling following small extracellular deposits of HRP has provided evidence that at least 60% of these interneurons project to the contralateral ventral horn of the same spinal segment (140). Kirkwood et al. (141), in a detailed description of these focal synaptic projections, interpreted them as showing either inhibitory (positive-going) or excitatory (negative-going) inputs from the respiratory interneurons to their target neurons (Fig. 14B). Comparison of the firing pattern of the presynaptic neuron and the polarity of the focal synaptic potential it produced showed that both inspiratory and expiratory interneurons with phasic discharge were principally inhibitory, while tonic interneurons with inspiratory or expiratory activity were principally excitatory. These results raise the intriguing possibility that respiratory modulation of intercostal motoneuron membrane potential may arise from "sculpting of tonic excitation by the phasic inhibition" (141). Such a possibility has previously been suggested based on the transition between phasic and tonic intercostal and phrenic nerve discharges with varying levels of chemical drive (299).

Nonrespiratory Inputs

The study of inputs to respiratory motoneurons has concentrated on inputs from respiratory neurons, in an effort to elucidate the basic neuronal circuitry involved in control of respiratory muscles during breathing. However, these same muscles are also involved in a myriad of other behavioral and voluntary acts requiring air movement, such as vocalization, coughing, sneezing, sighing, yawning, sniffing, and panting, or other nonrespiratory behaviors, such as posture, locomotion, intended movement, and digestion-related functions of swallowing, vomiting, and defecation. Many of these behaviors appear to be largely controlled by the forebrain, are independent of chemical control of respiration, and may involve integration at several levels of the neuraxis. Hugelin (300) provides a comprehensive review of respiratory effects evoked from fore- and midbrain areas. It is likely that neural subsystems controlling these behaviors modify respiratory output at both the brainstem and motoneuron levels.

Elucidation of the various pathways controlling these behaviors is, however, difficult and has often relied on relatively crude methods of electrical stimulation and lesion. A further difficulty is that many responses appear to be of long latency, indicating polysynaptic transmission, and that, more often than not, changes in output parameters whose underlying mechanisms are still ill-defined, such as the amplitude or timing of respiratory nerve discharges, have been used in attempts to deduce the central circuitry involved. Notwithstanding this, investigation of non-respiratory inputs to respiratory neurons and motoneurons is an important aspect of their responses and worthy of further attention. In this section, we will consider the current knowledge of inputs from the major descending spinal tracts to respiratory motoneurons via mono- or oligosynaptic pathways, with attention to areas in which we currently lack data.

Cortical

Cortical control of respiratory movements is prominent in voluntary breathing. There are clear premotor cortical potentials in humans during voluntary breathing, which disappear when the subject is distracted from thinking about breathing (301). In humans, cortical control seems to involve direct links to respiratory motoneurons, as the delay for transmission to the motoneuron pool is no longer than for voluntary finger movements (301).

Electrical stimulation of various areas of the cortex causes complex bilateral excitatory and inhibitory responses in phrenic and intercostal nerves and medullary respiratory neuron discharge (293,302–306). Longer-latency excitatory responses to cortical stimulation are most likely due to concurrent inhibition of propriobulbar respiratory neurons and activation of bulbospinal medullary neurons (305,307).

Neuroanatomical work indicates that spinal respiratory motoneuron pools may receive both direct and indirect corticospinal inputs. Injection of WGA-HRP into the pericruciate area of the sensorimotor cortex results in labeling of fibers and terminals in the spinal segments containing phrenic motoneurons and intercostal motoneurons (308). WGA-HRP injections into phrenic and intercostal motor nuclei also retrogradely label corticospinal neurons in the pericruciate sensorimotor cortex, with distinct but partially overlapping areas of distribution (309). Shinoda et al. (310) found that corticospinal axons predominantly projected to cervical segments, with a wide distribution of low threshold sites in the gray matter. These findings suggest that corticospinal projections may influence respiratory motoneuron pools, but are likely to do so through segmental interneurons, rather than synapsing directly with the motoneurons.

Pericruciate somatosensory cortical neurons also project to the reticular formation, where they collateralize extensively. A double-labeling study by Keizer and Kuypers (311) found that spinally projecting neurons of the pericruciate cortex, in particular, those located on the anterior sigmoid gyrus, also give off collaterals to the medial reticular formation. This is in accordance with electrophysiological findings, which show that reticulospinal neurons in these areas receive monosynaptic inputs from the contralateral sensorimotor cortex (312–314). Thus, input to phrenic motoneurons from the sensorimotor cortex could occur via a disynaptic corticobulbar-bulbospinal projection, with or without additional interneuronal relays at a spinal level. This dual control may be delivered by one and the same corticospinal neuron with collaterals to the reticulospinal systems (311,314).

Lipski et al. (306) showed that short-latency excitation and inhibition of phrenic nerve was due to evoked EPSPs and IPSPs in phrenic motoneurons. The EPSPs, evoked in 42% of phrenic motoneurons, had a mean latency of 4.7 ± 1.7

msec, mean rise times of 1.9 ± 1.1 msec, and amplitude ranging from 0.15 to 3.94 mV. These EPSPs are not the result of direct inputs from corticospinal axons of the pyramidal tract, as stimulation of the pyramidal tract at midmedullary levels could only evoke EPSPs with supramaximal currents that resulted in current spread outside of the pyramidal tract. Further to this, corticospinal pyramidal axons travel in the dorsolateral funiculus, and transection of this area at the C-2 to C-3 spinal segment does not abolish either phrenic nerve responses or PSPs in phrenic motoneurons (290). It is more likely that this excitatory pathway involves a corticobulbar-reticulospinal relay, as lower-intensity stimulation in the medial reticular formation dorsal to the pyramidal tract reliably evoked EPSPs with shorter latencies, faster rise times, and relatively reproducible amplitudes. This medial reticular area contains fibers of the reticulospinal, tectospinal, and vestibulospinal tracts (315). In the same study, cortically evoked IPSPs were seen in virtually all (98%) phrenic motoneurons. These IPSPs were readily reversed by diffusion or injection of Cl⁻ ions or hyperpolarizing current. Mean latency to onset and amplitude of IPSPs measured in cases where no early excitation was present were 4.9 ± 1.3 msec and 1.0 ± 0.6 mV during expiration and 5.8 ± 1.7 msec and 1.7 ± 1.1 mV during inspiration. Both excitation and inhibition were judged by these workers to be transmitted by at least disynaptic pathways.

The response of intercostal motoneurons to sensorimotor cortex stimulation in general consists of an excitatory expiratory intercostal nerve response and suppression of inspiratory intercostal nerve activity, although the latter is often preceded by a brief excitation (293,316). Stimulus sites producing responses are located in the motor cortex, around the cruciate sulcus. The latencies of the onset of excitatory responses range from 5 to 15 msec over the T-5 to T-10 levels.

Cortical neurons localized in the region of the pre- and postcentral gyri can be antidromically activated by stimulation of the hypoglossal nucleus in the monkey (316,317). However, in cat, Lund and Sessle (318) could not antidromically activate any of 273 neurons of the frontal cortex by stimulation in the hypoglossal nucleus. This is consistent with degeneration studies in the cat, which have also failed to demonstrate a corticobulbar projection to the hypoglossal nucleus (319,320) but did reveal a projection to the spinal trigeminal nucleus, where Porter (321) has reported the presence of neurons activated both by cortical stimulation at latencies of 5 msec and lingual nerve stimulation. In this latter study, similar cortical stimuli evoked EPSPs in hypoglossal motoneurons at latencies from 6 to 8 msec, depending on stimulus intensity.

The excitatory response seen by Porter (321) stands in contrast to extensive intracellular studies by Takata and others [see Takata (200) for a summary], which have characterized inhibitory inputs to cat hypoglossal motoneurons evoked by stimulation of a similar cortical area. These IPSPs have a short latency of 2–3 msec and consist of a fast chloride-dependent and strychnine-sensitive portion, a slower picrotoxin-sensitive IPSP, which could be reversed by injection of hyperpolarizing current, and a long-duration hyperpolarization, which could not be reversed. Blockade of the first glycinergic component revealed a cortically evoked EPSP of similar latency, whose duration could be increased by further blockade of the GABAergic second component.

Limb Muscle Afferents

Electrical stimulation of muscle or muscle nerves and physical stimulation of leg muscles have been shown to evoke a variety of effects on phrenic nerve discharge. Some of these effects are due to changes at the brainstem level, so that in intact animals, such stimuli results in facilitation of nerve discharge. However, evidence also exists for spinally mediated excitatory and inhibitory effects, which may in part be due to interactions between locomotor and respiratory pattern generators in the spinal cord (322,323). Electrical stimulation of hindlimb muscle afferents at levels that recruit group II and III afferents causes facilitation of phrenic nerve discharge in high-spinalized rabbits, after administration of nialamide and L-dopa, while physical or electrical stimulation of hind limb muscle afferents in high spinal cats results in inhibition of either evoked or spontaneous phrenic nerve discharge (171), which is due to glycinergic synaptic inhibition (324).

Other Input Systems

The descending axons of some other supraspinal systems, e.g., the reticulo-, vestibulo-, tecto-, raphe-, locus coeruleus, and rubrospinal neurons, are known to make monosynaptic or oligosynaptic connections to α-motoneuron groups in the cat spinal cord. The relative effect of monosynaptic excitation and inhibition of motoneurons from these descending pathways is quite small, and a larger proportion of the effect from these systems is mediated via common interneurons in which integration with input from peripheral afferents and intrinsic spinal systems takes place (275). The presence of inputs from these systems to phrenic motoneurons has not been extensively tested, data being limited to recordings of phrenic nerve discharge. While such inputs are unlikely to be directly involved in the transmission of respiratory drive to motoneuron pools, they have the potential to exert powerful effects in behavioral or voluntary control of respiration. In principle, the reticulo-, tecto- and vestibulospinal systems, which govern proximal muscle groups responsible for postural fixation and balance (325), are more likely to have effects on spinal respiratory motoneurons.

Reticulospinal Inputs. Findings from a number of studies make it highly likely that the reticular formation and reticulospinal neurons significantly influence the central control of respiration at both medullary and spinal levels. The reticulospinal system makes monosynaptic excitatory connections with a wide range of functional motoneuron groups, including cervical and thoracic motoneuron pools (275). This system also makes monosynaptic inhibitory connections with cervical neck muscle motoneurons (326). The cell bodies of origin of the descending reticulospinal axons are located in the nucleus reticularis gigantocellularis, nucleus reticularis pontis caudalis, and nucleus reticularis ventralis (326). These areas have been implicated in the control of respiratory rhythm by studies in which focal cooling of the nucleus reticularis gigantocellularis produced complete apnea or tonic inspiratory discharge (327,328). Electrical or chemical stimulation of this region depressed both respiratory and cardiac output (329).

Reticulospinal neurons receive collaterals from most of the other descending supraspinal systems; consequently, their effects on spinal interneurons and motoneurons may be spatially or temporally facilitated.

The lateral tegmental field also contains the majority of neurons premotor to hypoglossal motoneurons, as shown by retrograde (214,217,330,331) or transsynaptic labeling studies (216,250). These neurons are bilaterally distributed in the parvocellular reticular nucleus, mainly in its dorsal part, although at more rostral levels, these neurons are increasingly located more ventrally (330). A few cells are also found in the gigantocellularis nucleus. Recently, Manaker et al. (331) have demonstrated that lateral tegmental field and caudal raphe neurons (see below) can have axonal projections to both the hypoglossal nucleus and the spinal cord.

Electrical stimulation of the area lateral and ventrolateral to the hypoglossal nucleus in the rat brainstem slice preparation evokes a large compound EPSP in virtually all hypoglossal motoneurons, with a latency of 1–2 msec (F. Viana and M. Bellingham, unpublished observations).

Vestibulospinal Inputs. The vestibular nuclei and vestibulospinal systems are involved in the reflex control of equilibrium, postural adjustment, and locomotor control. The lateral and medial vestibulospinal tracts originate in the lateral and medial vestibular nuclei. Megirian (186) found that electrical stimulation of the vestibular nerve during inspiration resulted in excitation followed by a short period of inhibition in phrenic and recurrent laryngeal nerve discharge, while stimulation during expiration produced excitation at a latency of 20–25 msec. Bassal and Bianchi (332) also observed inhibition of phrenic nerve discharge with an average latency of 5.2 ± 1 msec and duration of 6–12 msec, after electrical stimulation of the vestibular nucleus. The vestibulospinal projection from the lateral vestibular nucleus has also been shown to produce monosynaptic EPSPs in neck and back extensor muscle motoneurons (333,334), while stimulation of the medial vestibular nucleus produces monosynaptic IPSPs in the same motoneuron groups (333). STA of the effects of single vestibular neurons on neck motoneurons has shown similar inputs (125).

Tectospinal Inputs. Electrical stimulation of the superior colliculus inhibits phrenic nerve discharge with a latency of 6.1 ± 1.7 msec (332,335). The tectospinal tract originates in the superior colliculus and is important in the coordinated movement of head and eyes directed toward visual targets. Stimulation of the superior colliculus also produces short-latency excitation in contralateral neck muscle motoneurons and short-latency inhibition in ipsilateral neck muscle motoneurons (336). These effects have been ascribed to tectobulbar projections from ipsi- and contralateral superior colliculus, which produce monosynaptic EPSPs in reticulospinal neurons (313,337,338). As injection of orthograde tracer into the superior colliculus reveals few tectospinal projections to the cervical spinal cord and no collateralization within cervical motoneuron pools (339), it is probable that tectal effects on cervical motoneurons are relayed either through reticulospinal neurons or, rarely, through segmental interneurons. Reticulospinal neurons receiving tectal inputs also frequently receive monosynaptic EPSPs from the cortex (313,337,340), suggesting that they may integrate both voluntary (cortical) and reflex (tectal) head-neck movements.

Raphe Nuclei Inputs. The caudal raphe nuclei including nucleus raphe pallidus and obscurus are the source of serotonergic inputs to various motoneuron pools (341). Along with substance P (SP) and thyrotropin-releasing hormone (TRH), these transmitters can be found localized in the same raphe neuron (342). Several studies have demonstrated the effects of serotonin on cat, rabbit, and rat phrenic motoneurons (343–348) and established the existence of serotonergic synaptic terminals within the phrenic nucleus and on phrenic motoneurons (349–352). The more caudal of these medullary serotonin-containing neuronal groups (B1–B3) project largely to the lower brainstem and spinal cord (353–355), consistent with the demonstration of terminal varicosities in the rat phrenic nucleus that were double-labeled for serotonin and SP or TRH (352). Electrical stimulation of the nucleus raphe obscurus results in a facilitation of phrenic motoneuron discharge that is mediated by serotonin (356,357).

Retrograde labeling studies have shown that neurons in the raphe nuclei project to the hypoglossal nucleus. While such neurons are present throughout the raphe nuclei, a larger proportion are located in the caudal parts of the raphe nuclei, and retrograde labeling is most frequent in raphe obscurus, followed by raphe magnus and then raphe pallidus (331). In contrast, injection of tritiated leucine into the raphe nuclei produces little anterograde labeling in the hypoglossal nucleus (358,359). Serotonin-containing axons and axon terminals have been demonstrated within the hypoglossal nucleus (360,361). The actions of 5-HT and TRH on hypoglossal motoneurons have been investigated (101,110).

Locus Coeruleus Inputs. Immunohistochemical labeling of rat spinal cord has revealed a dense plexus of fibers and varicosities containing dopamine-β-hydroxylase, the enzyme producing noradrenalin from dopamine, in the phrenic nucleus in the rat (349). The likely source of these projections is the locus coeruleus, a noradrenergic cell group in the caudal midbrain and upper pons, lateral to the periaqueductal gray matter (362). It has extensive axonal connections to the forebrain and contributes descending fibers to the motor nuclei of the trigeminal, facial, and hypoglossal nerves, and especially to the solitary nucleus, the commissural nucleus, the dorsal motor nucleus of the vagus, and the raphe nuclei. The locus coeruleus and the neighboring subcoeruleus are the major source of noradrenergic projections to all levels of the spinal cord (363). In addition, the area of the lateral ventral tegmentum surrounding the locus coeruleus also contains a large number of loosely scattered noradrenergic neurons; those lying more posterior project mainly to similar sites in the brainstem and spinal cord. In vitro studies using the neonatal rat brainstem–spinal cord preparation have demonstrated a depression of respiratory frequency mediated by α_2 receptors and induction of tonic spinal motoneuron discharge mediated by α_1 receptors, but both effects seem to be governed at supraspinal levels (364,365).

Rubrospinal Inputs. Similar to the lateral corticospinal pathway, the rubrospinal system serves to steer the extremities and plays a role in fine-motor control. However, in contrast to the corticospinal projection, rubrospinal fibers may preferentially control automatic or previously learned motions. The magno-cellular part of the red nucleus gives rise to both rubrospinal and rubrobulbar projections (325). The rubrospinal fibers descend in the contralateral ventral lateral medulla, continuing to the spinal cord in the dorsolateral funiculus, while the rubrobulbar fibers project to facial and hypoglossal motoneuron pools. Bassal and Bianchi (335) have reported a short-latency termination of phrenic nerve discharge, following electrical stimulation of the red nucleus or rubrospinal tract. Schmid et al. (366) studied the effects of rubrospinal tract stimulation on phrenic nerve and medullary respiratory neuronal discharge in the rabbit. They found phrenic nerve suppression of short latency (3 msec) and duration (29 msec) and were able to terminate inspiration by delivering single shocks during mid- to late inspiration. Discharge of inspiratory bulbospinal neurons was also suppressed at latencies ranging from 1.2 to 2.5 msec. After allowing for conduction time of 1.6 msec to the motoneuron pool, they concluded that nerve suppression was due to disfacilitation.

B. Recurrent Inhibition and Excitation

Phrenic Motoneurons

Recurrent axon collaterals, or recurrent inhibition via Renshaw interneurons (367), were thought not to be present in phrenic motoneurons, as Gill and Kuno (368) failed to record any recurrent IPSPs. More recently, morphological and electro-physiological evidence of phrenic motoneuron axon collaterals has been seen (16,18,22). Recurrent IPSPs have been recorded in 40% of phrenic motoneurons in a spinalized deafferented preparation (18), and extracellular discharges of Renshaw interneurons have been recorded near the phrenic nucleus (18,369). It has been reported that the recurrent IPSPs have amplitudes ranging from 45 to 260 μV (mean = 115 μV), a mean latency of 3.0 ± 0.6 msec, and duration of 12 to 25 msec (18). Stimulation of the C-5 phrenic root also caused inhibition of activity in the C-6 phrenic root, with a duration similar to that of both the recurrent IPSP and Renshaw interneuron discharge. Hilaire et al. (22) also recorded recurrent IPSPs in seven of 90 C-5 phrenic motoneurons. Extracellular records of Renshaw interneurons showed inspiratory-phase spike activity and increased spike frequency in inspiration following antidromic stimulation of the phrenic nerve, leading Hilaire et al. (22) to conclude that Renshaw interneurons associated with the phrenic nucleus receive central inspiratory drive. It is thus apparent that phrenic motoneurons do receive recurrent inhibition, although not to the same extent as lumbar hindlimb motoneurons (370) or intercostal motoneurons (32). The possibility of direct excitatory interactions between phrenic motoneurons by way of recurrent excitatory collaterals has also been raised by Hilaire's group. Stimulation of the phrenic nerve has been shown to evoke stable, shortlatency, orthodromic action potentials in unitary phrenic motoneuron axons in more than 60% of cases; this response could be blocked by a central nicotinic antagonist, mecamylamine (371). An attempt to substantiate this result by intracellular recording from phrenic motoneurons has been only partly successful, as few phrenic motoneurons showed short-latency excitatory responses (372). It has been suggested that a role of recurrent excitation might be to synchronize phrenic motoneuron discharge in the short term, as administration of mecamylamide results in slow reduction of the strength of such synchrony (373).

Intercostal Motoneurons

Recurrent inhibition was also thought not to exist in the intercostal motoneuron pools (162,374), despite the presence of neurons within thoracic segments that showed Renshaw cell–like discharge following intercostal nerve stimulation (162). More recently, recurrent inhibition has been unequivocally demonstrated by Kirkwood et al. (32). They confirmed the presence of Renshaw cells in deafferented thoracic segment and recorded IPSPs of up to 200 μV in inspiratory and expiratory intercostal motoneurons, following stimulation of intercostal motor axons with a delay consistent with disynaptic transmission. Poststimulus histograms of firing of inspiratory motoneurons of the same and adjacent segments showed a period of reduced firing probability that extended up to three segments distance, declining in intensity. Thus, Renshaw cells may have axons extending up to 30 mm, and although recurrent inhibition of individual intercostal motoneurons is weak in comparison to that of hindlimb motoneurons, its extent of spread of any one Renshaw cell's effect may compensate for this. The morphological basis for recurrent inhibition also exists, as axon collaterals are relatively common in inspiratory and expiratory intercostal motoneurons (25).

Kirkwood et al. (32) also noted that poststimulus histograms of intercostal nerve activity did not show any signs of short-latency excitation, suggesting that recurrent excitation or electrical coupling between intercostal motoneurons is not present in this motor pool.

Hypoglossal Motoneurons

IPSPs recorded in hypoglossal motoneurons following stimulation of the hypoglossal nerve are unlikely to be due to recurrent inhibition, as eliciting these responses generally requires stimuli 3 to 5 times greater than antidromic threshold (208,210) and there is no morphological evidence for recurrent axon collaterals in hypoglossal motoneurons (see above for references).

Laryngeal and Pharyngeal Motoneurons

The existence of recurrent collaterals in these motoneurons is still undecided. Grélot et al. (66) have described one instance of an axon collateral in an HRP-filled expiratory neuron of the retrofacial area, which they thought was a pharyngeal motoneuron, since its main axon joined the cranial nerve roots. Otake et al. (264) also described four expiratory neurons in the Böt complex, which could not be antidromically activated from the SLN or cervical vagus nerve, but whose axons had trajectories similar to those of vagal motoneurons but gave off collaterals. These neurons may have been pharyngeal motoneurons as well. Similarly, two inspiratory motoneurons of the r-VRG did not possess axon collaterals (375). Thus, if recurrent inhibition does exist in these motoneuron pools, it is probably rare.

C. Electrical Coupling

Phrenic Motoneurons

The close intertwining of phrenic motoneuron dendrites (17,18) has led to suggestions that phrenic motoneurons may be electrically coupled, thus accounting for some of their short-term firing synchrony. Lipski (23) investigated this by stimulating the phrenic nerve for one cervical segment and recording either action potential discharge in the phrenic nerve of an adjacent segment or phrenic motoneuron membrane potential. He did not observe any increase in firing probability of phrenic motoneurons and concluded that synchronization must occur through chemical synapses.

Hypoglossal Motoneurons

Electrical coupling exists between 10 and 40% of hypoglossal motoneurons in neonatal rats of less than 10 days age, as shown by dye or tracer coupling following intracellular injection of Lucifer Yellow or neurobiotin (376) or short-latency depolarizations elicited by stimulation of hypoglossal axons (Fig. 15) (376) (K. Ballanyi, personal communication). Similar phenomena have not been reported for adult hypoglossal motoneurons.

D. Origin of Central Respiratory Drive Potentials

It is highly probable that relatively synchronized and presumably phasic synaptic inputs impinge on respiratory motoneurons to produce their respiratory-related rhythmic fluctuations of membrane potential. The weight of evidence suggests

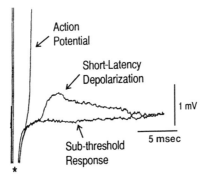

Figure 15 Short-latency depolarization observed in a neonatal hypoglossal motoneuron in response to subthreshold stimulation of the axon. Three different responses are shown, one of which is subthreshold; at a slightly higher stimulation intensity, there is an all-or-none short-latency depolarization response, and then with higher intensity a full antidromic action potential is generated whose peak is truncated in the illustration. Asterisk (*) indicates the stimulus artifact. Data obtained in an in vitro slice preparation from a 2-day-old rat. (Adapted from Ref. 376.)

that these respiration-related inputs derive either directly (i.e., monosynaptically) or indirectly (i.e., polysynaptically) from the descending axons of medullary respiratory neurons. We will now critically discuss the relative contribution of mono- versus polysynaptic inputs to the membrane potential fluctuations of respiratory motoneurons. Of necessity, our knowledge of cat phrenic motoneurons and their inputs will form the basis of this discussion.

The first intracellular recordings from phrenic motoneurons by Gill and Kuno (154,368) ascribed the slow inspiratory depolarizing shifts in phrenic motoneuron membrane potential to excitatory input, as synaptic noise was present during this phase. Since the expiratory hyperpolarization of phrenic motoneurons in their study lacked such noise, they postulated that it was due to disfacilitation of the descending excitatory inputs. Sears (24) also observed increased levels of synaptic noise during depolarization of expiratory and inspiratory intercostal motoneurons, but also reported that the hyperpolarizing phase of these motoneurons often changed to a depolarization when the recording electrode held chloride ions, presumably owing to the presence of chloride-dependent synaptic inhibition (Fig. 16A) (377). Since then, Berger (107) has shown that most phrenic motoneurons receive active inhibitory input during the expiratory phase under conditions of elevated respiratory drive, by reversal of the expiratory hyperpolarization using injection of hyperpolarizing current or Cl^- ions (Fig. 16B). A similar result has been observed by others (191,257), and Milano et al. (378) have extended this observation by recording multiphasic reversal of expiratory hyperpolarization in

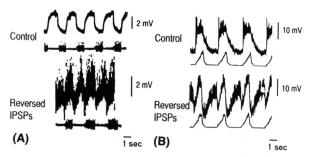

Figure 16 Respiratory-phase-related active inhibition in cat spinal respiratory moto-neurons. (A) Intracellular recording of an expiratory intercostal motoneuron shows reversal of inspiratory-phase hyperpolarization to a depolarizing wave following chloride injection into the motoneuron. (Adapted from Ref. 24.) (B) Intracellular recording of a phrenic motoneuron shows reversal of expiratory-phase hyperpolarization to a depolarizing wave during continuous passage of hyperpolarizing current through the microelectrode. (Adapted from Ref. 107.) In each panel, upper trace is the membrane potential and lower is the diaphragmatic EMG in A and the integrated phrenic neurogram in B.

all of a small number of phrenic motoneurons, following injections of Cl$^-$ ions. The time course and magnitude of this inhibitory synaptic input vary markedly (107,378). As other respiratory motoneurons also show phasic excitation and inhibition (54,95,379), it seems that alternating periods of excitation and inhibition are a general feature of respiratory motoneuron pools.

The question thus arises, "What are the sources of excitatory and inhibitory inputs to phrenic motoneurons?" The view has been advanced that respiratory motoneurons simply act as passive elements that translate the alternating rhythm of monosynaptic excitatory and inhibitory inputs from phasic bulbospinal pre-motor neurons to a motor output (222,380). This view has been challenged (1, 128,133). The recognized monosynaptic inputs from phasic neurons to phrenic motoneurons are those of the DRG inspiratory, inspiratory r-NRA, and Böt expiratory neurons, whereas only inputs from the DRG inspiratory neurons seem to make monosynaptic connections to inspiratory intercostal motoneurons with any frequency (see previous sections for references). The connectivity of these inputs to spinal respiratory motoneurons is 30–50% at most. Even without detailed knowledge of the cell numbers and spinal connectivity of these groups, it seems unlikely that they alone could provide sufficient synaptic input to produce the membrane potential shifts seen in these motoneurons, which typically vary from 5 to 12 mV.

A model of respiratory motoneuron firing developed by Tuck (381), cited by Davies et al. (128) and briefly described by Sears (382), calculated that a Poisson-distributed input rate of 20,000 EPSPs per second is required to bring a moto-neuron from a resting potential of -70 mV to a firing rate of 10–20 Hz with an input of 100 μV EPSPs. Davies et al. (127,128) have attempted to model the possible contribution of inspiratory monosynaptic drive on inspiratory motoneu-rons, using this model and the data derived from their cross-correlation studies of the connectivity between inspiratory bulbospinal neurons in the DRG or r-NRA and phrenic motoneurons. The mean firing rate of the bulbospinal neurons in Davies et al. (128) was 99 Hz, suggesting that 200 of these neurons producing 100 μV unitary EPSPs would provide sufficient inspiratory drive for a single moto-neuron. Although Davies et al. (127,128) were rigorous in excluding correlation peaks that could be due either to presynaptic synchronization of medullary neurons or to oligosynaptic transmission pathways (see discussion above), narrow-width cross-correlation histogram peaks, interpreted as monosynaptic connec-tions, were seen in 50% of cases. The magnitude of the EPSPs producing the narrow peaks seen was derived from the k ratio for the peaks (k is the ratio of the peak count in the cross-correlation histogram divided by the baseline count) (121,126,383), assuming that a k value of 1.5 for the cross-correlation histogram peaks corresponded to an EPSP amplitude of 100 μV. These assumed values were derived from the mean k value of 1.5 for cross-correlation histogram peaks produced by single Ia action potentials to single α-motoneuron unitary discharges in external intercostal nerve filaments (177), which gave a mean amplitude of 100 μV for STA Ia EPSPs in external intercostal motoneurons (176). As the mean k for phrenic motoneurons and intercostal motoneurons in Davies et al. (128) were 1.055 and 1.019, respectively, the number of bulbospinal neurons required to bring a single phrenic motoneuron to this firing rate would be 200 $\times$ (0.5/0.055) = 1818, while intercostal motoneurons would need 200 $\times$ (0.5/0.019) = 5263. The number of inspiratory bulbospinal neurons is uncertain, but may be ten-tatively put at about 400, based on the retrograde labeling studies of Rickard-Bell et al. (246) and of Onai and Miura (232). If this is assumed, then Davies et al. (128) calculated that bulbospinal inputs to phrenic and intercostal motoneurons produce approximately 3–4 mV and 1 mV of their inspiratory depolarization, respectively. They thus concluded that the majority of the inspiratory depolariza-tion in phrenic motoneurons is due to inputs from spinal interneurons. While these authors give several possible caveats for their conclusion, it remains to be tested.

The means by which expiratory hyperpolarization of respiratory moto-neurons is produced also remains unclear. An estimate similar to that of Davies et al. (128) has not been attempted. Indeed, we lack any quantitative measurement of the hyperpolarizing change due to active inhibition. The only expiratory-phase inhibitory input to phrenic motoneurons known is that from Böt expiratory neurons, and no bulbospinal source of monosynaptic inhibition has been described for intercostal motoneurons (133). Connectivity between Böt expiratory bulbo-spinal neurons and phrenic motoneurons is estimated to be about 30% (257). This study made no attempt to guard against presynaptic synchronization, and in our opinion, the true level of monosynaptic connectivity between Böt expiratory and phrenic motoneurons remains unknown. As only 25% of Böt expiratory neurons arborize in the phrenic nucleus, they are unlikely to be sufficient to provide enough inhibitory input to entirely account for the expiratory hyperpolarization of phrenic motoneurons.

V. Summary

Respiratory motoneurons are a diverse collection of brainstem and spinal neurons that innervate a number of widely separated groups of muscles involved in breathing. We can no longer simply consider respiratory motoneurons as simply linear follower cells. They have a rich palette of intrinsic voltage- and time-dependent conductances that contribute to their behavior. As discussed elsewhere in this book, neurotransmitters can modulate this behavior. The relevant output of a motoneuron, as far as the innervated muscle is concerned, is the spike-firing behavior. This is determined by both intrinsic properties and synaptic inputs to the motoneuron. A view has been advanced that respiratory motoneurons simply act to translate the alternating rhythm of monosynaptic excitatory and inhibitory inputs from respiratory medullary premotor neurons into a motor output. We regard this view as overly simplistic. As in other motor systems, interneurons function in conjunction with these inputs to drive motoneurons. We must consider also that respiratory motoneurons receive a rich innervation from nonrespiratory input systems. The future challenge is to determine how all of these features and properties, when combined, result in the observed behavior of the various respiratory motoneurons.

Acknowledgments

This work was supported by a Javits Neuroscience Investigator Award NS-14857 and Research Grant HL 49657 from the National Institutes of Health to A. J. Berger.

References

1. Monteau R, Hilaire G. Spinal respiratory motoneurons. Prog Neurobiol 1991; 37: 83–144.
2. Van Lunteren E, Dick TE. Intrinsic properties of pharyngeal and diaphragmatic respiratory motoneurons and muscles. J Appl Physiol 1992; 73:787–800.

3. Duron B, Jung-Caillol MC, Marlot D. Myelinated nerve fiber supply and muscle spindles in the respiratory muscles of cat: quantitative study. Anat Embryol 1978; 152:171–192.

4. Duron B. Postural and ventilatory functions of intercostal muscles. Acta Neurobiol Exp 1973; 33:355–380.

5. Duron B, Marlot D. Intercostal and diaphragmatic electrical activity during wakefulness and sleep in normal unrestrained adult cats. Sleep 1980; 3:269–280.

6. Sherrington CS. Remarks on some aspects of reflex inhibition. Proc Roy Soc Lond Ser B 1925; 97:519–545.

7. Burke RE. Motor units: anatomy, physiology, and functional organization. In: Brookhart JM, Mountcastle VB, eds. Handbook of Physiology. The Nervous System. Motor Control. Bethesda, MD: American Physiological Society, 1981: 345–422.

8. Duron B, Marlot D, Larnicol N, Jung-Caillol MC, Macron JM. Somatotopy in the phrenic motor nucleus of the cat as revealed by retrograde transport of horseradish peroxidase. Neurosci Lett 1993; 14:159–163.

9. Gordon DC, Richmond FJR. Topography in the phrenic motoneuron nucleus demonstrated by retrograde multiple-labelling techniques. J Comp Neurol 1990; 292:424–434.

10. Keswani NH, Hollinshead WH. Localization of the phrenic nucleus in the spinal cord of man. Anat Rec 1956; 125:683–699.

11. Berger AJ, Cameron WE, Averill DB, Kramis RC, Binder MD. Spatial distributions of phrenic and medial gastrocnemius motoneurons in the cat spinal cord. Exp Neurol 1984; 86:559–575.

12. Webber CL, Jr., Wurster RD, Chung JM. Cat phrenic nucleus architecture as revealed by horseradish peroxidase mapping. Exp Brain Res 1979; 35:395–406.

13. Kuzuhara S, Chou SM. Localization of the phrenic nucleus in the rat: a HRP study. Neurosci Lett 1980; 16:119–124.

14. Johnson SM, Getting PA. Phrenic motor nucleus of the guinea pig: dendrites are bundled without clustering of cell somas. Exp Neurol 1988; 101:208–220.

15. Sterling P, Kuypers HGJM. Anatomical organisation of the brachial spinal cord of the cat. II. The motoneurone plexus. Brain Res 1967; 4:16–32.

16. Webber CL, Jr., Pleschka K. Structural and functional characteristics of individual phrenic motoneurons. Pflügers Arch 1976; 364:113–121.

17. Cameron WE, Averill DB, Berger AJ. Morphology of cat phrenic motoneurons revealed by intracellular injection of horseradish peroxidase. J Comp Neurol 1983; 219:70–80.

18. Lipski J, Fyffe REW, Jodkowski J. Recurrent inhibition of cat phrenic motoneurons. J Neurosci 1985; 5:1545–1555.

19. Pilowsky PM, de Castro D, Llewellyn-Smith I, Lipski J, Voss MD. Serotonin immunoreactive boutons make synapses with feline phrenic motoneurons. J Neurosci 1990; 10:1091–1098.

20. Cameron WE, Averill DB, Berger AJ. Quantitative analysis of the dendrites of cat phrenic motoneurons stained intracellularly with horseradish peroxidase. J Comp Neurol 1985; 231:91–101.

21. Goshgarian HG, Rafols JA. The ultrastructure and synaptic architecture of phrenic motor neurons in the spinal cord of the adult rat. J Neurocytol 1984; 13:85–109.
22. Hilaire G, Khatib M, Monteau R. Central drive on renshaw cells coupled with phrenic motoneurons. Brain Res 1986; 376:133–139.
23. Lipski J. Is there electrical coupling between phrenic motoneurons in cats? Neurosci Lett 1984; 46:229–234.
24. Sears TA. The slow potentials of thoracic respiratory motoneurones and their relationship to breathing. J Physiol (Lond) 1964; 175:404–424.
25. Lipski J, Martin-Body RL. Morphological properties of respiratory intercostal motoneurons in cats as revealed by intracellular injection of horseradish peroxidase. J Comp Neurol 1987; 260:423–434.
26. Kirkwood PA, Sears TA. The synaptic connexions to intercostal motoneurones as revealed by the average common excitation potential. J Physiol (Lond) 1978; 275:103–134.
27. Lipski J, Duffin J. An electrophysiological investigation of propriospinal inspiratory neurons in the upper cervical cord of the cat. Exp Brain Res 1986; 61:625–637.
28. Le Bars P, Duron B. Are the external and internal intercostal muscles synergist or antagonist in the cat? Neurosci Lett 1984; 51:383–386.
29. Warwick R, Williams PL, eds. Gray's Anatomy, 35th ed. Philadelphia: Saunders, 1973.
30. Hilaire GG, Nicholls JG, Sears TA. Control and proprioceptive influences on the activity of levator costae motoneurones in the cat. J Physiol (Lond) 1983; 342:527–548.
31. Larnicol N, Rose D, Marlot D, Duron B. Anatomical organization of cat intercostal motor nuclei as demonstrated by HRP retrograde labelling. J Physiol (Paris) 1982; 78:198–206.
32. Kirkwood PA, Sears TA, Westgaard RH. Recurrent inhibition of intercostal motoneurones in the cat. J Physiol (Lond) 1981; 319:111–130.
33. Strohl KP, Mead J, Banzett RB, Loring SH, Kosch PC. Regional differences in abdominal muscle activity during various maneuvers. J Appl Physiol 1981; 51:1471–1476.
34. Miller AD. Localization of motoneurons innervating individual abdominal muscles of the cat. J Comp Neurol 1987; 256:600–606.
35. Holstege G, Van Neerven J, Evertse F. Spinal cord location of the motoneurons innervating the abdominal, cutaneous maximus, latissimus dorsi and lognissimus dorsi muscles in the cat. Exp Brain Res 1987; 67:179–194.
36. De Troyer A, Estenne M. Functional anatomy of the respiratory muscles. Clin Chest Med 1988; 9:175–193.
37. Rose PK, Keirstead SA, Vanner SJ. A quantitative analysis of the geometry of cat motoneurons innervating neck and shoulder muscles. J Comp Neurol 1985; 239:89–107.
38. Vanner SJ, Rose PK. Dendritic distribution of motoneurons innervating the three heads of the trapezius muscle in the cat. J Comp Neurol 1984; 226:96–110.
39. Decramer M. Respiratory muscle interaction. News Physiol Sci 1993; 8:121–124.

40. Lewis PR, Flumerfelt BA, Shute CC. The use of cholinesterase techniques to study topographical localization in the hypoglossal nucleus of the rat. J Anat 1971; 110: 203–213.

41. Krammer EB, Rath T, Lischka MF. Somatotopic organization of the hypoglossal nucleus: a HRP study in the rat. Brain Res 1979; 170:533–537.

42. Uemura M, Matsuda K, Kume M, Takeuchi Y, Matsushima R, Mizuno N. Typographical arrangement of hypoglossal motoneurons: an HRP study in the cat. Neurosci Lett 1979; 13:99–104.

43. Uemura-Sumi M, Itoh M, Mizuno N. The distribution of hypoglossal motoneurons in the dog, rabbit and rat. Anat Embryol (Berl) 1988; 177:389–394.

44. Takasu N, Hashimoto PH. Morphological identification of an interneuron in the hypoglossal nucleus of the rat: a combined Golgi–electron microscopic study. J Comp Neurol 1988; 271:461–471.

45. Davidoff MS, Schulze W. Coexistence of GABA- and choline acetyltransferase (ChAT)-like immunoreactivity in the hypoglossal nucleus of the rat. Histochemistry 1988; 89:25–33.

46. Boone TB, Aldes LD. The ultrastructure of two distinct neuron populations in the hypoglossal nucleus of the rat. Exp Brain Res 1984; 54:321–326.

47. Ramón y Cajal S. Histologie du systeme nerveux de l'homme et des vertebres. Tome I. Madrid: Instituto Ramón y Cajal, 1909.

48. Cooper MH. The hypoglossal nucleus of the primate: a Golgi study. Neurosci Lett 1981; 21:249–254.

49. Green JD, Negishi K. Membrane potentials in hypoglossal motoneurons. J Neurophysiol 1963; 26:835–856.

50. Sumi T. Functional differentiation of hypoglossal neurons in cats. Jpn J Physiol 1969; 19:55–67.

51. Mosfeldt Laursen A, Rekling JC. Electrophysiological properties of hypoglossal motoneurons of guinea-pigs studied in vitro. Neuroscience 1989; 30:619–637.

52. Viana F, Gibbs L, Berger AJ. Double- and triple-labeling of functionally characterized central neurons projecting to peripheral targets studied in vitro. Neuroscience 1990; 38:829–841.

53. Takasu N, Nakatani T, Arikuni T, Kimura H. Immunocytochemical localization of gamma-amino-butyric acid in the hypoglossal nucleus of the macaque monkey, *Macaca fuscata*: a light and electron microscopic study. J Comp Neurol 1987; 263: 42–53.

54. Withington-Wray DJ, Mifflin SW, Spyer KM. Intracellular analysis of respiratory-modulated hypoglossal motoneurons in the cat. Neuroscience 1988; 25:1041–1051.

55. Wan XST, Trojanowski JQ, Gonatas JO, Liu CN. Cytoarchitecture of the extra-nuclear and commissural dendrites of hypoglossal nucleus neurons as revealed by conjugates of horseradish peroxidase with cholera toxin. Exp Neurol 1982; 78: 167–175.

56. Gacek RR, Lyon MJ. Fiber components of the recurrent laryngeal nerve in the cat. Ann Otol 1976; 85:460–471.

57. Bartlett D. Upper airway motor systems. In: Cherniack NS, Widdicombe JG, eds.

Handbook of Physiology. Section 3: The Respiratory System. Vol. 2. Control of Breathing, Part 1. Bethesda, MD: American Physiological Society, 1986:223–245.

58. Bartlett D, Remmers JE, Gautier H. Laryngeal regulation of respiratory airflow. Respir Physiol 1973; 18:194–204.

59. Cohen MI. Phrenic and recurrent laryngeal discharge patterns and the Hering-Breuer reflex. Am J Physiol 1975; 228:1489–1496.

60. Megirian D, Sherrey JH. Respiratory functions of the laryngeal muscles during sleep. Sleep 1980; 3:289–298.

61. Sherrey JH, Megirian D. Spontaneous and reflexly evoked laryngeal abductor and adductor muscle activity of cat. Exp Neurol 1974; 43:487–498.

62. St. John WM, Bartlett D, Knuth KV, Hwang J-C. Brain stem genesis of automatic ventilatory patterns independent of spinal mechanisms. J Appl Physiol 1981; 51: 204–210.

63. Hairston LE, Sauerland EK. Electromyography of the human pharynx: discharge patterns of the superior pharyngeal constrictor during respiration. Electromyo Clin Neurophysiol 1981; 21:299–306.

64. Sherrey JH, Megirian D. Analysis of the respiratory role of pharyngeal constrictor motoneurons of cat. Exp Neurol 1975; 49:839–851.

65. Bianchi AL, Grélot L, Iscoe S, Remmers JE. Electrophysiological properties of rostral medullary respiratory neurones in the cat: an intracellular study. J Physiol (Lond) 1988; 407:293–310.

66. Grélot L, Bianchi AL, Iscoe S, Remmers JE. Expiratory neurones of the rostral medulla: anatomical and functional correlates. Neurosci Lett 1988; 89:140–145.

67. Davis PJ, Nail BS. On the location and size of laryngeal motoneurons in the cat and rabbit. J Comp Neurol 1984; 230:13–32.

68. Grélot L, Barillot JC, Bianchi AL. Central distributions of the efferent and afferent components of the pharyngeal branches of the vagus and glossopharyngeal nerves: an HRP study in the cat. Exp Brain Res 1989; 78:327–335.

69. Hinrichsen CFL, Ryan T. Localization of laryngeal motoneurons in the rat: morphologic evidence for dual innervation. Exp Neurol 1981; 74:341–355.

70. Kalia M, Mesulam M. Brainstem projections of sensory and motor components of the vagus complex in the cat. II. Laryngeal, tracheobronchial, pulmonary, cardiac and gastrointestinal branches. J Comp Neurol 1980; 193:467–508.

71. Kalia M, Mesulam M. Brainstem projections of sensory and motor components of the vagus complex in the cat. I. The cervical vagus and nodose ganglion. J Comp Neurol 1980; 193:435–465.

72. Kalia M, Sullivan M. Brain stem projections of sensory and motor components of the vagus nerve in the rat. J Comp Neurol 1982; 211:248–264.

73. Lawn AM. The localization, in the nucleus ambiguus of the rabbit, of the cells of origin of motor nerve fibers in the glossopharyngeal nerve and various branches of the vagus nerve by means of retrograde degeneration. J Comp Neurol 1966; 127: 293–306.

74. Pásaro R, Lobera B, González Barón S, Delgado García JM. Cytoarchitectonic organization of laryngeal motoneurons within the nucleus ambiguus of the cat. Exp Neurol 1983; 82:623–634.

75. Nunez-Abades PA, Pásaro R, Bianchi AL. Study of the topographical distribution of different populations of motoneurons within rat's nucleus ambiguus, by means of four different fluorochromes. Neurosci Lett 1992; 135:103–107.

76. Bieger D, Hopkins DA. Viscerotopic representation of the upper alimentary tract in the medulla oblongata in the rat: the nucleus ambiguus. J Comp Neurol 1987; 262: 546–562.

77. Barillot JC, Bianchi AL, Gogan P. Laryngeal respiratory motoneurones: morphology and electrophysiological evidence of separate sites for excitatory and inhibitory synaptic inputs. Neurosci Lett 1984; 47:107–112.

78. Kreuter F, Richter DW, Camerer H, Senekowitsch R. Morphological and electrical description of medullary respiratory neurons of the cat. Pflügers Arch 1977; 372: 7–16.

79. Hairston LE, Sauerland EK. Electromyography of the human palate: discharge patterns of the levator and tensor veli palatini. Electromyo Clin Neurophysiol 1981; 21:287–297.

80. St. John WM, Bledsoe TA. Comparison of respiratory-related trigeminal, hypoglossal and phrenic activities. Respir Physiol 1985; 62:61–78.

81. Taber E. The cytoarchitecture of the brain stem of the cat. I. Brain stem nuclei of cat. J Comp Neurol 1961; 116:27–70.

82. Mizuno N, Konishi A, Sato M. Localization of masticatory motoneurons in the cat and rat by means of retrograde axonal transport of horseradish peroxidase. J Comp Neurol 1975; 164:105–116.

83. Sasamoto K. Motor nuclear representation of masticatory muscles in the rat. Jpn J Physiol 1979; 29:739–747.

84. Travers JB. Organization and projections of the orofacial motor nuclei. In: Paxinos G, ed. The Rat Nervous System. Vol 2. Hindbrain and Spinal Cord. Sydney: Academic Press, 1985:111–128.

85. Keller JT, Rhoades RW, Enfiejian HL, Egger MD. Identification of motoneurons innervating the tensor tympani and tensor veli palatini muscles in the cat. Brain Res 1983; 270:209–215.

86. Jacquin MF, Rhoades RW, Enfiejian HL, Egger MD. Organization and morphology of masticatory neurons in the rat: a retrograde HRP study. J Comp Neurol 1983; 218: 239–256.

87. Moore JA, Appenteng K. The morphology and electrical geometry of rat jaw-elevator motoneurones. J Physiol (Lond) 1991; 440:325–343.

88. Shigenaga Y, Yoshida A, Tsuru K, Mitsuhiro Y, Otani K, Cao CQ. Physiological and morphological characteristics of cat masticatory motoneurons—intracellular injection of HRP. Brain Res 1988; 461:238–256.

89. Breuer J. Self-steering of respiration through the nervus vagus [trans. by E. Ullmann]. In: Porter R, ed. Breathing: Hering-Breuer Centenary Symposium. London: Churchill, 1970:365–394.

90. Ogawa T, Jefferson NC, Toman JE, Chiles T, Zambetoglou A, Necheles H. Action potentials of accessory respiratory muscles in dogs. Am J Physiol 1960; 199:569–572.

91. Hwang J-C, Chien C-T, St. John WM. Characterization of respiratory-related activity of the facial nerve. Respir Physiol 1988; 73:175–188.

92. Sherrey JH, Megirian D. State dependence of upper airway respiratory motoneurons: functions of the cricothyroid and nasolabial muscles of the unanesthetized rat. Electromyo Clin Neurophysiol 1977; 43:218–228.

93. Strohl KP. Respiratory activity of the facial nerve and alar muscles in anesthetized dogs. J Physiol (Lond) 1985; 363:351–362.

94. Strohl KP, Hensley MJ, Hallett M, Saunders NA, Ingram RH, Jr. Activation of upper airway muscles before onset of inspiration in normal humans. J Appl Physiol 1980; 49:638–642.

95. Huangfu D, Koshiya N, Guyenet PG. Central respiratory modulation of facial motoneurons in rats. Neurosci Lett 1993; 151:224–228.

96. Kume M, Uemura M, Matsuda K, Matsushima R, Mizuno N. Topographical representation of peripheral branches of the facial nerve within the facial nucleus: a HRP study in the cat. Neurosci Lett 1978; 8:5–8.

97. Martin MR, Lodge D. Morphology of the facial nucleus of the rat. Brain Res 1977; 123:1–12.

98. Watson CRR, Sakai S, Armstrong W. Organization of the facial nucleus in the rat. Brain Behav Evol 1982; 20:19–29.

99. Friauf E. Morphology of motoneurons in different subdivisions of the rat facial nucleus stained intracellularly with horseradish peroxidase. J Comp Neurol 1986; 253:231–241.

100. Haddad GG, Donnelly DF, Getting PA. Biophysical properties of hypoglossal neurons in vitro: intracellular studies in adult and neonatal rats. J Appl Physiol 1990; 69:1509–1517.

101. Bayliss DA, Viana F, Berger AJ. Mechanisms underlying excitatory effects of thyrotropin-releasing hormone on rat hypoglossal motoneurons in vitro. J Neurophysiol 1992; 68:1733–1745.

102. Viana F, Bayliss DA, Berger AJ. Multiple potassium conductances and their role in action potential repolarization and repetitive firing behavior of neonatal rat hypoglossal motoneurons. J Neurophysiol 1993; 69:2150–2163.

103. Viana F, Bayliss DA, Berger AJ. Calcium conductances and their role in the firing behavior of neonatal rat hypoglossal motoneurons. J Neurophysiol 1993; 69:2137–2149.

104. Takahashi T. Membrane currents in visually identified motoneurones of neonatal rat spinal cord. J Physiol (Lond) 1990; 423:27–46.

105. Berger AJ, Takahashi T. Serotonin enhances a low-voltage-activated calcium current in rat spinal motoneurons. J Neurosci 1990; 10:1922–1928.

106. Takahashi T. Inward rectification in neonatal rat spinal motoneurones. J Physiol (Lond) 1990; 423:47–62.

107. Berger AJ. Phrenic motoneurons in the cat: subpopulations and nature of respiratory drive potentials. J Neurophysiol 1979; 42:76–90.

108. Cameron WE, Jodkowski JS, Fang H, Guthrie RD. Electrophysiological properties of developing phrenic motoneurons in the cat. J Neurophysiol 1991; 65:671–679.

109. Staley KJ, Otis TS, Mody I. Membrane properties of dentate gyrus granule cells: comparison of sharp microelectrode and whole-cell recordings. J Neurophysiol 1992; 67:1346–1348.

110. Berger AJ, Bayliss DA, Viana F. Modulation of neonatal rat hypoglossal motoneuron excitability by serotonin. Neurosci Lett 1992; 143:164–168.

111. Brozanski BS, Guthrie RD, Volk EA, Cameron WE. Postnatal growth of genio-glossal motoneurons. Pediatr Pulmonol 1989; 7;133–139.

112. Smith JC, Liu G, Feldman JL. Intracellular recording from phrenic motoneurons receiving respiratory drive in vitro. Neurosci Lett 1988; 88:27–32.

113. Umemiya M, Berger AJ. Calcium currents and calcium channels in visually identified hypoglossal motoneurons. Soc Neurosci Abstr 1993; 19:988.

114. Bayliss DA, Viana F, Bellingham MC, Berger AJ. Characteristics and postnatal development of a hyperpolarization-activated inward current (I_h) in rat hypoglossal motoneurons in vitro. J Neurophysiol 1994; 71:119–128.

115. Viana F, Bayliss DA, Berger AJ. Postnatal changes in rat hypoglossal motoneuron membrane properties. Neuroscience 1994 (in press).

116. Jodkowski JS, Viana F, Dick TE, Berger AJ. Repetitive firing properties of phrenic motoneurons in the cat. J Neurophysiol 1988; 60:687–702.

117. Moore GE, Perkel DJ, Segundo JP. Statistical analysis and functional interpretation of neuronal spike data. Annu Rev Physiol 1966; 28:493–522.

118. Moore GE, Segundo JP, Perkel DJ, Levitan H. Statistical signs of synaptic inter-action in neurons. Biophys J 1970; 10:876–900.

119. Jankowska E, Roberts WJ. Synaptic actions of single interneurones mediating reciprocal Ia inhibition of motoneurones. J Physiol (Lond) 1972; 222:623–642.

120. Mendell LM, Henneman E. Terminals of single Ia fibers: location, density and distribution within a pool of 300 motor neurons. J Neurophysiol 1971; 34:171–187.

121. Kirkwood PA. On the use and interpretation of cross correlation measurements in the mammalian central nervous system. J Neurosci Meth 1979; 1:107–132.

122. Watt DGD, Stauffer EK, Taylor A, Reinking RM, Stuart DG. Analysis of muscle receptor connections by spike-triggered averaging. 1. Spindle primary and tendon organ afferents. J Neurophysiol 1976; 39:1375–1392.

123. Kirkwood PA, Sears TA. Monosynaptic excitation of motoneurones from secondary endings of muscle spindles. Nature 1974; 252:243–244.

124. Stauffer EK, Watt DGD, Taylor A, Reinking RM, Stuart DG. Analysis of muscle receptor connections by spike-triggered averaging. 2. Spindle group II afferents. J Neurophysiol 1976; 39:1393–1402.

125. Rapoport S, Susswin A, Uchino Y, Wilson VJ. Synaptic actions of individual vestibular neurones on cat neck motoneurons. J Physiol (Lond) 1977; 272:367–382.

126. Cope TC, Fetz EE, Matsumaura M. Cross-correlation assessment of synaptic strength of single Ia fibre connections with triceps surae motoneurones in cats. J Physiol (Lond) 1987; 390:161–188.

127. Davies JGM, Kirkwood PA, Sears TA. The detection of monosynaptic connexions from inspiratory bulbospinal neurones to inspiratory neurones. J Physiol (Lond) 1985; 368:33–62.

128. Davies JGM, Kirkwood PA, Sears TA. The distribution of monosynaptic connexions from inspiratory bulbospinal neurones to inspiratory motoneurones in the cat. J Physiol (Lond) 1985; 368:63–87.

129. Cohen MI, Piercey MF, Gootman PM, Wolotsky P. Synaptic connections between

medullary inspiratory neurons and phrenic motoneurons as revealed by cross-correlation. Brain Res 1974; 81:319–324.

130. Feldman JL, Speck DF. Interactions between inspiratory neurons in dorsal and ventral respiratory groups in cat medulla. J Neurophysiol 1983; 49:472–490.

131. Cohen MI, Feldman JL, Sommer D. Caudal medullary expiratory neurone and internal intercostal nerve discharges in the cat: effects of lung inflation. J Physiol (Lond) 1985; 368:147–178.

132. Hilaire G, Monteau R. Connections entre les neurones inspiratoires bulbaires et les motoneurones phréniques et intercortaux. J Physiol (Paris) 1976; 72:987–1000.

133. Merrill EG, Lipski J. Inputs to intercostal motoneurons from ventrolateral medullary respiratory neurons in the cat. J Neurophysiol 1987; 57:1837–1853.

134. Rall W. Distinguishing theoretical synaptic potentials computed for different soma-dendritic distributions of synaptic inputs. J Neurophysiol 1967; 30:1138–1168.

135. Rall W, Burke RE, Smith TG, Nelson PG, Frank F. Dendritic location of synapses and possible mechanisms for the monosynaptic EPSP in motoneurons. J Neurophysiol 1967; 30:1169–1193.

136. Jack JJB, Miller S, Porter R, Redman SJ. The time course of minimal excitatory post-synaptic potentials evoked in spinal motoneurones by group Ia afferent fibres. J Physiol (Lond) 1971; 215:353–380.

137. Berger AJ, Averill DB. Projection of single pulmonary stretch receptors to solitary tract region. J Neurophysiol 1983; 49:819–830.

138. Taylor A, Stephans JA, Somjen G, Appenteng K, O'Donovan MJ. Extracellular spike triggered averaging for plotting synaptic projections. Brain Res 1978; 140: 344–348.

139. Munson JB, Sypert GW. Properties of single central Ia afferent fibres projecting to motoneurones. J Physiol (Lond) 1979; 296:315–327.

140. Schmid K, Kirkwood PA, Munson JB, Shen E, Sears TA. Contralateral projections of thoracic respiratory interneurones in the cat. J Physiol (Lond) 1993; 461: 647–665.

141. Kirkwood PA, Schmid K, Sears TA. Functional identities of thoracic respiratory interneurones in the cat. J Physiol (Lond) 1993; 461:667–687.

142. Goshgarian HG, Roubal PJ. Origin and distribution of phrenic primary afferent nerve fibers in the spinal cord of the adult rat. Exp Neurol 1986; 92:624–638.

143. Conradi S. Ultrastructure of dorsal root boutons on lumbosacral motoneurons of the adult cat, as revealed by dorsal root section. Acta Physiol Scand 1969; 332(Suppl): 85–115.

144. Corda M, Euler C, Lennerstrand B. Proprioceptive innervation of the diaphragm. J Physiol (Lond) 1965; 178:161–177.

145. Macron J, Marlot D, Wallois F, Duron B. Phrenic-to-phrenic inhibition and excitation in spinal cats. Neurosci Lett 1988; 91:24–29.

146. Speck DF, Revelette WR. Attenuation of phrenic motor discharge by phrenic nerve afferents. J Appl Physiol 1987; 62:941–945.

147. Marlot D, Macron J, Duron B. Effects of ipsilateral and contralateral cervical phrenic afferent stimulation on phrenic motor unit activity in the cat. Brain Res 1988; 450:373–377.

148. Macron J, Marlot D, Duron B. Phrenic afferent input to the lateral medullary reticular formation of the cat. Respir Physiol 1985; 59:155–167.

149. Speck DF. Supraspinal involvement in the phrenic-to-phrenic inhibitory reflex. Brain Res 1987; 414:169–172.

150. Speck DF, Revelette WR. Excitation of dorsal and ventral respiratory group neurons by phrenic nerve afferents. J Appl Physiol 1987; 62:946–951.

151. Marlot D, Macron J, Duron B. Projection of phrenic afferents to the external cuneate nucleus in the cat. Brain Res 1985; 327:328–330.

152. Marlot D, Macron J, Duron B. Projections of phrenic afferences to the cat cerebellar cortex. Neurosci Lett 1984; 44:95–98.

153. Davenport PW, Thompson FJ, Reep RL, Freed AN. Projection of phrenic nerve afferents to the cat sensorimotor cortex. Brain Res 1985; 328:150–153.

154. Gill PK, Kuno M. Excitatory and inhibitory actions on phrenic motoneurones. J Physiol (Lond) 1963; 168:274–289.

155. Lewis LJ, Brookhart JM. Significance of the crossed phrenic phenomenon. Am J Physiol 1951; 166:241–254.

156. Goshgarian HG. The role of cervical afferent nerve fiber inhibition of the crossed phrenic phenomenon. Exp Neurol 1981; 72:211–225.

157. Downman CBB. Skeletal muscle reflex of splanchnic and intercostal nerve origin in acute spinal and decerebrate cats. J Neurophysiol 1955; 18:217–235.

158. Decima EE, Euler C. Excitability of phrenic motoneurones to afferent input from lower intercostal nerves in the spinal cat. Acta Physiol Scand 1969; 75:580–591.

159. Decima EE, Euler C. Intercostal and cerebellar influences on efferent phrenic activity in the decerebrate cat. Acta Physiol Scand 1969; 76:148–158.

160. Decima EE, Euler C, Thoden U. Intercostal-to-phrenic reflexes in the spinal cat. Acta Physiol Scand 1969; 75:568–579.

161. Remmers JE. Extra-segmental reflexes derived from intercostal afferents: phrenic and laryngeal responses. J Physiol (Lond) 1973; 233:45–62.

162. Sears TA. Some properties and reflex connexions of respiratory motoneurones of the cat's thoracic spinal cord. J Physiol (Lond) 1964; 175:386–403.

163. Bolser DC, Lindsey BG, Shannon R. Medullary inspiratory activity: influence of intercostal tendon organs and muscle spindle endings. J Appl Physiol 1987; 62:1046–1056.

164. Shannon R. Intercostal and abdominal muscle afferent influence on medullary dorsal respiratory group neurons. Respir Physiol 1980; 39:73–94.

165. Shannon R, Freeman DL. Nucleus retroambigualis respiratory neurons: responses to intercostal and abdominal muscle afferents. Respir Physiol 1981; 45:357–375.

166. Shannon R, Lindsey BG. Expiratory neurons in the region of the retrofacial nucleus: inhibitory effects of intercostal tendon organs. Exp Neurol 1987; 97:730–734.

167. Shannon R, Bolser DC, Lindsey BG. Medullary expiratory activity: influence of intercostal tendon organs and muscle spindle endings. J Appl Physiol 1987; 62:1057–1062.

168. Shannon R, Bolser DC, Lindsey BG. Medullary neurons mediating the inhibition of inspiration by intercostal muscle tendon organs? J Appl Physiol 1988; 65:2498–2505.

169. Bolser DC, Remmers JE. Synaptic effects of intercostal tendon organs on membrane potentials of medullary respiratory neurons. J Neurophysiol 1989; 61:918–926.

170. Shannon R. Reflexes from respiratory muscles and costovertebral joints. In: Cherniack NS, Widdicombe JG, eds. Handbook of Physiology, Section 3: The Respiratory System. Vol 2. Control of Breathing, Part 1. Bethesda, MD: American Physiological Society, 1986:431–447.

171. Eldridge FL, Gill-Kumar P, Millhorn DE, Waldrop TG. Spinal inhibition of phrenic motoneurones by stimulation of afferents from peripheral nerves. J Physiol (Lond) 1981; 311:67–79.

172. Bellingham MC. Synaptic inhibition of phrenic motoneurones by intercostal nerve stimulation. Neurosci Lett 1989; 34(Suppl):S59 (abstract).

173. Sears TA. Efferent discharges in alpha and fusimotor fibres of intercostal nerves of the cat. J Physiol (Lond) 1964; 174:295–315.

174. Sears TA. Activity of fusimotor fibres innervating muscle spindles in the intercostal muscles of the cat. Nature 1963; 197:1013–1014.

175. Eccles RM, Sears TA, Shealy CN. Intra-cellular recording from respiratory motoneurones of the thoracic spinal cord of the cat. Nature 1962; 193:844–846.

176. Kirkwood PA, Sears TA. Excitatory post-synaptic potentials from single muscle spindle afferents in external intercostal motoneurones of the cat. J Physiol (Lond) 1982; 322:287–314.

177. Kirwood PA, Sears TA. The effects of single afferent impulses on the probability of firing of external intercostal motoneurones in the cat. J Physiol (Lond) 1982; 322: 315–336.

178. Lowe AA. The neural regulation of tongue movements. Prog Neurobiol 1980; 15: 295–344.

179. O'Reilly PM, FitzGerald MJ. Fibre composition of the hypoglossal nerve in the rat. J Anat 1990; 172:227–243.

180. Nazruddin, Suemune S, Shirana Y, Yamauchi K, Shigenaga Y. The cells of origin of the hypoglossal afferent nerves and central projections in the cat. Brain Res 1989; 490:219–235.

181. Lodge D, Duggan AW, Biscoe TJ, Caddy KW. Concerning recurrent collaterals and afferent fibers in the hypoglossal nerve of the rat. Exp Neurol 1973; 41:63–75.

182. Bowman JP. The Muscle Spindle and Neural Control of the Tongue: Implications for Speech. Springfield, IL: Charles C Thomas, 1971:1–160.

183. Law ME. Lingual proprioception in pig, dog and cat. Nature 1954; 174:1107–1108.

184. Zapata P, Torrealba G. Reflex effects evoked by stimulation of hypoglossal afferent fibers. Brain Res 1988; 445:19–29.

185. Morimoto T, Kawamura Y. Inhibitory postsynaptic potentials of hypoglossal motoneurons of the cat. Exp Neurol 1972; 37:188–198.

186. Megirian D. Vestibular control of laryngeal and phrenic motoneurons of cat. Arch Ital Biol 1968; 106:333–342.

187. Biscoe TJ, Sampson SR. Analysis of the inhibition of phrenic motoneurones which occur on stimulation of some cranial nerve afferents. J Physiol (Lond) 1970; 209: 375–393.

188. Miller AJ, Loizzi R. Anatomical and functional differentiation of superior laryngeal nerve fibers affecting swallowing and respiration. Exp Neurol 1974; 42:369–389.

189. Jodkowski JS, Berger AJ. Influences from laryngeal afferents on expiratory bulbospinal neurons and motoneurons. J Appl Physiol 1988; 64:1337–1345.

190. Berger AJ. Respiratory gating of phrenic motoneuron responses to superior laryngeal nerve stimulation. Brain Res 1978; 157:381–384.

191. Bellingham MC, Lipski J, Voss MD. Synaptic inhibition of phrenic motoneurones evoked by stimulation of the superior laryngeal nerve. Brain Res 1989; 486:391–395.

192. Jiang C, Lipski J. Synaptic inputs to medullary respiratory neurons from superior laryngeal afferents in the cat. Brain Res 1992; 584:197–206.

193. Bellingham MC, Lipski J. Morphology and electrophysiology of superior laryngeal nerve afferents and postsynaptic neurons in the medulla oblongata of the cat. Neuroscience 1992; 48:205–216.

194. Berger AJ. Dorsal respiratory group neurons in the medulla of cat: spinal projections, responses to lung inflation and superior laryngeal nerve stimulation. Brain Res 1977; 135:231–254.

195. Sessle BJ, Greenwood F, Lund PJ, Lucier GE. Effects of upper respiratory tract stimuli on respiration and single respiratory neurons in the adult cat. Exp Neurol 1978; 61:245–259.

196. Donnelly DF, Sica AL, Cohen MI, Zhang H. Dorsal medullary inspiratory neurons: effects of superior laryngeal afferent stimulation. Brain Res 1989; 491:243–252.

197. McCrimmon DR, Speck DF, Feldman JL. Role of ventrolateral region of the nucleus of the tractus solitarius in processing respiratory afferent input from vagus and superior laryngeal nerves. Exp Brain Res 1987; 67:449–459.

198. Sumi T. Synaptic potentials of hypoglossal motoneurons and their relation to reflex deglutition. Jpn J Physiol 1969; 19:68–79.

199. Lowe AA. Excitatory and inhibitory inputs to hypoglossal motoneurons and adjacent reticular formation neurons in cats. Exp Neurol 1978; 62:30–47.

200. Takata M. Two types of inhibitory postsynaptic potentials in the hypoglossal motoneurons. Prog Neurobiol 1993; 40:385–411.

201. Duggan AW, Lodge D, Biscoe TJ. The inhibition of hypoglossal motoneurones by impulses in the glossopharyngeal nerve of the rat. Exp Brain Res 1973; 17:261–270.

202. Kerr FW. Structural relation of the trigeminal spinal tract to upper cervical roots and the solitary nucleus in the cat. Exp Neurol 1961; 4:134–148.

203. Porter R. Lingual mechanoreceptors activated by muscle twitch. J Physiol (Lond) 1966; 183:101–111.

204. Yamamoto T. Linguo-hypoglossal reflex: effects of mechanical, thermal and taste stimuli. Brain Res 1975; 92:499–504.

205. Blom S, Skoglund S. Some observations on the control of the tongue muscle. Experientia 1959; 15:12–13.

206. Hunter IW, Porter R. Glossopharyngeal influences on hypoglossal motoneurons in the cat. Brain Res 1974; 74:161–166.

207. Porter R. The synaptic basis of a bilateral lingual-hypoglossal reflex in cats. J Physiol (Lond) 1967; 190:611–627.

208. Porter R. Synaptic potentials in hypoglossal motoneurons. J Physiol (Lond) 1965; 180:209–224.

209. Sumino R, Nakamura Y. Synaptic potentials of hypoglossal motoneurons and a common inhibitory interneuron in the trigemino-hypoglossal reflex. Brain Res 1974; 73:439–454.

210. Morimoto T, Takata M, Kawamura Y. Effect of lingual nerve stimulation on hypoglossal motoneurons. Exp Neurol 1968; 22:174–190.

211. Woodburne RT. A phylogenetic consideration of the primary and secondary centers and connections of the trigeminal complex in a series of vertebrates. J Comp Neurol 1936; 65:403–501.

212. Stewart WA, King RB. Fibre projections from the nucleus caudalis of the spinal trigeminal nucleus. J Comp Neurol 1963; 121:271–286.

213. Borke RC, Nau ME. The ultrastructural morphology and distribution of trigemino-hypoglossal connections labeled with horseradish peroxidase. Brain Res 1987; 422: 235–241.

214. Borke RC, Nau ME, Ringler RL, Jr. Brain stem afferents of hypoglossal neurons of the rat. Brain Res 1983; 269:47–55.

215. Ungolini G, Kuypers HGJM, Simmons A. Retrograde transneuronal transfer of Herpes simplex virus type 1 (HSV 1) from motoneurones. Brain Res 1987; 422: 242–256.

216. Card JP, Rinaman L, Schwaber JS, et al. Neurotropic properties of pseudorabies virus: uptake and transneuronal passage in the rat central nervous system. J Neurosci 1990; 10:1974–1994.

217. Manaker S, Tischler LJ, Bigler TL, Morrison AR. Neurons of the motor trigeminal nucleus project to the hypoglossal nucleus in the rat. Exp Brain Res 1992; 90: 262–270.

218. Hwang J-C., St. John WM, Bartlett D, Jr. Respiratory-related hypoglossal nerve activity: influence of anesthetics. J Appl Physiol Respir Environ Exercise Physiol 1983; 55:785–792.

219. Hwang J-C, Bartlett D, Jr., St. John WM. Characterization of respiratory-modulated activities of hypoglossal motoneurons. J Appl Physiol Respir Environ Exercise Physiol 1983; 55:793–798.

220. Merrill EG. Where are the real respiratory neurons? Fed Proc 1981; 40:2389–2394.

221. Otake K, Sasaki H, Ezure K, Manabe M. Axonal trajectory and terminal distribution of inspiratory neurons of the dorsal respiratory group in the cat's medulla. J Comp Neurol 1989; 286:218–230.

222. Feldman JL. Neurophysiology of breathing in mammals. In: Bloom FE, ed. Handbook of Physiology. Section 1: The Nervous System. Vol IV. Intrinsic Regulatory Systems of the Brain. Bethesda, MD: American Physiological Society, 1986: 463–524.

223. Cohen MI. Neurogenesis of respiratory rhythm in the mammal. Physiol Rev 1979; 59:1105–1173.

224. Baumgarten R, Baumgarten C, Schaefer KP. Beitrag zur Lokalisationsfrage bulbo-reticularer respiratorischer Neurone de Katze. Pflügers Arch 1957; 264:217–227.

225. Mitchell RA, Herbert DA. The effect of carbon dioxide on the membrane potential of medullary respiratory neurons. Brain Res 1974; 75:345–349.

226. Richter DW, Camerer H, Meesmann M, Röhrig N. Studies on the synaptic interconnection between bulbar respiratory neurones of cats. Pflügers Arch 1979; 380: 245–257.

227. Lipski J, Kubin L, Jodkowski JS. Synaptic action of Rβ neurones on phrenic motoneurones studied with spike-triggered averaging. Brain Res 1983; 288: 105–118.

228. Fedorko L, Merrill EG, Lipski J. Two descending medullary inspiratory pathways to phrenic motoneurones. Neurosci Lett 1983; 43:285–291.

229. Monteau R, Khatib M, Hilaire G. Central determination of recruitment order: intracellular study of phrenic motoneurones. Neurosci Lett 1985; 56:341–346.

230. Berger AJ, Averill DB, Cameron WE. Morphology of inspiratory neurons located in the ventrolateral nucleus of the tractus solitarius of the cat. J Comp Neurol 1984; 224:60–70.

231. Fedorko L, Hoskin RW, Duffin J. Projections from inspiratory neurons of the nucleus retroambigualis to phrenic motoneurons in the cat. Exp Neurol 1989; 105:306–310.

232. Onai T, Miura M. Projections of supraspinal structures to the phrenic motor nucleus in cats studied by a horseradish peroxidase microinjection method. J Autonom Nerv Sys 1986; 16:61–77.

233. Yamada H, Ezure K, Manabe M. Efferent projections of inspiratory neurons of the ventral respiratory group. A dual labeling study in the rat. Brain Res 1988; 455: 283–294.

234. Howard BR, Tabatabai M. Localisation of the medullary respiratory neurons in rats by microelectrode recording. J Appl Physiol 1975; 39:812–817.

235. Saether K, Hilaire G, Monteau R. Dorsal and ventral respiratory groups of neurons in the medulla of the rat. Brain Res 1987; 419:87–96.

236. Zheng Y, Barillot JC, Bianchi AL. Patterns of membrane potentials and distributions of the medullary respiratory neurons in the decerebrate rat. Brain Res 1991; 546: 261–270.

237. Schwarzacher SW, Wilhelm Z, Anders K, Richter DW. The medullary respiratory network in the rat. J Physiol (Lond) 1991;435:631–644.

238. Ellenberger HH, Feldman JL. Monosynaptic transmission of respiratory drive to phrenic motoneurons from brainstem bulbospinal neurons in rats. J Comp Neurol 1988; 269:47–57.

239. Ellenberger HH, Feldman JL, Goshgarian HG. Ventral respiratory group projections to phrenic motoneurons: electron microscopic evidence for monosynaptic connections. J Comp Neurol 1990; 302:707–714

240. Rikard-Bell GC, Bystrzycka EK, Nail BS. The identification of brainstem neurones projecting to thoracic respiratory motoneurones in the cat as demonstrated by retrograde transport of HRP. Brain Res Bull 1985; 14:25–37.

241. Duffin J, Lipski J. Monosynaptic excitation of thoracic motoneurones by inspiratory neurones of the nucleus tractus solitarius in the cat. J Physiol (Lond) 1987; 390: 415–432.

242. Merrill EG. Finding a respiratory function for the medullary respiratory neurons. In: Bellairs R, Gray EG, eds. Essays on the Nervous System. Oxford: Clarendon Press, 1974:451–486.

243. Merrill EG. The lateral respiratory neurones of the medulla: their associations with nucleus ambiguus, nucleus retroambigualis, the spinal accessory nucleus and the spinal cord. Brain Res 1970; 24:11–28.

244. Miller AD, Ezure K, Suzuki I. Control of abdominal muscles by brain stem respiratory neurons in the cat. J Neurophysiol 1985; 54:155–167.

245. Dick TE, Berger AJ. Axonal projections of single bulbospinal inspiratory neurons revealed by spike-triggered averaging and antidromic activation. J Neurophysiol 1985; 53:1590–1603.

246. Rikard-Bell GC, Bystrzycka EK, Nail BS. Brainstem projections to the phrenic nucleus: an HRP study in the cat. Brain Res Bull 1984; 12:469–477.

247. Feldman JL, Loewy AD, Speck DF. Projections from the ventral respiratory group to phrenic and intercostal motoneurones in cat: an autoradiographic study. J Neurosci 1985; 5:1993–2000.

248. Sasaki H, Otake K, Mannen H, Ezure K, Manabe M. Morphology of augmenting inspiratory neurons of the ventral respiratory group in the cat. J Comp Neurol 1989; 282:157–168.

249. Ono T. Respiratory neurons in medullary reticular formation which directly project to hypoglossal motoneurons in cats. Kokubyo Gakkai Zasshi 1990; 57:370–384.

250. Dobbins EG, Feldman JL. Organization of the ventrolateral medulla: discrete projections to two respiratory nuclei in neonatal and adult rats. Soc Neurosci Abstr 1992; 18:124.

251. Ezure K. Synaptic connections between medullary respiratory neurons and considerations on the genesis of respiratory rhythm. Prog Neurobiol 1990; 35:429–450.

252. Ezure K, Manabe M. Monosynaptic excitation of medullary inspiratory neurons by bulbospinal inspiratory neurons of the ventral respiratory group in the cat. Exp Brain Res 1989; 74:501–511.

253. Ezure K, Manabe M. Otake K. Excitation and inhibition of medullary inspiratory neurons by two types of burst inspiratory neurons in the cat. Neurosci Lett 1989; 104:303–308.

254. Sasaki S, Uchino H, Imagawa M, Miyake T, Uchino Y. Lower lumbar branching of caudal medullary expiratory neurons of the cat. Brain Res 1991; 553:159–162.

255. Merrill EG. The descending pathways from the lateral respiratory neurones in the cat. J Physiol (Lond) 1971; 218:82–83P.

256. Arita H, Kogo N, Koshiya N. Morphological and physiological properties of caudal medullary expiratory neurons of the cat. Brain Res 1987; 401:258–266.

257. Merrill EG, Fedorko L. Monosynaptic inhibition of phrenic motoneurons: a long descending projection from Bötzinger neurons. J Neurosci 1984; 4:2350–2353.

258. Kirkwood PA, Munson JB, Sears TA, Westgaard RH. Respiratory interneurones in the thoracic spinal cord of the cat. J Physiol (Lond) 1988; 395:161–192.

259. Kirkwood PA, Sears TA. Monosynaptic excitation of thoracic expiratory motoneurones from lateral respiratory neurones in the medulla of the cat. J Physiol (Lond) 1973: 234:87–89P.

260. Lipski J, Merrill EG. Electrophysiological demonstration of the projection from expiratory neurones in rostral medulla to contralateral dorsal respiratory group. Brain Res 1980; 197:521–524.

261. Bianchi AL, Barillot JC. Respiratory neurons in the region of the retrofacial nucleus: pontile, medullary, spinal and vagal projections. Neurosci Lett 1982; 31:277–282.

262. Merrill EG, Lipski J, Kubin L, Fedorko L. Origin of the expiratory inhibition of nucleus tractus solitarius inspiratory neurones. Brain Res 1983; 263:43–50.

263. Fedorko L, Merrill EG. Axonal projections from the rostral expiratory neurones of the Bötzinger complex to medulla and spinal cord in the cat. J Physiol (Lond) 1984; 350:487–496.

264. Otake K, Sasaki H, Mannen H, Ezure K. Morphology of expiratory neurons of the Bötzinger complex: an HRP study in the cat. J Comp Neurol 1987; 258:565–579.

265. Ezure K, Manabe M. Decrementing expiratory neurons of the Bötzinger complex. II. Direct inhibitory synaptic linkage with ventral respiratory group neurons. Exp Brain Res 1988; 72:159–166.

266. Manabe M, Ezure K. Decrementing expiratory neurons of the Bötzinger complex. I. Response to lung inflation and axonal projection. Exp Brain Res 1988; 72:150–158.

267. Otake K, Sasaki H, Ezure K, Manabe M. Axonal projections from Bötzinger expiratory neurons to contralateral ventral and dorsal respiratory groups in the cat. Exp Brain Res 1988; 72:167–177.

268. Mateika JH, Duffin J. The connections from Bötzinger expiratory neurones to upper cervical inspiratory neurones in the cat. Exp Neurol 1989; 104:138–146.

269. Jiang C, Lipski J. Extensive monosynaptic inhibition of ventral respiratory group neurons by augmenting neurons in the Bötzinger complex in the cat. Exp Brain Res 1990; 81:639–648.

270. Bianchi AL, St. John WM. Medullary axonal projections of respiratory neurons of pontile pneumotaxic center. Respir Physiol 1982; 48:357–373.

271. Cohen MI. Switching of the respiratory phases and evoked phrenic responses produced by rostral pontine electrical stimulation. J Physiol (Lond) 1971; 217:133–158.

272. Holstege G, Kuypers HGJM. The anatomy of brainstem pathways to the spinal cord in cat. A labelled amino acid tracing study. Prog Brain Res 1982; 57:145–175.

273. Westlund KN, Coulter JD. Descending projections of the locus coeruleus and sub-coeruleus/medial parabrachial nuclei in monkey: axonal transport studies and dopamine-beta-hydroxylase immunocytochemistry. Brain Res Rev 1980; 2:235–264.

274. Wiberg M, Westman J, Blomqvist A. Somatosensory projection to the mesencephalon: an anatomical study in the monkey. J Comp Neurol 1987; 264:92–117.

275. Baldissera F, Hultborn H, Illert M. Integration in spinal neuronal systems. In: Brooks VB ed. Handbook of Physiology. Section 1: The Nervous System. Vol II. Motor Control, Part 1. Bethesda, MD: American Physiological Society, 1981: 509–595.

276. Aoki M, Mori S, Kawahara K, Watanabe H, Ebata N. Generation of spontaneous respiratory rhythm in high spinal cats. Brain Res 1980; 202:51–63.

277. Hoskin RW, Fedorko L, Duffin J. Projections from upper cervical inspiratory neurons to thoracic and lumbar expiratory motor nuclei in the cat. Exp Neurol 1988; 99:544–555.

278. Douse MA, Duffin J, Brooks D, Fedorko L. Role of upper cervical inspiratory neurons studied by cross-correlation in the cat. Exp Brain Res 1992; 90:153–162.
279. Hoskin RW, Duffin J. Excitation of upper cervical inspiratory neurons by inspiratory neurons of the nucleus retroambigualis in the cat. Exp Neurol 1987; 98:404–417.
280. Hoskin RW, Duffin J. Excitation of upper cervical inspiratory neurons by inspiratory neurons of the nucleus tractus solitarius in the cat. Exp Neurol 1987; 95: 126–141.
281. Duffin J, Hoskin RW. Intracellular recordings from upper cervical inspiratory neurons in the cat. Brain Res 1987; 435:351–354.
282. Keswani NH, Groat RA, Hollinshead WH. Localization of the phrenic nucleus in the spinal cord of the cat. J Anat Soc (India) 1954; 3:82–89.
283. Vascik DA, Maley BE, Holtman JRJ. GABA immunoreactive terminals contact phrenic motoneurons. Soc Neurosci Abstr 1988; 14:936.
284. Baumgarten R, Schmiedt H, Dodich N. Microelectrode studies of phrenic moto-neurones. Ann NY Acad Sci 1963; 109:536–546.
285. Dick TE, Jodkowski JS, Viana F, Berger AJ. Projections and terminations of single respiratory axons in the cervical spinal cord of the cat. Brain Res 1988; 449: 201–212.
286. Bellingham MC, Lipski J. Respiratory interneurons in the C_5 segment of the spinal cord of the cat. Brain Res 1990; 533:141–146.
287. Palisses R, Perségol L, Viala D. Evidence for respiratory interneurones in the C3–C5 cervical spinal cord in the decorticate rabbit. Exp Brain Res 1989; 78:624–632.
288. Cleland CL, Getting PA. Respiratory-modulated and phrenic afferent-driven neurons in the cervical spinal cord (C4–C6) of the fluorocarbon-perfused guinea pig. Exp Brain Res 1993; 93:307–311.
289. Satomi H, Takahashi K, Aoki M, Kasaba T, Kurosawa Y, Otsuki K. Localization of the spinal accessory motoneurons in the cervical cord in connection with the phrenic nucleus: an HRP study in cats. Brain Res 1985; 344:227–230.
290. Bellingham MC. Integration of inhibitory inputs to phrenic motoneurones. Ph.D. thesis, The Australian National University, Canberra, Australia; 1989.
291. Bellingham MC. Intracellular recordings from respiratory interneurons in the C_5 segment of the cat. Proceedings of the International Conference on Modulation of Respiratory Pattern: Peripheral and Central Mechanisms, Lexington, KY, 1990:77.
292. Douse MA, Duffin J. Axonal projections and synaptic connexions of C_5 segment expiratory neurons in the cat. J Physiol (Lond) 1993; 470:431–444.
293. Aminoff MJ, Sears TA. Spinal integration of segmental, cortical and breathing inputs to thoracic respiratory motoneurones. J Physiol (Lond) 1971; 215:537–575.
294. Sumi T. Spinal respiratory neurons and their reaction to stimulation of intercostal nerves. Pflügers Arch 1963; 278:172–180.
295. Sumi T. Organisation of spinal respiratory neurons. Ann NY Acad Sci 1963; 109: 561–570.
296. Cohen F. Responses of single thoracic respiratory neurons to electrical stimulation of suprasegmental respiratory areas. Exp Neurol 1975; 47:199–212.
297. Coffey GL. The distribution of respiratory motoneurones in the thoracic spinal cord of the cat. Ph.D. thesis, University of London, 1972.

298. Johnson IP, Sears TA. Ultrastructure of interneurons within motor nuclei of the thoracic region of the spinal cord of the adult cat. J Anat 1988; 161:171–185

299. Sears TA, Berger AJ, Phillipson EA. Reciprocal tonic activation of inspiratory and expiratory motoneurones by chemical drives. Nature 1982; 299:728–730.

300. Hugelin A. Forebrain and midbrain influence on respiration. In: Cherniack NS, Widdicombe JG, eds. Handbook of Physiology. Section 3: The Respiratory System. Vol II. Control of Breathing, Part 1. Betheseda, MD: American Physiological Society 1986:69–91.

301. Macefield G, Gandevia SC. The cortical drive to human respiratory muscles in the awake state assessed by premotor cerebral potentials. J Physiol (Lond) 1991; 439: 545–558.

302. Colle J, Massion J. Effet de la stimulation du cortex moteur sur l'activité électrique des nerfs phréniques et médians. Arch Int Physiol Biochem 1958; 66:496–514.

303. Plánche D. Effets de la stimulation du cortex cérébral sur l'activite du nerf phrénique. J Physiol (Paris) 1972; 64:31–56.

304. Bassal M, Bianchi AL. Effets de la stimulation des structures nerveuses centrales sur les activités respiratoires efférentes ches le chat. I. Résponses à la stimulation corticale. J Physiol (Paris) 1981; 77:741–757.

305. Bassal M, Bianchi AL, Dussardier M. Effets de la stimulation des structures nerveuses centrales sur l'activité des neurones respiratoires chez le chat. J Physiol (Paris) 1981; 77:779–795.

306. Lipski J, Bektas A, Porter R. Short latency inputs to phrenic motoneurones from the sensorimotor cortex in the cat. Exp Brain Res 1986; 61:280–290.

307. Plánche D, Bianchi AL. Modification de l'activité des neurones respiratoires bulbaires provoquée par stimulation corticale. J Physiol (Paris) 1972; 64:69–76.

308. Rikard-Bell GC, Törk I, Bystrzycka EK. Distribution of corticospinal motor fibres within the cervical spinal cord with special reference to the phrenic nucleus: a WGA-HRP anterograde transport study in the cat. Brain Res 1986; 379:75–83.

309. Rikard-Bell GC, Bystrzycka EK, Nail BS. Cells of origin of corticospinal projections to phrenic and thoracic respiratory motoneurones in the cat as shown by retrograde transport of HRP. Brain Res Bull 1985; 14:39–47.

310. Shinoda Y, Arnold AP, Asanuma H. Spinal branching of corticospinal axóns in the cat. Exp Neurol 1976; 26:215–234.

311. Keizer K, Kuypers HGJM. Distribution of corticospinal neurons with collaterals to lower brain stem reticular formation in cat. Exp Brain Res 1984; 54:107–120.

312. Magni F, Willis WD. Cortical control of brain stem reticular neurons. Arch Ital Biol 1964; 102:418–433.

313. Peterson BW, Anderson ME, Filion M. Responses of ponto-medullary reticular neurons to cortical, tectal and cutaneous stimuli. Exp Brain Res 1974; 21: 19–44.

314. He X, Wu C. Connections between pericruciate cortex and the medullary reticulospinal neurons in cat: an electrophysiological study. Exp Brain Res 1985; 61: 109–116.

315. Verhaardt WJC. A Stereotactic Atlas of the Brain Stem of the Cat. Assen: Van Gorcum, 1964.

316. Sirisko MA, Sessle BJ. Corticobulbar projections and orofacial and muscle afferent inputs of neurons in primate sensorimotor cerebral cortex. Exp Neurol 1983; 82:716–720.

317. Bowman JP, Combs CM. The cerebrocortical projection of hypoglossal afferents in the monkey as revealed by the evoked potential method. Exp Neurol 1969; 23:291–301.

318. Lund JP, Sessle BJ. Oro-facial and jaw muscle afferent projections to neurones in cat frontal cortex. Exp Neurol 1974; 45:314–331.

319. Walberg F. Do motor nuclei of the cranial nerves receive corticofugal fibres? An experimental study in the cat. Brain 1957; 80:597–605.

320. Kuypers HGJM. An anatomical analysis of corticobulbar connections to the pons and lower brain stem in the cat. J Anat 1958; 92:198–218.

321. Porter R. Cortical actions on hypoglossal motoneurons in cats: a proposed role for a common internuncial cell. J Physiol (Lond) 1967; 193:295–308.

322. Viala D, Freton E. Evidence for respiratory and locomotor pattern generators in the rabbit cervico-thoracic cord and for their interactions. Exp Brain Res 1983; 49: 247–256.

323. Viala D, Vidal C, Freton E. Coordinated rhythmic bursting in respiratory and locomotor muscle nerves in the spinal rabbit. Neurosci Lett 1979; 11:155–159.

324. Eldridge FL, Millhorn DE, Waldrop TG. Spinal inhibition of phrenic motoneurones by stimulation of afferents from leg muscles in the cat: blockade by strychnine. J Physiol (Lond) 1987; 389:137–146.

325. Kuypers HGJM. Anatomy of the descending pathways. In: Brooks VB, ed. Handbook of Physiology. Section 1: The Nervous System. Vol II. Motor Control. Bethesda, MD: American Physiological Society, 1981; 597–666.

326. Peterson BW, Pitts NG, Fukushima K, Mackel R. Reticulospinal excitation and inhibition of neck motoneurons. Exp Brain Res 1978; 32:471–489.

327. Búdzinska K, Euler C, Kao FF, Pantaleo T, Yamamoto Y. Effects of graded focal cold block in rostral areas of the medulla. Acta Physiol Scand 1985; 124:329–340.

328. Búdzinska K, Euler C, Kao FF, Pantaleo T, Yamamoto Y. Release of expiratory muscle activity by graded focal cold block in the medulla. Acta Physiol Scand 1985; 124:341–351.

329. Stremel RW, Waldrop TG, Richard CA, Iwamoto GA. Cardiorespiratory responses to stimulation of the nucleus reticularis gigantocellularis. Brain Res Bull 1990; 24:1–6.

330. Travers JB, Norgren R. Afferent projections to the oral motor nuclei in the rat. J Comp Neurol 1983; 220:280–298.

331. Manaker S, Tischler LJ, Morrison AR. Raphespinal and reticulospinal axon collaterals to the hypoglossal nucleus in the rat. J Comp Neurol 1992; 322:68–78.

332. Bassal M, Bianchi AL. Short-term effects of brain electrical stimuli on activities of the efferent respiratory nerves in cats. II. Responses to sub-cortical stimulation. J Physiol (Paris) 1981; 77:759–777.

333. Wilson VJ, Yoshida M, Schor RH. Supraspinal monosynaptic excitation and inhibition of thoracic back motoneurons. Exp Brain Res 1970; 11:282–295.

334. Wilson VJ, Yoshida M. Monosynaptic inhibition of neck motoneurons by the medial vestibular nucleus. Exp Brain Res 1969; 9:365–380.

335. Bassal M, Bianchi AL. Inspiratory onset or termination induced by electrical stimulation of the brain. Respir Physiol 1982; 50:23–40.

336. Anderson ME, Yoshida M, Wilson VJ. Influence of the superior colliculus on cat neck motoneurons. J Neurophysiol 1971; 34:898–907.

337. Iwamoto Y, Sasaki S, Suzuki I. Input-output organization of reticulospinal neurones, with special reference to connexions with dorsal neck motoneurones in the cat. Exp Brain Res 1990; 80:260–276.

338. Udo M, Mano N. Discrimination of different spinal monosynaptic pathways converging onto reticular neurons. J Neurophysiol 1970; 33:227–238.

339. Rose PK, MacDonald J, Abrahams VC. Projections of the tectospinal tract to the upper cervical spinal cord of the cat: a study with the anterograde tracer PHA-L. J Comp Neurol 1991; 314:91–105.

340. Alstermark B, Pinter MJ, Sasaki S. Tectal and tegmental excitation in dorsal neck motoneurones of the cat. J Physiol (Lond) 1992; 454:517–532.

341. Holstege JC, Kuypers HG. Brainstem projections to spinal motoneurons: an update. Neuroscience 1987; 23:809–821.

342. Johansson O, Hökfelt T, Pernow B, et al. Immunohistochemical support for three putative transmitters in one neuron: coexistence of 5-hydroxytryptamine, substance P and thyrotropin releasing hormone-like immunoreactivity in medullary neurons projecting to the spinal cord. Neuroscience 1981; 6:1857–1881.

343. Lalley PM. Serotoninergic and non-serotoninergic responses of phrenic motoneurones to raphe stimulation in the cat. J Physiol (Lond) 1986; 380:373–385.

344. Lalley PM. Responses of phrenic motoneurones of the cat to stimulation of medullary raphe nuclei. J Physiol (Lond) 1986; 380:349–371.

345. Schmid K, Bohmer G, Merkelbach S. Serotonergic control of phrenic motoneuronal activity at the level of the spinal cord of the rabbit. Neurosci Lett 1990; 116:204–209.

346. Mitchell GS, Sloan HE, Jiang C, Miletic V, Hayashi F, Lipski J. 5-Hydroxy-tryptophan (T-HTP) augments spontaneous and evoked phrenic motoneuron discharge in spinalized rats. Neurosci Lett 1992; 141:75–78.

347. Morin D, Monteau R, Hilaire G. Compared effects of serotonin on cervical and hypoglossal inspiratory activities: an in vitro study in the newborn rat. J Physiol (Lond) 1992; 451:605–629.

348. Lindsay AD, Feldman JL. Modulation of respiratory activity of neonatal rat phrenic motoneurones by serotonin. J Physiol (Lond) 1993; 461:213–233.

349. Zhan W, Ellenberger HH, Feldman JL. Monoaminergic and GABAergic terminations in phrenic nucleus of rat identified by immunohistochemical labeling. Neuroscience 1989; 31:105–113.

350. Pilowsky PM, de Castro D, Llewllyn-Smith I, Lipski J, Voss MD. Serotonin immunoreactive boutons make synapses with feline phrenic motoneurons. J Neurosci 1990; 10:1091–1098.

351. Holtman JRJ, Vascik DS, Maley BE. Ultrastructural evidence for serotonin-immunoreactive terminals contacting phrenic motoneurons in the cat. Exp Neurol 1990; 109:269–272.

352. Ellenberger HH, Vera PL, Feldman JL, Holets VR. Multiple putative neuro-messenger inputs to the phrenic nucleus in rat. J Chem Neuroanat 1992; 5:375–382.

353. Bowker RM, Westlund KN, Sullivan MC, Wilber JF, Coulter JD. Descending serotonergic, peptidergic and cholinergic pathways from the raphe nuclei: a multiple transmitter complex. Brain Res 1983; 288:33–48.

354. Holtman JRJ, Norman WP, Gillis RA. Projections from the raphe nuclei to the phrenic motor nucleus in the cat. Neurosci Lett 1984; 44:105–111.

355. Holtman JRJ, Skirbold L, Norman WP, et al. Evidence for 5-hydroxytryptamine, substance P, and thyrotropin-releasing hormone in neurons innervating the phrenic motor nucleus. J Neurosci 1984; 4:1064–1071.

356. Holtman JRJ, Anastasi NC, Norman WP, Dretchen KL. Effect of electrical and chemical stimulation of the raphe obscurus on phrenic nerve activity in the cat. Brain Res 1986; 362:214–220.

357. Holtman JRJ, Dick TE, Berger AJ. Involvement of serotonin in the excitation of phrenic motoneurons evoked by stimulation of the raphe obscurus. J Neurosci 1986; 6:1185–1193.

358. Basbaum AI, Clanton CH, Fields HL. Three bulbospinal pathways from the rostral medulla of cat: an autoradiographic study of pain modulating systems. J Comp Neurol 1978; 178:209–224.

359. Holstege G, Kuypers HG, Dekker JJ. The organization of the bulbar fibre connections to the trigeminal, facial and hypoglossal motor nuclei. II. An autoradiographic tracing study in cat. Brain 1977; 100:264–286.

360. Aldes LD, Chronister RB, Marco LA, Haycock JW, Thibault J. Differential distribution of biogenic amines in the hypoglossal nucleus of the rat. Exp Brain Res 1988; 73:305–314.

361. Aldes LD, Marco LA, Chronister RB. Serotonin-containing axon terminals in the hypoglossal nucleus of the rat. An immuno-electronmicroscopic study. Brain Res Bull 1989; 23:249–256.

362. Jones BE, Moore RY. Catecholamine-containing neurons of the nucleus locus coeruleus in the cat. J Comp Neurol 1974; 157:43–52.

363. Reddy VK, Fung SJ, Zhuo H, Barnes CD. Spinally projecting noradrenegic neurons of the dorsolateral pontine tegmentum: a combined immunocytochemical and retrograde labeling study. Brain Res 1989; 491:144–149.

364. Errchidi S, Hilaire G, Monteau R. Permanent release of noradrenaline modulates respiratory frequency in the newborn rat: an in vitro study. J Physiol (Lond) 1990; 429:497–510.

365. Errchidi S, Monteau R, Hilaire G. Noradrenergic modulation of the medullary respiratory rhythm generator in the newborn rat: an in vitro study. J Physiol (Lond) 1991; 443:477–498.

366. Schmid K, Bömher G, Fallert M. Influence of rubrospinal tract and the adjacent mesencephalic reticular formation on the activity of medullary respiratory neurons and the phrenic nerve discharge in the rabbit. Plüger's Arch 1988; 413:23–31.

367. Eccles JC, Fatt P, Koketsu K. Cholinergic and inhibitory synapses in a pathway from motor-axon collaterals to motoneurones. J Physiol (Lond) 1954; 126:524–562.

368. Gill PK, Kuno M. Properties of phrenic motoneurones. J Physiol (Lond) 1963; 168:258–273.

369. Hilaire G, Khatib M, Monteau R. Spontaneous respiratory activity of phrenic and intercostal Renshaw cells. Neurosci Lett 1983; 43:97–101.

370. Eccles JC, Eccles RM, Iggo A, Ito M. Distribution of recurrent inhibition among motoneurones. J Physiol (Lond) 1961; 159:479–499.

371. Khatib M, Hilaire G, Monteau R. Excitatory interactions between phrenic motoneurons in the cat. Exp Brain Res 1986; 62:273–280.

372. Khatib M, Hilaire G, Monteau R. Excitatory interactions between phrenic motoneurons: intracellular study in the cat. Exp Brain Res 1989; 74:131–138.

373. Hilaire G, Monteau R, Khatib M. Determination of recruitment order of phrenic motoneurons. In: Sieck GC, Gandevia SC, Cameron WE, eds. Respiratory Muscles and Their Neuromotor Control. New York: Alan R Liss, 1987:249–261.

374. Hultborn H, Jankowska E, Lindström S. Relative contribution from different nerves to recurrent depression of IA IPSP in motoneurones. J Physiol (Lond) 1971; 215: 637–664.

375. Otake K, Sasaki H, Ezure K, Manabe M. Medullary projection of nonaugmenting inspiratory neurons of the ventrolateral medulla in the cat. J Comp Neurol 1990; 302:485–499.

376. Mazza E, Nunez-Abades PA, Spielmann JM, Cameron WE. Anatomical and electrotonic coupling in developing genioglossal motoneurons of the rat. Brain Res 1992; 598:127–137.

377. Coombs JS, Eccles JC, Fatt P. The specific ionic conductances and the ionic movements across the motoneuronal membrane that produce the inhibitory postsynaptic potential. J Physiol (Lond) 1955; 130:326–373.

378. Milano S, Miller AD, Grélot L. Multi-phase expiratory inhibition of phrenic motoneurons in the decerebrate cat. Neuroreport 1992; 3:307–310.

379. Barillot JC, Grelot L, Reddad S, Bianchi AL. Discharge patterns of laryngeal motoneurones in the cat: an intracellular study. Brain Res 1990; 509:99–106.

380. Feldman JL, Smith JC, McCrimmon DR, Ellenberger HH, Speck DF. Generation of respiratory pattern in mammals. In: Cohen A, ed. Neural Control of Rhythmic Movements in Vertebrates. New York: Wiley, 1988:73–100.

381. Tuck DL. Investigation of intercostal neuronal intracellular processes and connectivity by signal analysis and computer simulation. Ph.D. thesis, University of London, 1977.

382. Sears TA. The respiratory motoneuron and apneusis. Fed Proc 1977; 36:2412–2420.

383. Sears TA, Stagg D. Short-term synchronization of intercostal motoneurone activity. J Physiol (Lond) 1976; 263:357–381.

384. Jodkowski JS, Viana F, Dick TE, Berger AJ. Electrical properties of phrenic motoneurons in the cat: correlation with inspiratory drive. J Neurophysiol 1987; 58: 105–124.

385. Bayliss DA, Viana F, Kanter RK, Szymeczek-Seay CL, Berger AJ, Millhorn DE. Early postnatal development of thyrotropin-releasing hormone (TRH) expression, TRH receptor binding and TRH responses in neurons of rat brainstem. J Neurosci 1994; 14:821–833.

386. Dick TE, Kon F-J, Berger AJ. Correlation of recruitment order with axonal conduction velocity for supraspinally driven diaphragmatic motor units. J Neurophysiol 1987; 57:245–259.

4

Glutamate, GABA, and Serotonin in Ventilatory Control

DONALD R. McCRIMMON

Northwestern University Medical School
Chicago, Illinois

GORDON S. MITCHELL

University of Wisconsin
Madison, Wisconsin

MICHAEL S. DEKIN

UMDNJ–Robert Wood Johnson Medical
    School
New Brunswick, New Jersey

I. Introduction

Neural network behavior is a function of its composite cellular, synaptic, and network elements (1). Thus, an understanding of any complex neural system, like the respiratory control system, requires an understanding of synaptic transmission: the identity of the chemical transmitters, associated receptors, and the second-messenger systems and ionic conductances that ultimately mediate the response. The characteristics of transmitter actions vary widely in their time course, spatial distribution, and mechanism of action; this heterogeneity is a function of both the neuroactive substance in question and the specific receptor subtypes that are activated by its release.

Numerous transmitter candidates and receptor subtypes have been identified in the central nervous system (CNS) (2). Each transmitter system that has been thoroughly studied mediates a number of different effector processes depending on the conditions of release and the postsynaptic receptors that are present. These fundamental processes include: (1) fast ("classical") synaptic transmission, characterized by rapid time course and ligand-gated ionic channels; (2) neuromodulation, generally characterized by a rather slow time course and ion channel effects that are mediated via second-messenger systems; (3) paracrine or endocrine functions in which the neuroeffector is released, but has a target action located some distance from the point of release; and (4) trophic/tropic influences, whereby neurotransmitters alter the phenotypic expression of the target neurons. Each transmitter may function in one or (simultaneously) in all of these modes. Furthermore, it is now apparent that several transmitters may coexist within the same neuron and be released from the same terminal ending. Thus, it is imperative to consider transmitter actions in the context of other neurochemicals that are operational at the same time.

In its simplest form, synaptic transmission may be regarded as a brief increase in ionic conductances, resulting in fast depolarization or hyperpolarization of the postsynaptic neuron. Such fast, "classic" neurotransmitter actions form the backbone of communication within a neural network, providing "throughput" (3) or sequential processing (2) of neuronal information. However, communication between system elements is not restricted to fast excitatory/inhibitory synaptic transmission. Neural system operation can be modified in a fundamental way by processes of modulation, altering cellular and synaptic properties over a time scale of several orders of magnitude. Modulation imparts a degree of plasticity to the system, potentially altering system function in both qualitative and quantitative terms (1,4,5).

Relatively little is known about the role of neurotransmitters in ventilatory control. Nevertheless, there is a substantial and growing body of literature concerning the roles of certain transmitters in some physiological conditions. Because it is difficult to cover the relevant literature for each of the transmitters that have been partially studied, our objective in this chapter is to provide more in-depth background concerning three specific transmitters with highly varied functions, and to review the literature concerning their roles in the control of breathing. These transmitters include: (1) excitatory amino acids (EAA), especially glutamate, which may be the dominant mediator of excitatory transmission in the CNS; (2) gamma-aminobutyric acid (GABA), a dominant mediator of inhibitory transmission; and (3) serotonin (5-hydroxytryptamine), a monoamine that typifies many important features of neuromodulators. Each of these transmitters is involved in a range of neuroeffector processes and should not be "pigeonholed" as a fast transmitter versus a modulator; nevertheless, it is useful to think about the most common forms of synaptic transmission mediated by each neurochemical.

Our hope is to provide a context in which to view these three important and relatively well-studied transmitter systems and their possible roles in the control of breathing. We do not intend to review the literature in which the effects of various pharmacological agents were studied on eupnic breathing; for this, we refer the reader to other, well-written reviews (6–10). Rather, we will attempt to restrict our attention to current literature concerning mechanisms of glutamate, GABA, and serotonin involvement in the central neural control of breathing. The focus will largely be on brainstem/spinal cord mechanisms since relatively little is known about suprapontine transmitters in ventilatory control.

II. Excitatory Amino Acids

EAAs are generally believed to be the principal mediators of excitatory synaptic transmission in the brain. Within this group, L-glutamate is the dominant candidate as an endogenous neurotransmitter, but other nominees include L-aspartate, L-cysteine sulfinate, L-cysteine, L-homocysteate, and even a dipeptide. N-acetyl-aspartylglutamate (NAAG) (11–16). However, some of these (e.g., homocysteate and cysteine sulfinate) are predominantly localized in glia, and their potential roles as transmitters are controversial (15,17,18). Independent of the identity of the transmitter, they share a mechanism of action mediated by the same groups of postsynaptic receptors. Hence, this review will focus on characterizing the postsynaptic response to activation of putative EAA pathways and a description of the receptors activated. We will begin with a general overview of EAA receptor subtypes and their pharmacology and then examine the suggested roles for EAA in the central neural control of breathing.

Most neurons in the CNS have receptors for, and are powerfully excited by, EAAs (19,20). Several EAA receptor subtypes exist; some open ion channels and mediate fast excitatory transmission, and others activate second-messenger systems to produce short- or long-term changes in response to other inputs. In the control of breathing, glutamate can mediate fast (millisecond) synaptic transmission, as may be employed between neurons within the circuitry generating the basic respiratory rhythm. Slower synaptic events (tens to hundreds of milliseconds or even longer) may allow temporal summation of synaptic inputs, potentially contributing to processes such as the development of the central respiratory drive potential. Thus, the diversity of EAA receptors provides mechanisms that underlie both fast transmission, generating basic respiratory patterns, and modulation of these patterns in both short and long time domains (21,22).

A. EAA Receptors

The characterization of EAA receptors is a fascinating, complex, and burgeoning field. Several gene families encode for multiple subunits of at least four different groups of EAA receptors (for reviews, see Refs. 23–25). Heteromeric combinations of these subunit proteins give rise to receptors that either incorporate ion channels or are linked via G-proteins to a variety of second-messenger systems. The functional variety of receptors appears to be further increased by post-transcriptional editing of subunit mRNA. A result of this extensive molecular heterogeneity is that even the designation of "excitatory" amino acid receptor can be questioned. For example, some of the G-protein-coupled receptors actually reduce excitatory neurotransmission. A further complication to understanding the functional consequences of activity at these synapses is the colocalization of multiple transmitters within a given presynaptic terminal and multiple subtypes of EAA receptor on the same postsynaptic membrane. It is easily recognized that this layered complexity can have a major impact on the computational powers at a single synapse (never mind an entire neural circuit). A major challenge of the future is the understanding of the rules by which the brain "decides" which receptors (and hence which currents) will be made available at which synapses so that its integrative/computational role can be effectively carried out.

At least two broad families of EAA receptors have been identified: iono-tropic receptors (iGluRs), which are ligand-gated, cation-selective ion channels, and metabotropic receptors (mGluRs), which are linked via GTP-binding proteins to several second-messenger systems. Ionotropic receptors consist of three major subgroups, named according to their preferred agonists: (1) α-amino-3-hydroxy-5-methyl-4-isoxazolepropionic acid (AMPA; previously referred to as quisqualate receptors), (2) kainic acid (KA), and (3) N-methyl-D-aspartic acid (NMDA). Antagonists have been identified that allow a clear distinction between NMDA receptors and the other two groups. Antagonists allowing as clear a distinction between the AMPA and KA receptors have not been identified, and these two groups are frequently referred to collectively as non-NMDA (or AMPA/kainate) receptors. Nevertheless, recent advances in the molecular biology of EAA receptors seem to support the existence of three iGluR families (23–25).

AMPA Receptor Properties

Synaptic activation of AMPA receptors gives rise to a large-amplitude, rapidly activated, and rapidly decaying current carried largely by monovalent cations (Na^+ and K^+). Agonists include AMPA, quisqualate, glutamate, and kainate. Competitive antagonists include the quinoxalinedione derivatives 6-cyano-7-nitroquinoxaline-2,3-dione (CNQX) and 6,7-dinitroquinoxaline-2,3-dione (DNQX) and the analog 2,3-dihydroxy-6-nitro-7-sulfamoylbenzo(F)quinoxaline (NBQX) (26,27). NBQX is the most selective of these; unlike CNQX and DNQX, it lacks significant activity at the glycine site (see below) on the NMDA receptor (27,28).

AMPA receptors appear to be pentameric proteins made up of a family of four related subunits designated GluR1 through GluR4 [or GluR-A through GluR-D (29)]. Expression of the cDNA for these subunits in cultured cells produces functional hetero- or homomeric receptors with the selective binding pharmacology of AMPA receptors (29,30). The subunit combinations of physiologically expressed channels are yet to be determined. The rank order of agonist potency for channels formed from these subunits in cultured mammalian cells is AMPA = quisqualate > glutamate > kainate (29).

Molecular biological approaches have revealed several additional aspects of

AMPA receptors. Rapid application of exogenous glutamate activates AMPA receptors and elicits an abruptly rising current, but the receptors rapidly desensitize and the current decays to a new plateau level despite continued agonist application (25,31). The magnitude of this desensitization is controlled by a 38-amino-acid segment for which two sequence versions (termed "flip" and "flop") exist. In the flop form, glutamate-activated currents rapidly decay to a low level, while in the flip form, there is much less decay of the elicited current (32). A differential expression of flip versus flop versions of the receptor has been identified in different regions of the CNS, suggesting selective control over receptor desensitization in different neural regions (25,32). In addition, the relative impermeability of AMPA receptor channels to divalent cations (Ca^{2+}, Mg^{2+}) is dictated by a single amino acid (arginine) in the GluR2 subunit (33,34). Since most native AMPA channels exhibit very low Ca^{2+} conductances, GluR2 appears to be a normal constituent of most AMPA channels. Nevertheless, AMPA receptors with significant Ca^{2+} permeability have been identified (35).

Kainate Receptor Properties

Protein subunits (GluR5–GluR7, KA1, KA2) with high affinity for KA and domoate, but low or negligible affinity for AMPA, have been identified (25). Homomeric expression of GluR5 produces channels with pharmacological properties similar to those of kainate-activated channels in dorsal root ganglion neurons (36), and the CNS distribution of GluR6 corresponds to that of the high-affinity kainate binding (25,37). It seems likely that GluR5–GluR7, KA1, and KA2 are subunits of a high-affinity kainate receptor, but the composition and properties of natural channels with these subunits have not yet been described (25).

NMDA Receptor Properties

NMDA receptor activation elicits a slower-rising, longer-lasting, and lower-amplitude potential when compared with the response to AMPA/kainate receptor activation (38,39). Even though NMDA receptors are present on postsynaptic membranes in several glutaminergic pathways, blockade of these receptors generally has only a minor effect on fast synaptic transmission (39–42). Nevertheless, the prolonged nature of the NMDA-mediated potential may contribute significantly to temporal summation of synaptic inputs or to generation of the central respiratory drive potential in spinal motor neurons (41–44). The long duration of the response to NMDA receptor activation also imparts a relatively long-lasting increase in neuronal excitability, potentially increasing the response evoked by other excitatory inputs (39). Thus, NMDA receptors may play a major role in the computational ability of the CNS. For example, NMDA receptors are necessary for the development of long-term potentiation, a long-lasting enhancement of synaptic efficacy most commonly studied in the hippocampus (45,46). On the other hand, excessive NMDA receptor activation can also lead to neurotoxic effects when glutamate release is excessive, as during brain ischemia (47). Finally, an important role for NMDA receptors occurs during development, when they contribute to the fundamental organization of CNS pathways (48–50).

NMDA channels, like AMPA/KA channels, are permeable to monovalent cations including Na^+ and K^+, but are also permeable to Ca^{2+}. The Ca^{2+} conductance is of particular relevance for synaptic integration (51) and plasticity (49,52). Mg^{2+} also imparts distinct properties to the NMDA channel: in normal physiological concentrations, Mg^{2+} causes a voltage-dependent block of the channel. The block occurs when the charged Mg^{2+} ion is drawn into the channel by the potential gradient across the membrane (39). However, the strongest effects occur near the resting membrane potential and decrease to negligible levels when the membrane is depolarized beyond -30 mV (39,53). In plots of current versus voltage, this voltage-dependent behavior imparts a region of negative slope at potentials more negative than about -30 mV. Thus, as discussed by Mayer et al. (39), activation of NMDA channels requires two conditions: (1) agonist (e.g., glutamate) binding, and (2) postsynaptic depolarization, relieving the Mg^{2+} block. This double control permits NMDA receptors to act as "Hebbian" switches, whereby excitatory input via one set of synapses on a neuron strengthens the response to a second set of synaptic inputs (39). This associative coupling is believed to underlie certain manifestations of associative long-term potentiation in the hippocampus (46,52).

Another novel aspect of NMDA receptors is the requirement for a coagonist, glycine (39). While the normal in vivo concentration of glycine in the extracellular space appears to be adequate for receptor activation, endogenous mechanisms may regulate activity at this site (39). Other extracellular modulators of the NMDA receptor include Zn^{2+} and polyamines such as spermine and spermidine. Endogenous Zn^{2+} may bind to a distinct extracellular site and exert a noncompetitive block of the NMDA receptor during synaptic transmission at some central synapses (54,55). Polyamines may allosterically modulate activity at the glycine site (39,56).

The availability of potent and highly selective antagonists have greatly facilitated investigations of the physiological roles of NMDA receptor activation. Competitive antagonists at the glutamate binding site include 2-amino-5-phosphonovalerate (AP5), 2-amino-7-phosphonoheptanoate (AP7), the conformationally restricted AP7 analog 3-(2-carboxypiperazin-4-yl)propyl-1-phosphonate (CPP), and the piperidine derivative *cis*-4-phosphonomethyl-2-piperidine carboxylate (CGS 19755) (57). Noncompetitive antagonists include Mg^{2+}, as well as the dissociative anesthetic ketamine and related drugs phencyclidine (PCP) and dizocilpine (MK-801), which are believed to bind within the NMDA ion channel (39). Several antagonists interact with the glycine site, including the pyrrolidone derivative 3-amino-1-hydroxy-2-pyrrolidone (HA-966), 5,7-dinitro-quinoxaline-2.3-dione (MNQX), and 7-chlorokynurenic acid (58,59).

Recently, NMDA receptor subunits have been cloned and termed NMDAR1 and NMDAR2A-D (60–63). Homomeric channels formed from NMDAR1 subunits exhibit many of the electrophysiological and pharmacological properties of native NMDA receptors (60). NMDAR2 subunits do not form functional homomeric channels, but in heteromeric combinations with NMDAR1, they enhance the responsiveness of NMDAR1 to NMDA (63). Different heteromeric combinations of NMDAR2A-D with NMDAR1 subunits confer different pharmacological properties to the resultant channels and may form the basis for the pharmacological variability reported for NMDA receptors in different brain regions (63).

Metabotropic Receptor Properties

These receptors form a heterogeneous class, distinguished from ionotropic receptors by their coupling to various second-messenger systems via GTP-binding proteins (64). To date, six members of this class have been cloned and designated mGluR1–6 (64). Depending on the receptor subtype, mGluRs have been linked to increases in phosphoinositide hydrolysis, either increases or decreases in cAMP formation, activation of phospholipase D, and altered conductance through various ion channels (64). Selective activation of mGluRs can be achieved with 1-aminocyclopentane-1,3-dicarboxylic acid (1S,3R-ACPD) (65). Other agonists include quisqualate and ibotenate, but these are also active at iGluRs (64). Activation of mGluR depolarizes many neurons by a variety of mechanisms. For example, 1S,3R-ACPD reduces current through a K^+ channel in neurons in the medial NTS (66), while in spinal dorsal horn neurons it increases calcium mobilization and the magnitude of currents induced by AMPA and NMDA (67). In contrast, 1S,3R-ACPD activates a Ca^{2+}-dependent K^+ conductance that reduces the excitability of cerebellar granule cells (68). Thus, the postsynaptic response can vary between neurons and is dependent on the cellular targets of the particular second-messenger system activated. In this context, the designation of an excitatory amino acid is something of a misnomer since activation of mGluR receptors can have either excitatory or inhibitory effects on the postsynaptic neuron (64). The recent description of two phenylglycine derivatives [(S)-4-carboxyphenylglycine and (RS)-α-methyl-4-carboxyphenylglycine; MCPG] as selective competitive antagonists of 1S,3R-ACPD in rat cortex and thalamus will greatly help with the characterization of the physiological roles of mGluRs (69).

The ability of L-2-amino-4-phosphonobutyrate (AP4) to reduce synaptic transmission by an apparent presynaptic mechanism led to the designation of an additional AP4 receptor type (70,71). However, the AP4 receptor may be synonymous with the mGluR4 receptor. Support for this possibility derives from the observation that AP4 receptors inhibit high-threshold calcium currents via a G-protein-coupled mechanism (72) and that AP4 is a potent agonist at the mGluR4 receptor (73). Regardless of the receptor activated, AP4 effectively inhibits EAA-mediated synaptic excitation within brain regions such as the hippocampus and spinal cord, including inputs to spinal respiratory motoneurons (41,44,74,75).

B. EAAs in the Control of Breathing

Like most other neurons within the CNS, the large majority of respiratory neurons increase their discharge rate in response to EAA application (76–84). A population of unresponsive respiratory neurons within the nucleus tractus solitarius (NTS) of cats has been reported (85), but this has not been confirmed by others. Given the extensive distribution of EAA receptors on respiratory neurons, it is not surprising that activation of these receptors has been implicated in both the generation of the basic respiratory pattern and its reflex modification (42,84, 86–89).

Respiratory Rhythm Generation

Brainstem respiratory neurons receive a significant excitatory synaptic input via activation of both NMDA and AMPA/kainate receptors. A role for mGluRs in respiratory control has yet to be identified. Iontophoretic or pressure application of antagonists for either AMPA/kainate or NMDA receptors to individual respiratory neurons decreased the discharge rate of all ventrolateral medullary neurons tested (82,90). Consistent with this finding, interruption of EAA neurotransmission within the ventrolateral medulla abolishes spontaneous respiratory motor output in anesthetized rats or cats (91–93). Thus, EAA neurotransmission is required for respiratory rhythm generation at least in anesthetized animals.

The relative roles of non-NMDA versus NMDA receptors in respiratory rhythm generation may depend on the preparation studied. In the in vitro neonatal rat brainstem–spinal cord preparation (94), rhythm generation is strongly dependent on activity at medullary non-NMDA receptors (42). In contrast, in vivo studies in both cats and rats indicate that activity at either NMDA or non-NMDA receptors is sufficient for respiratory rhythm generation (92,95).

In the in vitro preparation, respiratory burst frequency is increased by activating medullary non–NMDA receptors either by bath application of selective agonists (AMPA or kainate) or by blocking EAA reuptake in the presence of an NMDA receptor antagonist (42). Conversely, selective blockade of medullary non-NMDA receptors by CNQX causes a concentration-dependent decrease in respiratory burst frequency (42). NMDA receptors, on the other hand, are not likely to be required for respiratory rhythmogenesis in this in vitro preparation since selective NMDA receptor block had no discernible effect on respiratory burst frequency (42), although a slowing of respiratory frequency was found in one preliminary study (96).

The minimal circuitry required for respiratory rhythm generation may be localized within or near a limited region of the ventrolateral medulla termed the pre-Bötzinger complex (97,98) (and see Chapter 2). Injection of a selective non-NMDA receptor antagonist (CNQX) within this region of the in vitro preparation abolishes respiratory motor output (98), confirming that EAA neurotransmission is necessary for the expression of rhythm generation in this preparation. While the precise role of EAAs in generating respiratory rhythm is yet to be determined, possible roles include (but are not restricted to): (1) coordinating the period of excitation within or between subpopulations of neurons within the rhythm-generating network, (2) contributing to the buildup of activity within the network through recurrent excitatory connections, and (3) modulation of the oscillatory changes in membrane potential of neurons with pacemaker or conditional bursting behavior. Conditional bursting neurons develop pacemaker-like oscillatory changes in membrane potential in the presence of a depolarizing input (98). Recent evidence supports a role for neurons with pacemaker (97) or conditional bursting (98) properties in respiratory rhythm generation (see Chapter 2). Smith et al. (98) identified cells within the pre-Bötzinger complex that exhibit conditional bursting behavior. Activation of non-NMDA receptors on these cells could provide the requisite depolarization to elicit bursting behavior. Additionally, a group of respiratory neurons, termed Pre-I neurons, have been described with pacemaker-like behavior and which increase their burst rate during NMDA receptor activation (99). Taken together, these data suggest that EAAs, acting primarily (but not exclusively) via non-NMDA receptors, have an essential but as yet undefined role in respiratory rhythm generation.

In vivo, activation of either non-NMDA or NMDA receptors is adequate for respiratory rhythm generation (92,95). Independent injection of either an NMDA (CPP) or a non-NMDA (CNQX) receptor antagonist directly into a region proximal to the pre-Bötzinger region (recording of neuronal activity was not done and hence the exact relationship to the pre-Bötzinger region is not known) of spontaneously breathing cats elicits only modest changes in respiratory pattern (92). However, combining CPP and CNQX in the same injection markedly reduced tidal volume and resulted in apnea in most cats (92). A similar cooperativity between NMDA and non-NMDA receptor activation sustains respiratory rhythm generation in rats. Blockade of non-NMDA receptors by injections of antagonists within or proximal to the pre-Bötzinger complex of rats increased respiratory rate, but also increased variability of inspiratory timing and burst amplitude (95). However, if NMDA receptors were concomitantly blocked by intravenous dizocilpine (MK-801) or the injection of CPP from the same pipettes, most rats became apneic (95).

There are several possible reasons why non-NMDA receptor activation is required for respiratory rhythmogenesis in vitro but either non-NMDA or NMDA receptor activation is adequate in vivo. Included among these are the developmental differences between the neonatal rats used for in vitro studies compared to the more mature animals used for in vivo studies (100). Alternatively, there are presumably many fewer excitatory synaptic inputs to respiratory neurons in vitro compared to in vivo (100). The isolated brainstem and spinal cord are devoid of inputs from either sensory receptors (other than central chemoreceptors) or descending supramedullary structures. Activity in these ancillary pathways in vivo (many of which presumably utilize non-EAA neurotransmission) could provide a sufficient level of depolarization to remove the voltage-dependent inhibition of NMDA channels and thus provide the excitation necessary for rhythm generation. In contrast, the low level of activity in these non-EAA pathways in vitro may mean that activation of non-NMDA EAA receptors is required to produce the requisite depolarization for NMDA receptor activation.

NMDA Receptors Can Participate in Control of Inspiratory Duration

The timing of inspiratory termination is strongly influenced by sensory inputs, especially those arising from slowly adapting pulmonary stretch receptors (101). In the absence of these inputs, the CNS can still terminate inspiration using circuitry that, at least in anesthetized cats, requires neurons in the parabrachial region of the pons (102). In the absence of either sensory or parabrachial input in anesthetized cats, inspiration is prolonged and apneusis results (103–107). However, some species differences exist since removal of the pontine circuitry reportedly has much less impact on the respiratory pattern of rats (108), although in recent preliminary work, bilateral parabrachial pontine lesions quadrupled inspiratory duration in rats (109).

NMDA receptor blockade (by systemic administration of antagonists) lengthens inspiration in cats, newborn kittens, or monkeys deprived of vagal afferent feedback, similarly to lesions of the pontine parabrachial region (87,88,110–117). The similarity of these responses suggests that a major component of the pontine influence on respiratory control is mediated via NMDA receptor activation. However, the responses are not identical. While pontine lesions lengthen expiratory duration, NMDA receptor blockade has a more variable effect on expiratory duration—lengthening, shortening, and no net effect have all been reported (87,88,110–112,117). At least some of this variability may result from differential influences of the NMDA receptor blockade on the two phases of expiration (early or phase I, and late or phase II, expiration), phase I expiration being shortened, while phase II expiration is lengthened (88). NMDA receptor blockade also prolongs inspiratory duration in rats (100,118), but the effect is less marked than in cats and may even be strain dependent, being much greater in Sprague-Dawley than Wistar rats (100). This decreased sensitivity in rats is consistent with the reduced pontine role in the control of inspiratory duration in this species (108). Thus, NMDA receptor activation may mediate a subset of pontine influences on respiratory control, especially those controlling inspiratory duration, although species differences in the magnitude of these effects do exist.

The similar effects of pontine lesion and NMDA receptor blockade on inspiratory terminating mechanisms suggest the relevant NMDA receptors are on neurons within pontomedullary circuits controlling inspiratory duration. Localization of these receptors to medullary neurons is suggested by the observation that iontophoretic application of NMDA receptor antagonists decreases the discharge rate of all major classifications of medullary respiratory neurons (88,111). However, inspiratory termination elicited by electrical stimulation within the parabrachial pons is not prevented by prior systemic administration of an NMDA receptor antagonist (119), thereby implying the relevant receptors are located at a point prior to the pontine connection with medullary respiratory neurons. A pontine location is consistent with preliminary findings that MK-801 injected directly into the parabrachial pontine region elicits apneusis, mimicking the response to systemic administration of NMDA receptor antagonists (120). Interestingly, a link between pontine NMDA receptors and the intercellular, diffusible messenger nitric oxide is suggested by the observation that injection of a nitric oxide synthase inhibitor into the parabrachial pons also prolongs inspiratory duration when lung inflation is withheld (121). Nitric oxide synthase catalyzes the formation of nitric oxide, and nitric oxide may mediate some of the responses to NMDA receptor activation (122,123). Taken together, these findings are consistent with an obligate role for pontine NMDA receptors in inspiratory termination when lung-volume-related feedback is prevented, although a contribution from medullary NMDA receptors cannot be ruled out.

Since the production of apneusis presumably requires an alteration in the activity of neurons normally controlling inspiratory duration, studies of medullary respiratory neurons have been undertaken following global NMDA receptor blockade to identify neurons that may participate in respiratory rhythm generation. Following intravenous MK-801 administration of the NMDA receptor antagonist dizocilpine (MK-801), there is a prolongation of the discharge period of inspiratory neurons with a decrementing discharge pattern (I-Dec neurons) (87,88). I-Dec neurons begin to discharge coincident with, or slightly before, the onset of phrenic nerve activity. After reaching maximal activity, discharge rate progressively decreases to a low level before inspiratory termination. During NMDA receptor blockade, the rate of decline in discharge frequency of I-Dec neurons is slowed and their discharge period lengthened (87,88). One proposed role for I-Dec neurons is to control inspiratory duration by inhibiting neurons responsible for inspiratory termination (124,125). Thus, prolongation of I-Dec discharge is consistent with causing the lengthened inspiratory period (87,88). Pierrefiche et al. (88) also noted a decrease in the activity of neurons (termed "off-switch" neurons) that discharge briefly at inspiratory termination and neurons that begin discharging immediately after inspiratory termination and then exhibit a decrementing pattern during expiration (E-Dec neurons). However, Feldman et al. (87) did not confirm these changes when comparing neuronal activity between control respiratory cycles and apneustic cycles in which lung inflation was withheld from cats with intact vagi.

Sensory Afferent Transmission

Glutamate or a related EAA has been implicated as a transmitter for primary afferents arising from several sensory systems involved in respiratory control including: baroreceptors (126,127), slowly adapting pulmonary stretch receptors (83,84), peripheral chemoreceptors (89), and superior laryngeal nerve afferent fibers which elicit inspiratory termination during electrical stimulation (128). In addition, activation of EAA receptors within appropriate regions of the NTS elicits swallowing (129,130) or cardiorespiratory responses mimicking activation of pulmonary C-fiber afferents (131).

Glutamate is likely to be a transmitter of at least some cardiopulmonary afferents terminating in the NTS. It is present in high concentrations in the NTS, and levels are reduced following sectioning of the vagus and glossopharyngeal nerves (132). Furthermore, stimulation of the afferent fibers increases glutamate release within the NTS (133–135), and both non-NMDA and NMDA agonists elicit inward currents in isolated NTS neurons (136,137). However, studies on the high-affinity uptake system for glutamate have produced conflicting results. The presence of a high-affinity uptake system is used as an indicator of the presence of glutaminergic nerve terminals (138). Perrone (139) provided biochemical evidence for high-affinity glutamate uptake that was reduced by removing the nodose ganglion. However, decreased uptake following vagotomy could not be confirmed (140,141). In addition, retrograde transport of [^{3}H]D-aspartate from the NTS to nodose and petrosal ganglia, when used as an index of uptake mechanisms in vagal and glossopharyngeal afferents, has produced conflicting results. Sved and Backes (142) found no labeling in the ganglia of 50% of the rats studied, and less than 3% of neurons were labeled in the remaining animals. In contrast, Schaffar et al. (143) reported labeling about 5% of the neurons in the nodose ganglion and interpreted these findings as strong evidence for an EAA transmitter in at least some vagal afferent fibers.

Stronger support for EAA-mediated neurotransmission between primary afferent fibers and NTS neurons is provided by pharmacological studies of synaptic inputs to NTS neurons. Using in vitro NTS slice preparations, primary afferent fibers in the tractus solitarius can be electrically stimulated and the evoked, monosynaptic EPSP recorded in NTS neurons (144–147). Selective blockade of non-NMDA receptors or blockade of NMDA plus non-NMDA receptors markedly reduces or abolishes the presumed monosynaptic EPSP in most neurons within the medial or dorsomedial regions of the NTS (i.e., within areas where many of the cardiopulmonary afferents terminate) (144–147). Selective NMDA receptor blockade also reduced the amplitude of the evoked EPSP, but was much less effective (145). Taken together, the biochemical, neuroanatomical, and pharmacological data support a role for an EAA as a neurotransmitter of primary afferents terminating within the NTS, primarily via non-NMDA receptors.

Two lines of evidence support glutamate as a transmitter of slowly adapting pulmonary stretch receptor afferents. Pulmonary stretch receptor activation elicits the Breuer-Hering expiratory prolonging reflex (i.e., the prolongation of expiratory duration when lung inflation is maintained during the expiratory period). First, the Breuer-Hering reflex can be mimicked by the injection of EAAs into a region of the NTS where stretch receptor afferents are known to terminate (83,84). Second, EAA antagonists both markedly attenuate the Breuer-Hering reflex when injected into the NTS and block the monosynaptic excitation of "pump cells" (148,149) by pulmonary stretch receptor input (84). The reflex appears to be mediated primarily by non-NMDA receptor activation since NMDA receptor blockade by intravenous injection (86,87,115,118) or injection directly into the NTS (84) did not attenuate the reflex. However, in one recent study NTS injections of either NMDA or non-NMDA receptor antagonists blocked the reflex apnea resulting from electrical stimulation of the vagus nerves (150). The reason for this difference is unclear; the method of reflex activation (electrical stimulation in the latter study vs. lung inflation) may be an important consideration (150). Overall, the data are consistent with the hypothesis that slowly adapting pulmonary stretch receptors release an EAA transmitter that acts primarily on non-NMDA receptors, but that NMDA receptors may also participate, perhaps in a modulatory role.

Carotid chemoreceptor afferent processing in the NTS also appears to involve EAA neurotransmission (89). Injection of glutamate or related agonists into a midline region of the commissural NTS that contains terminal arborizations of carotid sinus nerve afferents (151,152) elicits an increase in minute ventilation, mimicking the response to carotid chemoreceptor activation (89). Blockade of either NMDA or non-NMDA receptors within the commissural NTS does not prevent the ventilatory response to carotid chemoreceptor activation (89); however, combined blockade of NMDA and non-NMDA receptors abolished the ventilatory response. Thus, EAA receptor activation within the NTS is required for the ventilatory response to carotid chemoreceptor activation, although the site of EAA neurotransmission could be at the synapse of primary afferent fibers or at a subsequent level of processing within the NTS.

Activation of a variety of sensory inputs elicits time-dependent changes in respiratory motor output. For example, brief activation of carotid chemoreceptors causes a short-term potentiation (afterdischarge) in respiratory motor output that outlasts the period of stimulation for several seconds to minutes (21). Similarly, pulmonary stretch receptor activation causes changes in respiratory pattern that outlast the period of stimulation (153). Recent data suggest that a component of these time-dependent responses may depend on EAA receptor activation. In a preliminary report, England et al. (154) note that NMDA receptor blockage by dizocilpine (MK-801) injections into the NTS reduced short-term potentiation by more than 50%. The cellular basis for this response may be similar to the NMDA receptor-mediated, frequency-dependent potentiation of synaptic transmission in the hippocampus (43). Repetitive activation of the Schaffer collateral input to hippocampal pyramidal neurons elicits a fast EPSP followed by a longer-lasting NMDA receptor-mediated depolarization. The amplitude of the slow component increases as the neuron depolarizes during high-frequency stimulation. The authors interpreted these data as suggesting that the depolarization during high-frequency stimulation reduced the Mg^{2+} block of the NMDA channels, thereby increasing channel conductance (43). A similar response of NTS neurons to repetitive activation of afferent fibers in the tractus solitarius has recently been described (147). Using an in vitro medullary slice preparation, short stimulus trains delivered to afferents in the tractus solitarius increased the magnitude of evoked EPSPs and caused a long-lasting depolarization of NTS neurons. Both the monosynaptic EPSP and an associated increase in spontaneous activity were suppressed by blockade of ionotropic EAA receptors. However, the depolarizing wave was not suppressed (147) and may result from activation of metabotropic glutamate receptors (155) (see below) or the release of another unidentified transmitter such as substance P.

Substance P may influence the Breuer-Hering reflex by a similar mechanism. Injection of small amounts of substance P into the NTS has no direct effect on respiratory motor output; however, the reflex apnea elicited by EAA injection is greatly potentiated by coadministration of substance P (84). The mechanism underlying this interaction has not been addressed, but it is consistent with the slow depolarization of NTS neurons following repetitive stimulation of tractus solitarius afferents (147). It is also consistent with the finding that substance P potentiates a glutamate induced inward current in rat spinal neurons (156). Whether substance P is coreleased with an EAA from primary afferent neurons or it has another source is not clear, but it is localized within the NTS (126,157), and iontophoretic application increases NTS neuron excitability (158). Hence, primary afferent input in several respiratory-related pathways is likely to be mediated via fast transmission at non-NMDA EAA receptors, but the gain of this response is susceptible to modulation by NMDA receptor activation and other transmitter systems, including peptides.

Metabotropic glutamate receptors also influence afferent processing in the NTS (89,155,159). The mGluR agonist 1S,3R-ACPD depolarizes neurons in the medial NTS by closing a K^+ channel, thereby mimicking the long-lasting depolarization in response to repetitive stimulation of the tractus solitarius in the in vitro medullary slice (66,147,155). Metabotropic receptors appear capable of modulating synaptic processing within the NTS in several ways. For example,

1S,3R-ACPD appears to act presynaptically to reduce the fast glutaminergic EPSP elicited by single pulse stimulation of the tractus solitarius, but it also potentiates the postsynaptic response to AMPA. In addition, 1S,3R-ACPD attenuated both the polysynaptic IPSP-associated currents elicited by single pulse stimulation of tractus solitarius stimulation and the current elicited by application of the GABA agonist muscimol (66,155). Thus, mGluR activation can have complex effects on synaptic processing within the NTS, and activation of both mGluR and NMDA receptors may contribute to many of the time-dependent changes in respiration elicited by sustained activation of afferent pathways such as those described by Eldridge and Millhorn (21) and England et al. (154).

Within the NTS, mGluR receptors are located on neurons in baroreceptor and chemoreceptor afferent pathways. Both the carotid chemoreflex-induced increase in minute ventilation and the arterial baroreflex-induced depressor response are mimicked by injection of 1S,3R-ACPD into the appropriate primary afferent terminal regions in rats (89,159). This depressor effect as well as those elicited by NTS injections of the mixed iGluR and mGluR agonists glutamate and quisqualate is not prevented by iGluR blockade (159,160). The recent development of selective mGluR antagonists may provide the key to unraveling the role played by mGluR in afferent processing (69).

Glutamate has also been identified *within* intrinsic NTS neurons (161) and has been suggested as a transmitter both within the NTS (147) and in efferent pathways to the ventrolateral medulla and pontine parabrachial region (162,163). Thus, glutaminergic neurotransmission may be involved both in the processing of respiratory-related sensory input within the NTS and in the transmission of this information to respiratory neurons in other brainstem regions.

In the spinal cord, glutamate and the related acidic amino acid aspartate are concentrated in, and released from, both unmyelinated C-fibers and myelinated dorsal root afferent neurons (164–168). EAA-mediated neurotransmission in spinal afferent pathways is strongly supported by an extensive literature (169). Primary afferent stimulation elicits NMDA- and non-NMDA-mediated EPSPs in motoneurons and dorsal horn neurons (170–173). Primary afferent inputs to spinal respiratory motoneurons also appear to utilize an EAA. The non-NMDA receptor antagonist DNQX markedly reduced or abolished focal synaptic potentials between individual intercostal spindle afferents and second-order interneurons, probably intercostal motoneurons (174). Thus, as in afferent input to other motoneurons, the transmitter of Ia afferent input to respiratory motoneurons is likely to be glutamate (174).

Transmission of Respiratory Drive to Motoneurons

EAA neurotransmission has a central role in communicating respiratory drive to motoneurons. This role of EAAs has been most clearly established in vitro using the neonatal rat brainstem–spinal cord preparation in which phrenic and intercostal motoneurons exhibit phasic inspiratory-related bursts of activity. In this preparation, a partition can be established separating the medium bathing the brainstem from that bathing the spinal motoneurons, allowing independent manipulations of the pharmacological environment surrounding the brainstem versus the spinal cord (175,176). Blockade of spinal EAA uptake in this preparation increases the availability of endogenously released EAA and increases the inspiratory discharge of phrenic nerves both in vivo and in vitro (41,42). Conversely, selective blockade of spinal non-NMDA receptors abolishes phasic respiratory activity on both the phrenic and intercostal motoneurons in vitro (41,42,44). Consistent with these in vitro findings, injection of either NMDA or non-NMDA receptor antagonists into the region of the phrenic motor nucleus of anesthetized rabbits reduced phrenic nerve activity (177), and whole-body blockade of non-NMDA receptors by intravenous administration of GYKI 52466 markedly reduced or abolished respiratory motor output in decerebrate cats (178). This latter effect is likely to have been mediated largely by disruption of bulbospinal input to phrenic motoneurons rather than by disrupting rhythm generation per se since there were minimal changes in respiratory frequency prior to abolition of motor output (178). Nevertheless, spinal NMDA receptors may contribute to descending respiratory drive since NMDA receptor blockade reduces respiratory motor output and the synaptic current recorded from individual phrenic motoneurons (41,42, 44,177). Expiratory bulbospinal neurons also appear to utilize an excitatory amino acid neurotransmitter. Iontophoretic application of a non-NMDA receptor antagonist, DNQX, significantly reduced the focal synaptic potential elicited by single identified bulbospinal expiratory neurons that make monosynaptic excitatory contacts with intercostal motoneurons (174).

Descending respiratory drive to spinal motoneurons also appears to be potently controlled by presynaptic receptors. The compound L-2-amino-4-phosphonobutyric acid (AP4) is believed to activate presynaptic receptors that decrease glutamate release, possibly by activating metabotropic GluR4 receptors (72,73). In the case of spinal respiratory motoneurons, AP4 decreases glutamate release from the in vitro neonatal brainstem–spinal cord preparation (179), and low concentrations abolish spinal respiratory motor output (41,42). In addition, the EPSP magnitude recorded in phrenic motoneurons is reduced, but the postsynaptic depolarization elicited by direct application of exogenous EAA agonists is unaffected (44). Taken together, these data strongly support a presynaptic site of action, but the physiological conditions under which these receptors are activated (e.g., eupnea vs. stimulated breathing) need to be established. Suggested physiological roles for this presynaptic regulation of glutamate release include: (1) the prevention of excessive glutamate release leading to excitotoxic depolarization of the phrenic motoneurons, or (2) an autoregulatory mechanism that establishes an upper limit to phrenic motoneuronal excitation, thereby reducing the maximal level of diaphragmatic motor activity and limiting fatigue (180).

III. GABA

γ-Aminobutyric acid (GABA) is the major inhibitory neurotransmitter in the vertebrate CNS. GABA receptors have been grouped into different classes on the basis of their pharmacology. These classes include $GABA_A$, $GABA_B$, and $GABA_C$ receptors. For $GABA_A$ receptors there appear to be several receptor subtypes (181,182), and this may also be true of $GABA_B$ receptors (183). Both $GABA_A$ and $GABA_C$ receptors are ionotropic, causing direct increases in membrane permeability to Cl^- ions. In contrast, $GABA_B$ receptors are metabotropic and exert their effects via G proteins that subsequently activate (or inhibit) second-messenger systems within the cell. There is compelling evidence for both $GABA_A$ and $GABA_B$ receptors in respiratory neurons. $GABA_C$ receptors have only recently been recognized as a unique receptor class and have been localized exclusively in the retina (184,185). The following discussion, therefore, will be limited to $GABA_A$ and $GABA_B$ receptors.

A. Overview of $GABA_A$ Receptors

The best-characterized receptor class is the ionotropic $GABA_A$ receptor responsible for fast inhibitory synaptic transmission. $GABA_A$ receptors are activated by muscimol and competitively inhibited by bicuculline. Picrotoxin acts as a noncompetitive inhibitor of the $GABA_A$ receptor by blocking its associated Cl^- ionophore. $GABA_A$ receptors are also well known for their interactions with benzodiazepines, barbiturates, and ethanol. Other pharmacological agents such as steroids (186,187) also modify $GABA_A$ receptor activity.

Structurally, $GABA_A$ receptors are hetero-oligomers assembled from four different subunit classes called α, β, γ, and δ (see Refs. 182 and 188 for reviews). This is in contrast to the $GABA_C$ receptor which appears to be a homomeric subunit channel (184). The gene family encoding for $GABA_A$ receptor subunits is large and consists of at least six α's, three β's, three γ's, and one δ in rodents. Recent studies have suggested that the specific "mix" of subunits and/or subunit variants contributing to the $GABA_A$ receptor allows for the expression of functional receptor subtypes in vivo (181,189–192). This hypothesis is exemplified by the differential expression of the γ subunit in different areas of the brain (190,192). The presence of the γ subunit confers benzodiazepine sensitivity to the $GABA_A$ receptor (193–195) and it is the most common $GABA_A$ receptor subtype in the vertebrate brain. Some areas of the CNS such as the thalamus, however, possess $GABA_A$ receptors lacking the γ subunit (196), and they may be insensitive to modulation by benzodiazepines (see Ref. 182). Splice forms of the γ subunit mRNA have also been associated with GABA$_A$ receptor sensitivity toward ethanol. One form, γ2L, contains a phosphorylation site for protein kinase C (190). Ethanol interferes with this phosphorylation site, leading to potentiation of the GABA$_A$ response (197). Another splice form, the γ2S subunit, lacks this phosphorylation site and is not affected by ethanol (197).

Mapping studies of the mRNAs for the γ2L and γ2S subunits have shown that they are also differentially expressed in the brain. For example, the γ2S mRNA predominates in the hippocampus whereas the γ2L mRNA subunit is highly localized in the striatum (190). There are many other examples of how different subunit combinations alter the activity of the GABA$_A$ receptor ionophore. Changes in single channel conductance, channel opening and closing kinetics, and susceptibility to desensitization have all been documented (194,195,198). Based on these studies, it has been suggested that at least four (181) and possibly six (182) GABA$_A$ receptor subtypes exist in vivo. In addition to the regional expression of GABA$_A$ receptor subtypes within the CNS, it has also been proposed that different receptor subtypes may be differentially expressed on individual neurons. For example, single channel studies of GABA$_A$ receptors on neurons often reveal channels with two unit conductances in the range of 15 and 25 pS, respectively (199). The most common interpretation of this observation is that a given GABA$_A$ ionophore displays subconductance states. The observation that the γ subunit increases the single channel conductance of GABA$_A$ receptors, however, has led to speculation that these two conductance states may represent a heterogeneous population of GABA$_A$ receptor subtypes on individual neurons (182). The mechanism(s) underlying the differential expression and localization of GABA$_A$ receptor subtypes remains unclear; however, recent studies have indicated that different subunit combinations carry a unique "sorting" signal that routes them to specific areas of the neuron (200).

Important differences have also been observed in GABA$_A$ receptors during development. In embryonic and early postnatal GABA$_A$ receptors, the "mix" of subunits and subunit variants differs from that in the adult (201,202). In addition, activation of the GABA$_A$ receptor Cl$^-$ ionophore often results in depolarization rather than the expected hyperpolarization of the membrane potential (203). This depolarization is believed to be caused by the presence of an inward Cl$^-$ pump in neonatal neurons that works against the outward Cl$^-$ pump normally found in adult neurons to set E$_{Cl}$ positive to the resting membrane potential (204). Often associated with this depolarization are increases in intracellular [Ca^{2+}] (205). The increases in intracellular [Ca^{2+}] that follow GABA$_A$ activation are thought to exert a trophic effect on the development of inhibitory synapses. In at least one instance, the depolarizing effect of GABA$_A$ receptors has been conserved in adult neurons. Michelson and Wong (206) demonstrated that some inhibitory hippocampal interneurons exhibit depolarization in response to GABA. The significance of conserving this novel $GABA_A$ response in the mature CNS is unknown, but it is interesting that, because these neurons are inhibitory interneurons, the net effect is still to inhibit hippocampal neuronal circuits.

B. Overview of $GABA_B$ Receptors

The $GABA_B$ receptor was first described by Bowery et al. (207) as a modulator of neurotransmitter release. $GABA_B$ receptors are not affected by either muscimol or bicuculline but are activated by the specific agonist ($\pm$)baclofen. Several $GABA_B$ receptor antagonists have also been identified but are limited in their effectiveness (i.e., mM concentrations are needed to elicit an effect). These antagonists include phaclofen (208) and saclofen (209), which are structural analogs of ($\pm$)baclofen. More recently, CGP-35348 [P-(3-aminopropyl)-P-diethoxymethyl-phosphinic acid] has been employed as a specific blocker of $GABA_B$ receptors and appears to be 20–30 times more potent than either saclofen or phaclofen in antagonizing $GABA_B$ responses in vitro (210). The major distinguishing feature of the $GABA_B$ receptor is its coupling to a second-messenger system (see Ref. 211 for review). Consequently, the effects of $GABA_B$ receptor activation are much more diverse than those for the $GABA_A$ ligand-activated Cl^- channel. Most of the actions of $GABA_B$ receptors have been associated with stimulation of guanosine 5'-triphosphate binding proteins (G proteins). These include both the opening of a Ba^{2+}-sensitive inward rectifying K^+ channel (212) and the closing of N-type Ca^{2+} channels (213). In both cases, intracellular injection of the stable GTP analog [guanosine-5'-O-(3-thiotriphosphate); GTPγS] mimics the effects of ($\pm$)baclofen, while pretreatment with pertussis toxin, an uncoupler of G proteins (specifically G_i and G_o) from their receptors, blocks the effects of ($\pm$)baclofen. Other actions of $GABA_B$ receptors have also been observed but have not as yet been associated with stimulation of G proteins. These include both potentiation of A-type K^+ currents by shifting their voltage dependence of activation in the positive direction (214) and the opening of a Ba^{2+}-insensitive outward rectifying K^+ channel (215) similar to the S-type K^+ conductance in *Aplysia* sensory neurons.

Owing to the diversity of ionic conductances coupled to the $GABA_B$ receptor, a number of different inhibitory processes can be affected. The Ba^{2+}-sensitive inward rectifying K^+ conductance activated by $GABA_B$ receptors has been shown to be responsible for a slow IPSP in several types of CNS neurons (216). $GABA_B$ receptors have also been associated with presynaptic inhibition throughout the CNS (207). In contrast to the slow IPSP, however, presynaptic inhibition mediated by $GABA_B$ receptors is insensitive to blockade by Ba^{2+} ions (217,218). Several ionic conductances have been implicated in this $GABA_B$ response. N-type calcium channels, which appear to have a role in neurotransmitter release (213) and have been shown to be inhibited by $GABA_B$ receptors, may participate in presynaptic inhibition. Recently, however, Scanziniani et al. (219) showed that presynaptic $GABA_B$ inhibition in the hippocampus was not necessarily dependent on blockade of Ca^{2+} channels. Saint et al. (214) have suggested that the enhancement of Ba^{2+}-insensitive A-type K^+ currents in presynaptic nerve terminals by $GABA_B$ would reduce excitability and diminish Ca^{2+} entry, thereby producing presynaptic inhibition. The Ba^{2+}-insensitive outward rectifying K^+ current recently described in putative premotor respiratory neurons (215) may also have a role in presynaptic inhibition, since this current would shorten calcium action potentials in the nerve terminal. The model that emerges for the role of $GABA_B$ in presynaptic inhibition is similar to that proposed for the control of neurotransmitter release in *Aplysia* sensory neurons where the neuropeptide FMRFamide simultaneously opens S-type K^+ channels and inhibits Ca^{2+} channels, resulting in an overall decrease in neurotransmitter release.

The various ionic conductances coupled to the $GABA_B$ receptor could also impact on how neurons sculpt their patterns of repetitive spike discharge. Decreases in input resistance (via activation of an outward rectifying K^+ conductance) could enhance spike frequency adaptation whereas inhibition of voltage-dependent conductances (i.e., Ca^{2+} and A-currents) could change the shape of the action potential and its undershoot. Since $GABA_B$-mediated effects such as these do not desensitize (214,215), it is tempting to speculate that GABA may exert a tonic modulation of neuronal membrane properties. Consistent with this hypothesis, it has recently been suggested that GABAergic interneurons, acting through the $GABA_B$ receptor, exert tonic presynaptic inhibition of mechanical afferents in the spinal cord (220).

An important consequence of the metabotropic actions of $GABA_B$ receptors is that it allows for "cross-talk" with other neurotransmitter systems. For example, the slow IPSP produced by serotonin (via IA receptors; $5\text{-}HT_{1A}$) in dorsal raphe neurons is identical to that produced by activation of $GABA_B$ receptors (221). The slow IPSPs produced by $5\text{-}HT_{1A}$ and $GABA_B$ receptors share the same Ba^{2+}-sensitive inward rectifying K^+ conductance, can be mimicked by intracellular injection of $GTP\gamma s$, and are inhibited by activation of protein kinase C (PKC). In addition, activation of the inward rectifying K^+ conductance by one transmitter occluded its activation by the other. Similar observations have been made for the slow IPSPs mediated by $5\text{-}HT_{1A}$ and $GABA_B$ receptors in hippocampal neurons (212). In substantia nigra neurons, $GABA_B$ and dopamine (acting at the D_2 receptor subtype) also activate a common G-protein-coupled Ba^{2+}-sensitive K^+ conductance (222). Similar cross-talk has been observed for the G-protein-mediated inhibition of Ca^{2+} currents by $GABA_B$ and adenosine (acting at the A_1 receptor subtype) on cultured sensory neurons from rat dorsal root ganglia (213). There is also evidence that different neurotransmitters antagonize $GABA_B$ actions. In cultured bulbospinal neurons from neonatal rats, the Ba^{2+}-insensitive outward rectifying K^+ conductance activated by ($\pm$)baclofen is shut down by thyrotropin-releasing hormone (TRH), which phosphorylates the channel via PKC (223,224). These observations suggest that neurotransmitter inputs from different CNS regions can converge on a single transduction mechanism, thereby providing a mechanism for "fine tuning" the activity of a neuron.

C. GABAergic Innervation of Respiratory Neurons

There is anatomical evidence for GABAergic inputs to major respiratory-related structures of the brainstem and spinal cord. In the phrenic motor nucleus, GABA immunoreactive boutons are observed in close apposition to both phrenic motoneuron cell bodies and dendrites (225). GABAergic innervation of the dorsal respiratory group (DRG) (102) has also been demonstrated (226,227). Within the ventral respiratory group (VRG) (102), GABAergic innervation has been inferred from a combination of observations, including: the presence of GABA-mediated inhibitory inputs to VRG neurons (228–230) and the presence of inhibitory connections arising from neurons in the region of the retrofacial nucleus (Bötzinger complex) (231–233), which contains GABAergic neurons (233,234). GABA immunoreactive boutons are also observed on presynaptic nerve terminals in both the phrenic motor nucleus and the DRG (225,227).

There are many potential sources for these GABAergic inputs since GABA-containing neurons are widely distributed throughout the CNS. In particular, GABAergic neurons are observed in the immediate vicinity of the DRG (236,237) and VRG (234,235) but their connections with other respiratory neurons are not known. The only identified GABAergic input to respiratory neurons derives from the retrofacial nucleus (RN; Bötzinger complex). Monosynaptic connections have been demonstrated from GABAergic RN neurons to DRG inspiratory neurons (226,231). A monosynaptic inhibitory connection has also been demonstrated from the RN to phrenic motoneurons (231,238).

GABAergic inputs from other brainstem respiratory areas may also exist. GABAergic cell bodies have been identified in the raphe nuclei (239), the parabrachial nucleus (240), and the nucleus ambiguus (234,235). These nuclei have extensive synaptic connections within the DRG and VRG, as well as bulbospinal projections to the phrenic motor nucleus. Although our knowledge of the source(s) of GABAergic input to respiratory neurons is limited, it is clear that GABA is a ubiquitous inhibitory neurotransmitter within the respiratory circuitry.

D. GABA$_A$ Receptors in Respiratory Control

Many studies have demonstrated a physiological role for GABA$_A$ receptors in the regulation of breathing. The central administration of GABA in eupnic animals causes respiratory depression (241–244), and these effects are mimicked by the GABA$_A$ agonist THIP (4,5,6,7-tetrahydroisoxazolo[5,4-c]pyridin-3-ol) (241).

The primary effect of $GABA_A$ receptor activation is to decrease phrenic nerve amplitude and tidal volume (241). However, in a recent study employing a perfused brainstem–spinal cord preparation from adult rats, activation of $GABA_A$ receptors depressed both respiratory frequency and phrenic nerve amplitude (245). Respiratory depression is also observed during the accumulation of endogenous GABA caused by treatment with aminooxoacetic acid, a GABA transaminase inhibitor (245,246). Studies employing $GABA_A$ antagonists such as bicuculline suggest that these receptors may exert a tonic depression of the respiratory circuit. Subseizure doses of bicuculline cause small, but consistent, increases in respiratory output (243–245,247). More dramatic effects on respiratory output are observed in hypoxic animals, where administration of bicuculline reverses the depression of respiration (247).

Studies employing intracellular recordings from respiratory neurons have provided insight into the role of inhibitory synaptic connections mediated by these $GABA_A$ receptors. Periodic synaptic inhibition mediated by fast IPSPs is observed in both inspiratory and expiratory premotor respiratory neurons of the DRG and VRG (248–251). In all cases, this synaptic inhibition is associated with an increase in membrane permeability to Cl^- ions and activation of $GABA_A$ receptors (81,228,229,252,253). $GABA_A$ receptors, however, are not the only Cl^- ionophore mediating fast synaptic inhibition in the respiratory circuit. The other major class of ligand-gated Cl^- ionophore in vertebrates, glycine receptors, has also been shown to depress brainstem respiratory neurons in the DRG and VRG (228,253,254). In contrast, periodic synaptic inhibition of phrenic motoneurons appears to be exclusively mediated by $GABA_A$ receptors (255).

Champagnat et al. (228) suggested that fast IPSPs mediated by $GABA_A$ and glycine receptors are spatially segregated in brainstem respiratory neurons. In inspiratory neurons, glycine-sensitive IPSPs are preferentially located on the soma and are responsible for rapid inhibition at the beginning of expiration. In contrast, $GABA_A$-mediated IPSPs are primarily located on distal dendrites and serve to maintain synaptic inhibition throughout the expiratory phase. The spatial segregation of "early" and "late" expiratory phase inhibition is consistent with electrophysiological recordings, where it was shown that reversal of late expiratory phase inhibition by intracellular Cl^- injection into the soma was associated with a long diffusion time (251).

Haji et al. (253,254) also observed that periodic synaptic inhibition in inspiratory and postinspiratory VRG neurons was mediated by both $GABA_A$ and glycine receptors. Their observations, however, differed from Champagnat et al. (228) in two important respects. First, they did not see a selective effect of glycine during stage I (i.e., early) expiration. Moreover, GABA exerted a tonic effect on membrane potential throughout the entire respiratory cycle, in addition to periodic synaptic inhibition (see Refs. 81 and 254). This latter action of GABA is consistent with animal studies using systemic injection or topical application of GABA analogs where a small tonic $GABA_A$ effect is observed (243–245,247) and electrophysiological studies of respiratory neurons in which Cl^- injection leads to a steady membrane potential depolarization spanning all phases of the respiratory cycle (251). One caveat with respect to a tonic $GABA_A$ input to respiratory neurons is that most $GABA_A$ responses exhibit pronounced desensitization during prolonged agonist exposure. However, there are isoforms of the $GABA_A$ receptor that do not desensitize. One can speculate that periodic inhibition is mediated by the desensitizing/benzodiazepine-sensitive $GABA_A$ receptor subtype whereas tonic control of membrane potential results from a different nondesensitizing $GABA_A$ receptor subtype.

Most contemporary models of the central respiratory circuitry recognize the importance of fast inhibitory synaptic connections. Periodic inhibition caused by fast IPSPs could contribute to *respiratory timing* by mediating phase termination and/or *burst pattern formation* via reciprocal inhibition between antagonists. In vivo studies in adult cats have demonstrated patterns of IPSPs consistent with both functions (248–251). More recently, Hayashi and Lipski (245) used a perfused brainstem preparation from adult rats to show that blockade of Cl^--dependent IPSPs completely suppressed respiratory rhythm generation. These observations are the opposite of those obtained in neonatal rats (176,180) (see also discussion in Ref. 98 and Chapter 2, this volume). In Cl^--free media or in the presence of $GABA_A$ and glycine receptor antagonists, the amplitude and duration of phrenic nerve burst activity are altered but respiratory timing is not affected. Although these data may reflect the removal of afferent input in the in vitro preparation, they may also be the result of developmental changes in which the contribution of fast IPSPs to the respiratory circuit is limited to burst pattern formation at this early developmental stage. Thus, these data highlight potential differences between respiratory rhythmogenesis in neonates and adults (see discussion in Refs. 125 and 245).

E. $GABA_B$ Receptors in Respiratory Control

The effects of the $GABA_B$ agonist ($\pm$)baclofen on rhythmic breathing movements are dependent on both dose and the route of administration. In cats, intravenous injections of low doses (<2 mg/kg) of ($\pm$)baclofen increase the activity of phrenic motoneurons (256), intercostal motoneurons (257), and both DRG and VRG respiratory neurons (230,258). Neither inspiratory (T_I) nor expiratory (T_E) timing is affected. Higher intravenous doses (>4 mg/kg) of ($\pm$)baclofen, as well as direct iontophoretic application of the drug, have the opposite effects on these neurons, leading to a decrease in respiratory activity (230,256,258). In addition, T_I is lengthened (256,258), leading to an overall decrease in respiratory rate. The combination of decreased phrenic nerve activity and respiratory rate leads to a profound depression of respiratory output. These results were obtained in ventilated animals where CO_2 was maintained constant. In spontaneously breathing cats, high doses of ($\pm$)baclofen caused an increase in tidal volume (241). Pierrefiche et al. (230) speculated that since ($\pm$)baclofen does not suppress chemosensory inputs (241), the increase in tidal volume may have been an indirect effect of raised CO_2 levels that masked the depression of phrenic nerve amplitude. Interestingly, the apneustic effect of ($\pm$)baclofen mimics that observed during application of the NMDA blocker dizocilpine (88). Thus, an important action of ($\pm$)baclofen may be the inhibition of glutamate release, which, in turn, depresses the inspiratory off-switch, leading to an increase in T_I.

There appear to be species differences with regard to ($\pm$)baclofen effects since a reduction in respiratory output is accomplished primarily through a reduction in phrenic nerve amplitude in rabbits (259) and rats (260). In the rabbit, high doses of ($\pm$)baclofen actually decreased T_I slightly, but this effect was paralleled by a similar increase in T_E, leading to no change in respiratory rate. Finally, in neonatal rats, ($\pm$)baclofen decreases respiratory frequency primarily through an increase in T_E alone (180), suggesting developmental differences may also be important.

Pharmacological studies with ($\pm$)baclofen have provided insight into connections between neurons within the respiratory circuit. In the cat, inverse effects on neuronal activity were observed in VRG expiratory neurons during intravenous administration of low versus high ($\pm$)baclofen doses. At low doses, VRG expiratory neurons were depressed while high doses caused them to fire tonically. Lalley (258) hypothesized that these effects reflected synaptic interactions with brainstem inspiratory neurons. At the low dose, inspiratory neurons were excited, thus inhibiting expiratory neurons; at the high dose, inspiratory neurons were themselves inhibited, thereby releasing expiratory neurons from inhibition and allowing them to fire continuously. Further support that circuit interactions are responsible for the effects of ($\pm$)baclofen on VRG expiratory neurons comes from the more recent study by Pierrefiche et al. (230) that showed that iontophoretic application of this drug directly onto expiratory neurons (comparable to a high systemic dose) causes only inhibition.

The excitatory effects of low ($\pm$)baclofen doses on respiratory neurons are accompanied by membrane potential depolarization and decreased conductance (256). These effects have been explained by disinhibition of a tonic inhibitory synaptic input such as that potentially mediated by $GABA_A$ receptors (243–245,247,253). Such disinhibition is most likely accomplished via presynaptic inhibition and demonstrates the potential for modulation of synaptic connections within the respiratory circuit. The inhibitory effects of high ($\pm$)baclofen doses are more complex. Part of this inhibition has been attributed to presynaptic inhibition of an excitatory neurotransmitter input (i.e., disfacilitation) because it is associated with both a conductance decrease and membrane hyperpolarization. Indeed, it has been suggested that $GABA_B$ receptors mediate presynaptic inhibition of glutamate release (230), which affects respiratory timing via NMDA receptors and phrenic nerve amplitude through non-NMDA receptors (41,42,86,178). The apparent dose dependence of ($\pm$)baclofen's ability to inhibit the release of inhibitory versus excitatory neurotransmitters is supported by direct observations in neurons of the NTS where IPSPs were more sensitive to $GABA_B$-mediated presynaptic inhibition than were EPSPs (261). In another report, Sun et al. (262) tested the ability of ($\pm$)baclofen and TRH to regulate neurotransmitter release in the phrenic motor nucleus of neonatal rats. As mentioned above, TRH closes a Ba^{2+}-insensitive outward rectifying K^+ channel activated by ($\pm$)baclofen. ($\pm$)Baclofen alone depressed an evoked non-NMDA-sensitive EPSP without altering the postsynaptic input resistance of phrenic motoneurons. TRH enhanced the evoked EPSP, again without any discernible effect on postsynaptic membrane properties. These drugs also cross-reacted; that is, ($\pm$)baclofen antagonized the facilitatory effects of TRH, and TRH antagonized the inhibitory effects of ($\pm$)baclofen. These data suggest that ($\pm$)baclofen and TRH mediated presynaptic inhibition and facilitation, respectively, and that they did so by modulating a common set of ionic conductances such as the Ba^{2+}-insensitive K^+ channel and/or Ca^{2+} channels.

The role of a direct effect of high ($\pm$)baclofen doses on respiratory neurons is less clear. Although $GABA_B$ receptor activation in many parts of the CNS is associated with a G-protein-dependent, Ba^{2+}-sensitive inward rectifying K^+ channel that gives rise to a slow IPSP, such IPSPs do not appear to be prevalent in areas containing respiratory neurons (261). It is possible, however, that ($\pm$)baclofen could modulate membrane excitability through a variety of other mechanisms. A Ba^{2+}-insensitive, outward rectifying K^+ channel activated by ($\pm$)baclofen has been described in the postsynaptic membrane of both DRG and VRG neurons and would lead to a decrease in action potential firing (215). Also, $GABA_B$ receptors are known to inhibit calcium channels (213), which are also present in these cells (264,265). Finally, many DRG and VRG neurons possess an A-type K^+ current (263–265) that, in hippocampal neurons, is enhanced by $GABA_B$ receptor activation (214). The interactions between ($\pm$)baclofen and these ionic conductances would all lead to a loss of membrane excitability. Nevertheless, receptor binding studies suggest that there is a relative paucity of postsynaptic $GABA_B$ receptors in respiratory areas such as the NTS, where presynaptic $GABA_B$ receptors are found in abundance (see discussion in Ref. 261). Along with the dose-dependent effects of ($\pm$)baclofen, such data support the hypothesis that the primary function of endogenously active $GABA_B$ receptors in the respiratory circuit is to regulate neurotransmitter release.

IV. 5-Hydroxytryptamine (Serotonin)

Serotonin is a neuroactive substance with interesting anatomical and physiological characteristics that in most respects typify important features of monoaminergic systems in general (e.g., norepinephrine and dopamine) (266). The serotonergic nervous system is characterized by discrete neuronal aggregates, the raphe nuclei of the brainstem, with highly divergent axonal arborizations projecting to virtually all regions of the CNS. Axons from serotonergic neurons terminate in both traditional (classical) synaptic specializations and nonsynaptic terminals that appear to function via "volume transmission" (267) or "nonsynaptic diffusion neurotransmission" (268). Specific actions on the postsynaptic site are determined by a range of receptor subtypes that act via ligand-gated ion channels or, indirectly, via second-messenger systems that open or close ion channels (269–271).

Other neuroactive substances (thyrotropin-releasing hormone, substance P, enkephalins, GABA) frequently coexist in the same neurons as serotonin. This neuronal system in fact provided one of the first examples of coexisting transmitters within a single neuron (3,272). Although the functional significance of this transmitter diversity remains obscure, it may contribute in important ways to the development and maintenance of proper system function.

The serotonergic nervous system exhibits considerable plasticity (273,274), and in turn, this system is sometimes thought to promote plasticity in other neuronal structures, acting as a trophic or tropic influence (275–277). Recent theories concerning the function of the raphe serotonergic system suggest that it may be critical in facilitating automatic rhythmic motor behaviors (274,278). Both sensory integration and motor output, including those involved in breathing, are modulated in this scheme (279). There are essential gaps in our understanding of the serotonergic nervous system and its role in respiratory motor control, yet sufficient information has emerged to formulate hypotheses concerning its basic functions in certain physiological conditions.

A. Control of Brain Serotonin Concentrations

Since the synthesis and degradation of serotonin are affected by a number of factors relevant to ventilatory control (e.g., Po_2, Pco_2, pH), we will briefly review the biochemistry of serotonin. The biosynthetic pathway of serotonin involves hydroxylation of the essential amino acid tryptophan to form 5-hydroxytryptophan, followed by decarboxylation to 5-hydroxytryptamine or serotonin (266). This synthetic pathway is tightly controlled by the activity of the rate-limiting enzyme, tryptophan hydroxylase (280). Tryptophan hydroxylase has an absolute requirement for molecular oxygen and for a reduced pteridine cofactor. Since the K_m values of tryptophan hydroxylase for tryptophan and oxygen and its pH optimum (7.2) are within observed physiological ranges, there is considerable potential to modify the biosynthesis of serotonin at this synthetic step. Under normal physiological circumstances, tryptophan hydroxylase is only half-saturated (281,282); thus, changes in tryptophan levels trigger changes in serotonin synthesis and metabolism. Indeed, changes in dietary tryptophan intake alter breathing (283).

Since the hydroxylation rate of tryptophan is directly dependent on molecular oxygen, serotonin levels fall during altitude exposure (284). However, because transmitter synthesis, storage, release, and response are dynamic processes under rigorous control, acute imbalances are often met with compensatory reactions, reestablishing normal function by increasing enzyme synthesis, up-regulating postsynaptic receptor densities, and so forth. Thus, it is found that brain serotonin concentration, after an initial decrease, returns toward (and actually exceeds) normal levels in rats exposed to hypoxia for 1 week (285). The rate of serotonin formation can also be increased by exposing rats to 100% oxygen (266), although this observation may not be reflected in serotonin release and utilization. Changes in pH and carbon dioxide tension also impact on 5-HT biosynthesis (285); the significance of these changes depends on the experimental paradigm being investigated (286).

Increased levels of brain tryptophan and increased serotonin synthesis have been observed during acute exercise (287) or following chronic endurance exercise in rats (288). Although increased brain serotonin concentrations do not necessarily lead to increased serotonin release and utilization, there is suggestive evidence that this is the case based on measurements of extracellular serotonin levels in the spinal ventral horn of exercising rats (289). Thus, serotonin may be important in regulating locomotor or respiratory motoneuron activity during exercise (279,290).

Stressful situations predispose to increased serotonin biosynthesis and turnover. For example, activation of the sympathetic nervous system increases brain tryptophan levels (via catecholaminergic effects). There are also important influences on the serotonergic nervous system mediated by glucocorticoids, sex hormones, and mineralocorticoids (291,292). Hormone-mediated changes in the serotonergic nervous system may play an important role in the plasticity of the ventilatory control system and its physiological responses to stress. This issue is of relevance to studies on serotonergic involvement in ventilatory control since many of these hormonal effects are sequelae to the experimental protocol used.

B. Anatomy of the Serotonergic Nervous System

Serotonin-containing cell bodies are mainly located in the brainstem, in discrete clusters along the midline of most mammalian species (274,293,294). These 5-HT clusters can be divided into superior (rostral) and inferior (caudal) groups. The superior group consists mainly of the caudal linear nucleus, the median raphe nucleus, neurons lying just lateral to the medial lemniscus, and the dorsal raphe nucleus. The superior group projects largely in a rostral direction, providing serotonergic input to forebrain structures. Although they are commonly regarded as diffuse and nonspecific in their projection patterns, it has become clear that these ascending axonal projections exhibit an intricate and orderly pattern (295,296). The inferior group consists of the nucleus raphe obscurus, raphe pallidus, raphe magnus, neurons in the ventrolateral medulla, the intermediate reticular nuclei, and the area postrema. The nuclei of the inferior group provide the major serotonergic innervation of the spinal cord and medulla. These descending projections exhibit a high degree of topographical arrangement (274,294,297). Fibers arising in the nucleus raphe magnus provide a dense serotonergic innervation in the superficial layers of the spinal dorsal horn; these serotonergic inputs are likely to be involved in modulating sensory processing, including pain. Recent evidence suggests that 60% of the serotonergic varicosities in the spinal dorsal horn do not form synaptic specializations (298,299), suggesting that serotonergic influences in this region occur via "volume transmission" or "nonsynaptic diffusion neurotransmission." Serotonergic innervation of the ventral horn largely arises from nucleus raphe pallidus or raphe obscurus (274,294,297). These fibers course throughout the ventrolateral or ventral funiculi and commonly form synaptic contacts with motoneurons (268). Many descending serotonergic fibers extend through the entire spinal cord, suggesting that they transmit information to postsynaptic sites at numerous segmental levels; this property may be of significance in coordinating complex physiological behaviors such as breathing (274).

Serotonergic neurons project to many regions of the CNS and innervate a number of structures of importance in ventilatory control. Serotonergic fibers arborize and terminate directly on or near medullary respiratory neurons of the dorsal (300) and ventral (301) respiratory groups and respiratory motoneurons, including: phrenic (225,302–304), intercostal (305), laryngeal (306,307), and hypoglossal (308,309) motoneurons. Serotonin immunoreactive varicosities form at least some synaptic specializations on phrenic motoneurons (302,310). Close appositions between immunoreactive varicosities and identified phrenic motoneurons are most dense in the region of the distal dendrites (302), suggesting that serotonergic influences on these motoneurons may affect primarily nonserotonergic synaptic inputs to the same dendritic arborization, allowing graded effects on the transmission of postsynaptic potentials to the soma (311,312).

The density of immunoreactive serotonergic varicosities appears to be heterogeneous among the various respiratory neurons studied to date. For example, serotonergic labeling in the vicinity of hypoglossal motoneurons, filled intracellularly with horseradish peroxidase, appears to be less dense (309) than labeling near similarly filled phrenic motoneurons (302). There also appears to be a greater density of serotonergic terminals near retrogradely labeled nucleus ambiguus (307) and inspiratory intercostal (305) motoneurons relative to phrenic motoneurons (225,303,304). The density and distribution of serotonergic contacts with DRG neurons can be characterized as lower and more diffuse than near phrenic motoneurons studied with the same techniques (300,302,313). The significance of this apparent heterogeneity in the density and distribution of serotonergic contacts with respiratory neurons is not clear, but it may impart a degree of functional differentiation among common targets of the same serotonergic axonal projection. This interesting possibility warrants further study.

It is important to know the degree of specificity in projections from raphe nuclei to respiratory neural structures: Do different populations of serotonergic raphe neurons (even within the same raphe nucleus) innervate different respiratory neuron types? Differential sensitivity of raphe serotonergic neurons to treatment with the tryptophan hydroxylase inhibitor para-chlorophenylalanine suggests at least two functionally distinct classes of serotonergic neurons with different projection patterns (314–316). Para-chlorophenylalanine-insensitive neurons project to CNS regions of interest in ventilatory control such as cranial motor and parasympathetic nuclei. In addition, populations of serotonergic neurons can be distinguished by the coexistence of neuropeptides (317). Serotonin colocalizes with TRH but not substance P in nerve terminals innervating spinal parasympathetic preganglionic motoneurons, with both TRH and substance P in terminals innervating somatic motoneurons, and with neither TRH nor substance P in terminals in the dorsal horn (317). Thus, the raphe-spinal serotonergic system may differentially modulate the excitability of these distinct spinal neuronal targets.

Serotonin may be of significance at other, less traditional locations in the respiratory control system. For example, Das and colleagues (318) reported that serotonin is present in the motor end-plates of the phrenic nerve-diaphragm; they suggest that it may play a modulatory role in acetylcholine release and, therefore, in neuromuscular transmission. There have been few studies concerning the role of serotonergic innervation of the spinal dorsal horn and its role in modulating sensory inputs of significance in ventilatory control. However, dorsal horn serotonin appears to mediate presynaptic inhibition of many classes of segmental sensory input to the spinal cord (274,319,320). For example, serotonin may simultaneously increase the excitability of intercostal respiratory motoneurons while inhibiting synaptic inputs from sensory receptors arising from respiratory muscles (279). The significance of this dual effect is not yet clear, but it may fit into a general hypothesis of serotonergic involvement in sensorimotor integration during automatic rhythmic motor acts including breathing (274,279). Little is known concerning the role of supramedullary serotonergic projections in ventilatory control, possibly involving neural structures in the pons, cerebellum, hypothalamus, or motor cortex.

C. Control of Serotonergic Neuron Activity

An understanding of the physiological roles played by any transmitter system requires knowledge of when the neurons are activated and, therefore, exert an influence on their postsynaptic targets. Since most studies on responses elicited in serotonergic raphe neurons have been conducted using in vitro or anesthetized in vivo preparations, they are of limited value in understanding the behavioral/ physiological functions of serotonergic neurons. Indeed, there are significant differences in the apparent responsiveness of rostral medullary raphe neurons (i.e., the inferior group) in anesthetized versus awake cats (274).

In in vitro slice preparations, raphe serotonergic neurons are intrinsically active, discharging at a highly regular, slow rate (321). This regularity has been regarded as a "signature" of serotonergic neurons (322,323). The steady discharge seems to arise from intrinsic pacemaker activity in serotonergic neurons since it persists even without afferent input (321). In vivo and in vitro (raphe slice), serotonergic neurons display a large afterhyperpolarization followed by a gradual depolarization without evidence of excitatory postsynaptic potentials, eventually leading to the next action potential (324,325). Under normal conditions, a slow calcium conductance initiates slow depolarization leading to spontaneous, regular discharge; a long refractory period associated with the potent afterhyperpolarization limits and stabilizes the rate of discharge. This slow, pacemaker activity is similar to pacemaker cells studied in other vertebrate and invertebrate systems and results in a rate of discharge that is typically as high as or higher than the highest levels recorded in vivo (274).

A major feature of serotonergic neurons in vivo is negative neuronal feedback or intraraphe coordination via axon collaterals; serotonin inhibits the activity of serotonergic neurons via 5-HT$_{1A}$ receptors. This feature provides a linkage between neighboring serotonergic neurons within a nucleus and may coordinate serotonergic neuronal discharge in different raphe nuclei (274). In addition to negative serotonergic feedback, serotonergic neurons receive a number of inhibitory synaptic inputs that are mediated by GABA, histamine, and glycine. On the other hand, facilitatory inputs from glutamatergic and noradrenergic synapses impinge on serotonergic neurons; the noradrenergic inputs seem to operate at near-maximal levels in vivo (274). The net result of these facilitatory and inhibitory synaptic inputs is that in vivo discharge frequencies of serotonergic neurons are slightly below their discharge rates in vitro, when the net inhibitory influence from other transmitters is minimal and the pacemaker activity continues at its intrinsic rate.

In anesthetized animals, many afferent inputs are reported to activate raphe neurons in the rostral medullary (inferior) group (278,326–331). Of particular relevance to ventilatory control, Lindsey and colleagues (332–334) provide evidence that many midline neurons in the raphe nuclei (many presumably serotonergic) form extensive interconnections with both inhibitory and excitatory effects. These interactions often occur with a temporal relationship that is phase-locked with respiration, suggesting that these neurons receive inputs from other medullary respiratory neurons. The functional significance of this coordination is not yet clear, but it may relate to the hypothesis that serotonergic neurons' primary role is to modulate and facilitate skeletal motor function (278), in this case, respiratory motor function. Other inputs of significance to respiratory control include augmentation of raphe discharge by activation of chemoreceptors and baroreceptor fibers in the carotid sinus nerve (67% of neurons) (331), inhibition and excitation (39%) due to vagal stimulation (329), and unspecified inputs from the medial parabrachial and Kölliker-Fuse nuclear complex (330).

It is difficult to interpret the significance of the many sensory inputs reported to activate or inhibit raphe neurons based on recordings in anesthetized animals. Literature accounts suggest that auditory, visual, nociceptive, thermoreceptive, stress-related, cardiovascular, respiratory, circadian, and other inputs all influence the activity of serotonergic raphe neurons (274,278,328). Individual raphe neurons are often reported to be multimodal, suggesting an integrative role in numerous physiological behaviors. However, these reports are at variance with the reports of presumptive serotonergic neurons in the major serotonergic cell groups in unanesthetized animals (274,278,335–337). In these experiments on unanesthetized cats, behavioral, physiological, and environmental challenges that would be expected to activate raphe neurons in anesthetized cats had scarcely any effect in any of the raphe nuclei investigated; specific challenges included: nociceptive inputs, fear, active restraint, cardiovascular challenge, thermal stress, auditory inputs, and others. Collectively, available data indicate that the activity of serotonergic neurons is difficult to perturb by strong challenges in unanesthetized cats. However, several important factors had powerful effects on serotonergic neuron discharge. Most notable was the sleep state of the animal. As the cats moved from active wakefulness to quiet wakefulness through the stages of slow-wave sleep, raphe neuron discharge progressively declined. During REM sleep, serotonergic neuronal discharge dropped precipitously. During wakefulness, the only factors with consistent effects on the discharge of cells in the dorsal raphe that could not be attributed to changes in sleep state were automatic, rhythmic motor behaviors such as grooming or mastication (excitatory) or alerting responses (inhibitory). Jacobs has formulated a general theory concerning the function of the serotonergic nervous system: "5-HT's primary role is to modulate and facilitate (automatic) skeletal motor function" (274,278,279). In this context, when the facilitatory influence of serotonin on motor systems is expressed, the serotonergic system simultaneously inhibits information processing in sensory systems. Thus, during rhythmic motor behaviors, such as chewing or breathing, the serotonergic system is activated, facilitating and coordinating the motor outflow while, at the same time, inhibiting unnecessary sensory feedback that might distract and disrupt the automated motor task. However, if the cat is alerted, drawing its attention to a novel stimulus, the cat will commonly sit, orient toward the novel stimulus, and focus its attention. During an alerting response, the cat's objective is to enhance sensory input, presumably via disinhibition by decreasing serotonergic neuron activity; the cost is diminished motor excitability. After the cat has been habituated to the (no longer) novel stimulus, it does not alert, the serotonergic neuron activity remains unaltered, and the motor behavior continues. Thus, serotonergic neurons may exert a gain control on sensory and motor activity in a reciprocal manner; the influence on target neurons is expressed in direct association with the motor behavior and the arousal/sleep state of the animal.

The disparate results arising from studies on anesthetized versus unanesthetized animals may be explained by recent observations of Grahn and Heller (328). These investigators demonstrated that urethane-anesthetized rats undergo electroencephalographic (EEG) changes reminiscent of the full range of sleep/ wakefulness stages in awake animals. Given the tight relationship between sleep state and the discharge of serotonergic raphe neurons, they hypothesized that many sensory inputs in urethane-anesthetized animals trigger changes in the EEG and mental state of the animal, thus indirectly altering raphe neuron discharge. Using thermoafferent stimulation, they demonstrated that changes in raphe neuronal activity were not specific to the afferent input, but related more closely to attendant changes in cortical activation (i.e., sleep state). Serotonergic neurons may not be multimodal in their receptivity to sensory input; it may be that the literature accounts suggesting this may reflect changes in arousal state, even in anesthetized animals.

D. Effects of Raphe Activation on Respiration

One method commonly used to simulate the physiological consequences of activating serotonergic raphe neurons is electrical or chemical stimulation of the raphe nuclei. The outcomes of these experiments are complicated and difficult to interpret. Electrical or chemical stimulation of the caudal raphe nuclei produces alterations in phrenic nerve activity, including both excitation [raphe obscurus and pallidus stimulation (306,338–341)] and inhibition [raphe magnus and obscurus stimulation (341,342)], depending on the preparation, the stimulus location, and its intensity. These excitatory and inhibitory influences are believed to be mediated indirectly via medullary premotoneurons and, at least in part, via serotonergic mechanisms (339,340,342). The effects of raphe stimulation on respiratory motor output have also been investigated in the recurrent laryngeal nerve [excitation by raphe obscurus stimulation (306)], in the hypoglossal nerve [depression by unspecified midline pontine neurons (343)], and in upper cervical inspiratory premotoneurons [inhibition by raphe magnus stimulation (344)].

Following a single shock to the raphe obscurus in anesthetized cats, two evoked responses are observed in the phrenic neurogram (339). The short-latency response was insensitive to methysergide (a serotonin receptor antagonist), whereas the longer-latency excitation was reduced or completely abolished with this treatment. Thus, both methysergide-sensitive and insensitive excitations can be observed in the phrenic neurogram, suggesting that only the longer-latency response requires activation of 5-HT$_1$ or 5-HT$_2$ receptor subtypes, i.e., those subtypes expected to be blocked by methysergide. Although it was argued that even the longer-latency, methysergide-sensitive response was too fast (ca. 7 msec) to be mediated via direct raphe serotonergic projections to motoneurons (339,340), recent evidence suggests that descending serotonergic neurons sometimes have higher conduction velocities than formerly believed (329,331). Thus, it remains possible that direct, descending serotonergic projections were involved in this stimulus-evoked response. It could be argued that, although the second excitation required serotonin, it may not have resulted directly from a serotonergic postsynaptic potential. Since spinal serotonin reveals previously ineffective non-serotonergic synaptic pathways to phrenic motoneurons (345,346), it is possible that serotonin, released in the phrenic nucleus, revealed a nonserotonergic synaptic input to phrenic motoneurons that accounted for the 7-msec excitation.

With longer stimulus trains applied to the raphe obscurus in cats, long-lasting facilitation of the phrenic burst amplitude continues for an hour or more after the stimulus train has ended (340). This long-lasting facilitation was sensitive to methysergide, indicating an involvement of serotonin receptors in the underlying mechanism. The effect is strikingly similar to that observed following direct microinjection of serotonin into the phrenic nucleus of anesthetized rabbits (347). Indeed, stimulation of raphe obscurus causes a two- to threefold increase in the release of serotonin within the cervical ventral horn of decerebrate cats (348), suggesting that spinal release of serotonin is at least partly responsible for the long-lasting facilitation of phrenic nerve activity following raphe obscurus stimulation.

Raphe stimulation is limited in its ability to simulate endogenous serotonergic neuron excitation since the raphe nuclei do not contain serotonergic neurons exclusively (274); thus, it cannot be assured that observed effects result from the serotonergic nervous system. Furthermore, most protocols investigating the effects of raphe stimulation on ventilation utilize stimulation frequencies in the range of 5 to over 100 Hz, a range seldom encountered under more physiological conditions (274). The particular stimulus characteristics used may have important implications in the differential, frequency-dependent release of coexisting transmitters from serotonergic projections (349), which in turn may contribute to variable responses.

E. Postsynaptic Actions of Serotonergic Neurons

Serotonin exerts postsynaptic influences on many types of neurons throughout the neuraxis at their cell bodies, on dendritic shafts (particularly distal dendrites), and on axon terminals. These influences are mediated via multiple categories of receptor subtypes (350–353), exerting their effects through a variety of ionic channels (269–271). Postsynaptic channels are ligand-gated or controlled by second-messenger systems that either open or close the channel (2,274). Thus, the postsynaptic actions of serotonin are complex and depend on many variables, such as: the status of other transmitter systems, the identity of postsynaptic receptors and their history of activation, the intensity and time course of serotonergic neuron activation, and reuptake mechanisms.

Postsynaptic receptors are generally categorized into four receptor families. Each family consists of multiple receptor subtypes that share similar properties. In general, members of the 5-HT$_1$ family (with the exception of the 5-HT$_{1c}$ subtype) are associated with the inhibition of adenylate cyclase and act to open a potassium channel, thereby hyperpolarizing the cell or axon terminal (350). Members of the 5-HT$_2$ family [including 5-HT$_{1c}$ receptors (350)] appear to be coupled with phosphatidyl inositol turnover; by stimulating phosphatidyl inositol, a slow depolarization is elicited, presumably by closing a potassium channel (271,350). 5-HT$_3$ receptors are an exception among monoamine neurotransmitter receptors in that they are ligand-gated and mediate fast synaptic transmission by opening a cationic channel (352). Recently, 5-HT$_4$ receptors have been identified; these receptors stimulate adenylate cyclase activity, thus increasing cAMP production and activating a cAMP-dependent protein kinase A. Depending on the intrinsic properties of the postsynaptic target, activation of 5-HT$_4$ receptors can lead to closure of a potassium channel, resulting in depolarization, or opening a voltage-sensitive Ca^{2+} channel on another presynaptic terminal, enhancing neuro-transmitter release (351). A new receptor nomenclature has recently been proposed by the Serotonin Club Receptor Nomenclature Committee (353). In particular, the new classifications are based on three types of criteria: operational, structural, and transductional. One consequence of this revision is that 5-HT$_{1c}$ receptors become 5-HT$_2$ receptors.

Experimental conditions such as body temperature can have a potent influence on the affinity constants of serotonin receptors for agonists or antagonists. For example, decreased temperature increases the affinity of 5-HT$_1$ and 5-HT$_2$ receptors for serotonin or selective agonists in frogs, but has no effect on receptor affinity for the antagonists studied (354).

The distribution of serotonin receptor subtypes in areas of interest to respiratory control is not well known. 5-HT$_3$ receptors are distributed widely throughout the NTS, area postrema, and vagus nerve (352); however, there is no known role as yet for these receptors in the control of breathing apart from an involvement in emesis. Autoradiographic mapping of serotonin receptors in the spinal cord indicates a preponderance of 5-HT$_{1A}$ receptors in the spinal dorsal horn, suggesting a role in modulating sensory input (see above). In the ventral horn, 5-HT$_2$ receptors predominate (355), suggesting an involvement in the regulation of motoneuron excitability.

Medullary Respiratory Neurons

Localized injections of serotonin or serotonin agonists elicit both facilitatory and inhibitory influences on several important classes of medullary respiratory neurons (77,78,356–359). However, very little is known about the specific receptor subtypes or cellular mechanisms involved. In inspiratory medullary neurons, iontophoretic application of serotonin had no effect on one-half of the cells studied, whereas the remaining half were excited (78). In contrast, these authors found that phase-spanning neurons were generally excited by serotonin. Cyproheptadin, a serotonin receptor antagonist, excited most medullary expiratory neurons, suggesting release from tonic serotonergic inhibition (77). Sessle and Henry (356) found that more than half of the inspiratory neurons studied in the NTS were excited by microiontophoretic application of serotonin. Although Champagnat et al. (357) and Jacquin et al. (358) report similar, but more consistent, results for NTS neurons studied in an in vitro slice preparation, their findings were complicated by the fact that the observed effects were highly modifiable when different transmitters were investigated simultaneously (358). In control conditions, serotonin had a uniformly excitatory effect via actions on 5-HT_2 receptors; when substance P was applied prior to serotonin administration, the excitatory 5-HT_2 effect was occluded and an inhibitory 5-HT_{1A}-mediated inhibition was revealed. It is likely that this occlusion involved different membrane permeabilities, resulting from an intracellular mechanism operating after receptor activation, but before channel modifications (357).

Arita and Ochiishi (359) investigated the effects of pressure microinjections of serotonin in the vicinity of inspiratory-augmenting and inspiratory-decrementing neurons of the nucleus ambiguus; no efforts were made to distinguish cranial motoneurons from propriobulbar or bulbospinal neurons. They found that a majority of the augmenting units (77%) were inhibited by serotonin whereas the majority of decrementing units (83%) were stimulated; these effects were characterized by a slow onset, suggesting a second-messenger-mediated effect via 5-HT_1 and 5-HT_2 receptors, respectively. In a recent study, Lalley and Richter (unpublished, personal communication) investigated the influence of 5-HT_{1A} receptor agonists on stage 2 medullary expiratory neurons in anesthetized cats. 8-OH-DPAT applied iontophoretically depressed the excitability of these expiratory neurons, causing hyperpolarization and decreased membrane input resistance.

Overall, the net influence of increased medullary serotonin in the in vitro neonatal rat brainstem–spinal cord preparation is an increase in respiratory frequency rather than nerve burst amplitude (360–362). On the other hand, global depletion of serotonin in awake adult animals also elicits hyperventilation via an increase in respiratory frequency (363,364), suggesting a release from net inhibition of ventilatory frequency. Both these experimental approaches suffer from the limitation that the application of drugs is nonspecific with respect to location and may be expected to elicit different results depending on the specific drug used, its distribution, and coincident conditions such as the presence of other synaptic inputs or neuromodulators (358,365).

Respiratory Motoneurons

Microinjections of serotonin into the phrenic nucleus of anesthetized rabbits augment phrenic burst amplitude without effects on burst frequency (347), suggesting that serotonin increases phrenic motoneuron excitability as it does in nonrespiratory motoneurons (274,366–373). The effects of a single injection of serotonin last for hours, suggesting that these effects may be mediated by second-messenger systems that exert effects beyond the period of direct agonist influence. Spinal serotonin causes two distinct effects on phrenic motoneurons studied in an in vitro neonatal rat brainstem–spinal cord preparation (362): (1) direct depolarization via $5\text{-}HT_{2,1c}$ receptors, possibly closing a potassium channel, and (2) a reduction of central respiratory drive potentials mediated via a distinct receptor subclass. The net result of these facilitatory and inhibitory effects is increased motoneuron excitability and respiration-related discharge. Thus, the effects, receptor subtypes, and underlying mechanisms of serotonergic influence on phrenic motoneurons appear to be similar to effects elicited in other nonrespiratory motoneurons (370,374). Serotonergic effects on phrenic motoneuron excitability most likely result from closure of a potassium channel, possibly mediated by G proteins but modulated negatively by protein kinase C (375). Inward calcium currents are also elicited by serotonin in some rat spinal motoneurons (369).

Lalley (342) observed only small excitations in phrenic motoneurons when serotonin was applied in their immediate vicinity via microiontophoretic application. This could be interpreted as indicating that spinal serotonergic effects on phrenic motoneurons are mostly mediated indirectly, via interneurons or synaptic inputs not exposed to the applied serotonin. On the other hand, this result may be equally well explained by application of serotonin near the soma, whereas most serotonergic inputs (and presumably receptors) are located on the distal dendrites (302).

Serotonin augments the excitability of hypoglossal motoneurons with respiratory inputs in decerebrate cats (376) via effects on $5\text{-}HT_{2/1c}$ receptors. In neonatal rat hypoglossal motoneurons (in vitro), serotonin caused motoneuron depolarization and decreased the amplitude of the postspike afterhyperpolarization, thereby increasing the slope of the relationship between steady-state firing frequency and injected current (377). In contrast, phrenic motoneurons from neonatal rats (362) exhibited depolarization and increased membrane resistance in response to serotonin, but there was no shift in the slope of the relationship between injected current and discharge frequency. The lack of effect on this slope was presumably due to the lack of an effect on the postspike afterhyperpolarization.

Some investigators have claimed that serotonin exerts inhibitory effects on hypoglossal motoneurons (360,373). However, these experiments on in vitro brainstem–spinal cord preparations from neonatal rats are complicated by bath application of the serotonin, making conclusions about the site of action difficult (360). In a more recent study (373), serotonin application was restricted to the hypoglossal motor nucleus, and similar results were found: depression of hypoglossal activity, membrane depolarization via 5-HT$_2$ receptors, and a decreased amplitude of the central respiratory drive potential. It remains possible that the inhibitory actions are indirect and are not mediated by the direct actions of 5-HT$_2$ receptors on hypoglossal motoneurons; the observed membrane depolarization is in support of direct excitatory actions and indirect inhibition or disfacilitation. The differences between these and other studies await resolution.

Neither phrenic motoneurons in neonatal rats (362) nor hypoglossal motoneurons in decerebrate adult cats (309) revealed bistable state behavior in response to injected current. This behavior, reported previously in lumbar motoneurons of decerebrate cats (378), requires a serotonin or norepinephrine-mediated decrease in the postspike afterhyperpolarization and is a manifestation of a calcium-channel-mediated plateau potential. Thus, it is possible that respiratory motoneurons either lack the 5-HT-mediated decrease in the afterhyperpolarizing current, the calcium channel, or both.

F. Effects of Serotonin on Nonserotonergic Synaptic Inputs

Little is known concerning the effects of serotonin on respiratory neurons and their responses to nonserotonergic synaptic inputs. In lumbar motoneurons, serotonin increases the response to pressure microinjections of glutamate without affecting basal discharge rate (379). In contrast, serotonin inhibits descending central respiratory drive to phrenic motoneurons in neonatal rats (362), an input mediated via glutamatergic synapses (44). Thus, the effects of spinal serotonin are complex and may involve presynaptic inhibition of glutamate release from axon terminals of medullary premotoneurons. The effects of serotonin on responses to exogenously applied glutamate or inhibitory transmitters such as GABA are not known for any class of respiratory motoneurons.

In recent studies on spinalized, anesthetized rats (345), systemic injections of 5-hydroxytryptophan (a serotonin precursor) and pargyline (a monoamine oxidase inhibitor) were used to increase spinal serotonin levels. Both spontaneous tonic phrenic nerve activity and responses evoked by single shocks applied to the C-2 lateral funiculus were enhanced. Although a short-latency (0.8 msec) evoked response in the ipsilateral phrenic neurogram was relatively unaffected by serotonin, a previously ineffective synaptic pathway mediating a longer-latency excitation (ca. 2.0 msec) was revealed following drug administration (345). In similar experiments on rats with spinal hemisection at C-1 to C-2, it was determined that pharmacological application of serotonin also reveals ineffective crossed spinal pathways to contralateral phrenic motoneurons (346). Prior to drug administration, there was little evidence for crossed spinal pathways to contralateral phrenic motoneurons when stimulating either the dorsolateral or ventrolateral funiculus at C-2. After drug administration, complex evoked responses were observed, including short (ca. 0.9 msec), medium (ca. 2.0 msec), and long (ca. 7.7 msec) latency excitations. Since these changes were antagonized by methysergide, it appears that spinal serotonin increases the efficacy of nonserotonergic synaptic inputs to phrenic motoneurons and converts functionally ineffective pathways to functionally effective pathways in the spinal cord. It remains to be determined whether serotonin is both necessary and sufficient in this modulatory process, or whether it is a nonspecific result of increased phrenic motoneuron excitability. The revelation of synaptic pathways in the spinal cord by serotonergic modulation may impart a degree of plasticity to the spinal integration of respiratory activity and may be involved in gating or controlling the information flow of spinal reflexes in relation to descending inputs to respiratory motoneurons.

Spinal serotonin may also control intrinsic membrane properties that contribute to processes of habituation or sensitization. In an in vitro brainstem–spinal cord preparation from adult frogs, repetitive activation of the lateral columns produces excitatory monosynaptic responses in the ipsilateral ventral roots that are depressed with an exponential time course (i.e., habituation (380)]. Application of serotonin or raphe stimulation reduced or eliminated the depression. Functionally, these actions of spinal serotonin would decrease spike frequency accommodation in response to descending inputs; the result may be an enhanced ability to respond in a sustained manner to supraspinal inputs.

G. Integrated Physiological Responses

Serotonergic raphe neurons are affected primarily by sleep state, but are also coactivated in association with automatic, rhythmic behaviors as well as by sensory inputs that facilitate such behaviors (274). Postsynaptic actions of serotonin are generally modulatory or "conditionally acting" (2,3) and may mediate changes in neuron excitability or the "gain" of neuronal responses to other synaptic inputs (297) (see above). In this context, respiration is the epitome of an automated rhythmic behavior and is facilitated by a number of different sensory inputs, most notably by chemoreceptors. These characteristics of serotonin have been implicated in several identified physiological mechanisms that represent degrees of plasticity or memory in ventilatory control. To identify a role for serotonin in any respiratory mechanism, it is not sufficient to observe only effects on eupnic breathing; it is often useful to evoke specific reflex or integrative pathways that may be associated with coactivation of serotonergic neurons (381).

Long-Term Facilitation of Respiration

Chemical or electrical stimulation of the peripheral chemoreceptors evokes an abrupt increase in ventilatory activity. However, after the stimulation ends, ventilatory output remains elevated in both anesthetized (21) and conscious animals (382,383). The decay of ventilatory activity following stimulation reflects at least two distinct mechanisms with time domains of minutes [*short-term potentiation* (384)] to hours [*long-term facilitation* (21,22)]. Short-term potentiation (formerly "afterdischarge") is elicited by a wider range of afferent inputs and does not require monoamine neurotransmitters (21,384). In contrast, long-term facilitation appears to be elicited uniquely by peripheral chemoreceptor stimulation, cannot be evoked following serotonin receptor antagonism with methysergide, and is impaired following application of the tryptophan hydroxylase inhibitor para-chlorophenylalanine or the serotonergic neurotoxin 5,7-dihydroxytryptamine (385,386).

Electrical stimulation of the carotid sinus nerve also elicits long-term facilitation of inspiratory activity in a parasternal branch of a T-5 to T-6 internal intercostal nerve (387). However, the effect appears to be more powerful in this neurogram, augmenting peak integrated nerve activity more than in the phrenic neurogram under the same experimental conditions. In contrast, Jiang et al. (309) failed to detect long-term facilitation in respiration-related hypoglossal motor output following carotid sinus or superior laryngeal nerve stimulation. Thus, there appears to be heterogeneity in the magnitude of long-term facilitation among different respiratory motoneuron pools. However, details in the experimental preparation, such as the prevailing level of arterial Pco_2 or decerebellation (22), may bias the experimental outcome, favoring or hindering manifestation of long-term facilitation in a given motor pool (22,309).

Episodic electrical stimulation of the carotid sinus nerve at 25 Hz for 2-min periods (22,309,385–387) is of questionable physiological relevance. Rarely do carotid chemoreceptors discharge at such a high frequency for prolonged periods, if at all, and seldom will chemoreceptor afferent fibers discharge in synchrony. However, Millhorn et al. (385) reported that one cat exhibited long-term facilitation following 10 min of moderately severe hypoxia. This essential observation has been confirmed using modified protocols that expose animals to repeated episodes of moderate to severe hypoxia. Long-term facilitation is now known to occur following repeated episodic hypoxia in anesthetized rats (22), awake rats (388), and awake dogs (382).

Millhorn et al. (385) and Millhorn (381) suggested that long-term facilitation may represent the mechanism underlying ventilatory acclimatization to chronic hypoxia (or deacclimatization from chronic hypoxia). However, at least three observations are inconsistent with this hypothesis. First, neither awake humans nor rats exhibit signs of deacclimatization after 1 hr of steady hypoxia followed by acute return to normoxia (389). Second, awake rats still exhibit ventilatory acclimatization to chronic hypoxia following whole-body serotonin depletion with para-chlorophenylalanine (390), a treatment that inhibits CSN-stimulation-induced long-term facilitation in anesthetized cats (386). Third, although repeated episodes of isocapnic hypoxia elicit long-term facilitation in anesthetized or awake animals (22,382), awake goats do not exhibit posthypoxic augmentation of ventilation following 4 hr of steady hypoxic exposure if arterial isocapnia is maintained, even though ventilatory acclimatization to chronic hypoxia is already evident at this time (391). Although interpretation of these studies is complicated by the different species and experimental paradigms used, collectively they suggest that long-term facilitation requires episodic hypoxia and is not elicited by the steady hypoxic exposures utilized in studies on ventilatory acclimatization to altitude. The basis for this difference remains unclear, but it may relate to differences in the intensity of afferent stimulation used or to differences between episodic versus steady hypoxia, such as processes of chemoreceptor adaptation or central neural habituation.

Since afferent fibers coursing through the carotid sinus nerve synapse predominantly in the vicinity of the NTS (151), and the cell bodies of serotonergic neurons are located in brainstem raphe nuclei (see above), long-term facilitation must involve brainstem neurons in its underlying mechanism. There is also presumptive evidence for an involvement of cerebellar structures since long-term facilitation could no longer be elicited in anesthetized rats following vermalectomy (22). This finding is difficult to interpret since vermalectomy reduced the CO_2-threshold for rhythmic phrenic activity and may have only indirectly abolished long-term facilitation; nevertheless, the cerebellum has been strongly implicated in the formation and storage of simple motor memories (392). The possible role of the cerebellum in long-term facilitation, a form of motor memory, is worthy of further investigation. Activation of carotid chemoreceptors stimulates raphe neurons (331,393,394), demonstrating a possible linkage for serotonergic involvement in long-term facilitation.

Based on the observation that long-term facilitation occurs via changes in both phrenic burst amplitude and frequency, Millhorn et al. (385) suggested that it operates via supraspinal mechanisms. However, the observed changes in frequency were rather small in their study, and subsequent studies indicate that long-term facilitation can occur without change in frequency (22,382,387). Thus, LTF occurs primarily via effects on burst pattern formation rather than rhythm generation, leaving open the possibility that at least some of the serotonergic effects occur at the spinal level via actions on spinal respiratory motoneurons.

Long-term facilitation may be significant in maintaining stable breathing during sleep since episodic hypoxia and hypercapnia often result from the unstable breathing patterns that characterize this physiological state. Serotonergic raphe neurons discharge at dramatically reduced rates during sleep (274), particularly stage IV and REM sleep. Repeated activation of these neurons by episodic hypoxia, and attendant arousal (328), could offset the withdrawal of serotonergic input to respiratory motoneurons, limiting or controlling the severity of respiratory muscle atonia (359,376). By thus controlling respiratory motoneuron excitability, long-term facilitation could assure adequate ventilatory efforts and ensure upper airway patency, thereby reducing obstructive episodes of sleep apnea. It would be intriguing to determine whether recurrent laryngeal motoneurons exhibit exaggerated long-term facilitation since they undoubtedly play a role in airway patency during sleep and receive a dense serotonergic innervation (307).

Heterogeneity in the magnitude of long-term facilitation between the phrenic and inspiratory intercostal motoneuron pools may serve to redistribute the work of breathing among the two muscle groups when posture is changed, or in conditions leading to respiratory insufficiency such as the onset of respiratory disease or diaphragmatic fatigue.

Short-Term Modulation of the Exercise Ventilatory Response

Small increases in respiratory dead space increase the exercise ventilatory response in goats and humans, maintaining Pa_{CO_2} regulation with respect to its resting level (395,396). Modulation of the exercise ventilatory response with increased dead space cannot be accounted for by changes in chemoreceptor feedback from rest to exercise and is similar to the modulation observed with several other experimental treatments that increase resting ventilation, including: acid-base changes, hormonal alterations, and manipulation of certain neurotransmitter systems (397). Because a wide range of experimental treatments elicits similar modulation, Mitchell and colleagues (397) postulated that a single mechanism links the exercise ventilatory response to resting ventilatory drive. This mechanism is referred to as short-term modulation (290) because the exercise ventilatory response is reversibly altered within a single exercise trial.

It was proposed that short-term modulation results from changes in the excitability of spinal respiratory motoneurons, resulting in greater motor output and ventilatory effort for a given stimulus associated with exercise. The overall excitability or "gain" of respiratory motoneurons results from a complex interplay between synaptic facilitation from spinal afferent inputs and brainstem–spinal cord projections from serotonergic neurons and other descending inputs. To test the hypothesis that serotonin is necessary for short-term modulation with in creased dead space in goats, experiments were conducted with intravenous administration of methysergide, a broad-spectrum serotonin receptor antagonist (290). Following methysergide, Pa_{CO_2} regulation during normal exercise was unchanged; however, during exercise with increased dead space, the goats exhibited graded ventilatory failure and hypercapnia. These results are consistent with the hypothesis that serotonin is necessary in short-term modulation, although systemic administration of the drug does not allow insight into the site or specificity of its effects. To minimize problems associated with systemic drug administration, a chronic catheter in the subarachnoid space of the thoracic spinal cord was used to administer methysergide or ketanserin directly into the spinal CSF of goats (398). The result was consistent with observations following systemic methysergide administration despite a total drug dose less than 2% of the effective systemic dose. Thus, *spinal* serotonin is necessary for short-term modulation of the exercise ventilatory response, probably acting via $5\text{-}HT_{2,1C}$ receptors.

Recovery of Ventilatory Function During Exercise After Thoracic Dorsal Rhizotomy

Following thoracic dorsal rhizotomy from T-2 to T-12, goats exhibit severe ventilatory failure during even mild treadmill exercise when wearing a respiratory mask, a mask easily tolerated prior to surgery (399). In subsequent exercise trials, functional recovery occurs despite evidence that dorsal rootlets have not regrown (400). The mechanism of functional recovery must overcome the persistent sensory deficit following dorsal rhizotomy by: (1) restoring motoneuron excitability, (2) overriding continued hypoexcitability by increasing descending central respiratory drive, or (3) altering the pattern of respiratory muscle recruitment. Functional recovery following thoracic dorsal rhizotomy almost certainly requires supraspinal involvement, producing greater descending central respiratory drive during exercise or increased descending control of spinal integration (401). Although there is some evidence for a mechanism that may enhance descending central ventilatory drive (402), immunocytochemical analysis of goat spinal cords following dorsal rhizotomy and recovery also provides evidence for spinal mechanisms that would alter or enhance the spinal integration of descending respiratory inputs (403). Greater numbers of serotonin-immunoreactive nerve terminals were observed in both the ventral and dorsal horns of the thoracic spinal cord (403) similar to reported enhancement of the serotonergic nervous system following dorsal rhizotomy in other experimental models (404). Recent evidence supports a role for serotonergic neurons in restoring motor function following spinal lesions in rats (405), leading us to speculate that serotonin also plays a role in restoring and/or maintaining ventilatory function following dorsal rhizotomy in goats.

V. Closing Thoughts

Although rapid progress is being made in understanding the role of neurotransmitters and neuromodulators in ventilatory control, there remains a great deal that is not yet understood. We have attempted to review current literature pertaining to the roles of only three neurotransmitters: glutamate, GABA, and serotonin. It should be apparent that, although there are clear differences among these neurochemicals, there are also many similarities; each has the potential (not always demonstrated in ventilatory control) to participate in a range of processes, including: fast (excitatory or inhibitory) synaptic transmission, neuromodulation, paracrine functions, and trophic or tropic interactions among neurons. There are no firm criteria that distinguish these transmitter substances since the functional roles of each will only be understood in the context of their specific neuronal projections, the pre- and postsynaptic receptor subtypes that they activate, the existence of cotransmitters within the specific pathway, and interactions among neurotransmitters in converging neuronal pathways that act in the fashion of a "committee" to determine postsynaptic effects. These properties determine the behavior of the neural ensemble that underlies the act of breathing. Even though glutamate, GABA, and serotonin are arguably the most thoroughly studied neurotransmitters from the perspective of ventilatory control, there remain large gaps in our fundamental understanding of many of these important issues and therefore of the role that these neurochemicals play in the control of breathing.

Thus, to further our understanding of neurotransmitters (generally) in ventilatory control, we must understand transmitter distribution and presence in specific neuronal projections. We must understand the circumstances of transmitter release, distribution, and duration of action. We must understand the receptor subtypes that are activated by transmitter release and the functions of the neuron on which the transmitter has its effect. We must understand the consequences of receptor coactivation: in the context of different receptors activated by the same neurotransmitter at the same synapse, by activation of receptors by different transmitters released at the same synapse (i.e., colocalization), by simultaneous activation of receptors responding to different transmitters at different synapses, or by shared second-messenger pathways, causing the same postsynaptic ionic conductance changes (or occluding them). In other words, it is critical that we understand interactions within and between different neurotransmitter systems. We must understand all these issues for an ever-increasing number of identified neurotransmitters/neuromodulators at all sites in the central nervous system that are relevant to ventilatory control. Finally, we must understand the translation of the cellular and synaptic events mediated by these neurotransmitter processes to animal behavior, in this case ventilatory behavior. This requires an understanding of the comprehensive neural network engaged in the central neural control of breathing and the emergent properties of that network. Only then will we understand the behavior of the respiratory control system in unanesthetized animals or human subjects, the ultimate objective of respiratory neurobiology. The task may appear daunting, but it is hoped that fundamental laws will become apparent that allow a conceptual framework within which to view this complex, integrative control system. An expectation that an understanding will emerge that is analogous to thermodynamics, a means of comprehending the physical/chemical behavior of molecules, does not seem unreasonable. We (respiratory neurobiologists) have much work to do.

Acknowledgments

We thank Dr. Simon Alford for helpful comments on the manuscript. This work was supported by National Institutes of Health Research Grants HL 40336, NS 17489 to D. R. McCrimmon, HL 36780 to G. S. Mitchell, and HL 40369, HL 02314 to M. S. Dekin.

References

1. Getting PA. Emerging principles governing the operation of neural networks. Annu Rev Neurosci 1989; 12;185–204.
2. Nicoll RA, Malenka RC, Kauer JA. Functional comparison of neurotransmitter receptor subtypes in mammalian central nervous system. Physiol Rev 1989; 70: 513–564.
3. Bloom FE. The functional significance of neurotransmitter diversity. Am J Physiol 1984; 246:C184–C194.
4. Dekin MS. Comparative neurobiology of invertebrate motor networks: implications for the control of breathing in mammals. In: Haddad GG, Farber JP, eds. Developmental Neurobiology of the Lung. New York: Marcel Dekker, 1991:111–154.
5. Harris-Warrick RM, Marder E, Selverston AI, Moulins M. Dynamic Biological Networks: The Stomatogastric Nervous System. Cambridge: MIT Press, 1992.
6. Eldridge FL, Millhorn DE. Central regulation of respiration by endogenous neurotransmitters and neuromodulators. Annu Rev Physiol 1981; 43:121–135.
7. Mueller RA, Lundberg BA, Breese GR, Hedner J, Hedner T, Jonason J. The neuropharmacology of respiratory control. Pharmacol Rev 1982; 34:255–280.
8. Dempsey JA, Olson EB, Jr., Skatrud JB. Hormones and neurochemicals in the regulation of breathing. In: Fishman AP, Cherniack NS, Widdicombe JG, eds. Handbook of Physiology: The Respiratory System, Section 3, Vol 2, Part 1. Bethesda, MD: American Physiological Society, 1986:181–221.
9. Kalia M, Viola JJ, Hudson ME, Fuxe K, Richter DW, Harfstrand A, Goldstein M. Chemical neuroanatomy of respiratory and cardiovascular nuclei in the medulla

oblongata. In: Euler C von, Lagercrantz H, eds. Neurobiology of the Control of Breathing. New York: Raven Press, 1986:165–173.

10. Moss IR, Denavit-Saubié M, Eldridge FL, Gillis RA, Herkenham M, Lahiri S. Neuromodulators and transmitters in respiratory control. Fed Proc 1986; 45:2133–2147.

11. Cuénod M, Do KQ, Grandes P, Morino P, Streit P. Localization and release of homocysteic acid, an excitatory sulfur-containing amino acid. J Histochem Cytochem 1990; 38:1713–1715.

12. Coyle JT, Stauch-Slusher B, Tsai G, Rothstein J, Meyerhoff JL, Simmons M, Blakely RD. N-Acetyl-aspartyl glutamate. Recent developments. In: Meldrum BS, Moroni F, Simon RP, Woods JH, eds. Fidia Research Foundation Symposium Series. Vol 5. Excitatory Amino Acids. New York: Raven Press, 1991:69–77.

13. Do KQ, Klancnik JM, Gähwiler B, Perschak H, Wieser H-G, Cuénod M. Release of excitatory amino acids. Animal studies and epileptic foci studies in humans. In: Meldrum BS, Moroni F, Simon RP, Woods JH, eds. Fidia Research Foundation Symposium Series. Vol. 5. Excitatory Amino Acids. New York: Raven Press, 1991;677–685.

14. Hicks TP, Kaneko T, Metherate R, Oka J-I, Stark CA. Amino acids as transmitters of synaptic excitation in neocortical sensory processes. Can J Physiol Pharmacol 1991; 69:1099–1114.

15. Streit P, Grandes P, Morino P, Tschopp P, Cuénod M. Immunohistochemical localization of glutamate and homocysteate. In Meldrum BS, Moroni F, Simon RP, Woods JH, eds. Fidia Research Foundation Symposium Series. Vol. 5. Excitatory Amino Acids. New York: Raven Press, 1991:61–67.

16. Zhang N, Ottersen OP. Differential cellular distribution of two sulphur-containing amino acids in rat cerebellum. An immunocytochemical investigation using antisera to taurine and homocysteic acid. Exp Brain Res 90:11–20.

17. Grieve A, Griffiths R. Simultaneous measurement by HPLC of the excitatory amino acid transmitter candidates homocysteate and homocysteine sulphinate supports a predominant astrocytic localisation. Neurosci Lett 1992; 145:1–5.

18. Tschopp P, Streit P, Do KQ. Homocysteate and homocysteine sulfinate, excitatory transmitter candidates present in rat astroglial cultures. Neurosci Lett 1992; 145:6–9.

19. Cotman CW, Monaghan DT, Ottersen OP, Storm-Mathisen J. Anatomical organization of excitatory amino acid receptors and their pathways. Trends Neurosci 1987; 7:273–280.

20. Mayer ML, Westbrook GL. The physiology of excitatory amino acids in the vertebrate central nervous system. Prog Neurobiol 1987; 28:197–276.

21. Eldridge FL, Millhorn DE. Oscillation, gating, and memory in the respiratory control system. In: Fishman AP, Cherniack NS, Widdicombe JG, eds. Handbook of Physiology: The Respiratory System, Section 3, Vol 2, Part 1. Bethesda, MD: American Physiological Society, 1986:93–114.

22. Hayashi F, Coles SK, Bach KB, Mitchell GS, McCrimmon DR. Time dependent phrenic nerve responses to carotid afferent activation: intact vs. decerebellate rats. Am J Physiol 1993; 265:R811–R819.

23. Gasic GP, Hollmann M. Molecular neurobiology of glutamate receptors. Annu Rev Physiol 1992; 54:507–536.

24. Nakanishi S. Molecular diversity of glutamate receptors and implications for brain function. Science 1992; 258:597–603.

25. Sommer B, Seeburg PH. Glutamate receptor channels: novel properties and new clones. Trends Pharmacol Sci 1992; 13:291–296.

26. Honoré T, Davies SN, Drejer J, Fletcher EJ, Jacobsen P, Lodge D, Nielsen FE. Quinoxalinediones: potent competitive non-NMDA glutamate receptor antagonists. Science 1988; 241:701–703.

27. Sheardown MJ, Nielsen EO, Hansen AJ, Jacobsen P, Honoré T. 2,3-Dihydroxy-6-nitro-7-sulfamoyl-benzo(F)quinoxaline: a neuroprotectant for cerebral ischemia. Science 1990; 247:571–574.

28. Harris KM, Miller RJ. CNQX (6-cyano-7-nitroquinoxaline-2,3-dione) antagonizes NMDA-evoked [^{3}H]GABA release from cultured cortical neurons via an inhibitory action at the strychnine-insensitive glycine site. Brain Res 1989; 489:185–189.

29. Keinänen K, Wisden W, Sommer B, Werner P, Herb A, Verdoorn TA, Sakmann B, Seeburg PH. A family of AMPA-selective glutamate receptors. Science 1990; 249:556–560.

30. Nakanishi N, Shneider NA, Axel R. A family of glutamate receptor genes: evidence for the formation of heteromultimeric receptors with distinct channel properties. Neuron 1990; 5:569–581.

31. Tang CM, Dichter M, Morad M. Quisqualate activates a rapidly inactivating high conductance ionic channel in hippocampal neurons. Science 1989; 243:1474–1477.

32. Sommer B, Keinänen K, Verdoorn TA, Wisden W, Burnashev N, Herb A, Kohler M, Takagi T, Sakmann B, Seeburg PH. Flip and flop: a cell-specific functional switch in glutamate-operated channels of the CNS. Science 1990; 249:1580–1585.

33. Hollmann M, Hartley M, Heinemann S. Ca^{2+} permeability of KA-AMPA-gated glutamate receptor. Science 1991; 252:851–853.

34. Hume RI, Dingledine R, Heinemann SF. Identification of a site in glutamate receptor subunits that controls calcium permeability. Science 1991; 253:1028–1031.

35. Burnashev N, Khodorova A, Jonas P, Helm PJ, Wisden W, Monyer H, Seeburg PH, Sakmann B. Calcium-permeable AMPA-kainate receptors in fusiform cerebellar glial cells. Science 1992; 256:1566–1570.

36. Huettner JE. Glutamate receptor channels in rat DRG neurons: activation by kainate and quisqualate and blockade of desensitization by Con A. Neuron 1990; 5:255–266.

37. Egebjerg J, Bettler B, Hermans-Borgmeyer I, Heinemann S. Cloning of a cDNA for a glutamate receptor subunit activated by kainate but not AMPA. Nature 1991; 351:745–748.

38. Dale N, Grillner S. Dual-component synaptic potentials in the lamprey mediated by excitatory amino acid receptors. J Neurosci 1986; 6:2653–2661.

39. Mayer ML, Benveniste M, Patneau DK, Vyklicky L, Jr. Pharmacologic properties of NMDA receptors. Ann NY Acad Sci 1992; 648:194–204.

40. Collingridge GL, Kehl SJ, McLennan H. The antagonism of amino acid-induced excitations of rat hippocampal CA1 neurones in vitro. J Physiol 1983; 334:19–31.

41. McCrimmon DR, Smith JC, Feldman JL. Involvement of excitatory amino acids in neurotransmission of inspiratory drive to spinal respiratory motoneurons. J Neurosci 1989; 9:1910–1921.

42. Greer JJ, Smith JC, Feldman JL. Role of excitatory amino acids in the generation and transmission of respiratory drive in neonatal rat. J Physiol 1991; 437:727–749.

43. Collingridge GL, Herron CE, Lester RAJ. Frequency-dependent N-methyl-D-aspartate receptor-mediated synaptic transmission in rat hippocampus. J Physiol 1988; 399:301–312.

44. Liu G, Feldman JL, Smith JC. Excitatory amino acid-mediated transmission of inspiratory drive to phrenic motoneurons. J Neurophysiol 1990; 64:423–436.

45. Landfield PW, Deadwyler SA. Long-Term Potentiation from Biophysics to Behavior. New York: Alan R Liss, 1988.

46. Bliss TVP, Collingridge GL. A synaptic model of memory: long-term potentiation in the hippocampus. Nature 1993; 361:31–39.

47. Meldrum B, Garthwaite J. Excitatory amino acid neurotoxicity and neurodegenerative disease. Trends Pharmacol Sci 1991; 11:379–387.

48. Cline HT, Debski EA, Constantine-Paton M. N-Methyl-D-aspartate receptor antagonist desegregates eye-specific stripes. Proc Natl Acad Sci USA 1987; 84:4342–4345.

49. Artola A, Singer W. NMDA receptors and developmental plasticity in visual neocortex. In: Watkins JC, Collingridge GL, eds. The NMDA Receptor. Oxford: Oxford University Press, 1989:153–166.

50. Komuro H, Rakic P. Modulation of neuronal migration by NMDA receptors. Science 1993; 260:95–97.

51. Dale N. The role of NMDA receptors in synaptic integration and the organization of complex neural patterns. In: Watkins JC, Collingridge GL, eds. The NMDA Receptor. Oxford: Oxford University Press, 1989:93–107.

52. Collingridge GL, Davies SN. NMDA receptors and long-term potentiation in the hippocampus. In: Watkins JC, Collingridge GL, eds. The NMDA Receptor. Oxford: Oxford University Press, 1989:123–135.

53. Watkins JC. The NMDA receptor concept: origins and development. In: Watkins JC, Collingridge GL, eds. The NMDA Receptor. Oxford: Oxford University Press, 1989:1–17.

54. Assaf SY, Chung SH. Release of endogenous Zn^{2+} from brain tissue during activity. Nature 1984; 308:734–736.

55. Legendre P, Westbrook GL. The inhibition of single NMDA-activated channels by zinc ions on cultured rat neurones. J Physiol 1990; 429:429–449.

56. Benveniste M, Clements J, Vyklicky L, Mayer ML. A kinetic analysis of the modulation of N-methyl-D-aspartic acid receptors by glycine in mouse cultured hippocampal neurones. J Physiol 1990; 428:333–357.

57. Olverman HJ, Watkins JC. NMDA agonists and competitive antagonists. In: Watkins JC, Collingridge GL, eds. The NMDA Receptor. Oxford: Oxford University Press, 1989:19–36.

58. Lodge D, Jones M, Fletcher E. Non-competitive antagonists of N-methyl-D-

aspartate. In: Watkins JC, Collingridge GL, eds. The NMDA Receptor. Oxford: Oxford University Press, 1989:37–51.

59. Sheardown MJ, Drejer J, Jensen LH, Stidsen CE, Honoré T. A potent antagonist of the strychnine insensitive glycine receptor has anticonvulsant properties. Eur J Pharmacol 1989; 174:197–204.

60. Moriyoshi K, Masu M, Ishii T, Shigemoto R, Mizuno N, Nakanishi S. Molecular cloning and characterization of the rat NMDA receptor. Nature 1991; 354:31–37.

61. Katsuwada T, Kashiwabuchi N, Mori H, Sakimura K, Kushiya E, Araki K, Meguro H, Masaki H, Kumanishi T, Arakawa M, Mishina M. Molecular diversity of the NMDA receptor channel. Nature 1992; 358:36–41.

62. Meguro H, Mori H, Araki K, Kushiya E, Kutsuwada T, Yamazaki M, Kumanishi T, Arakawa M, Sakimura K, Mishina M. Functional characterization of a heteromeric NMDA receptor channel expressed from cloned cDNAs. Nature 1992; 357:70–74.

63. Ishii T, Moriyoshi K, Sugihara H, Sakurada K, Kadotani H, Yokoi M, Akazawa C, Shigemoto R, Mizuno N, Masu M, Nakanishi S. Molecular characterization of the family of the N-methyl-D-aspartate receptor subunits. J Biol Chem 1993; 268:2836–2843.

64. Schoepp DD, Conn JP. Metabotropic glutamate receptors in brain function and pathology. Trends Pharmacol Sci 1993; 14:13–20.

65. Palmer E, Monaghan DT, Cotman CW. Trans-ACPD, a selective agonist of the phosphoinositide-coupled excitatory amino acid receptor. Eur J Pharmacol 1989; 166:585–587.

66. Glaum SR, Miller RJ. Activation of metabotropic glutamate receptors produces reciprocal regulation of ionotropic glutamate and GABA responses in the nucleus of the tractus solitarius of the rat. J Neurosci 1993; 13:1636–1641.

67. Bleakman D, Rusin KI, Chard PS, Glaum SR, Miller RJ. Metabotropic glutamate receptors potentiate ionotropic responses in the rat dorsal horn. Mol Pharmacol 1992; 42:192–196.

68. Fagni L, Bossu JL, Bockaert J. Activation of a large-conductance Ca^{++}-dependent K^+ channel by stimulation of glutamate phosphoinositide-coupled receptors in cultured cerebellar granule cells. Eur J Neurosci 1991; 3:778–789.

69. Eaton SA, Jane DE, Jones PL St J, Porter RHP, Pook PC-K, Sunter DC, Udvarhelyi PM, Roberts PJ, Salt TE, Watkins JC. Competitive antagonism at metabotropic receptors by (S)-4-carboxyphenylglycine and (RS)-α-methyl-4 carboxyphenylglycine. Eur J Pharmacol Mol Pharmacol 1993; 244:195–197.

70. Monaghan DT, McMillis MC, Chamberlin AK, Cotman CW. Synthesis of ^{3}H-2-amino-4-phosphonobutyric acid and characterization of its binding to rat brain membranes: a selective ligand for the chloride/calcium dependent class of L-glutamate binding sites. Brain Res 1983; 278:134–144.

71. Forsythe ID, Clements JD. Presynaptic glutamate receptors depress excitatory monosynaptic transmission between mouse hippocampal neurones. J Physiol 1990; 429:1–16.

72. Trombley PQ, Westbrook GL. L-AP4 inhibits calcium currents and synaptic transmission via a G-protein-coupled glutamate receptor. J Neurosci 1992; 12:2043–2050.

73. Thomsen C, Kristensen P, Mulvihill E, Haldeman B, Suzdak PD. L-2-Amino-4-phosphonobutyrate (L-AP4) is an agonist at the type IV metabotropic glutamate receptor which is negatively coupled to adenylate cyclase. Eur J Pharmacol Mol Pharmacol 1992; 227:361–362.

74. Koerner JF, Cotman CW. Micromolar L-2-amino-4-phosphonobutyric acid selectively inhibits perforant path synapses from lateral entorhinal cortex. Brain Res 1981; 216:192–198.

75. Davies J, Watkins JC. Action of d and l forms of 2-amino-5-phosphonovalerate and 2-amino-4-butyrate in the cat spinal cord. Brain Res 1982; 235:378–386.

76. Denavit-Saubié M, Champagnat J, Zieglgansberger W. Effects of opiates and methionine-enkephalin on pontine and bulbar respiratory neurones of the cat. Brain Res 1978; 155:55–67.

77. Böhmer G, Dinse HRO, Fallert M, Sommer TJ. Microelectrophoretic application of antagonists of putative neurotransmitters onto various types of bulbar respiratory neurons. Arch Ital Biol 1979; 117:13–22.

78. Fallert M, Böhmer G, Dinse HRO, Sommer TJ, Bittner A. Microelectrophoretic application of putative neurotransmitters onto various types of bulbar respiratory neurons. Arch Ital Biol 1979; 117:1–12.

79. Wang L, Boyarsky LL, Frazier DT. The effect of transmitter antagonists on phasic respiratory neurons. J Neurosci Res 1982; 8:657–664.

80. McCrimmon DR, Speck DF, Feldman JL. Respiratory motoneuronal activity is altered by injections of picomoles of glutamate into cat brain stem. J Neurosci 1986; 6:2384–2392.

81. Grélot L, Iscoe S, Bianchi AL. Effects of amino acids on the excitability of respiratory bulbospinal neurons in solitary and para-ambigual regions of medulla in cat. Brain Res 1988; 443:27–36.

82. Pierrefiche O, Schmid K, Foutz AS, Denavit-Saubié M. Endogenous activation of NMDA and non-NMDA glutamate receptors on respiratory neurones in cat medulla. Neuropharmacology 1991; 30:429–440.

83. Bonham AC, McCrimmon DR. Neurones in a discrete region of the nucleus tractus solitarius are required for the Breuer-Hering reflex in rat. J Physiol 1990; 427: 261–280.

84. Bonham AC, Coles SK, McCrimmon DR. Pulmonary stretch receptor afferents activate excitatory amino acid receptors in the nucleus tractus solitarii in rats. J Physiol 1993; 464:725–745.

85. Henry JL, Sessle BJ. Effects of glutamate, substance P and eledoisin-related peptide on solitary tract neurones involved in respiration and respiratory reflexes. Neuroscience 1985; 14:863–873.

86. Foutz AS, Champagnat J, Denavit-Saubié M. Involvement of *N*-methyl-D-aspartate (NMDA) receptors in respiratory rhythmogenesis. Brain Res 1989; 500:199–208.

87. Feldman JL, Windhorst U, Anders K, Richter DW. Synaptic interaction between medullary respiratory neurones during apneusis induced by NMDA-receptor blockade in cat. J Physiol 1992; 450:303–323.

88. Pierrefiche O, Foutz AS, Champagnat J, Denavit-Saubié M. The bulbar network of

respiratory neurons during apneusis induced by blockade of NMDA receptors. Exp Brain Res 1992; 89:623–639.

89. Vardhan A, Kachroo A, Sapru HN. Excitatory amino acid receptors in commissural nucleus of the NTS mediate carotid chemoreceptor responses. Am J Physiol 1993; 264:R41–R50.

90. Dogas Z, Tonkovic M, Stuth E, Bajic J, Hopp F, McCrimmon DR, Zuperku E. The role of excitatory amino acids in the pulmonary reflex control of expiratory bulbo-spinal (EBS) neurons. FASEB J 1993; 7:A399 (abstract).

91. Guyenet PG, Darnall RA, Riley TA. Rostral ventrolateral medulla and sympatho-respiratory integration in rats. Am J Physiol 1990; 259:R1063–R1074.

92. Abrahams TP, Hornby PJ, Walton DP, Taveira DaSilva AM, Gillis RA. An excitatory amino acid(s) in the ventrolateral medulla is (are) required for breathing to occur in the anesthetized cat. J Pharmacol Exp Ther 1991; 259:1388–1395.

93. Dillon GH, Welsh DE, Waldrop TG. Modulation of respiratory reflexes by an excitatory amino acid mechanism in the ventrolateral medulla. Respir Physiol 1991; 85:55–72.

94. Suzue T. Respiratory rhythm generation in the in vitro brain stem-spinal cord preparation of the neonatal rat. J Physiol 1984; 354:173–183.

95. Connelly CA, Feldman JL. Synergistic roles for NMDA and non-NMDA receptors in brainstem respiratory control in adult rats. Soc Neurosci Abstr 1992; 18:488 (abstract).

96. Onimaru H, Arata A, Homma I. The role of excitatory amino acid (EAA) transmitter in the generation of respiratory rhythm in medulla isolated from newborn rats. Jpn J Physiol 1989; 40:S55 (abstract).

97. Onimaru H, Arata A, Homma I. Firing properties of respiratory rhythm generating neurons in the absence of synaptic transmission in rat medulla in vitro. Exp Brain Res 1989; 76:530–536.

98. Smith JC, Ellenberger HH, Ballanyi K, Richter DW, Feldman JL. Pre-Bötzinger complex: a brainstem region that may generate respiratory rhythm in mammals. Science 1991; 254:726–729.

99. Kashiwagi M, Onimaru H, Homma I. Effects of NMDA on respiratory neurons in newborn rat medulla in vitro. Brain Res Bull 1993; 32:65–69.

100. Connelly CA, Otto-Smith MR, Feldman JL. Blockade of NMDA receptor-channels by MK-801 alters breathing in adult rats. Brain Res 1992; 596:99–110.

101. Clark FJ, Euler C von. On the regulation of depth and rate of breathing. J Physiol 1972; 222:267–295.

102. Feldman JL. Neurophysiology of breathing in mammals. In: Mountcastle VB, Bloom FE, eds. Handbook of Physiology. Section 1, The Nervous System. Vol 4, Intrinsic Regulatory Systems of the Brain. Bethesda, MD: American Physiological Society, 1986:463–524.

103. Bertrand F, Hugelin A. Respiratory synchronizing function of nucleus parabrachialis medialis: pneumotaxic mechanisms. J Neurophysiol 1971; 34:189–207.

104. St. John WM, Glasser RL, King RA. Apneustic breathing after vagotomy in cats with chronic pneumotaxic center lesions. Respir Physiol 1971; 12:239–250.

105. St. John WM, Glasser RL, King RA. Rhythmic respiration in awake vagotomized cats with chronic pneumotaxic area lesions. Respir Physiol 1972; 15:233–244.

106. Euler C von, Marttila I, Remmers JE, Trippenbach T. Effects of lesions in the parabrachial nucleus on the mechanisms for central and reflex termination of inspiration in the cat. Acta Physiol Scand 1976; 96:324–337.

107. Feldman JL, Gautier H. Interaction of pulmonary afferents and pneumotaxic center in control of respiratory pattern in cats. J Neurophysiol 1976; 39:31–44.

108. Monteau R, Errchidi S, Gauthier P, Hilaire G, Rega P. Pneumotaxic centre and apneustic breathing: interspecies differences between rat and cat. Neurosci Lett 1989; 99:311–316.

109. Morrison SF, Cravo SL. Respiratory modulation of splanchnic sympathetic nerve activity in rat after pontine lesions that prolong inspiration. Soc Neurosci Abstr 1993; 19:954 (abstract).

110. Foutz AS, Champagnat J, Denavit-Saubié M. Respiratory effects of the N-methyl-D-aspartate (NMDA) antagonist, MK-801, in intact and vagotomized chronic cats. Eur J Pharmacol 1988; 154:179–184.

111. Foutz AS, Champagnat J, Denavit-Saubié M. N-Methyl-D-aspartate (NMDA) receptors control respiratory off-switch in cat. Neurosci Lett 1988; 87:221–226.

112. Foutz AS, Denavit-Saubié M. Differentiation of phencyclidine and sigma receptor types affecting the central inspiratory termination mechanism in cat. Life Sci 1989; 45:1285–1292.

113. Schweitzer P, Pierrefiche O, Foutz AS, Denavit-Saubié M. Effects of N-methyl-D-aspartate (NMDA) receptor blockade on breathing pattern in newborn cat. Dev Brain Res 1990; 56:290–293.

114. Pierrefiche O, Foutz AS, Denavit-Saubié M. Pneumotaxic mechanisms in the non-human primate: effect of the N-methyl-D-aspartate (NMDA) antagonist ketamine. Neurosci Lett 1990; 119:90–93.

115. Karius DR, Ling L, Speck DF. Blockade of N-methyl-D-aspartate (NMDA) receptors has no effect on certain inspiratory reflexes. Am J Physiol 1991; 261:L443–L448.

116. Sica AL, Siddiqi ZA, Pisana FM. The effects of N-methyl-D-aspartate antagonism on the inspiratory activities of developing animals. Dev Brain Res 1992; 65:281–283.

117. Chae LO, Melton JE, Neubauer JA, Edelman NH. Phrenic and sympathetic nerve responses to glutamergic blockade during normoxia and hypoxia. J Appl Physiol 1993; 74:1954–1963.

118. Monteau R, Gauthier P, Rega P, Hilaire G. Effects of N-methyl-D-aspartate (NMDA) antagonist MK-801 on breathing pattern in rats. Neurosci Lett 1990; 109:134–139.

119. Ling G, Karius DR, Speck DF. Pontine-evoked inspiratory inhibitions after antagonism of NMDA, GABAa, or glycine receptor. J Appl Physiol 1993; 1265–1273.

120. Ling G, Karius DR, Speck DF. Role of NMDA receptors in the pontine pneumotaxic mechanism in the cat. FASEB J 1992; 6:A1825 (abstract).

121. Ling L, Karius DR, Fiscus RR, Speck DF. Endogenous nitric oxide required for an integrative respiratory function in the cat brain. J Neurophysiol 1992; 68:1910–1912.

122. Garthwaite J. Glutamate, nitric oxide and cell-cell signalling in the nervous system. Trends Neurosci 1991; 14:60–67.

123. Garthwaite J, Charles SL, Chess-Williams R. Endothelium-derived relaxing factor release on activation of NMDA receptors suggests a role as intercellular messenger in the brain. Nature 1988; 336:385–388.

124. Ezure K. Synaptic connections between medullary respiratory neurons and considerations on the genesis of respiratory rhythm. Prog Neurobiol 1990; 35:429–450.

125. Richter DW, Ballanyi K, Schwarzacher S. Mechanisms of respiratory rhythm generation. Curr Opin Neurobiol 1992; 2:788–793.

126. Van Giersbergen PLM, Palkovits M, De Jong W. Involvement in neurotransmitters in the nucleus tractus solitarii in cardiovascular regulation. Physiol Rev 1992; 72: 789–824.

127. Arnolda L, Minson J, Kapoor V, Pilowsky P, Llewellyn-Smith I, Chalmers J. Amino acid neurotransmitters in hypertension. Kidney Int 1992; 37(Suppl):S2–S7.

128. Karius DR, Ling L, Speck DF. Excitatory amino acid neurotransmission in superior laryngeal nerve-evoked inspiratory termination. J Appl Physiol 1993; 1840–1847.

129. Hashim MA, Bieger D. Excitatory amino acid receptor-mediated activation of solitarial deglutitive loci. Neuropharmacology 1989; 28:913–921.

130. Kessler J-P, Jean A. Evidence that activation of N-methyl-D-aspartate (NMDA) and non-NMDA receptors within the nucleus tractus solitarii triggers swallowing. Eur J Pharmacol 1991; 201:59–67.

131. Bonham AC, Joad JP. Neurones in commissural nucleus tractus solitarius required for full expression of the pulmonary C-fibre reflex in rat. J Physiol 1991; 441: 95–112.

132. Dietrich WD, Lowry OH, Loewy AD. The distribution of glutamate, GABA and aspartate in the nucleus tractus solitarius of the cat. Brain Res 1982; 237:254–260.

133. Granata AR, Reis DJ. Release of L-³H glutamic acid (L-Glu) and D-³H aspartic acid (D-Asp) in the area of nucleus tractus solitarius in vivo produced by stimulation of vagus nerve. Brain Res 1983; 259:77–95.

134. Granata AR, Sved AF, Reis DJ. In vivo release by vagal stimulation of L-[³H] glutamic acid in the nucleus tractus solitarius preloaded with L-[³H] glutamine. Brain Res Bull 1984; 12:5–9.

135. Meeley MP, Underwood MD, Talman WT, Reis DJ. Content and in vitro release of endogenous amino acids in the area of the nucleus of the solitary tract of the rat. J Neurochem 1989; 53:1807–1817.

136. Drewe JA, Miles R, Kunze DL. Excitatory amino acid receptors of guinea pig medial nucleus tractus solitarius neurons. Am J Physiol 1990; 259:H1389–H1395.

137. Nakagawa T, Shirasaki T, Wakamori M, Fukuda A, Akaike N. Excitatory amino acid response in isolated nucleus tractus solitarii neurons of rat. Neurosci Res 1990; 8:114–123.

138. McGeer PL, Eccles JC, McGeer EG. Molecular Neurobiology of the Mammalian Brain, 2nd ed. New York: Plenum Press, 1987:175–196.

139. Perrone MH. Biochemical evidence that L-glutamate is a neurotransmitter of primary afferent nerve fibers. Brain Res 1981; 230:283–293.

140. Simon JR, DiMicco SK, DiMicco JA, Aprison MH. Choline acetyltransferase and glutamate uptake in the nucleus tractus solitarius and dorsal motor nucleus of the vagus: effect of nodose ganglionectomy. Brain Res 1985; 344:405–408.

141. Sved AF. Lack of change in high affinity glutamate uptake in nucleus tractus solitarius following removal of the nodose ganglion. Brain Res Bull 1986; 16:325–329.

142. Sved AF, Backes MG. Neuroanatomical evidence that vagal afferent nerves do not possess a high affinity uptake system for glutamate. J Auton Nerv Syst 1992; 38:219–230.

143. Schaffar N, Pio J, Jean A. Selective retrograde labeling of primary vagal afferent cell-bodies after injection of [^{3}H]-aspartate into the rat nucleus tractus solitarii. Neurosci Lett 1990; 114:253–258.

144. Miller BD, Felder RB. Excitatory amino acid receptors intrinsic to synaptic transmission in nucleus tractus solitarii. Brain Res 1988; 456:333–343.

145. Andresen MC, Yang M. Non-NMDA receptors mediate sensory afferent synaptic transmission in medial nucleus tractus solitarius. Am J Physiol 1990; 259:H1307–H1311.

146. Paton JFR, Rogers WT, Schwaber JS. Tonically rhythmic neurons within a cardiorespiratory region of the nucleus tractus solitarii of the rat. J Neurophysiol 1991; 66:824–838.

147. Fortin G, Velluti JC, Denavit-Saubié M, Champagnat J. Responses to repetitive afferent activity of rat solitary complex neurons isolated in brainstem slices. Neurosci Lett 1992; 147:89–92.

148. Berger AJ. Dorsal respiratory group neurons in the medulla of cat: spinal projections, responses to lung inflation and superior laryngeal nerve stimulation. Brain Res 1977; 135:231–254.

149. Berger AJ, Dick TE. Connectivity of slowly adapting pulmonary stretch receptors with dorsal medullary respiratory neurons. J Neurophysiol 1987; 58:1259–1274.

150. Karius DR, Speck DF. NMDA receptors are involved in the inspiratory termination elicited by vagal stimulation in cats. FASEB J 1993; 7:A399 (abstract).

151. Housley GD, Martin-Body RL, Dawson NJ, Sinclair JD. Brain stem projections of the glossopharyngeal nerve and its carotid sinus branch in the rat. Neuroscience 1987; 22:237–250.

152. Finley JCW, Katz DM. The central organization of carotid body afferent projections to the brainstem of the rat. Brain Res 1992; 572:108–116.

153. Grippi MA, Pack AI, Davies RO, Fishman AP. Adaptation to reflex effect of prolonged lung inflation. J Appl Physiol 1985; 58:1360–1371.

154. England SJ, Melton JE, Pace P, Neubauer JA. NMDA receptors mediate respiratory short term potentiation in the nucleus tractus solitarius. FASEB J 1992; 6:A1826 (abstract).

155. Glaum SR, Miller RJ. Metabotropic glutamate receptors mediate excitatory transmission in the nucleus of the solitary tract. J Neurosci 1992; 12:2251–2258.

156. Randic M, Hecimovic H, Ryu PD. Substance P modulates glutamate-induced currents in acutely isolated rat spinal dorsal horn neurones. Neurosci Lett 1990; 117:74–80.

157. Palkovits M. Distribution of neuroactive substances in the dorsal vagal complex of the medulla oblongata. Neurochem Int 1985; 7:213–219.

158. Morin-Surun MP, Jordan D, Champagnat J, Spyer KM, Denavit-Saubié M. Excitatory effects of iontophoretically applied substance P on neurons in the nucleus tractus solitarius of the cat: lack of interaction with opiates and opioids. Brain Res 1984; 307:388–392.

159. Pawloski-Dahm C, Gordon FJ. Evidence for a kynurenate-insensitive glutamate receptor in nucleus tractus solitarii. Am J Physiol 1992; 262:H1611–H1615.

160. Talman WT. Kynurenic acid microinjected into the nucleus tractus solitarius of rat blocks the arterial baroreflex but not responses to glutamate. Neurosci Lett 1989; 102:247–252.

161. Kihara M, Kubo T. Immunocytochemical localization of glutamate containing neurons in the ventrolateral medulla oblongata and the nucleus tractus solitarius of the rat. J Hirnforsch 1991; 32:113–118.

162. Jhamandas JH, Harris KH. Excitatory amino acids may mediate nucleus tractus solitarius input to rat parabrachial neurons. Am J Physiol 1992; 263:R324–R330.

163. Takayama K, Miura M. Difference in the distribution of glutamate-immunoreactive neurons projecting into the subretrofacial nucleus in the rostral ventrolateral medulla. Brain Res 1992; 570:259.

164. Duggan AW, Johnston GAR. Glutamate and related amino acids in cat spinal roots, dorsal root ganglion, and peripheral nerves. J Neurochem 1970; 17:1205–1208.

165. Battaglia G, Rustioni A. Co-existence of glutamate and substance P in dorsal root ganglion neurons of the rat and monkey. J Comp Neurol 1988; 277:302–312.

166. Westlund KN, McNeill DL, Coggeshall RE. Glutamate-immunoreactive axons in normal rat dorsal roots. Neurosci Lett 1989; 96:13–17.

167. Westlund KN, McNeill DL, Patterson JT, Coggeshall RE. Aspartate immunoreactive axons in normal rat L4 dorsal roots. Brain Res 1989; 489:347–351.

168. Jeftinija S, Jeftinija K, Liu F, Skilling SR, Smullin DH, Larson AA. Excitatory amino acids are released from rat primary afferent neurons in vitro. Neurosci Lett 1991; 125:191–194.

169. Collingridge GL, Lester RAJ. Excitatory amino acid receptors in the vertebrate central nervous system. Pharmacol Rev 1989; 40:143–210.

170. Jahr CE, Jessel TM. Synaptic transmission between dorsal root ganglion and dorsal horn neurons in culture: antagonism of monosynaptic excitatory synaptic potentials and glutamate excitation by kynurenate. J Neurosci 1985; 5:2281–2289.

171. Jahr CE, Yoshioka K. Ia afferent excitation of motoneurones in the in vitro new born rat spinal cord is selectively antagonised by kynurenate. J Physiol 1986; 370:515–530.

172. Jessell TM, Yoshioka M, Jahr CE. Amino-acid receptor mediated transmission at primary afferent synapses in rat spinal cord. J Exp Biol 1986; 124:239–258.

173. Schneider SP, Pearl ER. Comparison of primary afferent and glutamate excitation of neurons in the mammalian spinal dorsal horn. J Neurosci 1988; 8:2062–2073.

174. Kirkwood PA, Schmid K, Otto M, Sears TA. Focal blockade of single unit synaptic transmission by iontophoresis of antagonists. NeuroReport 1991; 2:185–188.

175. Smith JC, Feldman JL. In vitro brainstem-spinal cord preparations for study of motor systems for mammalian respiration and locomotion. J Neurosci Meth 1987; 21:321–333.

176. Smith JC, Feldman JL. Central respiratory pattern generation studied in an in vitro mammalian brainstem-spinal cord preparation. In: Sieck GC, Gandevia SC, Cameron WE, eds. Neurology and Neurobiology. Vol. 26. Respiratory Muscles and Their Neuromotor Control. New York: Alan R Liss, 1987:27–36.

177. Böhmer G, Schmid K, Schauer W. Evidence for an involvement of NMDA and non-NMDA receptors in synaptic excitation of phrenic motoneurons in the rabbit. Neurosci Lett 1991; 130:271–274.

178. Pierrefiche O, Foutz AS, Denavit-Saubié M. Blockade of non-NMDA glutamate receptors by GYKI 52466 blocks respiratory output but not inspiratory off-switching mechanism in adult cat. Eur J Neurosci 1992; (Suppl 5):2195 (abstract).

179. Greer JJ, Smith JC, Feldman JL. Glutamate release and presynaptic action of AP4 during inspiratory drive to phrenic motoneurons. Brain Res 1992; 576:355–357.

180. Feldman JL, Smith JC. Cellular mechanisms underlying modulation of breathing pattern in mammals. Ann NY Acad Sci 1989; 563:114–130.

181. Olsen RW, McCabe RT, Wamsley JK. $GABA_A$ receptor subtypes: autoradiographic comparison of GABA, benzodiazepine, and convulsant binding sites in the rat central nervous system. J Chem Neuroanat 1990; 3:59–76.

182. Wisden W, Seeburg PH. $GABA_A$ receptor channels, from subunits to functional entities. Curr Opin Neurobiol 1992; 2:263–269.

183. Bonanno G, Raiteri M. Multiple $GABA_B$ receptors. Trends Pharmacol Sci 1993; 14: 259–261.

184. Cutting GR, Luo L, O'Hara BF, Kasch LM, Montrose-Rafizadeh C, Donovan DM, Shimada S, Antonarakis SE, Guggino WB, Uhl GR, Kazazian HH. Cloning of the GABA (rho1) cDNA: a novel $GABA_A$ receptor subunit highly expressed in the retina. Proc Natl Acad Sci USA 1991; 88:2673–2677.

185. Qian H, Dowling JE. Novel GABA responses from rod-driven retinal horizontal cells. Nature 1993; 361:162–164.

186. Purdy RH, Morrow AL, Moore PH, Paul SM. Stress induced elevations of γ-aminobutyric acid type A receptor-active steroids in the rat brain. Proc Natl Acad Sci USA 1991; 88:4318–4322.

187. Gee KW, Lan NC. γ-Aminobutyric acid$_a$ receptor complexes in rat frontal cortex and spinal cord show differential responses to steroid modulation. Mol Pharmacol 1991; 40:995–999.

188. Seeburg PH, Wisden W, Verdoorn TA, Pritchett DB, Werner P, Herb A, Luddens H, Sprengel R, Sakman B. The $GABA_A$ receptor family: molecular and functional diversity. Cold Spring Harbor Symp Quant Biol 1990; LV:29–40.

189. Bureau AN, Olsen RW. Multiple distinct subunits of the γ-aminobutyric acid-A receptor protein show different ligand binding affinities. Mol Pharmacol 1990; 37: 497–502.

190. Whiting P, McKernan RM, Iverson LI. Another mechanism for creating diversity in γ-aminobutyric acid type A receptors: RNA splicing directs expression of two forms of γ2-subunit. Proc Natl Acad Sci USA 1990; 87:9966–9970.

191. Kofuji P, Wang JB, Moss SJ, Huganir RL, Burt DR. Generation of two forms of the γ-aminobutyric acid$_A$ receptor γ2-subunit in mice by alternative splicing. J Neurochem 1991; 56:713–715.

192. Glencourse TA, Bateson AN, Darlison MG. Differential localization of two alternatively spliced GABA$_A$ receptor subunits mRNA's in the chick brain. Eur J Neurosci 1992; 4:271–277.

193. Pritchett DB, Luddens H, Seeburg PH. Type I and type II GABA$_A$-benzodiazepine receptors produced in transfected cells. Science 1989; 245:1389–1392.

194. Verdoorn TA, Draguhn A, Ymer S, Seeburg PH, Sakman B. Functional properties of recombinant rat GABA$_A$ receptors depend upon subunit composition. Neuron 1990; 4:919–928.

195. Puia G, Vicini S, Seeburg PH, Costa E. Influence of recombinant γ-aminobutyric acid$_a$ receptor subunit composition on the action of allosteric modulators of γ-aminobutyric acid-gated Cl⁻ currents. Mol Pharmacol 1991; 39:691–696.

196. Wisden W, Laurie DJ, Monyer H, Seeburg PH. The distribution of 13 GABA$_A$ receptor subunit mRNAs in the rat brain. I. Telencephalon, diencephalon, and mesencephalon. J Neurosci 1992; 12:1040–1062.

197. Wafford KA, Burnett DM, Leiedenheimer NJ, Burt DR, Wang JB, Kofuji P, Dunwiddie TV, Harris RA, Sikela JM. Ethanol sensitivity of the GABA$_A$ receptor expressed in *Xenopus* oocytes requires 8 amino acids contained in the γ2L subunit. Neuron 1991; 7:27–33.

198. Herb A, Wisden W, Luddens H, Puia G, Vicini S, Seeburg PH. The third γ subunit of the γ-aminobutyric acid type A receptor family. Proc Natl Acad Sci USA 1992; 89:1433–1437.

199. Edwards FA, Konnerth A, Sakman B. Quantal analysis of inhibitory transmission in the dentate gyrus of rat hippocampal slices: a patch clamp study. J Physiol 1990; 430:213–249.

200. Perez-Velazquez JL, Angelides KJ. Assembly of GABA$_A$ receptor subunits determines sorting and localization in polarized cells. Nature 1993; 361:457–460.

201. Killisch I, Dotti CG, Laurie DJ, Luddens H, Seeburg PH. Expression Patterns of GABA$_A$ receptor subtypes in developing hippocampal neurons. Neuron 1991; 7: 927–936.

202. MacLennan AJ, Brecha N, Khrestchatisky M, Sternini C, Tillakaratine NJK, Chaing MY, Anderson K, Lai M, Tobin AJ. Independent cellular and ontogenetic expression of mRNA's encoding three α polypeptides of the rat GABA$_A$ receptor. Neuroscience 1991; 43:369–380.

203. Cherubini E, Gaiarsa JL, Yehezkel B. GABA: an excitatory transmitter in early postnatal life. Trends Neurosci 14:1991; 515–519.

204. Misgeld U, Deisz RA, Dodt HU, Lux HD. The role of chloride transport in postsynaptic inhibition of hippocampal neurons. Science 1986; 232:1413–1415.

205. Yuste R, Katz LC. Control of postsynaptic Ca^{++} influx in developing neocortex by excitatory and inhibitory neurotransmitters. Neuron 1991; 6:333–344.

206. Michelson HB, Wong RKS. Excitatory synaptic responses mediated by GABA$_A$ receptors in the hippocampus. Science 1991; 253:1420–1423.

207. Bowery NG, Hill DR, Hudson AL, Doble A, Middlemiss JS, Turnbull M.

(−)Baclofen decreases neurotransmitter release in the mammalian CNS by an action at a novel GABA receptor. Nature 1980; 283:92–94.

208. Kerr DIB, Ong J, Prager RH, Gynther BD, Curtis DR. Phaclofen: a peripheral and central baclofen antagonist. Brain Res 1987; 405:150–154.

209. Kerr DIB, Ong J, Johnston GAR, Abbenante J, Prager RH. 2-Hydroxysaclofen: an improved antagonist at central and peripheral GABA$_B$ receptors. Neurosci Lett 1988; 92:92–96.

210. Olpe H, Karlsson G, Pozza MF, Brugger F, Steinmann M, Riezen H, Fagg G, Hall RG, Froestl W, Bittiger M. CGP 35348: a centrally active blocker of GABA$_B$ receptors. Eur J Pharmacol 1990; 187:27–38.

211. Bowery N. GABA$_B$ receptors and their significance in mammalian pharmacology. Trends Pharmacol Sci 1989; 10:401–407.

212. Andrade R, Malenka RC, Nicoll RA. A G-protein couples serotonin and GABA$_B$ receptors to the same channels in the hippocampus. Science 1986; 234:1261–1265.

213. Dolphin AC, Scott RH. Calcium channel currents and their inhibition by (−)-baclofen in rat sensory neurones: modulation by guanine nucleotides. J Physiol 1987; 386:1–17.

214. Saint DA, Thomas T, Gage PW. GABA$_B$ agonists modulate a transient potassium current in cultured mammalian hippocampal neurons. Neurosci Lett 1990; 118:9–13.

215. Wagner PG, Dekin MS. GABA$_b$ receptors are coupled to a barium-insensitive outward rectifying potassium conductance in premotor respiratory neurons. J Neurophysiol 1993; 69:286–289.

216. Newberry NR, Nicoll RA. Comparison of the action of baclofen with γ-aminobutyric acid on rat hippocampal pyramidal cells in vitro. J Physiol 1985; 360:161–185.

217. Allerton CA, Boden PR, Hill RG. Actions of the GABA$_B$ agonist (−)baclofen on neurons in deep dorsal horn of the rat spinal cord in vitro. Br J Pharmacol 1989; 96:29–38.

218. Lambert NA, Harrison NL, Teyler YJ. Baclofen-induced disinhibition in area CA1 of rat hippocampus is resistant to extracellular Ba^{++}. Brain Res 1991; 547:349–352.

219. Scanziniani M, Capogna M, Gahwiler BH, Thompson SM. Presynaptic inhibition of miniature excitatory synaptic currents by baclofen and adenosine in the hippocampus. Neuron 1992; 9:919–927.

220. Hao JX, Xu XJ, Yu YX, Seiger A, Wiesenfeld-Hallen Z. Baclofen reverses the hypersensitivity of dorsal horn wide dynamic range neurons to mechanical stimulation after transient spinal cord ischemia; implications for a tonic GABAergic inhibitory control of myelinated fiber input. J Neurophysiol 1992; 68:392–396.

221. Innis RB, Nestler EJ, Aghajanian GK. Evidence for G protein mediation of serotonin- and GABA$_B$-induced hyperpolarization of rat dorsal raphe neurons. Brain Res 1988; 459:27–36.

222. Lacey MG, Mercuri NB, North RA. On the potassium conductance increase activated by GABA$_B$ and dopamine D$_2$ receptors in rat substantia nigra neurones. J Physiol 1988; 401:437–453.

223. Dekin MS, Wagner PG. Thyrotropin-releasing hormone inhibits GABA$_B$ activated K$^+$ channels in cultured bulbospinal neurons of the neonatal rat. Soc Neurosci Abstr 1992; 18:488 (abstract).

224. Dekin MS, Sun Y, Wagner PG. Thyrotropin-releasing hormone (TRH) inhibits outward rectifying GABA$_B$ activated K$^+$ channels via a protein kinase C dependent pathway. Soc Neurosci Abstr 1993; 19:1194 (abstract).

225. Zhan W-Z, Ellenberger HH, Feldman JL. Monoaminergic and GABAergic terminations in phrenic motor nucleus of rat identified by immunocytochemical labeling. Neuroscience 1989; 31:105–113.

226. Livingston CA, Berger AJ. Immunocytochemical localization of GABA in neurons projecting to the ventrolateral nucleus of the solitary tract. Brain Res 1989; 494: 143–150.

227. Lipski J, Waldvogel HJ, Pilowski P, Jiang C. GABA-immunoreactive boutons make synapses with inspiratory neurons of the dorsal respiratory group. Brain Res 1990; 529:309–314.

228. Champagnat J, Denavit-Saubié M, Moyanova S, Rondouin G. Involvement of amino acids in periodic inhibitions of bulbar respiratory neurons. Brain Res 1982; 327: 351–365.

229. Takeda R, Haji A. Microiontophoresis of flurazepam on inspiratory and postinspiratory neurons in the ventrolateral medulla of cats: an intracellular study in vivo. Neurosci Lett 1989; 102:261–267.

230. Pierrefiche O, Foutz AS, Denavit-Saubié M. Effects of GABA$_B$ receptor agonists and antagonists on the bulbar respiratory network in cat. Brain Res 1993; 605:77–84.

231. Fedorko L, Merrill EG. Axonal projections from the rostral expiratory of the Bötzinger complex to medulla and spinal cord in the cat. J Physiol 1984; 350: 487–496.

232. Ezure K, Manabe M. Decrementing expiratory neurons of the Bötzinger complex. II. Direct inhibitory synaptic linkage with ventral respiratory group neurons. Exp Brain Res 1988; 72:159–166.

233. Jiang C, Lipski J. Extensive monosynaptic inhibition of ventral respiratory group neurons by augmenting neurons in the Bötzinger complex in the cat. Exp Brain Res 1990; 81:639–648.

234. Nagai T, Maeda T, Imai H, McGeer PL, McGeer EG. Distribution of GABA-T-intensive neurons in the rat hindbrain. J Comp Neurol 1985; 231:260–269.

235. Blessing WW. Distribution of glutamate decarboxylase-containing neurons in rabbit medulla oblongata with attention to intramedullary and spinal projections. Neurosci 1990; 37:171–185.

236. Maley B, Elde RE, Oertel WH, Schmechel DE. The localization of glutamic acid decarboxylase (GAD) immunoreactivity in the nucleus of the solitary tract. Soc Neurosci Abstr 1983; 9:1158 (abstract).

237. Maley B, Newton BW. Immunohistochemistry of γ-aminobutyric acid in the cat nucleus tractus solitarius. Brain Res 1985; 330:364–368.

238. Merrill EG, Fedorko L. Monosynaptic inhibition of phrenic motoneurons: a long descending projection from Bötzinger neurons. J Neurosci 1984; 4:2350–2353.

239. Millhorn DE, Hökfelt T, Seroogy K, Oertel W, Verhofstad AA, Wu JY. Immunohistochemical evidence for colocalization of gamma-aminobutyric acid and serotonin in neurons of the ventral medulla oblongata projecting to the spinal cord. Brain Res 1987; 410:179–185.

240. Mugnaini E, Oertel WH. An atlas of the distribution of GABA-ergic neurons and terminals in the rat CNS as revealed by GAD immunohistochemistry. In: Björklund A, Hökfelt T, eds. Handbook of Chemical Neuroanatomy, Vol. 4, Part 1. Amsterdam: Elsevier, 1985:436–608.

241. Da Silva AMT, Hartly B, Hamosh P, Quest J, Gillis RA. Respiratory depressant effects of GABA α- and β-receptor agonists in the cat. J Appl Physiol 1987; 62: 2264–2272.

242. Kneussl MP, Pappagianopoulos P, Hoop B, Kazemi H. Reversible depression of ventilation and cardiovascular function by ventriculocisternal perfusion with gamma-aminobutyric acid in dogs. Am Rev Respir Dis 1986; 133:1024–1028.

243. Yamada KA, Hamoush P, Gillis RA. Respiratory depression produced by activation of GABA receptors in hindbrain of cat. J Appl Physiol 1981; 5:1278–1286.

244. Yamada KA, Norman WP, Hamoush P, Gillis RA. Medullar ventral surface GABA receptors affect respiratory and cardiovascular function. Brain Res 1982; 248: 71–78.

245. Hayashi F, Lipski J. The role of inhibitory amino acids in the control of respiratory motor output in an arterially perfused rat. Respir Physiol 1992; 89:47–63.

246. Hedner J, Hedner T, Wessberg P, Jonason J. An analysis of the mechanisms by which γ-aminobutyric acid depresses ventilation in the cat. J Appl Physiol 1984; 56: 849–856.

247. Melton JE, Neubauer JA, Edelman NH. GABA antagonism reverses hypoxic respiratory depression in the cat. J Appl Physiol 1990; 69:1296–1301.

248. Ballantyne D, Richter DW. Postsynaptic inhibition of bulbar inspiratory neurons of cats. J Physiol 1984; 348:67–87.

249. Remmers JE, Richter DW, Ballantyne D, Bainton CR, Klein JP. Reflex prolongation of stage I of expiration. Pflügers Arch 1986; 407:190–198.

250. Richter DW. Generation and maintenance of the respiratory rhythm. J Exp Biol 1982; 100:93–107.

251. Richter DW, Camerer H, Meesman M, Rohrig N. Studies on the synaptic interconnection between bulbar respiratory neurons of cats. Pflügers Arch 1979; 380: 245–357.

252. Takeda R, Haji A, Hukuhara T. Diazepam potentiates postsynaptic inhibition in bulbar respiratory neurons of cats. Respir Physiol 1989; 77:173–186.

253. Haji A, Remmers JE, Connelly C, Takeda R. Effects of glycine and GABA on bulbar respiratory neurons of cat. J Neurophysiol 1990; 63:955–965.

254. Haji A, Takeda R, Remmers JE. Evidence that glycine and GABA mediate postsynaptic inhibition of bulbar respiratory neurons in the cat. J Appl Physiol 1992; 73:2333–2342.

255. Fedorko L, Connelly CA, Remmers JE. Neurotransmitter mediating synaptic inhibition of phrenic motoneurons. In: Sieck GC, Gandevia SC, Cameron WE, eds. Neurology and Neurobiology. Vol. 26. Respiratory Muscles and Their Neuromotor Control. New York: Alan R Liss, 1987:167–173.

256. Lalley PM. Biphasic effects of Baclofen on phrenic motoneurons: possible involvement of two types of γ-aminobutyric acid (GABA) receptors. J Pharmacol Exp Ther 1983; 226:616–624.

257. Lalley PM. Baclofen: unexpected disinhibitory effects of lioresal on cardiovascular and respiratory neurons. Brain Res Bull 1980; 5:565–573.

258. Lalley PM. Effects of baclofen and γ-aminobutyric acid on different types of medullary respiratory neurons. Brain Res 1986; 376:392–395.

259. Schmid K, Böhmer G, Gebauer K. GABA_B receptor mediated effects on the central respiratory system and their antagonism by phaclofen. Neurosci Lett 1989; 99: 305–310.

260. Hedner J, Hedner T, Jonason J, Lundberg D. GABAergic mechanisms in central respiratory control in the anesthetized rat. Naunyn-Schmiedeberg's Arch Pharmacol 1981; 317:315–320.

261. Brooks PA, Glaum SR, Miller RJ, Spyer KM. The actions of baclofen on neurons and synaptic transmission in the nucleus tractus solitarii of the rat in vitro. J Physiol 1992; 457:115–129.

262. Sun Y, Wagner PG, Dekin MS. Regulation of neurotransmitter release by GABA and TRH within the phrenic motor nucleus of neonatal rats. Soc Neurosci Abstr 1993; 19:1193 (abstract).

263. Dekin MS, Getting PA. Firing pattern of neurons in the nucleus tractus solitarius: modulation by membrane hyperpolarization. Brain Res 1984; 324:180–184.

264. Champagnat J, Jacquin T, Richter D. Voltage dependent currents in neurons of the nuclei of the solitary tract of rat brainstem slices. Pflügers Arch 1986; 406:272–379.

265. Dekin MS, Getting PA. In vitro characterization of neurons in the ventral part of the nucleus tractus solitarius. II. Ionic mechanisms responsible for repetitive firing activity. J Neurophysiol 1987; 58:215–229.

266. Cooper JR, Bloom FE, Roth RH. The Biochemical Basis of Neuropharmacology. New York: Oxford University Press, 1991.

267. Fuxe K, Agnati LF. Two principal modes of electrochemical communication in the brain: volume versus wiring transmission. In: Fuxe K, Agnati LF, eds. Volume Transmission in the Brain. New York: Raven Press, 1991:1–9.

268. Bach-Y-Rita P. Neurotransmission in the brain through the extracellular fluid. NeuroReport 1993; 4:343–350.

269. Anwyl R. Neurophysiological actions of 5-hydroxytryptamine in the vertebrate nervous system. Prog Neurobiol 1990; 35:451–468.

270. Bobker DH, Williams JT. Ion conductances affected by 5-HT receptor subtypes in mammalian neurons. Trends Neurosci 1990; 13:169–173.

271. Wallis DI, Elliott P. The electrophysiology of 5-HT. In: Fozard JR, Saxena PR, eds. Serotonin: Molecular Biology, Receptors and Functional Effects. Berlin: Birkhauser Verlag, 1991:203–219.

272. Hökfelt T, Johansson O, Ljungdahl A, Lundberg JM, Schultzberg M. Peptidergic neurones. Nature 1980; 284:515–521.

273. Azmitia EC, Whitaker-Azmitia PM. Awakening the sleeping giant: anatomy and plasticity of the brain serotonergic system. J Clin Psychiatry 1991; 52:4–16.

274. Jacobs BL, Azmitia EC. Structure and function of the brain serotonin system. Physiol Rev 1992; 75:165–229.

275. Whitaker-Azmitia PM, Azmitia EC. Serotonin trophic factors in development,

plasticity and aging. In: Fozard JR, Saxena PR, eds. Serotonin: Molecular Biology, Receptors and Functional Effects. Berlin: Birkhauser Verlag, 1991:43–49.

276. Bailey CH, Chen M, Keller F, Kandel ER. Serotonin-mediated endocytosis of apcam: an early step of learning-related synaptic growth in Aplysia. Science 1992; 256:645–649.

277. Mayford M, Barzilai A, Keller F, Schacher S, Kandel ER. Modulation of an NCAM-related adhesion molecule with long-term synaptic plasticity in *Aplysia*. Science 1992; 256:638–644.

278. Jacobs BL. Serotonin and behavior: emphasis on motor control. J Clin Psychiatry 1991; 52(suppl. 12):17–23.

279. Jacobs BL, Fornal CA. 5-HT and motor control: a hypothesis. Trends Neurosci 1993; 16:346–352.

280. Hamon M, Bourgoin S, Artaud F, El Mestikawy S. The respective roles of tryptophan uptake and tryptophan hydroxylase in the regulation of serotonin synthesis in the central nervous system. J Physiol 1981; 77:269–279.

281. Azmitia EC, Algeri S, Costa E. In vivo conversion of ^{3}H-L-tryptophan into ^{3}H-serotonin in brain areas of adrenalectomized rats. Science 1970; 169:201–203.

282. Friedman PA, Kappelman AH, Kaufman S. Partial purification and characterization of tryptophan hydroxylase from rabbit hind brain. J Biol Chem 1972; 247:4165–4173.

283. Armijo JA, Flórez J. The influence of increased brain 5-hydroxytryptamine upon the respiratory activity of cats. Neuropharmacology 1974; 13:977–986.

284. Davis N, Carlsson A, MacMillan V, Siesjo BK. Brain tryptophan hydroxylation: dependence on arterial oxygen tension. Science 1973; 182:72–74.

285. Olson EB, Jr, Vidruk EH, McCrimmon DR, Dempsey JA. Monoamine neurotransmitter metabolism during acclimatization to hypoxia in rats. Respir Physiol 1983; 54:79–96.

286. Mitchell GS. In vitro studies of respiratory control: an overview. In: Speck DF, Dekin MS, Revelette WR, Frazier DT, eds. Respiratory Control: Central and Peripheral Mechanisms. Lexington: University Press of Kentucky, 1993:30–33.

287. Chaouloff F. Physical exercise and brain monoamines: a review. Acta Physiol Scand 1989; 137:1–13.

288. Brown BS, Payne T, Kim C, Moore G, Krebs P, Martin W. Chronic response of rat brain norepinephrine and serotonin levels to endurance training. J Appl Physiol 1979; 46:19–23

289. Gerin C, Marlier L, Legrand A, Privat A. An in vivo microdialysis study of the release of serotonin in the spinal cord ventral horn of treadmill-running rats. Soc Neurosci Abstr 1992; 18:858 (abstract).

290. Bach KB, Lutcavage ME, Mitchell GS. Serotonin is necessary for short-term modulation of the exercise ventilatory response. Respir Physiol 1993; 91:57–70.

291. McEwen BS, Davis PG, Parsons B, Pfaff DW. The brain as a target for steroid hormone action. Annu Rev Neurosci 1979; 2:65–112.

292. Chaouloff F. Physiopharmacological interactions between stress hormones and central serotonergic systems. Brain Res Rev 1993; 18:1–32.

293. Fuxe K, Jonsson G. Further mapping of central 5-hydroxytryptamine neurons: studies with the neurotoxic dihydroxytryptamines. Adv Biochem Psychopharmacol 1974; 10:1–12.

294. Skagerberg G, Björklund A. Topographic principles in the spinal projections of serotonergic and non-serotonergic brainstem neurons in the rat. Neuroscience 1985; 15:445–480.

295. Molliver ME. Serotonergic neuronal systems: What their anatomic organization tells us about function. J Clin Psychopharmacol 1987; 7:3S–23S.

296. Parnavelas JG, Papadopoulos GC. The monoaminergic innervation of the cerebral cortex is not diffuse and nonspecific. Trends Neurosci 1989; 12:315–319.

297. Holstege JC, Kuypers HGJM. Brainstem projections to spinal motoneurons: an update. Neuroscience 1987; 23:809–821.

298. Marlier L, Sandillon F, Poulat P, Rajaofetra N, Geffard M, Privat A. Serotonergic innervation of the dorsal horn of rat spinal cord: light and electron microscopic immunocytochemical study. J Neurocytol 1991; 20:310–322.

299. Ridet J-L, Rajaofetra N, Teilhac J-R, Geffard M, Privat A. Evidence for nonsynaptic serotonergic and noradrenergic innervation of the rat dorsal horn and possible involvement of neuron-glia interactions. Neuroscience 1993; 52:143–157.

300. Voss MD, DeCastro D, Lipski J, Pilowsky PM, Jiang C. Serotonin immunoreactive boutons form close appositions with respiratory neurons of the dorsal respiratory group in the cat. J Comp Neurol 1990; 295:208–218.

301. Connelly CA, Ellenberger HH, Feldman JL. Are these serotonergic projections from raphe and retrotrapezoid nuclei to the ventral respiratory group in the rat? Neurosci Lett 1989; 105:34–40.

302. Pilowsky PM, de Castro D, Llewellyn-Smith I, Lipski J, Voss MD. Serotonin immunoreactive boutons make synapses with feline phrenic motoneurons. J Neurosci 1990; 10:1091–1098.

303. Holtman JR, Jr., Norman WP, Gillis RA. Projections from the raphe nuclei to the phrenic motor nucleus in the cat. Neurosci Lett 1984; 44:105–111.

304. Holtman JR, Jr., Norman WP, Skirboll L, Dretchen KL, Cuello C, Visser TJ, Hökfelt T, Gillis RA. Evidence for 5-hydroxytryptamine, substance P, and thyrotropin-releasing hormone in neurons innervating the phrenic motor nucleus. J Neurosci 1984; 4;1064–1071.

305. Jiang Z-H, Shen E. Synaptic connection between monoaminergic terminals and intercostal respiratory motoneurons in cats. Acta Physiol Sinica 1985; 37:479–485.

306. Holtman JR, Jr, Dick TE, Berger AJ. Serotonin-mediated excitation of recurrent laryngeal and phrenic motoneurons evoked by stimulation of the raphe obscurus. Brain Res 1987; 417:12–20.

307. Holtman JR, Jr. Immunohistochemical localization of serotonin- and substance P–containing fibers around respiratory muscle motoneurons in the nucleus ambiguus of the cat. Neuroscience 1988; 26:169–178.

308. Aldes LD, Marco LA, Chronister RB. Serotonin-containing axon terminals in the hypoglossal nucleus of the rat. An immuno-electronmicroscopic study. Brain Res Bull 1989; 23:249–256.

309. Jiang C, Mitchell GS, Lipski J. Prolonged augmentation of respiratory discharge in

hypoglossal motoneurons following superior laryngeal nerve stimulation. Brain Res 1991; 538:215–225.

310. Holtman JR, Jr., Vascik DS, Maley BE. Ultrastructural evidence for serotonin-immunoreactive terminals contracting phrenic motoneurons in the cat. Exp Neurol 1990; 109:269–272.

311. Vu Et, Krasne FB. Evidence for a computational distinction between proximal and distal neuronal inhibition. Science 1992; 255:1710–1712.

312. Arita H, Sakamoto M, Hirokawa Y, Odado N. Serotonin innervation patterns differ among the various medullary motoneuronal groups involved in upper airway control. Exp Brain Res 1993; 95:100–110.

313. Lipski J, Barton C, de Castro D, Jiang C, Llewellyn-Smith I, Mitchell GS, Pilowsky PM, Voss MD, Waldvogel HJ. Neurotransmitter content of respiratory neurons and their inputs: Double-labeling studies using intracellular tracers and immuno-histochemistry. In: Speck DF, Dekin MS, Revelette WR, Frazier DT, eds. Respiratory Control: Central and Peripheral Mechanisms. Lexington: University Press of Kentucky, 1993:60–65.

314. Carlton SM, Steinman JL, Hillman GR, Willis WD. Differential effects of p-chlorophenylalanine on indoleamines in brainstem nuclei and spinal cord of rats. II. Identification of immunohistochemically stained structures using computer-assisted image enhancement techniques. Brain Res 1987;426:310–322.

315. Steinman JL, Carlton SM, Haber B, Willis WD. Differential effects of p-chlorophenylalanine on indoleamines in brainstem nuclei and spinal cord of rats. I. Biochemical and behavioral analysis. Brain Res 1987; 426:297–309.

316. Tohyama I, Kameyama M, Kimura H. Quantitative morphometric analysis of two types of serotonin-immunoreactive nerve fibres differentially responding to p-chlorophenylalanine treatment in the rat brain. Neuroscience 1988; 26:971–991.

317. Wu W, Elde R, Wessendorf MW. Organization of the serotonergic innervation of spinal neurons in rats. III. Differential serotonergic innervation of somatic and parasympathetic preganglionic motoneurons as determined by patterns of co-existing peptides. Neuroscience 1993; 55:223–233.

318. Das M, Mohanakumar KP, Chauhan SPS, Ganguly DK. 5-Hydroxytryptamine in the phrenic nerve diaphragm: evidence for its existence and release. Neurosci Lett 1989; 97:345–349.

319. Riddell JS, Jankowska E, Eide E. Depolarization of group II muscle afferents by stimuli applied in the locus coeruleus and raphe nuclei of the cat. J Physiol 1992; 461:723–741.

320. Jankowska E, Riddell JS, Skoog B, Noga BR. Gating of transmission to moto-neurones by stimuli applied in the locus coeruleus and raphe nuclei of the cat. J Physiol 1993; 461:705–722.

321. Mosko SS, Jacobs BL. Recording of dorsal raphe unit activity in vitro. Neurosci Lett 1976; 2:195–200.

322. Aghajanian GK, Foote WE, Sheard MH. Lysergic acid diethylamide: sensitive neuronal units in the midbrain raphe. Science 1968; 161:706–708.

323. Aghajanian GK, Foote WE, Sheard MH. Action of psychotogenic drugs on single midbrain raphe neurons. J Pharmacol Exp Ther 1970; 171:178–187.

324. Aghajanian GK, VanderMaelen CP. Intracellular recordings from serotonergic dorsal raphe neurons: pacemaker potentials and the effect of LSD. Brain Res 1982; 238:463–469.

325. VanderMaelen CP, Aghajanian GK. Electrophysiological and pharmacological characterization of serotonergic dorsal raphe neurons recorded extracellularly and intracellularly in rat brain slices. Brain Res 1983; 289:109–119.

326. Moolenaar G-M, Holloway JA, Trouth CO. Responses of caudal raphe neurons to peripheral somatic stimulation. Exp Neurol 1976; 53:304–313.

327. Haselton JR, Winters RW, Liskowsky DR, Haselton CL, McCabe PM, Schneiderman N. Anatomical and functional connections of neurons of the rostral medullary raphe of the rabbit. Brain Res 1988; 453:176–182.

328. Grahn DA, Heller HC. Activity of most rostral ventromedial medulla neurons reflect EEG/EMG pattern changes. Am J Physiol 1989; 257:R1496–R1505.

329. Blair RW, Evans AR. Responses of medullary raphe spinal neurons to electrical stimulation of thoracic sympathetic afferents, vagal afferents, and to other sensory inputs in cats. J Neurophysiol 1991; 66:2084–2094.

330. Gang S, Mizuguchi A, Aoki M. Axonal projections from the pontine pneumotaxic region to the nucleus raphe magnus in cats. Respir Physiol 1991; 85:329–339.

331. Yates BJ, Goto T, Bolton PS. Responses of neurons in the caudal medullary raphe nuclei of the cat to stimulation of the vestibular nerve. Exp Brain Res 1992; 89: 323–332.

332. Lindsey BG, Hernandez YM, Morris KF, Shannon R. Functional connectivity between brain stem midline neurons with respiratory-modulated firing rates. J Neurophysiol 1992; 67:890–904.

333. Lindsey BG, Hernandez YM, Morris KF, Shannon R, Gerstein GL. Respiratory-related neural assemblies in the brain stem midline. J Neurophysiol 1992; 67:905–922.

334. Lindsey BG, Hernandez YM, Morris KF, Shannon R, Gerstein GL. Dynamic reconfiguration of brain stem neural assemblies: respiratory phase-dependent synchrony versus modulation of firing rates. J Neurophysiol 1992; 67:923–930.

335. Heym J, Steinfels GF, Jacobs BL. Activity of serotonin-containing neurons in the nucleus raphe pallidus of freely moving cats. Brain Res 1982; 251:259–276.

336. Heym J, Trulson ME, Jacobs BL. Raphe unit activity in freely moving cats: effects of phasic auditory and visual stimuli. Brain Res 1982; 232:29–39.

337. Fornal C, Auerbach S, Jacobs BL. Activity of serotonin-containing neurons in nucleus raphe magnus in freely moving cats. Exp Neurol 1985; 88:590–608.

338. Holtman JR, Jr., Anastasi NC, Norman WP, Dretchen KL. Effect of electrical and chemical stimulation of the raphe obscurus on phrenic nerve activity in the cat. Brain Res 1986; 362:214–220.

339. Holtman JR, Jr., Dick TE, Berger AJ. Involvement of serotonin in the excitation of phrenic motoneurons evoked by stimulation of the raphe obscurus. J Neurosci 1986; 6:1185–1193.

340. Millhorn DE. Stimulation of raphe (obscurus) nucleus causes long-term potentiation of phrenic nerve activity in cat. J Physiol 1986; 381:169–179.

341. Lalley PM. Responses of phrenic motoneurones of the cat to stimulation of medullary raphe nuclei. J Physiol 1986; 380:349–371.

342. Lalley PM. Serotoninergic and non-serotoninergic responses of phrenic motoneurones to raphe stimulation in the cat. J Physiol 1986; 380:373–385.

343. Morin D, Hennequin S, Monteau R, Hilaire G. Depressant effect of raphe stimulation on inspiratory activity of the hypoglossal nerve: in vitro study in the newborn rat. Neurosci Lett 1990; 116:299–303.

344. Aoki M, Fujito Y, Kurosawa Y, Kawasaki H, Kosaka I. Descending inputs to the upper cervical inspiratory neurons from the medullary respiratory neurons and the raphe nuclei in the cat. In: Sieck GC, Gandevia SC, Cameron WE, eds. Neurology and Neurobiology. Vol. 26. Respiratory Muscles and Their Neuromotor Control. New York: Alan R. Liss, 1987:73–82.

345. Mitchell GS, Sloan HE, Jiang C, Miletic V, Hayashi F, Lipski J. 5-Hydroxytryptophan (5-HTP) augments spontaneous and evoked phrenic motoneuron discharge in spinalized rats. Neurosci Lett 1992; 141:75–78.

346. Ling L, Bach KB, Mitchell GS. Serotonin reveals ineffective spinal pathways to contralateral phrenic motoneurons in hemisected rats. FASEB J 1993; 7:A401 (abstract).

347. Schmid K, Böhmer G, Merkelbach S. Serotonergic control of phrenic motoneuronal activity at the level of the spinal cord of the rabbit. Neurosci Lett 1990; 116:204–209.

348. Brodin E, Linderoth B, Goiny M, Yamamoto Y, Gazelius B, Millhorn DE, Hökfelt T, Ungerstedt U. In vivo release of serotonin in cat dorsal vagal complex and cervical ventral horn induced by electrical stimulation of the medullary raphe nuclei. Brain Res 1990; 535:227–236.

349. Iverfeldt K, Serfozo P, Arnesto LD, Bartfai T. Differential release of coexisting neurotransmitters: frequency dependence of the efflux of substance P, thyrotropin releasing hormone and [^{3}H]serotonin from tissue slices of rat ventral spinal cord. Acta Physiol Scand 1989; 137:63–71.

350. Schmidt AW, Peroutka SJ. 5-Hydroxytryptamine receptor "families." FASEB J 1989; 3:2242–2249 (abstract).

351. Bockaert J, Fozard JR, Dumuis A, Clarke DE. The 5-HT$_4$ receptor: a place in the sun. Trends Pharmacol Sci 1992; 13:141–145.

352. Peters JA, Malone HM, Lambert JJ. Recent advances in the electrophysiological characterization of 5-HT$_3$ receptors. Trends Pharmacol Sci 1992; 13:391–397.

353. Humphrey PPA, Hartig P, Hoyer D. A proposed nomenclature for 5-HT receptors. Trends Pharmacol Sci 1993; 14:233–236.

354. Prentice DJ, Barrett VJ, MacLennan SJ, Martin GR. Temperature dependence of agonist and antagonist affinity constants at 5-HT$_1$-like and 5-HT$_2$ receptors. In: Fozard JR, Saxena PR, eds. Serotonin: Molecular Biology, Receptors and Functional Effects. Berlin: Birkhauser Verlag, 1991:161–173.

355. Marlier L, Teilhac J-R, Cerruti C, Privat A. Autoradiographic mapping of 5-HT$_1$, 5-HT$_{1a}$, 5-HT$_{1b}$ and 5-HT$_2$ receptors in the rat spinal cord. Brain Res 1991; 550: 15–23.

356. Sessle BJ, Henry JL. Effects of enkephalin and 5-Hydroxytryptamine on solitary tract neurones involved in respiratory and respiratory reflexes. Brain Res 1985; 327:221–230.

357. Champagnat J, Branchereau P, Denavit-Saubié M, Fortin G, Jacquin T, Schweitzer P.

New insights on synaptic transmission in the nucleus tractus solitarius. In: Speck DF, Dekin MS, Revelette WR, Frazier DT, eds. Respiratory Control: Central and Peripheral Mechanisms. Lexington: University Press of Kentucky, 1993:15–20.

358. Jacquin T, Denavit-Saubié M, Champagnat J. Substance P and serotonin mutually reverse their excitatory effects in the rat nucleus tractus solitarius. Brain Res 1989; 502:214–222.

359. Arita H, Ochiishi M. Opposing effects of 5-hydroxytryptamine on two types of medullary inspiratory neurons with distinct firing patterns. J Neurophysiol 1991; 66:285–292.

360. Monteau R, Morin D, Hennequin S, Hilaire G. Differential effects of serotonin on respiratory activity of hypoglossal and cervical motoneurons: an in vitro study on the newborn rat. Neurosci Lett 1990; 111:127–132.

361. Morin D, Monteau R, Hilaire G. 5-Hydroxytryptamine modulates central respiratory activity in the newborn rat: an in vitro study. Eur J Pharmacol 1991; 192:89–95.

362. Lindsay AD, Feldman JL. Modulation of respiratory activity of neonatal rat phrenic motoneurones by serotonin. J Physiol 1993; 461:213–233.

363. Olson EB, Jr, Dempsey JA, McCrimmon DR. Serotonin and the control of ventilation in awake rats. J Clin Invest 1979; 64:689–693.

364. Mitchell GS, Smith CA, Jameson LC, Vidruk EH, Dempsey JA. Effects of p-chlorophenylalanine on ventilatory control in goats. J Appl Physiol 1983; 54:277–283.

365. Millhorn DE, Eldridge FL, Waldrop TG, Klinger LE. Centrally and peripherally administered 5-HTP have opposite effects on respiration. Brain Res 1983; 264: 349–354.

366. Anderson EG, Shibuya T. The effects of 5-hydroxytryptophan and l-tryptophan on spinal synaptic activity. J Pharmacol Exp Ther 1966; 153:352–360.

367. Myslinski NR, Anderson EG. The effect of serotonin precursors on α- and γ-motoneuron activity. J Pharmacol Exp Ther 1978; 204:19–26.

368. VanderMaelen CP, Aghajanian GK. Intracellular studies showing modulation of facial motoneurone excitability by serotonin. Nature 1980; 287:346–347.

369. Berger AJ, Takahashi T. Serotonin enhances a low-voltage-activated calcium current in rat spinal motoneurons. J Neurosci 1990; 10:1922–1928.

370. Jackson DA, White SR. Receptor subtypes mediating facilitation by serotonin of excitability of spinal motoneurons. Neuropharmacology 1990; 29:787–797.

371. Monteau R, Hilaire G. Spinal respiratory motoneurons. Prog Neurobiol 1991; 37: 83–144.

372. Elliott P, Wallis DI. Serotonin and l-norepinephrine as mediators of altered excitability in neonatal rat motoneurons studied in vitro. Neuroscience 1992; 47:533–544.

373. Morin D, Monteau R, Hilaire G. Compared effects of serotonin on cervical and hypoglossal inspiratory activities: an in vitro study in the newborn rat. J Physiol 1992; 451:605–629.

374. Rasmussen K, Aghajanian GK. Serotonin excitation of facial motoneurons: receptor subtype characterization. Synapse 1990; 5:324–332.

375. Aghajanian GK. Serotonin-induced inward current in rat facial motoneurons: evidence for mediation by G proteins but not protein kinase C. Brain Res 1990; 524: 171–174.

376. Kubin L, Tojima H, Davies RO, Pack AI. Serotonergic excitatory drive to hypoglossal motoneurons in the decerebrate cat. Neurosci Lett 1992; 139:243–248.

377. Berger AJ, Bayliss DA, Viana F. Modulation of neonatal rat hypoglossal motoneuron excitability by serotonin. Neurosci Lett 1992; 143:164–168.

378. Kiehn O. Plateau potentials and active integration in the "final common pathway" for motor behavior. Trends Neurosci 1991; 14:68–73.

379. White SR. A comparison of the effects of serotonin, substance P and thyrotropin-releasing hormone on excitability of rat spinal motoneurons in vivo. Brain Res 1985; 335:63–70.

380. Cardona A, Rudomin P. Activation of brainstem serotonergic pathways decreases homosynaptic depression of monosynaptic responses of frog spinal motoneurons. Brain Res 1983; 280:373–378.

381. Millhorn DE. Physiological significance of pharmacological studies of respiratory regulation. In: Euler C von, Lagercrantz H, eds. Neurobiology of the Control of Breathing. New York: Raven Press, 1986:89–95.

382. Cao K-Y, Zwillich CW, Berthon-Jones M, Sullivan CE. Increased normoxic ventilation induced by repetitive hypoxia in conscious dogs. J Appl Physiol 1992; 73:2083–2088.

383. Engwall MJA, Daristotle L, Niu WZ, Dempsey JA, Bisgard GE. Ventilatory afterdischarge in the awake goat. J Appl Physiol 1991; 71:1511–1517.

384. Wagner PG, Eldridge FL. Development of short-term potentiation of respiration. Respir Physiol 1991; 83:129–140.

385. Millhorn DE, Eldridge FL, Waldrop TG. Prolonged stimulation of respiration by a new central neural mechanism. Respir Physiol 1980; 41:87–103.

386. Millhorn DE, Eldridge FL, Waldrop TG. Prolonged stimulation of respiration by endogenous central serotonin. Respir Physiol 1980; 42:171–188.

387. Fregosi RF, Essif E, Mitchell GS. Long-term facilitation (LTF) of inspiratory intercostal (iic) nerve activities after carotid sinus nerve stimulation (CSN stim.). FASEB J 1992; 6:A1507 (abstract).

388. Powell FL, Aaron EA. Long-term facilitation of ventilation after hypoxia in awake rats. FASEB J 1993; 7:A397 (abstract).

389. Dempsey JA, Forster HV. Mediation of ventilatory adaptations. Physiol Rev 1982; 62:262–346.

390. Olson EB, Jr. Ventilatory adaptation to hypoxia occurs in serotonin-depleted rats. Respir Physiol 1987; 69:227–235.

391. Engwall MJA, Bisgard GE. Ventilatory responses to chemoreceptor stimulation after hypoxic acclimatization in awake goats. J Appl Physiol 1990; 69:1236–1243.

392. Krupa DJ, Thompson JK, Thompson RF. Localization of a memory trace in the mammalian brain. Science 1993; 260:989–991.

393. Erickson JT, Millhorn DE. Fos-like protein is induced in neurons of the medulla oblongata after stimulation of the carotid sinus nerve in awake and anesthetized rats. Brain Res 1991; 567:11–24.

394. Morris KF, Arata A, Shannon R, Lindsey BG. Concurrent effects of carotid chemoreceptor stimulation of distributed brain stem respiratory neural networks. Soc Neurosci Abstr 1991; 17:103 (abstract).

395. Mitchell GS. Ventilatory control during exercise with increased respiratory dead space in goats. J Appl Physiol 1990; 69:718–727.

396. Poon C-S. Potentiation of exercise ventilatory response by airway CO_2 and dead space loading. J Appl Physiol 1992; 73:591–595.

397. Mitchell GS, Smith CA, Dempsey JA. Changes in the VI:Vco$_2$ relationship during exercise in goats: role of carotid bodies. J Appl Physiol 1984; 57:1894–1900.

398. Mitchell GS, Bach KB, Martin PA, Foley KT. Modulation and plasticity of the exercise ventilatory response. Funct Biol Syst (in press).

399. Mitchell GS, Douse MA, Foley KT. Receptor interactions in modulating ventilatory activity. Am J Physiol 1990; 259:R911–R920.

400. Sloan HE, Miletic V, Bowen KK, Foley KT, Mitchell GS. Chronic thoracic dorsal rhizotomy alters immunoreactive CGRP and substance P in the dorsal horn of goats. Soc Neurosci Abstr 1990; 16:1072 (abstract).

401. Goldberger ME. Partial and complete deafferation of cat hindlimb: the contribution of behavioral substitution to recovery of motor function. Exp Brain Res 1988; 73:343–353.

402. Martin P, Mitchell GS. Long term modulation of the exercise ventilatory response. J Physiol 1993; 470:601–617.

403. Mitchell GS, Sloan HE, Foley KT, Brownfield MS, Miletic V. Increased serotonin in the thoracic spinal cord of goats following chronic thoracic dorsal rhizotomy (TDR). FASEB J 1992; 6:A1507 (abstract).

404. Murray M. Plasticity in the spinal cord: the dorsal root connection. Restor Neurol Neurosci 1993; 5:37–45.

405. Hashimoto T, Fukuda N. Contribution of serotonin neurons to the functional recovery after spinal cord injury in rats. Brain Res 1991; 539:263–270.

5

Central Pathways of Pulmonary and Airway Vagal Afferents

LESZEK KUBIN and RICHARD O. DAVIES

School of Veterinary Medicine, University of Pennsylvania
Philadelphia, Pennsylvania

I. Introduction

Three major receptor systems feed peripheral information to central respiratory neurons in the process of maintaining homeostasis: the peripheral arterial chemoreceptors, skeletal muscle and joint receptors, and the receptors distributed within the lungs and airways. Concerning the last system, several recent reviews cover the properties of individual receptor types (e.g., 1–4) and the input-output characteristics of the cardiorespiratory reflexes as tested by stimulation of selected subtypes of these receptors (e.g., 1,3,5–11; see also Chapter 2, this volume). However, the focus of these reviews did not allow them to provide an in-depth discussion of the knowledge that has accumulated over the last decade on the topic of central pathways of specific, modality-identified receptors important for the regulation of breathing. One notable exception is the review by Jordan and Spyer (12), which extensively covers the central pathways from arterial chemo- and baroreceptors. Consequently, we will focus on the corresponding pathways of vagal afferents from the lungs and airways. (See Chapter 4 for a review of the neurotransmitters involved in, and pharmacological aspects of, these pathways.)

In addition significant progress in their description and understanding over the last 10 years, there are other important reasons to focus on the central pathways of respiratory vagal afferents. First, they carry information about the physiological and pathophysiological processes in the lungs and airways that are critical for the homeostatic control of the cardiorespiratory system. Thus, as a guide for therapy, a detailed understanding of the neuroanatomy, physiology, and pharmacology of these pathways at the central level is highly desirable. Second, vagal afferents are capable of rapidly producing major adaptive changes in respiratory timing, tidal volume, and the pattern of breathing. This implies that some of them have a powerful and relatively direct access to the endogenous generator of the respiratory rhythm. Consequently, one can expect that the tracing of such pathways should lead to those brainstem sites that contain the central generator for breathing. Third, stimulation of some vagal afferents is known to trigger such stereotyped behaviors as coughing (6,10), swallowing (13–15), and vomiting (16–18), all of which involve, to a large extent, as their output the same muscles that are at other times controlled by the central generator for breathing. Thus, it seems that, by having access to several central pattern generators, vagal afferent pathways represent common components of an interesting assembly of several closely related central generators. As such, they provide a model system for the study of the mechanisms of adaptive redirecting and/or gating of the central effects of visceral afferent information. Finally, the relative contribution of some vagal afferent pathways to the control of breathing undergoes major quantitative, if not qualitative, changes with development, changes that may play a significant role in breathing disorders specifically associated with the early postnatal period (cf. 7,19,20; see also Chapter 16, this volume). A full understanding of the central mechanisms underlying these changes cannot be achieved without a satisfactory knowledge of the central pathways for vagal afferents in the mature central nervous system (CNS). Thus, it would be useful to have a comprehensive summary of our current knowledge of the central neurons and sites in the brain that relay and process the afferent information that originates in the lungs and airways.

An important caveat has to be made before attempting to analyze the central elements of a system comprising afferent pathways and an endogenous pattern generator such as the system of vagal afferents and the central respiratory rhythm generator: changes in the afferent input may produce reflex effects at the output through two distinct routes—those that do, and those that do not, pass through the central pattern generator (Fig. 1). In the case of central neurons that are a part of the pattern generator or its motor output (e.g., inspiratory Iα and Iβ cells), afferent input may reach them either directly or only through other elements of the generator network, or both ways. Consequently, elucidation of the connections and mechanisms that underlie changes in the activity of the pattern generator or motor output neurons in response to the afferent input is particularly difficult, if not impossible, with the present state of our knowledge. Progress in this regard can be made only after one gains a sufficient understanding of the organization of central pathways before they reach the central pattern generator, rather than by analysis of responses recorded on the motor side of the system. This should then allow one to

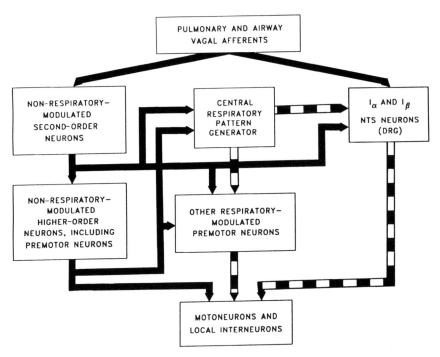

Figure 1 Framework for the approach used in this review indicating several confounding issues involved in studies of central pathways of vagal reflexes. Based on current information, it appears that vagal afferents terminate on second-order central neurons that are not modulated by the central respiratory rhythm, and they do not have direct access to those neurons that are the core of the central respiratory rhythm generator. Inspiratory cells of the dorsal respiratory group (DRG) are an exception to this rule and have been extensively studied in the cat [but their existence and premotor role in the rat are controversial (see 297,298)]. Therefore, they are represented separately and discussed in more detail in Section V.B. Furthermore, nonrespiratory-modulated second-order neurons are, in general, unlikely to act directly on motoneurons, while their connections with respiratory-modulated cells (represented by DRG) and nonrespiratory-modulated premotor neurons may be common. Thus, the position of second-order neurons is suitable for their involvement in processing and distributing the afferent information to higher-order central neurons, including those that are the core of the central respiratory generator, generators of other stereotyped motor functions (coughing, sneezing, etc.), and neurons involved in cardiovascular, somatic, and other regulations not represented here. The dashed and solid lines represent pathways in which the information arising from vagal afferent input is and is not, respectively, respiratory-modulated. This distinction, explained further in the text, emphasizes that once the afferent information becomes embedded into the circuits of the central pattern generator, the mechanisms and pathways involved in its further processing become difficult to study.

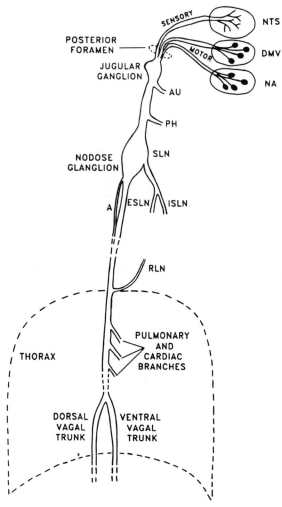

Figure 2 Supradiaphragmatic vagus and its branches (not to scale). The great majority of vagal afferents terminate in the nucleus of the solitary tract (NTS). Those of major importance for respiratory control are carried by the pulmonary branches of the intra-thoracic vagus [three distinct branches can be identified (23)], the internal branch of the superior laryngeal nerve (iSLN), and the recurrent laryngeal nerve (RLN). The latter two innervate primarily the larynx and supralaryngeal region (iSLN) and the trachea and sublaryngeal region (RLN), respectively (311). The pharyngeal (PH) and external laryngeal (eSLN) branches are primarily motor, with a small sensory component. Most of the cell bodies of the relevant pulmonary and airway vagal receptors are located in the nodose ganglion. Aortic (A) nerve afferents have their cell bodies in the nodose ganglion and, in most species, carry information from baro- and chemoreceptor afferents of the aortic arch. The sensory cells of the jugular ganglion and the auricular (AU) branch (Arnold's nerve) do not play a major role in respiratory regulation.

study how a given afferent input is fed into, and then processed by, the generator circuits. With such a strategy in mind, this review focuses primarily on those portions of the vagal afferent pathways relevant to the regulation of breathing for which the effects of the afferent input on central mechanisms are: (1) produced via defined neuronal pathways and (2) lie within our current ability to interpret the results. In addition, we chose to cover primarily studies published over the last 10 years; that is, since the first edition of this volume. Other studies from recent years dealing with the effects of vagal afferent input on breathing and central respiratory neurons in which a more general input-output approach was taken are discussed only as far as they can be specifically interpreted within the framework of the organization of vagal afferent pathways of known modalities controlling the act of breathing.

II. Vagal Afferent Innervation of the Lungs and Airways

In its peripheral course, the vagus nerve gives off separate branches that provide afferent innervation to distinct portions of the respiratory tract (Fig. 2). This permits studies of the central connectivities and functional roles of afferents in those individual branches. Unfortunately, each carries afferent fibers from receptors of several different modalities, which to a large degree confounds the interpretation of such studies.

The nodose (inferior) ganglion is the main sensory ganglion of the vagus nerve. There are about 30,000 afferent fibers in the cervical vagus nerve of the cat, which also gives a rough estimate of the number of cell bodies in the nodose ganglion (21). About 6000 cell bodies have afferent fibers that run in the pulmonary branches of each vagus nerve, which provides the sensory innervation to the lungs, bronchi, and intrathoracic trachea (22,23). In addition, the laryngeal and pharyngeal regions and the extrathoracic trachea are innervated by about 2000 nodose ganglion cells—an astoundingly large number given the relative size of the innervated regions, which points to their importance in respiratory regulation of visceral functions (24–27). The peripheral axons of these latter cells run in the superior laryngeal nerve (SLN) and recurrent laryngeal nerve (RLN). There are also a small number of vagal afferent fibers innervating the upper respiratory tract that may, at least in the rat, have their cell bodies in the glossopharyngeal (petrosal) ganglion (24,28). The jugular (superior) vagal ganglion contains afferent cells innervating the cerebral vasculature and meninges (29) and a few afferent cells of the glossopharyngeal (IX) and superior laryngeal nerves (28,30,31). Afferents with cell bodies in this ganglion appear to have no major role in respiratory control, although indirect anatomical data implicate the auricular branch of the vagus in occasionally evoking coughing, sneezing, and vomiting (see 32 for refs.). The great majority of the central axons of vagal afferent fibers terminate within the nucleus of the solitary tract (NTS) and the adjacent area postrema (AP), both in the region just dorsal to the dorsal motor nucleus of the vagus nerve (see Fig. 3).

Over 85% of the afferent fibers in the cervical vagus nerve are nonmyelinated and have conduction velocities of the order of 1 m/sec or less (C-fibers) (21–23). Receptors innervated by C-fibers usually have a very low level of spontaneous activity (less than 1 Hz) or are silent under typical experimental conditions (artificial ventilation at a low volume, often with pneumothorax) (33–35). The level of activity and the relative proportion of silent and active fibers strongly depend, however, on the experimental conditions (6,34,36) (see 3 for a review). The low level of activity in individual fibers of this group may be compensated for by their large number. Accordingly, they have a demonstrable effect on the pattern of breathing even under physiological conditions during eupneic breathing (37).

The remaining (less than 15%) vagal afferent fibers are myelinated, with the majority innervating supra- rather than subdiaphragmatic organs (21,33). Many have a substantial level of spontaneous activity during eupneic breathing; for example, activity in pulmonary stretch receptor (PSR) afferents often reaches 100 Hz at the peak of inspiration. The largest myelinated afferent fibers in the vagus nerve have conduction velocities of 35–60 m/sec (33,38). In contrast to the cervical vagus nerve, the SLN of adult animals contains relatively few nonmyelinated sensory fibers (27).

III. Receptor Modalities in the Pulmonary and Airway Vagal Branches and Their Reflex Effects

Many reviews provide extensive descriptions of the properties of vagal receptors and their morphology (2–4,33,38–40). Different mechanoreceptors, innervated by relatively fast-conducting, myelinated afferent fibers, relay to the CNS information about lung volume and intrathoracic airway distension, their rate of change, extrathoracic tracheal distension, and the tension and pressure developed in the larynx (Table 1). The slowly adapting PSRs, tracheal and bronchial stretch receptors, pulmonary rapidly adapting receptors (RARs), laryngeal pressure and "drive" (proprioceptors that are activated by contraction of intrinsic laryngeal muscles) receptors, and pulmonary slowly adapting deflation receptors [which are relatively numerous in the rat and rabbit (41–43), but rare in the cat and monkey] belong to this group. Although specific mechanical events are the primary stimuli for these receptors, the receptors often respond to other, sometimes subtle, changes in their chemical or physical microenvironment, or their sensitivity to the primary stimulus is modulated by such environmental changes. Thus, the sensitivity of PSRs to changes in lung volume decreases with an increase in the alveolar P_{CO_2} (see 44,45 for refs.) and the tone in airway smooth muscles (46,47) (see 48 for discussion); histamine sensitizes RARs both directly and through changes in airway mechanics (e.g., 49); the sensitivity of laryngeal mechanoreceptors is

Table 1   Major Pulmonary and Airway Receptors and Their Reflex Effects[a]

Receptor type	Reflex effects
PSR	Breuer-Hering reflex—inspiratory inhibition, expiratory facilitation Enhancement of inspiratory effort Bronchodilatation Tachycardia
RAR	Cough Broncho- and laryngoconstriction Augmented breath/gasp (on stimulation of RAR by a large, rapid lung inflation) Irregular, augmented inspiration and shortened expiration (on maintained airway deflation or inhalation of irritants) Airway mucus secretion Respiratory sensation
Bronchopulmonary C-fibers	Rapid, shallow breathing Apnea (on synchronous chemical stimulation) Broncho- and laryngoconstriction Airway mucus secretion Vasodilatation (pulmonary C-fibers only) Bradycardia Depression of somatic motoneurons (J-reflex) Respiratory sensation
Laryngeal receptors responding to[b]: Intraluminar pressure (decrease or increase) Cold Muscle strain [proprioceptors or "drive receptors"(120)] Osmotic and chemical stimuli CO_2 "Irritant" stimuli	Laryngo- and bronchoconstriction Apnea Cough Activation of upper airway dilators Swallowing Airway mucus secretion Respiratory sensation

[a]Many recent reviews have dealt with reflex effects of specific receptor modalities represented in the lungs and airways (e.g., 3,6,7,8,10,33,39,55–58).
[b]Although vagal receptors of many distinct modalities have been identified in the laryngeal region by recording from their afferent fibers in the SLN and RLN, their corresponding, presumably distinct, reflex effects are only beginning to be elucidated. In addition, many laryngeal receptors are polymodal. Thus, ascribing individual reflex effects to specific receptor types is still premature (see Section VII.B for more details).

CO_2- and temperature-dependent (50–52), and many of them respond to osmotic and chemical stimuli (53). All pulmonary receptors are stimulated to some degree by a sustained increase in pulmonary venous pressure, which indirectly affects the mechanical properties of the lung tissue and airway distensibility (54). The functional significance of receptor modulation by changes in their microenvironment, in most cases, still remains to be determined.

The term "pulmonary and bronchial C-fibers" has come into wide use over the last several years because it is general enough to include all afferents present in the lungs and airways, other than the distinctly defined mechanoreceptors. The name reflects the one major common feature of these receptors, the slow conduction velocity of their afferent fibers (<2.5 m/sec). These receptors are typically polymodal and frequently can be excited by large mechanical deformations (e.g., forceful inflations and deflations of other lungs), a variety of normal and abnormal chemical stimuli (e.g., capsaicin, phenylbiguanide, CO_2, autacoids) delivered through either the bronchial or pulmonary circulation, increased interstitial fluid volume (lung edema), and increased temperature (1,3,34,59). The subset of this broad group of receptors that are excited within 3–4 sec following an injection of capsaicin or phenylbiguanide into the pulmonary circulation is considered to be pulmonary C-fibers [originally termed pulmonary J-receptors (33)]. Those excited with longer latencies and more gradually are termed bronchial C-fibers. In contrast to pulmonary C-fibers, the bronchial ones are readily excited by chemical stimuli delivered into the bronchial circulation and are more sensitive than the former to autacoids such as histamine, bradykinin, and prostaglandins (3,56).

In addition to these pulmonary and airway receptors, vagal afferents carry information from laryngeal receptors (Table 1) (see 4,7,55 for reviews). Cardiac and aortic mechano- and chemoreceptors, whose properties, reflex effects, and central pathways have been extensively studied, are beyond the scope of this review (see 12,57,60 and Chapter 9, this volume).

Specific respiratory and cardiovascular reflex effects are associated with each of the pulmonary and airway receptor modalities identified so far. These are summarized in Table 1 and will be referred to in subsequent sections.

IV. Neuroanatomy of the Vagal Primary Afferent Pathways

A. Gross Neuroanatomy of Vagal Afferent Projections

Central afferent projections of the whole vagus nerve, its individual branches, and central sensory representations of individual organs innervated by the vagus nerve were studied extensively in many species using anterograde degeneration, amino acid autoradiography, or horseradish peroxidase (HRP) histochemistry. All these studies point to the NTS and the adjacent AP as the principal target sites. The projections are, as a rule, bilateral with a strong ipsilateral predominance (e.g., 61–64). Following their descending course within the solitary tract, most of the vagal afferent fibers that project to the contralateral NTS cross the midline caudal to obex through the commissural (*com*) portion of the nucleus. A smaller number of fibers may reach the contralateral NTS by crossing the midline under the floor of the fourth ventricle rostral to the obex (63). Since the NTS also receives major afferent projections from the IX, facial (VII), and trigeminal (V) nerves (65–69), it must be viewed as the single most important site of early integration of afferent input relevant to the control of the respiratory and other visceral systems.

Based on cytoarchitectonic features and some of the characteristic afferent and efferent projections, different subnuclei were distinguished within the NTS in many species, including the rat (28,61,70), cat (62,71), dog (72), sheep (73), hamster (74), and human (75,76). The subdivisions of the NTS in three representative species are shown in Figure 3. With the exception of the subnucleus centralis [identified, so far, only in the rat (77), hamster (74), and sheep (63) and involved in esophageal functions (78)], all other subnuclei were distinguished cytoarchitectonically in most vertebrate species studied, although the nomenclature still varies considerably among different authors (e.g., 74).

In addition to the NTS and AP, central terminations of the whole cervical vagus nerve, and of the SLN alone, have also been traced to the caudal portion of the principal trigeminal nucleus, the spinal trigeminal nucleus, and the dorsal horn of the first and second segments of the cervical spinal cord. These projections beyond the NTS region are, however, relatively weak (or absent) in the rat (24,28), rabbit (79), ferret (80), muskrat (81), primates (64), and probably dog (82) when compared to the cat (e.g., 30,62,83) and lamb (63,84).

With the exception of the aortic nerve, which innervates only aortic baroreceptors in some species, no single vagal afferent branch contains afferent fibers innervating a single receptor type. Consequently, the classical tracing studies cannot provide the much-needed information about the topographical distribution of central termination sites of afferent fibers that are localized to identified portions of the lungs or airways from receptors of known modalities. Nevertheless, these studies, particularly those in which the central projections of individual vagal branches or central representations of individual organs of the respiratory system were studied, provide evidence of an orderly topographical arrangement of vagal afferents to different portions (subnuclei) of the NTS.

B. Viscero- and Organotopic Organization of the Afferent Projections to NTS

Afferents of the V, VII, IX, and X cranial nerves have dense terminations in the NTS. Their projection patterns show a coarse somatotopic organization in that V

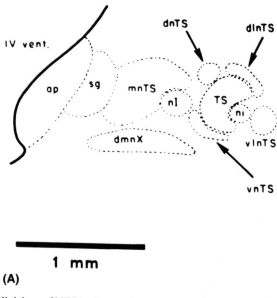

(A)

Figure 3 Subdivisions of NTS in the cat (A), rat (B), and human (C). Transverse sections taken from levels just cranial to the obex show that similar distributions of cytoarchitectonically distinct regions can be distinguished in these three species, although the relative proportions occupied by corresponding regions differ. The original labeling and nomenclature for different subnuclei have been retained to show the diversity among different neuroanatomists. Subnuclei in the cat: AP, area postrema; dlnTS, dorsolateral; dnTS, dorsal; dmnX, dorsal motor nucleus of the vagus; mnTS, medial; ni, interstitial; nI, intermediate; sg, gelatinosus [called also parvocellular (71)]; TS, solitary tract; vlnTS, ventrolateral; vnTS, ventral. Subnuclei in the rat: cen, centralis; dl, dorsolateral; DMV, dorsal motor nucleus of the vagus; gel, gelatinosus; int, intermediate; is, interstitial; vl, ventrolateral; v, ventral; XII, hypoglossal motor nucleus. Subnuclei in humans: AP, area postrema; *D*, dorsal; DMN, dorsal motor nucleus of the vagus; Gel, gelatinosus; INT, intermediate; IC, nucleus intercalatus; IS, interstitial; L, lateral; MVest, medial vestibular nucleus; SAP, area subpostrema; T, solitary tract; VL, ventrolateral; VM, ventromedial; 12, hypoglossal motor nucleus. (Reproduced with the permissions of the authors and the publishers: A from Ref. 62, *Journal of Comparative Neurology*, Vol. 193, copyright 1980 Alan R. Liss, Inc., by permission of Wiley-Liss, a division of John Wiley and Sons, Inc.; B from Ref. 28, *Journal of Comparative Neurology*, Vol. 283, copyright 1989 Alan R. Liss, Inc., by permission of Wiley-Liss, a Division of John Wiley and Sons, Inc.; C from Ref. 75, *Brain Research Bulletin*, Vol. 29, copyright 1992 Pergamon Press Ltd., with permission from Pergamon Press Ltd., Headington Hill Hall, Oxford OX3 0BW, UK.)

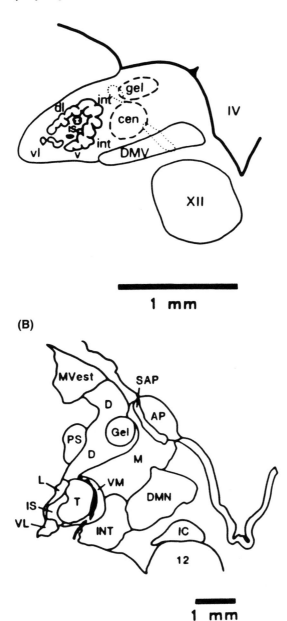

(B)

1 mm

(C)

1 mm

nerve afferents tend to have the highest density of terminations in the rostral portion of the nucleus, those of the X nerve in the caudal portion, and those of the IX and VII nerves in the intermediate zone (66,67,68,85). Consequently, the rostral half of the nucleus is commonly regarded as gustatory (special visceral) and the caudal half as general visceral in function (74,85). In agreement with anatomical studies, the appropriate rostrocaudal and mediolateral distribution of neurons excited by mechanical and chemical stimuli within the caudal oral cavity (innervated by the IX nerve) and epiglottis (innervated by the SLN) was observed in an electrophysiological study in lambs (86). For the IX and X nerves, a mediolateral gradient of projection densities for large, myelinated and small, unmyelinated afferents was observed, with the latter (originating in relatively smaller cells of the petrosal and nodose ganglia) terminating preferentially in the medial portion of the nucleus (87,88). A similar observation was made by recording the activities of individual cells in the NTS evoked by electrical stimulation of the vagus nerve with intensities appropriate for myelinated and unmyelinated vagal fibers (89).

The presence of a viscero- and organotopic organization of the vagal afferent pathway was searched for within the nodose ganglion and the NTS in many anatomical studies in which an anterograde tracer was applied to individual branches of the vagus nerve or organs innervated by vagal afferents. Most frequently, the focus of such studies was on either subdiaphragmatic (e.g., 90,91) or supradiaphragmatic (e.g., 24,81,83) vagal afferents alone. In the nodose ganglion, many anatomical studies revealed only a poorly developed (or no) viscerotopic distribution of cells (24,28,30,91,92). According to one extensive electrophysiological study, afferent cells of the SLN are concentrated around the nerve entry zone to the ganglion, and some preferential locations are observed for gastric, esophageal, and intestinal afferent cells; however, receptor cells of the pulmonary and cardiac regions are widely scattered throughout the ganglion (93).

In contrast to the generally poor viscerotopic organization within the nodose ganglion, projections to the NTS from different portions of the lungs and respiratory tract show a relatively orderly pattern and some organ specificity. It must be acknowledged, however, that only Kalia and Mesulam (62) have studied comprehensively the central projections from individual portions of the peripheral respiratory system. In this study, performed in the cat, the distribution of afferent fibers and terminals within the NTS was assessed following applications of HRP into the lung parenchyma, main bronchi, intrathoracic trachea, extrathoracic trachea, or larynx. After tracer injections into the lungs, the densest projections were observed within the dorsolateral (*d-l*) and ventrolateral (*v-l*) subnuclei, with less intense terminal densities in most other subnuclei, with the exception of gelatinosus (*gel*) and ventral (*v*) (see Fig. 3A for location of these subnuclei). After bronchial injections, the densest projections were again seen in the *v-l* subnucleus, with low and moderate projections to all other subnuclei except *gel*. Intrathoracic tracheal injections also led to labeling in most subnuclei, with that in the *d-l* being the densest, with no labeling in the AP and interstitial (*i*) subnuclei. In contrast, after injections in the extrathoracic trachea, the densest labeling occurred in the *v-l*, and weak or moderate projections were seen in all other subnuclei except the AP. Thus, only the *i* subnucleus received projections from the extra- but not intrathoracic trachea. These projections to *i* might have been carried by afferents in the RLN (see below). Finally, injections into intrinsic laryngeal muscles produced an intense labeling in the *i* and *d-l* subnuclei, no labeling in *gel*, AP, and intermediate (*I*), and weak or moderate labeling in the remaining subnuclei. Because the different organs selected in this study are innervated in different proportions by receptors of distinct modalities, the possibility exists that the apparent organ-specific projection patterns reflect, in fact, differences in the receptor modalities most abundant in these organs.

In contrast to the projections from specific portions of the lungs and lower airways, the projections of laryngeal vagal afferents have received much attention. Studies with tracer injections into the SLN, RLN, or laryngeal muscles were performed in the cat (30,83,92), rat (24,28,85,94), lamb (63,84), rabbit (79), and muskrat (81). In all species studied, the SLN afferents project to the *i* and medial (*m*) subnuclei. Substantial projections to other NTS subnuclei, the principal and spinal trigeminal nuclei, and the cervical dorsal horn are seen only in the cat and lamb; in the rat, rabbit, and muskrat such projections are very weak or absent. As shown by intra-axonal injections of HRP into individual SLN afferents within the NTS of the cat, a single laryngeal afferent can distribute terminal branches to several subnuclei (e.g., *d-l, i, v, v-l,* and *com*), although for any given afferent there seems to be only one site of particularly dense terminations (95). Afferent projections of the RLN are less dense than those of the SLN and are restricted to the *i* and *m* subnuclei in the rat (24,94) and to the *d-l* and *m* subnuclei in the cat (83).

The general picture emerging from these neuroanatomical studies of afferent projections from the laryngeal region to the NTS is that laryngeal afferents project to selected regions of the nucleus located adjacent to the solitary tract rather than to more peripheral portions of the nucleus, and that the contralateral projections are sparse or absent. Most, if not all, projections beyond the NTS originate in laryngeal afferents, not fibers supplying intrathoracic and subdiaphragmatic organs.

C. NTS Projections of Vagal Afferents of Identified Modalities

It takes a combination of neuroanatomical and physiological techniques to study central termination of afferents carrying information from receptors of specific, identified modalities. Therefore, there have been fewer studies employing such an approach. Nevertheless, very significant progress has been made over the last 10 years in elucidating the central projections of PSRs, RARs, and bronchopulmonary C-fibers. On the other hand, studies of the projections of laryngeal afferents of identified modalities have begun only recently (96).

Projections of PSRs

Because of the importance of the PSR input in the control of respiratory timing and pattern, and the relative ease of recording extracellularly from PSR afferent cells in the nodose ganglion (or, alternatively, from PSR axons within the NTS), the central projections of PSR afferents have been by far the most extensively studied of all vagal afferents. The sites of projection and the extent of ramification and termination of individual PSRs were determined by the techniques of antidromic mapping (97–99), spike-triggered averaging (100), and intra-axonal injections of HRP (101). All these studies show that PSRs project to the *l*, *v*, *v-l*, and *i* subnuclei of the NTS from the level of the obex to about 1.5 mm rostral. Projections to the *d* and medial portion of the *d-l* subnuclei were reported in the two electrophysiological studies (97,100) but were not observed in the HRP study. Because the activity of PSR fibers and neurons showing a strong PSR-related input (discussed in Section V.B) were recorded in the medial part of the *d-l* subnucleus (99), it is likely that a sampling bias or the inability to fill sufficiently with HRP those PSR branches that project to the dorsal aspects of NTS is responsible for the discrepancy between these studies. Figure 4A shows an example of branching within the NTS, seen in a dorsal view, of a single PSR afferent in a cat, as determined by antidromic mapping (98). No evidence of PSR projections to the contralateral NTS was obtained (99), in spite of the prominent excitatory responses of some NTS neurons to contralateral PSR inputs. No differences between cats and rabbits were reported for the central projections of PSRs (97).

The intramedullary conduction velocity of PSR central axons was estimated to be 4.6–12.6 m/sec (100), thus slightly faster than for major arborizations of these axons within the NTS [3.4–5.4 m/sec (98)] and less than half the velocity of the peripheral axons of PSR afferents [25–50 m/sec (33,100,102)]. No prominent slowing of conduction was detected in the PSR branches located within the presumed central termination zones (98), an observation consistent with anatomical data demonstrating that these branches are short and have myelin sheaths even on their preterminal portions (101). Ultrastructural examination of the terminal boutons of PSR afferents within the *v* and *v-l* subnuclei revealed that they make synaptic contacts with cell bodies, dendrites, dendritic spines, and other, unidentified, axon terminals. In addition, some of the PSR terminal boutons receive, in turn, axoaxonal synapses from unidentified terminal boutons (103).

No data are available on the projections of tracheal slowly adapting stretch receptors, particularly those of the extrathoracic trachea innervated by the RLN and SLN. On the basis of anatomical data (62) and the fact that stretch receptors of the trachea have different reflex effects from those of PSRs (104–106), the central projection patterns of tracheal stretch receptors and PSRs are likely to be different. Tracheal stretch receptors are not involved in Breuer-Hering reflexes, and their effects on breathing are relatively small compared to those of PSRs. This finding could be due to differences in the transmural pressure gradients that intrathoracic versus extrathoracic airway segments are subjected to during breath-

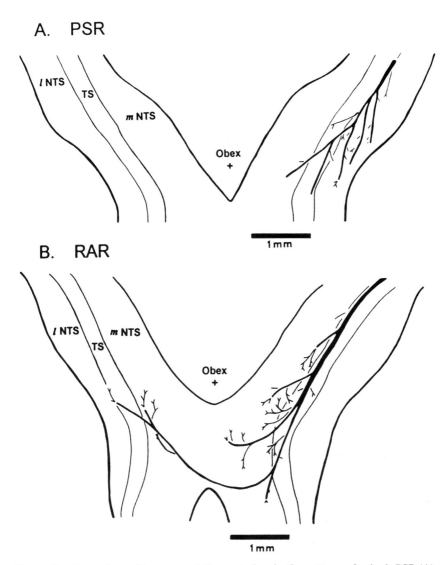

Figure 4 Comparison of the representative central projection patterns of a single PSR (A) and RAR (B), as determined by antidromic mapping. Each drawing represents a semi-schematic reconstruction of the ramification pattern within the NTS of a single afferent, as seen in a dorsal view of the caudal half of the NTS in the cat. The two receptor types show very different ramification patterns. For the PSR, most branches are localized in the lateral aspects of the NTS, rostral to the obex, and ipsilateral to the cell body in the nodose ganglion. In contrast, the RAR has most branches in the caudal, medial aspects of the nucleus (in fact, the majority are in *com*) with many reaching the contralateral medulla. (Modified and reproduced with the permission of the publisher from Ref. 98, *Journal of Physiology*, Vol. 373, copyright 1986 Physiological Society.)

ing (38), the number of receptors in the two segments (cf. 38,107), or their projection patterns, alone or in combination.

Projections of RARs

Although fewer studies of the projections of RARs have been done than of PSRs, detailed information is available about the central termination sites and patterns of RAR afferents (98,108–110). In many regards, the two projection patterns are strikingly different (Figs. 4 and 8). Individual RAR afferents consistently project to the NTS at levels caudal to the obex and cross the midline to reach the contralateral nucleus. The *commissural* and caudal *m* subnuclei are the primary termination sites bilaterally, with a slight ipsilateral predominance (98,108). Some branching is also observed rostral to the obex, both medial and (less frequently) lateral to the solitary tract. These lateral projections have also been directly visualized by means of intra-axonal injections of HRP and localized to the *d, d-l*, and dorsal aspects of *l* subnuclei (109). Projections to the inspiratory region of the NTS, the *v-l* subnucleus, are very weak or absent, suggesting that inspiratory neurons of the dorsal respiratory group (DRG) are not directly excited by RAR afferents (98,109). There is a remarkable consistency of the projections of individual, randomly sampled RAR afferents to several characteristic, yet widely separated, sites (98,109). The reason for this may be that projections of the same afferent to different loci are responsible for distinct aspects of the respiratory and cardiovascular reflexes characteristics of RARs (Table 1). Figure 4B shows one typical example of the central projection pattern of a single RAR afferent.

The conduction velocity of individual RAR main axons within the NTS is 6.2–9.7 m/sec, less than half that for the peripheral axons of RARs (33,98). In contrast to PSR afferents, the preterminal portions of RARs seem to travel over a relatively long distance, with a marked slowing of the conduction velocity (to less than 1 m/sec) (98). Thus, many preterminal branches of RARs must lose their myelin sheath. This feature, deduced from electrophysiological data obtained from RAR branches studied in different NTS subnuclei, was also seen in RAR terminals visualized around the level of the obex ipsilateral to the site of intra-axonal HRP injections (110). The latter morphological study also provides evidence that terminal boutons of RAR afferents form different synaptic contacts in the *d* and *I* subnuclei. The synapses in the *d* subnucleus are simple and consist of asymmetrical contacts with medium-size dendrites. In contrast, in the *I* subnucleus, RAR terminal boutons are in contact with several different neuronal profiles, thus forming a peculiar glomerulus-like structure that includes dendrites, other axon terminals, and dendritic spines. No axosomatic contacts made by RAR afferents were observed in either the *d* or *I* subnuclei.

Projections of Bronchopulmonary C-Fibers

There is, to date, only one study, in cats, of the central distribution of physiologically identified bronchopulmonary C-fibers (35). At levels from the obex to about

2 mm rostral, the typical projection sites occupy the dorsomedial portion of the NTS and AP in a pattern suggesting that the termination regions follow the outlines of the *gel* subnucleus. Caudal to the obex, the fibers terminate in the dorsal aspects of the *com* subnucleus. Projections are also observed in symmetrical locations within the contralateral nucleus, although their densities are appreciably weaker. No projections are observed within regions lateral, ventral, or immediately ventromedial to the solitary tract. Bronchial and pulmonary C-fibers, as distinguished by the latencies of their responses to a bolus injection of capsaicin into the pulmonary circulation, do not differ in terms of their central projection sites. Figure 5 shows the pooled distribution of central projection sites of 12 bronchopulmonary afferents.

The central axons of bronchopulmonary C-fibers had an average conduction velocity of about 0.5 m/sec, about 0.6 that of their peripheral axons. In contrast to a steep reduction in conduction velocity with the increasing order of central branching in RARs (98), the conduction velocities of the central branches of C-fibers are relatively uniform in branches of different orders (35).

A summary of the termination patterns within the NTS of PSR, RAR, and bronchopulmonary C-fibers is shown in Figure 8 and discussed in relation to the concept of modality-specific subdivisions of the nucleus in Section V.D.

V. Second-Order Afferent Neurons

Most of the work on the second-order neurons receiving information from respiratory vagal afferents has been done with neurons of the NTS. These studies can be divided into those in which electrical stimulation of the vagus nerve or its branches was performed and those in which stimuli that were relatively modality-specific were used.

A. Studies with Electrical Stimulation of the Vagus Nerve

Because of the mixed nature of all peripheral ramifications of the vagus nerve, afferent neuronal responses evoked in the brain by means of electrical stimulation cannot provide information about the modality of the receptor afferents reaching individual recording sites. Still, such studies are complementary to the classical tracing studies in that they often allow one to determine the patterns of spontaneous activities in the central neurons from which recordings were made. In addition, unlike the neuroanatomical tracing methods, mapping of the distribution of the evoked responses allows one to detect inputs beyond the first synaptic relay. One limitation to this is that with electrical stimulation one identifies the fastest pathways connecting the stimulation and recording sites. There are examples from many systems, however, in which the fastest pathways are not the ones that operate under physiological conditions, and the respiratory system is probably not different in this regard. Electrical stimulation has also been frequently used to assess the

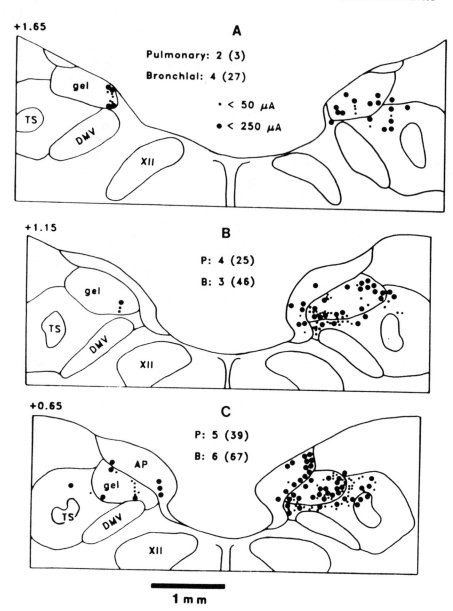

Figure 5 Central projections of pulmonary and bronchial C-fibers. Successive transverse sections through the NTS region show the distribution of low threshold points for antidromic stimulation of central branches of pulmonary and bronchial C-fibers. Data based on a study of 12 receptor cells recorded in the nodose ganglion. Projections of bronchial and pulmonary receptor cells did not differ and have been pooled. Numbers over

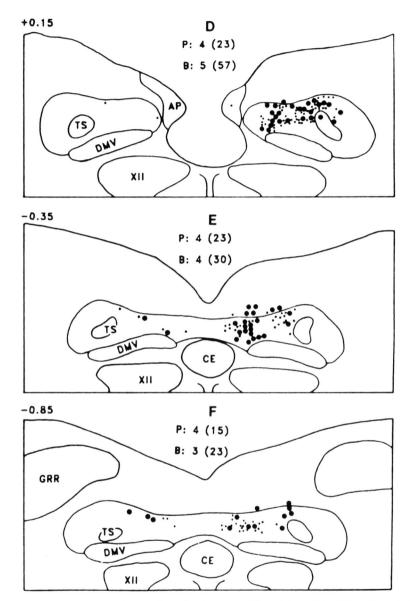

each cross-section show the number of pulmonary (P) and bronchial (B) cells and, in parentheses, the number of branches that contributed low threshold points to each cross-section. Two main projection regions were identified: around the *gel* subnucleus (rostral sections A–D) and in the dorsomedial portion of the *com* subnucleus (caudal sections E–F). (Modified and reproduced with permission of the publisher from Ref. 35, *Journal of Physiology*, Vol. 435, copyright 1991 Physiological Society.)

degree to which convergence from several distinct afferent nerves occurs in central neurons.

Despite the limited selectivity of electrical stimulation for fibers of different diameters, certain useful information can be derived from the fact that the threshold stimulus intensities for excitation of myelinated and nonmyelinated vagal afferent fibers differ by more than an order of magnitude (27,33). Thus, with the intensity of stimulation adequately controlled, and taking into account the very large difference in the conduction velocities of the two afferent fiber types, one can rather easily distinguish whether the evoked response is produced by myelinated or unmyelinated afferent fibers (cf. 89,111,112). Although the ability to obtain even better selectivity using electrical stimulation has been repeatedly questioned, the fact that PSR afferents have the largest diameter and the lowest threshold to electrical stimulation of all the afferent fibers of the cervical vagus has been successfully used, in combination with other physiological criteria, to make a convincing case for the PSR origin of evoked responses in individual NTS second-order neurons (102,113).

Specific data obtained from putative second-order neurons by means of electrical stimulation are presented in Section V.B for the SLN input and in Section V.C in relation to the issue of convergence of inputs from different peripheral and central afferents onto individual NTS neurons.

B. Second-Order Neurons with Modality-Specific Inputs

It is possible, under adequately controlled experimental conditions, to achieve a relatively selective stimulation of receptors of specific modalities located in a defined segment of the lungs or airways. A gradation of the stimulus intensity also can often be achieved. The recording from CNS neurons of responses whose magnitudes bear a consistent relationship to those of a specific afferent stimulation provides convincing evidence that neurons in a particular site in the brain are a part of the central pathway from the stimulated receptors. Additional criteria must be fulfilled, however, to determine whether a given central neuron receives the input of a specific modality directly (monosynaptically) from the corresponding peripheral afferents or, rather, through additional interneurons. Only carefully designed electrophysiological or anatomical (ultrastructural) studies can distinguish between these two possibilities.

Neurons in the Central Pathway from PSRs

PSRs can be rather selectively stimulated using lung inflations of sufficiently low volume and rate of rise. Such stimulation of PSRs produces changes in the depth and rate of breathing by shortening inspiration (Breuer-Hering inspiratory inhibitory reflex) and prolonging expiration (Breuer-Hering expiratory reflex), as well as other characteristic respiratory and cardiovascular reflex effects (see Table 1). These changes must obviously involve a host of central neurons, of which only a fraction are under the direct influence of pathways mediating the PSR-related activity, while the others have their pattern of activity changed secondarily to the PSR-induced changes in the activity of the central respiratory generator (cf. Fig. 1). Still, a modulation of the firing rate of central neurons induced by stimulation of PSR can be dissociated from that originating in the central respiratory drive by varying the magnitude of lung inflation and, in particular, omitting lung inflation in test respiratory cycles in paralyzed, artificially ventilated animals (48,114) (see 115 for refs.).

Within the NTS, two types of neurons with distinct firing patterns have been shown to be modulated by the PSR input (see Fig. 6). One, referred to as p-cells [p standing for (artificial ventilator) pump] (116), shows activity that faithfully parallels the activity of PSRs; the other, I-β cells, receives an excitatory input from both PSRs and the central inspiratory drive (117). Both cell types were originally found in the *v-l* NTS, and as required by the definition of a second-order neuron, both are monosynaptically excited by PSR afferents (102,113,118).

Some p-cells, like some PSRs, show a continuous (tonic) level of firing that increases with each lung inflation; others show only phasic bursts of activity coincident with increases in lung volume, also typical of many PSRs (33). The activity of p-cells is not modulated with the central respiratory rhythm; if spontaneously active, they will display a steady, tonic firing as long as the lung volume is kept constant, provided that the central respiratory modulation of the airway smooth muscle tone is prevented (e.g., with atropine). It is not clear how much of the tonic drive present in p-cells is derived from those PSRs that are active at end-expiratory lung volume and how much from other central or peripheral sources. Using the technique of spike-triggered averaging, excitatory postsynaptic potentials produced in individual p-cells by single PSR afferents were recorded (113). The latencies and fast-rising slopes of those unitary EPSPs indicated that the connection is monosynaptic. The range of EPSP amplitudes was 120–239 μV for the different pairs of PSR/p-cells studied. Based on their response latencies, many of the p-cells in the *v-l* NTS, and at least some of those in medial locations (see below), are monosynaptically excited by electrical stimulation of the SLN, in addition to their input from PSRs (116,119). The receptor modality of those SLN afferents remains unknown. Likewise, it is not known whether any of the tonic drive to p-cells originates in laryngeal afferents, some of which are spontaneously active under physiological conditions and show a pronounced respiratory modulation (4,120,121).

Since the first description of p-cell properties based on recordings in the most distinct respiratory region of the NTS, the *v-l* subnucleus (116), cells having a p-cell-type firing pattern have also been found in other locations within the nucleus; in particular, ventromedial and dorsal to the solitary tract (16,114,119,

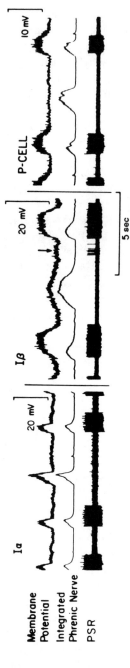

Figure 6 Intracellularly recorded responses to withholding lung inflation from an Iα, an Iβ, and a p-cell (top traces) during cycle-triggered ventilation in a paralyzed cat. The bursts of activity of a simultaneously recorded PSR afferent (bottom traces) mark the periods of lung inflations. In the middle of each record, lung inflation was omitted for one inspiratory period (marked by an increase in the integrated phrenic nerve activity in the middle traces). This maneuver reveals the presence of central inspiratory drive (depolarization) in the Iα and Iβ cells, but not the p-cell, as shown in the records of membrane potential. In the Iβ and p-cells, the cycles with no inflation result in less and no depolarization, respectively, when compared to control respiratory cycles with inflations occurring during inspiration. The arrow in the records from the Iβ cells marks an aberrant, small lung inflation that caused firing in the PSR cell and a depolarization of the Iβ cell. (Reproduced with permission of the authors and the publisher from Ref. 113, *Journal of Neurophysiology*, Vol. 58, copyright 1987 American Physiological Society.)

122), corresponding to the ventral *I* and dorsomedial portion of the *d-l* subnucleus, respectively. Although the monosynaptic connectivity of these cells with PSR afferents was not directly documented, their locations closely overlap the typical regions of projection and termination of PSR afferents (described in the preceding section) and some of them responded to electrical stimulation of the vagus nerve with a latency consistent with monosynaptic connectivity (119).

P-cells at different locations have distinct efferent projections. Those dorsal and ventrolateral to the solitary tract send their axons (or at least one of their axon collaterals) to the caudal and medial portion of the contralateral NTS (caudal *m* and *com* subnuclei), whereas the cells located ventromedial to the tract do not (99) (see Fig. 7). This suggests that p-cells do not represent a homogeneous group. The contralaterally projecting axons of the dorso- and ventrolateral p-cells have conduction velocities of 0.5–5.0 m/sec (99), these values being low and consistent with the presumably small size of the p-cell soma. Axonal projections of the ventromedial group of p-cells remain unknown. This lack of information is unfortunate as there is evidence suggesting that the latter cells are the ones mediating the Breuer-Hering inspiratory inhibitory reflex, whereas those located dorso- and ventrolaterally to the tract do not play a role in this reflex. Lesion experiments showed that the destruction of either the *v-l* NTS (123) or the caudal NTS, where the dorsal and ventrolateral p-cells send their axons, do not impair the Breuer-Hering reflex (99,124) (Kubin and Davies—unpublished data; see Figs. 8 and 9). In contrast, microinjections of excitatory amino acids or cobalt ions (to block synaptic transmission) into the medial NTS in rats, at sites where p-cell activity can be recorded, induce changes in the respiratory rhythm (prolongation of inspiration, slowing of breathing) compatible with those resulting from reductions in the PSR afferent input and the Breuer-Hering reflex (122). No data are available on the morphology of p-cells, and their axonal arborizations have not been visualized.

Iβ cells [or Rβ, as they were named at the time of their discovery (117)], the other second-order cells in the PSR pathway, are located mainly in the *v-l* NTS and are a part of the DRG (see 9,115 and Chapter 2, this volume). They show a ramp-like increase in firing during the inspiratory period of the respiratory cycle and are silent during expiration (Fig. 6). This phasic activity is reduced if lung inflation is withheld during the period of central inspiration and/or, in some Iβ cells, the onset of their firing is delayed from the onset of inspiration (113,114,125,126). These changes show that the cells are excited by lung inflation. Both cross-correlation analysis of spike trains recorded simultaneously from a PSR afferent and an Iβ cell (118) and intracellular spike-triggered averaging (102,113) have revealed a monosynaptic connection between PSR afferents and Iβ neurons. The amplitudes of the unitary EPSPs were 18–265 μV. A late excitatory component was also seen in some records, suggesting that the input from a single PSR can reach Iβ cells both monosynaptically and through interneurons or, alternatively,

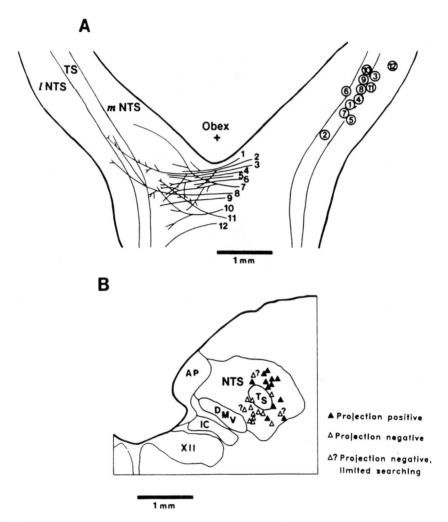

Figure 7   Distribution within the NTS of p-cells and some of their efferent projections. A dorsal view of the medial and lateral borders of the nucleus is shown in A with circles marking the location of cells for which axonal arborizations were found in the caudal, commissural portion of the nucleus (cell body locations, marked by circles, and their corresponding axons are labeled with the same numbers). (B) Only the p-cells located dorsal and some of those ventrolateral to the solitary tract had axons projecting to the *com* subnucleus (filled triangles). Thus, p-cells in different NTS subnuclei do not represent a homogeneous population in terms of their efferent projections. (Reprinted with the permission of the publisher from Ref. 99, *Journal of Physiology*, Vol. 383, copyright 1987 Physiological Society.)

that PSR afferent terminals are located on several compartments of the cell at different electrotonic lengths from the soma (102). In addition to a proven mono- and presumed paucisynaptic input from PSRs of the ipsilateral vagus nerve, a substantial PSR-related input reaches Iβ cells from PSR afferents of the contra-lateral vagus nerve. Both excitatory (127) and inhibitory (128) inputs from PSRs of the contralateral vagus have been reported, the direction of the effect probably being dependent on the experimental conditions. Because PSR afferents do not have contralateral projections, the PSR input reaching contralateral NTS neurons, including Iβ and p-cells, must be at least disynaptic. It is not known whether p-cells, like Iβ cells, also receive their PSR input through either ipsi- or contralateral paucisynaptic pathways, in addition to their monosynaptic connec-tions.

Most Iβ cells have spinal projections and make monosynaptic excitatory connections with phrenic and intercostal motoneurons (126,129), and at least some also have intramedullary collaterals (130). Thus, these cells combine features of second-order neurons, output neurons relaying the respiratory drive to respiratory motoneurons, and central neurons acting as elements of the central respiratory pattern generator. Consequently, it is not surprising that great effort has been devoted to elucidating the function of these neurons. In particular, Iβ cells seem to be well suited to serve as a necessary central element of the hypothetical inspiratory "off-switch" mechanism because of their ability to sum peripheral inputs from PSRs and inputs from the central inspiratory drive (see 9 for a review). Based on the magnitude of the delay of the firing onset of Iβ cells from the onset of inspiration in cycles with lung inflation, they have been classified as early or late (125). Such a distinction was, however, not seen when firing onsets of Iβ cells were analyzed during respiratory cycles without lung inflation (126), indicating that the PSR input may exaggerate the presence of functional subpopulations of Iβ cells. The late-onset Iβ cells were proposed to be the most likely ones to play a major role in the inspiratory termination by lung inflations. Iβ cells firing an abrupt and rather uniform burst of action potentials at the time of inspiratory termination ("off-switch" cells), a subpopulation with a particularly late firing onset time, have received particular attention (125,131). Accordingly, as an extension of the concept proposed by Clark and von Euler (132) that, owing to recruitment, PSR activity reaching the medulla increases nonlinearly toward the end of inspiration, Cohen (125) suggested that a nonlinear increase in the activity of Iβ cells toward the end of inspiration underlies inspiratory termination. Subsequently, however, by performing experiments discussed earlier by Wyman (133), Feldman et al. (134) determined that stimulation of the descending axons of bulbospinal Iβ cells does not cause major changes in respiratory rhythmicity, thus excluding the possibility that intramedullary collaterals of spinally projecting Iβ cells play an important role in respiratory rhythm generation. In fact, this eliminated most of the DRG cells (both Iα and Iβ type) from such considerations, as about 80% of them (at least in the cat) are bulbospinal (116,135,136). For any remaining cells of the DRG, this hypothetical function could be rejected on the basis of experiments in which extensive lesions of the *v-l* NTS had little effect on either respiratory rhythmicity (137) or the Breuer-Hering reflex (123).

Still, inspiratory, including Iβ, cells are present not just in the *v-l* NTS but in other regions of the nucleus (119,138). The relative abundance of these cells, their properties, and their connectivities have not been studied in any detail. Thus, a role for inspiratory-modulated cells located in regions of the NTS outside the DRG in processing the PSR input and in the inspiratory off-switch cannot be excluded. In addition, recent reports show that neurons (recorded in both the dorsomedial and ventrolateral medulla) that fire a burst of action potentials with a pattern that is independent of the input from PSRs at the time of inspiratory off-switch represent a class of cells that is distinct from the very late-onset Iβ cells (139,140).

Given their excitatory input from PSRs and excitatory connectivity with contralateral phrenic motoneurons, Iβ cells were expected to mediate a disynaptic excitatory effect of lung inflations to contralateral phrenic motoneurons (113). Although such a function of Iβ cells seems well founded in the cells' connectivity, the excitatory effect itself proved difficult to demonstrate and, if present, was relatively weak in most experimental designs utilized to date (141,142) (see 126 for refs.). It also proved difficult to demonstrate a lateralization of reflex effects of PSRs in phrenic motoneurons (142). This suggests that a number of second- and/or higher-order neurons relaying the input from PSRs have strong bilateral connections. The relatively small number of DRG cells in the cat, only a fraction being Iβs, compared with other sources of inspiratory inputs impinging on phrenic motoneurons, may explain the difficulty in demonstrating the role of Iβ cells in mediating the PSR excitatory effect (143). Thus, in contrast to a presumably prominent role of DRG cells in mediating the excitatory effects of the SLN input to contralateral phrenic motoneurons (discussed below), the role of Iβ cells in relaying the PSR input to phrenic motoneurons is as small as the effect itself.

Recordings have not yet been made from central neurons that specifically mediate the input from the tracheal slowly or rapidly adapting stretch receptors. Such studies would be of interest, as it has been proposed that the reflex effects elicited by activation of tracheal slowly adapting stretch receptors of the extrathoracic trachea may be different from those of PSRs (see, however, the discussion in Section IV.C).

In addition to receiving a monosynaptic input from PSRs, Iβ cells are monosynaptically excited by electrical stimulation of myelinated afferents of the SLN (116,144). Thus, they must also be regarded as second-order neurons in the afferent pathway from laryngeal afferents. This aspect of their function is discussed in more detail in Section V.B.

Neurons in the Central Pathway from RARs

Because a relatively large and rapid lung inflation is required to excite RARs, obtaining stable recordings from central neurons excited by RAR afferents is technically difficult owing to their small size (8–15 μm mean diameter) as estimated from the cytoarchitectonic data (62,71,72). In addition, large lung inflations will also excite many PSRs, confounding the interpretation of such an experiment. Consequently, there are fewer recordings from RAR-driven central cells. Excitatory postsynaptic potentials produced monosynaptically by individual pulmonary RAR afferents were recorded in the caudal *m* and *com* NTS subnuclei (108), thus proving that second-order cells were present at these locations, as expected from the study of the central projections of RAR afferents (98). The technique used did not permit a determination of the spontaneous activity patterns of the second-order cells in which these postsynaptic potentials were produced. Subsequently, however, neurons have been identified in the caudal *m* and *com* subnuclei that could be excited, with latencies compatible with the conduction time in RAR afferents, by electrical stimulation of both vagus nerves (145). This bilateral input is consistent with the strong bilateral projections of RAR afferents to the *com* subnucleus (98). The stimulus intensities required to produce these responses were higher than for PSR afferents, but below those necessary to excite nonmyelinated fibers. The cells having the appropriate bilateral input from myelinated vagal afferents also respond to ammonia inhalation, and some had a rapidly adapting response to rapid hyperinflations of the lungs. Thus, they have features expected of second-order cells excited by RAR afferents. Intracellular recordings obtained from a few of these neurons revealed EPSPs produced by electrical stimulation of both vagi and having shape indices consistent with monosynaptic projections from vagal afferents. Unlike primary RAR afferents, which are usually inactive under normal ventilatory conditions in the cat (98), about half of the second-order RAR cells displayed spontaneous activity (145). This might have been due to excitatory drive from sources other than RARs or because ammonia inhalations, used repeatedly to identify the cells excited by RAR, caused a maintained increase in activity in some RAR afferents. A variety of spontaneous activity patterns was observed, including modulation with pump-induced lung inflations or deflations, central respiratory drive, and cardiac rhythm in individual second-order RAR cells. However, the strong dependence of those patterns on FRC and lung compliance suggests that they reflect changes in the receptor environment in the periphery, rather than a convergence of PSR, central inspiratory drive, and baroreceptor inputs. In fact, other studies show that many of the variations of the activity patterns of second-order RAR cells described by Lipski et al. (145) could be elicited in RAR primary afferents by changing the magnitude of distension/collapse of the lungs or altering the lung compliance (146,147) (Kubin and Davies, unpublished observations).

Many of the second-order RAR neurons located in the *com* subnucleus can be antidromically activated from the ipsilateral dorsolateral pons (parabrachial region and Kölliker-Fuse nucleus) and have axonal ramifications in this region (124). In contrast, medullary projections of RAR neurons to the *v-l* subnucleus of the NTS, VRG, or Bötzinger complex are rare or absent; if present, no evidence of axonal branching has been obtained (124). Dense projections from *com* to the dorsolateral pons were revealed by both anterograde (148) and retrograde (71,149,150) axonal transport in the cat and rat (70). The morphology of cell bodies and axonal arborizations of electrophysiologically identified second-order RAR cells remain, however, unknown. In agreement with the presumed small size of the cells, the axonal conduction velocities determined by their antidromic activation from the pontine parabrachial region are less than 1 m/sec (145).

Consistent with the presence of both RAR primary afferents and their second-order neurons in *com* (98,108,145), lesions of this subnucleus abolished the reflex excitatory responses of the phrenic nerve to ammonia inhalation, rapid hyperinflations of the lungs, and mechanical stimulation of the mucosa near the tracheal bifurcation, without impairing the inspiratory inhibitory Breuer-Hering reflex (99,124) (Kubin and Davies, unpublished data; see Fig. 9).

Neurons in the Central Pathway from Laryngeal Receptors

The NTS receives vagal afferent input from the larynx via fibers of the SLN and RLN (Section IV.B). Few attempts have been made, however, to record from second-order neurons during stimulation of laryngeal receptors of specific modalities. Neurons in the intermediate third of the NTS (caudal part of the gustatory zone) were recorded during chemical (KCl, NH_4Cl, HCl, H_2O, etc.), thermal, and mechanical stimulation of the epiglottis in the lamb (86,151). Most of the neurons studied were localized in the medial NTS regions implicated in swallowing, yet some cells were located in the *d*, *v*, and *v-l* subnuclei and some had inspiratory modulation. [The relative potency of most chemical stimuli used was the same as for the chemosensitive afferents of the SLN in lambs (151,152). Because species differences exist in the sensitivity of SLN afferents to different chemicals (cf. 86,153), comparisons of data from different animals should be avoided or, at least, made with caution.] Most neurons (88%) responded to at least two modalities. This sensitivity of NTS neurons to stimuli of different modalities should not be interpreted, however, as indicative of convergence of SLN afferents of different modalities onto a single neuron because there is accumulating evidence that individual afferents are often polymodal. For example, "irritant" laryngeal receptors may be excited by smoke, water, mechanical stimulation, and CO_2, and "drive" receptors are also stimulated by solutions of low osmolarity and depressed by CO_2 (154,155). Thus, more information is needed about the prevalent patterns of response of individual laryngeal receptors to stimuli of different modalities in order to relate their behavior to that of second (and higher) order neurons. In addition, many of the neurons located in the gustatory zone of the NTS that show polymodal inputs may represent third- and higher-order afferent neurons excited by second-order neurons located in the oral portion of the trigeminal sensory nucleus. This possibility is supported by the studies in which polymodal neurons were much less frequently observed in the latter than in the NTS (86,156).

The relative lack of information about the central neurons mediating the effects of laryngeal receptors of specific modalities is compensated to some degree by the fact that different modalities of stimuli applied to the laryngeal region produce qualitatively similar reflex effects, at least in some respiratory motor outputs. Thus, apnea or a suppression of the phrenic nerve activity results from cooling of the laryngeal region (19,157), application of CO_2 (158,159), negative pressure in the upper airway (276), and instillation of water (246). (Responses in upper airway motoneurons are more complex; see section VII.B and 8,55 for refs.) Consequently, electrical stimulation of the SLN can be regarded as mimicking to some degree a combination of these afferent stimuli. Although these apparent similarities most likely reflect our still superficial knowledge of the details of the reflexes from laryngeal receptors, for the purpose of this review, they may justify including the effects of SLN electrical stimulation in a section dealing with second-order neurons of specific modalities.

As mentioned earlier, Iβ cells of the DRG are commonly excited by electrical stimulation of SLN afferents, as are Iα cells of the DRG. The latter also receive input from the central inspiratory drive (see 9 for refs.) and have monosynaptic efferent connections with contralateral phrenic motoneurons (160) (see 115 for earlier refs.), but no direct input from PSRs (see Fig. 6). Based on the response latency to SLN stimulation (116,144) and the shape indices of intracellularly recorded EPSPs evoked by SLN stimulation (161), the input to DRG inspiratory cells of both types is strong and monosynaptic. The shortest latencies are 2.1–2.3 msec in the cat. Interestingly, DRG cells with descending axons and positive cross-correlograms with the contralateral phrenic nerve activity have significantly shorter latencies to SLN stimulation than cells for which such evidence of spinal connections was absent (144). In this context, it is important to note that stimulation of the SLN evokes a distinct excitatory response in the contralateral phrenic nerve, with a latency consistent with a disynaptic pathway (141, 144,160,162). This excitation is abolished by lesions of the *v-l* NTS—the primary location of Iα and Iβ cells (123). Thus, both Iα and Iβ neurons probably act in concert and are of primary importance in mediating the excitatory input from laryngeal afferents to phrenic motoneurons.

Following an initial excitation, many Iα and Iβ cells are inhibited by ipsilateral SLN stimulation with latencies of 7–16 msec, while only a suppression of activity typically is observed following stimuli applied to the contralateral SLN.

However, a minority of Iα cells are excited with relatively short latencies (about 3 msec) from the contralateral SLN (163). Because laryngeal afferents do not have contralateral projections, central neurons (presumably located within the NTS but, to date, unknown) must mediate both contralateral excitation and inhibition. A portion of the inhibitory effects of SLN stimulation was shown to be chloride dependent and thus probably mediated by inhibitory amino acids (161).

Many nonrespiratory-modulated NTS cells are excited by SLN stimulation with latencies compatible with a monosynaptic connection and some are localized within or near the DRG (95,164). A few of the latter cells have axons projecting ventrolaterally and caudad, suggesting projections to the VRG and/or the spinal cord (95). One cell had an axon collateral within the NTS; thus it could serve as a local interneuron mediating the SLN input to other NTS cells. Three cells had descending axons at the level of the third cervical spinal segment bilaterally. Neurons in the rostral, gustatory region of the NTS project to the dorsomedial parabrachial region of the pons (70,165), an area distinct from the projection sites of *com* neurons.

Neurons in the Central Pathway from Bronchopulmonary C-Fibers

In a recent study in rats (166), reflex changes in breathing compatible with those produced by C-fiber stimulation were obtained by microinjections of excitatory amino acids into the dorsal portions of the *com* subnucleus, while microinjections of cobalt ions (to block synaptic transmission) impaired the respiratory effects of intra-atrial phenylbiguanide injections (166). This is consistent with one of the locations of second-order cells for bronchopulmonary C-fibers expected on the basis of mapping of their central projections in the cat (35). Thus, the microinjection data of Bonham and Joad (166) show that a synaptic relay relevant for respiratory and (at least in part) cardiovascular reflexes occurs in the *com* subnucleus. In the other characteristic C-fiber projection sites, the AP and the region surrounding the *gel* subnucleus, cells projecting to the pontine parabrachial area appeared to receive synaptic inputs from unidentified vagal afferents (167). Still, to date, there have been no recordings made from proven second-order cells of bronchopulmonary C-fibers in any of the NTS regions innervated by these fibers.

C. Convergence of Inputs onto Putative Second-Order Neurons

The interpretation of, and comparison of the evidence from, studies testing the presence of convergence of afferents of various modalities or peripheral locations onto different neurons of the central nervous system is not simple. Experimental results depend on the animal preparation, the type and level of anesthetic used (especially when looking at neurons beyond the site of the first sensory relay), conditions of stimulation (electrical vs. natural), its strength and selectivity, and so forth. In addition, most investigations used extracellular recordings to determine the presence of convergence, making weak excitatory and all inhibitory effects difficult to detect, especially when the spontaneous activity of the cell under study is not high.

The convergence of the PSR and SLN inputs onto p- and Iβ cells was discussed extensively in Section V.B. This, however, does not exhaust all the possibilities of convergence of vagal inputs, let alone other central and peripheral afferent pathways, on these neurons. Based on the changes in their firing characteristics during a rapid lung inflation, some Iβ cells may be excited by RARs, in addition to PSRs (116,131). However, a monosynaptic connection of RARs with Iβ cells is probably weak or absent because these afferents rarely project to the DRG region (Section IV.C). Similarly, indirect measurements of the changes in excitability of both Iα and Iβ cells induced in expiration by lung inflations of different rates did not provide unequivocal evidence of RAR input to DRG cells (168). Nevertheless, Iβ cells (and presumably some Iα) may receive their RAR-related input through interneurons, especially under conditions when lung hyperinflation is strong enough to produce the "gasp" reflex [i.e., the strong and abrupt burst in phrenic motoneuronal firing in response to a rapid hyperinflation of the lungs (cf. Fig. 9)]. In fact, DRG cells may mediate the "gasp" reflex under the latter conditions through their known connections with phrenic motoneurons (126,160). A rather widespread convergence of the effects of IX and SLN afferent volleys onto p-cells (the precise localization within the NTS was not provided) was reported, with a few also affected by afferents of the infraorbital nerve (169). A slightly higher incidence of convergence of the same three inputs was seen in the same study in NTS neurons whose firing was modulated with the central inspiratory drive. Still, such a triple (or even more numerous) convergent input appears to be more common in the reticular formation surrounding the NTS and in the VRG than in the NTS itself (170,171). NTS cells could be the source of some of the convergent connections onto reticular formation neurons; accordingly, neurons of the rostral portions of the NTS show heavy efferent projections to the parvicellular reticular formation (172). This difference highlights the need for precise identification of the recording sites in relation to the NTS and its subnuclei. The input from intercostal muscle afferents impinges on very few inspiratory neurons of the DRG (173), whereas silent neurons of the NTS frequently receive inputs from this source (11,174). In contrast, a large percentage of spontaneously active neurons (the character of activity was not described) located in the medial portion of the NTS is excited by both myelinated afferents of the cervical vagus nerve and group II and III afferents of the sural and peroneal nerves (175). Finally, a few (mostly silent) neurons in the medial NTS are activated by nonmyelinated afferents in both cardiac and pulmonary branches of the thoracic vagus (89,111).

Interestingly, an unidentified number of medial NTS cells show cardiac or respiratory rhythmicity but are not excited by either of the intrathoracic vagal branches.

In addition to the peripheral inputs discussed above, responses can be evoked in DRG cells by electrical stimulation of the motor cortex and midbrain regions (176) and the pontine parabrachial area (174) (see 9 for refs.). Direct projections to the NTS from these regions have been demonstrated anatomically (70,149,150,177,178). Similarly, nonrespiratory neurons excited by SLN afferents with latencies compatible with a monosynaptic connection are also excited by stimulation of the cortical regions involved with swallowing (179). Thus, many central inputs may modulate the effects of vagal afferents on putative second-order NTS neurons.

A convergent input from laryngeal and nasal (but not facial) afferents was reported for the cells of the rostral sensory trigeminal nucleus (180). Although SLN afferents project to this region (Section IV.B), the relatively long latencies of the responses to electrical stimulation of this nerve suggest that few of the studied neurons were second-order neurons for the SLN afferents.

Additional correlative evidence for the convergence of inputs of different modalities onto second-order cells of the NTS comes from neuroanatomical studies. For example, carotid sinus nerve afferents (arterial baro- and chemoreceptors) project, in different proportions, to the *com*, *d*, *d-l*, *l*, *i*, and *m* subnuclei (see 181–183 for refs.), and lesions of *com* interfere with reflexes from the carotid body chemoreceptors (184–186). It has not yet been demonstrated whether individual neurons in these subnuclei receive input from carotid sinus nerve afferents in addition to that from the pulmonary and airway receptors discussed in this review. Direct connectivity between carotid chemoreceptor afferents and inspiratory neurons of the DRG, which is a matter of controversy, has not been confirmed in the most recent study (187).

D. Modality-Specific Subdivisions of the NTS

The concept of a modality-specific organization at the NTS level that we propose (35) posits that, in principle, there is one primary receptor modality that directly reaches individual second-order neurons, and the neurons of specific modalities are spatially grouped in specific regions of the nucleus. In addition, the neurons are subjected to influences exerted by their central afferents (e.g., central respiratory pattern generator) and may receive inputs related to other peripheral receptor modalities through interneurons rather than directly from primary afferents. Such a system should provide for the necessary flexibility in using afferent information from specific receptors to meet the specific demands required for appropriate regulation.

Although the preceding section focused on the occurrence of convergence on second-order neurons, many studies provide ample evidence to the contrary, i.e., that the convergence of peripheral afferent information from functionally distinct sources occurs only in a minority of NTS neurons, the majority being affected by only one of the several afferent inputs tested in individual studies. Jordan and Spyer (12) have extensively reviewed studies published before 1986 from which it appears that the convergence of distinct afferent inputs onto putative second-order NTS neurons is not very common. Furthermore, electrophysiological studies in which NTS neurons are identified using "natural" rather than electrical stimuli do not reveal cells with pronounced inputs from combinations of distinct afferent systems. Rather, there is only one dominant modality characteristic of a given cell, and NTS neurons having similar discharge properties are usually encountered in clusters.

Figure 8 shows that the *major* projection sites of PSR, RAR, and bronchopulmonary C-fibers occupy separate portions of the NTS. The limited available evidence for the location of other physiologically identified second-order neurons also suggests that they are grouped in specific portions of the nucleus; e.g., second-order baroreceptor afferent neurons and their afferents were visualized using HRP in a region medial to the solitary tract and caudal to that occupied by p-cells and PSR afferents (188,189). Several anatomical studies also show that projections from individual organs that can be related to specific functions show very circumscribed projection patterns; e.g., gastric afferents project heavily to the center of the *gel* subnucleus (92,190), and esophageal afferents occupy a very restricted region of the medial NTS called the subnucleus centralis (78).

As discussed earlier, circumscribed lesions within the NTS can abolish selected reflexes. Figure 9 shows the effects of multiple electrolytic microlesions made within the *com* subnucleus on the reflex responses to a rapidly rising, then maintained lung inflation and to local mechanical stimulation within the region of the tracheal bifurcation. With lesions in this subnucleus, one can abolish reflexes that are characteristic of RARs without impairing the Breuer-Hering reflex. Conversely, lesions in the medial NTS rostral to the obex abolish the latter (122). Finally, synaptic transmission blockade in the dorsomedial *com* subnucleus impairs the respiratory effects of bronchopulmonary C-fiber stimulation without affecting the blood pressure response (166). These effects correlate with the distribution of major termination sites of the three groups of pulmonary afferents within the NTS (Fig. 8).

Data from immunocytochemical studies show that the distribution of certain transmitters within the NTS can be related to afferent pathways of specific modalities. For example, in the cat, substance P and its receptors are localized in sites that correspond well with the terminal projections of bronchopulmonary C-fibers (191–193). Aortic nerve afferents in the pigeon project to a discrete NTS region that is immunoreactive to catecholamines (194). The distributions within the NTS of the many neuropeptides (cholecystokinin, galanin, corticotropin-

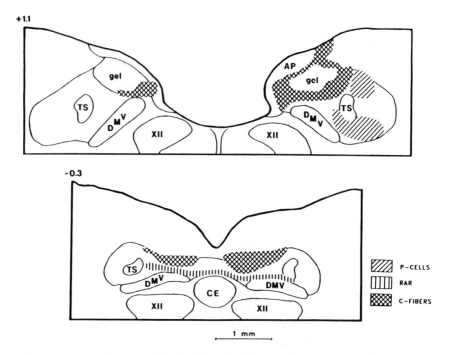

Figure 8   Distribution within the NTS of p-cells (which also marks projection sites of PSRs) and terminal ramification sites for RARs and bronchopulmonary C-fibers. The three afferent systems project to different portions of the nucleus with almost no overlap. This suggests a minimal convergence of primary afferents of the three systems on their second-order neurons, without, however, excluding the possibility that the three modalities may converge on some NTS neurons after passing through some central relays. The data represent a summary of three studies in which individual afferent cells of identified modalities were recorded in the right nodose ganglion and their central projections were determined by antidromic microstimulation in the NTS (35,98,99).

releasing factor, dynorphins, enkephalins, somatostatin, calcitonin gene-related peptide) (195–198) and enzymes (acetylcholinesterase, NADH dehydrogenase, cytochrome oxidase) (199) studied to date show differential localizations that often coincide with specific primary afferent projections to, and/or efferent projections from, the NTS, particularly to the pontine parabrachial area. Thus, it appears that the system consisting of vagal afferents and the pontine projections of their second-order cells is one in which an attempt to relate cytoarchitectural and immunohistochemical markers to the location and modality of the pathway should be particularly rewarding. An example of such an approach to afferent pathways in spinal nerves has recently been extensively discussed (200).

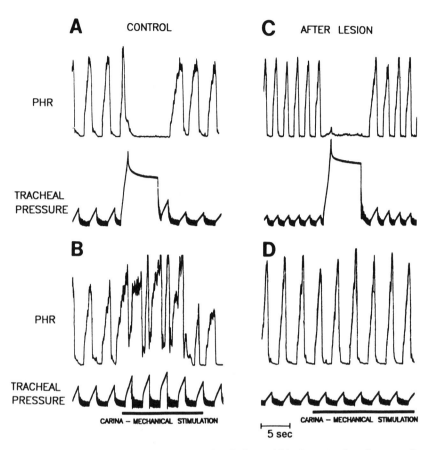

Figure 9 Effects of multiple electrolytic microlesions within the *com* subnucleus on reflex responses of the phrenic nerve to preferential stimulation of RARs or PSRs. Two test stimuli were used: a "ramp and hold" lung inflation of about three times normal tidal volume triggered from the onset of phrenic nerve activity, which will initially stimulate both RARs and PSRs and, after the former adapt, only PSRs (A and C), and local mechanical stimulation with a minibrush inserted into the region of tracheal bifurcation, which is likely to stimulate mainly RARs (B and D). After the lesion (C and D), the rapid burst of phrenic nerve activity occurring at the onset of lung inflation and the disturbance of phrenic nerve activity by local stimulation of the carina are abolished (cf. control records in A and B, respectively). The lesion also abolished the decreased lung compliance (increased tracheal pressure) seen during stimulation of the carina in B. The inhibition of phrenic nerve inspiratory activity for the duration of a steady lung inflation was not affected by the lesion. Thus, the *com* nucleus region plays a role in reflexes from RARs but not in the Breuer-Hering reflex. (Kubin and Davies, unpublished data from a decerebrate, paralyzed, artificially ventilated cat.)

Finally, while there is ample evidence of central interactions of different stimulus modalities in respiratory control (see 201 for a general discussion of interaction modes), there are also notable specific examples of the reflex effects, produced under condition of simultaneous stimulation of diverse respiratory afferents (under conditions such that occlusion is unlikely to play a role), that do not interact in a manner consistent with the presence of convergence and interaction of the corresponding afferent information. In particular, changes in CO_2 and O_2 do not affect either the threshold or the magnitude of the expiration reflex produced by mechanical stimulation of the vocal cords (202), changes in CO_2 do not have a significant effect of the magnitude of the suppression of activity in inspiratory motoneurons (phrenic, laryngeal, XII) by lung inflations (203), and cardiac and vascular responses to pulmonary C-fiber stimulation are not modified by a concomitant production of apnea by electrical stimulation of the SLN (204). In such cases, it appears unlikely that the two afferent inputs have common second- or even higher-order neurons.

VI. Central Control of Afferent Inflow

Vagal visceral receptors lack specialized efferent systems, such as that provided by gamma motoneurons to muscle spindles in skeletal muscles, that would allow for central control of the afferent receptor sensitivity. On the other hand, as mentioned in the Introduction, the sensitivity of individual pulmonary and airway receptors to their primary, specific stimuli can be modulated by other variables such as smooth muscle tone, airway wall compliance, volume of interstitial fluid, temperature, or CO_2. Although these modulatory influences are likely to play a physiological role, they are not sufficient to allow vagal afferents to exert their regulatory role with precision and specificity. Accordingly, the system is designed so that the activity of the second-order neurons is not a simple transformation of the primary afferent information and a large degree of central processing of the afferent information occurs at the level of the first central synaptic relay. The events occurring postsynaptically on second-order neurons were discussed in Sections V.C and V.D. In addition, there are effects exerted on the presynaptic terminals of the primary afferents that affect the excitability of the terminals and regulate the amount of transmitter released. In the older literature, this was referred to as primary afferent depolarization (PAD) (see 205 for refs). There is strong evidence for the presence of PAD in the central terminals of some vagal afferents. The role of PAD may be to not only control the magnitude of afferent inflow, but also act as a gate for specific afferent inputs, thereby permitting execution of central commands (e.g., during coughing, vomiting, etc.) undisturbed by peripheral events (cf. 206).

PAD in different vagal afferents is produced by both other peripheral afferents and central neurons. SLN and PSR afferents were most extensively studied as a peripheral source (207–210). Of the central sources, the motor cortex (208), raphe magnus and locus coeruleus (211), NTS (212), and the central inspiratory drive (anatomical origin undetermined) (210,213,214) produce PAD in various vagal afferents. PAD was found in the following respiratory vagal afferents in the NTS: SLN (207–209, 211,212), PSRs (208,210,214), and RARs (208). Various combinations of the source and the affected afferent type were reported, although not every possible combination has been studied (e.g., the central inspiratory drive acting on SLN afferents or raphe effects on PSR afferents). PAD is not uniformly present in vagal afferents of different origins and modalities [e.g., PAD from the central inspiratory drive is absent in aortic nerve afferents (210,213) and SLN input does not produce PAD in afferent fibers of the subdiaphragmatic vagus (208)]. When assessed by intra-axonal recordings within the NTS, the magnitude of the PAD occurring in synchrony with the central inspiratory drive in PSR afferents was of the order of 1–2 mV. That produced by electrical stimulation of the SLN was even larger and sufficient to generate action potentials in the afferents (210). These intra-axonal measurements were likely to have underestimated the effect as, for technical reasons, the recordings presumably were made at a distance from the terminals rather than from the terminals themselves, where the effects of PAD are expected to be the strongest. The duration of the PAD induced by SLN afferents in SLN (209) and PSR (210) afferents was 300–400 msec. Two components of the depolarization having different durations and magnitudes were observed in PSR afferents following SLN stimulation (210).

As in afferents of the somatic nervous system, PAD in vagal afferents is likely to be produced by two distinct mechanisms: changes in the extracellular concentration of potassium ions ($[K^+]$) around the terminals, and genuine axo-axonic synapses using specific neurotransmitters (see 215,216 for refs.). With respect to the former, substantial local increases in $[K^+]$ with each inspiration and following stimulation of myelinated vagal afferents (presumably originating in PSRs and RARs) were observed around respiratory-modulated neurons within the NTS (217). The authors argued that the increases were due to activity in presynaptic terminals rather than in the soma and dendrites of the respiratory neurons and estimated that they could account for several millivolts of depolarization in both terminals and their target neurons. However, in an in vitro study, 75% of the $[K^+]$ increase following a massive solitary tract stimulation in medullary slices was dependent on the presence of synaptic transmission, suggesting that post- rather than presynaptic elements were the major source of K^+ ions (218). Functionally, since PAD results in less transmitter release, the effects of K^+ ion-induced depolarizations exerted at both the pre- and postsynaptic sites of excitatory synapses may be mutually opposing, and the net effect on the excitability of postsynaptic neurons may be small. In fact, the functional significance of PAD resulting from changes in $[K^+]$ is relatively unimportant in the rubrospinal system compared to the transmitter-mediated PAD (215). Thus, the significance of the effect of $[K^+]$ on synaptic transmission between vagal afferents and their second-order neurons still has to be evaluated. The observation that the terminal potentials of PSR afferents are modulated with the central respiratory rhythm, while the postsynaptic potentials that these afferents produce in their target cells are not (214), may be related to the effects of K^+ ions that are significant at pre- but not postsynaptic sites.

With respect to synaptically mediated PAD, many studies have provided evidence of axoaxonic synapses on vagal afferents within different NTS subnuclei (e.g., 219,220). There is evidence that GABA, as in somatic afferents, is the transmitter mediating PAD produced by SLN stimulation (208). Although GABA-containing interneurons are present in the NTS (221), appropriate interneurons that could specifically mediate PAD within the NTS have not yet been systematically searched for. Axoaxonic synapses containing GABA have been observed in the NTS (222), yet were rarely seen on vagal afferents (223).

Most of the studies of the presynaptic mechanisms in the respiratory system were conducted when relatively little was known about specific transmitters and receptor subtypes that may be involved in the presynaptic control of transmitter release (e.g., adrenergic α_2, serotonergic 1B, and $GABA_B$ receptors) (see 224 and Chapter 4, this volume, for refs.). The availability of specific ligands for these receptors and a greatly improved understanding of the effects that they mediate should undoubtedly stimulate new experiments addressing the presynaptic mechanisms in respiratory control.

VII. Brain Distribution of Third- and Higher-Order Neurons Receiving Input from Pulmonary and Airway Receptors

Neuronal activities, including field potentials, related to inputs from vagal afferents have been recorded from many sites in the CNS beyond the NTS. However, as explained in the Introduction, our ability to interpret these data is limited by the fact that, once "embedded" into the networks of the respiratory pattern generator, vagal information may assume a number of parallel or interactive routes and these may change dynamically with the respiratory cycle. In addition, in many studies, electrical stimulation of the cervical vagus or the SLN, rather than a "natural" stimulation of specific receptors, was used, which left unresolved the physiological nature of the evoked responses. Consequently, in this section, we have chosen to minimize our discussion and interpretation of the data; instead, we merely denote in a systematic manner those recent studies that may have some bearing on the issue of central pathways from pulmonary and airway vagal afferents.

A. Studies with Electrical Stimulation

Following stimulation of the cervical vagus nerve, evoked responses are observed in (in addition to the NTS) neurons of the VRG (169,225), medullary reticular formation surrounding the NTS (170,171), inspiratory neurons of the upper cervical (C-1 to C-3) spinal cord (226), pontine parabrachial region (227), cerebellum (228,229), thalamus, hypothalamus, and several other forebrain sites (230–232), including the cerebral cortex (233,234). Because vagal afferents do not project to these regions (except for the parabrachial region in some species), all these responses must have involved two or more central synaptic relays.

By using electrical stimulation of large myelinated vagal fibers with pulses of constant strength but graded frequency (regarded as analogous to step inflations of the lung), Zuperku and Hopp (225) found that VRG neurons in halothane-anesthetized dogs show different response patterns that are related to the pattern of their spontaneous activity. About 50% of the VRG cells responded to this stimulus. Of those, inspiratory-augmenting and expiratory-decrementing cells were excited, while inspiratory-decrementing cells were suppressed. In addition, however, in a subsequent study from the same laboratory using a similar technique but thiopental anesthesia (235), an inhibition of both expiratory-augmenting and -decrementing cells was found and identified as originating predominantly from ipsilateral vagal afferents. In addition, an excitation of the decrementing neurons was produced from vagal afferents of either side. The shortest latencies, observed for the inhibitory responses in these neurons following single vagal stimuli, were of the order of 7–8 msec. Unfortunately, such latencies cannot provide any useful information about the pathways involved because they may result either from the presence of several synaptic relays or from just a disynaptic connectivity with an inhibitory neuron, located in the NTS, having a relatively slowly conducting axon. The identity of neurons transmitting the vagal input of any modality to the VRG remains, so far, unknown. The study of the projections from the NTS to VRG by Smith et al. (236) may provide an anatomical basis for a search for those particular cells mediating the responses to vagal input observed in the VRG region.

Regarding the pathways transmitting the PSR input to the pons, Cohen et al. (227) evaluated the responses of pontine, respiratory-modulated cells to vagal stimuli having an intensity just above the threshold for PSR afferents. Short latency responses were rare, the mean latency being 170 msec, suggesting that the afferent pathway involved is multisynaptic and diffuse. This awaits further confirmation as there is a relative paucity of information on the pontine, respiratory-modulated neuronal responses to electrical stimulation of myelinated afferents of the cervical vagus nerve.

Many studies have utilized single pulses or brief trains of stimuli to the SLN to assess the responses of neurons of the medullary reticular formation (169–171) and VRG neurons (237,238). Recently, Jiang and Lipski (161) recorded intracellularly from VRG neurons, including those in the Bötzinger complex, and attempted to relate the various patterns of evoked postsynaptic potentials in different neuronal types to the possible underlying pathways, a difficult task at the present state of knowledge. A respiratory modulation of the magnitude of the evoked responses was observed in all neuronal types. This could be due to respiratory changes in membrane resistance (and instantaneous membrane potential) of the neurons or a respiratory modulation of the presynaptic neurons mediating these responses. Since projections of DRG inspiratory neurons to the VRG are rare (239,240), Jiang and Lipski (161) proposed that the VRG cell responses to SLN stimulation are mediated by nonrespiratory NTS neurons. Interestingly, a few DRG neurons responded with an early, chloride-dependent IPSP. This, and the latency of these responses (about 3.2 msec), suggests the presence of a disynaptic pathway, which would mean that there exist inhibitory, amino-acid-containing, second-order NTS cells excited by SLN afferents.

Single shocks or trains of stimuli to the SLN at low intensities, sufficient to inhibit inspiration yet not strong enough to elicit swallowing (cf. 27), have been used in many studies because this afferent input halts the respiratory oscillator in its postinspiratory phase, i.e., one of the three distinct phases of the respiratory cycle (241,242). The effects of such stimulation on VRG neurons (238,243–246), upper airway motoneurons and muscles (247–249), and respiratory pump muscles and motoneurons (244,245,249) have been described. Different vagal afferents are thought to access different groups of medullary respiratory neurons at different times in expiration. In particular, SLN and high-threshold myelinated afferents of the cervical vagus (RARs?) preferentially excite postinspiratory neurons, whereas PSRs (activated by lung inflations) suppress activity in those neurons and augment the activity of late expiratory neurons (243,249,250). The concept that postinspiratory neurons exert a widespread inhibitory effect and are responsible for the distinct postinspiratory phase of the respiratory cycle has, however, been questioned on the grounds that there are insufficient experimental data supporting the proposed key inhibitory function of postinspiratory neurons in respiratory rhythmogenesis (130,161,244).

In many studies, evoked responses to stimulation of the vagus or the SLN are observed in various motoneurons with respiratory-modulated activity, including VII (251), XII (247,252–254), pharyngeal (248), laryngeal (161,237,238,255), and phrenic (141,162,247,256), as well as intercostal muscles (245). From the point of view of afferent control of upper airway motoneurons, an interesting finding was the long-lasting enhancement of XII nerve activity resulting from a brief train of stimuli to the SLN (257). [Activation of an inhibitory input to XII motoneurons by lingual nerve stimulation can reset this prolonged excitation (258).] This resembles the maintained increase in lumbar motoneuron excitability that can be demonstrated in the presence of activation of aminergic inputs (a phenomenon referred to as motoneuronal bistability) (259–261). However, the enhancement of XII nerve activity did not seem to be dependent on intrinsic membrane properties of the motoneurons and was not abolished after systemic application of methysergide, a broad-spectrum serotonin receptor antagonist (257). In addition, the records from the latter study (cf. also 252) suggest that the changes in XII motoneuron excitability parallel a long-lasting reduction in the respiratory rate and, as such, probably originate at a premotoneuronal level, at sites somehow related to the central respiratory rhythm generator. Thus, while bistability could not be demonstrated in XII motoneurons, these data suggest that, in other, so far unidentified, central neurons involved in shaping the respiratory rate and pattern, bistable properties may be revealed by stimulation of appropriate afferent inputs.

Single shock stimuli to the SLN, known for a long time to elicit a short-latency (disynaptic) excitation of contralateral phrenic motoneurons (162,262), produce an excitation in ipsi- rather than contralateral XII motoneurons (247). However, the relatively long latency of the XII motoneuron response (about 1.2 msec longer than in phrenic motoneurons) suggests that more than two synaptic relays are involved. Following the excitation, a period of suppressed activity occurs bilaterally in both phrenic and XII motoneurons; this also had a longer latency in XII than in phrenic motoneurons (247). The suppression in phrenic motoneurons is regarded as largely medullary in origin and disfacilitatory in character (123,141,162,262), although it may have a small postsynaptic inhibitory component at the motoneuronal level (256).

B. Studies with Stimulation of Specific Receptor Modalities

Central Neurons with PSR Input

NTS neurons with a tonic firing pattern that was phasically suppressed by lung inflations were observed in the medial portions of the NTS in the cat and tentatively labeled "inverted p" cells (119,263). Because slowly adapting deflation receptors, although present in the cat (41), are uncommon, the "inverted p" cell likely represents a third (or higher) order cell in the PSR pathway that is inhibited by p-cells, rather than a second-order neuron. Alternatively, some of these cells may have been driven by RAR afferents; under certain experimental conditions, second-order RAR cells in the caudal NTS show bursts of activity coincident with the termination of pump-induced lung inflations (145), and the same can be seen in RAR afferents (Kubin and Davies, unpublished data).

Responses of VRG cells to lung inflations are weaker and have been less frequently observed than in DRG cells. However, two recent studies of expiratory VRG cells reveal an interesting feature of response reversal with increasing lung inflations. In late expiratory cells in the cat, small inflations or deflations during expiration have a facilitatory, and larger inflations a depressant, effect (264). In dogs, a similar response reversal was observed for expiratory decrementing cells at tracheal pressures of about 4.6 mmHg, whereas the expiratory augmenting cells were suppressed at all tracheal pressures tested (3.3–12 mm Hg) (265). Both groups argued that PSRs alone mediated both effects, which posits that expiratory VRG cells are under two opposing effects of PSRs, presumably mediated by two different pathways.

Besides the NTS and VRG, the activities of central neurons modulated by PSR inputs have been recorded and studied consistently in only two sites: the pontine parabrachial region (266–268) and the midbrain (269). Tonically active neurons having an inspiratory modulation and phasic respiratory neurons with various activity patterns were described in the pontine medial parabrachial region and the Kölliker-Fuse nucleus (see 125 for refs.). The neurons are scattered rather widely throughout the region (266). The inspiratory modulation of these neurons is suppressed or abolished by lung inflations delivered in inspiration (267,268). Since the activity was never suppressed to a level below that seen during expiration, Feldman et al. (268) proposed that the PSR input acts presynaptically to reduce the amount of the central inspiratory drive reaching the pontine cells. The site of this presumed presynaptic action is unknown. The possibility that some p-cells of the NTS project to the pontine parabrachial region has not been investigated. An alternative argument, however, is that the enhancement of respiratory modulation of pontine neurons when lung inflation is withheld during inspiration may be due to an increased input from RARs resulting from lung collapse (266). Consistent with such a possibility, NTS cells located in the *com* subnucleus and having properties of putative second-order neurons in the RAR pathway project to the pontine parabrachial region (124). Thus, the issue of the source and mechanisms of the modulation of pontine neuronal activity with changes in lung volume needs further study.

Some neurons in the midbrain central tegmental field have a respiratory modulation of central origin; their activity, both tonic and respiratory-modulated, is suppressed by lung inflations (269). Based on the experimental design used in that study, the authors argued that the PSR input reached the midbrain neurons independently of the vagal effects on the central respiratory drive. The interposed pathway must have been, however, rather long, as the effects developed with a time constant appreciably longer than the duration of a single respiratory cycle.

PSR Inputs to Respiratory Motoneurons

The problem of the effects of changes in lung volume on motoneuronal activity is multidimensional and deserves a separate review. The dimensions that must be considered include at least the following: motoneuron type (inspiratory vs. expiratory with further subclassifications), function of the innervated muscle (e.g., respiratory pump vs. upper airway), direction and magnitude of the lung volume changes and the time of delivery during the respiratory cycle, the level of the central respiratory drive, and the level and type of anesthesia.

The reflex control of upper airway motoneurons by respiratory vagal afferents has been reviewed recently (8,55). The common generalization is that a transient activation of PSRs suppresses the inspiratory-related activity of upper airway motoneurons (e.g., 247,270,271), whereas it tends to enhance the expiratory-related activity of upper airway motoneurons. However, the latter effects are weaker, more variable, and sometimes opposite in direction, as in the case of motoneurons innervating the (early-expiratory) thyroarytenoid muscles, which are suppressed by expiratory lung inflations (250). Of the expiratory effects of lung inflations, those produced in early-expiratory upper airway motoneurons are of particular interest because they may be relevant to pathophysiological conditions associated with expiratory flow limitation.

In spinal respiratory motoneurons (phrenic, intercostal, abdominal), phasic lung inflations have a predominantly suppressant effect on the peak activity. With small lung inflations in expiration, however, expiratory motoneurons are excited, while with larger inflations, they are inhibited (e.g., 264,265,271,272). Thus, the current view is that there is a reversal of the effects of lung inflations on expiratory motoneurons similar to that seen in expiratory neurons of the VRG, many of which act as premotor neurons to spinal motoneurons. A reversal of the effect of both maintained lung inflation and its withdrawal is observed following microinjections of lidocaine into the region of the V motor nucleus (which is adjacent to the pontine parabrachial area) in anesthetized rabbits (273). This suggests that the reversal is central in origin, although one cannot exclude the possibility that a costimulation of other pulmonary receptors, in addition to PSRs, is necessary for the manifestation of this phenomenon. The latter is supported by recent experiments with vagal cooling in spontaneously breathing dogs that suggest that myelinated vagal afferents have an excitatory effect on abdominal expiratory muscle activity, while C-fibers have an inhibitory effect (274).

In contrast to the effects of a brief stimulation of PSRs, a steady elevation of the FRC results in only a transient suppression of XII and mylohyoid nerve activities (275), while a sustained lung deflation causes a maintained increase in the activity of both inspiratory and expiratory upper airway muscles (see 55 for refs.). These effects probably result from a combination of adaptations occurring at the receptor level and centrally and are impossible to interpret in terms of underlying pathways. Comparable studies in humans also yield conflicting results and are further complicated by the absence of evidence for a Breuer-Hering reflex at eupneic tidal volumes (132) despite the presence of activity in PSR afferents at FRC (277).

Vagotomy enhances the activity of orofacial motoneurons with inspiratory activity to a much greater degree than phrenic motoneurons, both in adult (e.g.,

275) and newborn (e.g., 278) animals. Figure 10 shows that, even with only one vagus nerve intact, vagal afferents exert a strong (and bilaterally symmetrical— not shown) suppressive effect on the activity recorded from the genioglossal branch of the XII nerve. Sectioning the remaining vagus nerve releases both the tonic and phasic inspiratory activities in the XII nerve, and the resulting increase is disproportionally large in the XII nerve when compared to the phrenic nerve output. Removal of the afferent activity originating in PSRs may be primarily responsible for this effect (203), yet a contribution from other afferent modalities is also likely; e.g., bronchopulmonary C-fibers may also exert suppressive effects on the motor output to genioglossal muscles (279). Regarding the central pathways of this effect, one possibility is that pontine parabrachial cells, in which respiratory modulation is released after vagotomy (see 115,267 for refs.) and some of which may project to the orofacial motor nuclei (280), provide a portion of the excitatory drive to upper airway motoneurons and thereby are responsible for the PSR-related suppression of the latter. [See Milsom (281) for an interesting discussion, from a comparative perspective, of the role of tonic and phasic inputs

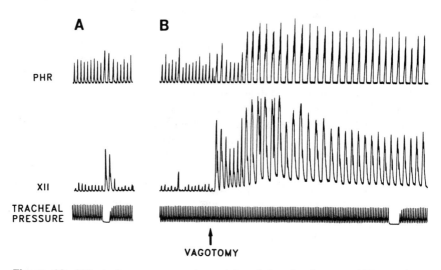

Figure 10 Effect of vagotomy on the activity of the phrenic nerve (PHR) and the genioglossal branch of the hypoglossal nerve (XII) in a paralyzed and artificially ventilated cat. (A) Moving averages of the two activities in a unilaterally vagotomized animal. (B) The remaining vagus nerve was cut (at arrow), which resulted in a disproportionate enhancement of XII nerve activity. This enhancement was much larger than that caused by stopping the ventilator for two respiratory cycles before vagotomy in A (see the tracheal pressure record at the bottom). Thus, the afferent activity present in the vagus at FRC suppresses both motor outputs, but especially XII activity. (Kubin and Davies, unpublished data.)

from mechanoreceptors in respiratory control and the differences between denervation and withholding of mechanoreceptor inputs.]

Neurons in the Central Pathway from Laryngeal Receptors

Although laryngeal vagal receptors of many distinct modalities have been described (Table 1), studies attempting to distinguish reflex respiratory effects of
stimulation of laryngeal receptors of specific modalities have only begun. To date,
they have focused on the characteristics of the reflex responses at the output,
motoneuronal, level rather than on central neurons. Accordingly, responses to
elevated CO_2 level in the larynx were studied in motor nerves innervating the
diaphragm, genioglossal, laryngeal, and triangularis sterni muscles (158,159).
The most pronounced effect was a suppression of phrenic and an increase in XII
nerve activity. Stimulation of laryngeal receptors by cold air suppresses phrenic
nerve activity, has mixed effects on XII motoneurons (19), and causes airway
smooth muscle contraction (282). The literature on the effects of upper airway
pressure changes on different respiratory motor outputs is extensive (see 8 for a
review). The membrane potential and firing rate changes in VRG neurons during
apnea induced by various "natural" laryngeal stimuli (ammonia, smoke, water)
have been described (246). Recently, in a study of the excitatory effect of negative
upper airway pressure pulses on genioglossal muscle activity in humans, the
relative contributions of supra- and subglottic receptors and superior laryngeal and
trigeminal afferents were evaluated (283,284). In this context, beneficial effects of
high-frequency oscillations (30 Hz, <1 cm H_2O) in upper airway pressure are now
being studied as a possible means of preventing airway occlusions characteristic of
the sleep apnea syndrome (285).

Lesions of the pontine parabrachial region, which increase the volume
threshold of inspiratory termination by lung inflations (see 9 for refs.), do not
affect the ability of the SLN input to terminate inspiration (139,286).

Neither acute (287) nor chronic (288,289) bilateral sections of the SLN have
major effects on the eupneic breathing pattern in several species. A comparable
result has been reported in humans by means of upper airway anesthesia (290).
This is difficult to reconcile with the known powerful reflex effects of the SLN
afferents on breathing and the reports showing substantial spontaneous activity
during baseline conditions in many SLN afferents (4,120,121) and suggests that
the activity in the afferent endings active during eupneic breathing has other
functions (and central connectivities) than the control of breathing.

Neurons Mediating Input from Other Pulmonary and Airway Receptors

The activity of inspiratory and expiratory neurons of the VRG was recorded during
bronchopulmonary C-fiber activation produced by capsaicin or phenylbiguanidine

injections into the pulmonary circulation (291). However, the observed changes in neuronal activity were likely to result from C-fiber input-mediated changes in central respiratory drive, rather than from effects exerted on VRG neurons through central pathways specific for C-fiber input. The recent descriptions of the effects of C-fiber stimulation by capsaicin on the activity of upper airway and spinal respiratory motoneurons (279,292), and bronchomotor activity (82,293), provide the necessary background for further elucidation of the central pathways of these reflexes.

VIII. Summary and Future Directions

In the decade in which the major interest and excitement in neuroscience has shifted from systems to in vitro studies of isolated cells and subcellular mechanisms, major progress has been made in the description and understanding of the central pathways that underlie the respiratory reflexes elicited by activation of vagal afferents of specific modalities. This is especially true in the case of the PSR and RAR pathways, which have been studied in great detail up to, or beyond, the termination sites of their corresponding second-order neurons. Logically, similar studies of the pathways from bronchopulmonary C-fibers and laryngeal afferents should follow because of the recognized importance of the receptor modalities that they mediate in pathological processes in the lungs and reflex control of upper airway patency, respectively. Recent advances in the understanding of the different receptor modalities represented in the laryngeal region have provided the necessary information to begin conducting systematic studies of the corresponding central pathways.

To better understand some of the organizing principles of vagal afferent pathways (and afferent systems in general), we need more information on the relationships among various immunocytochemical, electrophysiological, and anatomical markers that may be characteristic of pathways of physiologically identified modalities. The recent attempt by Carr and Nagy (200) to organize the information available at those various levels of analysis for afferent cells of dorsal root ganglia should be a useful guide for studies of vagal afferents. Unfortunately, there is, so far, little definite information on the transmitters utilized by modality-identified, vagal afferent neurons and their central targets (see Chapter 4). The correlative data discussed in Section V.D and recent studies of visceral sensory neurons strongly suggest that immunocytochemical (e.g., 31,294) and molecular (e.g., 295) markers can provide important distinguishing features for specific afferent pathways.

With regard to the ability of vagal afferents to trigger stereotyped responses (coughing, sneezing, etc.), more information is needed about the morphological and pharmacological bases of convergence and interaction (at both pre- and postsynaptic levels) of modality-identified afferents relevant for these behaviors. It has been proposed, for example, that stimuli acting on receptors of the laryngeal and pharyngeal regions and innervated by IX and X nerve afferents will produce different reflex responses depending on the combination of receptors stimulated simultaneously or in an appropriate sequence (14). If so, one should be able to identify specific spatial and pharmacological combinations of interacting central neurons and afferent fibers at or near the level of the first or second central relay that can be related to the corresponding stereotyped response at the output. Similarly, different dynamic characteristics have been reported for inspiratory termination by PSR and SLN afferents, with the latter being more rapid and powerful (141). Given the convergence of these two afferent systems on some second-order cells (p-cells and Iβ), one could hypothesize that the differences in inspiratory off-switch dynamics should be related to different input-output characteristics of the second-order cells to PSR versus laryngeal inputs. If so, there should be certain morphological and/or pharmacological differences between the synapses made by the two afferent systems on their common second-order neurons that can be related to these differences in off-switch dynamics. Alternatively, however, one could postulate the existence of separate pathways, one specific for PSR and another for SLN afferents, that have their own independent access to the system that terminates inspiration, with the SLN pathway being capable of overriding any effects mediated by PSR. Again, there should be an appropriate neuroanatomical and neuropharmacological basis for such an arrangement. Finally, the idea of a frequency-dependent release of colocalized transmitters (e.g., 296), derived from a nonrespiratory field of neuroscience, may prove useful in studies of vagal afferent pathways and the neural control of breathing (e.g., in explaining the mechanism of activation of different pattern generators by vagal afferents or of respiratory phase switching). Thus, with more information becoming available on the central pathways of vagal afferents of defined modalities, one can begin to formulate experimentally verifiable predictions of the expected features of the system.

　　Many studies and reviews (this one is no exception) devote considerable attention to the DRG neurons and p-cells, as they are defined in the cat. However, a number of recent studies of central respiratory regulation have used the rat as a model. Consequently, several important cautionary notes are justified. In the rat, the presence of a significant population of bulbospinal neurons corresponding to the DRG of the cat is still controversial (see 297,298); SLN afferents do not reach the *v-l* NTS (Section IV.B); slowly adapting PSRs excited by lung deflation are relatively common (42,43); and there are differences in the pontine mechanisms that control breathing (299). Consequently, it is important to determine in the rat the response of p-cells to SLN inputs, the presence of Iβ-like cells, and the phrenic nerve reflex responses to PSR and SLN inputs. In the meantime, these intriguing species differences should not impede studies of NTS cells and the processing of vagal afferent inputs in the cat, given the amount of information that has already been accumulated using this species.

New tools and techniques have become available and should prove useful in further studies of afferent pathways. Those include the use of viruses as trans-synaptically transported markers and vehicles delivering specific genetic material to selected populations of central neurons (e.g., 300–303), studies of the anatomical distribution of the loci of increased expression of c-*fos* and other early genes following selective stimulation of specific afferent pathways (e.g., 112,304,305), and antibody-coated probes ("transmitter traps") that can monitor transmitter release in very small, anatomically defined regions in response to specific afferent stimuli (e.g., 306).

A number of in vitro studies of synaptic transmission within the NTS have been initiated recently (e.g., 218,307,308). These studies are not yet capable of addressing the issue of synaptic transmission in modality-specific pathways. However, combined with neuroanatomy and immunocytochemistry, and equipped with more information derived from ultrastructural studies of physiologically identified cells and fibers, they have the potential of becoming critical in further advancing of our knowledge of the central processing of afferent information.

Finally, and on the other end of the spectrum of experimental approaches used, it must be acknowledged that relatively few studies were published in the last decade on the respiratory control exerted by pulmonary and airway vagal afferents in adult humans (e.g., 277,283–285,309,310). It may be hoped, however, that the progress made in this regard in animal studies will have a stimulatory effect on future studies in humans.

Acknowledgments

The authors' studies were supported in a large part by NIH Grant HL-36621. We are grateful to Dr. J. R. Romaniuk for a stimulating discussion of the effects of PSRs on motoneurons, Dr. S. Iscoe for his helpful comments on an earlier version of the manuscript, Ms. Rosemarie Cohen for her secretarial support, and Ms. Clotilde Reignier for assistance with the figures.

References

1. Coleridge JCG, Coleridge HM. Afferent vagal C fibre innervation of the lungs and airways and its functional significance. Rev Physiol Biochem Pharamcol 1984; 99:1–110.
2. Sant'Ambrogio G. Nervous receptors of the tracheobronchial tree. Annu Rev Physiol 1987; 49:611–627.
3. Coleridge HM, Coleridge JCG. Reflexes evoked from tracheobronchial tree and lungs. In: Cherniack NS, Widdicombe JG, eds. Handbook of Physiology. Section 3:

The Respiratory System. Vol II: Control of Breathing, Part 1. Bethesda, MD: American Physiological Society, 1986:395–429.

4. Widdicombe J, Sant'Ambrogio G, Mathew OP. Nerve receptors of the upper airway. In: Mathew OP, Sant'Ambrogio G, eds. Respiratory Function of the Upper Airway. New York: Marcel Dekker, 1988:193–231.

5. Monteau R, Hilaire G. Spinal respiratory motoneurons. Prog Neurobiol 1991; 37: 83–144.

6. Karlsson J-A, Sant'Ambrogio G, Widdicombe J. Afferent neural pathways in cough and reflex bronchoconstriction. J Appl Physiol 1988; 65:1007–1023.

7. Bartlett D Jr. Respiratory functions of the larynx. Physiol Rev 1989; 69:33–57.

8. Mathew OP, Sant'Ambrogio FB. Laryngeal reflexes. In: Mathew OP, Sant'Ambrogio G, eds. Respiratory Function of the Upper Airway, New York: Marcel Dekker, 1988: 259–302.

9. Euler C, von. Brain stem mechanisms for generation and control of breathing pattern. In: Cherniack NS, Widdicombe JG, eds. Handbook of Physiology. Section 3: The Respiratory System. Vol II: Control of Breathing, Part 1. Bethesda, MD: American Physiological Society, 1986:1–67.

10. Widdicombe JG. Reflexes from the upper respiratory tract. In: Cherniack NS, Widdicombe JG, eds. Handbook of Physiology. Section 3: The Respiratory System. Vol II: Control of Breathing, Part 1. Bethesda, MD: American Physiological Society, 1986:363–394.

11. Shannon R. Reflexes from respiratory muscles and costovertebral joints. In: Cherniack NS, Widdicombe JG, eds. Handbook of Physiology: Section 3: The Respiratory System. Vol II: Control of Breathing, Part 1. Bethesda, MD: American Physiological Society, 1986:431–447.

12. Jordan D, Spyer KM. Brainstem integration of cardiovascular and pulmonary afferent activity. Prog Brain Res 1986; 67:295–314.

13. Jean A. Control of the central swallowing program by inputs from the peripheral receptors. A review. J Auton Nerv Syst 1984; 10:225–233.

14. Miller AJ. Deglutition. Physiol Rev 1982; 62:129–184.

15. Altschuler SM, Davies RO, Pack AI. Role of medullary inspiratory neurones in the control of the diaphragm during gastrointestinal reflexes. J Physiol (Lond) 1987; 391:289–298.

16. Koga T, Fukuda H. Neurons in the nucleus of the solitary tract mediating inputs from emetic vagal afferents and the area postrema to the pattern generator for the emetic act in dogs. Neurosci Res 1992; 14:166–179.

17. Iscoe S, Grélot L. Regional intercostal activity during coughing and vomiting in decerebrate cats. Can J Physiol Pharmacol 1992; 70:1195–1199.

18. Miller AD, Nonaka S, Lakos SF, Tan LK. Diaphragmatic and external intercostal muscle control during vomiting: behavior of inspiratory bulbospinal neurons. J Neurosci 1990; 63:31–36.

19. Ukabam CU, Knuth SL, Bartlett D Jr. Phrenic and hypoglossal neural responses to cold airflow in the upper airway. Respir Physiol 1992; 87:157–164.

20. Haddad GG, Farber JP. Developmental Neurobiology of Breathing. New York: Marcel Dekker, 1991.

21. Mei N, Condamin M, Boyer A. The composition of the vagus nerve of the cat. Cell Tissue Res 1980; 209:423–431.
22. Agostoni E., Chinnock JE, Daly de Burgh M, Murray JE. Functional and histological studies of the vagus nerve and its branches to the heart, lung and abdominal viscera in the cat. J Physiol 1957; 135:182–205.
23. Jammes Y, Fornaris E, Mei N, Barrat E. Afferent and efferent components of the bronchial vagal branches in cats. J Auton Nerv Syst 1982; 5:165–176.
24. Patrickson JW, Smith TE, Zhou S-S. Afferent projections of the superior and recurrent laryngeal nerves. Brain Res 1991; 539:169–174.
25. Gacek RR, Lyon MJ. Fiber components of the recurrent laryngeal nerve in the cat. Ann Otol Rhinol Laryngol 1976; 85:460–471.
26. Murray JG. Innervation of the intrinsic muscles of the cat's larynx by the recurrent laryngeal nerve: a unimodal nerve. J Physiol (Lond) 1957; 135:206–212.
27. Miller AJ, Loizzi RF. Anatomical and functional differentiation of superior laryngeal nerve fibers affecting swallowing and respiration. Exp Neurol 1974; 42:369–387.
28. Altschuler SM, Bao X, Bieger D, Hopkins DA, Miselis RR. Viscerotopic representation of the upper alimentary tract in the rat: sensory ganglia and nuclei of the solitary and spinal trigeminal tracts. J Comp Neurol 1989; 283:248–268.
29. Keller JT, Beduk A, Saunders MC. Central brainstem projections of the superior vagal ganglion of the cat. Neurosci Lett 1987; 75:265–270.
30. Lucier GE, Egizii R, Dostrovsky JO. Projections of the internal branch of the superior laryngeal nerve of the cat. Brain Res Bull 1986; 16:713–721.
31. Finley JCW, Polak J, Katz DM. Transmitter diversity in carotid body afferent neurons: dopaminergic and peptidergic phenotypes. Neuroscience 1992; 51:973–987.
32. Nomura S, Mizuno N. Central distribution of primary afferent fibers in the Arnold's nerve (the auricular branch of the vagus nerve): a transganglionic HRP study in the cat. Brain Res 1984; 292:199–205.
33. Paintal AS. Vagal sensory receptors and their reflex effects. Physiol Rev 1973; 53:159–227.
34. Coleridge HM, Coleridge JCG. Afferent vagal C-fibers in the dog lung: their discharge during spontaneous breathing, and their stimulation by alloxan and pulmonary congestion. In: Paintal AS, Gill-Kumar P, eds. Respiratory Adaptations, Capillary Exchange and Reflex Mechanisms. Delhi: V. Patel Chest Institute, 1977: 397–406.
35. Kubin L, Kimura H, Davies RO. The medullary projections of afferent bronchopulmonary C fibres in the cat as shown by antidromic mapping. J Physiol (Lond) 1991; 435:207–228.
36. Delpierre S, Grimaud CH, Jammes Y, Mei N. Changes in activity of vagal bronchopulmonary C-fibres by chemical and physical stimuli in the cat. J Physiol (Lond) 1981; 316:61–74.
37. Pisarri TE, Yu J, Coleridge HM, Coleridge JCG. Background activity in pulmonary vagal C-fibers and its effects on breathing. Respir Physiol 1986; 64:29–43.
38. Sant'Ambrogio G. Information arising from the tracheobronchial tree of mammals. Physiol Rev 1982; 62:532–568.

39. Widdicombe JG. Pulmonary and respiratory tract receptors. J Exp Biol 1982; 100: 41–57.

40. Düring, M, von, Andres KH. Structure and functional anatomy of visceroreceptors in the mammalian respiratory system. Prog Brain Res 1988; 74:139–154.

41. Wei JY, Shen E. Vagal expiratory afferent discharges during spontaneous breathing. Brain Res 1985; 335:213–219.

42. Tsubone H. Characteristics of vagal afferent activity in rats: three types of pulmonary receptors responding to collapse, inflation, and deflation of the lung. Exp Neurol 1986; 92:541–552.

43. Bergren DR, Peterson DF. Identification of vagal sensory receptors in the rat lung: are these subtypes of slowly adapting receptors? J Physiol (Lond) 1993; 464: 681–698.

44. Schoener EP, Frankel HM. Effect of hyperthermia and $Paco_2$ on the slowly adapting pulmonary stretch receptor. Am J Physiol 1972; 222:68–72.

45. Green JF, Schertel ER, Coleridge HM, Coleridge JCG. Effect of pulmonary arterial Pco_2 on slowly adapting pulmonary stretch receptors. J Appl Physiol 1986; 60:2048–2055.

46. Mitchell RA, Herbert DA, Baker DG. Inspiratory rhythm in airway smooth muscle tone. J Appl Physiol 1985; 58:911–920.

47. Matsumoto S, Shimizu T, Kanno T, Yamasaki M, Nagayama T. Effects of histamine on slowly adapting pulmonary stretch receptor activities in vagotomized rabbits. Jpn J Physiol 1990; 40:737–752.

48. Iscoe S, Gordon SP. Chest wall distortion and discharge of pulmonary slowly adapting receptors. J Appl Physiol 1992; 73:1619–1625.

49. Yu J, Roberts AM. Indirect effect of histamine on pulmonary rapidly adapting receptors in cats. Respir Physiol 1990; 79:101–110.

50. Anderson JW, Sant'Ambrogio FB, Orani GP, Sant'Ambrogio G, Mathew OP. Carbon dioxide-responsive laryngeal receptors in the dog. Respir Physiol 1990; 82: 217–226.

51. Bartlett D Jr, Knuth SL. Responses of laryngeal receptors to intralaryngeal CO_2 in the cat. J Physiol (Lond) 1992; 457:187–193.

52. Sant'Ambrogio G, Sant'Ambrogio FB, Mathew OP. Effect of cold air on laryngeal mechanoreceptors in the dog. Respir Physiol 1986; 64:45–56.

53. Anderson JW, Sant'Ambrogio FB, Mathew OP, Sant'Ambrogio G. Water-responsive laryngeal receptors in the dog are not specialized endings. Respir Physiol 1990; 79:33–44.

54. Kappagoda CT, Man GCW, Teo KK. Behaviour of canine pulmonary vagal afferent receptors during sustained acute pulmonary venous pressure elevation. J Physiol (Lond) 1987; 394:249–265.

55. Iscoe SD. Central control of the upper airway. In: Mathew OP, Sant'Ambrogio G, eds. Respiratory Function of the Upper Airway. New York: Marcel Dekker, 1988: 125–192.

56. Coleridge HM, Coleridge JCG, Schultz HD. Afferent pathways involved in reflex regulation of airway smooth muscle. Pharmacol Ther 1989; 42:1–63.

57. Guyenet PG, Koshiya N. Respiratory-sympathetic integration in the medulla oblon-

gata. In: Kunos G, Ciriello J, eds. Central Neural Mechanisms in Cardiovascular Regulation, Vol 2. Boston: Birkhauser, 1991:226–247.

58. Green JF, Kaufman MP. Pulmonary afferent control of breathing as end-expiratory lung volume decreases. J Appl Physiol 1990; 68(5):2186–2194.

59. Roberts AM, Bhattacharya J, Schultz HD, Coleridge HM, Coleridge JCG. Stimulation of pulmonary vagal afferent C-fibers by lung edema in dogs. Circ Res 1986; 58:512–522.

60. Feldman JL, Ellenberger HH. Central coordination of respiratory and cardiovascular control in mammals. Annu Rev Physiol 1988; 50:593–606.

61. Kalia M, Sullivan JM. Brainstem projections of sensory and motor components of the vagus nerve in the rat. J Comp Neurol 1982; 211:248–264.

62. Kalia M, Mesulam M-M. Brain stem projections of sensory and motor components of the vagus complex in the cat. I. The cervical vagus and nodose ganglion. J Comp Neurol 1980; 193:435–465.

63. Martin Wild J, Johnston BM, Gluckman PD. Central projections of the nodose ganglion and the origin of vagal efferents in the lamb. J Anat 1991; 175:105–129.

64. Hamilton RB, Pritchard TC, Norgren R. Central distribution of the cervical vagus nerve in Old and New World primates. J Auton Nerv Syst 1987; 19:153–169.

65. Beckstead RM, Norgren R. An autoradiographic examination of the central distribution of the trigeminal, facial, glossopharyngeal, and vagal nerves in the monkey. J Comp Neurol 1979; 184:409–421.

66. Contreras RJ, Beckstead RM, Norgren R. The central projections of the trigeminal, facial, glossopharyngeal and vagus nerves: an autoradiographic study in the rat. J Auton Nerv Syst 1982; 6:303–322.

67. Torvik A. Afferent connections of the sensory trigeminal nuclei, the nucleus of the solitary tract and adjacent structures: An experimental study in the rat. J Comp Neurol 1956; 106:51–141.

68. Kerr FWL. Facial, vagal and glossopharyngeal nerves in the cat. Arch Neurol 1962; 6:264–281.

69. Ciriello J, Hrycyshyn AW, Calaresu FR. Glossopharyngeal and vagal afferent projections to the brain stem of the cat: a horseradish peroxidase study. J Auton Nerv Syst 1981; 4:63–79.

70. Herbert H, Moga MM, Saper CB. Connections of the parabrachial nucleus with the nucleus of the solitary tract and the medullary reticular formation in the rat. J Comp Neurol 1990; 293:540–580.

71. Loewy AD, Burton H. Nuclei of the solitary tract: efferent projections to the lower brain stem and spinal cord of the cat. J Comp Neurol 1978; 181:421–450.

72. Ruiz Pesini P, Cifuentes JM, Fernandez-Troconiz P. The nucleus of the tractus solitarius of the dog. A morphological and morphometric analysis. J Anat 1991; 176:113–132.

73. Störmer, R, Goller H. Zur finstrucktur des nucleus tractus solitarii von schaf und ziege. J Hirnforsch 1988; 29:633–641.

74. Whitehead MC. Neuronal architecture of the nucleus of the solitary tract in the hamster. J Comp Neurol 1988; 276:547–572.

75. Hyde TM, Miselis RR. Subnuclear organization of the human caudal nucleus of the solitary tract. Brain Res Bull 1992; 29:95–109.

76. McRitchie DA, Török I. The internal organization of the human solitary nucleus. Brain Res Bull 1993; 31:171–193.

77. Ross CA, Riggiero DA, Reis DJ. Projections from the nucleus tractus solitarii to the rostral ventrolateral medulla. J Comp Neurol 1985; 242:511–534.

78. Cunningham ET, Jr, Sawchenko PE. A circumscribed projection from the nucleus of the solitary tract to the nucleus ambiguus in the rat: anatomical evidence for somatostatin-28-immunoreactive interneurons subserving reflex control of esophageal motility. J Neurosci 1989; 9:1668–1682.

79. Hanamori T, Smith DV. Gustatory innervation in the rabbit: central distribution of sensory and motor components of the chorda tympani, glossopharyngeal, and superior laryngeal nerves. J Comp Neurol 1989; 282:1–14.

80. Odekunle A, Bower AJ. Brainstem connections of vagal afferent nerves in the ferret: an autoradiographic study. J Anat 1985; 140:461–469.

81. Panneton WM. Primary afferent projections from the upper respiratory tract in the muskrat. J Comp Neurol 1991; 308:51–65.

82. Chernicky CL, Barnes KL, Ferrario CM, Conomy JP. Afferent projections of the cervical vagus and nodose ganglion in the dog. Brain Res Bull 1984; 13: 401–411.

83. Nomura S, Mizuno N. Central distribution of efferent and afferent components of the cervical branches of the vagus nerve: a HRP study in the cat. Anat Embryol 1983; 166:1–18.

84. Sweazey RD, Bradley RM. Central connections of the lingual-tonsillar branch of the glossopharyngeal nerve and the superior laryngeal nerve in lamb. J Comp Neurol 1986; 245:471–482.

85. Hamilton RB, Norgren R. Central projections of gustatory nerves in the rat. J Comp Neurol 1984; 222:560–577.

86. Sweazey RD, Bradley RM. Responses of neurons in the lamb nucleus tractus solitarius to stimulation of the caudal oral cavity and epiglottis with different stimulus modalities. Brain Res 1989; 480:133–150.

87. Claps A, Torrealba F, Calderón F. Segregation of coarse and fine glossopharyngeal axons in the visceral nucleus of the tractus solitarius of the cat. Brain Res 1989; 489:80–92.

88. Torrealba F, Calderón F. Central projections of coarse and fine vagal axons of the cat. Brain Res 1990; 510:351–354.

89. Bennett JA, Goodchild CS, Kidd C, McWilliam PN. Neurones in the brain stem of the cat excited by vagal afferent fibres from the heart and lungs. J Physiol (Lond) 1985; 369:1–15.

90. Norgren R, Smith GP. Central distribution of subdiaphragmatic vagal branches in the rat. J Comp Neurol 1988; 273:207–223.

91. Altschuler SM, Ferenci DA, Lynn RB, Miselis RR. Representation of the cecum in the lateral dorsal motor nucleus of the vagus nerve and commissural subnucleus of the nucleus tractus solitarii in rat. J Comp Neurol 1991; 304:261–274.

92. Kalia M, Mesulam M-M. Brain stem projections of sensory and motor components of the vagus complex in the cat. II. Laryngeal, tracheobronchial, pulmonary, cardiac and gastrointestinal branches. J Comp Neurol 1980; 193:467–508.

93. Mei N. Disposition anatomique et propriétés électrophysiologiques des neurones sensitifs vagaux chez le chat. Exp Brain Res 1970; 11:465–479.

94. Hisa Y, Lyon MJ, Malmgren LT. Central projection of the sensory component of the rat recurrent laryngeal nerve. Neurosci Lett 1985; 55:185–190.

95. Bellingham MC, Lipski J. Morphology and electrophysiology of superior laryngeal nerve afferents and postsynaptic neurons in the medulla oblongata of the cat. Neuroscience 1992; 48:205–216.

96. Schwarzacher SW, Anders K, Richter DW. Central projections of laryngeal afferents in the cat. In: Proc Intern Conf on Modulation of Respiratory Pattern: Peripheral and Central Mechanisms, Lexington KY: University of Kentucky, 1990:59.

97. Donoghue S, Garcia M, Jordan D, Spyer KM. The brain-stem projections of pulmonary stretch afferent neurones in cats and rabbits. J Physiol (Lond) 1982; 322:353–363.

98. Davies RO, Kubin L. Projection of pulmonary rapidly adapting receptor neurones to the medulla of the cat: an antidromic mapping study. J Physiol (Lond) 1986; 373: 63–86.

99. Davies RO, Kubin L, Pack AI. Pulmonary stretch receptor relay neurones of the cat: location and contralateral medullary projections. J Physiol (Lond) 1987; 383:571–585.

100. Berger AJ, Averill DB. Projection of single pulmonary stretch receptors to solitary tract region. J Neurophysiol 1983; 49:819–830.

101. Kalia M, Richter D. Morphology of physiologically identified slowly adapting lung stretch receptor afferents stained with intra-axonal horseradish peroxidase in the nucleus of the tractus solitarius of the cat. I. A light microscopic analysis. J Comp Neurol 1985; 241:503–520.

102. Backman SB, Anders C, Ballantyne D, Röhrig N, Camerer H, Mifflin S, Jordan D, Dickhaus H, Spyer KM, Richter DW. Evidence for a monosynaptic connection between slowly adapting pulmonary stretch receptor afferents and inspiratory beta neurones. Pflügers Arch 1984; 402:129–136.

103. Kalia M, Richter D. Morphology of physiologically identified slowly adapting lung stretch receptor afferents stained with intra-axonal horseradish peroxidase in the nucleus of the tractus solitarius of the cat. II. An ultrastructural analysis. J Comp Neurol 1985; 241:521–535.

104. Lloyd TC Jr. Effects of extrapulmonary airway distension on breathing in anesthetized dogs. J Appl Physiol 1979; 46:890–896.

105. Lloyd TC Jr, Cooper JA. Failure of tracheal distension to inhibit breathing in anesthetized dogs. J Appl Physiol 1980; 48:794–798.

106. Agostoni E, Citterio G, Piccoli S. Reflex partitioning of inputs from stretch receptors of bronchi and thoracic trachea. Respir Physiol 1985; 60:311–328.

107. Ravi K. Distribution and location of slowly adapting pulmonary stretch receptors in the airways of cats. J Auton Nerv Syst 1986; 15:205–216.

108. Kubin L, Davies RO. Sites of termination and relay of pulmonary rapidly adapting receptors as studied by spike-triggered averaging. Brain Res 1988; 443:215–221.

109. Kalia M, Richter D. Rapidly adapting pulmonary receptor afferents. I. Arborization in the nucleus of the tractus solitarius. J Comp Neurol 1988; 274:560–573.

110. Kalia M, Richter D. Rapidly adapting pulmonary receptor afferents. II. Fine

structure and synaptic organization of central terminal processes in the nucleus of the tractus solitarius. J Comp Neurol 1988; 274:574–594.

111. Donoghue S, Fox RE, Kidd C, Koley BN. The distribution in the cat brain stem of neurones activated by vagal non-myelinated fibres from the heart and lungs. Q J Exp Physiol 1981; 66:391–404.

112. McCrimmon DR, Miller JF. Fos-like immunoreactivity in rat brainstem neurons following activation of large myelinated afferents in the vagus nerves. FASEB J 1992; 6:A1508.

113. Berger AJ, Dick TE. Connectivity of slowly adapting pulmonary stretch receptors with dorsal medullary respiratory neurons. J Neurophysiol 1987; 58:1259–1274.

114. Cohen MI, Feldman JM. Discharge properties of dorsal medullary inspiratory neurons: relation to pulmonary afferent and phrenic efferent discharge. J Neurophysiol 1984; 51:753–776.

115. Cohen MI. Neurogenesis of respiratory rhythm in the mammal. Physiol Rev 1979; 59:1105–1173.

116. Berger AJ. Dorsal respiratory group neurons in the medulla of cat: spinal projections, responses to lung inflation and superior laryngeal nerve stimulation. Brain Res 1977; 135:231–254.

117. Baumgarten R, von, Kanzow E. The interaction of two types of inspiratory neurons in the region of the tractus solitarius of the cat. Arch Ital Biol 1958; 96:361–373.

118. Averill DB, Cameron WE, Berger AJ. Monosynaptic excitation of dorsal medullary respiratory neurons by slowly adapting pulmonary stretch receptors. J Neurophysiol 1984; 52:771–785.

119. Pantaleo T, Corda M. Respiration-related neurons in the medial nuclear complex of the solitary tract of the cat. Respir Physiol 1986; 64:135–148.

120. Sant'Ambrogio G, Mathew OP, Fisher JT, Sant'Ambrogio FB. Laryngeal receptors responding to transmural pressure, airflow and local muscle activity. Respir Physiol 1983; 54:317–330.

121. Sant'Ambrogio FB, Mathew OP, Tsubone H, Sant'Ambrogio G. Afferent activity in the external branch of the superior laryngeal and recurrent laryngeal nerves. Ann Otol Rhinol Laryngol 1991; 100:944–950.

122. Bonham AC, McCrimmon DR. Neurones in a discrete region of the nucleus tractus solitarius are required for the Breuer-Hering reflex in rat. J Physiol (Lond) 1990; 427:261–280.

123. McCrimmon DR, Speck DF, Feldman JL. Role of the ventrolateral region of the nucleus of the tractus solitarius in processing respiratory afferent input from vagus and superior laryngeal nerves. Exp Brain Res 1987; 67:449–459.

124. Ezure K, Otake K, Lipski J, Wong She RB. Efferent projections of pulmonary rapidly adapting receptor relay neurons in the cat. Brain Res 1991; 564:268–278.

125. Cohen MI, Feldman JL. Models of respiratory phase-switching. Fed Proc 1977; 36:2367–2374.

126. Lipski J, Kubin L, Jodkowski J. Synaptic action of R_β neurons on phrenic motoneurons studied with spike-triggered averaging. Brain Res 1983; 288:105–118.

127. Kubin L, Davies RO. Bilateral convergence of pulmonary stretch receptor inputs on I-β neurons in the cat. J Appl Physiol 1987; 62:1488–1496.

128. Bajić J, Zuperku EJ, Hopp FA. Processing of pulmonary afferent input patterns by respiratory I-β neurons. Am J Physiol 1989; 256:R379–R393.

129. Duffin J, Lipski J. Monosynaptic excitation of thoracic motoneurones by inspiratory neurones of the nucleus tractus solitarius in the cat. J Physiol (Lond) 1987; 390: 415–431.

130. Ezure K. Synaptic connections between medullary respiratory neurons and considerations on the genesis of respiratory rhythm. Prog Neurobiol 1990; 35:429–450.

131. Marino PL, Davies RO, Pack AI. Responses of I-beta neurons to increases in the rate of lung inflation. Brain Res 1981; 219:289–305.

132. Clark FJ, Euler C, von. On the regulation of depth and rate of breathing. J Physiol (Lond) 1972; 222:267–295.

133. Wyman RJ. Neurophysiology of the motor output pattern generator for breathing. Fed Proc 1976; 35:2013–2023.

134. Feldman JL, McCrimmon DR, Speck DF. Effect of synchronous activation of medullary inspiratory bulbo-spinal neurones on phrenic nerve discharge in cat. J Physiol (Lond) 1984; 347:241–254.

135. Lipski J, Trzebski A, Kubin L. Excitability changes of dorsal inspiratory neurons during lung inflations as studied by measurement of antidromic invasion latencies. Brain Res 1979; 161:25–38.

136. Bianchi AL, St. John WM. Pontile axonal projections of medullary respiratory neurons. Respir Physiol 1981; 45:167–183.

137. Speck DF, Feldman JL. The effects of microstimulation and microlesions in the ventral and dorsal respiratory groups in the medulla of cat on respiratory outflow. J Neurosci 1982; 2:744–757.

138. Kubin L, Davies RO, Pack AI. Inspiratory neurons located in the medial part of the nucleus tractus solitarius (NTS) in cats. Fed Proc 1985; 44:1585.

139. Oku Y, Tanaka I, Ezure K. Possible inspiratory off-switch neurones in the ventrolateral medulla of the cat. NeuroReport 1992; 3:933–936.

140. Cohen MI, Huang W-X, Barnhardt R, See WR. Timing of medullary late-inspiratory neuron discharges: vagal afferent effects indicate possible off-switch function. J Neurophysiol 1993; 69:1784–1787.

141. Iscoe S, Feldman JL, Cohen MI. Properties of inspiratory termination by superior laryngeal and vagal stimulation. Respir Physiol 1979; 36:353–366.

142. Cross BA, Guz A, Jones PW. The summation of left and right lung volume information in the control of breathing in dogs. J Physiol (Lond) 1981; 321:449–467.

143. Berger AJ, Averill DB, Cameron WE. Morphology of inspiratory neurons located in the ventrolateral nucleus of the tractus solitarius of the cat. J Comp Neurol 1984; 224:60–70.

144. Donnelly DF, Sica AL, Cohen MI, Zhang H. Dorsal medullary inspiratory neurons: effects of superior laryngeal afferent stimulation. Brain Res 1989; 491:243–252.

145. Lipski J, Ezure K, Wong She RB. Identification of neurons receiving input from pulmonary rapidly adapting receptors in the cat. J Physiol (Lond) 1991; 443:55–77.

146. Jonzon A, Pisarri TE, Roberts AM, Coleridge JCG, Coleridge HM. Rapidly adapting receptor activity in dogs is inversely related to lung compliance. J Apply Physiol 1986; 61:1980–1987.

147. Armstrong DJ, Luck JC. A comparative study of irritant and type J receptors in the cat. Respir Physiol 1974; 21:47–60.

148. Otake K, Ezure K, Lipski J, Wong She RB. Projections from the commissural subnucleus of the nucleus of the solitary tract: an anterograde tracing study in the cat. J Comp Neurol 1992; 324:365–378.

149. King GW. Topology of ascending brainstem projections to nucleus parabrachialis in the cat. J Comp Neurol 1980; 191:615–638.

150. Kalia M. Neuroanatomical organization of the respiratory centers. Fed Proc 1977; 36:2405–2411.

151. Sweazey RD, Bradley RM. Responses of lamb nucleus of the solitary tract neurons to chemical stimulation of the epiglottis. Brain Res 1988; 439:195–210.

152. Bradley RM, Stedman HM, Mistretta CM. Superior laryngeal nerve response patterns to chemical stimulation of sheep epiglottis. Brain Res 1983; 276:81–93.

153. Dickman JD, Smith DV. Response properties of fibers in the hamster superior laryngeal nerve. Brain Res 1988; 450:25–38.

154. Tsubone H, Sant'Ambrogio G, Anderson JW, Orani GP. Laryngeal afferent activity and reflexes in the guinea pig. Respir Physiol 1991; 86:215–231.

155. Sant'Ambrogio G, Anderson JW, Sant'Ambrogio FB. Laryngeal sensory modalities and their functional significance. In: Speck DF, Dekin MS, Revelette WR, Frazier DT, eds. Respiratory Control: Central and Peripheral Mechanisms. Lexington: University Press of Kentucky, 1993:52–57.

156. Sweazey RD, Bradley RM. Response characteristics of lamb pontine neurons to stimulation of the oral cavity and epiglottis with different sensory modalities. J Neurophysiol 1993; 70:1168–1180.

157. Mathew OP, Anderson JW, Orani GP, Sant'Ambrogio FB, Sant'Ambrogio G. Cooling mediates the ventilatory depression associated with airflow through the larynx. Respir Physiol 1990; 82:359–368.

158. Bartlett D Jr, Knuth SL, Gdovin MJ. Influence of laryngeal CO_2 on respiratory activities of motor nerves to accessory muscles. Respir Physiol 1992; 90:289–297.

159. Bartlett D Jr, Knuth SL, Leiter JC. Alteration of ventilatory activity by intra-laryngeal CO_2 in the cat. J Physiol (Lond) 1992; 457:177–185.

160. Fedorko L, Merrill EG, Lipski J. Two descending medullary inspiratory pathways to phrenic motoneurones. Neurosci Lett 1983; 43:285–291.

161. Jiang C, Lipski. Synaptic inputs to medullary respiratory neurons from superior laryngeal afferents in the cat. Brain Res 1992; 584:197–206.

162. Berger AJ. Respiratory gating of phrenic motoneuron responses to superior laryngeal nerve stimulation. Brain Res 1978; 157:381–384.

163. Donnelly DF, Sica AL, Cohen MI, Zhang H. Effects of contralateral superior laryngeal nerve stimulation on dorsal medullary inspiratory neurons. Brain Res 1989; 505:149–152.

164. Mifflin SW. Laryngeal afferent inputs to the nucleus of the solitary tract. Am J Physiol 1993; R269–R276.

165. Travers JB. Efferent projections from the anterior nucleus of the solitary tract of the hamster. Brain Res 1988; 457:1–11.

166. Bonham AC, Joad JP. Neurones in commissural nucleus tractus solitarii required for

full expression of the pulmonary C fibre reflex in rat. J Physiol (Lond) 1991; 441: 95–112.

167. Strain SM, Gwyn DG, Rutherford JG, Losier BJ. Direct vagal input to neurons in the area postrema which project to the parabrachial nucleus: an electron microscopic-HRP study in the cat. Brain Res Bull 1990; 24:457–463.

168. Davies RO, Metzler J, Silage DA, Pack AI. Effects of lung inflation on the excitability of dorsal respiratory group neurons. Brain Res 1986; 366:22–36.

169. Sessle BJ, Greenwood LF, Lund JP, Lucier GE. Effects of upper respiratory tract stimuli on respiration and single respiratory neurons in the adult cat. Exp Neurol 1978; 61:245–259.

170. Sessle BJ. Excitatory and inhibitory inputs to single neurones in the solitary tract nucleus and adjacent reticular formation. Brain Res 1973; 53:319–331.

171. Biscoe TJ, Sampson SR. Responses of cells in the brain stem of the cat to stimulation of the sinus, glossopharyngeal, aortic and superior laryngeal nerves. J Physiol (Lond) 1970; 209:359–373.

172. Beckman ME, Whitehead MC. Intramedullary connections of the rostral nucleus of the solitary tract in the hamster. Brain Res 1991; 557:265–279.

173. Iscoe S, Grélot L, Bianchi AL. Responses of inspiratory neurons of the dorsal respiratory group to stimulation of expiratory muscle and vagal afferents. Brain Res 1990; 507:281–288.

174. Shannon R, Bolser DC, Lindsey BG. Medullary neurons mediating the inhibition of inspiration by intercostal muscle tendon organs? J Appl Physiol 1988; 65:2498–2505.

175. Person RJ. Somatic and vagal afferent convergence on solitary tract neurons in cat: electrophysiological characteristics. Neuroscience 1989; 30:283–295.

176. Bassal M, Bianchi AL, Dussardier M. Effets de la stimulation des structures ner-veuses sur l'activite des neurones respiratoires chez le chat. J Physiol (Paris) 1981; 77:779–795.

177. van der Kooy D, Koda LY, McGinty JF, Gerfen CR, Bloom FE. The organization of projections from the cortex, amygdala, and hypothalamus to the nucleus of the solitary tract in rat. J Comp Neurol 1984; 224:1–24.

178. Willett CJ, Gwyn DG, Rutherford JG, Leslie RA. Cortical projections to the nucleus of the tractus solitarius: an HRP study in the cat. Brain Res Bull 1986; 16:497–505.

179. Jean A, Car A. Inputs to the swallowing medullary neurons from the peripheral afferent fibers and the swallowing cortical area. Brain Res 1979; 178:567–572.

180. Jordan D, Wood, LM. A convergent input from nasal receptors and the larynx to the rostral sensory trigeminal nuclei of the cat. J Physiol (Lond) 1987; 393:147–155.

181. Torrealba F, Claps A. The carotid sinus connections: a WGA-HRP study in the cat. Brain Res 1988; 455:134–143.

182. Claps A, Torrealba F. The carotid body connections: a WGA-HRP study in the cat. Brain Res 1988; 455:123–133.

183. Donoghue S, Felder RB, Jordan D, Spyer KM. The central projections of carotid baroreceptors and chemoreceptors in the cat: a neurophysiological study. J Physiol (Lond) 1984; 347:397–409.

184. Kubin L, Trzebski A, Lipski J. Descending pathways utilized by chemoreceptor and

baroreceptor sympathetic reflexes in the lower medulla. In: Belmonte C, Pallot DJ, Acker H, Fidone S, eds. Arterial Chemoreceptors. Proceedings of the 6th International Meeting. Leicester: Leicester University Press, 1980:481–490.

185. Kubin L, Trzebski A, Lipski J. Split medulla preparation in the cat: arterial chemoreceptor reflex and respiratory modulation of the renal sympathetic nerve activity. J Auton Nerv Syst 1985; 12:211–225.

186. Housley GD, Sinclair JD. Localization by kainic acid lesions of neurones transmitting the carotid chemoreceptor stimulus for respiration in rat. J Physiol (Lond) 1988; 406:99–114.

187. Lawson EE, Richter DW, Ballantyne D, Lalley PM. Peripheral chemoreceptor inputs to medullary inspiratory and postinspiratory neurons of cats. Pflügers Arch 1989; 414:523–533.

188. Czachurski J, Lackner KJ, Ockert D, Seller H. Localization of neurones with baroreceptor input in the medial solitary nucleus by means of intracellular application of horseradish peroxidase in the cat. Neurosci Lett 1982; 28:133–137.

189. Czachurski J, Dembowsky K, Seller H, Nobiling R, Taugner R. Morphology of electrophysiologically identified baroreceptor afferents and second order neurones in the brainstem of the cat. Arch Ital Biol 1988; 126:129–144.

190. Shapiro RE, Miselis RR. The central organization of the vagus nerve innervating the stomach of the rat. J Comp Neurol 1985; 238:473–488.

191. Maley B, Elde R. Immunohistochemical localization of putative neurotransmitters within the feline nucleus tractus solitarii. Neuroscience 1982; 7:2469–2490.

192. Baude A, Lanoir J, Vernier P, Puizillout JJ. Substance P-immunoreactivity in the dorsal medial region of the medulla in the cat: effects of nodosectomy. J Chem Neuroanat 1989; 2:67–81.

193. Maley BE, Sasek CA, Seybold VS. Substance P binding sites in the nucleus tractus solitarius of the cat. Peptides 1989; 9:1301–1306.

194. Katz DM, Karten HJ. The discrete anatomical localization of vagal aortic afferents within a catecholamine-containing cell group in the nucleus solitarius. Brain Res 1979; 171:187–195.

195. Lee HS, Basbaum AI. Immunoreactive pro-enkephalin and pro-dynorphin products are differentially distributed within the nucleus of the solitary tract of the rat. J Comp Neurol 1984; 230:614–619.

196. Torrealba F. Calcitonin gene-related peptide immunoreactivity in the nucleus of the tractus solitarius and the carotid receptors of the cat originates from peripheral afferents. Neuroscience 1992; 47:165–173.

197. Riche D, DePommery J, Menetrey D. Neuropeptides and catecholamines in efferent projections of the nuclei of the solitary tract in the rat. J Comp Neurol 1990; 293:399–424.

198. Herbert H, Saper CB. Cholecystokinin-, galanin-, and corticotropin-releasing factor-like immunoreactive projections from the nucleus of the solitary tract to the parabrachial nucleus in the rat. J Comp Neurol 1990; 293:581–598.

199. Barry MA, Halsell CB, Whitehead MC. Organization of the nucleus of the solitary tract in the hamster: acetylcholinesterase, NADH dehydrogenase, and cytochrome oxidase histochemistry. Microsc Res Technol 1993; 26:231–244.

200. Carr PA, Nagy JI. Emerging relationships between cytochemical properties and sensory modality transmission in primary sensory neurons. Brain Res Bull 1993; 30: 209–219.

201. Mitchell GS, Douse MA, Foley KT. Receptor interactions in modulating ventilatory activity. Am J Physiol 1990; 259:R911–R920.

202. Nishino T, Honda Y. Time-dependent responses of expiration reflex in cats. J Appl Physiol 1986; 61:430–435.

203. Kuna ST. Interaction of hypercapnia and phasic volume feedback on motor control of the upper airway. J Appl Physiol 1987; 63:1744–1749.

204. Daly M de B, Kirkman E. Cardiovascular responses to stimulation of pulmonary c fibres in the cat: their modulation by changes in respiration. J Physiol (Lond) 1988; 402:43–63.

205. Schmidt RF. Presynaptic inhibition in the vertebrate central nervous system. Rev Physiol Biochem Pharmacol 1971; 63:20–101.

206. Hildebrandt JR. Gating: a mechanisms for selective receptivity in the respiratory center. Fed Proc 1977; 36:2381–2385.

207. Rudomin P. Presynaptic inhibition induced by vagal afferent volleys. J Neurophysiol 1967; 30:964–981.

208. Barillot JC. Dépolarisation présynaptique des fibres sensitives vagales et laryngées. J Physiol (Paris) 1970; 62:273–294.

209. Sessle BJ. Presynaptic excitatory changes induced in single laryngeal primary afferent fibres. Brain Res 1973; 53:333–342.

210. Richter DW, Jordan D, Ballantyne D, Meesmann M, Spyer KM. Presynaptic depolarization in myelinated vagal afferent fibres terminating in the nucleus of the tractus solitarius in the cat. Pflügers Arch 1986; 406:12–19.

211. Lucier GE, Sessle BJ. Presynaptic excitability changes induced in the solitary tract endings of laryngeal primary afferents by stimulation of nucleus raphe magnus and locus coeruleus. Neurosci Lett 1981; 26:221–226.

212. Rudomin P. Excitability changes of superior laryngeal, vagal and depressor afferent terminals produced by stimulation of the solitary tract nucleus. Exp Brain Res 1968; 6:156–170.

213. Jordan D, Donoghue S, Spyer KM. Respiratory modulation of afferent terminal excitability in the nucleus tractus solitarius. J Auton Nerv Syst 1981; 3:291–297.

214. Kubin L. Respiratory modulation of the pulmonary stretch receptor (PSR) input to dorsal respiratory group (DRG) neurons in the cat. Acta Physiol Pol (Warsaw) 1987; 30:128–129.

215. Rudomin P, Engberg I. Jankowska E. Jiménez I. Evidence of two different mechanisms involved in the generation of presynaptic depolarization of afferent and rubrospinal fibers in the cat spinal cord. Brain Res 1980; 189:256–261.

216. Jiménez I, Rudomin P, Solodkin M, Vyklicky L. Specific and potassium components in the depolarization of the Ia afferents in the spinal cord of the cat. Brain Res 1983; 272:179–184.

217. Richter DW, Camerer H, Sonnhof U. Changes in extracellular potassium during the spontaneous activity of medullary respiratory neurones. Pflügers Arch 1978; 376: 139–149.

218. Ballanyi K, Branchereau P, Champagnat J, Fortin G, Velluti J. Extracellular potassium, glial and neuronal potentials in the solitary complex of rat brainstem slices. Brain Res 1993; 607:99–107.

219. Chazal G, Baude A, Barbe A, Puizillout JJ. Ultrastructural organization of the interstitial subnucleus of the nucleus of the tractus solitarius in the cat: identification of vagal afferents. J Neurocytol 1991; 20:859–874.

220. Kawai Y, Mori S, Takagi H. Vagal afferents interact with substance P–immunoreactive structures in the nucleus of the tractus solitarius: immunoelectronmicroscopy combined with an anterograde degeneration study. Neurosci Lett 1989; 101:6–10.

221. Meeley MP, Ruggiero DA, Ishitsuka T, Reis DJ. Intrinsic gamma-aminobutyric acid neurons in the nucleus of the solitary tract and the rostral ventrolateral medulla of the rat: an immunocytochemical and biochemical study. Neurosci Lett 1985; 83–88.

222. Lipski J, Waldvogel HJ, Pilowsky P, Jiang C. GABA-immunoreactive boutons make synapses with inspiratory neurons of the dorsal respiratory group. Brain Res 1990; 529:309–314.

223. Maqbool A, Batten TFC, McWilliam PN. Ultrastructural relationships between GABAergic terminals and cardiac vagal preganglionic motoneurons and vagal afferents in the cat: a combined HRP tracing and immunogold labelling study. Eur J Neurosci 1991; 3:501–513.

224. Starke K, Göthert M, Kilbinger H. Modulation of neurotransmitter release by presynaptic autoreceptors. Physiol Rev 1989; 69:864–989.

225. Zuperku EJ, Hopp FA. Control of discharge patterns of medullary respiratory neurons by pulmonary vagal afferent inputs. Am J Physiol 1987; 253:R809–R820.

226. Dawkins MA, Foreman RD, Farber JP. Short latency excitation of upper cervical respiratory neurons by vagal stimulation in the rat. Brain Res 1992; 594:319–322.

227. Cohen MI, Shaw C-F, Barnhardt R. Connectivity of rostral pontine inspiratory-modulated neurons as revealed by responses to vagal and superior laryngeal afferent stimulation. In: Speck DF, Dekin MS, Revelette WR, Frazier DT, eds. Respiratory Control: Central and Peripheral Mechanisms. Lexington: University Press of Kentucky, 1993:91–94.

228. Perrin J, Crousillat J. The projection of vagal afferents on the cerebellar vermis of the cat. J Auton Nerv Syst 1985; 13:175–177.

229. Tong G, Robertson LT, Brons J. Vagal and somatic representation by the climbing fiber system in lobule V of the cat cerebellum. Brain Res 1991; 552:58–66.

230. Radna RJ, MacLean PD. Vagal elicitation of respiratory-type and other unit responses in basal limbic structures of squirrel monkeys. Brain Res 1981; 213:45–61.

231. Radna RJ, MacLean PD. Vagal elicitation of respiratory-type and other unit responses in striopallidum of squirrel monkeys. Brain Res 1981; 213:29–44.

232. Barone FC. Effects of neurotransmitters and vagus nerve stimulation of diencephalic and mesencephalic neuronal activity. Brain Res Bull 1984; 13:565–571.

233. Bassal M, Bianchi AL. Effets de la stimulation des structures nerveuses centrales sur les activités respiratoires efférentes chez le chat. I. Réponses à la stimulation corticale. J Physiol (Paris) 1981; 77:741–757.

234. Ito S-i. Multiple projection of vagal non-myelinated afferents to the anterior insular cortex in rats. Neurosci Lett 1992; 148:151–154.

235. Tonković-Ćapin M, Zuperku EJ, Bajić J, Hopp FA. Expiratory bulbospinal neurons of dog. II. Laterality of responses to spatial and temporal pulmonary vagal inputs. Am J Physiol 1992; 262:R1087–R1095.

236. Smith JC, Morrison DE, Ellenberger HH, Otto MR, Feldman JL. Brainstem projections to the major respiratory neuron populations in the medulla of the cat. J Comp Neurol 1989; 281:69–96.

237. Bianchi AL, Grélot L, Iscoe S, Remmers JE. Electrophysiological properties of rostral medullary respiratory neurones in the cat: an intracellular study. J Physiol (Lond) 1988; 407:293–310.

238. Czyżyk-Krzeska MF, Lawson EE. Synaptic events in ventral respiratory neurones during apnoea induced by laryngeal nerve stimulation in neonatal pig. J Physiol (Lond) 1991; 436:131–147.

239. Otake K, Sasaki H, Ezure K, Manabe M. Axonal trajectory and terminal distribution of inspiratory neurons of the dorsal respiratory group in the cat's medulla. J Comp Neurol 1989; 286:218–230.

240. Duffin J, Brooks D, Fedorko L. Paucity of dorsal inspiratory neuron collateral projections to ventral inspiratory neurons. NeuroReport 1991; 2:225–228.

241. Richter DW. Generation and maintenance of the respiratory rhythm. J Exp Biol 1982; 100:93–107.

242. Remmers JE, Richter DW, Ballantyne D, Bainton CR, Klein JP. Reflex prolongation of stage I of expiration. Pflüger's Arch 1986; 407:190–198.

243. Ballantyne D, Richter DW. The non-uniform character of expiratory synaptic activity in expiratory bulbospinal neurones of the cat. J Physiol (Lond) 1986; 370: 433–456.

244. Jodkowski JS, Berger AJ. Influences from laryngeal afferents on expiratory bulbospinal neurons and motoneurons. J Appl Physiol 1988; 64:1337–1345.

245. Bongianni F, Corda M, Fontana G, Pantaleo T. Influences of superior laryngeal afferent stimulation on expiratory activity in cats. J Appl Physiol 1988; 65:385–392.

246. Lawson EE, Richter DW, Czyżyk-Krzeska MF, Bischoff A, Rudesill RC. Respiratory neuronal activity during apnea and other breathing patterns induced by laryngeal stimulation. J Appl Physiol 1991; 70:2742–2749.

247. Sica AL, Cohen MI, Donnelly DF, Zhang H. Hypoglossal motoneuron responses to pulmonary and superior laryngeal afferent inputs. Respir Physiol 1984; 56:339–357.

248. Grélot L, Barillot JC, Bianchi AL. Pharyngeal motoneurones: respiratory-related activity and responses to laryngeal afferents in the decerebrate cat. Exp Brain Res 1989; 78:336–344.

249. St. John WM, Zhou D. Differing control of neural activities during various portions of expiration in the cat. J Physiol (Lond) 1989; 418:189–204.

250. St. John WM, Zhou D. Discharge of pulmonary vagal receptors differentially alters neural activities during various stages of expiration in the cat. J Physiol (Lond) 1990; 424:1–12.

251. Tanaka T, Asahara T. Synaptic actions of vagal afferents on facial motoneurons in the cat. Brain Res 1981; 212:188–193.

252. Withington-Wray DJ, Mifflin SW, Spyer KM. Intracellular analysis of respiratory-modulated hypoglossal motoneurons in the cat. Neuroscience 1988; 25:1041–1051.

253. Lowe AA. Excitatory and inhibitory inputs to hypoglossal motoneurons and adjacent reticular formation neurons in cats. Exp Neurol 1978; 62:30–47.

254. Tomomune N, Takata M. Excitatory and inhibitory postsynaptic potentials in cat hypoglossal motoneurons during swallowing. Exp Brain Res 1988; 71:262–272.

255. Lucier GE, Daynes J, Sessle BJ. Laryngeal reflex regulation: peripheral and central neural analyses. Exp Neurol 1978; 62:200–213.

256. Bellingham MC, Lipski J, Voss MD. Synaptic inhibition of phrenic motoneurones evoked by stimulation of the superior laryngeal nerve. Brain Res 1989; 486: 391–395.

257. Jiang C, Mitchell GS, Lipski J. Prolonged augmentation of respiratory discharge in hypoglossal motoneurons following superior laryngeal nerve stimulation. Brain Res 1991; 538:215–225.

258. Tojima H, Kubin L, Davies RO, Pack AI. Reflex control of upper airway patency: role of serotonin (5HT). Am Rev Respir Dis 1992; 145:A212.

259. Crone C, Hultborn H, Kiehn O, Mazieres L, Wigström H. Maintained changes in motoneuronal excitability by short-lasting synaptic inputs in the decerebrate cat. J Physiol (Lond) 1988; 405:321–343.

260. Hounsgaard J, Hultborn H, Jespersen B, Kiehn O. Bistability of α-motoneurones in the decerebrate cat and in the acute spinal cat after intravenous 5-hydroxytryptophan. J Physiol (Lond) 1988; 405:345–367.

261. Kiehn O. Plateau potentials and active integration in the "final common pathway" for motor behavior. Trends Neurosci 1990; 13:367–373.

262. Berger AJ, Mitchell RA. Lateralized phrenic nerve responses to stimulating respiratory afferents in the cat. Am J Physiol 1976; 230:1314–1320.

263. Shannon R. Intercostal and abdominal muscle afferent influence on medullary dorsal respiratory group neurons. Respir Physiol 1980; 39:73–94.

264. Cohen MI, Feldman JL, Sommer D. Caudal medullary expiratory neurone and internal intercostal nerve discharges in the cat: effects of lung inflation. J Physiol (Lond) 1985; 368:147–178.

265. Bajić J, Zuperku EJ, Tonković-Ćapin M, Hopp FA. Expiratory bulbospinal neurons of dogs. I. Control of discharge patterns by pulmonary stretch receptors. Am J Physiol 1992; 262:R1075–R1086.

266. St. John WM. Influence of pulmonary inflations on discharge of pontile respiratory neurons. J Appl Physiol 1987; 63:2231–2239.

267. Shaw C-F, Cohen MI, Barnhardt R. Inspiratory-modulated neurons of the rostrolateral pons: effects of pulmonary afferent input. Brain Res 1989; 485:179–184.

268. Feldman JL, Cohen MI, Wolotsky P. Powerful inhibition of pontine respiratory neurons by pulmonary afferent activity. Brain Res 1976; 104:341–346.

269. Eldridge FL, Chen Z. Respiratory-associated rhythmic firing of midbrain neurons is modulated by vagal input. Respir Physiol 1992; 90:31–46.

270. Sica AL, Cohen MI, Donnelly DF, Zhang H. Responses of recurrent laryngeal motoneurons to changes of pulmonary afferent inputs. Respir Physiol 1985; 62: 153–168.

271. Hwang J-C, St. John WM. Alterations of hypoglossal motoneuronal activities during pulmonary inflations. Exp Neurol 1987; 97:615–625.

272. Fregosi RF, Bartlett D Jr, St. John WM. Influence of phasic volume feedback on abdominal expiratory nerve activity. Respir Physiol 1990; 82:189–200.

273. Gromysz H, Karczewski WA. Motor nucleus of the V-th nerve and the control of breathing (Hering-Breuer reflex and apneustic breathing). Acta Physiol Pol (Warsaw) 1990; 41:147–155.

274. Hollstien SB, Carl ML, Schelegie ES, Green JF. Role of vagal afferents in the control of abdominal expiratory muscle activity in the dog. J Appl Physiol 1991; 71:1795–1800.

275. Bartlett D Jr, St. John WM. Influence of lung volume on phrenic, hypoglossal and mylohyoid nerve activities. Respir Physiol 1988; 73:97–110.

276. Hwang J-C, St. John WM, Bartlett D Jr. Afferent pathways for hypoglossal and phrenic responses to changes in upper airway pressure. Respir Physiol 1984; 55: 341–354.

277. Hamilton RD, Horner RL, Winning AJ, Guz A. Effect on breathing of raising end-expiratory lung volume in sleeping laryngectomized man. Respir Physiol 1990; 81: 87–98.

278. Watchko JF, O'Day TL, Brozanski BS, Vazquez RL, Guthrie RD. Control of gengioglossal muscle activity in the anesthetized piglet: the role of vagal afferents. Biol Neonate 1992; 61:366–373.

279. van Lunteren E, Cherniack NS, Dick TE. Upper airway pressure receptors alter expiratory muscle EMG and motor unit firing. J Appl Physiol 1988; 65:210–217.

280. Travers JB, Norgren R. Afferent projections to the oral motor nuclei in the rat. J Comp Neurol 1983; 220:280–298.

281. Milsom WK. Mechanoreceptor modulation of endogenous respiratory rhythms in vertebrates. Am J Physiol 1990; 259:R898–R910.

282. Jammes Y, Barthelemy P, Delpierre S. Respiratory effects of cold air breathing in anesthetized cats. Respir Physiol 1983; 54:41–54.

283. Horner RL, Innes JA, Murphy K, Guz A. Evidence for reflex upper airway dilator muscle activation by sudden negative airway pressure in man. J Physiol (Lond) 1991; 436:15–29.

284. Horner RL, Innes JA, Holden HB, Guz A. Afferent pathway(s) for pharyngeal dilator reflex to negative pressure in man: a study using upper airway anaesthesia. J Physiol (Lond) 1991; 436:31–44.

285. Henke KG, Sullivan CE. Effects of high-frequency oscillating pressures on upper airway muscles in humans. J Appl Physiol 1993; 75:856–862.

286. Karius DR, Ling L, Speck DF. Lesions of the rostral dorsolateral pons have no effect on afferent-evoked inhibition of inspiration. Brain Res 1991; 559:22–28.

287. Citterio G, Mortola JP, Agostoni E. Reflex effects on breathing of laryngeal denervation, negative pressure and SO$_2$ in upper airways. Respir Physiol 1985; 62: 203–215.

288. Mortola JP, Piazza T. Breathing pattern in rats with chronic section of the superior laryngeal nerves. Respir Physiol 1987; 70:51–62.

289. Mortola JP, Rezzonico R. Ventilation in kittens with chronic section of the superior laryngeal nerves. Respir Physiol 1989; 76:369–382.

290. Easton PA, Jadue C, Arnup ME, Meatherall RC, Anthonisen NR. Effects of upper or

lower airway anesthesia on hypercapnic ventilation in humans. J Appl Physiol 1985; 59:1090–1097.

291. Koepchen HP, Kalia M, Sommer D, Klüssendorf D. Action of type J afferents on the discharge pattern of medullary respiratory neurons. In: Paintal AS, Gill-Kumar P, eds. Respiratory Adaptations, Capillary Exchange and Reflex Mechanisms, Delhi: V. Patel Chest Institute, 1977; 408–426.

292. Haxhiu MA, van Lunteren E, Deal EC, Cherniack NS. Effect of stimulation of pulmonary C-fiber receptors on canine respiratory muscles. J Appl Physiol 1988; 65:1087–1092.

293. Haxhiu MA, Deal EC, Cherniack NS. Influence of respiratory drive on airway responses to excitation of lung C-fibers. J Appl Physiol 1989; 67:203–209.

294. Ichikawa H, Rabchevsky A, Helke CJ. Presence and coexistence of putative neurotransmitters in carotid sinus baro- and chemoreceptor afferent neurons. Brain Res 1993; 611:67–74.

295. Czyżyk-Krzeska MF, Bayliss DA, Seroogy KB, Millhorn DE. Gene expression for peptides in neurons of the petrosal and nodose ganglia in rat. Exp Brain Res 1991; 83:411–418.

296. Iverfeldt K, Serfözö P, Arnesto LD, Bartfai T. Differential release of coexisting neurotransmitters: frequency dependence of the efflux of substance P, thyrotropin releasing hormone and [³H]serotonin from tissue slices of rat ventral spinal cord. Acta Physiol Scand 1989; 137:63–71.

297. Portillo F, Núñez-Abades PA. Distribution of bulbospinal neurons supplying bilateral innervation to the phrenic nucleus in the rat. Brain Res 1992; 583:349–355.

298. Castro D de, Lipski J, Kanjhan R. Electrophysiological study of dorsal respiratory neurons in the medulla oblongata of the rat. Brain Res 1994 (in press).

299. Monteau R, Errchidi S, Gauthier P, Hilaire G, Rega P. Pneumotaxic centre and apneustic breathing: interspecies differences between rat and cat. Neurosci Lett 1989; 99:311–316.

300. Ugolini G, Kuypers HGJM, Strick PL. Transneural transfer of herpes virus from peripheral nerves to cortex and brainstem. Science 1989; 243:89–91.

301. Card JP, Rinaman L, Schwaber JS, Miselis RR, Whealy ME, Robbins AK, Enquist LW. Neurotropic properties of pseudorabies virus: uptake and transneuronal passage in the rat central nervous system. J Neurosci 1990; 10:1974–1994.

302. Blessing WW, Li Y-W, Wesselingh SL. Transneuronal transport of herpes simplex virus from the cervical vagus to brain neurons with axonal inputs to central vagal sensory nuclei in the rat. Neuroscience 1991; 42:261–274.

303. Haxhiu MA, Jansen ASP, Cherniack NS, Loewy AD. CNS innervation of airway-related parasympathetic preganglionic neurons: a transneuronal labeling study using pseudorabies virus. Brain Res 1993; 618:115–134.

304. Herdegen T, Kummer W, Fiallos CE, Leah J, Bravo R. Expression of c-JUN, JUN B and JUN D proteins in rat nervous system following transection of vagus nerve and cervical sympathetic trunk. Neuroscience 1991; 45:413–422.

305. Erickson JT, Millhorn DE. Fos-like protein is induced in neurons of the medulla oblongata after stimulation of the carotid sinus nerve in awake and anesthetized rats. Brain Res 1991; 567:11–24.

306. Duggan AW, Morton CR, Zhao ZQ, Hendry IA. Noxious heating of the skin releases immunoreactive substance P in the substantia gelatinosa of the cat: a study with antibody microprobes. Brain Res 1987; 403:345–349.

307. Miles R. Frequency dependence of synaptic transmission in nucleus of the solitary tract in vitro. J Neurophysiol 1986; 55:1076–1090.

308. Fortin G, Velluti JC, Denavit-Saubié M, Champagnat J. Responses to repetitive afferent activity of rat solitary complex neurons isolated in brainstem slices. Neurosci Lett 1992; 147:89–92.

309. Strobel RJ, Daubenspeck JA. Early and late respiratory-related cortical potentials evoked by pressure pulse stimuli in humans. J Appl Physiol 1993; 74:1484–1491.

310. Sanders MH, Costantino JP, Owens GR, Sciurba FC, Rogers RM, Reynolds CF, Paradis IL, Griffith BP, Hardesty RL. Breathing during wakefulness and sleep after human heart-lung transplantation. Am Rev Respir Dis 1989; 140:45–51.

311. Lee B-P, Sant'Ambrogio G, Sant'Ambrogio FB. Afferent innervation and receptors of the canine extrathoracic trachea. Respir Physiol 1992; 90:55–65.

6

Mechanisms and Analysis of Ventilatory Stability

EUGENE N. BRUCE

Center for Biomedical Engineering
University of Kentucky
Lexington, Kentucky

J. ANDREW DAUBENSPECK

Dartmouth Medical School
Lebanon, New Hampshire

I. Introduction

The pattern of the respiratory cycle, as well as the resulting ventilation, shows variations on many time scales. Over the course of days ventilation exhibits circadian variations, while over the course of hours there are periodic fluctuations in ventilatory and gas exchange variables (1,2). Some of these variations may be due to thermoregulation or to circadian oscillations in metabolism, in addition to fluctuations related to sleep-waking cycles. Over the course of minutes respiratory pattern may vary owing to such factors as transient metabolic changes, speech, postural changes, rapid alterations in state of consciousness, or effects related to pathological disturbances (e.g., periodic breathing of the Cheyne-Stokes type). Over the course of seconds (i.e., on a breath-by-breath basis) respiratory pattern may vary as a result of these longer-term factors or consequent to short-lived (but perhaps continual) disturbances from regions within the central nervous system that are not primarily related to respiratory function. For a normal subject it is only in the deep stages of non-rapid eye movement (NREM) sleep or under anesthesia that respiration becomes regular, in the sense that the patterns of all respiratory cycles are very similar. Yet even in these states there is some breath-to-breath variability in the respiratory pattern. On the other hand, in some circum-

285

stances respiration is so variable that the high degree of irregularity (albeit sometimes a very regularly recurring irregularity) is considered abnormal and indicative of morbidity. In this chapter we will attempt to analyze, characterize, and interpret the degree of regularity of the respiratory pattern using the concept of stability.

Stability has various definitions in the engineering literature and not all will suffice for the present purpose. The common usage of *stability* to mean that a measurable behavior remains "within finite bounds" seems inappropriate for physiological systems since all physiological behavior is bounded by saturation phenomena. We will define stability implicitly by defining instability: Physiological behavior is considered unstable if, in response to a brief disturbance, it fails to approach a *constant* steady-state value or, for naturally oscillatory behavior, it fails to approach a state in which every cycle is identical to every other cycle. By this definition, breathing is never truly stable, although it approximates this state in deep NREM sleep and in deep anesthesia. On the other hand, the advantage of this viewpoint will be that it encompasses recent suggestions that irregularity (and instability) can take forms other than periodic oscillations in ventilation.

Instability in respiratory pattern does not necessarily imply instability in gas exchange since fluctuations in pattern variables can be offsetting with respect to alveolar ventilation. The more general viewpoint, however, would focus on instabilities in respiratory pattern irrespective of their effects on gas exchange variables on the assumption that any instability in pattern may provide insight into potentially abnormal behavior. This viewpoint will be taken in this chapter.

It is well recognized that *periodic* instabilities in ventilation can be diagnostic for physiological abnormality, and it has been suggested that weak periodic oscillations in ventilation may presage impending respiratory dysfunction. On the other hand, *nonperiodic* breath-to-breath variability in respiratory cycle parameters and ventilation may have unrecognized implications for respiratory performance. Fluctuations in motor outflow may produce variability in chest wall and pulmonary mechanoreceptor feedback, and fluctuations in ventilation will lead to variability in blood gas tensions that may be sensed by chemoreceptors. Whether the reflex ventilatory consequences of these effects are trivial or substantial will depend on both the characteristics of the breath-to-breath variability and the properties of the receptors and feedback loops. The initial disturbances in blood gases may be exaggerated or buffered as a consequence of reflex responses. In addition, variability in motor activation of upper airway muscles could alter airway resistance and introduce further disturbances to ventilation (3–5). Fluctuations in motor activities may lead to breath-to-breath changes in end-expiratory lung volume (1), which could affect arterial blood gases. All of these effects are in addition to the potential primary interpretation that a sufficiently irregular breathing pattern may imply neurological dysfunction.

Another important issue is that conclusions about the functional importance of observed respiratory variations have been drawn in the absence of information about respiratory neurochemical control system reactions to random disturbances. For example, the respiratory variability in REM sleep (6) and wakefulness (6,7) is assumed to result from respiratory responses to stimuli having large random fluctuations unrelated to the respiratory cycle. Also, the influence of random disturbances is implicit in some hypotheses regarding the onset of periodic breathing (8,9). Yet the expected reactions of the respiratory neurochemical control system to random fluctuations in physiological variables are not at all obvious, because this nonlinear system comprises multiple neuromechanical, chemical, and central neural feedback loops, which, under different circumstances, could either exaggerate or attenuate responses to random fluctuations.

II. Measurement of Respiratory Pattern Stability

Assessment of the stability of respiratory pattern generally proceeds from measurement of the usual respiratory variables (e.g., tidal volume, V_T; inspiratory and expiratory durations, T_I and T_E; ventilation, $\dot{V}_I$) on a breath-by-breath basis. (Such analysis requires computer processing of data records in order to handle a meaningful number of breaths.) Many studies have utilized standard deviations or coefficients of variation as the measure of variability of respiratory pattern. In a "steady state" of waking respiration, the coefficients of variation of breath-to-breath values of tidal volume and inspiratory and expiratory times are typically 10–30%, with V_T/T_I being somewhat less variable (10–13). Sleep state, anesthesia, chemical drive, and cortical activity all have profound influences on respiratory variability (6,13–19). For resting, awake human subjects these standard deviations are relatively reproducible from day to day (12). It is well known that the respiratory pattern is more variable during REM sleep and wakefulness than during NREM sleep. (See Chapter 22.)

An extreme form of instability in respiratory pattern is the occurrence of apneas, and a common measure of instability applied to neonates is the percentage of time spent apneic. Because the duration of an apnea is itself quite variable (20) and the rate of occurrence of apneas depends on sleep state (17,20), simply counting the number of apneas is a poor measure of the degree of instability. Although apnea may develop as a consequence of the hypoventilatory phase of periodic breathing, the percentage of time spent in apnea does not represent the full contribution of periodic breathing to respiratory pattern instability. In this case a modulation index, M, has been proposed for quantifying the variability in ventilation (8); M reflects both the periodic contribution and the apneic period.

Histograms of breath-by-breath values of respiratory cycle variables reflect the contributions of all factors that influence respiratory pattern instability.

Histograms of V_T, T_I, and T_E often deviate from that of a Gaussian-distributed variable (13,14,18,19), and the shape of these distributions may change with chemical drive (14). Irrespective of whether or not these are Gaussian, changes in the corresponding standard deviations would express changes in stability. The advantage of a histogram is that it differentiates situations that a single measure (such as standard deviation) may not distinguish. For example, an instability that produces a histogram with entries scattered uniformly over a large range probably is different from one that produces a few very scattered values on a background of regularity. The statistical measures of skewness and kurtosis can begin to quantify such differences. What is more difficult to ascertain from histograms is the time structure of the respiratory cycle variability, e.g., periodic versus random variations. Therefore, while the approaches discussed so far can provide an initial insight into the question of respiratory pattern stability, use of other techniques that can incorporate both the amplitude range and the time structure of breath-by-breath changes in the respiratory cycle is essential.

   Analysis of amplitudes and frequencies of oscillatory instabilities in respiration has received considerable attention, and a variety of techniques for identifying oscillations have been utilized. Typically, breath-by-breath values of a respiratory variable are formed into a time series and analyzed. The autocorrelation function of a time series can detect regular oscillations (21,22), and the cross-correlation between two time series can reveal phase relationships (21,23). When a time series contains oscillations at more than one frequency, correlation functions are harder to interpret because the superimposed oscillations impair visual identification of individual frequencies. This limitation is overcome if a correlation function is converted to a frequency-domain representation by computing its Fourier transform. Localized peaks in this representation, which is the autopower spectrum of the time series (or the cross-power spectrum of two time series), reveal both strong oscillations and weak ones that might be overshadowed by strong ones in the correlation function representation (21,24). Statistical confidence limits on spectra, however, are often quite large (25). Identification of a localized peak requires knowledge of both the confidence limits and the mean level of the spectrum on either side of the peak. Strictly speaking, the usual types of spectral analysis require that the first- and second-order statistical properties of the data be consistent and unvarying across the entire record being analyzed. Comb filtering (26) can be applied to data whose properties are time-varying (i.e., nonstationary), but the time resolution of this technique diminishes directly with the center frequency of each filter. Furthermore, the published confidence limits on filter outputs, which are used for detecting when the output of a given filter is greater than would occur if random noise were its input, do not consider that the nonoscillatory variations in respiratory variables may not be white noise. Therefore, although this method can be useful, every oscillation reportedly found by comb filter analysis may not be unique.

The tradeoff between time resolution and frequency resolution is inherent in methods for analyzing nonstationary signals. Some newer methods can be "tuned" a priori to provide adequate resolution of a few time-varying signal components that do not overlap much in time or frequency. On the other hand, these methods, such as the smoothed pseudo-Wigner distribution and the wavelet transform (27), tend to produce artifacts when signal components overlap in time or frequency; therefore, their application to tracking time-varying respiratory stability will require considerable care.

So far we have addressed the two extremes of unstable behavior: periodic oscillations, for which respiratory cycle variables for each breath follow those of the preceding breath in a regular (essentially predictable) manner, and totally random and unpredictable variations from breath to breath. Instability also may exhibit as breath-to-breath changes that are partly predictable; e.g., an increase on one breath may be more likely to be followed by another increase. Such breath-to-breath *correlated variability* can be identified from autocorrelation functions (i.e., one that is not periodic and decays to zero over several or many lags) and autopower spectra (i.e., one that does not have distinct peaks but also is not uniform across a broad frequency range) (28,29). Although seemingly easy to detect, the importance of instability due to correlated variability has been unclear until recently (see below).

To this point we have ignored the important issue of how to construct a time series for analysis. The techniques discussed above all assume that the data are generated by discretizing a waveform using a constant sampling interval. Since breath duration, T_{TOT}, is not constant, and since only one value of a respiratory cycle variable is available per breath, this assumption is not valid. Many investigators either presume that the T_{TOT} variations are sufficiently small that the techniques are not invalidated, or that "the breath" is a biological unitary event or unit of time. Other investigators construct a continuous-time waveform by first holding each variable constant throughout the duration of each breath and then resampling this waveform using a constant sampling interval. Often it is said that analyses done both without and with resampling provide essentially similar results. This issue has received greater attention relative to analysis of heart rate variations, and some differences have been noted (30), although for identification of periodic oscillations in heart rate, resampling seems not to be strictly necessary. It is not clear whether analyses for correlated variations in respiratory variables would be biased by the choice to resample or not. It would seem that the accumulating evidence that the respiratory pattern is generated by a continuously modulatable nonlinear oscillator (31–33) is incompatible with the idea that "the breath" is a unitary event. Furthermore, respiratory pattern is modulated by continuous-time feedback. Therefore, it is likely that resampling should be done, although the specific distortions produced by not resampling need to be elucidated.

290 Bruce and Daubenspeck

The techniques discussed above provide the means to detect and quantify respiratory pattern instability. Many physiological mechanisms can contribute to instability, and the above techniques cannot inherently differentiate them. Thus identifying a cause of instability requires prudent use of these techniques combined with judiciously designed experimentation.

III. Instability in Spontaneous Breathing

Periodic instabilities in spontaneous breathing have been described in many pathological and normal situations. Periodic ventilatory oscillations of the Cheynes-Stokes type often are associated with corresponding periodicities in tidal volume (7,34). Such pronounced periodicities have been attributed to a variety of pathological causes, such as increased circulation delay and altered chemosensitivities (34). (These mechanisms are examined in a later section.) Periodic oscillations in ventilation that do not include an apneic phase are seen commonly in the breathing of premature infants (26), of normal adults in wakefulness and non-REM sleep (35), at altitude (36), and at the onset of sleep (37,38). A variety of conditions produce periodic instability in respiration in anesthetized animals— e.g., increased peripheral relative to central chemosensitivity, as in hypoxia or cooling of central chemoreceptors, circulation delays, and lung deflation (39)—as well as in mathematical models of respiratory control (40–42). All of these periodic behaviors have cycle times on the order of a few seconds to a few minutes. Oscillations having longer cycle times, on the order of tens of minutes or hours, have been described in humans (1,2) but these oscillations have received little additional study.

The report of cyclical variations in FRC (1) in adult humans raises the question whether end-expiratory lung volume (EEV) is a controlled respiratory variable. EEV appears to be controlled actively in human neonates (43,44), adult mice (45), and adult rats (46), all of which are species whose chest walls are more compliant than their lungs. However, relaxed breathing in humans appears to maintain EEV at the passive FRC. A transition from the upright to the supine posture decreases EEV and elicits an alteration in diaphragm activation that seems aimed at maintaining tidal volume constant (47,48), but there has been no suggestion that the decrease in EEV is actively opposed. It may be that in adult humans cyclical variations in EEV are merely secondary to periodic variations in other respiratory cycle variables.

Nonperiodic breath-to-breath variations in respiratory cycle parameters typically have been ascribed to uncorrelated random noise superimposed on true respiratory behavior, the latter estimated by averages over many cycles. Priban (49) and Bolton and Marsh (50) showed that in selected records of resting breathing in awake humans, the deviations of tidal volume and respiratory timing parameters about their average levels were not uncorrelated random variations, but the parameters exhibiting correlated variations were not consistent from subject to subject. Breath-to-breath correlations of tidal volume and cycle duration were reported (28) in data from eight eupneic human subjects, but the analyses did not distinguish between correlations produced by noncorrelated random variations about a mean level and those produced by slow, semiperiodic fluctuations of the mean level itself, which may result from similar variations in chemical reflex inputs. From such findings it was proposed that unknown nonrandom influences may be "an inherent property of the central respiratory oscillator" (28). This conclusion, however, ignores the potential of producing correlated changes in the respiratory pattern through interactions of random disturbances anywhere in the respiratory system with the dynamic response properties of the respiratory chemical, neural, and mechanical feedback pathways. A "short-term memory" in phrenic neurogram parameters from paralyzed, vagotomized, ventilated cats with T-1 spinal section has been reported (22), but the one example in this paper appears to be nonstationary (and therefore the analysis is not reliable). Furthermore, this result was not confirmed in a recent study in anesthetized rats (51). On the other hand, breath-to-breath correlations of V_I, V_T, and T_I have been reported in *spontaneous breathing* of awake and sleeping humans and anesthetized rats (29,51–53). Thus, in the absence of periodic breathing a given respiratory state appears to comprise: (1) a mean behavior dictated by chemical and nonchemical drives; (2) uncorrelated random variations from breath to breath; and (3) an adjustment of each breath correlated with the deviations of one or more previous breaths from the mean behavior.

Both periodic and nonperiodic respiratory irregularities are commonly observed in neonates, and it is likely that there are many causes, including periodic breathing, immature central neural mechanisms, and discoordination of upper airway and chest wall muscles. Recent studies in adult rats suggest that control of EEV in a species with a compliant chest wall can lead to breath-to-breath irregularities in respiratory phase switching at both the inspiratory-expiratory (I-E) and expiratory-inspiratory (E-I) transitions (46,54). Analyses of these behaviors in rats using techniques from nonlinear dynamics imply that this irregularity in respiratory pattern is due to inherent nonlinear properties of phase-switching dynamics and not to random disturbances. Applicability of these findings to human neonates is speculative but the resting breathing patterns of neonates are similar to those of anesthetized rats (unpublished observations).

It is important to recognize that apparent instability of the ventilatory control system might originate from long-lasting or repeated disturbances of this system due to nonrespiratory factors. For example, respiratory disturbances due to speech (55) or to conditioned responses (56) could be considered as instabilities of the respiratory pattern according to the definition given above. Likewise, the irregularities associated with "wakefulness drive" and with REM sleep (6) may be instabilities that are imposed on the respiratory system rather than inherent to its functioning. In all these cases, however, respiratory pattern and ventilatory irregularities may elicit neuromechanical reflex or chemoreflex responses that further alter respiratory behavior, and differentiation between the imposed and the reflex-induced irregularities becomes difficult. The importance of this differentiation is that one probably is more concerned with characterizing the properties of the respiratory system, which will be manifest in the reflex responses, than those of the disturbance. With periodic instabilities it is usually assumed that the frequency and amplitude of the oscillation are functions strictly of the properties of the respiratory system (40,57), although some periodicities may have a central neural origin (34,35). However, nonperiodic instabilities may evoke periodicities (58), as discussed below. The situation is more complicated with nonperiodic instabilities, as these behaviors may entirely reflect the characteristics of imposed disturbances or may entirely reflect respiratory responses to truly random disturbances, or both. We believe that the mere observation of any of the types of respiratory pattern instability is not sufficient to provide an interpretation of its cause. This point is elaborated later.

IV. Mechanisms of Ventilatory Instability

A. Nonperiodic Instabilities

On a breath-by-breath basis, respiratory variability may be uncorrelated or correlated. In either case, this variability must originate from disturbances to the respiratory neurochemical control system—for example, variations in discharge of chemoreceptors or of respiratory-related neurons, variations in "nonspecific" or "wakefulness" suprabulbar inputs (59–61), alterations in cardiac output or cerebral blood flow (62). Such disturbances might be correlated with the respiratory cycle but need not be; uncorrelated disturbances applied to a dynamic system can produce correlated behavior at other points in the system (25). The potential involvement of several mechanisms can be proposed based on existing knowledge.

Substantial evidence indicates that variations in peripheral chemoreceptor stimuli can be sensed and alter the ongoing breath (63–65) and perhaps subsequent breaths (66). Additional variability can be introduced by chemoreceptor rate sensitivity (67) or if the within-breath timing of chemoreceptor afferent impulses changes—e.g., because respiratory rate or cardiac output fluctuates (68,69). The net effect on ventilation depends on the phase between the original disturbances to ventilation and the reflex responses mediated by peripheral chemoreceptor afferent activity. Both uncorrelated and correlated breath-by-breath changes in respiratory pattern could be introduced by such mechanisms.

In nonhuman species, or possibly with large tidal volumes in men, vagal afferent activity may modify both the current and the next breath (70–73). This mechanism may influence variability both as a feedback path sensing variations in tidal volume and as a source of random neural input to the respiratory pattern generator.

Central chemoreceptors may have only a small role in responses to blood gas fluctuations introduced by breath-to-breath variability in respiratory cycle parameters. Despite the possibility of altering ventral medullary pH within a few seconds of a change in $Paco_2$ (74), the gain (tonically only about 0.01 pH unit/torr) and the frequency of these variations mitigate against significant pH changes. Thus when ventilation is primarily dependent on central drive, fluctuations in blood gases will be less effective in producing ventilatory variability. On the other hand, the recent demonstration in awake humans that a single-breath inhalation of 2% CO_2 on a background of >95% O_2 produces a demonstrable ventilatory response suggests that the central pathway is not completely unresponsive (75). This report also showed that three consecutive breaths of 2% CO_2 could cause a transient change in $Petco_2$ comparable to what might occur during spontaneous breathing. This stimulus produced a centrally mediated ventilatory change of 0.25 LPM.

Variations in brain blood flow may alter central chemoreceptor environment and discharge rate and thus induce fluctuations in respiratory pattern (6,62). Nonrespiratory central mechanisms—e.g., hypothalamic, raphe, cerebellar— may interact with respiratory mechanisms in the vicinity of central chemoreceptor sites in the ventral medullary shell (76) and introduce variability in respiration.

Suprabulbar and "wakefulness" inputs (61,77,78) seem likely to be uncorrelated with the respiratory cycle and therefore are logical candidates as sources of white-noise disturbances. Wakefulness seems to provide two types of inputs—a "tonic" respiratory drive (6,16,79), which exhibits as an increase in ventilation during the transition from sleep to waking (80,81) and probably involves the reticular activating system (61), and "behavioral" inputs that are consequences of volitional and other behavioral acts (6). Even subtle behaviors during wakefulness—such as closing the eyes, performing mental activity, anxiety, or auditory stimulation—alter ventilation and respiratory pattern (15,18,60). Furthermore, a variety of evidence supports the concept of neural interactions between suprabulbar mechanisms and brainstem respiratory neurons. Anatomical pathways from the cortex to respiratory regions of the brainstem and spinal cord have been mapped (82,83), and brainstem respiratory neuronal activities change with behavioral acts (56). Brainstem respiratory activity may also affect cortical activity (60,84) by neural pathways, creating the possibility of feedback loops. An intriguing finding is that electroencephalographic fluctuations can be correlated qualitatively with ventilatory fluctuations (23,37,81,84). It is unclear, however, whether this finding represents an action of suprabulbar mechanisms on brainstem mechanisms, or vice versa, or results from the actions of a third mechanism at both the suprabulbar and bulbar levels.

The exaggerated respiratory variability in REM has been attributed to "random" (7) or "behavioral" (6,77) suprabulbar inputs, coupled with greatly diminished CO_2 and O_2 sensitivities (6,7). The separate contributions of (1) changes in random disturbances and (2) changes in breath-to-breath correlations produced by respiratory responses to random disturbances, to state-related alteration of respiratory variability, have not been considered. It is likely that uncorrelated disturbances to respiratory pattern change with sleep state, but correlated variability probably also changes, at least as a consequence of changes in respiratory system dynamic properties. Thus, while sleep-state factors do alter respiratory variability, it is likely that other factors besides increased "random" stimulation of breathing are involved. Recently it has been demonstrated that the pattern of a breath is influenced by the concurrent presence of eye movements in REM (85,86), with ventilation being more depressed in association with longer bursts of eye movements. Although the distribution of eye movements within a burst can be described as a Markov process, the distribution of bursts across breaths has been described as an uncorrelated random process (87); therefore, these disturbances to respiratory pattern are of the white-noise type.

Variations in activation of upper airway muscles from whatever mechanism— e.g., spontaneous variability in recruitment, unequal effects of peripheral chemoreceptor drive variability on upper airway (UAW) and chest wall muscles (88–90) [a debated factor in humans (91)]—may contribute additional variability either via actions on UAW mechanoreceptors or indirectly through influences on airflow and ventilation. UAW mechanoreceptors can alter the breathing pattern of anesthetized animals (92), but natural stimuli in awake rats (93) and dogs (94) were reported to have little or no effect. Recent studies indicate that the effects of airway anesthesia on breathing pattern in humans may not be due to blockade of UAW mechanoreceptors (95). Thus changes in airway resistance seem more likely to affect respiratory variability through indirect effects on ventilation than through UAW mechanoreceptors. We recently analyzed respiratory pattern variations in anesthetized rats using techniques from nonlinear dynamics and found that the pattern is more variable in rats with an intact airway than in tracheotomized rats (96).

Disturbances in cardiac output and brain blood flow can influence respiration substantially (97). Variations in the former may alter gas exchange at the lung and also influence the time delays between pulmonary ventilatory responses and detection of their consequences by chemoreceptors. Variations in the latter can modulate CO_2/H^+ levels at central chemosensitive sites (76). Disturbances to these cardiovascular variables may be uncorrelated with the respiratory cycle and appear random even if they are not random relative to the cardiac cycle. Cardiac output disturbances are predicted to be influential in promoting both nonperiodic and periodic instabilities in respiratory pattern (97,98). At the same time, respiratory modulation of cardiac output, both via respiratory sinus arrhythmia and via effects on blood gases and peripheral chemosensory afferent activity, will itself disturb the cardiovascular system. These interactions may be important in explaining respiratory behaviors in sleep.

B. Periodic Instabilities

Much has been written about periodic breathing, and we shall discuss primarily some recent concepts that emphasize the complexity of this behavior. Periodicities are attributed typically to unstable operation of neurochemical feedback loops, and numerous experimental findings demonstrate that the chemical feedback mechanisms that control ventilation can be made to oscillate, or to cease oscillating, under appropriate conditions (8,24,34). Numerous mathematical modeling studies have predicted these behaviors (40,41,99). At issue is not the potential for chemoreflex loop-mediated oscillations to occur, but the actual applicability of this concept in individual cases. Because of the diverse physiological parameters that influence the chemoreflex loop gains and phase shifts (which are the determinants of an oscillation), recent efforts have striven to develop a subset of parameters that could be measured from individual subjects and used to predict periodic instability (24,41). Most approaches have emphasized the potential contributions of the following factors: peripheral chemosensitivity, lung-to-chemoreceptor transport delay, lung gas stores, metabolic rate, CO_2 capacity of blood, and mean levels of Pa_{CO_2} and Pa_{O_2}. There has been emphasis as well on CO_2-mediated oscillations, with the primary effect of hypoxia assumed to be a modulation of CO_2 chemosensitivity. This emphasis may be misleading, since the response to a single breath of hypoxia in humans has been shown to be different when $P_{ET}CO_2$ is maintained constant than when it is allowed to vary (98). In particular, the overdamped ventilatory response to single-breath hypoxia became underdamped when $P_{ET}CO_2$ was uncontrolled. Thus there is a dilemma: The complex mathematical models that include extensive physiological details are more likely to represent CO_2-O_2 interactions correctly, but their many parameters hinder application of the specific simulation results to *individual* subjects.

A potentially fruitful approach, in which ventilatory stability is assessed from the response to a transient disturbance, was suggested by Fleming et al. (100) and further developed by Carley and Shannon (9,24). These latter authors proposed to quantify the ventilatory response to a brief CO_2 stimulus by measuring the amplitude of the resulting oscillation in tidal volume. This approach is essentially a direct implementation of the definition of stability given earlier, and those subjects who respond to a CO_2 disturbance with strong oscillations should exhibit periodicities during spontaneous breathing. The quantitative relationships presented showed a great deal of scatter, but the qualitative relationships were "in the right direction." This concept was extended by Modarreszadeh et al. (101), who used the pseudorandom stimulation method of Sohrab and Yamashiro (102) to estimate the respiratory responses to a single breath of hypercapnia and then fitted a second-order transfer function to the estimated response to quantify the damping factor of the response (98). Centrally mediated ventilatory responses to CO_2 were found to be overdamped in most awake, normal human subjects; these responses were due entirely to the response of tidal volume, as breath timing was unchanged. This approach was applied also to the ventilatory responses to a single breath of hypoxia during mild hypercapnia (inhalation of 2.5% CO_2). Hypercapnia was necessary to permit use of an adaptive technique for maintaining $P_{ET}CO_2$ essentially constant (103). This single-breath response was much faster than the central response to CO_2 but also was overdamped *when $P_{ET}CO_2$ was prevented from changing* but was underdamped when $P_{ET}CO_2$ was allowed to change (98). Thus this method seems able to provide a useful index of respiratory stability in individual subjects in the face of chemical disturbances; its weakness is that there has not yet been any demonstration of a direct correspondence between features of the measured responses and individual physiological parameters.

Other factors besides CO_2 and O_2 chemosensitivities (and their interactions) are now recognized as potential contributors to respiratory periodicities; thus these factors constrain conclusions from previous studies (both experimental and mathematical) that focused exclusively on chemoreflex control of ventilation. A major factor is UAW resistance (R_{UAW}), which can fluctuate during periodic breathing (4,104). The potentially significant effect of changes in UAW resistance on alveolar ventilation is seen during the transition from wakefulness to sleep, when an increase in this resistance contributes to a rise in Pa_{CO_2} (3). The exact relationship between chemical drives and R_{UAW} is probably nonlinear (105). It is likely that variations in R_{UAW} affect ventilation during periodic breathing; it may be possible that a transient increase in R_{UAW} could disturb blood gases and initiate periodicity, which is sustained by the feedback effect of blood gases on R_{UAW}.

Another potential contributor is the rate of loss of "wakefulness drive" at sleep onset. Khoo (38) has shown that loss of this drive can disturb respiratory chemoreflex control sufficiently to initiate several cycles of oscillatory ventilation, even in subjects whose respiration is stable (by our definition). Another mechanism related to sleep state transitions involves recurring changes in sleep state. It is proposed that the decrease in minute ventilation at sleep onset may lead to blood gas changes that produce central nervous system arousal. Chemoreflex gains are larger awake and therefore ventilation increases due to arousal. As blood gases are restored to normal, the subject returns to sleep and the process repeats itself (38).

Another factor that is often minimized is the dynamic responsiveness of central chemoreflex pathways. Several studies have argued that this pathway responds too slowly and too little to contribute to the development of periodicities in respiration (40,120). In awake humans, this pathway does respond to a single breath of hypercapnia, and it can show slight underdamping in some subjects.

While not the major contributor in most circumstances, the central pathway might sustain a very-low-frequency oscillation in respiratory pattern (101).

Similarly lacking in many considerations of the mechanisms of periodicities is the effect of central nervous system dynamics on oscillatory behavior. It is clear that part of chemoreflex ventilatory responses in anesthetized animals is due to slow central dynamics (i.e., afterdischarge) (106) and also that central responses to presumed mechanoreceptor inputs exhibit slow adaptations (33,70–72). Therefore, these factors likely influence the conditions that lead to periodic breathing in these experimental models. Afterdischarge may be a factor in respiratory responses of humans as well (107,108), but adaptations to mechanoreceptor inputs have not been described in humans. It is thought that afterdischarge would tend to stabilize respiration.

Random disturbances to respiratory pattern may be important also in the development of respiratory periodicities, especially small-amplitude ones of the type detected by comb filters or spectral analysis. On the one hand, white-noise disturbances may lead to correlated breath-to-breath variations in respiratory pattern which contain periodic components that directly induce similar periodicities in blood gases. The latter will elicit further fluctuations in respiratory pattern. On the other hand, continuous random excitation of a system having even a slight tendency for damped oscillations (but not truly unstable) likely will excite these oscillations, perhaps intermittently, depending on the properties of the random disturbances. Figure 1 shows an example of this effect. Thus changes in respiratory periodicities may reflect either: (1) changes in random disturbances to respiratory pattern (and the resulting effects on chemoreflex loops), or (2) changes in system properties such as chemoreflex gains or circulatory delays, or (3) both types of mechanisms. Because some investigators have hypothesized that small-amplitude periodicities precede gross respiratory instability and pathophysiology (7,26), it will be important to distinguish whether the former are indeed due to incipient changes in mechanisms that will lead, for example, to pronounced periodic breathing.

Longobardo et al. (57) have emphasized the potential for complex interactions between central and obstructive apneas and periodic breathing (26,104). These interactions will be influenced by concurrent nonperiodic respiratory pattern instabilities in at least two ways. First, "memory" of past behavior implicit in correlated breath-to-breath variations in respiratory pattern may decrease the potential for apnea but also delay recovery from apnea. Second, fluctuations in UAW muscle activity may increase the chances of hypopnea or UAW obstruction, even when mean UAW activity levels would otherwise maintain patency.

Figure 2 summarizes our concepts regarding the interactions of periodic and nonperiodic instabilities in respiratory pattern and how these effects lead to either normal or abnormal breath-to-breath fluctuations in pattern. The horizontal axis qualitatively represents the net effect of those factors that determine chemoreflex

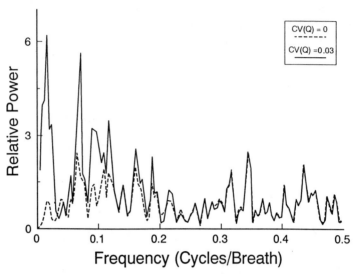

Figure 1.   Uncorrelated (white) noise added to a nonlinear feedback system can produce both correlated variability and apparent periodic fluctuations in its output, as seen in this example showing power spectra of ventilation obtained from a model of chemical control of ventilation in an awake human (similar to Ref. 40) when different levels of white-noise random disturbances were added to cardiac output (Q). CV, coefficient of variation. When CV = 0, ventilation power is not uniform because a small white noise is also added directly to ventilation to simulate breathing during wakefulness. In this case, note how the presence of chemoreflex feedback enhances the ventilation power around 0.07–0.20 cycle per breath. With noise also added to Q, definite peaks suggestive of periodic oscillations appear in the ventilation power spectrum below 0.10 cycle per breath.

loop propensity to oscillate, and the first row of ventilatory waveform responses to a brief respiratory disturbance shows the effect of increasing oscillatory tendency moving from left to right. Movement down the vertical axis represents increasing levels of externally imposed random disturbances to respiratory pattern. (The first row represents a single disturbance.) The resulting ventilatory waveforms reflect both the direct effects of the disturbances and the respiratory chemoreflex (and possibly neuromechanical reflex) responses to them. Because of these feedback loops, ventilation will exhibit correlated instabilities at higher disturbance levels. Furthermore, in the middle column the slight oscillatory tendency in response to a single disturbance becomes a sustained, small-amplitude oscillation at higher disturbance levels. In this case the resulting ventilatory pattern has both oscillatory and correlated, nonperiodic behaviors, much like resting breathing in wakefulness (unpublished observations).

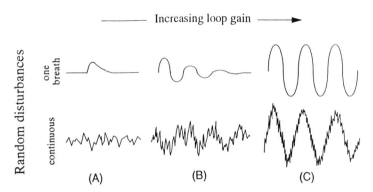

Figure 2. Cartoon showing the joint influences of chemoreflex loop gains and random disturbances on ventilatory stability. Each tracing is a hypothetical sketch of ventilation versus time under conditions of increasing loop gain (A–C). (Top row) In the noise-free case, a single-breath disturbance (e.g., to $Paco_2$) causes a transient, damped disturbance in ventilation (A), a damped ventilatory oscillation (B), or a sustained oscillation (C). (Bottom row) For A and C, continuous random disturbances primarily just add to the underlying noise-free behavior, but for B the disturbances elicit continual damped oscillations that appear to be due to a sustained oscillation.

V. Time-Varying Effects of Afferent Inputs on Respiratory Pattern

Two groups of experimental findings suggest that respiratory pattern instability can be induced via the responses of the respiratory central pattern generator (RCPG) to neuromechanical afferent inputs. The first group of studies has demonstrated that modulation of the central respiratory pattern by afferent inputs can outlast the input itself. The second group provides a growing body of evidence that *nonlinear* dynamical mechanisms underlie respiratory pattern generation and that these mechanisms can produce variable behavior that is not stochastic. (In the present context, a "dynamic" mechanism is one that produces a response to a stimulus that continues beyond any instantaneous effect of the stimulus. In general, such a system could be linear or nonlinear.)

The effects of low-threshold vagal and superior laryngeal nerve (SLN) afferent inputs to respiratory rhythm-generating and pattern-forming neural circuits can long outlast the stimulus (32,71,72,109,110). Furthermore, the respiratory pattern responses to continuous stimulation of vagal pulmonary stretch receptor (PSR) afferents partly adapt to this input over the first 20 sec or more of stimulation (72,111). Electrical stimulation of the SLN that is repeated every breath, or every second breath, or every third breath, and so on, does not elicit the same response with every stimulus (32) unless the stimuli are separated by nine or more breaths. Indeed, applying a constant stimulus to the SLN on every third or fourth breath, and so on, can induce variability in the respiratory pattern. Furthermore, differences between first-breath and steady-state phase response curves also demonstrate the presence of such aftereffects (112). The implication of such findings is that even if low-threshold pulmonary vagal or SLN afferent feedback were exactly the same on two consecutive breaths (which is unlikely), the central mechanisms would be in different states and the reflex responses might be different. Nonetheless, one might expect that the respiratory pattern would not become variable because eventually a "balance" would be reached between the afferent feedback effects on central respiratory pattern and the efferent effects of pattern on mechanoreceptor afferent activity, whereupon all breaths would become identical. This expectation is not necessarily valid for a nonlinear dynamic system.

Key to interpreting these time-dependent effects of afferent inputs to the RCPG is an understanding of its basic oscillatory mechanisms. (We include both central respiratory rhythm generation and pattern formation in the inclusive phrase "RCPG.") The concept that respiratory-phase transitions occur via instantaneous switches (113) is a simplification of the actual dynamic processes that occur at the I-E and E-I transitions. Apparent discontinuities in phase response curves (31,112,114) support this statement, but it is difficult to distinguish dynamic oscillators from those with instantaneous phase switching (115), and it is valid to question such interpretations of experimental findings (32,112,116). On the other hand, reversible "graded" inhibition at I-E (54,117) and temporal changes in the inhibitory effect of a vagal or pontine stimulus (70,118) must signify a dynamic (not instantaneous) phase-switching process. Less direct evidence supports a similar conclusion regarding the E-I transition, i.e., unpredictability of E-I in some situations (54,119,120), an apparent "mobilization" time for E-I (121), and graded diaphragm EMG responses due to low-intensity vagal electrical stimulation in late expiration (54).

The importance of the above findings is that, unlike instantaneous processes, dynamic processes can continue to be modified by afferent feedback after they have been initiated. In the case of respiratory phase switching, there are at least two important consequences of this continued sensitivity to the afferent inputs. First, the time courses of RCPG neural activities during the phase transition are likely to be modulated by the continuing afferent input; consequently, respiratory muscle activities during the phase transition might well be continuously graded. Second, it is conceivable that the onset of the subsequent respiratory phase might be somewhat altered if the RCPG activities during the transition are altered, and that this effect might change the respiratory pattern of that phase.

Given that dynamic processes almost certainly underlie the progressive changes in central neural activities within each respiratory phase (113) and the evidence that I-E and E-I transitions are dynamic processes, it seems likely that the

RCPG can be characterized globally as a nonlinear dynamic oscillator. This viewpoint provides a consistent framework for interpreting all the above studies regarding time-dependent effects of afferent inputs, phase-transition dynamics, and phase response data and establishes the possibility of further global characterizations of respiratory pattern using techniques for analysis of nonlinear systems (122,123). These techniques include: phase plots, which plot the variables of a system versus one another; correlation dimension (DC), a geometric measure related to the space-filling nature of the phase plot (DC = 1.0 for a regular oscillation; DC > 1 for complex signals); Lyapunov exponents and entropy, which both relate to whether nearby points in phase plots converge (not chaotic) or diverge with time (chaotic); a first-return map geometrically provides similar information to Lyapunov exponents (for a noisy oscillator it is a single cluster of points). To the extent that these methods can be correlated with and provide insight into physiological mechanisms, they become useful tools. One should not lose sight of the fact that the actual RCPG is a complex neural network and that any model (conceptual or mathematical) of its behavior is an abstraction that attempts to capture the essence of that behavior in representative circumstances.

From the nonlinear systems framework, variability in respiratory pattern may be due to the intrinsic, nonstochastic nature of the system rather than due to "noise." It is difficult to conclude with certainty that data from a laboratory measurement represent nonlinear deterministic variability rather than noise (122,124,125), but several findings regarding respiratory pattern have been so interpreted. Observations of "1/f" spectra (126) of respiratory pattern variables without other results are not very conclusive. A rescaled range analysis suggests that variability in tidal volume is not simply due to random noise (127). Calculations of correlation dimension, Lyapunov exponents, and entropy from tidal volume records of awake humans (128) and flow patterns of anesthetized and awake rats (33) suggest that the respiratory pattern is not a noisy one-dimensional oscillation. Although such calculations based on noisy data must be interpreted with considerable caution, horseshoe-shaped first-return maps from rats strengthened the suggestion of nonlinear dynamic variability (33).

On the other hand, two recent studies have shown that the degree of respiratory pattern variability of anesthetized rats can be changed reversibly by brief electrical stimulation of the afferent vagus (54) and by continuous negative airway pressure (CNAP) (46). In the first study a short stimulus train (three to seven shocks at 10-msec intervals, at the threshold voltage for PSR effects) was applied at the same time in every inspiration. When applied early in inspiration, it caused a brief transient depression of inspiratory airflow. When applied near the end of inspiration, it caused rapid cessation of that phase. When the stimulus was applied at a fixed intermediate time, the response varied from breath to breath, including both of the above responses and a continuum of responses between them. That is, even though the afferent feedback was the same on every breath, the respiratory pattern response was highly variable. Analogous findings were ob-

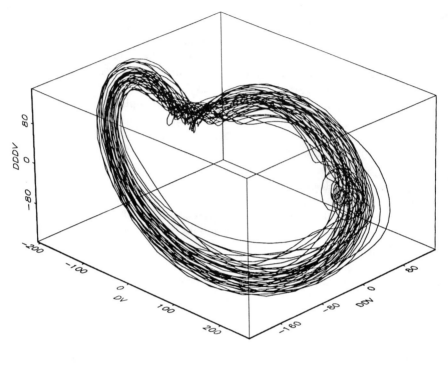

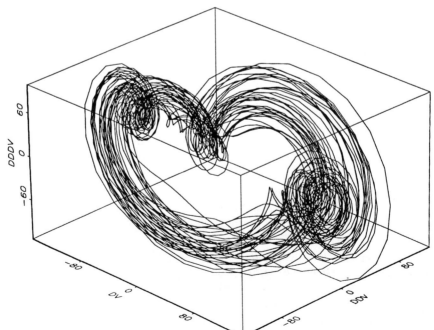

tained when the stimulus was delivered in the second half of expiration. In both cases the qualitative behavior of the respiratory pattern was reversibly dependent on the time into the phase at which the stimulus train was presented. Although the reported calculations of correlation dimension must be interpreted cautiously, it was quite clear that the degree of respiratory pattern instability could be changed by the timing of the afferent input.

In the second study it was shown that CNAP caused an increase in instability of the respiratory pattern of anesthetized tracheotomized rats (Fig. 3) whereas continuous positive airway pressure (CPAP) promoted a highly regular and stable pattern. The degree of instability was graded with the level of CNAP, and the pattern changes were reversible when CNAP was lowered to zero. Because these responses were absent after bilateral vagotomy, it was hypothesized that the reduced end-expiratory volume during CNAP elicited vagally mediated afferent activity that interacted with the RCPG to cause respiratory pattern instability. This afferent activity may have originated from slowly adapting lung deflation receptors, which are common in the rat (129). It was further proposed that the elicited responses were an attempt to maintain dynamic EEV above static FRC.

A. Hypothesized Interactions of EEV Control with Chemical Drive

We expect that the variations in breathing pattern caused by the mechanisms described above will affect blood gases. If these mechanisms do function to control EEV, a low EEV may impair pulmonary gas exchange compared to a higher EEV and may also produce larger within-breath variations in blood gases, leading to somewhat greater chemoreflex stimulation with low EEV. This stimulation of breathing may alter UAW braking effects (through effects on tidal volume, T_E, or UAW muscle activities), possibly helping to raise EEV and regularize the breathing pattern. Over several breaths, the elevated EEV may improve gas exchange enough that blood gases improve and reduce the chemical drive, reversing the above processes and leading to a reduction of EEV. Such a pattern, with slow changes in EEV and in the complexity of respiratory pattern, are seen often in the breathing of awake and even of anesthetized rats. Thus, it may be worth considering whether mechanisms for control of EEV may be a major contributor to breath-to-breath respiratory instability during wakefulness (and possibly during sleep), not only through direct effects on breathing pattern, but

---

Figure 3. Phase portraits of respiration from an anesthetized rat breathing 100% O_2. Portraits were constructed by plotting the first three derivatives (DV, DDV, DDDV) of a plethysmographic volume measurement in three dimensions. (Top) Resting breathing. (Bottom) During steady lung deflation due to a mean transrespiratory pressure of -6.5 cm H_2O. Deflation results in a much more complex and variable respiratory pattern.

also via interactions with chemoreflexes. In humans, such a mechanism is likely to be more important in infants than in adults.

VI. Spontaneous Breathing as Dynamic Homeostasis

It is apparent that there are many opportunities for nonlinear dynamic interaction among feedback processes in the normal physiological regulation of the respiratory pattern. As discussed in the Introduction, these feedback loops encompass time scales ranging from seconds to days, yet all influence to some extent the instantaneous neural excitation of muscles that serves to drive the respiratory mechanical system to produce airflow. That the confluence of this variety of nonlinear interactions should result in structured variability is not unexpected; rather, it would be surprising if this were not so. Although some degree of randomness always exists, the case has been made above that stochastic input perturbations affecting these interacting feedback loops might well induce correlated or periodic variability in the respiratory pattern.

Earlier, the point was made that respiration is rarely completely stable, except under deep anesthesia, in deep NREM sleep, and in certain reduced and deafferented preparations. In light of these observations, and with regard for the many neurochemical, neuromechanical, and central neural mechanisms that can elicit instability in respiratory pattern, we suggest that the common perspective that the object of respiratory control is to regularize breathing pattern (and gas exchange) may be too restrictive. The average ventilation over a few tens of seconds will be influenced by many factors that can either stabilize or destabilize the respiratory pattern, and it may be inappropriate to assume that the long-term average of the destabilizing factors is zero even when their effects "look" like random disturbances. Examples for which this assumption may be invalid include respiratory variability caused by nonlinear dynamic feedback mechanisms or by nonperiodic disturbances to chemoreflex loops. Thus instead of considering a given state of the respiratory pattern to comprise a completely reproducible respiratory cycle (i.e., an "average" breath) plus a variety of disturbances to the cycle, we would consider the "state" to comprise all of the respiratory patterns that are observed and would argue that the characteristics of the respiratory variability are inherent properties of the respiratory state. From this perspective homeostasis is a dynamic (i.e., moment to moment) balancing act among all of the stabilizing and destabilizing factors affecting respiratory pattern. Under certain abnormal experimental conditions (e.g., deep anesthesia and deafferentation), this dynamic homeostasis becomes static (having long-term constancy), but under normal conditions breath-to-breath change is expected owing to the dynamic balancing (in addition to any truly random, extrinsic disturbances present).

The "dynamic balance" perspective has been discussed previously (without being called such) by Glass (123) as a framework for understanding "dynamic diseases." A dynamic disease is one in which the dynamic balance shifts toward one or more of the destabilizing factors, causing either abnormal variability (such as periodic breathing) or an abnormal time course of a response to a provocative stimulus. In either case, the *average* levels of respiratory behavior may not reflect the disease process to the same extent as dynamic respiratory behaviors. Furthermore, it is possible that changes in parameters of a dynamic balance of nonlinear mechanisms could produce abrupt changes in behavior (i.e., bifurcations). In this case, the concept that a disease process should manifest a slow, progressive deterioration of behavior would be inappropriate.

If it is allowed that structured, nonperiodic variability is a reasonable consequence of the previously discussed feedback loop interactions, it stands to reason that reduction in the strength of any of these feedback pathways relative to the remainder might alter the observed variability of the respiratory pattern. For example, the normal electroencephalogram (EEG) reflects the activity of a mass of neurons connected in vastly complex spatiotemporal patterns, interacting through a multitude of nonlinear connections. It has been shown that the EEG shows diminishing dynamic complexity as the observed state of consciousness proceeds from wakefulness through deep sleep to coma (130). One interpretation of this finding is that the EEG signals become more coherent or synchronized and show variation more periodic in character as the normal, diffuse range of cerebral activity becomes more constrained. With regard to the control of breathing, the respiratory pattern is less variable in deep NREM sleep than in wakefulness (131). A decrease in cortical information processing following the transition from wakefulness to deep NREM sleep, as well as a reduction of cortical input, may contribute to the increased regularity of breathing in the latter condition.

This is not to say that biological rhythms become obviously less variable with reduced feedback strengths, since one effect of having many competent and competing feedback loops would be to make the influence of any one such pathway less than if it acted alone. Thus the attenuation of feedback influences from one or a variety of compensating and decompensating reflexes may leave the closed-loop response determined by the strongest remaining loop. This might result in greater apparent variability than in the normal state, albeit with diminished complexity. For example, epileptic seizure activity provides EEG traces that are much greater in magnitude and variability to the eye than the normal EEG, yet this seizure EEG signal demonstrates reduced dynamic complexity compared even to normal deep sleep (132). With respect to breathing, it seems likely that the complexity of the effective RCPG (including feedback loop reflexes) may determine the character of the observed pattern variability.

The hypothesis that the healthy physiological state is characterized by complex variability has been put forth by several authors and summarized by Pool (133), considering evidence related to a variety of physiological systems. The putative value to a control system of structured, nonrandom variability may lie in the fact that this characteristic reflects a rich background of competing interactions based in part on feedback regulatory loops involved in a variety of processes. That these loops are effective is demonstrated by the resultant complexity in the physiological responses. This is the basis for the supposition (as yet unproven) that a state characterized by relatively high structured variability is more capable to meet changing environmental stresses than a state with reduced variability.

Disease processes and the process of aging have interesting and similar aspects with respect to the complexity of the underlying systems. Lipsitz and Goldberger (134) recently reviewed some anatomical and physiological consequences of aging in humans. Their conclusion that "aging can be defined by a progressive loss of complexity in the dynamics of all physiological systems" is supported indirectly by a variety of anatomical and physiological data (135–137). These authors infer reduced feedback responsiveness with aging and have hypothesized that reduced variability of many physiological variables with aging is due to age-related reductions in systems complexity and feedback sensitivity. The applicability of this hypothesis to the respiratory system is a completely open question.

It was suggested recently that the human resting breathing pattern itself shows variability characteristics consistent with deterministic chaos (128). It is not easy to definitely establish the existence of deterministic, nonperiodic variability in noisy, nonstationary behavior such as that seen in the normal, wakeful state in humans, and the conclusions from this paper must be considered tentative. A better approach may be to use a variety of techniques as outlined by Denton et al. (138) to estimate changes in complexity of the structure of respiratory pattern variability as a function of state of consciousness, level of activity and respiratory drive, aging, and pathology. The hope is that these results may provide insights for predicting future changes in respiratory pattern regulation in ways analogous to what has been proposed for the regulation of the heartbeat, where a decline in the complexity of variability of the heart rate has been correlated with subsequent severe cardiac arrhythmias (139,140). Whether changes in respiratory pattern variability (of any of the types discussed in this chapter) correlate to the future appearance of respiratory dysrhythmias such as sleep apnea is an interesting topic for future research.

References

1. Hlastala MP, Wranne B, Lenfant C. Cyclical variation in FRC and other respiratory variables in resting man. J Appl Physiol 1973; 34(5):670–676.
2. Lenfant C. Time-dependent variations of pulmonary gas exchange in normal man at rest. J Appl Physiol 1967; 22(4):675–684.
3. Wiegand DA, Latz B, Zwillich CW, Wiegand L. Upper airway resistance and genio-

hyoid muscle activity in normal men during wakefulness and sleep. J Appl Physiol 1990; 69:1252–1261.

4. Hudgel DW, Chapman KR, Faulks C, Hendricks C. Changes in inspiratory muscle electrical activity and upper airway resistance during periodic breathing induced by hypoxia during sleep. Am Rev Respir Dis 1987; 135:899–906.

5. Remmers JE, DeGroot WJ, Sauerland EK, Anch AM. Pathogenesis of upper airway occlusion during sleep. J Appl Physiol Resp Environ Exercise Physiol 1978; 44(6):931–938.

6. Phillipson EA. Control of breathing during sleep. Am Rev Respir Dis 1978; 118: 909–939.

7. Cherniack NS. Sleep apnea and its causes. J Clin Invest 1984; 73:1501–1506.

8. Waggener TB, Brusil PJ, Kronauer RE, Gabel RA, Inbar GF. Strength and cycle time of high-altitude ventilatory patterns in unacclimatized humans. J Appl Physiol Respir Environ Exercise Physiol 1984; 56(3):576–581.

9. Carley DW, Shannon DC. A minimal mathematical model of human periodic breathing. J Appl Physiol 1988; 65:1400–09.

10. Winning AJ, Hamilton RD, Shea SA, Knott C, Guz A. The effect of airway anaesthesia on the control of breathing and the sensation of breathlessness in man. Clin Sci 1985; 68:215–225.

11. Kay J, Strange-Petersen E, Vejby-Christensen H. Mean and breath-by-breath pattern of breathing in man during steady-state exercise. J Physiol 1975; 251:657–669.

12. Tobin MJ, Mador M, Guenther S, Lodato RF, Sackner MA. Variability of resting drive and timing in healthy subjects. J Appl Physiol 1988; 65:309–317.

13. Kelsen SG, Shustack A, Hough W. The effect of vagal blockade on the variability of ventilation in the awake dog. Respir Physiol 1982; 49:339–353.

14. Newsom Davis J, Stagg DT. Analysis of breathing patterns in man. J Physiol 1975; 245:481–49.

15. Bechbache RR, Chow HHK, Duffin J, Orsini EC. The effects of hypercapnia, hypoxia, exercise and anxiety on the pattern of breathing in man. J Physiol 1979; 293:285–300.

16. Orem JM. Central neural interactions between sleep and breathing. In: Saunders NA, Sullivan CE, eds. Sleep and Breathing. New York: Marcel Dekker, 1984.

17. Shore ET, Millman RP, Silage DA, Chung D-C, Pack AI. Ventilatory and arousal patterns during sleep in normal young and elderly subjects. J Appl Physiol 1985; 59(5):1607–1615.

18. Shea SA, Walter J, Murphy K, Guz A. Evidence for individuality of breathing patterns in resting healthy man. Respir Physiol 1987; 68:331–344.

19. Daubenspeck JA, Farnham MW. Temporal variation in the V_T-T_I relationship in humans. Respir Physiol 1982; 47:97–106.

20. Read DJC, Henderson-Smart D. Regulation of breathing in the newborn during different behavioral states. Annu Rev Physiol 1984; 46:675–85.

21. Hathorn MKS. Analysis of periodic changes in new-born infants. J Physiol 1978; 285:85–99.

22. Benchetrit G, Bertrand F. A short-term memory in the respiratory centers: statistical analysis. Respir Physiol 1975; 23:147–158.

23. Pack AI, Cola MF, Goldszmidt A, Ogilive MD, Gottschalk A. Correlation between oscillations in ventilation and frequency content of the electroencephalogram. J Apply Physiol 1992; 72:985–992.

24. Carley DW, Shannon DC. Relative stability of human respiration during progressive hypoxia. J Appl Physiol 1988; 65:1389–1399.

25. Priestley MB. Spectral Analysis and Time Series. London: Academic Press, 1981.

26. Waggener TB, Frantz ID, Stark AR, Kronauer RE. Oscillatory breathing patterns leading to apneic spells in infants. J Appl Physiol Respir Environ Exercise Physiol 1982; 52(5):1288–1295.

27. Hlawatsch F, Bourdreaux-Bartels GF. Linear and quadratic time-frequency signal representations. IEEE Sig Proc 1992; 9:21–68.

28. Benchetrit G, Pham Dinh T. Analyse d'une etude statisque de la ventilation cycle par cycle chez l'homme au repos. Biomet Hum 1973; 8:7–19.

29. Modarreszadeh M, Bruce EN. Nonrandom variability in respiratory cycle parameters of humans during stage 2 sleep. J Appl Physiol 1990; 69:630–639.

30. DeBoer RW, Karemaker JM, Strackee J. Comparing spectra of a series of point events particularly for heart rate variability data. IEEE Trans Biomed Engin 1984; BME-31:384–387.

31. Paydafar D, Eldridge F, Kiley J. Resetting of mammalian respiratory rhythm: existence of a phase singularity. Am J Physiol 1986; 19:R721–R727.

32. Lewis J, Bachoo M, Polosa C, Glass L. The effects of superior laryngeal nerve stimulation on the respiratory rhythm: phase-resetting and aftereffects. Brain Res 1989; 517:44–50.

33. Sammon MP, Bruce EN. Pulmonary vagal afferent activity increases dynamical dimension of respiration in rats. J Appl Physiol 1991; 70:1748–1762.

34. Cherniack NS, Longobardo GS. Abnormalities in respiratory rhythm. In: Handbook of Physiology. Section 3: The Respiratory System. Bethesda, MD: American Physiological Society, 1987.

35. Pack AI, Silage DA, Millman RP, Knight H, Shore ET, Chung D-C. Spectral analysis of ventilation in elderly subjects awake and asleep. J Apply Physiol 1988; 64:1257–1267.

36. Brusil PJ, Waggener TB, Kronauer RE, Gulesian Jr. P. Methods for identifying respiratory oscillations disclose altitude effects. J Appl Physiol 1980; 28: 545–556.

37. Bulow K. Respiration and wakefulness in man. Acta Physiol Scand 1963; 51:230–238.

38. Khoo MCK, Gottschalk A, Pack AI. Sleep-induced periodic breathing and apnea: a theoretical study. J Apply Physiol 1991; 70:2014–2024.

39. Cherniack NS, von Euler C, Homma I, Kao FF. Experimentally induced Cheyne-Stokes breathing. Respir Physiol 1956; 187:395–398.

40. Khoo MC, Kronauer RE, Strohl KP, Slutsky AS. Factors inducing periodic breathing in humans: a general model. J Appl Physiol Respir Environ Exercise Physiol 1982; 53(3):644–659.

41. Elhefnawy A, Saidel G, Bruce EN, Cherniack NS. Stability analysis of CO_2 control of ventilation. J Appl Physiol 1990; 69:498–503.

42. Milhorn HT, Guyton AC. An analog computer analysis of Cheyne-Stokes breathing. J Appl Physiol 1965; 20:328–333.

43. Kosch P, Stark A. Dynamic maintenance of end-expiratory lung volume in full-term infants. J Appl Physiol 1984; 57:1125–1133.

44. Kosch P, Hutchinson A, Wozniack J, Carlo W, Stark A. Posterior cricoarytenoid and diaphragm activities during tidal breathing in neonates. J Appl Physiol 1988; 64: 1968–1978.

45. Vinegar A, Sinnett E, Leith D. Dynamic mechanisms determine functional residual capacity in mice, *Mus musculus*. J Appl Physiol 1978; 46:867–871.

46. Sammon MP, Romaniuk JR, Bruce EN. Bifurcations of the respiratory pattern associated with reduced lung volume in the rat. J Appl Physiol 1993; 75:887–901.

47. Green M, Mead J, Sears TA. Muscle activity during chest wall restriction and positive pressure breathing in man. Respir Physiol 1978; 25:283–300.

48. Begle RL, Skatrud JB, Dempsey JA. Ventilatory compensation for changes in functional residual capacity during sleep. J Appl Physiol 1987; 62:1299–1306.

49. Priban IP. An analysis of some short-term patterns of breathing in man at rest. J Physiol 1963; 166:425–424.

50. Bolton DPG, Marsh J. Analysis and interpretation of turning points and run lengths in breath-by-breath ventilatory variables. J Physiol 1984; 351:451–459.

51. Khatib M, Oku Y, Bruce EN. Contribution of chemical feedback loops to breath to breath variability of tidal volume. Respir Physiol 1991; 83:115–128.

52. Bruce EN. Breath to breath correlation of respiratory cycle parameters of anesthetized rats. FASEB J 1988; 2:A1289.

53. Modarreszadeh M, Bruce EN, Hudgel D, Gothe B. Nonperiodic correlations of respiratory cycle parameters are increased in REM. FASEB J 1990; 4:A539.

54. Sammon MP, Romaniuk JR, Bruce EN. Bifurcations of the respiratory pattern produced with phasic vagal stimulation in the rat. J Appl Physiol 1993; 75:912–926.

55. Warner RM, Waggener TB, Kronauer RE. Synchronized cycles in ventilation and vocal activity during spontaneous conversational speech. J Apply Physiol 1983; 54: 1324–1334.

56. Orem J, Netick A. Behavioral control of breathing in the cat. Brain Res 1986; 366: 238–253.

57. Longobardo GS, Gothe B, Goldman MD, Cherniack NS. Sleep apnea considered as a control system instability. Respir Physiol 1982; 50:311–333.

58. Modarreszadeh M, Kump KS, Chizeck HJ, Hudgel DW, Bruce EN. Adaptive buffering of breath-by-breath variations in end-tidal CO_2 of humans. J Appl Physiol 1993; 75:2003–2012.

59. Fink BR. Influence of cerebral activity in wakefulness on regulation of breathing. J Appl Physiol 1961; 16:15–20.

60. Asmussen E. Regulation of respiration: "the black box." Acta Physiol Scand 1977; 99:85–90.

61. Hugelin A. Forebrain and midbrain influence on respiration. In: Handbook of Physiology. Section 3: The Respiratory System. Bethesda, MD: American Physiological Society, 1987.

62. Parisi RA, Neubauer JA, Frank MM, Santiago TV, Edelman NH. Linkage between brain blood flow and respiratory drive during rapid-eye-movement sleep. J Appl Physiol 1988; 64:1457–1465.

63. Cunningham DJC, Howson MG, Metias EF, Petersen ES. Patterns of breathing in response to alternating patterns of alveolar carbon dioxide pressures in man. J Physiol 1986; 376:31–45.
64. Takahashi E, Menon AS, Kato H, Slutsky AS, Phillipson EA. Control of expiratory duration by arterial CO_2 oscillations in vagotomized dogs. Respir Physiol 1990; 79:45–56.
65. Cunningham DJC, Robbins PA. The pattern of breathing in man in response to sine waves of alveolar carbon dioxide and hypoxia. J Physiol 1984; 350:475–486.
66. Jennett S, McKay FC, Moss VA. The human ventilatory response to stimulation by transient hypoxia. J Physiol 1981; 315:339–351.
67. Cross BA, Leaver KD, Semple SJG, Stidwill RP. The effect of small changes in arterial carbon dioxide tension on carotid chemoreceptors activity in the cat. J Physiol 1986; 380:415–427.
68. Kumar P, Nye P, Torrance R. Effect of waveforms of inspired gas tension on the respiratory oscillations of carotid body discharge. Am J Physiol 1991; 259:R911–R920.
69. Bowes G, Andrey SM, Kozar LF, Phillipson EA. Role of the carotid chemoreceptors in regulation of inspiratory onset. J Appl Physiol Respir Environ Exercise Physiol 1982; 52(4):863–868.
70. Younes M, Baker J, Remmers JE. Temporal changes in effectiveness of an inspiratory inhibitory electrical pontine stimulus. J Appl Physiol 1987; 62(4):1502–1512.
71. Zupurku EJ, Hopp FA. On the relation between expiratory duration and the subsequent inspiratory duration. J Appl Physiol 1985; 58:419–430.
72. Younes M, Polachek J. Central adaptation to inspiratory-inhibiting expiratory-prolonging vagal input. J Appl Physiol 1985; 59:1072–1084.
73. Younes M, Polachek J. Temporal changes in effectiveness of a constant inspiratory-terminating vagal stimulus. J Appl Physiol 1981; 50:1183–1192.
74. Eldridge FL, Kiley JP, Paydarfar D. Dynamics of medullary hydrogen ion and respiratory responses to square-wave change of arterial carbon dioxide in cats. J Physiol 1987; 385:627–642.
75. Modarreszadeh M, Bruce EN. Long-lasting ventilatory response of humans to a single breath of hypercapnia in hyperoxia. J Appl Physiol 1992; 72:242–250.
76. Bruce EN, Cherniack NS. Central chemoreceptors. J Appl Physiol 1987; 62:389–402.
77. Lydic R. State-dependent aspects of regulatory physiology. FASEB J 1987; 1:6–15.
78. Orem J, Netick A. Behavioral control of breathing in the cat. Brain Res 1986; 366: 238–253.
79. Cherniack NS. Breathing disorders during sleep. Hosp Pract 1986; 81–104.
80. Skatrud JB, Dempsey JA. Interaction of sleep state and chemical stimuli in sustaining ventilation. J Appl Physiol Respir Environ Exercise Physiol 1983; 55: 813–822.
81. Colrain IM, Trinder J, Fraser G, Wilson GV. Ventilation during sleep onset. J Appl Physiol 1987; 63(5):2067–2074.
82. Rikard-Bell GC, Bystrzycka EK, Nail BS. Cells of origin of corticospinal projections to phrenic and thoracic respiratory motoneurons in the cat as shown by retrograde transport of HRP. Brain Res Bull 1985; 14:39–47.

83. Gandevia SC, Rothwell JC. Activation of the human diaphragm from the motor cortex. J Physiol 1987; 384:109–118.

84. Kumagai H, Sakai F, Sakuma A, Hukuhara T. In: Tokizane, Schade, eds. Progr. in Brain Res. Correl Neurosciences. Fundamental Mechanisms. Vol 21A. Amsterdam: Elsevier, 1966;88.

85. Gould GA, Gugger M, Molloy J, Tsara V, Shapiro C, Douglas NJ. Breathing pattern and eye movement density during REM sleep in humans. Am Rev Respir Dis 1988; 138:874–877.

86. Millman RF, Knight H, Kline LR, Shore ET, Ching D-C, Pack AI. Changes in compartmental ventilation associated with eye movements during REM sleep. J Appl Physiol 1988; 65:1196–1202.

87. Boukadam AM, Ktonas PY. Non-random patterns of REM occurrences during REM sleep in normal human subjects: an automated second-order study using Markovian modeling. Electroenceph Clin Neurophysiol 1988; 70:404–416.

88. Bruce EN, Mitra J, Cherniack NS. Central and peripheral chemoreceptor inputs to phrenic and hypoglossal motoneurons. J Appl Physiol 1982; 53:1504–1511.

89. Bonora M, St. John WM, Bledsoe TA. Differential elevation by protriptyline and depression by diazepam of upper airway respiratory motor activity. Am Rev Respir Dis 1985; 131:41–45.

90. Haxhiu MA, van Lunteren E, Mitra J, Cherniack NS. Comparison of the response of diaphragm and upper airway dilating muscle activity in sleeping cats. Respir Physiol 1987; 70:183–193.

91. Onal E, Lopata M, O'Connor TD. Diaphragmatic and genioglossus electromyogram responses to CO_2 rebreathing in humans. J Appl Physiol 1981; 50:1052–1055.

92. Mathew O, Farber J. Effect of upper airway negative pressure on respiratory timing. Respir Physiol 1984; 54:259–268.

93. Mortola JP, Piazza T. Breathing pattern in rats with chronic section of the superior laryngeal nerves. Respir Physiol 1987; 70:51–62.

94. Stradling JR, England SJ, Harding R, Kozar LF, Andrey S, Phillipson EA. Role of upper airway in ventilatory control in awake and sleeping dogs. J Appl Physiol 1987; 62(3):1167–1173.

95. Hamilton RD, Winning AJ, Perry A, Guz A. Aerosol anesthesia increases hypercapnic ventilation and breathlessness in laryngectomized humans. J Appl Physiol 1987; 63:2286–2292.

96. Bruce EN. Upper airway and postural influences on complexity of breathing pattern of anesthetized rats. FASEB J 1993.

97. Bruce EN, Modarreszadeh M. Chemoreceptive contribution to periodic breathing. In: Kuna ST, Suratt PM, Remmers JE, eds. Sleep and Respiration in Aging Adults. New York: Elsevier 1991:279–283.

98. Bruce EN, Modarreszadeh M, Kump K. Identification of closed-loop chemoreflex dynamics using pseudorandom stimuli. In: Honda Y, et al, eds. Control of Breathing and Its Modeling Perspective. New York: Plenum Press (in press).

99. Saunders KB, Bali HN, Carson ER. A breathing model of the respiratory system: the controlled system. J Theor Biol 1980; 84:135–161.

100. Fleming PJ, Goncalves AL, Levine MR, Woolard S. The development of stability of

respiration in human infants: changes in ventilatory responses to spontaneous sighs. J Physiol 1984; 347:1–16.

101. Modarreszadeh M, Bruce EN. Long-lasting ventilatory response of humans to a single breath of hypercapnia in hypoxia. J Appl Physiol 1992; 72:242–250.

102. Sohrab S, Yamashiro S. Pseudorandom testing of ventilatory response to inspired carbon dioxide in man. J Appl Physiol 1980; 49:1000–1009.

103. Modarreszadeh M, Kump K, Chizeck HJ, Hudgel DW, Bruce EN. Adaptive buffering of breath-by-breath variations of end-tidal CO_2 of humans. J Appl Physiol 1993; 75:2003–2012.

104. Warner G, Skatrud J, Dempsey JA. Effect of hypoxia-induced periodic breathing on upper airway obstruction during sleep. J Appl Physiol 1987; 62:2201–2211.

105. Bartlett D Jr. Respiratory functions of the larynx. Physiol Rev 1989; 69:33–57.

106. Eldridge FL, Millhorn DE. In: Fisherman AP, ed. Handbook of Physiology. Respiration. Section 3. Vol II. 1986:93–113.

107. Fregosi RF. Short-term potentiation of breathing in humans. J Appl Physiol 1991; 71:892–899.

108. Georgopoulos D, Bshouty Z, Younes M, Anthonisen NR. Hypoxic exposure and activation of the afterdischarge mechanism in conscious humans. J Appl Physiol 1990; 69:1159–1164.

109. Jiang C, Mitchell G, Lipski J. Prolonged augmentation of respiratory discharge in hypoglossal motoneurons following superior laryngeal nerve stimulation. Brain Res 1991; 538:215–225.

110. D'Angelo E. Effects of single breath in lung inflation on the pattern of subsequent breaths. Brain Res 1977; 31:1–18.

111. Grippi M, Pack AI, Davies R, Fishman AP. Adaptation to reflex effects of prolonged lung inflation. J Appl Physiol 1985; 58:1360–1371.

112. Kitano S, Komatsu A. Central respiratory oscillator: phase-response analysis. Brain Res 1988; 439:19–30.

113. von Euler C. Brain stem mechanisms for generation and control of breathing pattern. In: Handbook of Physiology. The Respiratory System II. Bethesda, MD: American Physiological Society. 1986:1–76.

114. Paydafar D, Eldridge F. Phase resetting and dysrhythmic responses of the respiratory oscillator. Am J Physiol 1987; 21:R55–R62.

115. Glass L, Winfree A. Discontinuities in phase-resetting experiments. Am J Physiol 1984; 15:R251–R258.

116. Lewis J, Bachoo M, Glass L, Polosa C. Complex dynamics resulting from repeated stimulation of nonlinear oscillators at a fixed phase. Physics Lett A 1987; 125: 119–122.

117. Younes M, Remmers J, Baker J. Characteristics of inspiratory inhibition by phasic volume feedback in cats. J Appl Physiol 1978; 45:80–86.

118. Younes M, Baker J, Remmers J. Temporal changes in effectiveness of an inspiratory inhibitory electrical pontine stimulus. J Appl Physiol 1987; 62:1502–1512.

119. Romaniuk J, Dick T, Bruce E, Supinski G, DiMarco A. Shortening of the expiratory phase by lung inflation (LI) in dogs. Soc Neurosci Abstr 1990.

120. Mathew O. Upper airway negative-pressure effects on respiratory activity of upper airway muscles. J Appl Physiol 1984; 56:500–505.

121. Cohen M, Feldman J, Sommer D. Caudal medullary expiratory neurone and internal intercostal nerve discharges in the cat: effects of lung inflation. J Physiol 1985; 368:147–178.

122. Thompson J, Stewart H. Nonlinear Dynamics and Chaos. New York: Wiley, 1988.

123. Glass L, Mackey M. From Clocks to Chaos: The Rhythms of Life. Princeton, NJ: Princeton University Press, 1988.

124. Albano A, Mees A, de Guzman G, Rapp P. Data requirements for reliable estimation of correlation dimension. In: Chaos on Biological Systems, New York: Plenum Press, 1987:207–220.

125. Osborne A, Provenzale A. Finite correlation dimension for stochastic systems with power-law spectra. Physica D 1989; 35:357–381.

126. Kawahara K, Yamauchi Y, Nakazono Y, Miyamoto Y. Spectral analysis on low frequency fluctuation in respiratory rhythm in the decerebrate cat. Biol Cybern 1989; 61:265–270.

127. Hoop B. Rescaled range analysis of resting respiration. Workshop on Models of Complex Respiratory Dynamics in Sleep and Wakefulness, Los Angeles, CA, May 11, 1991.

128. Donaldson G. The chaotic behavior of resting human respiration. Respir Physiol 1992; 88:313–321.

129. Tsubone H. Characteristics of vagal afferent activity in rats: three types of pulmonary receptors responding to collapse, inflation, and deflation of the lungs. Exp Neurol 1986; 92:541–552.

130. Gallez D, Babloyantz A. Predictability of human EEG: a dynamical approach. Biol Cybern 1991; 64:381–91.

131. Mador MJ, Tobin MJ. Effect of alterations in mental activity on the breathing pattern in healthy subjects. Am Rev Respir Dis 1991.

132. Babloyantz A, Destexhe A. Low-dimensional chaos in an instance of epilepsy. Proc Natl Acad Sci USA 1986; 83:3513–3517.

133. Pool R. Is it healthy to be chaotic? Science 1989; 243:604–607.

134. Lipsitz LA, Goldberger AL. Loss of 'complexity' and aging. Potential applications of fractals and chaos theory to senescence. JAMA 1992; 267:1806–1809.

135. Scheibel AB. Falls, motor dysfunction, and correlative neurohistological changes in the elderly. Clin Geriatr Med 1985; 1:671–676.

136. Frolkis VV, Bezrukov VV. Aging of the central nervous system. Interdiscip. Topics Gerontol 1979; 16:87–89.

137. Wei JY, Gersh BJ. Heart disease in the elderly. Curr Prob Cardiol 1987; 12:7–65.

138. Denton TA, Diamond GA. Can the analytic techniques of nonlinear dynamics distinguish periodic, random and chaotic signals? Comput Biol Med 1991; 21: 243–63.

139. Goldberger AL. Nonlinear dynamics, fractals and chaos: applications to cardiac electrophysiology. Ann Biomed Eng 1990; 18:195–198.

140. Goldberger AL, West BJ. Applications of nonlinear dynamics to clinical cardiology. Ann NY Acad Sci 1987.

7

Hypothalamic Involvement in Respiratory and Cardiovascular Regulation

TONY G. WALDROP

University of Illinois College of Medicine
Urbana, Illinois

JAMES P. PORTER

University of Louisville School of Medicine
Louisville, Kentucky

I. Introduction

The hypothalamus has long been known to be involved in the regulation of a number of physiological functions, including thermoregulation, hormonal control, and central arousal. In fact, areas in the hypothalamus exert an influence over most, if not all, systems in the body. It is obvious that normal body functions as well as responses to stress require the interaction of many organ systems. Several sites in the hypothalamus likely serve as integrative areas that coordinate the activity of a number of systems such that body homeostasis is maintained. Regulation of some functions, such as temperature and sexual behavior, is totally dependent on the integrity of the hypothalamus. In contrast, many cardiovascular and respiratory reflexes are modulated by descending input from hypothalamic sites but do not require an intact hypothalamus for the reflex to be active. The focus of this review will be on the role of hypothalamic areas in regulating cardiorespiratory function.

   Involvement of the hypothalamus in cardiovascular control was shown in experiments performed in the first part of this century (92). A number of early studies used electrical stimulation to demonstrate that activation of hypothalamic structures elicits changes in both cardiovascular and respiratory function. These

315

experiments linked sites in the rostral hypothalamus with vasodepressor responses; the caudal hypothalamus was shown to exert an excitatory influence on the cardiorespiratory system. Furthermore, the perifornical region of the hypothalamus was shown to be capable of eliciting the full components of the rage reaction, or fight-or-flight response (104). Subsequent experiments focused on hypothalamic involvement in cardiovascular reflexes with a focus on the baroreceptor reflex. However, far fewer studies were conducted to ascertain the role of the hypothalamus in respiratory regulation. This neglect of respiratory activity was noted in an excellent review written by Mancia and Zanchetti in 1981 (104). These investigators stated that "respiratory reactions obtained with electrical stimulation of the hypothalamus were considered in detail by Kabat in 1936, with little additional work having been done thereafter" (86).

The last decade has seen a heightened focus on the role of hypothalamic structures in regulating both cardiovascular and respiratory activity. These recent studies have supported most of the older findings evoked by electrical stimulation of hypothalamic structures and have utilized new techniques for examining the role of the hypothalamus in cardiorespiratory regulation. In addition, strong evidence now exists that altered activity in hypothalamic sites is associated with hypertension (155,156). Moreover, recent studies suggest that individual neurons may function as central chemoreceptors sensitive to hypoxia and hypercapnia (38,39).

II. Rostral Hypothalamus

A. Anatomy

Several regions of the rostral hypothalamus have been implicated in control of cardiovascular and/or respiratory function. The rostral hypothalamus can be generally defined as the hypothalamic structures that extend from the lamina terminalis anteriorly to the caudal aspect of the paraventricular nucleus posteriorly. Structures of importance include the median preoptic nucleus, the organum vasculosum of the lamina terminalis, the anterior hypothalamic area, and the paraventricular nucleus (PVN). All of these structures are known to be involved in cardiorespiratory control, but the PVN has received by far the most attention. Because of the potential to affect both neural and hormonal (oxytocin and vasopressin) outflow, the PVN is ideally situated to subserve an integrative function. Most of the following discussion will focus on the involvement of the PVN in cardiopulmonary control mechanisms. However, where appropriate, data concerning other rostral hypothalamic areas will also be presented.

Efferent Connections

In the mid-1970s, investigators began to use agents such as horseradish peroxidase or fluorescent dyes to trace the neural pathways with potential for involvement in autonomic and respiratory control. These techniques take advantage of the axoplasmic transport that occurs naturally within neurons. The agents typically were injected into the area where a presumed terminal field existed, and through the process of retrograde transport, the cell bodies giving rise to the terminal fields could subsequently be identified.

In 1976, Saper et al. injected horseradish peroxidase into the spinal cord or dorsal medulla of rats, cats, and monkeys (145). Many cells in the rostral hypothalamus, including the PVN, and the caudal hypothalamus, including the posterior hypothalamic nucleus, were labeled with the retrograde tracer. To confirm the presence of pathways from the hypothalamus to the medulla and spinal cord, these investigators subsequently injected tritiated amino acids into the hypothalamus. Cell bodies in the hypothalamus presumably "took up" the tritiated amino acids for protein synthesis and through the process of anterograde transport moved the label to the area of the neuron terminals. Using autoradiography, it was confirmed that many of the neurons in the rostral hypothalamus did send projections to the medulla and spinal cord. These data provided the first definitive evidence that the hypothalamus might influence autonomic functions through long descending monosynaptic pathways, rather than the short polysynaptic organization that was typically envisioned.

In subsequent studies, the existence of these hypothalamic projections onto medullary and spinal neurons was confirmed (21,73,150). In addition, it was shown that it is the parvocellular neurons in the PVN that contribute the majority of the rostral hypothalamic outflow with presumed autonomic function (163). Using double-labeling techniques, it was shown that a portion of the parvocellular neurons in the PVN send collateral projections to both the medulla and the spinal cord. When retrograde tracing techniques were combined with immunocytochemistry, it was shown that a significant portion of the long descending neurons contained material that was immunoreactive for oxytocin and vasopressin and other putative peptide neurotransmitters (147).

A weakness of the retrograde transport techniques is that the exact location of the terminal neurons cannot be identified. Injections into the terminal field are typically fairly large; thus, uptake and retrograde transport by damaged axons in the area cannot be ruled out. However, the detailed identification of terminal fields became possible as new anterograde transport agents began to be employed. For example, the leukoagglutinin *Phaseolus vulgaris*, when injected into the area of the PVN, is subsequently transported to the neuron terminal. Immunocytochemical techniques can then be used to identify the distribution of the agglutinin. Neurons originating in the PVN were shown to descend through two different pathways, one medial and one lateral (103). In the pons, the lateral pathway had some neurons that terminated in medial and lateral parabrachial nuclei, areas that are known to subserve both cardiovascular and respiratory functions. In the medulla, both pathways converged to the surface of the ventrolateral medulla. Here some neurons terminated while others swept dorsally to terminate in the area of the nucleus of the tractus solitarius (NTS) and dorsal nucleus of the vagus while others continued down into the intermediolateral column of the spinal cord, all areas with known autonomic function.

Although the existence of connections between the PVN and the medulla and spinal cord was clearly demonstrated, the studies outlined above still failed to definitively show that the long descending neurons actually terminated on sympathetic preganglionic neurons. Several newer techniques have recently been employed to show the actual connection with the sympathetic nervous system. In one technique, anterograde transport of agglutinins injected into the rostral hypothalamus is combined with retrograde transport of cholera toxin. The cholera toxin is injected into a sympathetic ganglion so that cell bodies and dendrites of the spinal preganglionic neuron can be labeled. The presence of terminal buttons containing immunoreactivity for the agglutinins, juxtaposed to the sympathetic preganglionic dendrites containing immunoreactivity for the cholera toxin, would provide strong evidence of synaptic arrangement. Hosoya et al. showed that in the intermediolateral column of the spinal cord, the labeling of terminals and dendrites was too dense to identify individual connections (76). However, in other autonomic areas of the spinal cord, that is, the nucleus intercalatus and the central autonomic nucleus, fibers from the PVN were visualized that wound around dendrites containing cholera toxin and appeared to make synaptic contact. In a different technique, inactive pseudorabies virus was injected into different sympathetic ganglia. The virus was presumably retrogradely transported to the cell body of origin in the spinal cord and then carried transsynaptically to neurons innervating that particular sympathetic preganglionic neuron. The virus could then be transported back to the cell body providing the innervation to the spinal cord. Using this technique, Strack et al. have identified only five areas in the brain that provide monosynaptic input to sympathetic preganglionic neurons (162). The PVN was the only hypothalamic nucleus with substantial input to the sympathetic nervous system. In certain cases, depending on which ganglion was injected, neurons in the lateral hypothalamus and zona incerta were also labeled with the virus. In the medulla, cell bodies in the caudal raphe nuclei, the ventromedial medulla, and the ventrolateral medulla were labeled. All three of these areas are known to affect cardiovascular and respiratory function. Hypothalamic influences on these functions, other than some from the PVN, must involve synapses at these medullary or other brainstem sites.

Another approach to show which pathways function in cardiovascular or respiratory control has been to inject retrograde tracing agents into areas known to be involved in cardiorespiratory regulation. For example, cardiorespiratory effects produced by electrical stimulation of the NTS could be divided into three distinct categories depending on the area of stimulation. Once a site was identified functionally, horseradish peroxidase was injected for retrograde tracing of the efferent inputs to the area. The PVN was shown to be connected to all three areas of the NTS (121).

As a whole, these anatomical studies suggest that the PVN can influence cardiorespiratory function through several different pathways. Inputs from this nucleus to the parabrachial nucleus, the ventromedial medulla, the ventrolateral medulla, and the dorsal medulla all have the potential to modulate cardiovascular or respiratory function (101). The long descending neurons from the PVN to autonomic centers in the spinal cord also have the potential to regulate autonomic functions.

Afferent Connections

Over the past 20 years, the notion has arisen that the PVN is an important site for integration of cardiorespiratory function. The efferent connections outlined above provide the anatomical substrate by which this nucleus could function to modulate sympathetic or respiratory activity. However, to serve an integrative function, the PVN would also have to be situated anatomically to receive significant sensory input concerning the cardiovascular or respiratory state of the whole organism. In this light, it is not surprising that neuroanatomical techniques have identified numerous afferent inputs to the PVN that originate from central areas that are known to receive baroreceptor and chemoreceptor inputs.

In 1982, Sawchenko and Swanson presented a detailed description of the noradrenergic connections between the caudal medulla and the PVN (148). They combined retrograde and anterograde transport techniques with immunocyto-chemistry to show that the noradrenergic input to magnocellular (vasopressin-secreting) cells in the PVN arose exclusively from the A1 area in the rostral ventrolateral medulla. On the other hand, ascending inputs to parvocellular divisions of the PVN arose from both the A1 area and the A2 area of the dorsal medulla. Given the critical location of these areas in relation to baro- and chemoreceptor input, it is not surprising that these authors postulated that the ascending noradrenergic pathways were important for integrating cardiorespira-tory function. In a recent study in which anterograde transport of *P. vulgaris* injected into the area of A1 was used to identify ascending projections, the strong projection to the PVN was confirmed (186). In addition, terminals were found in the lateral hypothalamus, perifornical region, and zona incerta.

B. Functional Studies

Given the evidence that neurons of the PVN are interconnected with brainstem and spinal autonomic centers, it is not surprising that many studies have addressed potential functional roles for the PVN, especially with regard to cardiovascular control. One approach has been to activate cells in the PVN using either electrical or chemical stimulation and to monitor changes in blood pressure, heart rate, respiration rate, plasma catecholamine levels, and/or directly recorded sympa-thetic nerve activity. Because of the complexity of the PVN, this approach has often produced conflicting results. Complications produced by the use of anesthesia have also contributed to the confusion. Nevertheless, electrical or chemical activation studies have provided a great deal of information regarding possible involvement of the PVN in regulation of cardiorespiratory functions. In a second approach, electrical or chemical lesions in the PVN have been used to assess the contribution of this nucleus to various cardiorespiratory control mechanisms.

Electrical Stimulation

In 1980, Ciriello and Calaresu reported that electrical stimulation of the PVN in anesthetized cats produced increases in arterial pressure and heart rate (23). Since these animals were artificially ventilated, the effect of the stimulation on respiratory functions was not addressed. These authors also provided evidence that PVN neurons could modulate baroreflex function. The bradycardia produced by stimulation of the carotid sinus nerve was diminished by stimulation of the PVN, and lesion of this nucleus augmented the bradycardia.

In subsequent years, because of the explosion of neuronal tracing techniques performed mostly in rats, studies employing electrical stimulation of the PVN were also done primarily in rats. Studies that used anesthetized rats reported conflicting information regarding the cardiovascular effects of electrical stimulation of the PVN. In some studies, the stimulations produced increases in arterial pressure and heart rate, while in others, the response was depressor and sympathoinhibitory (90,129,187). A study by Porter and Brody, where a small monopolar electrode was used to activate different subnuclei within the PVN, showed that stimulation sites in the medial and anterior (magnocellular) portion of the PVN tended to be depressor and vasodilatory (hindquarter), while stimulation sites in the posterior and lateral (parvocellular) portion of the PVN were pressor and vasoconstrictor (Fig. 1) (130). These data raised the possibility that within the PVN there may be a complex arrangement of neurons, with some subserving depressor and some subserving pressor functions.

The electrical stimulation studies mentioned above were all performed using anesthetized animals. Some of the differences in the responses to stimulation could have been due to the different anesthetics used. Several electrical stimulation studies have now been reported in which conscious animals were used. In conscious rats, electrical stimulation of the PVN has always been associated with increases in blood pressure and sympathoexcitation (89,131). In one interesting report by Kannan et al., electrical stimulation of the PVN in conscious rats produced an increase in arterial pressure and renal nerve activity, but when the animals were subsequently anesthetized with pentobarbital, stimulation of the PVN produced a decrease in blood pressure and sympathetic nerve activity (89).

Taken together, these reports suggest that activation of neurons in the PVN can produce a variety of cardiovascular responses. Current evidence indicates that

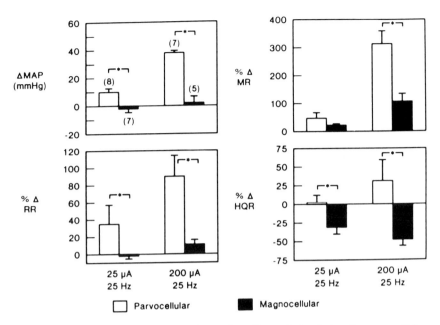

Figure 1 Blood pressure and regional vascular effects of stimulating the parvocellular and magnocellular divisions of the paraventricular nucleus. MAP = mean arterial pressure; RR = renal resistance; MR = mesenteric resistance; HQR = hindquarter resistance. *$p < 0.05$. (From Ref. 130.)

the more posterior parvocellular neurons mediate a pressor function while more anterior neurons can produce a decrease in blood pressure. Differences in sensitivity to electrical current and differences in responsiveness to anesthetics may also contribute to the different functional responses. It should be noted that in the studies outlined above, the effect of electrical stimulation of PVN on respiration was not investigated. Hence, our understanding of the contribution of the PVN to respiratory function is very limited.

Chemical Stimulation

A weakness that is always raised with electrical stimulation studies is that both cell bodies and fibers of passage within the affected area are stimulated. Hence, an effect produced by electrical stimulation of the PVN could be mediated not only by cell bodies within the nucleus, but also by ascending or descending neurons that originate elsewhere and send projections through the area of the PVN. In recent years, investigators have begun to use chemical substances to activate neurons within the central nervous system. Since these chemical neuromodulators presumably act through a receptor-mediated event, an effect would be limited to dendrites and cell bodies where the receptors are located. Axons of passage, which lack the appropriate receptor, would not be affected.

Most neurons in the central nervous system can be activated with excitatory amino acids such as glutamate or kainic acid. Hence, it was anticipated that some of the confusion that arose with electrical stimulation of the PVN might be cleared up by using chemical activation. However, conflicting data continued to be presented. In rats anesthetized with ketamine or urethane-chloralose, injections of glutamate into the PVN produced decreases in arterial pressure and renal nerve activity (93,187). Only the activity of the adrenal nerve was increased by the chemical activation. In rats anesthetized with urethane, injection of kainic acid or another excitatory amino acid, D,L-homocysteate, produced increases in blood pressure, heart rate, and respiration rate (56,139). Because of the potential confounding effects of anesthesia, Jin and Rockhold injected kainic acid into the PVN of conscious rats (82). They found that mean arterial pressure, heart rate, urine volume, and sodium excretion were all increased by kainic acid. In addition, baroreflex function was inhibited. Finally, Martin and Haywood used very small injections (50 nl) of glutamate into the PVN of conscious rats and found that blood pressure, heart rate, and circulating catecholamines were all increased (107).

Thus, as with the electrical stimulation studies, chemical activation of the PVN with excitatory amino acids confirmed the complex nature of the neuronal circuits originating from this important hypothalamic nucleus. It appears that both sympathoexcitatory and sympathoinhibitory outputs can arise from the PVN. The excitatory output seems to be more sensitive to the effects of anesthesia. The limited data that are available concerning respiratory function suggest that the PVN may be stimulatory.

The anterior hypothalamus and PVN are known to be major termination sites for neurons containing endogenous opioids (95,109). There is some suggestion that the central opioid system may be important in blood pressure control since intracerebroventricular (icv) administration of opioid agonists produced an increase in blood pressure and plasma catecholamines and a decrease in respiration rate (109). Since intracisternal injections were less effective, it was suggested that the important opioid receptors were located in the hypothalamus. Subsequent studies where opioid agonists have been injected directly into the anterior hypothalamus or PVN of conscious rats have also reported increases in blood pressure and plasma catecholamines (94,128). In two studies using anesthetized rats, injection of opioid agonists into the anterior hypothalamus or PVN was reported to decrease blood pressure, heart rate, and respiration rate, again pointing to the potential confounding effects of anesthesia (133,169). In this regard, Jin and Rockhold showed that injection of β-endorphin into the PVN of conscious rats produced increases in blood pressure, heart rate, and plasma epinephrine (83). When these animals were subsequently anesthetized with chloralose, the effects of the β-endorphin were greatly reduced.

It has long been recognized that angiotensin II can act within the central nervous system to increase arterial pressure. The effect on blood pressure is mediated by angiotensin-induced vasopressin release and sympathoexcitation. Given the importance of magnocellular neurons in the PVN with regard to synthesis and secretion of vasopressin, it is not surprising that an action of angiotensin within this nucleus has been postulated. Immunocytochemical studies have confirmed the presence of angiotensin in the PVN, and tracing studies have shown that angiotensin-containing neurons may innervate this nucleus (99). However, studies that have investigated the cardiovascular effects of injections of angiotensin II into the PVN do not always agree. Shoji et al. reported that injections of angiotensin II into the PVN of conscious rats did not affect blood pressure or vasopressin release (154). Rather, injections into the area anterior to the PVN were effective in increasing both vasopressin secretion and blood pressure. On the other hand, Jensen et al. reported that injections of angiotensin II or angiotensin III into the PVN of anesthetized or conscious rats produced increases in blood pressure (81). In a recent study, Ambühl et al. investigated the effects of iontophoretic application of angiotensin II or angiotensin-(1–7) on extracellular recordings of spontaneously active neurons in the PVN (2). Both these agents had a predominantly excitatory effect. It is not known how these studies relate to actual cardiovascular function. The neural activity recorded in the PVN did not exhibit the bursting pattern typical of vasopressin-secreting cells. Hence, the neurons that responded with excitation were probably not magnocellular. If the responsive neurons are those that send projections to autonomic neurons in the brainstem or spinal cord, then they might represent the substrate for the increases in blood pressure observed by Jensen et al. after injections of angiotensin II into the PVN (81).

There is another route by which intracerebroventricular injections of angiotensin II could affect the activity of neurons in the PVN. A recent report used microdialysis techniques to show that icv injection of angiotensin II increased the release of norepinephrine in the area of the PVN (161). A dense noradrenergic projection from the A1 region of the brainstem to the PVN is known to exist. The angiotensin in the ventricle system may have activated this ascending projection and produced an increase in neurotransmitter release in the PVN. Direct injections of norepinephrine into the PVN have been associated with increases in blood pressure and plasma vasopressin (13). Furthermore, the increase in blood pressure could be blocked by administration of a peripheral vasopressin receptor antagonist. Hence, the vasopressin-dependent portion of the central angiotensin II pressor response could result, not from an action of angiotensin II directly within the PVN, but through the ability of angiotensin II to increase the release of norepinephrine from neurons that innervate magnocellular cell bodies.

Respiratory effects of infusing norepinephrine into the rostral hypothalamus have been examined in anesthetized rats. Microinfusions of norepinephrine as well as thyrotropin-releasing hormone elicited increases in breathing frequency without any significant effects on tidal volume. Since the administration of lidocaine had effects similar to those of the other two chemicals, it was concluded that the observed respiratory responses were due to depression of an inhibitory pathway in the rostral hypothalamus (49).

Progesterone is a potential endogenous hypothalamic agent that can affect breathing. Early studies demonstrated that progesterone stimulates breathing in humans and may explain the hyperventilation present in women during pregnancy (12). It has also been argued that progesterone can alter the respiratory responses to hypoxia and hypercapnia (12).

Recent studies by Balis and Millhorn have identified the mechanism of stimulation and potential sites at which progesterone acts to stimulate breathing (11,12). In a first set of studies, a progesterone agonist, promegestone, was administered systemically to anesthetized cats. Promegestone elicited a dose-dependent stimulation of phrenic nerve activity, which could be blocked by a progesterone receptor antagonist. Further experiments indicated that this respiratory stimulation was dependent on an estrogen-dependent, progesterone-receptor-inducing gene expression. Ablative experiments indicated that the locus of action was in the hypothalamus; additional in situ hybridization experiments localized the site of action to anterior hypothalamic structures.

Substance P is a putative central neurotransmitter that is known to produce increases in blood pressure and sympathetic nervous activity when injected into the cerebral ventricles (170). In a recent study, small amounts of substance P were injected into different hypothalamic nuclei to determine the sites of its sympatho-excitatory action (80). Interestingly, injections in the anterior hypothalamic area (including the PVN) produced the expected increase in blood pressure and heart rate. On the other hand, injections into the posterior hypothalamus were without effect.

As a whole, the studies outlined above suggest that the rostral hypothalamus, especially the PVN, may be an important central site for control of the cardiovascular system. Its potential contribution to the control of respiration is less well established since only a few studies have even addressed the role of the PVN in this regard. It should be pointed out that the studies with electrical or chemical stimulation of the PVN cannot definitively identify a physiological function for this nucleus. Other studies, such as those that utilize selective ablation of neurons or injection of specific receptor antagonists into this area, can help to address the question of actual involvement in physiological control mechanisms.

Ablation Studies

Several studies have examined the contribution of the PVN to cardiovascular responses that are produced by acute stress. Callahan et al. showed that the increase in heart rate that is produced by a foot-shock stress was markedly reduced in rats that had electrolytic lesions in the PVN. The stress also increased arterial pressure, but the lesion did not reduce the pressor response (20).

Stress is also known to increase the secretion of renin by renal juxtaglomerular cells. The subsequent generation of angiotensin II can then influence the cardiovascular system. Electrical stimulation of the PVN has been shown to evoke an increase in plasma renin activity in conscious rats (132). However, the involvement of the PVN in stress-induced increases in renin secretion is a subject of controversy. Gotoh et al. showed that lesions in the PVN resulted in a long-term decrease in circulating angiotensinogen, but the lesions did not prevent the increase in plasma renin concentration that is produced by immobilization stress (59). On the other hand, Richardson Morton et al. reported that both electrolytic and ibotenic acid (cell body specific) lesions in the PVN attenuated the increase in plasma renin concentration and corticosterone produced by a conditioned emotional response paradigm (137). It should be noted that blood pressure was not measured in either study. Hence, more work is necessary before an involvement of the PVN in stress-induced renin release is established.

Darlington et al. performed studies in conscious and anesthetized rats to determine the contribution of the PVN to cardiovascular and hormonal responses that result from a hypotensive hemorrhage (34). The PVN was isolated from afferent and efferent connections using a triangular knife. In both anesthetized and conscious rats, the knife cut prevented the rise in ACTH that accompanied the hypotension, but had little effect on the compensatory increase in plasma renin and norepinephrine or on cardiovascular variables.

C. Baro- and Chemoreflex Control

There is ample electrophysiological data to suggest that the rostral hypothalamus, especially the PVN, is involved in modulation of the baro- or chemoreflexes. Neurons that project to the PVN have been antidromically identified in both the ventrolateral and dorsomedial (NTS) area of the medulla oblongata. A significant number of these medullary neurons showed altered firing rates following activation of the baroreflex by increasing pressure in the carotid sinus or by stimulation of the carotid sinus or aortic depressor nerves (19,24,88,91). Electrical stimulation of these afferent nerves does not allow a determination of separate baro- or chemoreceptor activation. However, Banks and Harris specifically explored the effect of chemoreceptor activation (injection of saline equilibrated with 100% CO_2 into the area of the carotid body) on the firing of neurons in the PVN or anterior hypothalamus (6). Of the 157 cells identified in these areas, none were affected by chemoreceptor activation. Hence, the rostral hypothalamus may play no role in modulating the peripheral chemoreflex; the observed activation most likely was due to baroreceptor input.

As mentioned previously, one of the earliest studies to examine the cardiovascular effects of electrical stimulation of the PVN showed that activation of this nucleus inhibited the reflex bradycardia induced by stimulation of the carotid sinus nerve in anesthetized cats (23). Conversely, lesions in the PVN resulted in an enhanced baroreflex-induced bradycardia. Jin and Rockhold showed a similar inhibition of baroreflex control of heart rate with activation of the PVN using kainic acid injections in conscious rats (82). On the contrary, Patel and Schmid reported that focal anesthesia of the PVN with microinjections of lidocaine in anesthetized rabbits had no effect on reflex bradycardia induced by acute increase in arterial pressure with injections of phenylephrine (126). However, the lidocaine did enhance the reflex-induced decrease in directly recorded lumbar sympathetic activity. In conscious rats, complete deafferentation and deefferentation of the PVN actually produced a slight, but significant, attenuation of baroreflex control of heart rate, and of course, as mentioned above, lesions in the PVN prevent the sympathoexcitation that results from aortic barodenervation (34,192). However, when cell-body-specific lesions were made in the PVN (with the excitotoxic neurotransmitter agonist NMDA), baroreflex sensitivity was unaffected even 5 weeks after the lesions (138).

Taken together, these studies suggest that neurons in the PVN may be involved in modulating baroreflex function, although the relative importance of this involvement is not clear. The contribution of the rostral hypothalamus to modulation of chemoreflexes appears to be minimal.

D. Hypertension

There is now evidence that neurons in the PVN contribute to the development and maintenance of genetic and neurogenic forms of experimental hypertension. In the spontaneously hypertensive rat (SHR), a genetic model, electrolytic lesions in the PVN prevented any elevation in arterial pressure from age 4 to 8 weeks; thereafter, although blood pressure began to rise, even by 16 weeks it was still significantly lower than in sham-lesion control animals (25). In a separate study, the contribution of the sympathetic nervous system and/or vasopressin to resting blood pressure in the SHR with PVN lesions was investigated (164). Ganglionic blockade produced a greater decrease in blood pressure in the sham-lesion animals than in the lesion animals, suggesting that ablation of the PVN had removed a neurogenic component of blood pressure maintenance. On the other hand, peripheral administration of a vasopressin receptor antagonist did not affect blood pressure in either group. These data support the notion that neurons in the PVN are involved in the full expression of the neurogenic component of hypertension in SHR.

Electrolytic lesions in the PVN have also been shown to prevent or reverse the hypertension that is produced by denervation of the aortic depressor nerves, figure-8 wrapping of the kidney (one-kidney preparation), and feeding a high salt diet to Dahl salt-sensitive rats (58,64,192). All these models of hypertension are known to exhibit at least a partial neurogenic component to the elevation in arterial pressure. Whether ablation of the PVN affects the hypertension through a common mechanism is not presently known.

The PVN is not the only nucleus in the rostral hypothalamus that has been implicated in the development of hypertension. In 1975, Nathan and Reis reported that electrolytic lesions in the anterior hypothalamic area of rats produced a fulminating hypertension that was accompanied by pulmonary edema (115). These authors concluded that neural pathways that originated in or passed through the anterior hypothalamus had a tonic inhibitory influence on sympathetic outflow to the cardiovascular system. However, in a subsequent study, it was shown that electrical stimulation in the anterior hypothalamic area produced the same sort of cardiovascular response and respiratory stimulation that was evoked by the lesions (induced using anodal current and stainless steel electrodes) (53). When lesions were made using platinum electrodes and cathodal current, no hypertension was observed. Hence, the hypertension resulting from lesions in the anterior hypothalamus may have actually occurred because of a stimulatory "irritative action of the metallic ions deposited at the lesion sites."

In summary, the role of the rostral hypothalamus in the control of cardiovascular function has received a great deal of attention, while effects on respiratory function have been less well studied. In the rostral hypothalamus, the PVN appears to be the major forebrain site for control of the cardiovascular system. This nucleus has the potential to produce both sympathoexcitatory and sympathoinhibitory influences. Additional research is required to determine the actual respiratory influences of this brain site; initial studies indicate that the PVN can elicit minor changes in respiratory drive. Clearly, baroreflex input is integrated in the PVN; however, the contribution of the PVN to chemoreflexes is less well documented. The PVN may also be involved in integration of other sensory afferent inputs such as those originating from the kidney. Finally, the PVN appears to play a contributing role in the development and maintenance of several forms of experimental hypertension, especially those with a neurogenic component.

III. Caudal Hypothalamus

A. Anatomy

Various sites in the caudal hypothalamus, including the dorsomedial nucleus, the posterior hypothalamic area, and the lateral hypothalamic area, are involved in cardiorespiratory regulation. The caudal hypothalamus can be defined as the hypothalamic structures that extend from the caudal aspects of the paraventricular nucleus to the perifornical areas of the hypothalamus dorsal and dorsolateral to the medial mammillary nucleus. The area contained in the region between the third ventricle, the fornix, and the mammillothalamic tract is the most important location in the caudal hypothalamus that modulates respiratory and cardiovascular activity. This area has long been known to exert an excitatory influence on arterial pressure, heart rate, and respiration.

Efferent Connections

A variety of techniques have been utilized for determining the efferent connections of neurons located in the caudal hypothalamus. In early studies, Wang and Ranson used electrical stimulation of the caudal hypothalamus to evoke increases in arterial pressure in the intact, anesthetized cat that were compared to the response seen after *extensive* sectioning of various sites in the central nervous system (182). The rise in pressure elicited by hypothalamic stimulation was not substantially altered by large lesions that destroyed most of the dorsal medulla. However, lesions that extended through the reticular formation in the ventral medulla produced a large attenuation of the pressor response to hypothalamic stimulation. Similar results were obtained with sections of the ventrolateral columns of the cervical spinal cord. Schramm and Bignall subsequently demonstrated that smaller electrolytic lesions in the ventrolateral medulla also abolished the atropine-sensitive vasodilation elicited by hypothalamic stimulation (149). Extensive lesions of the "vasomotor" areas in the dorsal pons and medulla did not prevent the vasodilation produced by stimulating the caudal hypothalamus. Even though these two studies used nonspecific lesions, the results suggest that the cardiovascular responses originating from hypothalamic stimulation involve a descending pathway through areas in the ventral medulla. These findings were supported by studies performed by Ciriello and Calaresu, who made unilateral lesions in hypothalamic sites from which electrical stimulation increased arterial pressure and heart rate (22). Histological analyses were performed after the animals were allowed to survive for 5–11 days in order to identify locations containing degenerating axons and terminals. Their results described a pathway from the hypothalamus that courses down to the periaqueductal gray, through the midbrain, pons, and medulla, and terminates in the ventrolateral medulla in a region dorsolateral to the superior olivary nucleus.

Retrograde and anterograde tracings with horseradish peroxidase (HRP), fluorescent tracers, and tritiated amino acids have been used as more refined techniques for establishing efferent connections of the caudal hypothalamus. Investigators have made injections of HRP into presumed projection sites of the hypothalamus and then examined hypothalamic sections for retrograde labeling of cell bodies (73,123,145). Using this technique, neurons in the caudal hypothalamus have been shown to send descending projections to a number of CNS sites involved in cardiorespiratory regulation, including the nucleus of the solitary tract, the dorsal motor nucleus of the vagus, the raphe magnus, the raphe pallidus, reticular formation of the caudal medulla, the parabrachial nucleus, and various levels of the spinal cord. Projections to areas in the ventrolateral medulla were also identified in several studies (102,158). In addition, efferent projections from the caudal hypothalamus were identified in such diverse locations as the locus coeruleus, the hippocampus, and the insular cortex (3,29,189). Baev et al. have shown that the "locomotor region" in the caudal hypothalamus sends projections to other locomotor sites in the mesencephalon and the medial brainstem reticular formation (3). Injections of anterograde tracers into the caudal hypothalamus have revealed a distribution of efferent connections similar to that obtained with HRP (73,96,145).

Electrophysiological studies have also been utilized to determine the efferent connections of caudal hypothalamic neurons. An advantage of these techniques over neuroanatomical tracing studies is that one can provide some functional information about the connections. For example, it has been possible to determine efferent connections of hypothalamic sites that when stimulated electrically produce a cardiovascular, respiratory and locomotor activation. Orlovskii reported that stimulation of caudal hypothalamic areas that elicit locomotion evokes excitatory postsynaptic potentials in dorsal pontine and medullary neurons that project to the spinal cord (123). Connections have also been shown electrophysiologically to exist between locomotor regions in the hypothalamus and the mesencephalon (110). Evidence for both monosynaptic and polysynaptic connections was presented. Li and Lovick provided electrophysiological support for the neuroanatomical studies that showed projections from the caudal hypothalamus to the ventrolateral medulla (98). In their study, stimulation of the "defense area" of the hypothalamus evoked an excitatory response in neurons located in the nucleus paragigantocellularis lateralis. In addition, neurons located in the hypothalamus were antidromically activated by stimulation in the ventrolateral medulla. A recent study has shown that neurons in the lateral tegmental field that receive baroreceptor input are affected by electrical stimulation of the caudal hypothalamus in rabbits (185). However, it was not determined in this study whether this was a direct or polysynaptic connection.

Direct connections between the caudal hypothalamus and other areas involved in cardiorespiratory regulation have been demonstrated. The most complete study was performed by Barman, who used signal averaging to classify the basal discharge of hypothalamic neurons (7). A small number of sympathoexcitatory neurons in the hypothalamus, including the perifornical region, were shown to project to the ventrolateral medulla and a slightly greater number to the lateral tegmental fields. However, over 30% of the caudal hypothalamic neurons tested were shown to have axons in the periaqueductal gray (PAG). Antidromic mapping techniques indicated that many of the axons from the hypothalamus branched or terminated in the PAG. Only one caudal hypothalamic neuron was found that sent a direct projection to the thoracic spinal cord.

Both the anatomical and electrophysiological studies have shown that caudal hypothalamic neurons send direct projections to other areas involved in respiratory and cardiovascular regulation. The PAG, the nucleus tractus solitarius, and the ventrolateral medulla appear to be the most directly connected with the caudal hypothalamus. Thus, the caudal hypothalamus affects cardiovascular and respiratory output to the spinal cord by impinging monosynaptically on medullary neurons and/or by direct projections to the PAG, which in turn is connected with the ventrolateral medulla.

Afferent Connections

The caudal hypothalamus receives afferent input from most of the cardiorespiratory areas that receive projections from the hypothalamus. Injection of HRP into areas of the caudal hypothalamus that, when stimulated electrically, elicit locomotion results in retrograde labeling of numerous brainstem sites (14). This study demonstrated that the caudal hypothalamus receives input from the anterior hypothalamus, the parabrachial nucleus, the nucleus of the tractus solitarius, the lateral tegmental fields, and the ventrolateral medulla. Similar afferent connections of the caudal hypothalamus have been elucidated in studies utilizing anterograde tracers (29,136). The caudal hypothalamus also receives input from forebrain regions such as the amygdala, basal ganglia, and cortical areas (4,191). These connections are probably related to the locomotor and/or integrative autonomic functions of the caudal hypothalamus.

Thus, the afferent input to and the efferent output from the caudal hypothalamus is organized in a reciprocal manner that would suggest an important role of this hypothalamic area in cardiovascular, respiratory, and locomotor function. This hypothalamic connectivity suggests a strong integrative function for this brain area. Even though most of the above studies did not determine the functional significance of the pathways, physiological studies described below will highlight the importance of the caudal hypothalamus in cardiorespiratory integration.

B. Functional Studies

Electrical Stimulation

It has long been known that electrical stimulation in the caudal hypothalamus elicits an increase in cardiovascular and respiratory activity. Early studies utilized electrical stimulation of various brain sites in an attempt to ascribe physiological function to active sites. In 1935, Kabat and colleagues demonstrated that stimulation in the caudal hypothalamus produces pronounced increases in arterial pressure (87). It was noted that the largest pressor responses were elicited by stimulation in the subfornical region, the lateral hypothalamic area, and the H1 field of Forel. An increase in the rate and depth of breathing was evoked by stimulation in the same areas (86).

Subsequent experiments revealed that caudal hypothalamic stimulation elicits elaborate changes in autonomic and respiratory function (1,15,35,47,74, 105,141,177,190). Associated with activation of this area are increases in arterial pressure, heart rate, ventricular contractility, tidal volume, respiratory frequency, sympathetic nerve discharge, and other autonomic changes such as pupillary dilation, retraction of the nictitating membrane, piloerection, and release of catecholamines from the adrenal gland. A redistribution of blood flow also occurs, which includes sympathetic-mediated vasodilation in skeletal muscles and vasoconstriction in the skin and intestines. It is interesting that stimulation of this general region in the human during surgery has been reported to have respiratory effects (151).

These coordinated responses elicited by caudal hypothalamic stimulation resemble the autonomic and respiratory changes that occur during the "defense" or "fight or flight" reaction in awake animals that encounter a threatening environment (104). For this reason, the perifornical area of the hypothalamus from which electrical stimulation evokes this response has been labeled the defense area by Hilton and colleagues (65). The function of these autonomic responses is to prepare the animal for aggressive behavior since stimulation of this defense area in unanesthetized cats elicits a rage response (104).

It was originally argued that the pathway for the vasodilation elicited by stimulation in the perifornical hypothalamus originates in the motor cortex. Since electrical stimulation in the motor cortex produced an atropine-sensitive vasodilation in skeletal muscles of anesthetized animals, it was suggested that the motor cortex could elicit the motor response in limb skeletal muscles as well as the circulatory changes needed for the increased work (28,48). In this hypothesis, the caudal hypothalamus would serve as part of the pathway responsible for eliciting increased sympathetic outflow to skeletal muscle vasculature. However, careful experiments by Hilton et al. demonstrated that the vasodilation elicited by cortical stimulation is simply a postcontraction hyperemia. The vascular response to cortical stimulation was shown to disappear after muscular paralysis with gallamine as well as after sectioning of the motor fibers to the skeletal muscles (71).

Hilton et al. have provided evidence that the outflow of the defense region in the hypothalamus involves a synapse in the ventrolateral medulla (68). These investigators used electrical stimulation to trace an efferent pathway from the hypothalamus to the superficial ventrolateral medulla. In addition, they found that bilateral lesions or placement of glycine onto a small region of the surface of the ventrolateral medulla produced a pronounced fall in arterial pressure as well as a concomitant attenuation of the autonomic and respiratory responses elicited by hypothalamic stimulation. It was concluded that the caudal hypothalamus normally provides a tonic drive to this medullary region involved in maintenance of vasomotor tone. This hypothesis is consistent with the known connections between the hypothalamus, the PAG, and the ventrolateral medulla. Moreover, stimulation of the caudal hypothalamus evokes an excitatory response in neurons located in this area of the ventrolateral medulla (70).

Chemical Stimulation

The observed responses evoked by electrical stimulation could be due to stimulation of fibers originating outside the caudal hypothalamus instead of the local cell bodies. This hypothesis has been tested by several investigators who used microinjection of chemicals that activate cell bodies and do not affect axons (57). In most of these cases, neurotransmitter agonists or antagonists were microinjected to stimulate or disinhibit cell bodies located in the caudal hypothalamus.

Several studies that used chemical stimulation of the caudal hypothalamus were unable to elicit the same cardiorespiratory responses as that produced by electrical stimulation. Hilton and Redfern reported that microinjection of the excitatory amino acid, D,L-homocysteic acid (DLH) evoked a rise in breathing but a fall in arterial pressure when injected into the caudal hypothalamus of the anesthetized rat (69). Electrical stimulation at the same site produced a pressor response. Locomotor responses associated with electrical stimulation in the unanesthetized rat were also not produced by microinjection of DLH. Neither Tan and Dampney nor Spencer et al. were able to elicit pressor responses when they injected glutamate into the caudal hypothalamus of anesthetized animals (160, 165). Therefore, they concluded that the cardiovascular responses produced by electrical stimulation in the caudal hypothalamus are due to activation of fibers of passage. A similar conclusion was reached by Bandler, who was unable to elicit rage responses with glutamate microinjections in the unanesthetized cat (5).

In contrast to the above studies, several investigators have reported that chemical stimulation or disinhibition of caudal hypothalamic neurons elicits all the cardiorespiratory and locomotor responses that follow electrical stimulation. Ohta et al. found that microinjection of glutamate into the posterior hypothalamus of the unanesthetized rat caused increases in arterial pressure and heart rate that were accompanied by behavioral excitation (119). All these responses were reduced by prior injection of propranolol, hexamethonium, and phentolamine, indicating involvement of catecholaminergic and/or cholinergic systems in the hypothalamus. Microinjection of GABA antagonists or synthesis inhibitors has been used to "disinhibit" neurons in the posterior hypothalamus. DiMicco and colleagues reported that injections of the GABA antagonist bicuculline into the posterior hypothalamus of the anesthetized rat produced large increases in heart rate with small elevations in arterial pressure (40,184). Similar results were obtained with microinjection of an inhibitor of GABA synthesis. No attempt was made to determine whether the observed responses could have been due to feedback from contraction of skeletal muscles produced by the injections.

Subsequent experiments by Waldrop and colleagues expanded the findings obtained with chemicals that alter GABAergic function (10,174,175). In their studies, microinjection of GABA antagonists (bicuculline or picrotoxin) into the caudal hypothalamus produced pronounced increases in arterial pressure, heart rate, sympathetic nerve activity, and respiratory activity accompanied by locomotor movements of the limbs of anesthetized cats and rats. All the observed responses were reversed by microinjection of the GABA agonist muscimol. These responses could be obtained with microinjections as small as 40 nl, a volume that spreads less than 1 mm in the brain (152). Microinjection of the GABA synthesis inhibitor 3-mercaptopropionic acid produced similar responses (37,127). The respiratory and cardiovascular stimulation produced by the microinjections were not prevented by muscular paralysis, indicating that the responses were not produced by the movement elicited by the GABA antagonists (175).

Microinjection of other chemicals besides those that alter GABAergic function has also been shown to exert an excitatory effect on the cardiovascular system. Microinjection of excitatory amino acids (N-methyl-D-aspartic acid and kainic acid) into the caudal hypothalamus elevates arterial pressure and heart rate (159). In addition, microinjection of carbachol and cholinesterase inhibitors into the posterior hypothalamus of anesthetized rats produces an elevation in arterial pressure and tachycardia (17). Similar changes have been evoked by microinjection of neuropeptide Y into the posterior hypothalamus (108). Thus, it appears that a number of neurotransmitter systems exert an influence on neurons in the caudal hypothalamus. In addition, it is clear that activation of neurons in the caudal hypothalamus, without affecting fibers of passage, provides an activation of the respiratory and cardiovascular systems.

It has not been resolved why some investigators have not elicited a cardiovascular activation with chemical stimulation of caudal hypothalamic neurons. A number of possibilities can be considered, including differences in anesthetic state, concentration of the chemicals utilized, volume of injectate, and microinjection site (100). The anesthetic state of an animal can have a pronounced effect on the cardiovascular and respiratory systems; different anesthetics have differing effects. It is also known that excitatory amino acids can produce a depolarization blockade at the site of injection (100). Moreover, injection of large volumes can spread to other sites in the surrounding brain such that any observed responses are a balance between those elicited by the brain sites stimulated. Any of these factors may explain the lack of effect seen by some investigators.

Modulation of Basal Respiratory and Cardiovascular Activity

Early studies by Redgate and Gellhorn examined the effects of chemical or electrolytic depression of neurons in the caudal hypothalamus on breathing and blood pressure in anesthetized cats (55,134,135). Electrolytic lesions produced an immediate fall in the rate and depth of breathing that was accompanied by slight decreases in arterial pressure and heart rate. Bilateral injections of barbiturates into the caudal hypothalamus produced a reversible fall in breathing. Waldrop et al. also reported that bilateral lesions in the posterior hypothalamus evoke a fall in the resting levels for respiratory frequency, minute ventilation, heart rate, and arterial pressure (178). It was concluded from these results that the posterior hypothalamus exerts a tonic facilitatory effect on brainstem cardiovascular and respiratory neurons. These findings support the hypothesis of Hilton et al., who have proposed that this facilitatory effect from the hypothalamus is mediated through a synapse in the ventrolateral medulla (68). They demonstrated that blockade of a superficial area of the ventrolateral medulla produces a fall in arterial pressure and heart rate and abolishes the cardiorespiratory responses to stimulation in the caudal hypothalamus.

Evidence has also accumulated that hypothalamic and other forebrain areas contribute to basal sympathetic nerve discharge. Midbrain transections of the neuroaxis have been shown by Huang et al. to elicit falls in sympathetic nerve discharge and arterial pressure (77). This fall in activity was prevented by first placing lesions in the medial diencephalon. The transection-induced fall in sympathetic nerve activity was not likely due to surgical trauma since a subsequent lower transection had no effect on resting sympathetic activity. Even though these initial experiments did not locate the actual neuroanatomical site responsible for the effect on sympathetic discharge, it was concluded that a significant portion of sympathetic activity originates in the forebrain. Subsequent experiments localized the site in the forebrain by making more precise lesions (78). Lesions in the caudal hypothalamus and in the medial thalamus prevented the fall in arterial pressure and sympathetic discharge produced by transection of the neuroaxis. Lesions of the anterior hypothalamus did not have any effects on the responses elicited by subsequent midbrain transection. Thus, it was concluded that both the caudal hypothalamus and medial thalamus contribute to the origination of sympathetic nerve discharge in anesthetized cats.

Electrophysiological studies have provided additional support for a role of caudal hypothalamic neurons in cardiorespiratory control. Barman and Gebber as well as Dillon and Waldrop have used signal averaging techniques to relate the discharge of neurons in the caudal hypothalamus to the cardiac cycle, sympathetic nerve discharge, and/or the respiratory cycle (7,8,39,171). Both laboratories identified neurons in the caudal hypothalamus that possess a basal discharge related to the cardiac cycle and sympathetic nerve discharge. Dillon and Waldrop found that approximately half of the hypothalamic neurons tested had a cardiac-related discharge and 38% had a discharge related to sympathetic nerve activity (Fig. 2) (39). In addition, a small percentage (19%) of neurons in the caudal hypothalamus had a discharge temporally related to phrenic nerve discharge. These experiments indicate that cardiovascular, sympathetic, and respiratory neurons exist in the hypothalamus; however, these experiments do not allow one to determine whether this discharge is due to origination within the hypothalamus or to feedback from other brain sites and/or peripheral receptors.

C. Baroreceptor Reflex

Numerous studies have concluded that the caudal hypothalamus plays an important modulatory role in the baroreceptor reflex. Involvement of the caudal hypothalamus in the baroreceptor reflex was suggested by Gellhorn et al. in 1956 (55). They demonstrated that the baroreceptor-mediated fall in heart rate following a rise in arterial pressure, evoked by intravenous adrenaline, was accentuated after bilateral lesions were made in the posterior hypothalamus. This finding indicates that the caudal hypothalamus exerts at tonic inhibitory effect on the baroreceptor reflex. This hypothesis was supported by a subsequent report by Hilton (66). He found that the decreases in heart rate and arterial pressure elicited by increasing the pressure in an isolated carotid sinus were abolished by electrical stimulation of the defense areas of the hypothalamus. Hilton's preliminary findings prompted a number of investigators to test the role of caudal hypothalamic neurons, both within and outside the defense areas, in the functioning of the baroreceptor reflex (30,41,54,79). Most of these studies reported that the magnitude of the baroreceptor-mediated bradycardia is reduced by electrical stimulation in the posterior hypothalamus. However, some investigators concluded that caudal hypothalamic stimulation did not alter the depressor response to baroreceptor stimulation. Coote et al. have explained these divergent findings by arguing that both the baroreceptor-mediated bradycardia and depressor response are altered by stimulation only within the defense areas of the hypothalamus and not by stimulation in surrounding areas (30).

A major problem with these earlier studies that demonstrated an alteration of the baroreceptor reflex is that techniques were used that are not specific for cell bodies. Bauer et al. addressed this problem by using GABA antagonists to disinhibit neurons in the posterior hypothalamus (10). The heart rate and arterial pressure responses to baroreceptor stimulation were attenuated following microinjection of a GABA antagonist into the posterior hypothalamus of anesthetized cats and rats. This depression of the baroreceptor reflex could be reversed by microinjection of a GABA agonist into the same hypothalamic site. Thus, it was concluded that depression of the bradycardia produced by hypothalamic stimulation results from activation of cell bodies in the caudal hypothalamus. Moreover, this hypothalamic alteration of the baroreceptor reflex may involve a GABAergic mechanism.

Subsequent experiments by Dillon et al. examined the effects of hypothalamic stimulation on the respiratory responses to baroreceptor stimulation in anesthetized rats (37). Baroreceptor stimulation during control conditions pro-

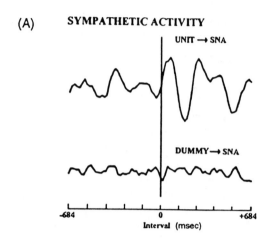

(A)   SYMPATHETIC ACTIVITY

UNIT → SNA

DUMMY → SNA

-684   0   +684
Interval (msec)

Figure 2   Neurons located in the posterior hypothalamus that possess basal discharge patterns related to sympathetic nerve discharge (A), the cardiac cycle (B), and the respiratory rhythm (C). A and B are from anesthetized cats (39); C is from an anesthetized rat. All of these represent signal-averaged data.

duced a fall in both tidal diaphragmatic activity and respiratory frequency. These respiratory responses to baroreceptor activation were blocked by microinjections into the caudal hypothalamus of either GABA receptor antagonists or an inhibitor of GABA synthesis. Microinjection of a GABA agonist into the same caudal hypothalamus sites as the GABA antagonists restored the baroreceptor-mediated respiratory responses. It was concluded that a GABAergic mechanism in the caudal hypothalamus modulates the respiratory responses to baroreceptor activation.

The neural circuitry by which the hypothalamus modulates the respiratory response to stimulation of the baroreceptors was not determined in the above study. However, both electrophysiological and neuroanatomical studies have demonstrated that connections exist between this area of the hypothalamus and the area of the nucleus tractus solitarius that receives afferents from carotid baroreceptors (14,19,84). Noteworthy studies conducted by Spyer and colleagues suggest that the defense region of the caudal hypothalamus exerts an inhibitory effect on neurons in the NTS (84,111). Their studies found that all the neurons in the NTS excited by baroreceptor activation are inhibited by stimulation in the hypothalamus. The inhibitory effect was determined to be mediated via a GABAergic mechanism. Thus, this circuitry may be responsible for the hypothalamic depression of the respiratory responses to baroreceptor stimulation.

Additional support for hypothalamic influence on the baroreceptor reflex has

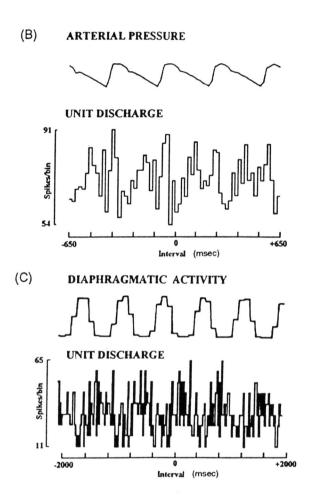

been provided in electrophysiological and in anatomical studies. Frazier et al. reported two populations of baroreceptor-sensitive neurons in the posterior hypothalamus (52). Activation of the baroreceptors by abdominal aortic occlusion stimulated 15 and inhibited five neurons located in the posterior hypothalamus. Barman subsequently expanded these findings in studies in which recordings were made from hypothalamic neurons that had a sympathetic and/or cardiac-related discharge. Many of these neurons were inhibited by baroreceptor stimulation (7). Thus, it appears that activation of baroreceptors leads to a depression of neuronal activity in an area of the hypothalamus that normally provides a tonic drive to the cardiovascular system. Ciriello et al. have used [³H]2-deoxyglucose as a metabolic marker of neuronal activity to determine whether aortic baroreceptor stimulation affects neurons in various brain sites in the anesthetized rat (26). They demonstrated that physiological stimulation of the baroreceptors alters the labeling of neurons in many structures including the posterior hypothalamus. This labeling of the caudal hypothalamus was not observed with electrical stimulation of the aortic nerve.

D. Chemoreception

Hypercapnia

Diencephalic involvement in the cardiorespiratory responses to hypercapnia has been examined by several investigators. Fink et al. reported in 1962 that removal of the diencephalon attenuates the respiratory response to CO_2 (50). Based on other studies, it was concluded that this altered response was due to removal of hypothalamic structures. Similar findings were obtained later by Nielson et al. in the anesthetized dog (117). Both of these studies indicate that diencephalic structures exert an excitatory influence on the respiratory response to CO_2. In neither case, however, was an attempt made to determine the actual neuroanatomical site responsible for this attenuation of the hypercapnic response.

Strong evidence that the caudal hypothalamus modulates the respiratory responses to increases in inhaled CO_2 has been provided by Waldrop, who found that microinjection of GABA antagonists into the caudal hypothalamus of the anesthetized cat greatly accentuates the phrenic nerve response to hypercapnia (173). This potentiation was reversed by microinjection of a GABA agonist into the same site (Fig. 3). A similar effect was observed with microinjections of a GABA synthesis inhibitor or $CoCl_2$ into the posterior hypothalamus of the anesthetized rat (75,127). These findings indicate that a GABAergic mechanism in the caudal hypothalamus modulates the respiratory response to hypercapnia.

Cross and Silver reported in 1963 that over 50% of hypothalamic neurons recorded were responsive to systemic hypercapnia in rabbits (31). However, two major problems make their findings difficult to interpret. First, the magnitude of the hypercapnic stimulus (80% CO_2) presented to the animals was far outside of a physiological range. Therefore, it is possible that the observed neuronal effect was due to nonspecific damage rather than to a direct response to hypercapnia. Moreover, no attempt was made to determine the type (cardiovascular, respiratory, or sympathetic) of neuron that was being recorded in the hypothalamus. Therefore, it is not possible to make any statements about the physiological significance of the responses to CO_2 in their study.

A recent study that avoided these problems found that increases in inspired CO_2 stimulate neurons in the caudal hypothalamus of anesthetized cats (Fig. 4) (39). Thirty-two percent of the caudal hypothalamic neurons studied were stimulated by a physiological hypercapnic stimulus (5% CO_2). Moreover, all of the CO_2-activated neurons had a discharge pattern related to cardiovascular and/or respira-

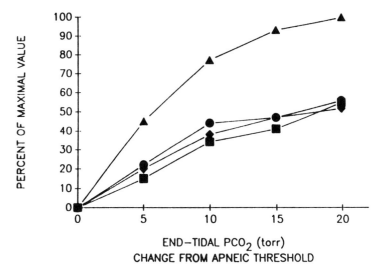

Figure 3 Phrenic nerve (% of maximal) responses to step increases in end-tidal CO_2 in an anesthetized cat. The control responses (boxes) were obtained prior to any microinjections. Microinjection of Ringer's solution did not alter the response to CO_2 (diamonds), but a subsequent microinjection of the GABA antagonist picrotoxin greatly increased the CO_2 response (triangles). Note that microinjection of a GABA agonist, muscimol, restored the response to control levels (circles). (From Ref. 173.)

tory rhythms as revealed by signal-averaging analyses. Dillon and Waldrop also provided evidence that this response was not dependent on input from peripheral chemoreceptors; a similar percentage of neurons were stimulated by hypercapnia in sinoaortic denervated cats (39). Thus, it was concluded that these electrophysiological findings support the possibility that neurons in the caudal hypothalamus play a role in the cardiorespiratory responses to hypercapnia.

At least two mechanisms could be responsible for the stimulation of hypothalamic neurons observed by Dillon and Waldrop (39). The first possibility is that these neurons were activated by other neurons in other brain sites that are responsive to CO_2. Recent experiments have provided convincing evidence that CO_2-sensitive neurons exist in both the dorsal and ventrolateral medulla (36,116,118). Connections are known to exist between these sites and the area of the caudal hypothalamus examined by Dillon and Waldrop. A second possibility is that the caudal hypothalamic neurons have an inherent responsiveness to CO_2. Dillon and Waldrop as well as Bauer and Waldrop have tested this latter hypothesis by recording from hypothalamic neurons in a rat brain slice preparation (9,38). Extracellular recordings from these neurons in both studies revealed that approx-

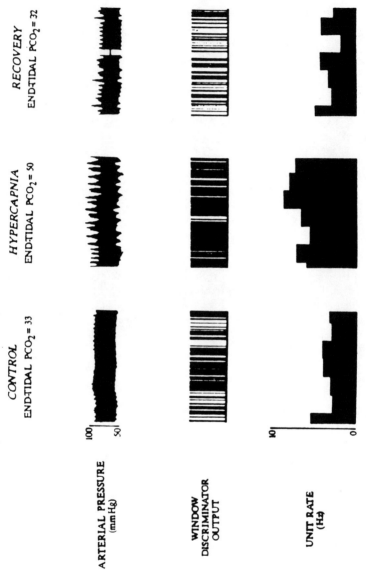

Figure 4 Response of a caudal hypothalamic neuron to hypercapnia in an anesthetized cat. (From Ref. 39.)

imately 25% of the tested neurons increased their discharge frequency when the brain slices were exposed to a hypercapnic gas. Further characterization of these neurons with whole-cell patch recordings revealed that hypercapnia elicits a depolarization and/or increase in discharge frequency in 35% of the neurons (Fig. 5). Similar responses to CO_2 were also observed during blockade of chemical transmission by perfusing the slices with a medium containing high Mg^{2+} and low Ca^{2+} concentrations. These findings suggest that hypercapnia can exert a direct effect on caudal hypothalamic neurons and, thereby, influence cardiorespiratory function.

Hypoxia

Strong evidence supports the hypothesis that suprapontine sites modulate the cardiorespiratory responses to hypoxia. Tenney and Ou demonstrated that the respiratory response to hypoxia was larger after decortication than in the intact, unanesthetized cat (166). Furthermore, this potentiated response returned to control levels after a subsequent decerebration. These authors suggested that some unidentified site in the diencephalon exerted an excitatory effect on the response to hypoxia after removal of forebrain inhibitory influences. This hypothesis has recently been supported by Hayashi and Sinclair, who found that anemic decerebration attenuates the hypoxia-induced increase in respiration (63). However, neither of these studies identified the actual neuroanatomical site responsible for this modulation.

Activation of neurons in the caudal hypothalamus have been shown to alter some of the cardiorespiratory responses to stimulation of the peripheral chemoreceptors. Preliminary findings by Hilton and Joels indicated that stimulation in the defense area of the caudal hypothalamus enhances the increase in arterial pressure and ventilation evoked by cyanide stimulation of the carotid body (67). In addition, the bradycardia elicited by selective stimulation of the carotid body has also been shown to be inhibited by stimulation in the posteriomedial hypothalamus (168).

The hypothalamus is known to receive input from peripheral chemoreceptors. Thomas and Calaresu reported that electrical stimulation of the carotid sinus nerve effects the firing frequency of 45% of neurons located in the medial hypothalamus (167). Selective stimulation of the peripheral chemoreceptors and the arterial baroreceptors also altered the discharge frequency of hypothalamic neurons located in a region that when stimulated produced increases in arterial pressure and heart rate. A stimulation of caudal hypothalamic neurons by systemic hypoxia was observed in earlier studies by Cross and Silver (31). These investigators found that all the neurons stimulated by hypoxia were affected by other stimuli such as noxious stimulation and hypercapnia. A serious problem with this latter

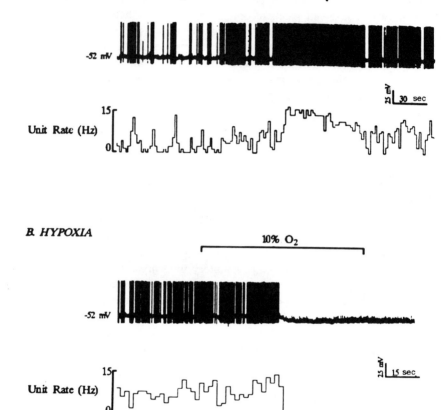

Figure 5   Whole-cell patch recording of a caudal hypothalamic neuron studied in a rat brain slice preparation. This neuron was stimulated by hypercapnia (A) but inhibited by hypoxia (B). (From Ref. 38.)

study is that the hypoxic stimulus (100% N_2 or N_2O) used was nonphysiological and may have resulted in a stimulation unrelated to the direct actions of hypoxia.

A recent study has demonstrated that a physiological hypoxic stimulus (10% O_2) excites approximately 20% of the caudal hypothalamic neurons tested in anesthetized cats (39). Ryan and Waldrop recently reported that some of these hypoxia-sensitive neurons in the caudal hypothalamus project to the PAG (143). Moreover, these neurons have a basal discharge correlated temporally with cardiovascular and/or respiratory activity. Furthermore, this effect on hypothalamic neurons does not require input from peripheral chemoreceptors since a similar proportion of hypothalamic neurons were stimulated following inhalation of 10% O_2 in peripherally chemodenervated animals (39). The responses of the same neurons to hypercapnia were also studied; only 13% of the neurons that were studied responded to both hypoxia and hypercapnia. Thus, it appears that separate populations of neurons in the caudal hypothalamus are involved in hypercapnic and hypoxic responses (39).

A direct effect of hypoxia on caudal hypothalamic neurons has been demonstrated in experiments performed by Dillon and Waldrop in a rat brain slice preparation (38). Approximately 80% of the caudal hypothalamic neurons tested in this in vitro preparation were stimulated by hypoxia; this response persisted during synaptic blockade (Fig. 6). These findings suggest that neurons in the caudal hypothalamus serve as central hypoxic chemoreceptors. A number of whole animal experiments have previously suggested that hypoxia can exert a central excitatory influence on cardiorespiratory activity. Hypoxia evokes a tachypnea in unanesthetized cats and rats that have been peripherally chemodenervated (16,112). Moreover, increases in breathing and sympathetic outflow to the heart and peripheral vasculature can be elicited with hypoxia isolated to the brain (33,42). The caudal hypothalamic neurons studied by Dillon and Waldrop are located in an area that, when activated, produces a cardiorespiratory stimulation (Fig. 7). Thus, the possibility exists that these neurons when stimulated by central hypoxia elicit a cardiorespiratory activation.

E. Hering-Breuer Reflex

Redgate used injections of thiopental into the caudal hypothalamus to examine the possibility that the Hering-Breuer reflex is modulated by this brain site (134). The injection resulted in a decrease in the resting level of respiration and arterial pressure. In addition, the respiratory inhibition produced by lung inflation was markedly enhanced after administration of thiopental. Romaniuk et al. found that the Hering-Breuer reflex was attenuated during locomotion produced by stimulation in the caudal hypothalamus (140). It was not determined whether the observed alteration of the Hering-Breuer reflex was due to the direct effects of hypothalamic stimulation or to feedback elicited by the locomotion. Thus, the role the caudal hypothalamus plays in the Hering-Breuer reflex is uncertain; additional experiments are needed to address this issue.

F. Exercise

Two major neural mechanisms are believed to regulate cardiorespiratory activity during exercise (46,172). One mechanism involves the activation of mechanically and/or metabolically sensitive receptors located in contracting skeletal muscles. This afferent input ascends through spinal pathways to impinge on cardiorespira-

A. *EXTRACELLULAR*

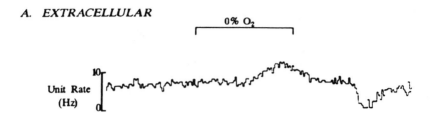

B. *INTRACELLULAR*

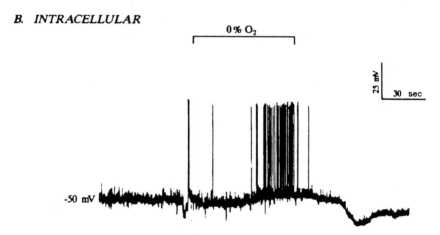

Figure 6 Two caudal hypothalamic neurons that were stimulated by hypoxia in a rat brain slice preparation. (From Ref. 38.)

tory neurons in the brainstem. The other mechanism is a feedforward drive that has been termed "central command." This mechanism is thought to originate from the same central sites that are responsible for generation of descending drive to spinal locomotor neurons. Thus, cardiorespiratory function is increased in parallel with the exercise that is being performed.

Considerable evidence supports the hypothesis that the locomotor region of the caudal hypothalamus is important in the central command control of locomotion, circulation, and respiration. In 1940, Waller reported that electrical stimulation of this area elicits locomotion in decorticate cats and in lightly anesthetized cats with intact brains (181). The area of the hypothalamus from which locomotion

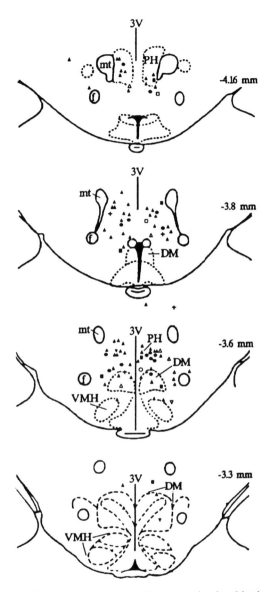

Figure 7 Location of hypothalamic neurons that were stimulated by hypoxia or hypercapnia in a rat brain slice preparation. (Filled triangles) Hypoxia stimulated; (filled circles) hypercapnia stimulated; (filled boxes) stimulated by both hypoxia and hypercapnia; (open triangles) inhibited by hypoxia; (open circles) inhibited by CO_2; (inverted filled triangles) unaffected by hypercapnia and unaffected by CO_2; (inverted open triangles) inhibited by CO_2 and unaffected by hypoxia; (open boxes) unaffected by CO_2; (+) unaffected by hypoxia and hypercapnia. (From Ref. 38.)

can be induced includes the posterior hypothalamic area and adjacent lateral areas. The locomotion elicited by hypothalamic stimulation is similar to that observed during voluntary exercise. These findings were subsequently corroborated and expanded by Grossman and by Orlovski and co-workers (60,124,153). It was also shown that unanesthetized decorticate cats can locomote spontaneously, indicating that the motor cortex is not requisite for the generation of descending motor signals.

Rushmer and colleagues were the first to propose that the hypothalamic locomotor region is involved in central command control of cardiorespiratory activity during exercise (142,157). They demonstrated that electrical stimulation of the fields of Forel in the caudal lateral hypothalamus produces running movements that are accompanied by changes in cardiovascular function similar to those observed in dogs running on a treadmill. Since these cardiovascular responses persisted after muscular paralysis, descending motor signals must be responsible for the parallel activation of the cardiovascular system during hypothalamic stimulation. Similar results were reported in an abstract by Marshall and Timms, who studied anesthetized cats (106). These investigators found that stimulation in the hypothalamus evoked running movements that were accompanied by increases in ventilation, arterial pressure, heart rate, and renal and mesenteric vasoconstriction. All the autonomic responses persisted during muscular paralysis. It was suggested that this hypothalamic site participates in the generation of locomotion and the accompanying cardiovascular and respiratory responses.

A more complete characterization of the role of the hypothalamic locomotor region in controlling cardiorespiratory activity during exercise has been provided by Eldridge and co-workers, who studied both anesthetized brain-intact and unanesthetized decorticate cats (44,45,113). These investigators demonstrated that electrical stimulation in the hypothalamic locomotor region (HLR) produces locomotion accompanied by proportional increases in respiration and arterial pressure. Moreover, stimulation in paralyzed animals produced "fictive locomotion" (recorded as motor nerve activity) and increases in phrenic nerve activity and arterial pressure. Furthermore, these responses persisted even after prevention of feedback from peripheral chemoreceptors, baroreceptors, lung receptors, and central chemoreceptors. It was also noted that spontaneous bursts of actual and fictive locomotion with concomitant increases in respiratory activity and arterial pressure occurred in the unanesthetized decorticate cats. These findings indicate that neither feedback from peripheral receptors nor input from cortical regions is requisite for parallel activation of cardiorespiratory and locomotor activity. Thus, it was concluded that command signals emanating from the hypothalamus are the major cause for the changes in respiration and circulation that occur during exercise. This conclusion suggests that activation of neurons in this hypothalamic region provides a model for central command and simulates the central neural mechanism that controls the cardiorespiratory systems during exercise. Additional support for this hypothesis has been provided recently by other investigators (61,176).

In addition to the cardiorespiratory responses reported by Eldridge et al., Waldrop et al. have demonstrated that electrical stimulation of the hypothalamic locomotor region in anesthetized cats produces a redistribution of blood flow similar to that seen during voluntary exercise in awake cats (177). These changes, which were measured using the radioactive microsphere technique, include increased blood flow to the heart, diaphragm, and limb skeletal muscles and a concomitant decrease in blood flow to the kidneys. In addition, the vascular resistance of the intestines, gallbladder, and stomach increased during stimulation. These blood flow changes are similar to those reported by other investigators who stimulated in hypothalamic areas probably, including the hypothalamic locomotor region (27,51).

Since the above studies used electrical stimulation of the hypothalamic locomotor region, the observed responses could have resulted from stimulation of axons whose cell bodies were located distant to the hypothalamic locomotor region. Eldridge et al. addressed this possibility by injecting a GABA antagonist into the locomotor regions of the hypothalamus (44). Injections elicited all the responses seen with electrical stimulation, suggesting that the observed responses are due to stimulation of cell bodies alone in the hypothalamic locomotor region. However, relatively large volumes were injected in this study, and thus, the responses could have resulted from spread of the antagonist to sites outside of the hypothalamic locomotor region. Waldrop et al. and Bauer et al. subsequently reported that microinjections of small volumes of GABA antagonists into the posterior hypothalamus produce increases in arterial pressure, heart rate, and minute ventilation, which are accompanied by locomotor movements of the limbs of both cats and rats (Fig. 8) (10,175). Moreover, these responses were reversed by microinjections of a GABA agonist (Fig. 9). Similar cardiovascular responses have been obtained by DiMicco and colleagues (40,184). These results indicate that stimulation of cell bodies alone in the hypothalamic locomotor region produces all the cardiorespiratory and locomotor responses evoked by electrical stimulation and that a GABAergic mechanism exerts a tonic depressive influence over the cardiorespiratory and locomotor systems by an action in the posterior hypothalamus. Moreover, it is possible that a lifting (or disinhibition) of the GABAergic inhibition exerted on the posterior hypothalamus is responsible for locomotion and the cardiorespiratory responses to exercise. The site of origin of the neurons that produce the GABAergic inhibition is not known; however, a number of brainstem and more rostral sites are known to project to the HLR.

The effects on the cardiovascular responses to voluntary exercise of destroying the hypothalamic locomotor region have been examined in three studies. In experiments from Rushmer's laboratory, bilateral lesions were placed in the fields

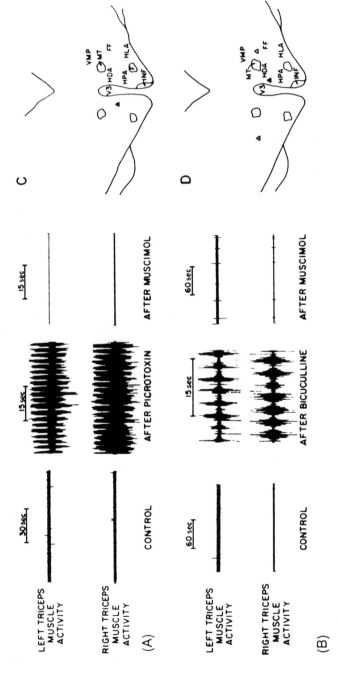

Figure 8 Microinjection of GABA antagonists into the caudal hypothalamus evokes running movements as indicated by bursts of electromyographic activity in the left and right triceps of an anesthetized cat. Notice that the effects of picrotoxin (A) and bicuculline (B) were reversed by microinjection of a GABA agonist, muscimol, at the same site. The injection sites for picrotoxin and bicuculline are denoted by filled triangles in panels C and D, respectively. (From Ref. 175.)

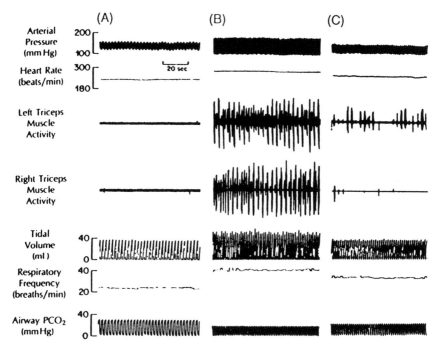

Figure 9 Microinjection of a GABA antagonist elicits locomotor activity accompanied by cardiovascular and respiratory responses. (A) Control levels; (B) changes that occurred after the microinjection; (C) a GABA agonist reverses the responses evoked by the GABA antagonist. (From Ref. 172.)

of Forel of dogs that had been instrumented for chronic cardiovascular monitoring (142). No cardiovascular responses to treadmill exercise were observed in one of the dogs with the bilateral lesions. However, this experiment has been reported only in a textbook by Rushmer, and the data from only one of the dogs were given. Similar experiments have been conducted subsequently in baboons performing isometric exercise (72). This preliminary study reported that diencephalic lesions reduced the cardiovascular responses to isometric exercise in only two of the five baboons that were studied. In a recent experiment, Ordway et al. examined the effects of lesioning the HLR on the cardiovascular responses of dogs running on a treadmill (122). Bilateral lesions did not alter the cardiovascular responses to exercise in any of the dogs studied. Thus, at present, evidence suggests that conscious animals deprived of the locomotor areas in and adjacent to the posterior hypothalamus display normal cardiovascular responses to dynamic exercise. The possibility exists that other areas in the brain assume the functions of this area when animals are deprived of structures that normally modulate cardiovascular responses to exercise.

Both central command and feedback originating from contracting muscles are known to produce increases in cardiovascular function. Moreover, both these mechanisms are probably active in generating the appropriate responses to voluntary exercise. Mitchell has pointed out that these are redundant control mechanisms operative during exercise and that neural occlusion occurs (114). Evidence supporting neural occlusion in the cardiovascular responses to exercise has been presented to support this contention. Waldrop et al. demonstrated that putative central command (elicited by hypothalamic stimulation) and reflexes evoked by muscular contraction exert smaller cardiorespiratory effects when activated simultaneously than when activated individually (179). These findings have been corroborated by Rybicki et al., who also showed that the reduced responses during simultaneous activation of both the central and reflex mechanisms do not result from saturation of the involved neuronal circuitry (144).

Since both central command and peripheral feedback are likely to be active simultaneously during exercise, central neural sites must exist that integrate information from both these mechanisms to provide the appropriate cardiovascular responses to exercise. Only a few studies have sought to locate such central nervous system areas. One site that has been considered is the hypothalamic locomotor region. Bilateral lesions of the HLR in anesthetized cats accentuate the heart rate response to muscular contraction (178). In addition, Waldrop and Stremel have shown that the majority of neurons recorded from in the hypothalamic locomotor region are stimulated by muscular contraction (Fig. 10) (180). Since the HLR is thought to play a role in the central command mechanisms, these results suggest that this hypothalamic region may serve as an integrative region for cardiovascular control during exercise.

G. Hypertension

The spontaneously hypertensive rat (SHR) was developed by Okamoto and co-workers as an experimental genetic model for investigating essential hypertension (120,188). These investigators provided initial evidence that a hypothalamic area may contribute to the elevated arterial pressure present in these animals. Transection of connections between the mesencepalon and the caudal hypothalamus produced a much larger fall in arterial pressure in the SHR than in normotensive rats (188). Others have demonstrated that electrical stimulation in the caudal hypothalamus evokes a larger pressor and sympathetic nerve response in hypertensive than in normotensive rats (18,85). Strong additional evidence for hypothalamic involvement in hypertension was provided recently by Eilam et al. (43). These investigators evoked hypertension by implanting hypothalamic grafts from SHR into the hypothalamus of normotensive rats.

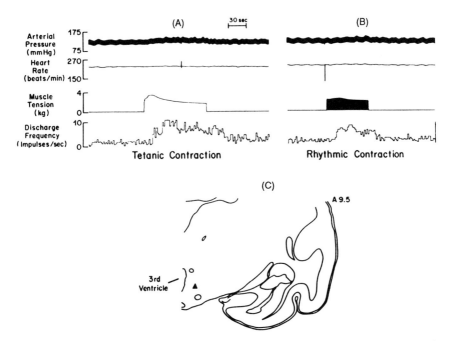

Figure 10 Neuron that was stimulated by muscular contraction elicited by stimulation of the L-7 and S-1 ventral roots. Both tetanic (A) and rhythmic (B) contractions stimulated this neuron located in the caudal hypothalamus (C; triangle). (From Ref. 180.)

Considerable evidence supports the hypothesis that an alteration of GABA-ergic function in the caudal hypothalamus contributes to the high blood pressure present in the SHR. Biochemical studies have revealed that the concentration of GABA and the number of GABA receptors is reduced in the posterior hypothalamus of the SHR (32,62). Moreover, there is also a reduction in the activity of the enzyme glutamic acid decarboxylase, which is responsible for GABA synthesis in this area of the brain (32). Saski et al. have shown that the elevated pressor response to electrical stimulation of the hypothalamus of SHRs is reduced to that evoked in the normotensive animal after ventricular administration of GABA (146). In addition, microinjection of a GABA agonist into the posterior hypothalamus of the SHR produces a much larger fall in arterial pressure in the hypertensive than in the normotensive rat (183). Additional support for decreased GABAergic activity in the caudal hypothalamus of the hypertensive rat was provided recently by Shonis et al. (156). They found that microinjection of an inhibitor of GABA synthesis into the posterior hypothalamus of two different strains of normotensive rats produced a rise in arterial pressure and heart rate. In contrast, microinjection of the synthesis inhibitor into the adult SHR had no effect on heart rate or arterial pressure. It was concluded that the SHR has a deficiency in the GABAergic input onto the caudal hypothalamus. Thus, loss of this inhibition onto a known pressor area permits a rise in arterial pressure.

Additional support for the above hypothesis suggesting a loss of inhibitory input onto caudal hypothalamic neurons has been provided by studies that have shown that caudal hypothalamic neurons in the hypertensive rat have an elevated activity. Krukoff and Weigel used hexokinase histochemistry to compare the metabolic activity of various brain regions of both hypertensive and normotensive rats (97). They reported that the caudal hypothalamus of the SHR had a significantly larger amount of labeling than that of the normotensive rat, indicating an elevated metabolic rate. Thus, they concluded this elevated activity plays a role in the etiology of hypertension. Recent electrophysiological studies by Shonis and Waldrop have shown that neurons in the hypothalamus of the SHR have both an elevated discharge rate and altered discharge pattern compared to those in normotensive controls (155). In addition, it was shown that this alteration in neuronal activity was present in a brain slice preparation (155). Therefore, the elevated neuronal activity observed in the SHR hypothalamus cannot be due to input from other brain sites or from peripheral feedback.

IV. Summary

Sites in both the rostral and caudal hypothalamus play an important role in cardiovascular and respiratory modulation. In fact, almost all aspects of the tonic and reflex regulation are affected by neurons in the hypothalamus. The importance of the hypothalamus is not lessened by the fact that cardiovascular and respiratory reflexes persist in the absence of an intact hypothalamus. Modulation and fine tuning of cardiorespiratory control by the hypothalamus is necessary for meeting the demands of an organism in an ever-changing environment. The hypothalamus provides strong input onto medullary neurons that are ultimately responsible for neural outflow to the cardiovascular and respiratory systems. Thus, the medullary outflow to sympathetic preganglionic neurons in the intermediolateral columns of the spinal cord and to respiratory motoneurons is strongly influenced by descending input from sites in the hypothalamus. Disruption of this hypothalamic influence may well explain several autonomic disorders, including hypertension.

Even though the hypothalamus is known to be involved in numerous reflexes, almost no one has evaluated the overlap of function that may exist in various hypothalamic sites. Evidence has been offered that the baroreceptor reflex, peripheral chemoreceptor reflex, and exercise are all modulated by areas in the hypothalamus. Experiments need to be conducted to determine whether individual neurons are segregated according to these different reflexes. A likely possibility is that an individual neuron in the hypothalamus may be involved in a number of different aspects of cardiorespiratory regulation. Integration of cardiorespiratory activity along with other functions, including temperature regulation and behavior, may be the most important role of the hypothalamus. Future experiments may reveal that the hypothalamus serves as an integrative center necessary for the coordination of all body functions such that an animal can survive and function in a normal physiological manner.

Acknowledgments

The research from the authors' laboratories was supported by funds from the National Institutes of Health and the American Heart Association. TGW was an Established Investigator of the American Heart Association during these studies.

References

1. Abrahams VC, Hilton SM, Zbrozyna A. Active muscle vasodilation produced by stimulation of the brain stem: its significance in the defence reaction. J Physiol 1960; 154:491–513.
2. Ambühl P, Felix D, Imboden H, Khosla MC, Ferrario CM. Effects of angiotensin analogues and angiotensin receptor antagonists on paraventricular neurones. Reg Pept 1992; 38:111–120.
3. Baev KV, Berezovskii VK, Kebkalo TT, Savos'kina LA. Projections of neurons of the hypothalamic locomotor region to some brainstem and spinal cord structures in the cat. Neurophysiology (English translation) 1985; 17:595–600.
4. Baev KV, Berezovskii VK, Kebkalo TT, Savos'kina LA. Forebrain projections to the hypothalamic locomotor region in cats. J Neurophysiol (English translation) 1985; 17:183–189.
5. Bandler R. Induction of "rage" following microinjections of glutamate into midbrain but not hypothalamus of cats. Neurosci Lett 1982; 30:183–188.
6. Banks D, Harris MC. Activation of hypothalamic arcuate but not paraventricular neurons following carotid body chemoreceptor stimulation in the rat. Neuroscience 1988; 24:967–976.
7. Barman SM. Descending projections of hypothalamic neurons with sympathetic nerve-related activity. J Neurophysiol 1990; 64:1019–1032.
8. Barman SM, Gebber GL. Hypothalamic neurons with activity patterns related to sympathetic nerve discharge. Am J Physiol 1982; 242:R34–R43.
9. Bauer RM, Waldrop TG. Excitation of posterior hypothalamic neurons by hypercapnia in a rat brain slice preparation. FASEB J 1990; 4:A406.
10. Bauer RM, Vela MB, Simon T, Waldrop TG. A GABAergic mechanism in the posterior hypothalamus modulates baroreflex bradycardia. Brain Res Bull 1988; 20: 633–641.

11. Bayliss DA, Millhorn DE. Chronic estrogen exposure maintains elevated levels of progesterone receptor mRNA in guinea pig hypothalamus. Mol Brain Res 1991; 10:167–172.

12. Bayliss DA, Millhorn DE. Central neural mechanisms of progesterone action: application to the respiratory system. J Appl Physiol 1992; 73:393–404.

13. Benetos A, Gavras I, Gavras H. Norepinephrine applied in the paraventricular hypothalamic nucleus stimulates vasopressin release. Brain Res 1986; 381: 322–326.

14. Berezovskii VK, Kebkalo TG, Savos'kina LA. Afferent brainstem projections to the hypothalamic locomotor region of the cat brain. J Neurophysiol 1984; 16:279–286.

15. Bolme P, Ngai SH, Uvnas B, Wallenberg LR. Circulatory and behavioral effects on electrical stimulation of the sympathetic vasodilator areas in the hypothalamus and the mesencephalon in unanesthetized dogs. Acta Physiol Scand 1967; 70:334–346.

16. Bonora M, Gautier H. Influence of dopamine and norepinephrine on the central ventilatory response to hypoxia in conscious cats. Respir Physiol 1988; 71:11–24.

17. Brezenoff HE. Cardiovascular responses to intrahypothalamic injections of carbachol and certain cholinesterase inhibitors. Neuropharmacology 1972; 11: 637–644.

18. Bunag RD, Eferakeya AE, Langdon DS. Enhancement of hypothalamic pressor responses in spontaneously hypertensive rats. Am J Physiol 1975; 228:217–222.

19. Calaresu FR, Ciriello J. Projections to the hypothalamus from buffer nerves and nucleus tractus solitarius in the cat. Am J Physiol 1980; 239:R130–R136.

20. Callahan MF, Kirby RF, Cunningham JT, Eskridge-Sloop SL, Johnson AK, McCarty R, Gruber KA. Central oxytocin systems may mediate a cardiovascular response to acute stress in rats. Am J Physiol 1989; 256:H1369–H1377.

21. Cechetto DF, Saper CB. Neurochemical organization of the hypothalamic projection to the spinal cord in the rat. J Comp Neurol 1988; 272:579–604.

22. Ciriello J, Calaresu FR. Descending hypothalamic pathways with cardiovascular function in the cat: a silver impregnation study. Exp Neurol 1977; 57:561–580.

23. Ciriello J, Calaresu FR. Role of paraventricular and supraoptic nuclei in central cardiovascular regulation in the cat. Am J Physiol 1980; 239:137–R142.

24. Ciriello J, Caverson MM. Ventrolateral medullary neurons relay cardiovascular inputs to the paraventricular nucleus. Am J Physiol 1984; 246:R968–R978.

25. Ciriello J, Kline RL, Zhang T-X, Caverson MM. Lesions of the paraventricular nucleus alter the development of spontaneous hypertension in the rat. Brain Res 1984; 310:355–359.

26. Ciriello J, Rohlidcek CV, Polosa C. Aortic baroreceptor reflex pathway: a functional mapping using [^{3}H]2-deoxyglucose autoradiography in the rat. J Auton Nerv Sys 1983; 8:111–128.

27. Clarke NP, Rushmer RF. Tissue uptake of ^{86}Rb with electrical stimulation of hypothalamus and midbrain. Am J Physiol 1967; 213:1439–1444.

28. Clarke NP, Smith OA, Shearn DW. Topographical representation of vascular smooth muscle of limbs in primate motor cortex. Am J Physiol 1968; 214:122–129.

29. Clasca F, Llamas A, Reinoso-Suarez F. Hypothalamic connections of the insular cortex in the cat. Brain Res 1989; 490:361–366.

30. Coote JH, Hilton SM, Perez-Gonzalez JF. Inhibition of the baroreceptor reflex on stimulation in the brain stem defence centre. J Physiol 1979; 288:549–560.

31. Cross BA, Silver IA. Unit activity in the hypothalamus and the sympathetic response to hypoxia and hypercapnia. Exp Neurol 1963; 7:375–393.

32. Czyzewska-Szafran H, Wutkiewicz M, Remiszewska M, Jastrazebski Z, Czarnecki A, Danysz A. Down-regulation of the GABAergic system in selected brain areas of spontaneously hypertensive rats (SHR). Pol J Pharmacol Pharm 1988; 41:619–627.

33. Daristotle L, Engwall MJ, Niu W, Bisgard GE. Ventilatory effects and interactions with change in Pao$_2$ in awake goats. J Appl Physiol 1991; 71:1254–1260.

34. Darlington DN, Shinsako J, Dallman MF. Paraventricular lesions: hormonal and cardiovascular responses to hemorrhage. Brain Res 1988; 439:289–301.

35. Dean C, Coote JH. Discharge patterns in postganglionic neurones to skeletal muscle and kidney during activation of the hypothalamic and midbrain defence areas in the cat. Brain Res 1986; 377:271–278.

36. Dean JB, Lawling WL, Millhorn DE. CO$_2$ decreases membrane conductance and depolarizes neurons in the nucleus tractus solitarii. Exp Brain Res 1989; 76: 656–661.

37. Dillon GH, Shonis CA, Waldrop TG. Hypothalamic GABAergic modulation of respiratory responses to baroreceptor stimulation. Respir Physiol 1991; 85: 289–304.

38. Dillon GH, Waldrop TG. In vitro responses of caudal hypothalamic neurons to hypoxia and hypercapnia. Neuroscience 1992; 51:941–950.

39. Dillon GH, Waldrop TG. Responses of feline caudal hypothalamic cardiorespiratory neurons to hypoxia and hypercapnia. Exp Brain Res 1993; 96:260–272.

40. DiMicco JA, Abshire VM, Hankins KD, Sample RHB, Wible JH. Microinjection of GABA antagonists into posterior hypothalamus elevates heart rate in anesthetized rats. Neuropharmacology 1986; 25:1063–1066.

41. Djojosugito AM, Folkow B, Kylstra PH, Lisander B, Tuttle RS. Differentiated interaction between the hypothalamic defence reaction and baroreceptor reflexes. I. Effects on heart rate and regional flow resistance. Acta Physiol Scand 1970; 78: 376–385.

42. Downing SE, Mitchell JH, Wallace AG. Cardiovascular responses to ischemia, hypoxia and hypercapnia of the central nervous system. Am J Physiol 1963; 204: 881–887.

43. Eilam R, Malach R, Bergmann F, Segal M. Hypertension induced by hypothalamic transplantation from genetically hypertensive to normotensive rats. J Neurosci 1991; 11:401–411.

44. Eldridge FL, Millhorn DE, Kiley JP, Waldrop TG. Stimulation by central command of locomotion, respiration and circulation during exercise. Respir Physiol 1985; 59:313–337.

45. Eldridge FL, Millhorn DE, Waldrop TG. Exercise hyperpnea and locomotion: Parallel activation from the hypothalamus. Science 1981; 211:844–846.

46. Eldridge FL, Waldrop TG. Neural control of breathing during exercise. In: Whipp B, Wasserman K, eds. Exercise: Pulmonary Physiology and Pathophysiology. New York: Marcel Dekker, 1991:309–360.

47. Eliasson S, Folkow B, Lindgren P, Uvnas B. Activation of sympathetic vasodilator nerves to the skeletal muscles in the cat by hypothalamic stimulation. Acta Physiol Scand 1951; 23:333–351.

48. Eliasson S, Lindgren P, Uvnas B. Representation in the hypothalamus and the motor cortex in the dog of the sympathetic vasodilator outflow to the skeletal muscles. Acta Physiol Scand 1952; 27:18–27.

49. Farber JP, Connors AF, Gisolfi CV, McCaffree DR, Smith RM. Effects on breathing of putative neurotransmitters in the rostral hypothalamus of the rat. Brain Res Bull 1981; 6:13–17.

50. Fink BR, Katz R, Reinhold H, Schoolman A. Suprapontine mechanisms in regulation of respiration. Am J Physiol 1962; 202:217–220.

51. Forsyth RP. Hypothalamic control of the distribution of cardiac output in the unanesthetized Rhesus monkey. Circ Res 1970; 26:783–794.

52. Frazier DT, Tzauini C, Boyarsky LL, Wilson MF. Hypothalamic unit responses to increases in arterial blood pressure. Proc Soc Exp Biol Med 1965; 120:450–454.

53. Gauthier P, Reis DJ, Nathan MA. Arterial hypertension elicited either by lesions or by electrical stimulation of the rostral hypothalamus in the rat. Brain Res 1981; 211:91–105.

54. Gebber GL, Synder DW. Hypothalamic control of baroreceptor reflexes. Am J Physiol 1969; 218:214–231.

55. Gellhorn E, Nakao H, Redgate ES. The influence of lesions in the anterior and posterior hypothalamus on tonic and phasic autonomic reactions. J Physiol 1956; 131:402–423.

56. Gelsema AJ, Roe MJ, Calaresu FR. Neurally mediated cardiovascular responses to stimulation of cell bodies in the hypothalamus of the rat. Brain Res 1989; 482: 67–77.

57. Goodchild AK, Dampney RAL, Bandler R. A method for evoking physiological responses by stimulation of cell bodies but not axons of passage within a localized region of the central nervous system. J Neurosci Meth 1982; 6:351–363.

58. Goto A, Ikeda T, Tobian L, Iwai J, Johnson MA. Brain lesions in the paraventricular nuclei and catecholaminergic neurons minimize salt hypertension in Dahl salt-sensitive rats. Clin Sci (Lond) 1981; 61:53S–55S.

59. Gotoh E, Murakami K, Bahnson TD, Ganong WF. Role of brain serotonergic pathways and hypothalamus in regulation of renin secretion. Am J Physiol 1987; 253: R179–R185.

60. Grossman RG. Effects of stimulation of non-specific thalamic system on locomotor movements in cat. J Neurophysiol 1958; 21:85–93.

61. Hajduczok G, Hade JS, Mark AL, Williams JL, Felder RB. Central command increases sympathetic nerve activity during spontaneous locomotion in cats. Circ Res 1991; 69:66–75.

62. Hambley JW, Johnston GAR, Shaw J. Alterations in a hypothalamic GABA system in the spontaneously hypertensive rat. Neurochem Int 1984; 6:813–822.

63. Hayashi F, Sinclair JD. Respiratory patterns in anesthetized rats before and after anemic decerebration. Respir Physiol 1991; 84:61–76.

64. Herzig TC, Buchholz RA, Haywood JR. Effects of paraventricular nucleus lesions on chronic renal hypertension. Am J Physiol 1991; 261:H860–H867.

65. Hilton SM. The defence-arousal system and its relevance for circulatory and respiratory control. J Exp Biol 1982; 100:159–174.

66. Hilton SM. Inhibition of baroreceptor reflexes on hypothalamic stimulation. J Physiol 1963; 165:56P–57P.

67. Hilton SM, Joels N. Facilitation of chemoreceptor reflexes during defence reaction. J Physiol 1964; 176:20P–22P.

68. Hilton SM, Marshall JM, Timms RJ. Ventral medullary relay neurones in the pathway from the defence areas of the cat and their effect on blood pressure. J Physiol 1983; 345:149–166.

69. Hilton SM, Redfern WS. A search for brain stem cell group integrating the defence reaction in the rat. J Physiol 1986; 378:213–228.

70. Hilton SM, Smith PR. Ventral medullary neurones excited from the hypothalamic and mid-brain defence areas. J Auton Nerv Sys 1984; 11:35–42.

71. Hilton SM, Spyer KM, Timms RJ. The origin of the hind limb vasodilatation evoked by stimulation of the motor cortex in the cat. J Physiol 1979; 287:545–557.

72. Hobbs SF. Central command during exercise: parallel activation of the cardiovascular and motor systems by descending command signals. In: Smith OA, Galosy RA, Weiss SM, eds. Circulation, Neurobiology and Behavior. Amsterdam: Elsevier, 1982:217–231.

73. Holstege G. Some anatomical observations on the projections from the hypothalamus to brainstem and spinal cord: an HRP and autoradiographic tracing study in the cat. J Comp Neurol 1987; 260:98–126.

74. Horeyseck G, Janig W, Kirchner F, Thamer V. Activation and inhibition of muscle and cutaneous postganglionic neurones to hindlimb during hypothalamically induced vasoconstriction and atropine-sensitive vasodilation. Pflügers Arch 1976; 361:231–240.

75. Horn EM, Waldrop TG. Modulation of the respiratory responses to hypoxia and hypercapnia by synaptic input onto caudal hypothalamic neurons. Soc Neurosci Abstr 1992; 18:827.

76. Hosoya Y, Sugiura Y, Okado N, Loewy AD, Kohno K. Descending input from the hypothalamic paraventricular nucleus to sympathetic preganglionic neurons in the rat. Exp Brain Res 1991; 85:10–20.

77. Huang Z-S, Gebber GL, Barman SM, Varner KJ. Forebrain contribution to sympathetic nerve discharge in anesthetized cats. Am J Physiol 1987; 252:R645–R652.

78. Huang Z-S, Varner KJ, Barman SM, Gebber GL. Diencephalic regions contributing to sympathetic nerve discharge in anesthetized cats. Am J Physiol 1988; 254:R249–R256.

79. Humphreys PW, Joels N, McAllen RM. Modification of the reflex response to stimulation of carotid sinus baroreceptors during and following stimulation of the hypothalamic defence area in the cat. J Physiol 1971; 216:461–482.

80. Itoi K, Jost N, Badoer E, Tschöpe C, Culman J, Unger T. Localization of substance

P-induced cardiovascular responses in the rat hypothalamus. Brain Res 1991; 558: 123–126.

81. Jensen LL, Harding JW, Wright JW. Role of paraventricular nucleus in control of blood pressure and drinking in rats. Am J Physiol 1992; 262:F1068–F1075.

82. Jin C, Rockhold RW. Effects of paraventricular hypothalamic microinfusions of kainic acid on cardiovascular and renal excretory function in conscious rats. J Pharmacol Exp Ther 1989; 251:969–975.

83. Jin C, Rockhold RW. Sympathoadrenal control by paraventricular hypothalamic β-endorphin in hypertension. Hypertension 1991; 18:503–515.

84. Jordan D, Mifflin SW, Spyer KM. Hypothalamic inhibition of neurones in the nucleus tractus solitarius of the cat is GABA mediated. J Physiol 1988; 399:389–404.

85. Juskevich JC, Robinson DS, Whitehorn D. Effect of hypothalamic stimulation in spontaneously hypertensive and Wistar-Kyoto rats. Eur J Pharm 1978; 51:429–439.

86. Kabat H. Electrical stimulation of points in the forebrain and midbrain: the resultant alterations in respiration. J Comp Neurol 1936; 64:187–208.

87. Kabat H, Magoun HW, Ranson SW. Electrical stimulation of points in the forebrain and midbrain: the resultant alterations in blood pressure. Arch Neurol Psych 1935; 34:931–955.

88. Kannan H, Yamashita H. Electrophysiological study of paraventricular nucleus neurons projecting to the dorsomedial medulla and their response to baroreceptor stimulation in rats. Brain Res 1983; 279:31–40.

89. Kannan H, Hayashida Y, Yamashita H. Increase in sympathetic outflow by paraventricular nucleus stimulation in awake rats. Am J Physiol 1989; 256:R1325–R1330.

90. Kannan H, Niijima A, Yamashita H. Inhibition of renal sympathetic nerve activity by electrical stimulation of the hypothalamic paraventricular nucleus in anesthetized rats. J Auton Nerv Sys 1987; 21:83–86.

91. Kannan H, Osaka T, Kasai M, Okuya S, Yamashita H. Electrophysiological properties of neurons in the caudal ventrolateral medulla projecting to the paraventricular nucleus of the hypothalamus in rats. Brain Res 1986; 376:342–350.

92. Karplus JP, Kreidl A. Zwischenhirnbasis und halssympathicus. Pflügers Arch 1909; 129:138–144.

93. Katafuchi T, Oomura Y, Kurosawa M. Effects of chemical stimulation of paraventricular nucleus on adrenal and renal nerve activity in rats. Neurosci Lett 1988; 86:195–200.

94. Kiritsy-Roy JA, Appel NM, Bobbitt FG, Van Loon GR. Effects of Mu-opioid receptor stimulation in the hypothalamic paraventricular nucleus on basal and stress-induced catecholamine secretion and cardiovascular responses. J Pharmacol Exp Ther 1986; 239:814–822.

95. Kiss JZ, Cassell MD, Palkovits M. Analysis of the ACTH/β-end/-MSH-immunoreactive afferent input to the hypothalamic paraventricular nucleus of rat. Brain Res 1984; 324:91–99.

96. Kooy D van der, Koda LY, McGinty JF, Gerfen CR, Bloom FE. The organization of projections from the cortex, amygdala, hypothalamus to the nucleus of the solitary tract in the rat. J Comp Neurol 1984; 224:1–24.

97. Krukoff TL, Weigel MA. Metabolic alterations in discrete regions of the rat brain during development of spontaneous hypertension. Brain Res 1989; 499:1–6.

98. Li P, Lovick TA. Excitatory projections from hypothalamic and midbrain defense regions to nucleus paragigantocellularis lateralis in the rat. Exp Neurol 1985; 89:543–553.

99. Lind RW, Swanson LW, Bruhn T, Ganten D. The distribution of angiotensin II–immunoreactive cells and fibers in the paraventriculo-hypophysial system of the rat. Brain Res 1985; 338:81–89.

100. Lipski J, Bellingham MC, West MJ, Pilowsky P. Limitations of the technique of pressure microinjection of excitatory amino acids for evoking responses from localized regions of the CNS. J Neurosci Meth 1988; 26:169–179.

101. Loewy AD. Forebrain nuclei involved in autonomic control. Prog Brain Res 1991; 87:253–268.

102. Lovick TA. Projections from the diencephalon and mesencephalon to nucleus paragigantocellularis lateralis in the cat. Neuroscience 14:853–861, 1985.

103. Luiten PGM, Horst GJ ter, Karst H, Steffens B. The course of paraventricular hypothalamic efferent to autonomic structures in the medulla and spinal cord. Brain Res 1985; 329:374–378.

104. Mancia G, Zanchetti A. Hypothalamic control of autonomic functions. In: Morgane PJ, Panksepp J, eds. Handbook of the Hypothalamus, Vol 3, part B: Behavioral Studies of the Hypothalamus. New York: Marcel Dekker, 1981:147–202.

105. Markgraf CG, Winters RW, Liskowsky DR, McCabe PM, Green EJ, Schneiderman N. Hypothalamic, midbrain and bulbar areas involved in the defense reaction in rabbits. Physiol Behav 1991; 49:493–500.

106. Marshall JM, Timms RJ. Experiments on the role of the subthalamus in the generation of the cardiovascular changes during locomotion in the cat. J Physiol 1980; 301:92P–93P.

107. Martin DS, Haywood JR. Sympathetic nervous system activation by glutamate injections into the paraventricular nucleus. Brain Res 1992; 577:261–267.

108. Martin JR, Beinfeld M, Westfall TC. Blood pressure increases after injection of neuropeptide Y into posterior hypothalamic nucleus. Am J Physiol 1988; 254: H879–H888.

109. May CN, Dashwood MR, Whitehead CJ, Mathias CJ. Differential cardiovascular and respiratory responses to central administration of selective opioid agonists in conscious rabbits: correlation with receptor distribution. Br J Pharmacol 1989; 98:903–913.

110. Mel'nikova ZL. Connections of the subthalamic and mesencephalic "locomotor regions" in rats. Neurophysiology (English translation) 1977; 9:214–218.

111. Mifflin SW, Spyer KM, Withington-Wray DJ. Baroreceptor inputs to the nucleus tractus solitarius in the cat: modulation by the hypothalamus. J Physiol 1988; 399: 369–387.

112. Miller MJ, Tenney SM. Hypoxia-induced tachypnea in carotid-deafferented cats. Respir Physiol 1975; 23:31–39.

113. Millhorn DE, Eldridge FL, Waldrop TG, Kiley JP. Diencephalic regulation of

respiration and arterial pressure during actual and fictive locomotion in cat. Circ Res 1987; 61(Suppl I):I53–I59.

114. Mitchell JH. Cardiovascular control during exercise: central and reflex neural mechanisms. Am J Cardiol 1985; 55:34D–41D.

115. Nathan MA, Reis DJ. Fulminating arterial hypertension with pulmonary edema from release of adrenomedullary catecholamines after lesions of the anterior hypothalamus in the rat. Circ Res 1975; 37:226–235.

116. Neubauer JA, Gonsalves SF, Chou W, Geller HM, Edelman NH. Chemosensitivity of medullary neurons in explant tissue cultures. Neuroscience 1991; 45:701–708.

117. Nielsen AM, Bisgard GE, Mitchell GS. Phrenic nerve responses to hypoxia and CO_2 in dogs. Respir Physiol 1986; 65:267–283.

118. Nolan PC, Waldrop TG. In vivo and in vitro responses of neurons in the ventrolateral medulla to hypoxia. Brain Res 1993; 630:101–114.

119. Ohta M, Nakamura S, Watanabe S, Ueki S. Effect of L-glutamate, injected into the posterior hypothalamus, on blood pressure and heart rate in unanesthetized and unrestrained rats. Neuropharmacology 1985; 24:445–451.

120. Okamoto K. Spontaneous hypertension in rats. Int Rev Exp Pathol 1969; 7: 227–270.

121. Onai T, Takayama K, Miura M. Projections to areas of the nucleus tractus solitarii related to circulatory and respiratory responses in cats. J Auton Nerv Sys 1987; 18: 163–175.

122. Ordway GA, Waldrop TG, Iwamoto GA, Gentile BJ. Hypothalamic influences on cardiovascular response of beagles to dynamic exercise. Am J Physiol 1989; 257: H1247–H1253.

123. Orlovskii GN. Connexions of the reticulo-spinal neurones with the "locomotor sections" of the brain stem. Biophysics (English translation) 1970; 15:171–177.

124. Orlovskii GN. Spontaneous and induced locomotion of the thalamic cat. Biophysics (USSR—English translation) 1969; 14:1154–1162.

125. Pare D, Smith Y, Parent A, Steriade M. Neuronal activity of identified posterior hypothalamic neurons projecting to the brainstem peribrachial area of the cat. Neurosci Lett 1989; 107:145–150.

126. Patel KP, Schmid PG. Role of paraventricular nucleus (PVH) in baroreflex-mediated changes in lumbar sympathetic nerve activity and heart rate. J Auton Nerv Sys 1988; 22:211–219.

127. Peano CA, Shonis CA, Dillon GH, Waldrop TG. Hypothalamic GABAergic mechanism involved in the respiratory response to hypercapnia. Brain Res Bull 1992; 28:107–113.

128. Pfeiffer A, Feuerstein G, Zerbe RL, Faden AI, Kopin IJ. μ-Receptors mediated opioid cardiovascular effects at anterior hypothalamic sites through sympatho-adrenomedullary and parasympathetic pathways. Endocrinology 1983; 113:929–938.

129. Porter JP, Brody MJ. Neural projections from paraventricular nucleus that subserve vasomotor functions. Am J Physiol 1985; 248:R271–R281.

130. Porter JP, Brody MJ. A comparison of the hemodynamic effects produced by electrical stimulation of subnuclei of the paraventricular nucleus. Brain Res 1986; 375:20–29.

131. Porter JP, Bonham AC, Mangiapane ML, Webb RL, Brody MJ. The cardiovascular effects of centrally and peripherally administered indoramin in conscious rats. Eur J Pharmacol 1985; 109:9–17.

132. Porter JP. Electrical stimulation of the paraventricular nucleus increases plasma renin activity. Am J Physiol 1988; 254:R325–R330.

133. Rabkin SW. Cardiorespiratory effects of D-ala-2-me-phe-4-met-(o)-ol enkephalin in the third ventricle, and in anterior hypothalamic and paraventricular areas of the rat brain. Cardiovasc Res 1989; 23:904–912.

134. Redgate ES. Hypothalamic influence on respiration. Ann NY Acad Sci 1963; 109: 606–618.

135. Redgate ES, Gellhorn E. Respiratory activity and the hypothalamus. Am J Physiol 1958; 193:189–194.

136. Ricardo JA, Koh ET. Anatomical evidence of direct projections from the nucleus of the solitary tract to the hypothalamus, amygdala, and other forebrain structures in the rat. Brain Res 1978; 153:1–26.

137. Richardson Morton KD, Van de Kar LD, Brownfield MS, Bethea CL. Neuronal cell bodies in the hypothalamic paraventricular nucleus mediate stress-induced renin and corticosterone secretion. Neuroendocrinology 1989; 50;73–80.

138. Rockhold RW, Acuff CG, Clower BW. Excitotoxic lesions of the paraventricular hypothalamus: metabolic and cardiac effects. Neuropharmacology 1990; 29: 663–673.

139. Rockhold RW, Jin C, Huang H-M, Farley JM. Acute tachycardia and pressor effects following injections of kainic acid into the antero-dorsal medial hypothalamus. Neuropharmacology 1987; 26:567–573.

140. Romaniuk JR, Kasicki S, Borecka U. The Breuer-Hering reflex at rest and during electrically induced locomotion in decerebrate cat. Acta Neurobiol Exp 1986; 46: 141–151.

141. Rosen A. Augmented cardiac contraction, heart acceleration and skeletal muscle vasodilatation produced by hypothalamic stimulation in cats. Acta Physiol Scand 1961; 52:291–308.

142. Rushmer RF. Structure and Function of the Cardiovascular System. Philadelphia: Saunders, 1972:94–97, 142–144, 220–243.

143. Ryan J, Waldrop TG. Descending projections to the periaqueductal gray from caudal hypothalamic neurons that are stimulated by hypoxia or hypercapnia. Soc Neurosci Abstr 1993; 19:319.

144. Rybicki KJ, Stremel RW, Iwamoto GA, Mitchell JH, Kaufman MP. Occlusion of pressor responses to posterior diencephalic stimulation and muscular contraction. Brain Res Bull 1989; 22:305–312.

145. Saper CB, Loewy AD, Swanson LW, Cowan WM. Direct hypothalamo-autonomic connections. Brain Res 1976; 117:305–312.

146. Sasaki S, Lee L, Iyota I, Kambara S, Okajima H, Inou A, Takahashi H, Takeda K, Youshimura M, Nakagawa M, Ijichi H. Central GABA-ergic stimulation attenuates hypertension and hypothalamic hyperactivity in spontaneously hypertensive rats. J Hyperten 1986; 4:S171–S174.

147. Sawchenko PD, Swanson LW. Immunohistochemical identification of neurons in the

paraventricular nucleus of the hypothalamus that project to the medulla or to the spinal cord in the rat. J Comp Neurol 1982; 205:250–272.

148. Sawchenko PE, Swanson LW. The organization of noradrenergic pathways from the brainstem to the paraventricular and supraoptic nuclei in the rat. Brain Res Rev 1982; 4:275–325.

149. Schramm LP, Bignall KE. Central neural pathways mediating active sympathetic muscle vasodilation in cats. Am J Physiol 1971; 221:754–767.

150. Schwanzel-Fukuda M, Morrell JI, Pfaff DW. Localization of forebrain neurons which project directly to the medulla and spinal cord of the rat by retrograde tracing with wheat germ agglutinin. J Comp Neurol 1984; 226:1–20.

151. Segundo JP, Arana R, Migliaro E, Villar JE, Garcia-Guelfi A, Garcia Austt E. Respiratory responses from fornix and wall of third ventricle in man. J Neurophysiol 1955; 18:96–101.

152. Segura T, Martin DS, Sheridan PJ, Haywood JR. Measurement of the distribution of [^{3}H]bicuculline microinjected into the rat hypothalamus. J Neurosci Meth 1992; 41:175–186.

153. Shik ML, Severin FV, Orlovskii GN. Control of walking and running by means of electrical stimulation of the midbrain. Biofizika 1966; 11:659–666.

154. Shoji M, Share L, Crofton JT. Effect on vasopressin release of microinjection of angiotensin II into the paraventricular nucleus of conscious rats. Neuroendocrinology 1989; 50:327–333.

155. Shonis CA, Waldrop TG. Augmented neuronal activity in the hypothalamus of the spontaneously hypertensive rats. Brain Res Bull 1993; 30:45–52.

156. Shonis CA, Peano CA, Dillon GH, Waldrop TG. Cardiovascular responses to blockade of GABA synthesis in the hypothalamus of the spontaneously hypertensive rat. Brain Res Bull 1993; 31:493–499.

157. Smith OA, Rushmer RE, Lasher EP. Similarity of cardiovascular responses to exercise and to diencephalic stimulation. Am J Physiol 1960; 198:1139–1142.

158. Sofroniew MV, Schrell U. Hypothalamic neurons projecting to the rat caudal medulla oblongata, examined by immunoperoxidase staining of retrogradely transported horseradish peroxidase. Neurosci Lett 1980; 19:257–263.

159. Soltis RP, DiMicco JP. GABA$_A$ and excitatory amino acid receptors in dorsomedial hypothalamus and heart rate in rats. Am J Physiol 1991; 260:R13–R20.

160. Spencer SE, Sawyer WB, Loewy AD. L-Glutamate mapping of cardioreactive areas in the rat posterior hypothalamus. Brain Res 1990; 511:149–157.

161. Stadler T, Veltmar A, Qadri F, Unger T. Angiotensin II evokes noradrenaline release from the paraventricular nucleus in conscious rats. Brain Res 1992; 569:117–122.

162. Strack AM, Sawyer WB, Hughes JH, Platt KB, Loewy AD. A general pattern of CNS innervation of the sympathetic outflow demonstrated by transneuronal pseudorabies viral infections. Brain Res 1989; 491:156–162.

163. Swanson LW, Kuypers HGJM. The paraventricular nucleus of the hypothalamus: cytoarchitectonic subdivisions and organization of projections to the pituitary, dorsal vagal complex, and spinal cord as demonstrated by retrograde fluorescence double-labeling methods. J Comp Neurol 1980; 194:555–570.

164. Takeda K, Nakata T, Takesako T, Itoh H, Hirata M, Kawasaki S, Hayashi J, Oguro

M, Sasaki S, Nakagawa M. Sympathetic inhibition and attenuation of spontaneous hypertension by PVN lesions in rats. Brain Res 1991; 543:296–300.

165. Tan E, Dampney RAL. Cardiovascular effects of stimulation of neurones within the "defence area" of the hypothalamus and midbrain of rabbits. Clin Exp Pharm Physiol 1983; 10:299–303.

166. Tenney SM, Ou LC. Ventilatory response of decorticate and decerebrate cats to hypoxia and CO_2. Respir Physiol 1977; 29:81–92.

167. Thomas MR, Calaresu FR. Responses of single units in the medial hypothalamus to electrical stimulation of the carotid sinus nerve in the cat. Brain Res 1972; 44: 49–62.

168. Thomas MR, Calaresu FR. Hypothalamic inhibition of chemoreceptor-induced bradycardia in the cat. Am J Physiol 1973; 225:201–208.

169. Tsushima H, Mori M, Matsuda T. Effects of fentanyl, injected into the hypothalamic supraoptic and paraventricular nuclei, in a water-loaded and ethanol-anesthetized rat. Neuropharmacology 1990; 29:757–763.

170. Unger Th, Becker H, Petty M, Demmert G, Schneider B, Ganten D, Lang RE. Differential effects of central angiotensin II and substance P on sympathetic nerve activity in conscious rats. Circ Res 1985; 56:563–575.

171. Varner KJ, Barman SM, Gebber GL. Cat diencephalic neurons with sympathetic nerve-related activity. Am J Physiol 1988; 254:R257–R267.

172. Waldrop TG. Respiratory responses and adaptations to exercise. In: Scientific Foundations of Sports Medicine. Teitz CC, ed. Philadelphia: BC Decker, 1989:59–76.

173. Waldrop TG. Posterior hypothalamic modulation of the respiratory response to CO_2 in cats. Pflügers Arch 1991; 418:7–13.

174. Waldrop TG, Bauer RM. Modulation of sympathetic discharge by a hypothalamic GABAergic mechanism. Neuropharmacology 1989; 28:263–269.

175. Waldrop TG, Bauer RM, Iwamoto GA. Microinjection of GABA antagonists into the posterior hypothalamus elicits locomotor activity and a cardiorespiratory activation. Brain Res 1988; 444:84–94.

176. Waldrop TG, Bauer RM, Iwamoto GA, Stremel RW. Hypothalamic modulation of cardiovascular, respiratory and locomotor activity. In: Koepchen HP, Huopaniemi T, eds. Cardiorespiratory and Motor Coordination. Berlin: Springer, 1991:208–214.

177. Waldrop TG, Henderson MC, Iwamoto GA, Mitchell JH. Regional blood flow responses to stimulation of the subthalamic locomotor region. Respir Physiol 1986; 64:93–102.

178. Waldrop TG, Mullins DC, Henderson MC. Effects of hypothalamic lesions on the cardiorespiratory responses to muscular contraction. Respir Physiol 1986; 66: 215–224.

179. Waldrop TG, Mullins DC, Millhorn DE. Control of respiration by the hypothalamus and by feedback from contracting muscles in cats. Respir Physiol 1986; 64: 317–328.

180. Waldrop TG, Stremel RW. Muscular contraction stimulates posterior hypothalamic neurons. Am J Physiol 1989; 256:R348–R356

181. Waller WH. Progression movements elicited by subthalamic stimulation. J Neurophysiol 1940; 3:300–307.

182. Wang SC, Ranson SW. Descending pathways from the hypothalamus to the medulla and spinal cord. Observations on blood pressure and bladder responses. J Comp Neurol 1939; 71:457–472.

183. Wible JH, DiMicco JA, Luft FC. Hypothalamic GABA and sympathetic regulation in spontaneously hypertensive rats. Hypertension 1989; 14:623–628.

184. Wible JH, Luft FC, Dimicco JA. Hypothalamic GABA suppresses sympathetic outflow to the cardiovascular system. Am J Physiol 1988; 254:R680–R687.

185. Winters RW, McCabe PM, Green EJ, Duan Y-F, Schneiderman N. Electrophysiological evidence for hypothalamic defense area input to cells in the lateral tegmental field of the medulla of rabbits. Brain Res 1991; 558:171–175.

186. Woulfe JM, Flumerfelt BA, Hrycyshyn AW. Efferent connections of the A1 noradrenergic cell group: a DBH immunohistochemical and PHA-L anterograde tracing study. Exp Neurol 1990; 109:308–322.

187. Yamashita H, Kannan H, Kasai M, Osaka T. Decrease in blood pressure by stimulation of the rat hypothalamic paraventricular nucleus with L-glutamate or weak current. J Auton Nerv Sys 1987; 19:229–234.

188. Yamori Y, Okamoto D. Hypothalamic tonic regulation of blood pressure in spontaneously hypertensive rats. Jpn Circ J 1969; 33:509–519.

189. Yanagihara M, Niimi K. Substance P-like immunoreactive projection to the hippocampal formation from the posterior hypothalamus in the cat. Brain Res Bull 1989; 22:689–694.

190. Yardley CP, Hilton SM. The hypothalamic and brainstem areas from which the cardiovascular and behavioural components of the defence reaction are elicited in the rat. J Auton Nerv Sys 1986; 15:227–244.

191. Yoshimoto Y, Sakai K, Luppi PH, Fort P, Salvert D, Jouvet M. Forebrain afferents to the cat posterior hypothalamus: a double labeling study. Brain Res Bull 1989; 23: 83–104.

192. Zhang T-X, Ciriello J. Effect of paraventricular nucleus lesions on arterial pressure and heart rate after aortic baroreceptor denervation in the rat. Brain Res 1985; 341:101–109.

8

Cerebral Cortex and Respiration

PAUL W. DAVENPORT and ROGER L. REEP

University of Florida
Gainesville, Florida

I. Introduction

Humans can easily sense and control their breathing pattern. This conscious awareness can produce distressing sensations in many pathological conditions. While it is generally recognized that humans and animals (1) can consciously sense their breathing and behaviorally control breathing pattern, the cortical mechanisms are unknown. The activation of neurons in the forebrain by stimulation of respiratory afferents has been studied primarily in cats. Cortical neural activity has been elicited by stimulation of the cervical vagus, superior laryngeal, intercostal, and phrenic nerves. Respiratory mechanics are transduced into a sensory neural code by afferents in these nerves supplying the airway, lung, and respiratory muscles. Airflow, volume, and pressure are encoded by afferents that project to the central nervous system via the cranial nerves, especially the vagus and its branches. Respiratory muscle mechanics are encoded by diaphragm and intercostal muscle mechanoreceptors. Small-diameter myelinated and nonmyelinated afferents provide additional afferent information.

Recording cortical evoked potentials (CEP) with electrodes placed on the surface of the cerebral cortex has been the principal method for identifying cortical sites activated by respiratory afferents in experimental animals. The surface

365

recording site with the shortest latency, largest amplitude, initially positive potential indicates that the surface electrode is over the cortical region first to receive activation from the stimulated afferents, the primary site. The positive potential is produced by a dipole generated by depolarization of a group of neurons in a cortical column below the surface. Scalp surface electrodes have been used in humans to identify regions activated by respiratory afferents. Efferent projections from the cerebral cortex have also been studied with surface electrodes to electrically stimulate the underlying neurons in experimental animals. It is clear that respiratory afferents activate neurons in the forebrain and cerebral cortical efferents alter respiratory neural activity, but understanding of the afferent and efferent mechanisms is incomplete.

II. Afferent Activation of Cerebral Cortex

A. Vagal and Superior Laryngeal Afferents

Stimulation of the cervical vagi elicits surface CEPs in the cerebral cortex of cats and monkeys. Primary contralateral cortical sites for vagal stimulation were located in the orbital cortex of the cat (Fig. 1), based on cortical surface identification (2). The stimulus parameters used in that study, 1 msec pulse width, activate the large- and small-diameter myelinated fibers. The latency for the CEP was 15–25 msec, which also suggests activation of myelinated afferents. Korn and Massion (3) used electrical stimulus trains applied to the cat cervical vagus to activate group I, II, and III fibers but insufficient to activate group IV nonmyelinated afferents. They recorded primary CEPs in the contralateral cortex in four frontal cortical sites: the motor precruciate region, a region caudal to the ansate sulcus, and the two fronto-orbital regions found by Siegfried (2). Aubert and Legros (4) found similar results using single pulse stimulation of the cat cervical vagus nerve. In addition to the four cortical regions reported previously, they found a wider distribution of contralateral cortical activity elicited by stimulation of group I and II afferents. The regions activated were in the area of the posterior sigmoid gyrus, anterior suprasylvian gyrus, anterior ectosylvian gyrus, anterior sylvian gyrus, cruciate gyrus, and orbital cortex. Adjustment of the stimulus parameters to recruit group III afferents additionally activated the regions of the anterior sigmoid gyrus and marginal gyri. Vagal stimulation also elicited activity in the ipsilateral cortex in the same regions activated by contralateral vagal stimulation. The ipsilateral CEP had a longer latency, suggesting a corticocortical pathway. The specific identification of the cortical areas activated by vagal stimulation can only be inferred from the surface recording sites, as histological identification of the regions was not reported.

  Aubier and Guilhen (5) stimulated the superior laryngeal nerve (SLN) and recorded the surface CEP. The cortical regions activated by SLN afferents were also activated by vagal afferents. The SLN projection sites were more focal and comprised a subgroup of the larger vagal representation. SLN stimulation elicited primary CEPs in the regions of the cruciate sulcus, anterior ectosylvian sulcus, anterior sylvian sulcus, suprasylvian sulcus, and orbital cortex.

Similar studies of vagal afferent activation of the cerebral cortex were performed in monkeys (6). The contralateral cervical vagus was electrically stimulated with two to three shock trains. In addition, the SLN and recurrent laryngeal nerve (RLN) were stimulated. Cortical activity was recorded with surface electrodes and microelectrodes. The specific cortical regions were identified histologically. Vagal stimulation elicited activity in the sensory and motor cortices. Single pulse electrical stimulation produced large-amplitude, short-latency responses in the postrolandic sensory cortex. Stimulus trains were more effective in eliciting activity in the motor cortex. There was significant convergence in the motor cortex from vagal, SLN, hands, face, and tongue afferents. The motor region activated in the monkey is homologous to Broca's area in the human for vocalization. No cortical response was recorded with stimulation of RLN afferents. However, microstimulation of the motor region activated by vagal afferents elicited a motor response recorded in the RLN.

Very little is known about the vagal and SLN afferent pathways to the cerebral cortex. Hallowitz and MacLean (7) recorded neurons responsive to vagal afferent stimulation in the thalamus. They recorded neurons in the anterior medial, paracentral, lateral dorsal, central lateral, and medial dorsal nuclei that had either initial excitatory or inhibitory responses to vagal afferent stimulation. They also found units in part of the ventral lateral nucleus responding to vagal afferents. Paracentral and anterior nuclei project to the cingulate and supracingulate regions of the mesocortex. The medial dorsal nucleus is connected to the orbital region of the mesocortex. The ventral lateral and central lateral nuclei, however, have connections with the motor cortex.

These studies in the cat and monkey demonstrate short latency activation of the somatosensory, motor, and mesocortex. The specific source of the afferents mediating the vagal and SLN sensory activation of the cortex is unknown. Respiratory-related afferents from the larynx, pharynx, airways, and lungs are found in these nerves. It is likely vagal respiratory afferents are responsible for a portion of the cortical activation. It is apparent that there are at least two vagal and SLN afferent pathways to the cerebral cortex. One pathway projects to the somatosensory and motor cortex. A second pathway projects to the mesocortex. Little anatomical and physiological information exists, however, on the role of SLN and vagal afferents in the cortical control of respiration.

B. Respiratory Muscle Afferents

Electrical stimulation of myelinated phrenic afferents has been shown to elicit evoked potentials in the somatosensory region of the cat cerebral cortex (8,9).

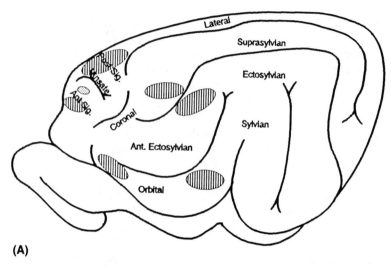

(A)

Figure 1   Schematic surface representation of the respiratory afferent projection sites in the cat cerebral cortex. (A) Lateral cerebral cortex. The surface locations of the primary afferent activated areas are indicated. The major cortical gyri (sig. = sigmoid) and the ansate sulcus are labeled. (B) Dorsal cerebral cortex. The cruciate and ansate sulci are labeled. PCD = postcruciate dimple. The respiratory afferent-activated areas are based on the reports of Refs. 2–5,8–11,13,16.

Davenport et al. (9) mapped the cat sensorimotor region and found the majority of the phrenic afferent evoked activity in areas 3a and 3b (Fig. 1). Electric stimulation of the whole phrenic nerve in the thorax predominantly activated group I and II and to a lesser extent group III afferents. Shortening the pulse width to selectively stimulate group I and II afferents, the projection loci are confined to areas 3a/3b in the trunk region on the rostral medial edge of the cat postcruciate dimple. Davenport et al. (10) subsequently recorded phrenic afferent–activated neurons in this region. They observed focal localization of the phrenic afferent cortical neurons from 400 to 1500 μm in depth. These neurons were located within lamina III of area 3b.

The CEP elicited by fast-conducting, low-threshold phrenic afferents (activated by 0.1 msec stimulus pulse widths) was compared to the CEPs elicited by slow-conducting, high-threshold phrenic afferents activated by stimulus trains (11). Stimulation of the large myelinated, fast-conducting type I and II phrenic afferents elicited an evoked potential in the region of the postcruciate dimple in area 3a on the border of 3a–3b of the sensorimotor cortex. When stimulus trains were applied, a longer-latency evoked potential was found more laterally in the cortex in the forelimb region of area 4γ (Fig. 1). The conduction velocity to the

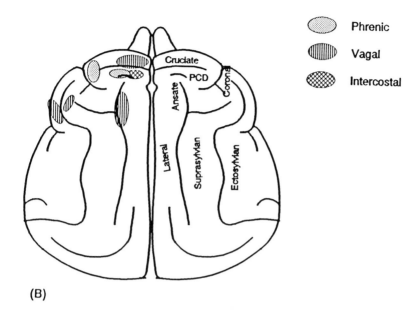

Phrenic

Vagal

Intercostal

Cruciate

PCD

Coronal

Ansate

Lateral

SuprasyMan

EctosyMan

(B)

cerebral cortex is consistent with group III afferent activation, but no evidence of group IV afferent projections was found. The cortical neurons activated by high-threshold phrenic afferent stimulation were also deeper in the cortex at 2.0–2.3 mm depth.

Bolser et al. (12) recorded spinothalamic tract neurons activated by group II or III phrenic afferents. The phrenic-activated spinothalamic tract neurons were in the cervical cord and also responded to shoulder afferents. The group III afferent-elicited CEP in the lateral forelimb region activated neurons in the motor area 4γ (11). The activated site was lateral to the short-latency, group I and II mediated activation of the 3a/3b phrenic afferent cortical locus. These observations suggest a second projection pathway via the spinothalamic tract for small myelinated, high-threshold phrenic group III afferents to the cerebral cortex.

The physiological role of respiratory muscle afferent (RMA) activation of the cerebral cortex remains unknown. Respiratory muscle mechanics change over the ventilatory cycle. These changes are transduced into a neural code by respiratory muscle mechanoreceptors. These afferents project to the sensorimotor cortex. Studies on the cortical representation of RMAs relate directly to cortical proprioceptive control of respiratory muscles and the perception of respiratory loads in humans. The results of animal studies provide evidence that the neural substrate for RMA projections to the somatosensory regions is present.

Intercostal muscle afferent projections to the cerebral cortex have been identified by both electrical and mechanical stimulation (13). Both methods of intercostal afferent activation resulted in localization of cortical foci in area 3a medial (2–3 mm) to the phrenic foci. The intercostal and phrenic afferents do not colocalize. A primary CEP was found with only 50 μm stretch of the intercostal space. Low-amplitude stretch of the intercostal space selectively stimulated intercostal muscle spindles (Bolser). The CEP elicited by 50 μm stretch was, thus, due to muscle spindle stimulation. The CEP amplitude increased with increasing stretch to a plateau at 300 μm. Little increase in CEP amplitude was noted with stretch magnitudes greater than 300 μm, suggesting that tendon organs add little to the observed CEP response. Group III and IV afferents and costovertebral joint receptors have much higher thresholds for mechanical stimulation and are unlikely to be activated with this mechanical stimulation (14,15).

Thalamic neurons activated by phrenic nerve electrical stimulation, mechanical stimulation of the diaphragm, and mechanical probing of the intercostal muscle have been recorded (Davenport PW, unpublished results). The low-threshold phrenic afferents activated neurons in the thalamus with latencies for the initial thalamic spike of 8–10 msec. The phrenic stimulation was accompanied by a 10–15 msec burst of thalamic neuron activity. Mechanical probing of the diaphragm elicited activity in a few thalamic neurons. The body surface was probed and shoulder afferents were found to also stimulate thalamic neurons in the recording area. This suggests that the phrenic afferents in the thalamus are represented in the same thalamic projection for shoulder afferents (C_5–C_7 dermatome). These thalamic neurons are probably the relay neurons projecting to 3a/3b cortical loci.

A population of phrenic-activated neurons was also located in the ventral lateral nucleus of the rostral thalamus. These neurons were stimulated only by high-threshold, slow-conducting phrenic afferents. Mechanical probing of the diaphragm did not stimulate these thalamic neurons. The same neurons were also activated by mechanical probing of shoulder cutaneous afferents. Thus, this region of the thalamus contains neurons that have a dual sensitivity to slow-conducting phrenic afferents and shoulder cutaneous afferents.

C. Anatomical Pathways

In cats, CEPs related to respiratory muscle afferents have been recorded from the somatic motor and sensory areas of the anterior and posterior sigmoid gyri. The majority of short-latency potentials are found in area 4γ at the lateral margin of the cruciate sulcus and in the region of area 3a immediately rostral to the postcruciate dimple (8,9,13). The somatic motor and sensory areas are arranged as a series of mediolaterally oriented bands, each having a distinct cytoarchitectural structure, pattern of thalamic connections, and functional role. The most rostral of these is the motor area 4γ, which extends from the surface of the anterior sigmoid gyrus down into the cruciate sulcus and out onto the surface of the posterior sigmoid gyrus. It lacks a granular layer IV and has large pyramidal cells in layer V (16). The ventral, anterior–ventral lateral complex is the principal source of thalamic afferents to area 4γ, with additional inputs arising from the ventromedial, dorsomedial, intralaminar, and posterior nuclei (17,18). Area 3a borders the caudal margin of area 4γ and contains a thin granular layer IV with a well-developed pyramidal layer V (16,19). Prominent thalamic afferents to area 3a originate from the oralis portion (VPO) of the ventroposterior nuclear complex (20). Area 3a contains a topographically organized body map of deep tissue receptors, with the forelimb region represented laterally, the hindlimb medially, and the trunk between them (20,21). Area 3b lies caudal and adjacent to area 3a. The postcruciate dimple is a shallow depression found near the border between these areas and is located approximately halfway from the midline to the lateral edge of the hemisphere at this rostrocaudal level (Fig. 1). Area 3b is characterized by a well-developed granular layer IV and very sparse pyramidal layer V (16). Its primary thalamic input arises from the lateral portion (VPL) of the ventroposterior nuclear complex (20). Area 3b contains a topographically organized body map for the representation of skin receptors, organized in the same mediolateral fashion as the map in area 3a for deep receptors (20–22).

Thalamocortical projections activated by respiratory afferents were recently identified in cats (23). CEPs were recorded in the right somatosensory cortex following phrenic nerve stimulation of the left C-5 root. Retrograde fluorescent tracers were then injected at the site of primary activation and in adjacent cortical areas that were not activated by phrenic stimulation. The majority of primary CEPs were found in the vicinity of the postcruciate dimple, in area 3a near the 3a/3b border, corresponding to the trunk region of the cortical body map. Within the thalamus, nucleus VPO contained labeled neurons following injections in the sites of primary activation (Fig. 2). Control injections produced thalamic labeling that did not overlap with injections of phrenic primary activation sites. These findings indicate that activity in phrenic nerve respiratory afferents projects to the trunk region of primary somatosensory cortex via specific thalamocortical projections originating in VPO. It seems likely that representation in area 3a of muscle afferents originating in the intercostal muscles (13) is also relayed via nucleus VPO, but this remains to be demonstrated. It is also possible that cortical regions in addition to area 3a also receive respiratory muscle afferent signals.

These animal studies demonstrate that afferents in the respiratory tract and muscle have projection pathways to the cerebral cortex. The regions predominantly activated by these afferents are the somatosensory-motor cortex and the mesocortex. The respiratory pattern is transduced into a sensory neural code by respiratory mechanoreceptors. The changes in pressure, volume, airflow, and muscle mechanics are encoded by these afferents. This neural code is then transmitted to the central nervous system by the nerve fibers of these afferents via

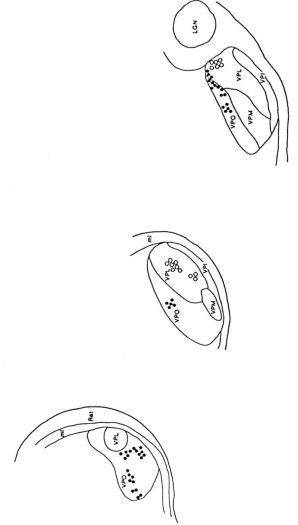

Figure 2 Three serial coronal sections illustrating retrogradely labeled neurons in the thalamus from florescent injections in the phrenic afferent-activated regions of the cerebral cortex. (Closed circles) Neurons that were retrogradely labeled from the phrenic activated site in area 3a. (Open circles) Neurons retrogradely labeled by control injections in area 3b. VPO = ventroposterior oralis nucleus; VPL = ventroposterior lateralis nucleus; VPM = ventroposterior medialis nucleus; LGN = lateral geniculate nucleus; ML = medial lemniscus. (Adapted from Ref. 23.)

spinal and brainstem pathways. There is also evidence for a separate cortical projection from small-diameter afferents that may be involved in respiratory nociception. The physiological role of these cortical sensory systems remains to be determined.

D. Respiratory-Related Evoked Potentials

Activation of cortical neurons by respiratory afferents has been studied in humans using scalp surface recording electrodes. The transduction of mechanical events related to breathing produces a change in the pattern of sensory information projecting to the cortex. The activation of cortical neurons by mechanical loads has been studied using evoked potential techniques similar to those routinely used in other somatosensory systems. Inspiratory occlusions were applied while recording from the somatosensory region of the cortex in the adult human (24). This load was presented at the onset of an inspiration. Electroencephalographic activity was recorded from scalp electrodes placed over the frontal (F_Z) and somatosensory (C_Z, C_3) regions of the cerebral cortex. Bipolar recordings were obtained with a cephalic reference, C_Z. The inspiratory occlusion pressure was used to synchronize the occlusions and trigger the signal averager. The inspiration preceding each occlusion was averaged as the control. A specific occlusion-related evoked potential (RREP) was recorded. The evoked potential was absent in unoccluded averages. The RREP pattern was recorded from the electrodes, C_Z–C_3, over the somatosensory region (Fig. 3). The evoked potential was similar to somatosensory evoked potentials reported for the hand and leg. Four voltage peaks were observed in all subjects. The first peak, P_1, was a positive voltage due to the dipole occurring when a cerebral cortical column was depolarized by the arrival of activity from a population of afferents activated by the occlusion stimulus. This first peak signals the arrival of the afferent information at the somatosensory cortex. The peak latencies varied between subjects, but the P_1 latency was related to the $P_{0.1}$, i.e. decreased P_1 latency with increased $P_{0.1}$. This suggests that with larger driving pressures the stimulus threshold will be exceeded sooner with a shorter latency for the onset of the sensory signal. This will result in a shorter P_1 latency because of a decrease in the transduction time for generating the sensory signal to the cortex.

The RREP was subsequently recorded bilaterally from the somatosensory region of the cortex with a cephalic reference, C_Z–C_3 and C_Z–C_4 (25). It was elicited by occlusions at that beginning of the breath and by an occlusion interruption of the breath at approximately midinspiration. The interruption of inspiration produced a larger-amplitude RREP with a shorter latency than the onset occlusion (Fig. 2). The interrupted breath methodology is easier to use and is the preferred method for eliciting the RREP.

The relationship between inspiratory drive and P_1 latency was studied by

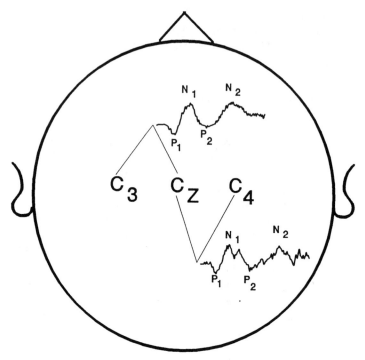

Figure 3 Respiratory-related evoked potentials recorded from C_Z–C_3 and C_Z–C_4 electrode pairs. The RREP was elicited with midinspiratory occlusions. The major peaks are labeled according to Ref. 24.

comparing the RREP with steady-state hypercapnia and normocapnia (26). The RREP was initially recorded with normocapnia. The subjects were then exposed to steady-state hypercapnia, which produced a fourfold increase in the occlusion pressure elicited with onset and midinspiratory occlusions. The P_1 amplitude was not significantly different between normocapnic and hypercapnic conditions. The only parameter of the evoked potential that changed was a small, but significant, decrease in the P_1 latency that is related to the increase in $P_{0.1}$. This decrease in latency can be explained by an increase in the rate at which the stimulus will reach threshold because of the increase of respiratory drive going to the respiratory pump. The amplitude of the P_1 potential in other sensory systems is directly related to the stimulus magnitude (27). That would suggest that if the mouth pressure was the source of the afferent information, the increases in mouth pressure during hypercapnia should have produced an increased amplitude for the P_1 potential. The lack of change in the RREP P_1 amplitude suggests that mouth pressure is not the source of the afferent information mediating the RREP elicited by inspiratory occlusion.

There is, however, the possibility that nonrespiratory artifacts contaminate the RREP. The occlusion elicited RREP was recorded from C_Z–C_3 and C_Z–C_4. In addition, C_3 and C_4 were referenced to electrodes placed over the lower cervical spine and the lower leg. The electrocardiogram (ECG) was recorded separately (Hill PMcN, Davenport PW, unpublished results). The average RREP was obtained by averaging all the occlusion presentations, averaging only those occlusion presentations that occurred during the isovoltage phase of the ECG between the T and P waves, and averaging the same number of presentations with ECG activity related to the QRS wave occurring during the first 200 msec of the occlusion. The RREP was unaffected by ECG activity when C_3 and C_4 were referenced to C_Z. However, large-voltage peaks in the RREP average due to ECG transients were found with noncephalic references, especially with the leg reference. These results demonstrate that the RREP recorded from the C_Z–C_3 and C_Z–C_4 electrode pairs is not contaminated with ECG or motion artifact and is of cephalic origin.

The RREP had been previously recorded primarily from only two scalp sites with a cephalic reference, C_Z, and the scalp distribution of the RREP remained unknown. The scalp topographical distribution of the RREP was studied in 10- to 13-year-old children (28). Using electrocaps, occlusion interruption of inspiration-elicited scalp activity was recorded from 17 electrode sites referenced to the joined earlobes. C_3 and C_4 were also recorded with the C_Z reference. The RREP was found in the C_Z–C_3 and C_Z–C_4 electrode pairs in all of the children. The P_1 peak was found in the postcentral electrodes C_3, C_4, P_3, P_4, and to a lesser extent T_3 and T_4 when referenced to the joined earlobes. This suggested a source in the somatosensory cortex, which may be best recorded with electrodes intermediate between the C and P locations (the C′ site). A negative peak, N_f, not found with the C_Z reference, was observed in the precentral electrodes: F_3, F_4, F_7, F_8, and to a lesser extent C_3 and C_4. This N_f peak had a peak latency approximately 13 msec after P_1. The source of this peak was separate from P_1 and may be associated with the motor cortex. The P_1 and N_f peaks were not observed in the midline electrodes. These results demonstrate that the early components of the RREP are of cephalic origin and the signal-to-noise ratio is greatly improved with the C_Z reference. There are probably two sources of occlusion-elicited cortical activity in the somatosensory and motor cortices.

The RREP has also been correlated with the perception of resistive loads in adult humans (29). The RREP was recorded bilaterally from C_Z–C_3 and C_Z–C_4 with graded resistive loads of 2, 9, and 21 $cmH_2O/L/sec$. The three load magnitudes and no-load presentation sets were randomized to remove order effects. The RREP was obtained by averaging the presentations for each load magnitude. The averaged control, no-load presentations were subtracted from each averaged load magnitude. The subjects also provided a magnitude estimation of the load on the 5th presentation of each load set. The log of the P_1 peak amplitude was linearly correlated with the log of the magnitude estimation of the loads and the log of the resistive load magnitude. These results demonstrate that the P_1 amplitude is a function of the stimulus magnitude and may be related to the resultant perceptual estimation of the load. This is consistent with other somatosensory systems that have similar correlations (27).

The application of negative mouth pressure pulses to adult subjects was reported to elicit an evoked potential similar to the RREP (30). The pressure pulses ranged from -2 to -25 cmH$_2$O. The evoked potential was recorded from a midline C_Z electrode referenced to the right earlobe. A positive peak was observed with a latency of approximately 20 msec. The negative pressure stimulus provided a mouth pressure change with a reproducible onset that aided in signal averaging. This type of stimulus also has a more rapid onset than the occlusion method. The early positive peak is probably the result of the initial activation of the cortex, similar to the P_1 peak of the occlusion-elicited RREP. The difference in latency may be due in part to the larger magnitude and rapid onset of the stimulus.

The RREP has also been recently recorded during non-REM sleep in normal adult humans (31). The RREP was initially elicited in awake subjects respiring through a face mask with occlusions that interrupted inspiration. The RREP was observed bilaterally (C_Z–C_3 and C_Z–C_4). The peak amplitudes were similar to those of previous reports, but the latencies were longer. During non-REM sleep, the RREP waveform was altered. The P_1 peak had a longer latency but there was no significant difference in amplitude. The N_1 and P_2 peaks also had longer latencies and there was a significant increase in peak amplitude. The N_1–N_2 peak during non-REM sleep had the waveform and latency similar to those of a K-complex. It is apparent that the RREP is present but significantly altered when subjects sleep. These changes may reflect sleep-dependent alterations in the cortical processing of respiratory afferent information. Future studies on the changes in the RREP during sleep will be essential.

The afferents mediating the RREP are unknown. The intercostal muscles are one source of afferents that can elicit evoked potentials in the cerebral cortex (32). An evoked potential was recorded at C_Z with electrical stimulation of the intercostal muscles. Thus, respiratory muscle afferents project to the somatosensory region in the human, a finding supported by animal studies.

The human studies performed to date demonstrate that the RREP can be recorded in adults and children. The afferents mediating the RREP remain unknown. If this respiratory-related cortical activity is similar to evoked potentials for other sensory systems, then the P_1 potential represents the arrival of the sensory signal in the somatosensory region of the cerebral cortex, similar to the primary evoked potential found with cortical surface recordings in the cat. The later peaks are related to the cortical processing of the respiratory afferent stimuli. Determination of the relationship between the components of the RREP and the perception of changes in breathing pattern must be studied. One role for the activation of the somatosensory region of the cerebral cortex may be in respiratory muscle proprioception. Respiratory muscle afferents have transduction properties and cortical projection pathways consistent with their hypothesized role in respiratory load sensation. The correlation of the P_1 peak of the RREP with the magnitude estimation of resistive loads suggests that conscious humans may use cerebral cortical somatosensory and motor systems as one response mechanism to respiratory loads.

III. Respiratory Efferent Responses from Cerebral Cortex

Electrical stimulation of the cerebral cortex increased respiratory rate and modulated the response amplitude in monkeys, cats, and dogs (33). Studies using stimulation of the cerebral cortex have suggested a respiratory excitatory zone in the cingulate cortex of the cat, dog, and human (33–35). Planche (36) recorded phrenic nerve activity with cortical stimulation in the cat. Single shock stimulation of the cerebral cortex produced a complex phasic response. Separate excitatory and inhibitory zones were observed. An excitatory zone was localized in the thoracic field of SII somatosensory cortex and in the primary and secondary visual projection areas (Fig. 4). Orbital gyrus stimulation, however, produced a burst of activity with an onset latency of 7–11 msec., followed by a 5–25 msec. inhibition of phrenic activity. Single shock cortical stimulation has also been shown to exert an excitatory influence on respiratory bulbospinal neurons (37). It was suggested that descending activity from the cortex to the brainstem respiratory centers excites both phrenic motor neurons while inhibiting oscillator activity (36). Single shock cortical stimulation in the pericruciate cortex also produces inhibition or off-switching of contralateral C5 phrenic root inspiratory activity.

Lipski et al. (38) found that short-latency excitatory inputs to phrenic motoneurons from pericruciate cortex in the cat were mediated by extrapyramidal descending pathways, which were faster-conducting than inhibitory pathways (Fig. 4). It has been suggested that the transmission of cortically evoked responses involves reticulospinal pathways (38–41). Regions producing phrenic nerve excitation include cingulate cortex, SII somatosensory cortex, primary and secondary visual areas, and pericruciate cortex (33–35). Thompson et al. (42) identified cerebral cortical regions producing short-latency contralateral C5 phrenic compound action potentials with a localization lateral to the cruciate sulcus in the cerebral cortex (Fig. 4). This localization was in cytoarchitectonic areas 3, 1, and 2 (16), distinct from the pericruciate motor cortex localization suggested by Lipski et al. (38). This was in part the result of differences in methodology, which included shorter-duration stimulus pulses (0.2 msec) presented as single shocks

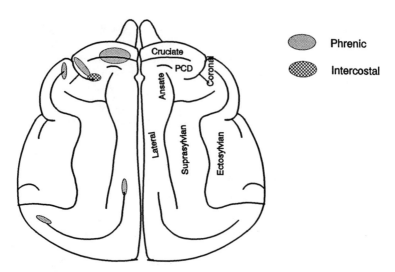

Figure 4 Schematic dorsal surface representation of the respiratory efferent projection sites in the cat cerebral cortex. The cortical areas that elicit phrenic efferent activity with surface stimulation are indicated. The locations of the cortical sites are based on the reports of Refs. 36–38,41,47.

or up to three pulse trains, lower stimulus intensity, and stimulation spanning both inspiratory and expiratory phases. The regions identified as phrenic motor cortex produced low-threshold, short-latency contralateral phrenic action potentials, including the banks of the coronal sulcus and areas of the posterior sigmoid gyrus, rostral to the ansate sulcus. Lipski et al. (38) localized the lowest-threshold points to areas 3, 4, and 6. Thompson et al. (42) found that the regions that elicited inhibition or off-switching of the phrenic inspiratory burst with single shock stimulation were also localized in areas, 3, 1, and 2. This suggests the presence of a region in the sensorimotor cortex of the cat that produces short-latency activation of phrenic motor neurons. This region may also provide cortical modulation of brainstem inspiratory activity. Stimulation of neurons in the subsurface layers of the phrenic motor cortex with microelectrodes (followed by histological analysis) demonstrated that activation intracortical neurons in layer V, rather than spread to subcortical white matter, produced the phrenic nerve activation observed in these experiments.

Cortical projections to the phrenic motor nucleus and brainstem dorsal respiratory group have been identified anatomically. Rickard-Bell et al. (43) utilized horseradish peroxidase (HRP) techniques in the cat to identify cells of origin of corticospinal projections to the 5th and 6th cervical segment phrenic motorneurons. Following identification of phasic inspiratory activity, iontophoretic injections of HRP were made in the phrenic motor nucleus. Labelled cortical cells projecting to the phrenic motor nucleus in cats originate from the portion of motor area 4γ located around the lateral margin of the cruciate sulcus, in the anterior and posterior sigmoid gyri (43,44). Stimulation of this portion of area 4γ is known to produce an acceleration of respiratory movements (45). Projections to the region of the dorsal respiratory group have been reported to originate in the sigmoid, anterior ectosylvian, anterior sylvian, and anterior suprasylvian gyri (46), but no maps of these findings were presented.

The phrenic sensory sites in the cortex were, however, not colocalized with the motor loci (47). This means separate cortical columns are receiving the sensory information from phrenic afferents and projecting a motor output to the phrenic spinal neurons. The means by which phrenic afferent activity in area 3a influences the output of motor area 4γ is not known. If there is a link between cortical loci activated by phrenic afferents and the subsequent motor response, that connection must be a cortical or subcortical link. Until recently, it was suspected from evidence in monkeys that area 3a exerts its primary influence on motor area 4γ via projections to area 2, which in turn projects to area 4γ (48,49), and these pathways have also been identified in cats (50,51). However, recent anatomical and electrophysiological findings have demonstrated direct projections from area 3a to area 4γ in cats (52–55) and monkeys (56,57).

Motor area 4γ is not the only cortical area that influences respiratory behavior. In a variety of mammalian species, respiratory movements are influenced by the cingulate, subcallosal, posterior orbital, insular, and temporal pole regions of cerebral cortex (45). These cortical areas also modulate other autonomic responses, including cardiovascular function, gastric motility, peristaltic activity, piloerection, pupillary dilation, and adrenaline secretion (45,58–67). In primates and cats, electrical stimulation in these cortical regions produces respiratory inhibition. In cats, acceleration of respiratory movements occurs upon stimulation of the motor, secondary somatic sensory (anterior ectosylvian), and posterior cingulate cortical areas (45).

Respiratory events do not occur in isolation. Newman (68) noted that emotional expression often involves respiratory responses occurring together with one or more of the other autonomic responses mentioned above that are influenced by these same cortical areas. Electrical stimulation of the above-mentioned cortical areas produces respiratory effects, often in conjunction with cardiovascular changes. As emphasized by Kaada (45), the cortical areas having these effects are contiguous and are part of a continuous ring of mesocortex (see 69). They have robust connections with the hypothalamus, amygdala, and visceral brainstem centers (70–84).

Cortical activation of respiratory muscles has been reported in human subjects (85). Electrical stimulation was applied through the scalp and the respiratory motor response was assessed by recording diaphragm electromyographic (EMG) activity and transdiaphragmatic pressure. Stimulation of the motor cortex produced short-latency excitation of the human diaphragm. The mean latency of 12.3 msec was consistent with a relatively direct motor projection to the motoneurons. Magnetic stimulation of the cortex was also found to elicit short-latency EMG excitation of the diaphragm (87). The stimulating coils used in these studies were not selective for the diaphragm and produced bilateral activation of several muscle groups. The diaphragm was included in the thoracic region in the human motor cortex homunculus (88). Future studies using paired magnetic stimulating coils, which produces more focal and isolated activation of the underlying cortical neurons, may be useful for more selective identification of the cortical regions with efferent projections to respiratory motor neurons.

The implication from these stimulation studies is that these regions of the cerebral cortex projection to respiratory neurons are involved in the behavioral control of breathing. Electrical and magnetic stimulation of specific areas of the cerebral cortex provides essential evidence for afferent and efferent connections between cortical neurons and respiratory brainstem and spinal neurons. However, these studies do not provide information on cortically mediated reflex and behavioral control of breathing. It is obvious that respiratory pattern can be controlled by volitional and behavioral influences. Animals have been behaviorally conditioned to change breathing pattern in response to nonrespiratory stimuli (89) and to signal the detection of respiratory loads (1). Behavioral conditioning in the cat produces well-documented changes in brainstem respiratory neuronal activity (89–92). It is reasonable that some of the behavioral changes in breathing pattern are mediated by cortical mechanisms. However, it is difficult in these conscious animal studies to identify the underlying specific cortical processes. Identification of the specific cerebral cortical mechanisms mediating the sensory and motor control of breathing will require future application of multiple methodologies.

IV. Conclusion

It appears that two relatively independent cortical systems influence respiratory movements. One is the pathway (Fig. 5) for respiratory muscle afferents. These afferents enter the spinal cord and ascend in the dorsal and/or dorsolateral columns. The afferent activity is relayed in the brainstem, presumably by the external cuneate nucleus, the projects to VPO nucleus in the thalamus via the medial lemniscal tract. The thalamic afferent activate neurons in area 3a and influence the output of motor area 4γ. The descending activity from the motor area projects to spinal respiratory muscle motorneurons and may have a brainstem connection. Afferent projections from the vagus and its branches may also use a similar thalamocortical pathway (with initial activation in the brainstem) to this region of the cortex.

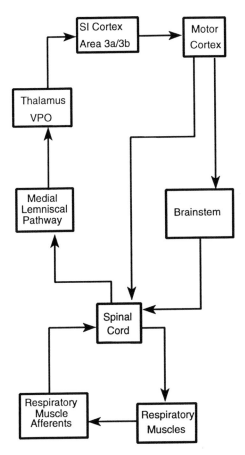

Figure 5   Afferent and efferent projection sensorimotor cortical pathway for respiratory muscle afferents. The lack of detail in this diagram and Figure 6 underscores the need for future studies to define the specific components of cortical pathways.

The cortical projection site of group I and II phrenic afferents in areas 3a and 3b of the postcruciate dimple region of the cortex (9), has been described to be transitional in cytoarchitecture containing characteristics of both motor and sensory cortex (93). Within the 3a cortex, the group I afferents from limb muscles influence neurons found between 500 and 1500 m beneath the cortical surface, i.e., laminae III and IV (94,95). Phrenic nerve afferents similarly activate neurons at depths of 400–1500 m, in lamina III of this region. The function of the group I input to the 3a cortex neurons is presumed to be used in the integration of movements elicited from the cortex. Phillips (96) proposed a cortical load compensation mechanism, which acts through a transcortical servoloop. This loop adjusts the output of the motor cortex, in response to changing afferent signals from peripheral sense organs during the course of movement. The lack of a spinal load compensation mechanism for the diaphragm may make this transcortical mechanism of increased importance.

The second cortical system (Fig. 6) involves ascending afferent information from the vagus nerve and its branches (and possibly phrenic afferents), relayed from the brainstem to the amygdala. The neurons in the amygdala relay the information to its mesocortical targets and the medial dorsal nucleus. The output from the mesocortex is relayed through the amygdala and hypothalamus to the brainstem respiratory centers. This circuit may deal with the affective components of respiratory behavior. In addition, the mesocortex has connections with the motor cortex, which provides a link between the two respiratory cortical pathways and a common output pathway to the respiratory pump.

The ability of humans to produce volitional alterations in respiratory rhythm

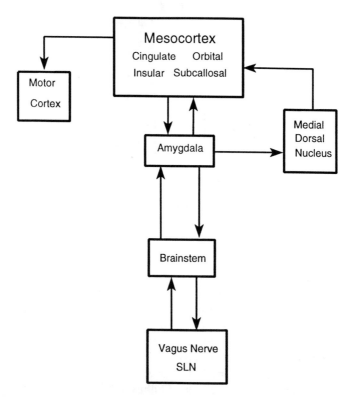

Figure 6 Afferent and efferent mesocortical pathway for vagal afferents.

and drive in association with speech, singing, and other similar activities suggests the existence of a cortical center capable of inhibiting the pattern generator and activating the muscles of respiration, including the diaphragm. The dual actions of cortical stimulation indicate that activation of cerebral cortical neurons can inhibit brainstem respiratory drive and directly activate spinal respiratory muscle motorneurons. It is apparent that the neural substrate is present in the cerebral cortex for motor control of ventilation.

References

1. Davenport PW, Dalziel DJ, Webb B, Bellah JR, Vierck, Jr. CJ. Inspiratory resistive load detection in conscious dogs. J Appl Physiol 1991; 70(3):1284–1289.

2. Siegfried J. Topographie des projections corticales du nerf vague chez le chat. Helv Physiol Acta 1961; 19:269–278.

3. Korn H, Massion J. Origine et topographie des projections vagales sur le cortex anterieur chez le Chat. C R Acad Sci Paris 1964 259:4373–4375.

4. Aubert M, Legros J. Topographie des projections de la sensibilite viscerale sur l'ecorce cerebrale du chat I. Etude des projections corticales du vague cervical chez le chat anesthesie. Arch Ital Biol 1970; 109:423–446.

5. Aubert M, Guilhen C. Topographie des projections de la sensibilite visverale sur l'ecorce cerebrale du chat. III. Etude des projections corticales du nerf larynge superieur. Arch Ital Biol 1971; 109:236–252.

6. O'Brien JN, Pimpaneau A, Albe-Fessard D. Evoked cortical responses to vagal, laryngeal and facial afferents in monkeys under chloralose anesthesia. Electroenceph Clin Neurophysiol 1971; 31:7–20.

7. Hallowitz RA, MacLean PD. Effects of vagal volleys on units of intralaminar and juxtalaminar thalamic nuclei in monkeys. Brain Res 1977; 130:271–286.

8. Frankstein SI, Smolin LN, Segeeva ZN, Sergeeva TI. Cortical representation of the phrenic nerve. Exp Neurol 1979; 63:447–449.

9. Davenport PW, Thompson FJ, Reep RL, Freed AN. Projection of phrenic nerve afferents to the cat sensorimotor cortex. Brain Res 1985; 328:150–153.

10. Davenport PW, Reep RL, Thompson FJ. Projection of phrenic nerve afferents to the cat sensorimotor cortex: laminar analysis. Fed Proc 1985; 44(5):1586.

11. Davenport M. Projection of slow conducting phrenic afferents to the cerebral cortex. B.A. thesis, Spring Arbor College, Spring Arbor, MI, 1989.

12. Bolser DC, Hobbs SF, Chandler MJ, Ammons WS, Brennan TJ, Foreman RD. Convergence of phrenic and cardiopulmonary spinal afferent information on cervical and thoracic spinothalamic tract neurons in the monkey: implications for referred pain from the diaphragm and heart. J Neurophysiol 1991; 65(5):1042–1054.

13. Davenport PW, Shannon R, Mercak A, Reep RL, Lindsey BG. Cerebral cortical evoked potentials elicited by cat intercostal muscle mechanoreceptors. J Appl Physiol 1993; 74(2):799–804.

14. Bolser DC, Lindsey BG, Shannon R. Medullary inspiratory activity: influence of intercostal tendon organs and muscle spindle endings. J Appl Physiol 1987; 62(3): 1046–1056.

15. Godwin-Austen RB. The mechanoreceptors of the costovertebral joints. J Physiol Lond 1969; 202:737–753.

16. Hassler R, Muhs-Clement K. Architektonischer aufbau des sensomotorischen und parietalen cortex der katze. J Hirnforsch 1964; 6:377–420.

17. Morán A, Avendaño C, Reinoso-Suárez F. Thalamic afferents to the motor cortex in the cat. A horseradish peroxidase study. Neurosci Lett 1982; 33:229–233.

18. Morán A, Reinoso-Suárez F. Topographical organization of the thalamic afferent connections to the motor cortex in the cat. J Comp Neurol 1988; 270:64–85.

19. Avendaño C, Verdu A. Area 3a in the cat. I. A reevaluation of its location and architecture on the basis of Nissly, myelin, acetylcholinesterase, and cytochrome oxidase staining. J Comp Neurol 1992; 321:357–372.

20. Dykes RW, Herron P, Lin C-S. Ventroposterior thalamic regions projecting to cyto-architectonic areas 3a and 3b in the cat. J Neurophysiol 1986; 56:1521–1541.

21. Dykes RW, Rasmusson DD, Hoeltzell PB. Organization of primary somatosensory cortex in the cat. J Neurophysiol 1980; 43:1527–1546.

22. Felleman DJ, Wall JT, Cusick CG, Kaas JH. The representation of the body surface in S-I of cats. J Neurosci 1983; 3:1648–1669.

23. Yates JS, Davenport PW, Reep RL. Thalamocortical projections activated by phrenic nerve afferents in the cat (submitted to Brain Res 1993).

24. Davenport PW, Friedman WA, Thompson FJ, Franzén O. Respiratory related cortical evoked potentials in humans. J Appl Physiol 1986; 60:1843–1848.

25. Revelette WR, Davenport PW. Effects of timing of inspiratory occlusion on cerebral evoked potentials in humans. J Appl Physiol 1990; 68(1):282–288.

26. Davenport PW, Holt GA, Hill PMcN. The effect of increased inspiratory drive on the sensory activation of the cerebral cortex by inspiratory occlusion. In: Speck DF, Dekin MS, R. Revelette WR, Frazier DT, eds. Respiratory Control: Central and Peripheral Mechanisms. Lexington: University Press of Kentucky, 1992:216–221.

27. Franzén O, Offenloch K. Evoked response correlates of psychophysical magnitude estimates for tactile stimulation in man. Exp Brain Res 1969; 8:1–18.

28. Davenport PW, Colrain I, Hill PMcN. Scalp topography of the short latency components of the respiratory related evoked potential in children. Biol Psychol Abstr 1993 (in press).

29. Knafelc ME. Effect of ventilatory loads on respiratory mechanics and dyspnea. Ph.D. dissertation, University of Florida, Gainesville, FL, 1992.

30. Strobel RJ, Daubenspeck JA. Early and late respiratory-related cortical potentials evoked by pressure pulse stimuli in humans. J Appl Physiol 1993; 74(4):1484–1491.

31. Wheatlet JR, White DP. Influence of NREM sleep on respiratory-related cortical evoked potentials in normal humans. J Appl Physiol 1993; 74(4):1803–1810.

32. Gandevia SC, Macefield G. Projection of low-threshold afferents from human intercostal muscles to the cerebral cortex. Respir Physiol 1989; 77:203–214.

33. Kaada BR. A study of responses from the limbic, subcallosal, orbito-insular, piriform and temporal cortex, hippocampus-fornix and amygdala. Acta Physiol Scand 1951; 24 (Suppl 83):1–285.

34. Kremer WF. Autonomic and somatic reactions induced by stimulation of the cingular gyrus in dogs. J Neurophysiol 1974; 10:371–392.

35. Pool JL, Ransohoff J. Autonomic effects on stimulating rostral portion of cingulate gyri in man. J Neurophysiol 1949; 12:385–392.

36. Planche D. Effets de la stimulation du cortex cerebral sur l'activité du nerf phréniques. J Physiol Paris 1972; 64:31–56.

37. Planche D, Bianche AL. Modification de l'activité des neurons respiratoires bulbaires provoqueé par stimulation corticale. J Physiol Paris 1972; 64:69–76.

38. Lipski J, Bektas A, Porter R. Short latency inputs to phrenic motorneurons from the sensorimotor cortex in the cat. Exp Brain Res 1986; 61:280–290.

39. Peterson BW. Reticulospinal projections to spinal motor nuclei. Annu Rev Physiol 1979; 41:127–140.

40. Holstege G, Kuypers HGJM, Boer RC. Anatomical evidence for direct brain stem projections to the somatic motoneuronal cell groups and autonomic preganglionic cell groups in cat spinal cord. Brain Res 1979; 171:329–333.

41. Kuypers HGJM, Huisman AM. The new anatomy of descending brain pathways. In: Sjolund B, Bjorklund A, eds. Brain Stem Control of Spinal Mechanisms. Amsterdam: Elsevier Biomedical, 1982:29–54.

42. Thompson FJ, Davenport PW, Warner JJ. Phrenic inspiratory activity modulated by stimulation of phrenic sensorimotor cortex. Neurosci Abstr 1987; 13:1639.

43. Rickard-Bell GC, Bystrzycka, EK, Nail BS. Cells of origin of corticospinal projections to phrenic and thoracic respiratory motoneurones in the cat as shown by retrograde transport of HRP. Brain Res Bull 1985; 14:39–47.

44. Rickard-Bell GC, Törk, Nail BS. Distribution of corticospinal motor fibers within the cervical spinal cord with special reference to the phrenic nucleus: a WGA-HRP anterograde transport study in the cat. Brain Res 1986; 379:75–83.

45. Kaada BR. (1960). Cingulate, posterior orbital, anterior insular and temporal pole cortex. In: Field J, Magoun HW, Hall VE, eds., Handbook of Physiology. 1. Neurophysiology, Vol II. Bethesda, MD: American Physiological Society, 1960:1345–1372.

46. Onai T, Takayama K, Miura M. Projections to areas of the nucleus tractus solitarii related to circulatory and respiratory responses in cats. J Auton Nerv Syst 1987; 18:163–175

47. Warner JJ, Coffey JP, Thompson FJ, Davenport P, Davda M, Schrimsher G. Afferent-efferent organization and cytoarchitecture of phrenic sensorimotor cortex in the cat. Neuroscience Abs 1988; 14:462.

48. Jones EG, Porter R. What is area 3a? Brain Res Rev 1980; 2:1–43.

49. Jones EG. (1986). Connectivity of the primate sensory-motor cortex. In: Jones EG, Peters A, eds. Cerebral Cortex, Vol 5. New York: Plenum Press, 1986:118–134.

50. Porter LL, Sakamoto T, Asanuma H. Morphological and physiological identification of neurons in the cat motor cortex which receive direct input from the somatic sensory cortex. Exp Brain Res 1990; 80:209–212.

51. Waters RS, Favorov O, Asanuma H. Physiological properties and pattern of projection of cortico-cortical connections from the anterior bank of the ansate sulcus to the motor cortex, area 4γ, in the cat. Exp Brain Res 1982; 46:403–412.

52. Asanuma H, Waters RS, Yumiya H. Physiological properties of neurons projecting from area 3a to area 4γ of feline cerebral cortex. J Neurophysiol 1982; 48:1048–1057.

53. Avendaño C, Isla AJ, Rausell E. Area 3a in the cat. II. Projections to the motor cortex and their relations to other corticocortical connections. J Comp Neurol 1992; 321: 373–386.

54. Porter LL. Patterns of connectivity in the cat sensory-motor cortex: a light and electron microscopic analysis of the projection arising from area 3a. J Comp Neurol 1991; 312:404–414.

55. Zarzecki P. Influence of somatosensory cortex on different classes of cat motor cortex output neuron. J Neurophysiol 1989; 62:487–494.

56. Ghosh S, Brinkman C, Porter R. A quantitative study of the distribution of neurons projecting to the precentral motor cortex in the monkey (M. fascicularis). J Comp Neurol 1987; 259:424–444.

57. Huerta MF, Pons TP. Primary motor cortex receives input from area 3a in macaques. Brain Res 1990; 537:367–371.

58. Cechetto DF. Central representation of visceral function. Fed Proc 1986; 46:17–23.

59. Delgado JMR. Circulatory effects of cortical stimulation. Physiol Rev 1960; 40: 146–171.

60. Hall RE, Livingston RB, Bloor CM. Orbital cortical influences on cardiovascular dynamics and myocardial structure in conscious monkeys. J Neurosurg 1977; 46: 638–647.

61. Hoff EC, Kell JF, Carroll MN. Effects of cortical stimulation and lesions on cardiovascular function. Physiol Rev 1963; 43:68–114.

62. Hoffman BL, Rasmussen T. Stimulation studies of insular cortex of *Macaca mulatta*. J Neurophysiol 1953; 16:343–351.

63. Krushel LA, van der Kooy D. Visceral cortex: integration of the mucosal senses with limbic information in the rat agranular insular cortex. J Comp Neurol 1988; 270: 39–54.

64. Penfield W, Faulk ME. The insula: further observation of its function. Brain 1955; 78:445–470.

65. Ruggiero DA, Mraovitch S, Granata AR, Anwar M, Reis DJ. A role of insular cortex in cardiovascular function. J Comp Neurol 1987; 257:189–207.

66. Von Euler US, Folkow B. The effect of stimulation of autonomic areas in the cerebral cortex upon the adrenaline and noradrenaline secretion from the adrenal gland in the cat. Acta Physiol Scand 1958 42:313–320.

67. Wall PD, Davis GD. Three cerebral cortical systems affecting autonomic function. J Neurophysiol 1951; 14:507–517.

68. Newman PP. Visceral Afferent Functions of the Nervous System. London: Edward Arnold, 1974.

69. Reep RL. Relationship between prefrontal and limbic cortex: a comparative anatomical review. Brain Behav Evol 1984; 25:5–80.

70. Allen GV, Saper CB, Hurley KM, Cechetto DF. Organization of visceral and limbic connections in the insular cortex of the rat. J Comp Neurol 1991; 311:1–16.

71. Barbas H, De Olmos J. Projections from the amygdala to basoventral and mediodorsal prefrontal regions in the rhesus monkey. J Comp Neurol 1990; 300:549–571.

72. Hurley KM, Herbert H, Moga MM, Saper CB. Efferent projections of the infralimbic cortex of the rat. J Comp Neurol 1991; 308:249–276.

73. Moga MM, Herbert H, Hurley KM, Yasui Y, Gray TS, Saper CB. Organization of cortical, basal forebrain, and hypothalamic afferents to the parabrachial nucleus in the rat. J Comp Neurol 1990; 295:624–661.

74. Neafsey EJ, Hurley-Gius KM, Arvanitis D. The topographical organization of neurons in the rat medial frontal, insular and olfactory cortex projecting to the solitary nucleus, olfactory bulb, periaqueductal gray and superior colliculus. Brain Res 1986; 377:261–270.

75. Room P, Russchen FT, Groenewegen HJ, Lohman AHM. Efferent connections of the prelimbic (area 32) and the infralimbic (area 25) cortices: an anterograde tracing study in the cat. J Comp Neurol 1985; 242:40–55.

76. Russchen FT. Amygdalopetal projections in the cat. I. Cortical afferent connections. A study with retrograde and anterograde tracing techniques. J Comp Neurol 1982; 206:159–179.

77. Shipley MT. Insular cortex projection to the nucleus of the solitary tract and brainstem visceromotor regions in the mouse. Brain Res Bull 1982; 8:139–148.

78. Shipley MT, Sanders MS. Special senses are really special: evidence for a reciprocal, bilateral pathway between insular cortex and nucleus parabrachialis. Brain Res Bull 1982; 8:493–501.

79. Smith OA, De Vito JL. Central neural integration for the control of autonomic responses associated with emotion. Annu Rev Neurosci 1984; 7:43–65.

80. Terreberry RR, Neafsey EJ. The rat medial frontal cortex projects directly to autonomic regions of the brainstem. Brain Res Bull 1987; 19:639–649.

81. van der Kooy D, McGinty JF, Koda LY, Gerfen CR, Bloom FE. Visceral cortex: a direct connection from prefrontal cortex to the solitary nucleus in rat. Neurosci Lett 1982; 33:123–127.

82. van der Kooy D, Koda LY, McGinty JF, Gerfen CR, Bloom FE. The organization of projections from the cortex, amygdala, and hypothalamus to the nucleus of the solitary tract in rat. J Comp Neurol 1984; 224:1–24.

83. Yasui Y, Breder CD, Saper CB, Cechetto DF. Autonomic responses and efferent pathways from the insular cortex in the rat. J Comp Neurol 1991; 303:355–374.

84. Yasui Y, Itoh K, Kaneko T, Shigemoto R, Mizuno N. Topographical projections from the cerebral cortex to the nucleus of the solitary tract in the cat. Exp Brain Res 1991; 85:75–84.

85. Gandevia SC, Rothwell JC. Activation of the human diaphragm from the motor cortex. J Physiol (Lond) 1987; 384:109–118.

86. Similowski T, Launois S, Carthala HP, Bouche P, Derenne J-Ph. Activation of the diaphragm from magnetic stimulation of the motor cortex in man. Am Rev Respir Dis 1989; 139:A500 (abstract).

87. Murphy K, Mier A, Adams L, Guz A. Putative cerebral cortical involvement in the ventilatory response to inhaled CO_2 in conscious man. J Physiol (Lond) 1990; 420:1–8.

88. Foerster D. Motorische felder und bahen. In: Bumke A, Foerster D, ed. Handbuch der Neurologie, Band 6. Berlin: Springer, 1936:50–51.

89. Orem J, Netick A. Behavioral control of breathing in the cat. Brain Res 1986a; 366:238–253.

90. Orem J, Brooks EG. The activity of retrofacial expiratory cells during behavioral inhibition of inspiration. Brain Res 1986b; 374:409–412.

91. Orem J. The activity of late inspiratory cells during the behavioral inhibition of inspiration. Brain Res 1988; 458:224–230.

92. Orem J. Behavioral inspiratory inhibition: inactivated and activated respiratory cells. J Neurophysiol 1989; 62(5):1069–1078.

93. Jones EG, Powell TPS. The ipsilateral cortical connections of the somatic sensory areas in the cat. Brain Res 1968; 9:71–94.

94. Oscarsson O, Rosen I. Projection to cerebral cortex of large muscle spindle afferents in forelimb nerves of the cat. J Physiol (Lond) 1963; 169:924–945.

95. Oscarsson O, Rosen I, Sulg I. Organization of neurons in the cat cerebral cortex that are influenced from group I muscle afferents. J Physiol (Lond) 1966; 183:189–220.

96. Phillips CG. Motor apparatus of the baboon's hand. Proc Roy Soc London Ser B 1969; 173:141–153.

Part Three

AFFERENT SYSTEMS

9

Mechanisms of Carotid Body Chemoreception

CONSTANCIO GONZALEZ

University of Valladolid
Valladolid, Spain

BRUCE G. DINGER and
SALVATORE J. FIDONE

University of Utah School of Medicine
Salt Lake City, Utah

I. Introduction

A. General

The initiation and regulation of ventilation in lung-breathing creatures are controlled by special chemoreceptor organs that sense changes in body fluid composition (e.g., oxygen, carbon dioxide, and pH). Principal among these specialized chemosensory organs are the peripheral arterial chemoreceptors and the central chemoreceptors. This chapter is devoted to the arterial chemoreceptors of the mammalian carotid body, an organ that detects blood levels of O_2, CO_2, and pH. This specialized chemoreceptor organ is primarily responsible for the hyperventilation that occurs during hypoxia, but it is also involved in the hyperventilatory response accompanying respiratory or metabolic acidosis. Respiratory drive during hypoxia can also be attributed to the aortic chemoreceptors, and during acidosis to the central chemoreceptors.

Current concepts view the chemoreceptors of the carotid body as composite sensory receptors, consisting of specialized preneural (glomus or type I) cells, which are able to detect blood gas and pH levels and transduce these stimuli into neurosecretory responses leading to activation of closely apposed sensory terminals of the carotid sinus nerve (CSN). This chapter will focus on recent findings related to the mechanisms involved in the conversion of chemoreceptor stimuli (decreased P_{O_2} or pH, or increased P_{CO_2}) into nerve impulse activity on the CSN. Chemosensory transduction and transmission are thus the two principal subjects of this chapter.

B. Basic Anatomy and Structure of the Carotid Body

The carotid bodies are paired organs located in the vicinity of the bifurcations of the common carotid arteries. The carotid body is irrigated by one or more small arteries and drained by a small vein that originates from a dense vascular plexus on the surface of the organ. The CSN, a branch of the IXth cranial nerve, provides the sensory innervation to the carotid body, as well as components of the organ's sympathetic and parasympathetic innervation. Another nerve, the ganglio-glomerular nerve from the nearby superior cervical ganglion (SCG), also carries a large contingent of sympathetic fibers destined primarily to innervate the carotid body vasculature (Fig. 1A).

The parenchymal cells of the carotid body are grouped together into islets of cells (also referred to as cell clusters, lobules, or glomoids), which are separated by interstitial connective tissue elements containing nerve fiber bundles and numerous blood vessels (Fig. 1B; Kohn, 1900). The parenchymal cell lobules are composed of two cell types, the "chemoreceptor" or type I cell (also called glomus, chief, or principal cell), and the "sustentacular" or type II cell (also capsule or sheath cell; De Kock, 1951, 1954). Type I cells are approximately five times more abundant than type II cells in most species (see McDonald, 1981), although larger and smaller ratios have been reported (Pequignot et al., 1984; Hansen, 1985).

A conspicuous histological trait of the perfusion-fixed carotid body is the large cross-sectional area occupied by blood vessel lumena (De Castro, 1940, 1951; Verna, 1975, 1979; McDonald, 1981). According to De Castro and Rubio (1968), one-quarter to one-third of the volume of the cat carotid body is occupied by capillaries and venules, a figure confirmed by more recent morphometric studies (see McDonald, 1981; Pallot, 1987). Such vascular volume ratios exceed that for brain by a factor of 5–6 (Kety, 1987). Relatively extensive arteriovenous anastomoses are also characteristic of the carotid body vasculature (McDonald and Larue, 1983; McDonald and Haskell, 1984).

At the ultrastructural level, chemoreceptor type I cells appear round to ovoid, with a diameter of 8–12 μm, and are readily distinguished from the slender encapsulating processes of the sustentacular type II cells (Fig. 2). The distinctive morphological characteristics of type I cells include the presence of numerous cytoplasmic organelles, most notably large numbers of mitochondria and dense-core vesicles, the latter being likened to those of adrenal medullary cells; clear-

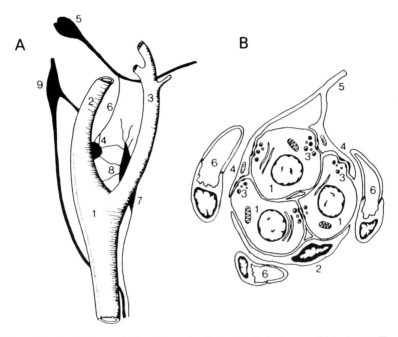

Figure 1 Carotid artery bifurcation and cellular lobule in the carotid body. (A) Frontal view of the right carotid artery bifurcation in the rabbit. The common carotid artery (1) gives rise to the internal (2) and external (3) carotid arteries. The carotid body (4) is located on the internal carotid artery close to the bifurcation. Sensory fibers from the petrosal ganglion (5) reach the carotid body via the carotid sinus nerve (6). The superior cervical ganglion (7) also innervates the bifurcation area, including the carotid body, via the ganglioglomerular nerves (8). The nodose ganglion (9) is situated externally to the internal carotid artery (B) Lobule of parenchymal cells of the carotid body, comprised of chemoreceptor cells (1) partly surrounded by sustentacular cells (2). The proportion of chemoreceptor to sustentacular cells is approximately 3–5 to one. Chemoreceptor cells have in their cytoplasm a heterogeneous population of synaptic vesicles (3), some of which are located near the contacts with the sensory nerve endings (4) of the carotid sinus nerve (5). The lobules are surrounded by a dense network of capillaries (6). (From Gonzalez et al., 1992.)

core vesicles are much less numerous and considerably smaller than the dense-core vesicles (Lever and Boyd, 1957). These dense-core vesicles of type I cells are not uniform in size, and some investigators have reported that vesicle-size distribution allows subclassification of rat type I cells into small versus large vesicle-containing cells (McDonald and Mitchell, 1975; Hellstrom, 1975; see McDonald, 1981). Other studies, on the contrary, have found a unimodal size

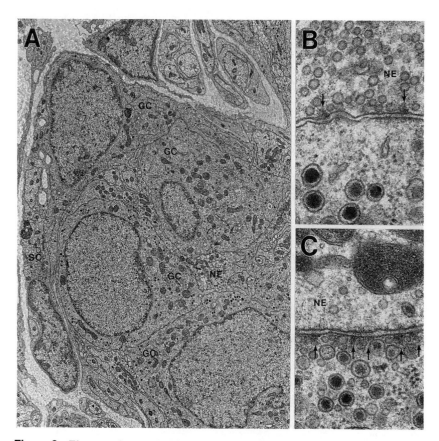

Figure 2   Electron micrographs of rat carotid body. (A) Portion of a calyx-shaped sensory nerve ending (NE) in contact with three glomus cells (GC). Note the extensive area of apposition of the nerve ending and one of the glomus cells ($\sim 7000\times$). Processes of a type II or sustentacular cell (SC) envelop nerve endings and glomus cells. Sensory nerve endings in the rat are presynaptic (B) and postsynaptic (C) to glomus cells. Arrows designate presynaptic dense projections. Note that small, clear-cored vesicles and large, dense-cored vesicles are present in glomus cells near presynaptic sites ($\sim 75,000\times$). (From McDonald, 1981.)

distribution for dense-core vesicles of type I cells in rat, rabbit, and cat carotid bodies (Verna, 1979; Pallot, 1987). Moreover, recent studies have shown that chemoreceptor cells exhibit a continuous gradation in a number of immunocyto-chemical, neurochemical, and electrophysiological properties, leaving doubtful the existence of different subclasses of these cells (Gomez-Nino et al., 1990; Schamel and Verna, 1992a,b; Wang et al., 1991, 1992; Perez-Garcia et al., 1992).

These cells are known to contain multiple putative neurotransmitter substances, including biogenic amines and neuropeptides (see below), and while vesicular costorage of catecholamines and opioid peptides is known (Kobayashi et al., 1983; Gonzalez-Guerrero et al., 1993a), the profile of neurotransmitter costorage is incompletely understood (Wang et al., 1992). Finally, it is important to note that clusters of type I cells exhibit gap junctions and electrical coupling (Monti-Bloch et al., 1993).

Type I cells are innervated by sensory fibers of the CSN, which have their cell bodies located almost exclusively in the petrosal ganglion of the glosso-pharyngeal (IXth cranial) nerve. The terminals of these sensory fibers end in synaptic-like apposition with the type I cells, forming terminal enlargements varying in shape from bouton to calyciform. Based on morphological criteria, these synaptic contacts have been described as polarized from cell to nerve, from nerve to cell, or reciprocally polarized with bidirectional synaptic contacts (McDonald, 1981). The carotid body is innervated from the CSN by medium- to small-diameter myelinated fibers, as well as by unmyelinated chemosensory fibers (Fidone and Sato, 1969). A given fiber may undergo multiple branching as it penetrates the cell lobules en route to innervating numerous (as many as 20 or more) type I cells. The sustentacular cells encapsulating the cellular lobules appear to lack any specialized contact with the type I cells or the nerve fibers and are thought to represent glial-like supporting elements for the chemoreceptor lobules (Kondo et al., 1982).

II. Functional Properties of Chemoreceptor Cells

The energetic metabolism and the electrical properties of chemoreceptor cells are important elements for any model of chemosensory transduction in the carotid body. The available data pertaining to the energetic metabolism of the carotid body deal primarily with studies of O_2 consumption in the whole organ; however, recent experimental evidence supports the notion that the type I, or glomus, cells are the principal determinants of carotid body O_2 consumption and therefore justify ascribing whole-organ O_2 measurements to the chemoreceptor type I cells.

A. Biochemical Properties: O_2 Sensing Versus O_2 Consumption

In the intact animal, the carotid body chemoreceptors are activated by a reduction of arterial Po_2 below the normal resting levels (80–100 mmHg) and are maximally driven at a Po_2 near the P_{50} for hemoglobin (26 mmHg). Thus, the chemoreceptor cells must mount an increasing physiological response in the face of a dwindling O_2 supply to the tissue. This peculiar interactive state, whereby low O_2 is the physiological signal for the cellular response, yet at the same time is a limiting ingredient triggering higher energy demands by the chemoreceptive tissue, has been viewed differently by several groups of investigators and has led to opposing views of the chemoreception process.

Oxygen Delivery to the Carotid Body: Carotid Body Blood Flow

The first measurement of carotid body blood flow was carried out by Daly et al. (1954), who reported a value for the cat carotid body of 2000 ml/100 g/min, with an arteriovenous difference of 2.2%; O_2 consumption was 9 ml/100 g/min, under conditions of normal blood P_{O_2} and P_{CO_2}. Comparable values for the cat under similar resting conditions were later reported by Purves (1970a,b). Other investigators (Acker and Lubbers, 1975, 1977; O'Regan, 1981; Acker and O'Regan, 1981) also found similar values for cat carotid body blood flow, employing a gravidimetric method for the measurement of the venous effluent. The radioactive microsphere method has also been used to measure cat carotid body blood flow, yielding values that are likewise high (1417 ml/100 g/min; Barnett et al., 1988).

While there is apparent unanimity regarding the high value for carotid body blood flow, the actual amount of O_2 available to the tissue is in doubt because of the possible presence of arteriovenous anastomoses that shunt the blood to bypass the chemoreceptor cell lobules. Acker and co-workers have suggested that local intraglomic blood flow is only a small percentage of total organ flow (Acker and Lubbers, 1977; Acker, 1989; but also see Keller and Lubbers, 1972; Acker and Lubbers, 1975). But Torrance (1974), on the basis of functional considerations, claimed there is insufficient evidence for substantial shunting through such arteriovenous anastomoses. It has also been proposed that plasma skimming (and, therefore, decreased O_2 delivery to the tissue) is quantitatively significant in the carotid body (Acker, 1980), but Verna (1981) has presented convincing morphological evidence against plasma skimming, at least in the rabbit carotid body. Consequently, it would appear that the intraglomic tissue is perfused at the rate of 1500 ml/100 g/min, a value that exceeds human cerebral blood flow by more than 15 times (Kety, 1987; Hornbein, 1991). As a result, the O_2 supply to the carotid body is high enough to support a very active metabolic rate, even under conditions of severe hypoxia.

Carotid Body Oxygen Consumption

As mentioned above, initial studies of carotid body O_2 consumption yielded rates of 9 ml/100 g/min, or about three times that of human brain (Kety, 1987; Hornbein, 1991). However, as pointed out by Torrance (1974), these figures should be viewed with caution because they were derived from extremely small values for arteriovenous oxygen differences and consequently are subject to large potential inaccuracies. In fact, Whalen and Nair (1977, 1983) concluded that when perfusing the cat carotid body with blood, arteriovenous O_2 differences were meaningless and could not be used to calculate O_2 consumption. In a series of reports, Whalen and co-workers measured the kinetic parameters of the O_2 disappearance curves that resulted from stopping carotid body blood flow and obtained O_2 consumption rates between 1 and 1.5 ml/100 g/min during perfusion of the organs with either blood or balanced saline at a P_{O_2} near 100 mmHg (Whalen and Nair, 1975, 1976, 1977, 1983; Whalen et al., 1981; Nair et al., 1986; Buerk et al., 1989a,b).

Several other groups have measured O_2 consumption in the carotid body and have reported values ranging from 1 to 9 ml/100 g/min. The scatter among these reported values can be attributed, at least in part, to differences in the estimation of carotid body weight, to the nature of the experimental perfusate (blood vs. saline), and to the coefficients chosen for O_2 solubility. In an important review on this subject, Whalen and Nair (1983) estimated that under resting conditions, the O_2 consumption of the carotid body is 1.3 ml/100 mg/min, and that this value held true for both the in vivo and the in vitro carotid body preparations.

Using a completely different approach, Obeso et al. (1989, 1993) obtained similar values for resting carotid body O_2 consumption. These workers studied rabbit carotid bodies incubated in solutions equilibrated with 100% O_2 and containing tracer concentrations of ^{3}H-2-deoxyglucose. They found a rate of 2-deoxyglucose phosphorylation equal to 61 nmole/g/min (Fig. 3A), which, after application of lumped constants similar to those found for brain and muscle tissue (Sokoloff, 1982; Meszaros et al., 1987), yielded a rate of glucose consumption of 120 nmole/g/min. Assuming that 60% of the glucose consumed is fully oxidized, CO_2 production was estimated at 1.1 ml/100 g/min, yielding an O_2 consumption of 1.2–1.3 ml/100 g/min (Horowitz and Larrabee, 1962). Comparable values have been obtained for the cat carotid body using ^{14}C-U-glucose (unpublished observations). Autoradiographic analysis of the carotid bodies revealed that over 90% of the 2-deoxyglucose phosphorylation occurred within the carotid body parenchymal tissue (Fig. 3B).

Using both the tracer ^{3}H-2-deoxyglucose method and the ^{14}C-U-glucose method, Obeso et al. (1993) observed that exposure of the in vitro carotid body preparation to a moderate hypoxic stimulus (20% O_2) resulted in a 45% increase in glucose consumption and oxidation (Fig. 3A). Thus, increased chemoreceptor activity of the carotid body is accompanied by higher energy demands and increased metabolism by the tissue. These investigators also reported that blockade of the Na^+-K^+ pump prevented this low P_{O_2}-induced increase in glucose consumption. This observation is consistent with that observed for other excitable tissues, where the stimulus-related increase in energy demand results primarily from the Na^+-K^+ pump activity necessary to maintain the cell's ionic gradients and excitability (Fig. 3A; see Yarowsky and Ingvard, 1981, for review). Strangely,

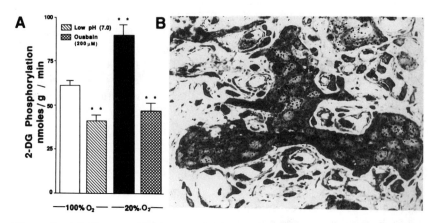

Figure 3 (A) Glucose utilization in the rabbit carotid body as indicated by the phosphorylation of (tritiated) 2-deoxyglucose (2-DG) in vitro. Basal 2-DG phosphorylation was established in 100% O_2-equilibrated media at pH 7.42. Lowering pH to 7.0 significantly reduces glucose uptake ($p < 0.01$). Hypoxia (20% O_2-equilibrated media) elevates 2-DG phosphorylation above control values ($p < 0.01$), and the presence of the sodium-potassium ATPase inhibitor ouabain prevents the hypoxia-induced increase ($p < 0.01$ compared to 20% O_2-equilibrated media without drug). (B) Autoradiograph showing localization of ^{3}H-2DG in lobules of type I/type II cells in the rabbit carotid body. Tissue was incubated for 10 min in 20% O_2-equilibrated media prior to freeze drying/vacuum fixation-embedding. (From Obeso et al., 1993.)

most studies on the carotid body have shown either no change (Starlinger and Lubbers, 1976) or a decrease in O_2 consumption upon exposure to low Po_2 (Purves, 1970; Acker and Lubbers, 1975; Whalen and Nair, 1983; Nair et al., 1986; Buerk et al., 1989a,b). Rumsey et al. (1991), however, did find that after the flow of perfusate through the in vivo carotid body preparation stopped, the rate of O_2 disappearance from the tissue began to increase at the same time as the CSN discharge became elevated. This study, taken together with that of Obeso et al. (1993), makes it unlikely that the carotid body undergoes a shutdown of its O_2 consumption and energy expenditure, while responding maximally and without adaptation to hypoxic stimulus.

Carotid Body Tissue Po_2

Knowledge of the tissue Po_2 in the carotid body is integral to understanding the O_2-sensing capacity of this tissue. It has been known for many years that there is not an absolute physiological threshold for initiation of carotid chemoreceptor activity, and that even at a Po_2 of 600 mmHg, there is a finite probability for chemoreceptor discharge. At an arterial Po_2 of about 75 mmHg, chemoreceptor discharge rises abruptly and reaches maximum activity at a Po_2 of 10–20 mmHg (Hornbein, 1968; Biscoe et al., 1970; see Fidone and Gonzalez, 1986). Unfortunately, the literature regarding carotid body tissue Po_2 is replete with disagreement. Thus, while Whalen and co-workers have consistently reported mean resting tissue Po_2 values around 70 mmHg for the cat carotid body (arterial Po_2 near 100 mmHg; Nair et al., 1986; Buerk et al., 1989a,b; see Whalen and Nair, 1983), Acker's group found mean values of 25 mmHg for the cat and 7 mmHg for the rabbit (Degner and Acker, 1985, 1986; Acker, 1987; see Acker et al., 1983). More recently, Rumsey et al. (1991) found Po_2 values in carotid body exchange vessels to be 23 and 74 mmHg during perfusion of the organ with saline equilibrated at 111 and 131 mmHg Po_2, respectively.

The extensive vascularization of the carotid body and its reported high rate of organ blood flow would seem to favor the larger values for tissue Po_2. In fact, Torrance (1974) has estimated that the Po_2 drop between the capillaries and the core of the parenchymal cell lobules should be in the range of 20 mmHg. However, Acker and co-workers (Acker, 1980, 1987; Acker et al., 1983; Degner and Acker, 1985, 1986) have set forth a mathematical analysis that assumes both a large shunting of blood and plasma skimming. The values reported by this group (see Fig. 9 in Acker et al., 1983) suggest that under resting conditions, most of the carotid body in the rat and a significant portion of that in the cat have a Po_2 below 10 mmHg. According to other studies (Wilson et al., 1988; Rumsey et al., 1991), this Po_2 value would force the chemoreceptor cells into anaerobic metabolism. When the Po_2 in the perfusate (whether blood or saline) is lowered to the chemoresponse threshold of 75 mmHg or below, the tissue Po_2 would drop off abruptly, leaving the chemoreceptor cells in anaerobic metabolism throughout the range of their physiological response. The effect would be exacerbated if organ blood flow was also decreased during hypoxia (Acker and Lubbers, 1975, 1977).

The mean resting tissue Po_2 reported by Whalen and co-workers is approximately 70 mmHg, which agrees with the estimates for the drop in Po_2 between the capillaries and the core of the parenchymal cell clusters (Torrance, 1974). The threshold for chemoreceptor discharge was reported to occur at a tissue Po_2 between 50 and 65 mmHg, with peak CSN activity at a tissue Po_2 of 3–5 mmHg (Whalen and Nair, 1977a,b; Whalen et al., 1981; Nair et al., 1986; Buerk et al., 1989). The tissue P_{50} for chemoreceptor activity has been estimated at 15 mmHg (Nair et al., 1986) and 32 mmHg (Buerk et al., 1989). This latter value is not too dissimilar from the $P_{50} = 40$ mmHg for CSN discharge reported by Lahiri and Delaney (1976). Considering the O_2 dependence of mitochondrial function (Wilson et al., 1988; Rumsey et al., 1991), these values for tissue Po_2 would meet the energetic demands required for full expression of chemoreceptor function throughout the pathophysiological range of hypoxic stimulation. These data may also provide clues to the oxygen affinity of the presumptive O_2 sensor (see below).

Rumsey et al. (1991) measured carotid body intravascular Po_2 utilizing a recently developed method based on the oxygen-dependent quenching of Pd-coproporphyrin phosphorescence (Rumsey et al., 1988; Wilson et al, 1988). They reported that the threshold CSN response to hypoxia occurred at an intravascular Po_2 of 17 mmHg; the P_{50} of the response was 8 mmHg, and maximal CSN activity was achieved at 3 mmHg. Based on these observations, they concluded that oxygen metabolism determines the expression of carotid body chemoreception; that is, the greater the compromise of oxidative phosphorylation with decreasing PO_2, the greater is the chemoreceptor discharge of the CSN. It is intriguing, however, that two values (23 and 74 mmHg) were reported for the resting preocclusion intravascular Po_2 during perfusion with saline at Po_2 levels of 111 and 131 mmHg, respectively. These differences were attributed to differences in saline flow through the carotid bodies (but the perfusion pressure was constant in all experiments). The authors equated intravascular Po_2 with mitochondrial Po_2. Previous estimates (Torrance, 1974), as well as the microelectrode measurements of tissue Po_2, indicated a drop of about 20 mmHg between the capillaries and the core of the cell lobules. If the lower values for intravascular Po_2 are assumed to be correct, as the authors suggest in their article, mitochondrial function would be seriously compromised even under resting conditions. On the other hand, if the higher values for intravascular Po_2 are considered valid, the results would appear to coincide in many quantitative aspects with the above-described data of Whalen and co-workers.

B. Electrical Properties of Chemoreceptor Cells

Chemoreceptor type I cells, once considered inexcitable and having a membrane potential independent of K^+ ions (Baron and Eyzaguirre, 1977; Eyzaguirre et al., 1977, 1983; Oyama et al., 1986), have been studied in recent years using the patch-clamp technique, which has revealed that these cells are indeed excitable, with voltage-dependent Na^+, K^+, and Ca^{2+} channels (Lopez-Barneo et al., 1988). The resting membrane potential measured with conventional intracellular microelectrodes has usually been reported as very low, averaging between -20 and -30 mV, but with a broad range from -8 to -80 mV (Baron and Eyzaguirre, 1977; Eyzaguirre et al., 1983, 1989, 1990; Pang and Eyzaguirre, 1992). Changes in membrane potential during natural and pharmacological stimulation of the organ were variable in amplitude and sign, and consequently it was not possible to correlate membrane potential with chemoreceptor cell function or activity. However, this problem of variability could be traced in part to those cells having very low resting membrane potentials. Thus, in a short note, Hayashida and Eyzaguirre

(1979) reported that pharmacological stimulation with acetylcholine (ACh) produced consistent and marked depolarization in two cat chemoreceptor cells having resting membrane potentials of -52 mV and -56 mV; other publications from this group showed small and variable responses to ACh in chemoreceptor cells with lower membrane potentials (Eyzaguirre et al., 1990). Moreover, Matsumoto et al. (1982) reported a mean resting potential for rabbit chemoreceptor cells of -52 mV and observed that cyanide, ACh, and dopamine (DA) produced consistent membrane potential changes only in those cells with resting potentials greater than -37 mV.

With respect to the contribution of K^+ to the membrane potential of chemoreceptor cells, it was shown in neurochemical experiments that high $[K^+]_e$ released DA from the cat carotid body; the threshold for this effect appeared at 17 mM $[K^+]_e$ and increased sigmoidally with increasing $[K^+]_e$ between 20 and 80 mM, with the effect being wholly dependent on extracellular Ca^{2+} (Almaraz et al., 1986). DA release elicited by 60 mM $[K^+]_e$ declined within 2 min; later studies showed this was due to a depolarization-induced cessation of Ca^{2+} entry into the chemoreceptor cells (Almaraz et al., 1986; Obeso et al., 1992). Consequently, it was concluded that the membrane potential is indeed dependent on K^+ ions and that these cells possess voltage-dependent Ca^{2+} channels. These Ca^{2+} channels appear to be of the L type, because dihydropyridines are excellent blockers of the high K^+-induced release of DA (Obeso et al., 1987, 1992; Shaw et al., 1989, 1990). Furthermore, in newborn rabbit chemoreceptor cells, elevation of $[Ca^{2+}]_i$ mediated by these channels is blocked by D600 (Sato et al., 1991). Also, the open probability of Ca^{2+} channels in cultured adult rat chemoreceptor cells is enhanced by the dihydropyridine Ca^{2+} channel agonist BayK 8644 and is decreased by nifedipine (Fieber and McCleskey, 1993). The presence of voltage-dependent Na^+ channels in chemoreceptor cells was also inferred from neurochemical experiments. It was shown that veratridine promoted a Na^+- and Ca^{2+}-dependent release of DA that could be blocked by tetrodotoxin (Rocher et al., 1988; see also Sato et al., 1989); tetrodotoxin also reduced by about 30% the release of DA produced by low Po_2 stimulation (Gonzalez et al., 1990). In sum, by the late 1980s, the available data suggested that chemoreceptor cells are excitable cells, with a K^+-dependent resting potential and both Na^+- and Ca^{2+}-dependent voltage-gated channels.

The whole-cell patch-clamp experiments using isolated adult rabbit chemoreceptor cells confirmed these observations and showed further that chemoreceptor cells exhibit a unique K^+ current that is reversibly inhibited upon lowering the Po_2 in the bathing media (Lopez-Barneo et al., 1988). Finally, the passive electrical properties of chemoreceptor cells from adult rabbits included an average input resistance of 4.6 GΩ and a capacitance of 6–7 pF, which is consistent with a specific membrane capacitance of about 1 $\mu F/cm^2$ (Duchen et al., 1988; Ureña et al., 1989).

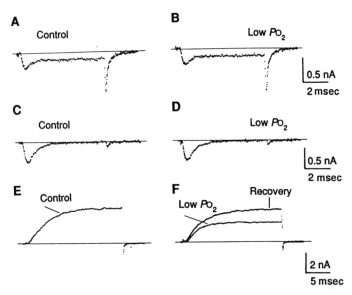

Figure 4   Effect of low Po_2 on the voltage-dependent ionic currents of chemoreceptor cells. (A and B) Na^+ and Ca^{2+} currents recorded by voltage steps to 20 mV from a holding potential of -80 mV in an external solution with a Po_2 of 150 mmHg (control) (A) and 3 min after switching to a solution of the same composition but equilibrated with a Po_2 of 10 mmHg (low Po_2) (B). External solution: 140 mM NaCl, 10 mM $CaCl_2$, 2.7 mM KCl, and 10 mM Hepes; internal solution: 80 mM potassium glutamate, 30 mM KCl, 20 mM KF, 2 mM $MgCl_2$, 10 mM Hepes, and 1 mM EGTA. K^+ currents were abolished by replacement of internal K^+ with Cs^+. Internal solution also contained 3 mM ATP. (C and D) Na^+ currents recorded after depolarization to 10 mV from a holding potential of -80 mV at a Po_2 of 150 and 10 mmHg. Solutions were as in (A) and (B) except for the different external Ca^{2+} concentration (1.5 mM) and the addition of 0.5 mM $CdCl_2$ to block Ca^{2+} channels. (E and F) K^+ currents during 20-msec voltage steps to 40 mV from a holding potential of -80 mV recorded in an external solution with 150 mmHg Po_2 and 10 mmHg Po_2. A reduction in current amplitude of about 45% was observed, which reverted after the reintroduction of the control solution (recovery). Solutions contained 5 mM $CaCl_2$ and TTX (1 µg/ml) externally. The internal solution had 3 mM ATP and 0.5 µM Ca^{2+} (5 mM EGTA plus 4.44 mM $CaCl_2$). (From Lopez-Barneo et al., 1988.)

Properties of Na^+, K^+, and Ca^{2+} Channels in Chemoreceptor Cells from Adult Animals (Fig. 4)

The following presentation of the biophysical properties of ion-selective channels in chemoreceptor cells and their involvement in chemotransduction focuses on data obtained from cultured adult rabbit cells. Studies using other species and/or different developmental stages have confirmed many of these findings, although important differences appear to exist. Except for a limited discussion on ion channel properties in neonatal animals, any comprehensive presentation of such comparative data is considered beyond the scope of this review.

Sodium Currents

The Na$^+$ current of chemoreceptor cells exhibits a fast activation and inactivation, is selectively carried by Na$^+$ ions, and is blocked by nanomolar concentrations of tetrodotoxin. The activation threshold is ≈ -40 mV, with peak current at $+10$ mV and 50% steady-state inactivation at -50 mV (Duchen et al., 1988; Ureña et al., 1989). The average peak Na$^+$ current amplitude recorded from cells without internal Na$^+$ is 0.5 nA, and the calculated Na$^+$ current density is 0.15 mA/cm^2; this Na$^+$ current density is about one-tenth of that for the squid giant axon (Ureña et al., 1989). On switching to current-clamp recording, chemoreceptor cells exhibit spontaneous Na$^+$ potentials, sometimes as trains of spikes, with overshoots between $+15$ mV and $+30$ mV (Duchen et al., 1988; Ureña et al., 1989).

Potassium Currents

Following a depolarizing pulse to $+40$ mV from a holding potential of -80 mV, all chemoreceptor cells generate an outward current that is almost completely blocked by 40 mM tetraethylammonium and that disappears with dialyzing solutions containing 140 mM CsCl in place of KCl (Ureña et al., 1989). Whole-cell K$^+$ currents, identified by these criteria, exhibit a variable Ca^{2+}-dependent component, which declines with time, and which is partly blocked by apamin and nearly completely blocked in the presence of 2 mM Co^{2+} (Ureña et al., 1989; Duchen et al., 1988; Perez-Garcia et al., 1992). The Ca^{2+}-independent component of the K$^+$ current exhibits a threshold of ≈ -30mV. The amplitude of this component increases linearly up to $+60$ to $+70$ mV and shows a tendency to saturate; K$^+$ current amplitude at $+40$ mV is in the range of 1.5–3.5 nA. Activation exhibits a sigmoidal time course (at $+40$ mV, half-maximal amplitude is achieved at 3.9 msec); inactivation occurs with prolonged depolarization (Ureña et al., 1989).

Further analysis of the Ca^{2+}-independent component of the whole-cell K$^+$ current showed that it was composed of two different currents: (1) a transient inactivating current, which represents the largest component ($\approx 90\%$) of the whole-cell outward current in most chemoreceptor cells, and which corresponds to the K$^+$ current that is reversibly inhibited by low PO$_2$, and (2) a residual component that is not inactivating (Lopez-Lopez et al., 1993). The transient K$^+$ current exhibits a threshold at -40 mV, a mean rise time of 4.8 msec at $+60$ mV, and a time course for inactivation that can be described by exponentials with time constants of 80 and 800 msec at $+40$ mV. Steady-state inactivation is absent at -80 mV; inactivation is 50% at -41 mV and complete at -10 mV. Recovery from inactivation has at least two components; i.e., at -100 mV, about 80% of the current recovers in 2 sec, but full recovery requires more than 30 sec (Lopez-Lopez et al., 1993).

The P_{O_2}-sensitive, transient K^+ current in chemoreceptor cells is selectively and completely blocked by 1 mM 4-aminopyridine, with an IC_{50} of 0.2 mM; this drug also augments the duration of action potentials from 2.3 to 7 msec (Lopez-Lopez et al., 1993). Thus, it appears that the P_{O_2}-sensitive, transient K^+ current of chemoreceptor cells shares the properties of transient currents recorded in many other cells (Rudy, 1988) in that it exhibits delayed rectification and A-type K^+ currents. The mixed properties of the O_2-sensitive transient K^+ current allow it to play a role both in action potential repolarization and in the putative pacemaker activity of the chemoreceptor cells (Lopez-Lopez et al., 1989; see Rudy, 1988). In fact, it has been observed that the firing frequency of dialyzed cells increases with decreasing P_{O_2} in the bathing media (Lopez-Lopez et al., 1989). Single channel recordings from isolated membrane patches of adult rabbit chemoreceptor cells have shown that Ca^{2+}-independent channels with conductances of 20 pS reduced their opening probability when the bath P_{O_2} was lowered (Ganfornina and Lopez-Barneo, 1991). It was shown further that the addition of GTP-γ-S, which is known to inhibit the G-protein modulation of ion channels, failed to affect the reversible response to low P_{O_2}. More recently, these authors have carried out a detailed analysis of K^+ channels at the single-channel level and have found that chemoreceptor cells have three types of K^+ channels (Ganfornina and Lopez-Barneo, 1992a,b). In addition to the O_2-sensitive K^+ channel, the cells exhibit Ca^{2+}-dependent K^+ channels with high conductance (≈ 210 pS) and Ca^{2+}-independent K^+ channels with low conductance (≈ 16 pS), which do not show inactivation; neither of these two channels is sensitive to P_{O_2}. It is important to stress the correlation between the findings from the single-channel studies with those obtained from the whole-cell recordings described above. In their single-channel study, Ganfornina and Lopez-Barneo (1992b) kinetically modeled the O_2-sensitive K^+ channel, and according to their construct, low P_{O_2} would tend to maintain the channel in a closed state and drive those channels that do open into a permanent state of inactivation.

Calcium Currents

Ca^{2+} currents have their threshold at ≈ -40 mV, reach a peak at $+20$ mV, and are blocked by 10 mM Mg^{2+}, 2 mM Co^{2+}, and submillimolar Cd^{2+}. Current amplitude is doubled when Ba^{2+} is used as the charge carrier. Ca^{2+} currents are slowly activating (time to peak ≈ 8 msec), slowly inactivating (27% in 300 msec at $+40$ mV), and rapidly deactivating currents (time constant, 0.16 msec at -80 mV); such properties are characteristic features of L-type Ca^{2+} currents (Duchen et al., 1988; Ureña et al., 1989). Peak Ca^{2+} current amplitudes have been found to vary from cell to cell. Thus, Ureña et al. (1989) reported an average peak amplitude of 0.4 nA from eight cells bathed in 10 mM external Ca^{2+}, but a later study observed that it was common to find cells with peak currents near 1 nA (Lopez-Lopez et al., 1993).

Ionic Channels in Chemoreceptor Cells of Neonatal Animals

The electrical properties of chemoreceptor cells have also been studied in dispersed cell preparations from neonatal rats and from rabbit embryos. Peers and coworkers (Peers 1990a,b,c,d; Peers and O'Donnell, 1990a,b; Peers and Green, 1991) found that chemoreceptor cells from neonatal rats lack Na^+ currents, but do exhibit K^+ currents and small Ca^{2+} currents. The Ca^{2+} currents also have the characteristics of L-type currents, including their sensitivity to the dihydropyridines. The I/V relationship for the K^+ current showed a prominent outward shoulder between $+10$ mV and $+30$ mV, which was enhanced both by BayK8644 and by increased extracellular Ca^{2+}, but was insensitive to apamin and reversibly inhibited by charybdotoxin. Superfusion of the dispersed cell preparations with N_2-equilibrated media containing 1 mM sodium dithionite selectively reduced certain K^+ currents, with the greatest effect seen on the Ca^{2+}-dependent component of the K^+ current. Stea and Nurse (1991), on the other hand, observed that chemoreceptor cells from neonatal rats had small tetrodotoxin-sensitive Na^+ currents (usually 50–100 pA), which were usually incapable of generating action potentials; also observed were small Ca^{2+} currents and a K^+ current with a significant Ca^{2+}-dependent component (Stea et al., 1991). Low Po_2 (20–30 mmHg) reversibly inhibited K^+ currents at all the voltages tested. More recently, Nurse and co-workers (Stea et al., 1992) have reported that chemoreceptor cells cultured in low Po_2 atmospheres exhibit increased Na^+ currents, and that cAMP analogs mimic the effects of hypoxia. Chemoreceptor cells from rabbit embryo likewise had high membrane resistances, as well as Ca^{2+} and K^+ voltage-dependent currents, but these were of smaller amplitude than those found in the adult rabbit (Hescheler et al., 1989). It is unknown whether embryonic rabbit chemoreceptor cells express Na^+ currents, but in newborn rabbits Sato et al. showed that a Na^+ channel activator, veratridine, elevates intracellular Ca^{2+} in chemoreceptor cells, an effect that is blocked by tetrodotoxin. Ca^{2+} currents from rabbit embryos were augmented by BayK8644, but were insensitive to Po_2 in the bathing media, while K^+ currents were reversibly inhibited at all the tested voltages when the bath Po_2 was lowered (Hescheler et al., 1989; Hescheler and Delpiano, 1990). Rabbit embryo cells also have a poorly defined, inwardly rectifying K^+ current, which seems to be active at -50 mV and is also reversibly inhibited by low Po_2 (Delpiano and Hescheler, 1989, 1990).

In summary, it is evident that there are differences in the electrical properties of chemoreceptor cells from embryos or neonatal animals and those from adult animals. These developmental differences in the properties of isolated chemo receptor cells may be correlated with the established differences in the functional parameters observed with the intact organs (see Lagercrantz et al., 1991) and undoubtedly reflect the course of postnatal maturation of these chemoreceptor elements. An important common finding is that independent of age, carotid bodies that respond to hypoxia possess chemoreceptor cells with low P_{O_2}-sensitive K^+ currents.

III. Chemosensory Transduction in Carotid Body Chemoreceptor Cells

Chemoreceptor cells are receptor-effector units, which respond to chemoreceptor stimuli by initiating secretory activity involving the release of neurotransmitters and the subsequent activation of CSN sensory terminals. This stimulus-induced release of neurotransmitters, exemplified by the release of DA, depends on the presence of extracellular Ca^{2+} (Obeso et al., 1992; Fishman et al., 1985). In this sense, sensory transduction of chemoreceptor stimuli into a neurosecretory response of these cells is Ca^{2+}-dependent, comparable to the process of stimulus-secretion coupling present in other synapses or secretory cells (see Grundfest, 1971, and Rubin, 1982).

A. Low P_{O_2} Transduction

Based on the above concept of sensory transduction, it is clear that an understanding of the pathways for Ca^{2+} entry into the chemoreceptor cells is a central feature for any description of transductive mechanisms in this arterial chemoreceptor organ.

A Plasma Membrane Model of Low P_{O_2} Transduction

Dihydropyridine blockers of L-type Ca^{2+} channels markedly inhibit the high $[K^+]_e$ and low P_{O_2}-induced release of DA from the cat, rabbit, and rat carotid body, but are without effect on DA release induced by high P_{CO_2}/low pH (Obeso et al., 1987, 1992; Shaw et al., 1989, 1990). The high $[K^+]_e$ and low P_{O_2}-induced release of DA are potentiated by BayK8644, a dihydropyridine agonist of L-type Ca^{2+} channels (Obeso et al., 1992). Consequently, chemosensory transduction of low P_{O_2} stimuli likely involves depolarization of chemoreceptor cells as a necessary step to activate Ca^{2+} channels (see Shirahata and Fitzgerald, 1991), whereas transduction of acidic stimuli may not require chemoreceptor cell depolarization.

It was proposed by Lopez-Barneo et al. (1988) that low P_{O_2} acts on the O_2-sensitive K^+ channel, leading to inhibition of K^+ currents and depolarization of the chemoreceptor cells. Activation of Ca^{2+} channels would trigger neurotransmitter release, thereby initiating chemotransmission in the organ. According to this proposal, inhibition of the transient K^+ current represents the initial electrical event in the cascade of low P_{O_2} transduction (Lopez-Barneo et al., 1988; Lopez-Lopez et al., 1989; Gonzalez et al., 1990; Ganfornina and Lopez-Barneo, 1991, 1992a,b; Gonzalez et al., 1992).

The low P_{O_2} inhibition of the K^+ current develops more rapidly than the tetrodotoxin-mediated inhibition of the Na^+ current, which is known to occur in a few hundred milliseconds. The apparent half-times for inhibition, which include time for arrival of the solutions into the recording chamber, mixing and diffusion times, were 3.68 sec and 7.14 sec for the K^+ and Na^+ currents, respectively (Lopez-Lopez and Gonzalez, 1992). Therefore, contrary to the criticism of Biscoe and Duchen (1990), inhibition of the K^+ currents by low P_{O_2} temporally matches the known dynamic properties of the hypoxic response of the in situ carotid body preparation (Ponte and Purves, 1974; Fig. 5).

The relationship between K^+ current inhibition and the opening probability of K^+ channels to low P_{O_2} does not, however, show obvious correlations with the responses obtained from the intact carotid body preparation. The maximum inhibition of the K^+ current by low P_{O_2} in whole-cell recordings was observed at ≈ 85 mmHg P_{O_2}, and the same degree of inhibition was observed at 10, 65, and 110 mmHg P_{O_2} (Lopez-Lopez et al., 1989); in single-channel recordings from isolated membrane patches, the maximum decrease in the opening probability was seen at a P_{O_2} of 100 mmHg, and the same decrease was observed at 50 and 130 mmHg P_{O_2} (Ganfornina and Lopez-Barneo, 1991). Thus, neither the threshold responses nor the peculiar shapes of these relationships are correlated with the observed tissue P_{O_2}, the CSN discharges, or the release of DA that occurs during hypoxic stimulation. One possibility, however, is that the lack of feedback modulation by released neurotransmitters (Gomez-Niño et al., 1989) from the isolated chemoreceptor cell preparation may contribute to a low P_{O_2} hypersensitivity by these cells, distorting the normal relationship between P_{O_2} and K^+ current inhibition (see Fuortes, 1971). In addition to the possible need for extracellular messengers, the lack of intracellular (e.g., second) messengers in dialyzed cells or isolated patches may also alter the relationship between P_{O_2} and K^+ current inhibition. In this regard, it is noteworthy that a cell-permeant analog of cAMP inhibited the transient K^+ current in a manner strikingly similar to that for low P_{O_2} (Lopez-Lopez et al., 1993). This observation gains physiological significance from the finding that low P_{O_2} increases cAMP levels in the carotid body (Perez-Garcia, 1990; Wang et al., 1991; Delpiano and Acker, 1991), and that the shape of the relationship between P_{O_2} and cAMP content is very similar to that between P_{O_2} and K^+ current inhibition, except for a displacement to the left by about 40 mmHg (Perez-Garcia et al., 1990; see Fig. 7A). Thus, it is conceivable that cAMP modulation of the K^+ current shifts the P_{O_2}-dependent inhibition to a physiologically relevant P_{O_2} and smooths the humps in the curve that relate P_{O_2} and K^+ current inhibition; this suggestion, however, must await experimental verification.

To establish that inhibition of the O_2-sensitive K^+ current is the initial

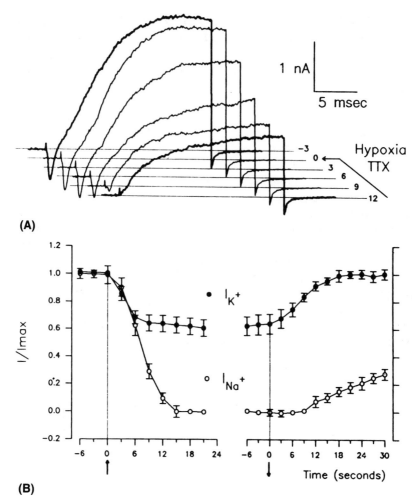

(A)

(B)

Figure 5   Time course of the inhibition of the Na^+ and K^+ currents in hypoxic TTX-containing solution. (A) Whole-cell clamp records of Na^+ and K^+ currents from a chemoreceptor cell before and after the application of a hypoxic N_2-equilibrated solution (bath $Po_2 \approx 5$ mmHg) containing 0.1 μm TTX. The currents were elicited by test pulses (20 msec; +20 mV) applied every 3 sec. Leak substraction pulses to −120 mV were applied between test pulses. (B) Average time courses of the inhibition of K^+ and Na^+ currents by the hypoxic TTX-containing solution (left) and of their recovery on returning to control solution (right). Solutions were changed as indicated by arrows. The amplitudes of both currents were normalized. Values are means ± SEM of six individual data. (From Lopez-Lopez and Gonzalez, 1992.)

electrical event in chemotransduction of low P_{O_2} stimuli, it is necessary to show that these K^+ channels are active at the normal resting membrane potential of the chemoreceptor cells. A comparison has been made between carotid body chemoreceptor cells and gustatory taste cells (see Lopez-Barneo et al., 1988). However, the sugar-transducing K^+ channel of taste cells is not voltage dependent, but is active at the resting membrane potential, and therefore the sugar-triggered kinase-A-dependent phosphorylation of the K^+ channel closes the channel and depolarizes the taste cells (Avenet et al., 1988; Tonosaki and Funakoshi, 1988; Kinnamon, 1988). In chemoreceptor cells, the O_2-sensitive K^+ current is voltage dependent, with an apparent activation threshold of ≈ -40 mV, and the resting membrane potential is likely in the range of -55 mV (see earlier). Consequently, it remains to be shown how inhibition of the K^+ current by low P_{O_2} leads to depolarization of the chemoreceptor cells. However, a factor that should be considered here is that chemoreceptor cells may exhibit spontaneous action potentials. These cells possess the required conductances for action potential generation, and it has been found that dialyzed cells do generate spontaneous action potentials, the frequency of which increases when the bath P_{O_2} is lowered (Lopez-Lopez et al., 1989). Additionally, it has been shown that tetrodotoxin partially inhibits the low P_{O_2}-induced release of DA (Gonzalez et al., 1990), and that the release of DA induced by 4-aminopyridine at normal P_{O_2} is partly inhibited by tetrodotoxin (Gonzalez, Lopez-Lopez, and Perez-Garcia, unpublished). These data suggest that chemoreceptor cells generate Na^+-dependent action potentials. Thus, if chemoreceptor cells in situ do in fact elicit spontaneous action potentials, then the inhibition of the K^+ current by low P_{O_2} should increase their firing frequency, as occurs in dialyzed chemoreceptor cells (Lopez-Lopez et al., 1989). The tentative conclusion here is that there exists a reasonable experimental basis on which to propose that the low P_{O_2} inhibition of the transient K^+ current may indeed represent the initial electrical event in the chemosensory transduction of hypoxic stimuli.

This proposed mechanism for O_2 chemotransduction does not address the issues of where in the chemoreceptor cells the low P_{O_2} stimulus is detected, or how the detected signal reduces the open probability of the O_2-sensitive K^+ channel. As stated earlier, the O_2 chemosensor must have a moderate affinity for O_2 in order to account for the well-known relationship among P_{O_2}, CSN discharge, and DA release. Thus, the O_2 chemosensor should have a lower affinity for O_2 than does hemoglobin, in order to account for an apparent P_{50} for CSN discharge at about 40 mmHg P_{O_2} (Lahiri and Delaney, 1976). In proposing the above-described mechanism for O_2 chemotransduction, Gonzalez et al. (1992, 1993) have incorporated into the model a notion originally put forth by Lloyd and co-workers (1968) and later revived by Lahiri and co-workers (Lahiri and Delaney, 1976; Lahiri, 1977, 1981), namely, that chemoreceptor cells have a hemoglobin-like O_2-sensor molecule that reports the P_{O_2} level to the cellular machinery as the degree of the molecule's O_2 saturation.

The idea that chemoreceptor cells may have a hemoglobin-like O_2 chemosensor gained support from data obtained from another O_2-sensitive cell line, i.e., human hepatoma cells, which increase their production of erythropoietin upon exposure to lowered P_{O_2} (Goldberg et al., 1988). Inhibition of heme synthesis either by chelating iron in the culture medium or by blocking δ-aminolevulinate reductase blocks this response to low P_{O_2}. The response to low O_2 is also blocked when carbon monoxide is introduced into the culture medium to balance the decrease in P_{O_2} (Goldberg et al., 1988); the rationale here is that carbon monoxide reacts only with iron-containing proteins, which appears to be the case for most biological systems (Coburn and Forman, 1987). In the carotid body, carbon monoxide is also able to prevent (and reverse) the effects of low P_{O_2} on the chemoreceptor cells; thus, the inhibition of the O_2-sensitive K^+ current produced when the P_{O_2} in the bathing solution is decreased from 150 mmHg to ≈33 mmHg was reduced by 70% in the presence of 70 mmHg carbon monoxide (Lopez-Lopez and Gonzalez, 1992). This finding strongly suggests that an iron protein, probably a hemeprotein, is involved in sensing P_{O_2}. Furthermore, the fact that low P_{O_2} reduces the open probability of K^+ channels in isolated patches of chemoreceptor cell membrane localizes the O_2 sensor to the plasma membrane (Ganfornina and Lopez-Barneo, 1991, 1992a,b). While Ganfornina and Lopez-Barneo (1991) suggested that the O_2-sensitive K^+ channel itself is the O_2 chemosensor, Lopez-Lopez and Gonzalez (1992) favored the notion that the O_2 chemosensor was a molecule independent of the K^+ channel, but at present, there are no experimental data to distinguish between these possibilities.

Another chemosensor mechanism has been proposed by Acker and his co-workers (Acker et al., 1989; Cross et al., 1990), who have suggested that the O_2 sensor in chemoreceptor cells could be a heme-linked NADPH oxidase. According to this proposal, hypoxia would reduce the amount of H_2O_2 generated by the oxidase, thereby leading to changes in the redox state of glutathione. Transitional changes in oxidized/reduced glutathione would alter the configuration of cell membrane proteins and hence the membrane ionic conductances. Moreover, it has recently been reported that transient K^+ channels are selectively affected by H_2O_2 (Vega-Saenz de Miera and Rudy, 1992). However, it should be recalled that isolated membrane patches from chemoreceptor cells, which are presumably devoid of any intracellular cofactors, nonetheless exhibit K^+ channels whose open probability is decreased when the P_{O_2} in the bathing media is lowered (Ganfornina and Lopez-Barneo, 1991).

Mitochondrial Model of P_{O_2} Transduction

Other proposed mechanisms of chemotransduction, which may be grouped collectively under the term "metabolic hypotheses," have suggested that O_2 sensing by chemoreceptor cells is linked to mitochondrial structure and function.

A metabolic hypothesis was first put forth by Anichkov and Belenki'i (1963) and was based on the observation that metabolic poisons known to decrease ATP levels in other structures produced excitation of the carotid chemoreceptors. It was reasoned that low P_{O_2} should likewise decrease ATP levels in the carotid body, leading to chemoreceptor activation. The validity of this hypothesis was later questioned on theoretical grounds (Forster, 1968), because the estimated decay in P_{O_2} between the tissue capillaries and the core of the parenchymal cell lobules, at a blood P_{O_2} where the carotid body is discharging at more than half its maximal rate, was too small to achieve the required decrease in electron transport along the respiratory chain (and hence ATP production; Coxon, 1968). Later, a low O_2-affinity cytochrome oxidase was reported for chemoreceptor cells, leading to a reappraisal of the metabolic hypothesis (Mills and Jobsis, 1972; Mills, 1972, 1975; but see also Acker and Eyzaguirre, 1987). In the early 1980s, Lahiri and co-workers used the drug oligomycin in a series of experimental studies that revitalized the concept that a decrease in the phosphate potential i.e., the [ATP]/[ADP][P_i] quotient, might trigger the O_2 response by the chemoreceptor cells. The presence of a low O_2-affinity cytochrome oxidase meant that the decrease in phosphate potential could occur at a blood P_{O_2} of 70 mmHg (Mulligan et al., 1982; Mulligan and Lahiri, 1981; Shirahata et al., 1987). More recently, these investigators have proposed a similar model that is not dependent on the presence of a unique low O_2-affinity cytochrome oxidase, but rather relies on modern concepts of mitochondrial respiration (Wilson et al., 1988; Rumsey et al., 1991). All the various versions of metabolic hypotheses depart from the premise stated earlier that chemoreceptor cells must maintain an adequate energy supply throughout their full range of physiological function. Independent of the relationship between the decrease in ATP and the increase in chemoreceptor response, it is clear that the greater the chemoresponse, the higher are the energetic requirements of the chemoreceptor cell, which must be met in the face of an ever-decreasing supply of ATP. Another difficulty with the metabolic hypothesis is that the link between a decrease in ATP and the Ca^{2+}-triggered release of neurotransmitters has remained unclear.

Variants of the metabolic hypothesis have been advanced by Leitner and co-workers (Roumy and Leitner, 1977; Bernon et al., 1983) and more recently by Biscoe and co-workers (Biscoe and Duchen, 1989, 1990a,b,c; Biscoe et al., 1989). Leitner's group used ruthenium red and Ca^{2+}-containing liposomes in their experiments, and concluded that cytoplasmic Ca^{2+} in carotid body cells increased in parallel with the level of CSN discharge. Ruthenium red was thought to act by blocking the Ca^{2+}-buffering capacity of mitochondria, thereby leading to increased cytoplasmic Ca^{2+} and the release of neurotransmitters from the chemoreceptor cells; low P_{O_2} might presumably act in a similar manner. From the experiments of Biscoe and co-workers, it was proposed that low P_{O_2} would slow electron transfer through the mitochondrial respiratory chain of chemoreceptor cells, leading to an immediate decrease in the proton electrochemical gradient of the mitochondria. This would result in the release of mitochondrial Ca^{2+}, leading to an increase in $[Ca^{2+}]_i$ and the release of neurotransmitters from the cells. In addition, the low O_2-affinity cytochrome oxidase was incorporated into this model, which allowed it to operate over the full physiological range of the chemoreceptor response to low Po_2. Problems with this model have been discussed at length by Gonzalez et al. (1992, 1993). Furthermore, Duchen and Biscoe (1992) have recently concluded that mitochondria are not the source of Ca^{2+} required for the neurosecretory response, which they concluded must come instead from some other intracellular source. Whatever the intracellular Ca^{2+} source proposed for this model, it remains to be considered that the low Po_2-induced release of DA is greatly ($\approx 95\%$) dependent on extracellular Ca^{2+} and is markedly inhibited by blockers of voltage-dependent Ca^{2+} channels (Fidone et al., 1982; Obeso et al., 1987, 1992; Shaw et al., 1989). Yet another view regarding the role of cytoplasmic Ca^{2+} during hypoxia was presented by Donnelly and Kholwadwala (1992); these workers reported a decrease in Ca^{2+}_i in acutely isolated adult rat chemoreceptor cells exposed to hypoxia.

Another important point recently addressed by Biscoe and Duchen (1992a,b) relates to the nature and/or location of the O_2 sensor in the chemoreceptor cells. These authors undertook an extensive analysis of the Po_2 dependence of mitochondrial membrane potential and NADH autofluorescence in chemoreceptor cells and compared these parameters with measurements made in adrenomedullary cells and dorsal root ganglion neurons. In chemoreceptor cells, it was observed that at a bath Po_2 of about 60 mmHg, which resulted in a tissue Po_2 very close to threshold for the carotid body hypoxic response (see earlier; Whalen et al., 1983), the mitochondrial membrane potential decreased while the NADH signal increased. Below this threshold Po_2 of 60 mmHg, the relationship between the mitochondrial parameters and Po_2 was very similar to that relating Po_2 to CSN discharge. In contrast, the same mitochondrial parameters for nonchemoreceptor cells remained unaltered until the bath Po_2 was lowered to 10 mmHg. Based on these apparent unique properties of chemoreceptor cell mitochondria, it was proposed that the Po_2 chemosensors are the mitochondria themselves.

A possible problem with this interpretation, however, arises from a comparison of the Po_2 dependence of mitochondrial parameters in resting cells (i.e., the sensory neurons and adrenomedullary cells) with the same parameters in activated cells (i.e., chemoreceptor cells in low Po_2). It is important to compare these mitochondrial parameters when nonchemoreceptor excitable cells become activated. Judging from the literature, they likely would behave similarly to chemoreceptor cells exposed to low Po_2 (see Erescinka and Wilson, 1982; Erescinka and Dagani, 1989). Thus, activation of excitable cells results in increased K^+ efflux and increased Na^+ and Ca^{2+} influx. Increased Na^+ influx leads to activation of the Na^+/K^+ pump, which in turn increases the expenditure of ATP, producing a drop in the phosphate potential, ($[ATP]/[ADP][P_i]$). In other cells, it has been demonstrated that the Na^+/K^+-triggered decrease in the phosphate potential is primarily responsible for the increase in metabolic rate observed during cell activation, and furthermore that inhibition of the Na^+/K^+ pump completely blocks the metabolic response (Mata et al., 1980; Yarowsky and Ingvar, 1981; Erescinka et al., 1990). Increase in the metabolic rate means an increase in the transference of equivalents of reduction through the respiratory chain and consequently an increase in the NADH/NAD ratio. The ensuing increase in ATP synthesis implies increased entry of H^+ ion at the ATPase site of the mitochondria, leading to a drop in the mitochondrial potential (i.e., mitochondrial depolarization). Increased influx of Ca^{2+} during cell activation would enhance metabolism by activating mitochondrial dehydrogenases (McCormack et al., 1990). Such sequelae to cell activation are well established in many cell types, but only partially explored for the carotid body (but see below). Nonetheless, it appears that these changes in mitochondrial parameters associated with hypoxic stimulation of the carotid body reflect a series of second- or third-order events that are universal mechanisms in the activation of any cell type and necessarily follow the primary events associated with cell depolarization. Support for this conclusion has recently been obtained for the carotid body in experiments demonstrating that low Po_2 stimulation increases glucose consumption by the organ; as in other excitable tissues, this increased metabolic response is completely blocked by ouabain, but only marginally reduced by removal of extracellular Ca^{2+} (Obeso et al., 1993; compare with Mata et al., 19890, and Erescinka et al., 1990).

B. High Pco_2/Low pH Chemotransduction

Intracellular Hydrogen Concentration: The Sensed Parameter Is Acidosis

It had been debated for many years whether CO_2 activates the carotid chemoreceptors exclusively via its acidifying action or involves in addition pH-independent effects on the receptor. At present, the general consensus is that CO_2 activates chemoreceptor cells through intracellular acidification (see Fidone and Gonzalez, 1986). Likewise, extracellular changes in pH perturb the chemoreceptor cells by concomitantly affecting intracellular pH (Hanson et al., 1981; Rocher et al., 1991; Rigual et al., 1991, 1985; Buckler et al., 1991a,b). On this basis, the transduction of hypercapnic/low pH stimuli by chemoreceptor cells corresponds to the series of receptor-effector events associated with an increase in intracellular hydrogen ion concentration.

To consider first how a decrease in pH_i might be generated, it is well known that three simultaneous processes help maintain steady-state pH_i: metabolic H^+ production, H^+ efflux, and H^+ influx (Roos and Boron, 1981). A modification in any of these processes alters pH_i. When pH_e is decreased, the electrochemical

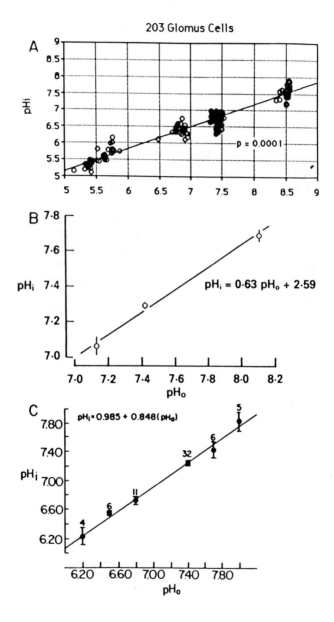

203 Glomus Cells

gradient causes increased H^+ influx. At a pH_e of 7.4, chemoreceptor cells with a membrane potential at ≈ -55 mV reach H^+ equilibrium when pH_i falls to 6.48; that is, under resting conditions, there is a net tendency for H^+ to enter the cells, a tendency that increases with decreasing pH_e, and vice versa. The passive membrane permeability of chemoreceptor cells to H^+ appears to be high, as evident from the step dependence of pH_i on pH_e and the rapid change in pH_i when pH_e is modified (He et al., 1990; Buckler et al., 1991; Wilding et al., 1992). The decrease in pH_e may inhibit H^+ extrusion mechanisms (Boron 1986; Boron and Knakal, 1992), but at the same time these mechanisms become activated by the concomitant decrease in pH_i (Boron, 1986; Grinstein and Rothstein, 1986; Clark and Limbird, 1991). Finally, intracellular acidification reduces metabolic acid production as a mechanism of defense against acid load (Roos and Boron, 1981); thus, rabbit carotid bodies incubated in HEPES-buffered media at pH_e of 7 and 6.8 lowered their glucose consumption by 30% and 40%, respectively (Obeso et al., 1993; see above, Fig. 3A). The net result of these several processes is that a unit change in pH_e in the range 5.5–8.5 produces a directional steady-state change in pH_i of the chemoreceptor cells equal to 0.7–0.8 pH unit, independent of whether the bathing solution is buffered with HEPES or CO_2/bicarbonate (He et al., 1990; Buckler et al., 1991; Wilding et al., 1992; Fig. 6).

Elevation of PCO_2 decreases pH_i by producing a net injection of H^+ into the cells, as CO_2 diffuses inside and becomes hydrated, liberating H^+ ions; this hydration is greatly accelerated by the presence of carbonic anhydrase in the chemoreceptor cells (Rigual et al., 1985). Under conditions of simulated noncompensated respiratory acidosis (increased PCO_2 and decreased pH_e), the above arguments hold; the only difference for simulated metabolic acidosis (normal PCO_2 and reduced bicarbonate and pH_e) is the half-time for the change in pH_i, which was found to be almost instantaneous for respiratory acidosis, but about 1 min for metabolic acidosis. A controversial point here is the time course of pH_i under conditions of isohydric hypercapnia. Gray (1968) observed that CSN discharge was not sustained under these conditions, but other investigators reported the contrary for both in vivo and in vitro preparations (Biscoe et al., 1970; Rigual

---

Figure 6   (A) Effects of changing extracellular pH (pH_o) on intracellular pH (pH_i). As the medium becomes acidic (pH < 7.43), pH_i follows. When the medium is alkaline (pH > 7.43), pH_i increases but to levels lower than pH_o. P = significance level of regressions. (From He et al., 1990.) (B) Effects on pH_i of changing pH_o (by altering PCO_2 at constant $[HCO_3^-]_o$). Data are means ± SEM from seven experiments. Line of best fit determined by linear regression; regression coefficient = 0.95. (From Wilding et al., 1992.) (C) Relationship between pH_i and pH_o in the nominal absence of CO_2. Means ± SEM; 32 cells. Correlation coefficient = 0.995. Each experiment was started at pH_o 7.40. (From Wilding et al., 1992.)

et al., 1991; Iturriaga et al., 1991). Buckler et al. (1991) and Wilding (1992) measured pH_i in isolated chemoreceptor cells from neonatal and adult rats, and found, in agreement with Gray's earlier observations, that isohydric hypercapnia produces a transient decrease in pH_i, which subsequently returns to near-normal levels within a few minutes; however, some dependence of steady-state pH_i on P_{CO_2} was observed. In view of these apparently contradictory experimental data, the issue remains unresolved at the present time (but see below).

Other experimental maneuvers, including superfusion with solutions containing weak acids, protonophores, or 2-deoxyglucose, have been used to produce intracellular acidification of chemoreceptor cells at normal pH_e, to test the notion that an increase in $[H^+]_i$ stimulates these cells. Weak acids permeate the cells in their protonized form but dissociate inside the cells, releasing H^+ and decreasing pH_i (Roos and Boron, 1981; Boron, 1986). Protonophores, such as dinitrophenol, greatly increase H^+ membrane permeability and allow H^+ ions to distribute across the cell membrane in electrochemical equilibrium, thereby driving pH_i of the chemoreceptor cells to 6.48 without any change in membrane potential (Grinstein and Cohen, 1987). The glucose analog, 2-deoxyglucose, also produces intracellular acidification when applied at millimolar concentrations, by yet unknown mechanisms (Grinstein and Furuya, 1986). Each of these maneuvers activates the carotid body chemoreceptors, producing proportional increases in both the release of DA and CSN discharge (Fidone et al., 1990).

A Model Explaining the Coupling Between Increased Intracellular Hydrogen Ion Concentration and the Activation of Chemoreceptor Cells

Having defined the chemosensory parameter for acidic/hypercapnic stimulation to be an increase in $[H^+]_i$, it remains to be shown how this increase in $[H^+]_i$ leads to the release of neurotransmitters from the chemoreceptor cells. Interestingly, the final proposal by Torrance and co-workers (Hanson et al., 1981) regarding the acidic hypothesis of chemoreception acknowledged the importance of this question, but could provide no answer at that time. It is now known from studies of cellular pH regulation that when cells are challenged by an intracellular acid load, they respond by extruding H^+, which eventually leads to partial or total recovery of the original intracellular pH and a net gain of intracellular Na^+. Thus emerged the notion of Na^+-dependent mechanisms for proton extrusion (see Roos and Boron, 1981; Thomas, 1984; Aronson, 1985; Boron, 1986; Grinstein and Rothstein, 1986; Wray, 1988; Clark and Limbird, 1991). Rather than considering all the possible mechanisms involved in pH_i homeostasis, suffice it to state here that the Na^+/H^+ and Na^+/H^+-HCO_3^-/Cl^- exchangers belonging to the category of Na^+-dependent H^+ extruding mechanisms are the most important systems for maintaining pH_i during acid challenge (Boron, 1986; Ganz et al., 1989; Boron et al.,

1989). In regard to the net Na^+ gain during acid load, if the cells have a Na^+/Ca^{2+} exchanger it is possible to reverse its resting function, so that Na^+ is extruded instead and there is a net influx of Ca^{2+}, thereby triggering $[Ca^{2+}]_i$-dependent cellular responses (Mullins, 1984; Grinstein and Rothstein, 1986; Blaustein, 1988). Such appears to be the case in cardiac muscle cells, where it has been shown that an acid challenge is associated with an increase both in $[Na^+]_i$ and in the Ca^{2+}-dependent generation of muscle tension (Bountra and Vaughan-Jones, 1989).

Experiments designed to explore these relationships in the carotid body demonstrated that intracellular acidifying stimuli such as high P_{CO_2}/low pH, weak acids, 2-deoxyglucose, and dinitrophenol induced a release of DA from chemoreceptor cells that was Ca^{2+} dependent and insensitive to the dihydropyridines (Obeso et al., 1986, 1989, 1992; Rigual et al., 1991; Rocher et al., 1990, 1991). Experimental maneuvers that tested for the presence of a Na^+/Ca^{2+} exchanger in chemoreceptor cells (e.g., Na^+_e removal and Na^+/K^+ pump inhibition by ouabain or K^+_e removal) produced an intense release of DA, which was Ca^{2+}_e- and Na^+_e-dependent and insensitive to Ca^{2+} channel blockers. Such findings clearly indicated that the chemoreceptor cells possess a strong Na^+/Ca^{2+} exchanger (Rocher et al., 1991). A link between the increase in $[H^+]_i$ and the influx of Ca^{2+} via the Na^+/Ca^{2+} exchanger was established in further experiments that showed that DA release induced by acidic stimuli was Na^+-dependent and sensitive to the blockade of H^+ extrusion mechanisms.

Based on these observations, the following sequence of events was proposed for chemosensory transduction of acidic stimuli: on exposure to the acidic stimulus, pH_i falls and the Na^+/H^+ and Na^+-dependent anion exchanger becomes activated, resulting in H^+ extrusion and the influx and Na^+; an increase in $[Na^+]_i$ modifies the reversal potential of the Na^+/Ca^{2+} exchanger, so that at normal resting potential the exchanger extrudes Na^+ in exchange for Ca^{2+} influx. The influx of Ca^{2+} triggers the exocytosis of neurotransmitters (Rocher et al., 1991; Gonzalez et al., 1992, 1993). Simple calculations show that a minimal gain of Na^+_i can alter the operational direction of the exchanger (Gonzalez et al., 1990; see Mullins, 1984).

Evidence from isolated chemoreceptor cells supports this model of chemosensory transduction of acidic stimuli. Thus, adult rabbit chemoreceptor cells have been shown to possess a strong Na^+/Ca^{2+} exchanger (Biscoe et al., 1989), and the presence of Na^+/H^+ and Na^+-dependent anion exchangers has been demonstrated for neonatal rat chemoreceptor cells (Buckler et al., 1991). In addition to Na^+-dependent H^+ extrusion mechanisms, adult rat chemoreceptor cells may also possess a K^+/H^+ exchanger (Wilding et al., 1991). Although an increase in $[Ca^{2+}]_i$ during acidic stimulation has been questioned (Biscoe et al., 1989), two recent studies have reported an increase in $[Ca^{2+}]_i$ during superfusion with low pH solutions buffered with CO_2/bicarbonate or HEPES (Buckler and Vaughan-Jones, 1992; Sato et al., 1993). Exposure to isohydric-hypercapnic solutions also increases $[Ca^{2+}]_i$; following an initial spike-like increase, $[Ca^{2+}]_i$ adapts but does not return to basal levels. Thus, it appears that a sustained increase in $[Ca^{2+}]_i$ capable of driving the release of neurotransmitters occurs during isohydric-hypercapnic stimulation.

Some aspects of this model for chemosensory transduction of acidic stimuli need to be explored in greater depth. For example, the kinetic properties of the exchangers should be studied, to determine whether their operation matches the characteristic rapid onset of the chemoreceptor response to acidic stimuli (Ponte and Purves, 1974). The effects of simultaneous low P_{O_2} stimulation should be examined to verify that exchanger functions can account for the known inter-actions between acidic and hypoxic stimuli (see Fidone and Gonzalez, 1986). Finally, the model should operate at the resting membrane potential of the chemoreceptor cells and undergo increased activation on depolarization. However, it has been reported that low pH_e inhibits K^+ currents in adult chemoreceptor cells (Lopez-Lopez et al., 1989; Stea et al., 1991), and that in neonatal rats, low pH_e or selective intracellular acidification inhibits Ca^{2+}-dependent K^+ currents without affecting Ca^{2+} (Peers, 1990; Peers and O'Donnell, 1990a,b; Peers and Green, 1991); such findings suggest that transduction of acidic stimuli might involve significant changes in the membrane potential of chemoreceptor cells. In recent experiments exploring the pH dependence of the three principal ionic currents in adult rabbit chemoreceptor cells, it was found that low pH inhibited these currents with the same pK, making it unlikely that membrane potential plays a key role in the response to acidic stimuli (Lopez-Lopez, Ganfornina, and Lopez-Barneo, unpublished; see also Kinnamon, 1988). For many different tissues, low pH on either side of the cell's plasma membrane reduces the peak amplitude of Na^+, K^+, and Ca^{2+} currents (Brown and Noble, 1978; Hagiwara et al., 1978; Yatani and Goto, 1983; Krafte and Kass, 1988; see Hille, 1984).

In conclusion, the experimental evidence suggests that low P_{O_2} and high P_{CO_2}/low pH are independent, but interacting, stimuli that have fundamentally different mechanisms for chemotransduction in adult mammalian chemoreceptor cells. This viewpoint is contrary to earlier proposals (Torrance, 1974; Hanson et al., 1981), but receives convincing experimental support from the observed differences in the effects of low P_{O_2} and acidic stimuli on the ionic currents of chemoreceptor cells, as well as from the differences in time course and pharmaco-logical properties of carotid body responses to low P_{O_2} versus high P_{CO_2}/low pH (Rocher et al., 1981; Obeso et al., 1992; Iturriaga et al., 1991).

C. Second Messengers and Chemoreceptor Cell Function

For the most part, the literature on the role of second messengers in carotid body chemoreception has evolved during the last 5 years, and only limited aspects of their functional biology and significance in this organ are known at the present time.

Cyclic AMP

Joels and Neil (1968) first suggested a role for cAMP in the excitation of chemoreceptor discharge by adrenaline. They observed that perfusion of the carotid bifurcation with 10^{-4} M cAMP increased CSN discharge and potentiated the response to cyanide. A decade later, the levels of cAMP were measured in rat and cat carotid bodies. In the rat, basal cAMP levels were 45 pmole/pair of carotid bodies ($\approx$400 pmole/mg), and this was increased to $\approx$510 pmole/mg following exposure to severe hypoxia (two 20-min periods at 5% O_2 with 1 hr interim at room air; Hanbauer, 1977). In the cat, incubation of the carotid body for 15 min in 10 mM theophyline yielded cAMP levels of 20 pmole/carotid body ($\approx$40 pmole/ mg), while incubation in 200 μM DA elevated the nucleotide levels between 20 and 30% (Fitzgerald et al., 1977). A later study also in the cat reported seasonal fluctuations in basal cAMP levels in the carotid body, ranging between 0.1 and 1.5 pmole/carotid body ($\approx$0.2–3 pmole/mg); exposure of the cats to an atmosphere of 5% O_2 for 3, 10, or 20 min yielded an average cAMP level (pooled samples from all time groups) that was significantly higher than in the control carotid bodies (Delpiano et al., 1984). Basal cAMP levels in rabbit and rat carotid bodies incubated in IBMX were reported to be 0.69 and 0.59 pmole/carotid body ($\approx$1.7 and 9.83 pmole/mg), respectively (Mir et al., 1983, 1984). It was also observed in this study that isoproterenol (10^{-5} M) boosted cAMP levels 10-fold, but that NE, serotonin, DA, and adenosine had no effect on the nucleotide levels. Furthermore, hypoxic exposure to an atmosphere of 5% O_2 for 2–5 min failed to alter cAMP levels in the rat carotid body. Taken together, data from these earlier studies were inconclusive in establishing a significant role for cAMP in carotid body chemoreception.

More recent publications (Wang et al., 1989, 1991; Perez-Garcia et al., 1990a,b, 1991, 1992; Almaraz et al., 1991; Delpiano and Acker, 1991), while still sharing discrepancies, are nonetheless consistent in demonstrating that low P_{O_2} stimulation increased cAMP content in rabbit and cat carotid bodies incubated under a variety of conditions, including Ca^{2+}-free media. In two of these studies (Wang et al., 1991; Delpiano and Acker, 1991), it was found that basal cAMP levels, as well as low P_{O_2}-elevated cAMP levels, were both increased in Ca^{2+}-free media, which suggests that Ca^{2+}_i may activate phosphodiesterases (Hanbauer, 1977). This latter suggestion is supported by the observation that in Ca^{2+}-free media, and in the presence of a phosphodiesterase inhibitor (IBMX), basal and low P_{O_2}-stimulated carotid bodies showed reduced cAMP levels compared to their controls in Ca^{2+}- and IBMX-containing media, although the average ratio for basal/stimulated cAMP levels were similar to those found with normal Ca^{2+} media

(Perez-Garcia et al., 1990a,b; Fig. 7A). The observed difference in cAMP levels in control versus Ca^{2+}-free media at any P_{O_2} (test range 5–660 mmHg) was attributed to the suppression of neurotransmitter release by the zero Ca^{2+} media. This in turn would result in the loss of feedback effects on adenylate cyclase activity mediated by neurotransmitter autoreceptors located on the chemoreceptor cells. In support of this interpretation, it was shown that exogenously applied NE and DA augmented cAMP levels in the carotid body (Perez-Garcia et al., 1990, 1993). Other stimuli, such as high P_{CO_2}/low pH, cyanide, and high $[K^+]_e$, increased cAMP levels only in Ca^{2+}-containing media, thereby reinforcing the above interpretation and indicating further that low P_{O_2} was the only chemoreceptor stimulus capable of activating adenylate cyclase independent of feedback effects via released neurotransmitters (Perez-Garcia et al., 1990a,b). It was also shown that forskolin (an activator of adenylate cyclase), IBMX, and dibutyryl-cAMP increased the stimulus-induced release of catecholamines from the carotid body (Perez-Garcia et al., 1991; Wang et al., 1991); forskolin also augmented the low P_{O_2}-induced increase in CSN discharge (Wang et al., 1991; Fig. 7B). It appears that cAMP may function to inhibit the O_2-sensitive K^+ current in the carotid body (Lopez-Lopez et al., 1993; see above), yet the nucleotide is not necessary for the inhibition of the transductive current (Ganfornina and Lopez-Barneo, 1991, 1992a,b). It may be through this mechanism that cAMP potentiates the low P_{O_2}-induced release of DA. A direct action of cAMP on the exocytotic machinery would explain the effect of the nucleotide on DA release evoked by other stimuli, and perhaps also for that evoked by low P_{O_2}. Forskolin, probably acting through cAMP, has been shown to selectively increase DA synthesis (Perez-Garcia et al., 1991), which suggests that tyrosine hydroxylase in the chemoreceptor cells is modulated by kinase-A-dependent phosphorylation.

Cyclic GMP

cGMP levels in the carotid body are decreased by hypoxic stimulation and are increased by high K^+_e and sodium nitroprusside; these effects were immuno-histochemically demonstrated to occur both within the parenchymal cell lobules and in carotid body blood vessels (Fidone et al., 1990; Wang et al., 1991). Marked increases in cGMP levels in the carotid body are produced by exogenous administration of atrial natriuretic peptide (ANP) or its analogs, and it has been shown in immunocytochemical experiments that the increase in nucleotide levels occurs in the chemoreceptor cells (Wang et al., 1991, 1993). It was also shown that ANP could inhibit CSN discharge evoked by hypoxia or nicotine, and that these effects were mimicked by cell-permeant analogs of cGMP. However, in Ca^{2+}-free media, ANP failed to alter CSN discharge elicited by 20 mM K^+ (Wang et al., 1993). Additionally, it was observed that neither ANP nor cell-permanent analogs of cGMP had any affect on the release of DA elicited by hypoxia. Thus, it appears

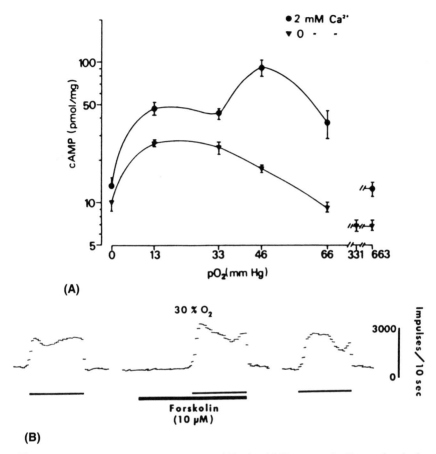

(A)

(B)

Figure 7 (A) Effects of O_2 tension on carotid body cAMP content. In all cases incubation lasted 10 min and the Po_2 was assessed with an O_2 electrode in replicate samples. The media contained 0.5 mM IBMX. The effects of Po_2 in Ca^{2+}-free medium were evaluated in tissues preincubated and incubated in the absence of Ca^{2+}. The data are means ± SEM of 8–10 CBs (From Perez-Garcia et al., 1990b.) (B) Effect of forskolin on CSN activity evoked in a superfusion drop chamber by media equilibrated with 30% O_2 (balance N_2). The three consecutive traces show the basal (100% O_2 media) and stimulus-evoked discharge during 5-min stimulus periods. The introduction of forskolin for 5 min before stimulation did not alter the basal discharge, but the drug augmented the response to the lowered O_2 tension. After the preparation was washed for 40 min, the response to 30% O_2 media was smaller. (From Wang et al., 1991.)

that cGMP inhibition of carotid body chemoreceptor activity is mediated via a DA-independent mechanism, perhaps involving modulation of release of inhibitory neurotransmitter(s).

Prostaglandins

The potentiating effect of acetylsalicylic acid on the respiratory drive evoked by hypoxia or high CO_2 has been well known for many years (Samet et al., 1962; Riley et al., 1977). More recently, McQueen et al. (1989) suggested that these effects may be mediated in part by the carotid body, because in the rat they disappeared following CSN transection, and administration of salicylate to the animals increased CSN discharge. These investigators proposed that the effects of salicylate on the carotid body might result from the uncoupling properties of this anti-inflammatory agent. However, it was also possible that salicylate actions on the chemoreceptors were due not to their uncoupling potency, but rather to their ability to inhibit prostaglandin synthesis. Exploring this possibility, Gonzalez and co-workers (Gomez-Niño et al., 1992; Perez-Garcia et al., 1993; Gomez-Niño, Almaraz, Lopez-Lopez, and Gonzalez, in preparation) found that indomethacine and acetylsalicylic acid at concentrations that did not affect basal DA release, and hence lacked significant uncoupling actions, nonetheless strongly potentiated the low Po_2- and high Pco_2/low pH-induced release of this catecholamine. Prostaglandin E_2 reversed the effect of the anti-inflammatory drugs and, when administered alone, inhibited in a dose-dependent manner the low Po_2- and high K^+-induced release of DA. Furthermore, it was observed that low Po_2, high K^+, and acidic stimulation augmented the production of prostaglandin E_2 by the carotid body. Whole-cell patch-clamp recording of chemoreceptor cells revealed that prostaglandin E_2 produced a dose-dependent inhibition of Ca^{2+} currents, which could be blocked by the inclusion of GDPβS in the micropipette solution, indicating a G-protein mediation of prostaglandin E_2 actions. Taken together, these findings suggest that prostaglandin E_2 is a physiologically significant inhibitory modulator of chemoreceptor cell function. In fact, McQueen and Belmonte (1974) had earlier reported that prostaglandin E_2 inhibited CSN discharge in a dose-dependent manner, although they attributed this finding to a direct action of the prostanoid on carotid body blood vessels.

IV. Neurotransmission

A. General Considerations

During the last decade or more, it has become clear that neurotransmission at the chemoreceptor cell-sensory nerve ending synapse involves a complex interplay between multiple neuroactive agents and, like neurotransmission at many CNS synapses, has many unexplored and ill-defined characteristics. One problem is that physiological studies aimed at functional descriptions of chemotransmission in the organ invariably lag behind morphological studies, which reveal ever-increasing assortments of neuroactive substances in the organ. Furthermore, studies of synaptic neurotransmission quite frequently lack the ideal characteristics of well-conceived investigations: generation of complete dose-response curves, choice of appropriate physiological levels of stimulation, and selection of the simplest available preparation (see Kupfermann, 1991). These limitations notwithstanding, carotid body researchers enjoy today much greater insight into the mechanisms of chemotransmission than was appreciated in the past.

It is relevant here to consider the concept of neurotransmission. Potter et al. (1981) defined a neurotransmitter as any substance secreted by a neuron that controls a target cell, including the secreting neuron; Kupfermann (1991) set forth a common definition for neurotransmitters, messengers, and modulators alike, as being any molecules that upon release transmit information. Such a broad definition encompasses the classical neurotransmitters and peptides, as well as many other substances released during neuronal activity, such as ions, purines, ascorbate, and products of phospholipid metabolism. Yet, both Potter et al. (1981) and Kupfermann (1991) excluded trophic substances from their definition of neurotransmitter, but duly noted that many neurotransmitters may also have trophic effects. Certainly all these characteristics and definitions have merit; the problem for the carotid body, as for any other synapse, lies with their experimental elucidation and verification.

It is well established that multiple neurotransmitters coexist within the chemoreceptor cells of the carotid body (Fidone et al., 1990; Gonzalez et al., 1991), but it is important to distinguish between transmitter coexistence and synaptic cotransmission. Transmitter coexistence, as demonstrated for example by immunohistochemical techniques, implies colocalization within the same neuron or even within the same population of storage vesicles (Lundber and Hökfelt, 1985; Campbell, 1987; Bartfai et al., 1988; Kupfermann, 1991). Transmitter storage in different vesicles or cellular compartments allows for different ratios of corelease, which might be regulated by the stimulus parameters (Lundberg et al., 1986; Bartfai et al., 1988; Kupfermann, 1991); thus, it is known that some neuroactive peptides are differentially released at high stimulus intensities. Cotransmission usually implies corelease, but is not a necessary consequence of coexistence. Transmitters that are coreleased may have varying degrees of inter-action. At one extreme, they may act only on their separate and specific receptor populations, interacting to the extent that the target cell integrates their net effects. At the other extreme, the sole action of one coreleased transmitter may be to modulate the receptor sensitivity of the other coreleased transmitter (e.g., VIP modulation of muscarinic ACh receptors in the salivary gland; Potter et al., 1981; Lundberg and Hökfelt, 1985; Campbell, 1987). Finally, cotransmitter modulation of synaptic activity can be exerted presynaptically and/or postsynaptically. Interactions at the presynaptic level act to modulate the ongoing release of the neurotransmitter. Presynaptic receptors for a given neurotransmitter (i.e., "autoreceptors") usually exhibit higher affinities for the transmitter molecule than do the corresponding postsynaptic receptors (Siggins, 1986). It is important to consider this fact when designing pharmacological experiments involving exogenous administration of putative transmitter substances or their agonist and antagonists. The observed effects may be attributable to presynaptic receptor modulation of ongoing transmitter release, which might have greater effects on net synaptic activity than the direct action of the administered drug on the postsynaptic receptors. In the carotid body, for example, it is known that presynaptic DA receptors are present on the chemoreceptor cells, as well as postsynaptically on the apposed sensory terminals of CSN fibers (Fidone et al., 1980; Dinger et al., 1981; Mir et al., 1984; Schamel and Verna, 1992). It is therefore important to construct complete dose-response curves when examining the pharmacological actions of exogenously applied dopaminergic agents in the carotid body preparation.

With the above considerations in mind, the following description of neurotransmission in the carotid body will primarily emphasize an in-depth treatment of the role of catecholamines (CA) in chemoreceptor function. CA are present in this tissue at much higher concentrations than any other putative neurotransmitters, and a wealth of experimental studies implicate CA as key transmitters or modulators of the chemoresponse. Other important putative neurotransmitters, in particular substance P and the opiates, will also be considered for their role in chemoreception, but because of the limited scope of this review, these agents will be dealt with primarily for their cotransmitter interactions with CA.

B. Catecholamines

*Diversity and Content of Catecholamines in
Chemoreceptor Cells*

The earlier literature describing the histochemical demonstration of CA in chemoreceptor cells, based on their chromaffin or fluorescent reaction products, has been reviewed in detail in several previous publications (Kobayashi, 1971a,b; Verna, 1979; Pallot, 1987), including one by McDonald (1981) in the first edition of this book. The more recent immunohistochemical studies of carotid body CA have been primarily directed at distinguishing subpopulations of chemoreceptor cells based on their differential content of DA vs. NE.

Bolme et al. (1977) first reported for the rat carotid body that only a few chemoreceptor cells were positive for dopamine-β-hydroxylase (DβH), the enzyme responsible for conversion of DA to NE; all the cells, on the other hand, were positive for tyrosine hydroxylase (TH), the rate-limiting enzyme for CA synthesis, and also for dopa decarboxylase, the ubiquitous enzyme that converts dopa to DA.

Later, Chen and co-workers (Chen and Yates, 1984; Chen et al., 1985) observed a higher proportion (30%) of DβH-positive chemoreceptor cells in the rat, and they suggested on the basis of other experimental evidence that these presumed NE-containing cells corresponded to the "small vesicle" (type B) subpopulation of chemoreceptor cells earlier described by Hellstrom (1975) and by McDonald and Mitchell (1975). However, this notion that rat chemoreceptor cells are divisible into "large vesicle" (type A) and "small vesicle" (type B) cells has been challenged (Verna, 1979; Pallot, 1987). Nonetheless, there is good evidence that chemoreceptor cells in the rat carotid body do in fact contain NE, because a significant fraction of the NE content (10–50%) of the carotid body remains after sympathectomy of the organ by removal of the superior cervical ganglion (Hanbauer and Hellstrom, 1978; Chiochio et al., 1981; Mir et al., 1982; Pequignot et al., 1986), indicating the presence of NE stores outside of sympathetic nerve endings, and most probably in the chemoreceptor cells (Fig. 8B).

The rabbit carotid body, like that in the rat, is mostly a dopaminergic organ, containing nearly five times more DA than NE (Dearnaley et al., 1968; Mir et al, 1982; Leitner et al., 1986; Gonzalez-Guerrero et al., 1993a,b) and synthesizing DA at a rate 10 times higher than that for NE (Fidone and Gonzalez, 1982; Fidone et al., 1980, 1982; Rigual et al., 1987; Almaraz et al., 1992; Gonzalez-Guerrero et al., 1993a,b). As in the rat, about 50% of the NE content and synthesis disappears after removal of the superior cervical ganglion (Fig. 8B; Fidone and Gonzalez, 1982; Gonzalez-Guerrero, 1993a). Schamel and Verna (1992a,b) performed a quantitative autoradiographic assessment of ^{3}H-NE uptake in combination with a morphometric analysis of dense-core vesicle size, chromaffin reaction product, and immunohistochemical staining for DβH and NE. They reported that about 1% of the chemoreceptor cells accumulated labeled NE, were DβH- and NE-positive, and exhibited chromaffin reaction product. The intensity of the immunohistochemical staining of the cells varied considerably, and the morphometric analysis revealed a dense-core vesicle size larger than average. But a considerable gradation of the measured parameters was observed, so the interesting conclusion was made that these apparently noradrenergic cells evolve somehow from precursor dopaminergic chemoreceptor cells. This concept that chemoreceptor cells evolve through different phases of development was first put forth by Stensaas et al. (1981) in studies performed with the cat carotid body, and a similar notion was suggested by Pallot (1987). Recent electrophysiological studies using isolated adult rabbit chemoreceptor cells have revealed K^+ currents that exhibit a continuum of properties among the cells: most cells have a characteristically small Ca^{2+}-dependent component and a very high transient Ca^{2+}-independent component, but a continuous gradation in the shape of the recorded currents was observed (Perez-Garcia et al., 1992). Finally, in a neurochemical study by Gomez-Niño et al. (1990), it was found that different carotid body stimuli can elicit differential release of CA from the organ; i.e., low Po_2 stimulation

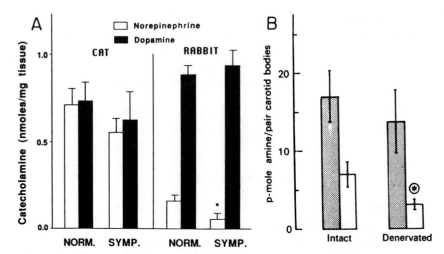

Figure 8 (A) Endogenous catecholamine levels in normal and chronically sympathec-tomized (12–14 days) carotid bodies from cat and rabbit, measured using HPLC with electrochemical detection. (Fidone and Gonzalez, unpublished.) (B) Effect of removal of superior cervical ganglion on the dopamine and noradrenaline concentrations in rat carotid body. The catecholamine levels are expressed as mean ± SD pmole/pair carotid bodies. Statistical significance of experimental changes was calculated using Student's *t*-test. *$p <$ 0.05 when compared with the controlateral intact side. ■, dopamine; □, noradrenaline. (From Hanbauer and Hellstrom, 1978.)

preferentially released DA while nicotinic agonists preferentially released NE from the rabbit carotid body. This finding also suggests that nicotinic receptors may be located on noradrenergic cells in the carotid body, which is reminiscent of a study by Chen and Yates (1984) that showed that HRP-conjugated α-bungaro-toxin preferentially bound to a subpopulation of chemoreceptor cells containing small-diameter, dense-core vesicles (type B). It was this subpopulation of chemo-receptor cells that they presumed corresponded to the DβH-positive subpopulation of cells they described in another study (Chen et al., 1985; see earlier).

The cat carotid body contains approximately equivalent amounts of DA and NE (Fig. 8B), although there is some disagreement among the various studies (see Fidone and Gonzalez, 1986). The rate of DA synthesis is more than 10 times higher than NE synthesis, indicating important differences in the turnover of these two CA (Rigual et al., 1986, 1987). Immunohistochemical studies have revealed varying levels of DβH among the chemoreceptor cells (Varndell et al., 1982; Chen et al., 1985; Wang et al., 1991, 1992). Less than 5% of the chemoreceptor cells were immunopositive only to TH, prompting the conclusion that in the cat, DA and NE may coexist in the same cells (Wang et al., 1991, 1992; Fig. 9). In other species, including dogs, humans, and guinea pigs, chemoreceptor cells have been reported immunopositive to DβH and NE (Varndell et al., 1982; Kobayashi et al., 1983; Fried et al., 1989).

Catecholamine Metabolism

The above findings suggest that the carotid body is primarily a dopaminergic organ, which in some species also contains high levels of NE. The carotid bodies of the three species most commonly used for chemoreceptor studies (i.e., rat, rabbit, and cat) have DA levels 5–10 times higher than those reported for the corpus striatum (Mefford et al., 1982). Among peripheral nervous system structures, the carotid body has the highest DA levels (Lackovick and Neff, 1983).

Consistent with its high CA levels, the carotid body contains high levels of the rate-limiting enzyme, TH. The levels of TH activity in the rat and rabbit carotid body are 5.2 and 1.3 μmole/g/hr, respectively, which are comparable to the levels found for the adrenal medulla of these same species (Gonzalez et al., 1979, 1981); cat carotid body TH activity was found to be similar to that for the rabbit (Gonzalez et al., 1981a,b). However, markedly lower values for TH activity in some of these species has also been reported (Hanbauer et al., 1977; Starlinger, 1980).

As in the brain, the level of TH activity in the carotid body of a given species is reflected in the turnover rate of DA in the organ. In the rat, DA turnover has been estimated to be about 3–5 pmole/CB/hr ($\approx$67 nmole/g/hr; Hanbauer and Hellstrom, 1978; Brokaw et al., 1985; Pequignot et al., 1987), yielding a total DA turnover time of 3–5 hr. In the rabbit, DA turnover was estimated to be 12–15 nmole/g/hr and was derived from the rate of ^{3}H-DA synthesis in carotid bodies incubated in HEPES-buffered saline with physiological levels of the precursor, ^{3}H-tyrosine (Fidone and Gonzalez, 1982). The turnover time for DA in the rabbit has been calculated to be 50–60 hr (Rigual et al., 1987). However, Leitner et al. (1987) and Roumy et al. (1986) found a DA turnover rate in vivo four times higher, based on the rate of DOPAC disappearance following inhibition of monoamine oxidase. There is no ready explanation for this marked difference, but Gonzalez et al. (1979) measured DA turnover rates for rat striatum with the same in vitro conditions used for the carotid body measurements and found identical values for this brain structure to those measured previously under in vivo conditions (Bacopoulos and Bathnagar, 1977). In the cat, DA turnover rates were found to be similar to those for the rabbit (Rigual et al., 1986, 1987).

The activity of the enzyme aromatic amino acid decarboxylase (dopa decarboxylase) has not been directly measured in the carotid body, but it has been demonstrated immunocytochemically to be present in all chemoreceptor cells of the rat carotid body (Bolme et al., 1977). Its existence in the rabbit and cat carotid

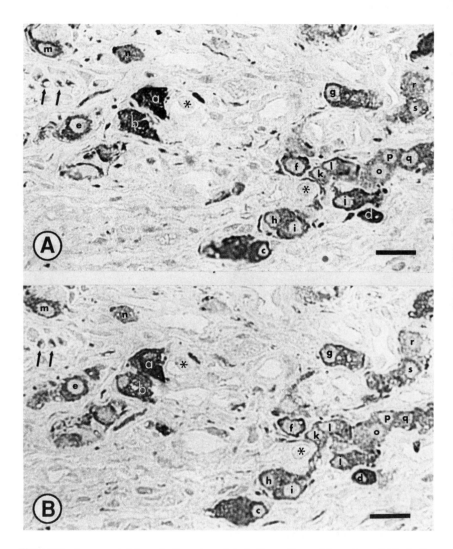

Figure 9 Immunostaining of adjacent, serial plastic sections of the cat carotid body for TH (A) and DβH (B) delineates a high incidence of colocalized reaction product. Type I cells with equivalent levels of reaction product are readily distinguished, and there are few unstained type I cells (asterisk). Some myelinated nerve fibers (arrows) are also doubly labeled. Bar = 20 μm. (From Wang et al., 1991.)

body is implied from the ability of these organs to synthesize DA from their precursor molecules, tyrosine and dopa (Fidone and Gonzalez, 1982; Rigual et al., 1986).

The activity of dopamine beta hydroxylase (DβH), the enzyme that converts DA to NE, has been measured in the rat and cat carotid body; the level of the enzyme in the rat was found to be 78 pmole/pair CBs/hr ($\approx$650–700 nmole/g/hr; Hanbauer, 1977; Hanbauer et al., 1977), and that for the cat varied considerably between a low of 50 nmole/g/hr (Morgado et al., 1976; Starlinger, 1977) to a high of 1400 nmole/g/hr (Starlinger, 1979). Belmonte et al. (1977), on the other hand, determined activities of 550 and 350 nmole/g/hr in control and sympathectomized carotid bodies, respectively. A comparison of the ratios for DβH/NE and TH/DA in the carotid bodies of these species suggests a slower turnover rate for NE than DA, a prediction that has been experimentally confirmed by numerous investigators (Hanbauer and Hellstrom, 1978; Brokaw et al., 1985; Pequignot, 1987; Gonzalez and Fidone, 1982; Rigual et al., 1987). However, the turnover rate for NE in the sympathetic neurons innervating the organ is considerably higher than that for NE present in the chemoreceptor cells (Fidone and Gonzalez, 1982; Rigual et al., 1986; Rigual et al., 1987).

In general, the regulation of CA synthesis and turnover in the carotid body is similar to that described for other catecholaminergic structures. Thus, short-term activation of TH, as well as long-term induction of this enzyme following hypoxic stimulation of the carotid body, has been described for both the rat and rabbit (Hanbauer et al., 1977; Gonzalez et al., 1979, 1981; Fidone et al., 1982; Brokaw et al., 1985; Gonzalez-Guerrero et al., 1993a). More recently, experimental verification of this TH induction has been obtained by in situ hybridization of TH mRNA in rat carotid bodies following exposure of the animals to 10% O_2 for periods of 1–48 hr (Czyzyk-Krzeska et al., 1992). In the cat, acute exposure to hypoxia produces short-term activation of TH and increased DA synthesis (Rigual et al., 1986), but the delayed induction of TH following hypoxia was not observed in this animal (Gonzalez et al., 1981). Among the mechanisms that influence short-term regulation of TH, one of the most important is the removal of feedback inhibition consequent to the release of CA; consequently, increased DA synthesis by hypoxia should imply stimulus-induced release of this CA from the chemoreceptor cells, and such has been inferred from a large number of in vivo studies (Hellstrom et al., 1976; Hellstrom, 1977; Hanbauer, 1977; Hanbauer and Hellstrom, 1978; Chiochio, 1981; Fitzgerald et al., 1983; Pallot and Al-Neamy, 1983; Brokaw et al., 1985; Pallot, 1987). The release of DA by hypoxia was first directly measured in studies in vitro by Gonzalez and Fidone (1977) and later verified in numerous investigations. Finally, it has been suggested that this short-term regulation of TH involves a cAMP-dependent phosphorylation (Perez-Garcia et al., 1991).

In contrast to TH and DA, the activity of DβH and the levels of NE in the carotid body seem to be less affected by natural chemoreceptor stimulation. Thus in the rat, DβH was not induced nor were NE levels and turnover rates modified by acute hypoxic stimulation (Hanbauer et al., 1977; Hellstrom et al., 1976; Hanbauer and Hellstrom, 1978; Brokaw et al., 1985). Likewise in the cat, NE levels were unchanged by hypoxia (Fitzgerald et al., 1983; Starlinger et al., 1983), although a decrease in NE levels has been observed following intense hypoxic stimulation (Starlinger and Acker, 1986). Using a combined in vivo/in vitro experimental protocol, in which the animals are first exposed to hypoxic atmospheres and then the carotid bodies quickly removed for in vitro assessments of CA synthesis, it has likewise been found that hypoxic stimulation fails to alter the rate of NE synthesis in either the cat or rabbit carotid bodies (Rigual et al., 1986; Gonzalez et al., 1981; Fidone et al., 1982; Gonzalez-Guerrero et al., 1993a). Although the above experiments suggest that NE is not released by hypoxic stimulation, in fact the contrary has been shown in experiments that directly measured NE release; in these studies, NE was released by hypoxic stimulation but in much lower amounts than DA (Gomez-Niño et al., 1990; Perez-Garcia et al., 1991). Finally, chronic hypoxic stimulation also modifies CA levels in the carotid body: tissue levels and turnover rates for DA are increased simultaneously (Hanbauer et al., 1981; Pequignot et al., 1987, 1990; Gonzalez-Guerrero et al., 1993b), and tissue levels for NE are increased but with a delayed time course (Pequignot et al., 1987).

The effects of acidic/hypercapnic stimulation on CA synthesis and turnover in the carotid body are somewhat different than those resulting from hypoxic stimulation. For one thing, acidic stimuli are much less potent in evoking DA release than even mild hypoxic stimuli. However, the same may be said for chemoreceptor activity; CSN discharge provoked by either stimulus is proportional to the accompanying release of DA (e.g., compare Rigual et al., 1986, and Rigual et al., 1991; Fitzgerald and Parks, 1971). Yet despite minimal evoked release, incubation of cat carotid bodies at pH 7 markedly increases both DA and NE synthesis, a finding largely attributable to the activation of TH by intracellular acidification. Taken together, these data suggest that short-term acidic/hypercapnic stimuli should increase, rather than decrease, CA levels in the carotid body; in fact, this has been confirmed for the cat (Fitzgerald et al., 1983) and the rat (Pallot, 1987). Chronic hypercapnic stimulation of the rat also produced increased levels of DA (15%) and NE (50%), which likewise can be interpreted as nonspecific activation of CA synthesis (Pequignot et al., 1990).

The processes involved in chemoreceptor cell inactivation of released CA also incorporate the general mechanisms described for other catecholaminergic systems; namely, reuptake, enzymatic degradation, and washout. In one study that examined these aspects of CA metabolism in the carotid body, it was apparent that there is not a kinetically demonstrable high-affinity uptake system for DA in the rabbit carotid body (Gonzalez et al., 1987). This finding, which is similar to that reported for the adrenal medulla (Wakade and Wakade, 1984), explains the lack of sensitivity of carotid chemoreceptor cells to the neurotoxin 6-hydroxydopamine (Hess, 1976; Suazo and Zapata, 1978; Hansen and Ord, 1978), a substance that requires a concentrative, high-affinity uptake for its selective action. DOPAC has been identified as the principal CA catabolite in the carotid body, although methylated catabolites are also present (Gonzalez et al., 1987). Thus, during basal or low levels of chemoreceptor stimulation, ^{3}H-DOPAC is the principal species appearing in the washout from carotid bodies incubated with the CA precursor, ^{3}H-tyrosine; at high intensities of chemoreceptor stimulation, on the other hand, over 80% of the tritium in the washout media appears as unmetabolized ^{3}H-DA (Obeso et al., 1992). Under resting conditions then, the low-affinity uptake and degradation of DA by monoamine oxidase and catechol-O-methyltransferase is the predominant mechanism for CA inactivation, while overflow and washout of undegraded DA from the tissue would terminate the action of this CA during chemoreceptor stimulation.

Release of Catecholamines

Although the release of DA in response to natural stimulation has been indirectly inferred from numerous in vivo studies, the most detailed characterization of this release response has been achieved with the in vitro experimental preparation, where simultaneous measurements can be made of stimulus intensity, DA release, and CSN discharge. These experiments usually involved preincubating carotid bodies with the catecholamine precursor, ^{3}H-tyrosine, and then mounting the organ-nerve preparation in an in vitro chamber where it could be superfused with physiological media containing chemoreceptor stimuli. In the initial studies performed with rabbit carotid bodies (Fidone et al., 1981, 1982), the organs were superfused with media equilibrated at a Po_2 between 0 and 630 mmHg. It was observed that the release of labeled DA (collected as DA plus DOPAC in the superfusates) increased quasilinearly with decreasing Po_2 between 300 and 0 mmHg; the chemoreceptor discharge recorded simultaneously from the CSN increased in parallel with the release of DA (Fig. 10). This low Po_2-induced release of DA was blocked by more than 95% in Ca^{2+}-free media, while the CSN discharge was reduced by only 55%. Carotid bodies that had been chronically denervated by CSN section (Fidone et al. 1982) also released DA in direct proportion to the hypoxic stimulus intensity, as did type I cells maintained in culture (Fishman et al., 1985).

In the above studies, the nearly linear relationship observed among the parameters of Po_2 stimulation, CSN discharge, and DA release differed from the sigmoidal or exponential relationship between Po_2 and CSN discharge reported in earlier in vivo and in vitro studies (Hornbein, 1968; Eyzaguirre and Koyano, 1965; Biscoe et al., 1970). These differences may be due in part to variations in the

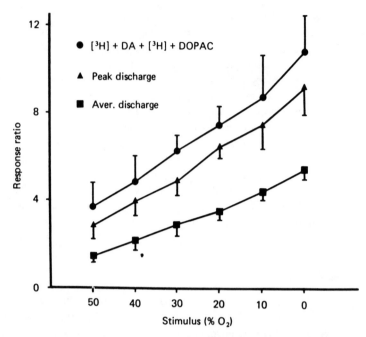

Figure 10   Relationship between total [³H]DA release ([³H]DA + [³H]DOPAC), peak chemoreceptor discharge, and average chemoreceptor discharge during the stimulus conditions indicated. (From Fidone et al., 1982a.)

experimental apparatus used in these studies: different chamber configurations and materials for superfusion lines allowed for different rates of diffusional gas exchange and permeation, leaving uncertain the actual Po_2 of a superfusate presented to the organ itself. In recent experiments using an in vitro experimental arrangement that permitted accurate control and measurement of the Po_2 bathing the preparation, the relationship between Po_2 and DA release was identical to that observed in vivo between Po_2 and CSN discharge (Perez-Garcia, 1991). This close correlation of DA release and CSN discharge implies a tight coupling between these two chemoreceptor processes. It was also found in later studies that there was a small, but clear, increase in NE release during low Po_2 stimulation (Gomez-Niño et al., 1990; Obeso et al., 1992).

Thus, despite certain shortcomings, the early experiments established the following points: (1) Chemoreceptor cells can detect and transduce low Po_2 stimuli into an observable release of putative neurotransmitter substances; (2) the release of DA is an accurate measure of chemoreceptor drive; and (3) the full expression of the chemoreceptor response to low Po_2, including the release of DA and CSN discharge, is Ca^{2+}-dependent, but basal release and CSN activity are relatively insensitive to zero Ca^{2+} media, as is commonly the case with other catecholaminergic systems. These initial experiments obtained using the rabbit carotid body have recently been repeated in the cat (Rigual et al., 1986) and the rat (Shaw et al., 1989, 1990).

The effects of acidic stimulation on CA release have been studied in both the rabbit (Rocher et al., 1991) and the cat (Rigual et al., 1984, 1991) carotid bodies, but only in the latter species has the release been correlated with the simultaneous recording of CSN discharge. Although the relative magnitude of release and nerve discharge evoked by acidic stimuli was much smaller than that evoked by low Po_2, there nonetheless was observed a close linear relationship between the decrease in pH and the increase in DA release and CSN discharge. A similar relationship between pH and CSN discharge was described earlier for in vivo experiments (Fitzgerald and Parks, 1971), and consequently DA release may also be a valid measure of acidic chemotransduction by the carotid body. As was shown for low Po_2 stimuli, the low pH-induced release of DA was unaltered by chronic CSN denervation, but was reduced by 80% in Ca^{2+}-free media; likewise, the low pH-evoked CSN discharge was only moderately reduced in the absence of Ca^{2+}. Release was also greater at any given extracellular pH if the superfusion media also contained CO_2, and superfusates at pH 7.4 equilibrated with $Pco_2 = 80$ mmHg, or containing weak acids, were also effective in promoting DA release and increased CSN discharge (Rigual et al., 1991). Additionally, it was observed that inhibition of carbonic anhydrase produced proportional reductions in both DA release and CSN discharge. This latter finding demonstrates that the parameter sensed by the chemoreceptor cells during acidic stimulation is the intracellular pH, rather than the extracellular pH, as had been proposed many years earlier (Torrance, 1974, 1977).

Pharmacological studies with the in vitro cat carotid body preparation using chemoexcitant drugs such as 2-deoxyglucose, cyanide, or dinitrophenol have revealed similar relationships between the intensity of stimulation (drug concentration), on the one hand, and DA release and CSN discharge, on the other (Obeso et al., 1986, 1989). Again, Ca^{2+}-free media reduced the evoked release of DA by $\approx 80\%$, whereas the evoked CSN discharge was reduced by a much smaller percentage. A similar Ca^{2+} dependence for the DA release induced by these pharmacological stimuli has been demonstrated for the in vitro rabbit carotid body preparation as well (Obeso et al., 1992).

The experimental findings described above clearly show that the normally close correlation between the magnitude of the stimulus-evoked release of DA and the frequency of CSN discharge is dramatically altered in Ca^{2+}-free media, and that the effects are similar whether the chemoreceptor stimulus is low Po_2, high Pco_2/low pH, or pharmacological stimulants. Thus, the common observation is a marked reduction in release (80->95%) accompanied by only a moderate reduction in CSN discharge (30–55%). Factors contributing to this apparent dissociation between release and discharge might include: an increase in receptor-transmitter affinity in Ca^{2+}-free media (Paiva and Paiva, 1975; van Buskirk and Dowling, 1982); an increase in transmitter-mediated ionic conductances in low Ca^{2+} solutions (Kanno et al., 1976; Kato and Narahashi, 1982); and finally, a large "safety factor" at the sensory synapse between the chemoreceptor cell and CSN terminal, which acts to preserve chemotransmission under conditions of reduced transmitter release; such appears to be the case at certain other catecholaminergic synapses, where marked reductions in the evoked release of CA (>90%) following reserpinization are accompanied by more moderate reductions (30–50%) in the evoked postsynaptic response (Lee, 1967; Wakade and Krusz, 1972).

The pharmacological effects of a variety of neurotransmitter agonists and antagonists on the release of CA have been examined in experimental preparations of the cat and rabbit carotid body. These studies have attempted to assess the modulatory action of neurotransmitters on CA release by the chemoreceptor cells and consequently are important for interpreting the pharmacological actions of exogenously administered neurotransmitter agents on CSN chemoreceptor discharge. The net effect of any drug or neurotransmitter agent is thus the resultant of both its presynaptic and postsynaptic effects. As we will see below, much of the interactive pharmacological effects reported thus far can be attributed to presynaptic actions on the chemoreceptor cells.

It is well known that nicotinic agonists provoke the release of CA and increased CSN discharge from both the rabbit and cat carotid bodies, and that these effects are larger in the cat because of the relative predominance of nicotinic receptors in this species (Dinger et al., 1985; Gomez-Niño, 1989; Gomez-Niño et al., 1990; Dinger et al., 1991). The release of CA by nicotinic agonists is completely blocked by mecamylamine, hexamethonium, and *d*-tubocurarine, but only partly inhibited by saturating concentrations of α-bungarotoxin (Dinger et al., 1985; Gomez-Niño, 1989). Analysis of the released CA revealed that nicotinic agents preferentially release NE. Taken together with the apparent absence of nicotinic receptors on the sensory nerve endings (Dinger et al., 1985; Hirano et al., 1992), these findings indicate that the effects of nicotinic agents are likely mediated primarily via the chemoreceptor cells. In fact, it had been noted many years earlier by Eyzaguirre and co-workers (1975) that the excitatory actions of ACh in the cat carotid body were reduced in Ca^{2+}-free, Mg^{2+}-rich media, a finding that is consistent with a mechanism involving presynaptic Ca^{2+}-dependent release of a neurotransmitter.

In contrast to the actions of nicotinic agents, muscarinic agonists such as bethanechol and oxotremorine partially block the ACh- and nicotine-induced release of CA from the rabbit carotid body, indicating negative coupling of muscarinic receptors to this exocytotic process (Dinger et al., 1991). Muscarinic receptors may also be negatively coupled to adenylate cyclase, because it has been observed that bethanechol reduces cAMP content in the rabbit carotid body (Perez-Garcia et al., 1993). Like nicotinic receptors, muscarinic receptors appear to be localized to the chemoreceptor cells and absent from the sensory nerve endings, as determined from experiments that localized ^{3}H-QNB (a muscarinic ligand) binding in normal and chronically CSN-denervated carotid bodies (Hirano et al., 1992; Dinger et al., 1986, 1991).

It has been found that adrenergic agonists and antagonists modulate both the basal and low Po_2-induced release of CA from the carotid body, indicating that NE receptors are likely also present on the chemoreceptor cells. It has been observed that isoproterenol augments both the basal- and stimulus-induced release of DA in a propranolol-sensitive manner (Perez-Garcia et al., 1993). Use of selective α_2-agonists (for example, UK-14304) reduced the low Po_2-evoked release of CA, and this effect was reversed by α_2-antagonists (e.g., yohimbine and SKF-86466); administration of the antagonists alone increased the low Po_2-induced release, indicating that NE released by natural stimuli acts on α_2-receptors to negatively modulate the response of the chemoreceptor cells (Almaraz, Perez-Garcia, Gomez-Niño, and Gonzalez, unpublished). These findings complement those of Prabhakar and co-workers (Kou et al., 1991; Prabhakar et al., 1992; see also Pizarro et al., 1992) obtained with CSN recordings of chemoreceptor activity and confirm that the effects of adrenergic agents on CSN discharge are mediated in part by the chemoreceptor cells.

The neuroleptic drugs haloperidol and spiroperidol were found to augment both the resting and low Po_2-induced release of DA from the rabbit carotid body, while selective DA-1 agonists and antagonists were without effect (Fig. 11; Fidone et al., 1991; Almaraz et al., 1991). These findings suggest that DA-2 receptors in the carotid body that survive chronic CSN denervation are very likely DA autoreceptors located on the chemoreceptor cells and are involved in the feedback modulation of DA release (Dinger et al., 1981; Mir et al., 1984). Electrophysiohlogical patch-clamp experiments have revealed that DA inhibits Ca^{2+} currents in chemoreceptor cells (Benot and Lopez-Barneo, 1990). Thus, any interpretation of the effects of dopaminergic blockers on CSN discharge, or ventilation, must consider that DA blockers (at low doses) may augment discharge or ventilation by preferential blockade of presynaptic DA autoreceptors, leading to increased DA release and postsynaptic action (Siggins, 1986; see above). Finally, although DA-1 receptors appear not to be involved in regulation of CA release from chemoreceptor cells, these receptors have been shown to be present in the carotid body and apparently are located on blood vessels in the organ (Almaraz et al., 1991). Consequently, they may participate in the overall chemoreceptor response through vasodilatory regulation of carotid body blood flow. DA released from chemoreceptor cells, as well as exogenously administered dopaminergic agents, might also influence these vascular DA-1 receptors.

Finally, it has recently been observed that selective δ-opioid, but not μ,

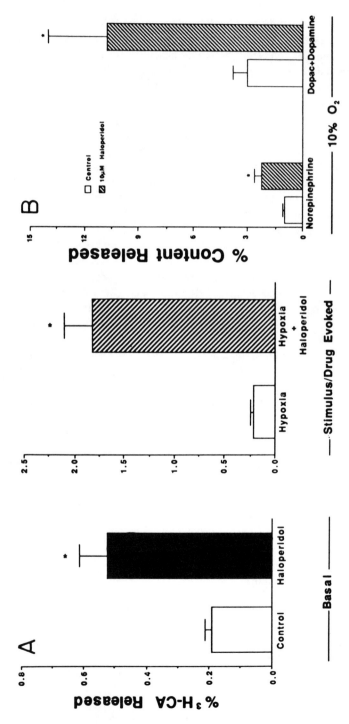

Figure 11 (A) Effect of haloperidol (10 μM) on ³H-CA synthesized from ³H-tyrosine) release from cat carotid bodies superfused in vitro. Haloperidol elevates ³H-CA release (expressed as percent of tissue content) in media equilibrated with 100% O_2 (basal; $p <$ 0.002) and 10% O_2 (hypoxia; $p < 0.001$). (B) HPLC analysis of hypoxia- (10% O_2) evoked ³H-CA release shows that haloperidol promotes a large increase in the release of dopamine and its metabolite dihydroxyphenylacetic acid along with a modest elevation of norepinephrine release. *$p < 0.02$.

agonists inhibit the release of DA induced by several chemoreceptor stimuli, including low P_{O_2}; naloxone, a broad-spectrum opioid antagonist, augments the low P_{O_2}-induced release of DA (Gonzalez-Guerrero et al., 1993b). These studies also demonstrated that some of the opioid receptors in the carotid body are located on the chemoreceptor cells. This suggests that opioid peptides (e.g., met-enkephalin) that are released from the chemoreceptor cells by natural stimuli (Hanson et al., 1986; Gonzalez-Guerrero et al., 1993b) might negatively modulate the release of DA from these cells and thereby account for the δ-opioid, receptor-mediated inhibition of DA release (Gonzalez-Guerrero et al., 1993b) and CSN discharge (Kirby and McQueen, 1986).

At the beginning of this section, it was noted that adaptive changes in the ventilatory response to chronic hypoxia that are mediated by the carotid body (Weil, 1986; West, 1991) might be reflected in functional modifications at the chemoreceptor cell/sensory nerve ending synapse. Chronic exposure of rabbits to hypoxia is accompanied by a time-dependent increase in carotid body DA content, but opioid peptide levels remain unchanged (Gonzalez-Guerrero et al., 1993a). Because DA and opioid peptides are thought to be costored in the same vesicles, it appears that chronic hypoxia modifies the ratio of these transmitters in the secretory vesicles and, upon release, their concentrations within the synaptic cleft. This "imbalance" in DA/opioid release may contribute to changes in the hypoxic ventilatory and chemoreceptor response observed during acclimatization to hypoxia and upon return to normal O_2 atmospheres.

The Response of the Carotid Sinus Nerve to Catecholaminergic Agonists and Antagonists

In examining the actions of CA in the carotid body, it should be recalled that both presynaptic and postsynaptic CA receptors (and perhaps also nonchemosynaptic receptors, e.g., on blood vessels) may be involved in mediating the transmitters' effects, especially those for DA, and further, that presynaptic and extrasynaptic CA receptors usually exhibit higher affinities for their transmitters than do postsynaptic receptors (Siggins, 1986).

It has been established for a number of animal species (e.g., cat, rabbit, and dog) that intravascular administration of NE and epinephrine (E) increases both CSN discharge and ventilation, and that the increase in nerve discharge is frequently preceded by a transient inhibition (Eldridge and Gill-Kumar, 1980; Joels and Neil, 1968; Llados and Zapata, 1978; Folgering et al., 1982; Prabhakar et al., 1993; Sampson et al., 1976; Bisgard et al., 1979; Milsom and Sadig, 1983). A similar increase in ventilation has been reported in humans, which is unaffected by adrenergic blockade (Heistad et al., 1972; Patrick et al., 1978).

Pharmacological studies of the effects of adrenergic agents on CSN discharge have revealed that the inhibitory component of the nerve response is resistant to dibenamine (Llados and Zapata, 1978b), but sensitive to phenoxybenzamine (Sampson et al., 1976), haloperidol (Folgering et al., 1982), and SKF-86466 (a specific α_2-noradrenegic blocker; Prabhakar et al., 1993). Prabhakar and co-workers (Prabhakar et al., 1993; Kou et al., 1991) showed further with receptor-binding studies that α_2 receptors are present in the carotid body, and that the specific α_2 agonist guanabenz mimics the inhibitory effects of NE on both basal- and hypoxia-evoked CSN discharge, and conversely, that the α_2 antagonist SKF-86466 augments basal- and hypoxia-evoked CSN responses. These observations point to a physiologically relevant inhibitory component for NE actions in the carotid body.

The excitatory component of NE actions on CSN discharge was shown in the cat and rabbit to be blocked by propranolol and metoprolol, suggesting mediation by β_1-adrenergic receptors. However, a contribution from α_1 receptors to the excitatory component also seemed to be present because phenylephrine (an α_1 agonist) was shown to increase CSN discharge (Folgering et al., 1982). Isoproterenol, a nonspecific β-adrenergic agonist, as well NE and E, potentiated the CSN response to hypoxia and hypercapnia (Lahiri et al., 1981; Folgering et al., 1982; Milsom and Sadig, 1983), while β_1-adrenergic blockers produced the opposite effects (Folgering et al., 1982). Based on these experimental observations, it was proposed that NE might mediate the hypoxic response in the carotid body (Folgering et al., 1982; Milsom and Sadig, 1983). However, this notion has been contested by several groups of investigators (Gonsalves et al., 1984; Hudgel et al., 1986; Mulligan et al., 1986). It is important to note that receptor-binding studies have revealed the presence of β-adrenergic receptors in the rabbit carotid body (Mir et al., 1984), at least some of which appear to be located on the chemoreceptor cells, because β agonists increase both the basal- and low P_{O_2}-evoked release of DA (Perez-Garcia et al., 1993). The general conclusion emerging from these data is that adrenergic mechanisms very likely participate in the overall chemoresponse of the carotid body, but it is clear that knowledge of the precise location of adrenergic receptors in the organ, as well as a thorough characterization of the actions of selective agonists and antagonists, will be necessary before the role of NE in carotid chemoreception is fully characterized.

The first account of the effects of DA on CSN discharge was by Comroe and his co-workers (Jacobs and Comroe, 1968; Black et al., 1972), who reported that DA increased chemoreceptor activity in the dog. However, Bisgard et al. (1979) later showed in the dog that low doses of DA depressed CSN discharge, whereas chemoexcitation was consistently observed only at higher doses. Using the in vivo cat carotid body preparation, numerous investigators have shown that the predominant action of DA and its agonists is inhibition of basal- and stimulus-evoked CSN discharge (Sampson, 1972; Sampson et al., 1976a,b; Docherty and McQueen, 1968; Llados and Zapata, 1968; Lahiri and Nishino, 1980; Zapata et al., 1983, 1984; Zapata and Torrealba, 1984; Nishi, 1977; Zapata and Llados, 1977; McQueen, 1984; Okajima and Nishi, 1981; Shirahata et al., 1987; Ponte and

Sadler, 1989). Likewise in the in vivo rabbit carotid body preparation, DA has been found to inhibit CSN discharge (Docherty and McQueen 1979; McQueen et al., 1984; Ponte and Sadler, 1989). Comparable results have also been obtained in other species, including humans, where it was observed that phrenic output or ventilation was depressed following administration of DA. Consistent with these findings, the most common effect reported for dopaminergic antagonists is an increase in CSN discharge or ventilation.

It was cautioned by McQueen (1983), however, that most of the above studies tested only a single dose or a narrow dose range for the given dopaminergic agent. Thus, Ward (1984) reported that administration of 2.5 mg (i.e., $\approx$35 μg/kg) of droperidol, a dopaminergic blocker, increased the hypoxic ventilatory response in humans and prevented the inhibitory effects of DA infusion. Aminoff et al. (1978), working in the cat, administered droperidol at two dose levels: the low dose (20–50 μg) increased both basal and asphyxia-evoked CSN discharge, while the higher dose (100–300 μg) produced a short-lasting (about 40 sec) increase in basal discharge, followed by abolition of basal- and stimulus-evoked nerve activity; also, high doses of chlorpromazine and pimozide reduced or abolished spontaneous CSN discharge. In studies where dose-response curves were generated, it was commonly observed that high doses of DA produced either immediate excitation of CSN discharge or an initial short-lasting inhibition followed by sustained excitation (Docherty and McQueen, 1968; Llados and Zapata, 1968; Zapata and Llados, 1977; Okajima and Nishi, 1981). Furthermore, it was observed that DA blockers (including haloperidol, spiroperidol, α-flupen-thixol, domperidone, and sulpiride) converted the inhibitory response for exogenous DA into one of excitation (Nishi, 1977; Zapata and Llados, 1977; Llados and Zapata, 1978; Docherty and McQueen, 1968; Okajima and Nishi, 1981; Lahiri and Nishino, 1980; Fig. 12A). However, in a study by McQueen et al. (1984), DA blockade by domperidone or sulpiride failed to reveal chemoexcitation in the rabbit and cat carotid body. The conclusion from these studies, most of which were performed in the cat, can only be that two sets of DA receptors are present in the carotid body, each with different apparent accessibility and/or affinity for DA. The more accessible and/or higher-affinity DA receptors apparently mediate the observed inhibitory effects, whereas the less accessible/lower-affinity receptors account for the excitatory actions of DA. As pointed out earlier, separate populations of DA receptors localized to the nerve terminals and probably the chemoreceptor cells have been biochemically identified in the rabbit carotid body. Relevant to this point is the study by Okajima and Nishi (1981), which showed that DA produced only a dose-dependent increase in CSN discharge in reserpinized cats. One possible interpretation of these findings is that depletion of CA stores from the chemoreceptor cells minimizes presynaptic DA actions, leading to the loss of the inhibitory DA component.

Using the in vitro cat carotid body preparation, Zapata (1975) reported a

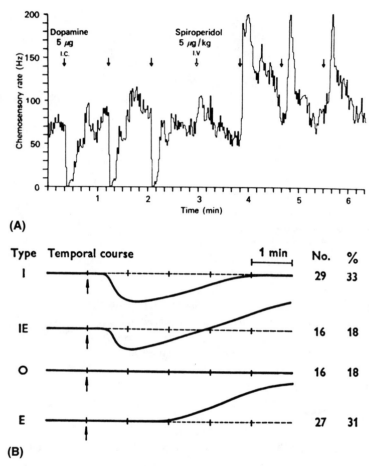

Figure 12   (A) Changes in chemosensory activity elicited by 5 μg dopamine hydro-
chloride i.c. (solid arrows) injected at ca. 1-min intervals, before and after spiroperidol, 5
μg/kg (open arrow). Ordinate: frequency of carotid nerve discharges, in Hz (impulses/sec).
In each horizontal trace, frequency was counted for 1-sec period and obtained through an
electronic counterdigital printer system operating continuously. (From Llados and Zapata,
1978a.) (B) Summary of effects of DA on frequency of chemoreceptor discharges. Doses
between 5 and 200 μg. Arrows, intrastream injections. Time, 1 min. In I (inhibition), there
is a transient decrease of frequency; in IE, inhibition is followed by excitation; in O, there
is no effect of DA on frequency; in E (excitation), there is only a late increase in frequency.
(From Zapata, 1975.)

variety of excitatory/inhibitory CSN responses to exogenous DA; at low doses, both excitatory and inhibitory components occurred with approximately equal frequency, whereas at higher doses excitation of slow onset, or preceded by a short inhibition, was more common than inhibition (Fig. 12B). Monti-Bloch and Eyzaguirre (1980), on the other hand, used a similar experimental preparation and observed a dose-dependent inhibition of CSN discharge in response to exogenous DA. In still another study, Donnelly and co-workers (Nolan et al., 1985) found that haloperidol (0.13–5.32 μM) reduced or abolished spontaneous activity in single chemoreceptor fibers recorded in vitro. The effect had a peculiarly long time course, requiring 8–10 min of superfusion for maximal effect; it was also observed that haloperidol abolished the CSN response to ACh. Finally, Leitner and Roumy (1986) showed that cat carotid bodies from reserpinized animals exhibited lower basal CSN discharge, as well as a slower onset and a marked reduction in the response to both low P_{O_2} and high P_{CO_2}.

In contrast to their findings in the cat, Monti-Bloch and Eyzaguirre (1980) showed that DA produced a dose-dependent increase in CSN discharge in the in vitro rabbit carotid body preparation. Leitner and Roumy (1985) later confirmed these results and reported also that DA increased the response to high P_{CO_2}. Administration of the DA blocker (+)-butaclamol at low doses (0.2–0.5 μM) failed to affect either the basal- or low P_{O_2}-evoked CSN discharge, but at higher doses (1 μm) this drug markedly reduced the hypercapnic response. Similarly, chlorpromazine increased basal CSN discharge at low doses, inhibited discharge at intermediate doses, and produced an anesthetic-like blockade of discharge at higher doses. These workers also examined the effects of catacholaminergic agents in reserpinized rabbit carotid bodies (Leitner et al., 1983; Leitner and Roumy, 1986), and made observations similar to those they reported for the reserpinized cat carotid body.

In conclusion, this section on neurotransmission presents data pertinent to the role of CA, and especially DA, in the chemoreceptor responses of the carotid body. Clearly, many of the experimental observations cited here permit only uncertain interpretations. Consequently, any hypothesis or proposal based on such incomplete data must be considered tentative and viewed more as a starting point for further experimental inquiry than as an established theoretical framework. Such limitations notwithstanding, it must be conceded that a wealth of experimental data suggest, at a minimum, that DA participates somehow in the ongoing chemoresponses of the carotid body; it is the equivocal actions of DA as an excitatory/inhibitory transmitter or modulator that remain the principal unexplained and perplexing problem. Furthermore, the presence of multiple putative transmitters within the chemoreceptor cell presents the possibilities for numerous transmitter interactions, compounding the complexities of the chemoresponse. Ultimately, experimental clarification of chemotransmission in the carotid body must follow from a detailed microelectrophysiological analysis of the chemoreceptor cell-sensory nerve ending synapse, which up to now has resisted experimental feasibility.

From the available experimental evidence, it seems reasonable to conclude that endogenously released DA should act on both presynaptic and postsynaptic DA receptors at the chemoreceptor cell-sensory nerve ending synapse. DA might also act on vascular DA receptors, during chemoreceptor stimulation, when DA overflow from the chemoreceptor synapse is high. Administration of exogenous DA in the in vivo carotid body preparation should act on both vascular and chemosynaptic DA receptors. In low doses, exogenous DA might preferentially target high-affinity presynaptic receptors, leading to decreased DA release from the chemoreceptor cells and, as the data show, a decrease in CSN discharge. Activation of vascular DA receptors would promote vasodilatation of carotid body blood vessels, adding to the inhibitory effects in the in vivo preparation. The experimental findings from reserpinized carotid bodies support this interpretation: depletion of DA stores minimizes ongoing presynaptic actions of DA, leaving the postsynaptic facilitatory actions of exogenous DA as the dominant pharmacological effect at any dose level. In the normal animal, high doses of administered DA effectively activate all DA receptors; activation of postsynaptic DA receptors would directly excite CSN discharge, despite autoreceptor shutdown of DA release and any accompanying vascular effects of DA action. The observation that DA-induced excitation of CSN discharge is commonly preceded by a transient inhibition might be explained by sequential dose-gradient effects on vascular, presynaptic, and postsynaptic DA receptors. The observed effects of dopaminergic blockers can be interpreted similarly: in low doses, preferential blockade of presynaptic DA receptors results in increased DA release, and consequently increased CSN discharge; at higher doses, blockade of postsynaptic DA receptors on the sensory nerve terminal reduces or abolishes CSN discharge, irrespective of the effects of the blocking agent on other DA receptors.

C. Other Neurotransmitters: Metabolism, Effects on CSN Discharge, and Possible Functional Roles

Acetylcholine

Chemoreceptor cells accumulate ^{3}H-choline via a high-affinity, Na^+-dependent uptake system (Fidone et al., 1977), and choline acetyltransferase, the ACh-synthesizing enzyme, has been biochemically detected in the rat carotid body (Hanbauer et al., 1977) and immunocytochemically located in chemoreceptor cells of the rabbit and cat carotid body (Wang et al., 1989). Acetylcholinesterase, the ACh-degrading enzyme, also is abundant in the tissue (Jones, 1975; Nurse, 1987). There has been controversy regarding the levels of ACh in this organ. Thus, Eyzaguirre et al. (1965) and Jones (1975), using bioassays, and Gual and Marsal

(1987), using the choline oxidase method, have reported a content of 20–30 μg/g tissue for the cat carotid body. In contrast, Fidone et al. (1976) and Hellstrom (1977) used the highly sensitive method of gas chromatography–mass spectrometry and found ACh levels 10 times lower than those cited above for the cat and rat, respectively. The turnover rate for ACh in the carotid body appears to be relatively fast; Fidone et al. (1977) reported a turnover time for acetylcholine of 90 min for the cat carotid body.

Nicotinic and muscarinic receptors have been studied in the carotid body using radiolabeled α-bungarotoxin and quinuclidinylbenzilate, respectively, as ligands. Biochemical and autoradiographic data suggest that the number of putative nicotinic sites in the cat carotid body (Dinger et al., 1985; but see Carbonetto et al., 1978) and muscarinic sites in the rabbit organ (Dinger et al., 1986, 1991) remains constant after chronic CSN denervation. As mentioned earlier, muscarinic receptors predominate in the rabbit carotid body, whereas nicotinic receptors are more prevalent in the cat (Hirano et al., 1992).

The first indication that chemoreceptor cells might release an ACh-like substance was obtained by Schweitzer and Wright (1938), who found that prostigmine, an inhibitor of acetylcholinesterase, augmented ventilation in a manner similar to that produced by injections of ACh. This observation was soon confirmed by other researchers, and the theme was further developed years later by Eyzaguirre et al. (1965) and Eyzaguirre and Zapata (1968a,b,c). In an elegant series of in vitro experiments, these investigators used a Loewi-type superfusion chamber to demonstrate that an ACh-like substance released from an upstream carotid body could excite a downstream organ. The upstream organ was stimulated either electrically or with asphyxia (by lifting the preparation into the overlying layer of mineral oil) while CSN discharge was recorded from the downstream organ. The increased discharge from the downstream organ could be blocked by addition of mecamylamine or acetylcholinesterase to the bathing solution, and the discharge was augmented further in the presence of eserine. Although later criticized (Paintal, 1967, 1972), these experiments nonetheless strongly suggested that a nicotinic ACh-like substance, degradable by acetylcholinesterase, was released from carotid body chemoreceptor cells during intense stimulation. However, the asphyxic stimulus was probably too intense and too long in duration to discriminate between the unique O_2 chemosensitivity of chemoreceptor cells and a generalized cellular response to marked O_2 deprivation. Also, it could not be determined from these experiments whether ACh released from the upstream carotid body directly activated CSN discharge in the downstream organ or acted instead by modifying the release of other neurotransmitters from the downstream organ, which in turn increased CSN activity. In fact, the later observation by Eyzaguirre et al. (1975) that the chemoexcitatory properties of ACh in the cat carotid body are attenuated in Ca^{2+}-free or Mg^{2+}-rich superfusion solutions favors the notion that ACh actions in the carotid body are mediated by release of other neurotransmitters. This interpretation gains further support from more recent experiments demonstrating the presence of putative nicotinic receptors on chemoreceptor cells and their absence from sensory nerve endings in the cat carotid body (Dinger et al., 1985), and also from the potent depolarizing actions of nicotinic agents on chemoreceptor cells (Eyzaguirre et al., 1990) which can provoke release of CA from these cells (Gomez-Niño et al., 1990).

Although originally proposed as the principal chemosensory transmitter in the carotid body, acting between the chemoreceptor cell and the sensory nerve ending (see Eyzaguirre and Zapata, 1968), the data currently available suggest instead that ACh is released from these cells to modify the ongoing release of other transmitters. As mentioned above, putative nicotinic receptors predominate in the cat carotid body and provoke cell depolarization and CA release, followed by chemoexcitation. Muscarinic receptors are likewise localized to the chemoreceptor cells and are undetectable on the sensory nerve terminals; these receptors predominate in the rabbit carotid body and mediate inhibition of CSN discharge and CA release in this species (Monti-Bloch and Eyzaguirre, 1980; Dinger et al., 1991; Hirano et al., 1992). Thus, depending on the receptor and animal species, ACh appears to act either as a positive or negative feedback modulator or neurotransmitter release from the chemoreceptor cells.

Serotonin

Serotonin has been measured biochemically in the carotid bodies of rat, cat, and humans (Chiochio et al., 1967; Hellstrom and Koslow, 1975; Hellstrom, 1977; Perrin et al., 1990) and immunocytochemically identified in the chemoreceptor cells of these species (Grönblad et al., 1983; Perrin et al., 1986; Abramovici et al., 1991). The metabolism of serotonin in the carotid body has not been extensively studied and the available data are not consistent. Thus, although no measurable serotonin synthesis was observed in rabbit carotid bodies incubated with the labeled natural precursor ^{3}H-tryptophan (Gonzalez and Fidone, unpublished), Fishman et al. (1985) reported that serotonin was nonetheless present in media bathing cultured type I cells.

The pharmacology of serotonin actions in the carotid body also fails to clarify its role in the organ. When injected into the carotid artery of the rat and dog, serotonin produces a hyperventilation that is abolished by CSN section (Sapru and Krieger, 1977; Black et al., 1972). In the cat, however, serotonin produces apnea that persists after CSN transection but disappears with vagotomy (Black et al., 1972). Intracarotid injections of serotonin in the cat, dog, and rabbit produce a transient increase followed by a decrease in CSN discharge that is unaffected by conventional serotonin antagonists (Nishi, 1975; Bisgard et al., 1979; Docherty and McQueen, 1979). In the cat, more specific blockers of 5-HT$_2$ and 5-HT$_3$ receptors selectively block the different components of the CSN response to exogenously applied serotonin, but fail to modify the low P_{O_2}-induced CSN activity (Kirby and McQueen, 1984). A recent autoradiographic study of ^{3}H-serotonin binding in normal and CSN-denervated cat carotid bodies showed that serotonin receptors persist (or even increase) after CSN denervation, and that selective 5-HT$_3$ antagonists in high doses reduce both the basal- and hypoxia-evoked CSN discharge (Dashwood et al., 1990; McQueen and Evrard, 1990); similar results were reported for the rat carotid body (Yoshioka, 1989). The general sentiment from these studies is that serotonin may not be of paramount importance in the immediate chemoexcitation process.

Opioid Peptides

The chemoreceptor cells of the carotid body contain opioid peptides (Lundberg et al., 1979; Wharton et al., 1980) that are apparently colocalized with CA in dense-core granules (Hansen et al., 1982; Varndell et al., 1982; Kobayashi et al, 1983). More recent studies reveal greater immunoreactivity of chemoreceptor cells to met-enkephalin than leu-enkephalin (Heym and Kummer, 1989; Abramovici et al., 1991; Smith et al., 1990) and an absence of prodynorphin and β-endorphin immunoreactivity in the carotid bodies of the cat, rabbit, dog, and monkey (Heym and Kummer, 1989).

Consistent with the immunohistochemical findings, a number of laboratories have demonstrated with radioimmunoassay of carotid body homogenates that met-enkaphalin is present in much higher concentrations than leu-enkephalin (Wharton et al., 1980; Smith et al., 1990; Gonzalez-Guerrero et al., 1993b). Hanson et al. (1986) reported that strong hypoxic stimulation (5% O_2 in N_2; 1 hr) of the rabbit carotid body markedly reduced the normal levels of met-enkephalin-like immuno-reactivity in the organ (63 ng/mg prot, or ca. 15 nmole/g). Using a radioreceptor assay specific for δ-opioid ligands, Rigual et al. (1990) and Gonzalez-Guerrero et al. (1993b) found 248 pmole/mg prot of total opioid activity in the rabbit carotid body, most (86%) of which was of low-molecular-weight activity. HPLC fractiona-tion of the tissue extracts followed by radioreceptor assay of the fractions revealed that the met- to leu-enkephalin ratio was 5.86, indicating that the precursor molecule for carotid body opioid peptides is proenkephalin A. The unusually high level of opioid processing in the normal carotid body compared with other peripheral structures suggests that opioids may have a prominent role in the physiology of this organ (Rigual et al., 1990). Moderate hypoxic stimulation of the carotid body (8% O_2; 3 hr) reduced DA levels as well as the various molecular species of opioids by 40% (Gonzalez-Guerrero et al., 1993b). These data suggest, in agreement with the immunocytochemical findings, that DA and opioid peptides are costored in the same secretory vesicles, which release their contents upon natural stimulation. When rabbits were chronically exposed to an hypoxic atmo-sphere (11% O_2), opioid species of all molecular weights are decreased by day 2, but gradually returned to control levels between days 4 and 8. During recovery in air, high-molecular-weight species initially increased and then returned to control levels by the 8th day; low-molecular-weight species, on the other hand, did not change during the recovery period. The changes observed for the opioid peptides and for DA revealed a progressively increasing ratio of DA/low-molecular-weight species during the hypoxic exposure, which reached a maximum by the second day of recovery and returned to normal by day 8 (Gonzalez-Guerrero et al., 1993a).

Pharmacological studies of the effects of opioid peptides on CSN discharge indicate that inhibition is the primary action of this class of putative neurotransmitter. In the in vivo cat carotid body preparation, met-enkephalin depresses the resting CSN discharge in a dose-dependent and naloxone-sensitive manner (McQueen, 1983). In vitro experiments in this same species have revealed that met-enkephalin (10^{-6} M) decreases the chemoreceptor responses to low P_{O_2}, high P_{CO_2}, low pH, cyanide, and ACh, although the dose-dependent inhibition was sometimes followed by a rebound increase in CSN resting discharge (Monti-Bloch and Eyzaguirre, 1985). However, it was observed in this study that naloxone depressed resting CSN discharge, whereas simultaneous administration of both naloxone and met-enkephalin increased the nerve activity. On the other hand, more recent and detailed pharmacological studies have demonstrated that opioid agonists active at δ-opioid receptors reduce the CSN response to both hypoxia and hypercapnia, and conversely that the corresponding antagonists increase the nerve response (Kirby and McQueen, 1986; McQueen and Evrard, 1990). These findings agree with earlier reports showing that naloxone augments the low P_{O_2}-induced hyperventilation (Pokorski and Lahiri, 1981) and suggest that opioids released in response to natural chemoreceptor stimulation act to inhibit CSN activity (Hanson et al., 1986; Gonzalez-Guerrero et al., 1993b).

As mentioned above, the low P_{O_2}-induced release of DA is inhibited by δ (but not μ) opioid agonists, and is potentiated by naloxone (Gonzalez-Guerrero et al., 1993b). This observation, coupled with the pharmacological effects of opioids on CSN discharge, indicates that opioid peptides are coreleased with DA from the chemoreceptor cells and that δ-opioid receptors located on these cells mediate a feedback inhibition of DA release. This mechanism is only one possible explanation for the inhibition of CSN discharge by opioid peptides, because it is not known whether δ-opioid receptors are also located on other carotid body elements, in particular the sensory nerve endings.

Substance P

Substance P and neurokinin A have been immunocytochemically identified in nerve fibers and chemoreceptor cells of the carotid body (Cuello and McQueen, 1980; Scheibner et al., 1988; Prabhakar et al., 1989; Smith et al., 1990). Carotid body substance P levels have been measured in the cat (54–57 pmole/g; Wharton et al., 1980; Prabhakar et al., 1989), the rabbit (ca. 295 pmole/g; Hanson et al., 1986), and the human (15 pmole/g; Smith et al., 1990). It has been reported that acute hypoxic stimulation reduces substance P levels in the rabbit carotid body (Hanson et al,. 1986), but increases the peptide levels in the cat carotid body (Prabhakar et al., 1989); in this latter study, basal levels of neurokinin A (85 pmole/g) were reduced nearly 60% after the animals were exposed for 1 hr to 100% O_2, but exposure to hypoxia had no effect.

The pharmacology of substance P actions in the carotid body indicates that this peptide is primarily excitatory to the chemoreceptor response. Intracarotid injections of substance P produce a prolonged dose-dependent increase in basal CSN discharge and an augmentation of the response to cyanide, but depression of the acetylcholine response (McQueen, 1983). In the in vitro preparation, the effect was the same on basal CSN discharge, but opposite effects were observed for the responses to cyanide and ACh (Monti-Bloch and Eyzaguirre, 1985). Prabhakar et al. (1984, 1987, 1989, 1990, 1992) confirmed the excitatory effects of substance P and neurokinin A on basal CSN discharge, but, more important, demonstrated that certain substance P antagonists abolished or reduced the natural chemoreceptor response to low P_{O_2}, and high P_{CO_2}. However, other pharmacological studies with these substance P antagonists could not confirm their blocking effect on the response to low P_{O_2} (Shirahata, 1989; McQueen and Evrard, 1990), high P_{CO_2}, or cyanide (McQueen and Evrard, 1990). Consequently, at the present time, although substance P remains an attractive candidate as a putative excitatory neurotransmitter in the carotid body, knowledge of the release dynamics and site(s) of action of this peptide in the carotid body are still lacking.

Vasoactive Intestinal Polypeptide and Neuropeptide Y

Both these peptides are contained primarily in the sympathetic innervation of the carotid body vasculature (Wharton et al., 1980; Fitzgerald et al., 1981; Smith et al., 1990; Kondo et al., 1986; Kummer, 1990), and their exogenous administration provokes an increase in CSN discharge in vivo (Fitzgerald et al., 1981; McQueen and Ribeiro, 1981; Potter and McCloskey, 1987). Their effects can likely be attributed to changes in carotid body blood flow; also, these peptides may account for the increase in CSN discharge produced by the component of sympathetic ganglioglomerular nerve stimulation that is resistant to adrenergic blockade (Potter and McCloskey, 1987).

Adenosine

Adenosine triphosphate is a normal constituent of dense-core vesicles in the carotid body (Böck, 1980a,b) and consequently should be released with CA during exocytosis. Prompt degradation by ectonucleotidases presumably yields free adenosine. Pharmacological studies show that adenosine increases CSN discharge from the cat carotid body both in vivo (McQueen and Ribeiro, 1983) and in vitro (Runold et al., 1990). The nucleotide has been shown to activate ventilation in a number of species (Watt et al., 1987; Griffths et al., 1990; Reid et al., 1991; Monteiro and Ribeiro, 1987, 1989a,b, 1990; but see McQueen, 1992), an effect that is potentiated by adenosine uptake blockers (Monteiro and Ribeiro, 1989b). It is likely, then, that adenosine derived from vesicular exocytosis contributes to the overall chemoresponse.

Acknowledgments

This work was supported by USPHS Grants NS12636 and NS07938 and DGICYT (Spain) Grant 89/0358.

References

Abramovici A, Pallot DJ, Polak JM. Immunohistochemical approach to the study of the cat carotid body. Acta Anat Basel 1991; 140:70–74.

Acker H. The meaning of tissue P_{O_2} and local blood flow for the chemoreceptive process of the carotid body. Fed Proc 1980; 39:2641–2647.

Acker H. Importance of oxygen supply in the carotid body for chemoreception. Biomed Biochim Acta 1987; 46:885–898.

Acker H. P_{O_2} chemoreception in arterial chemoreceptors. Annu Rev Physiol 1989; 51: 835–844.

Acker H, Eyzaguirre C. Light absorbance changes in the mouse carotid body during hypoxia and cyanide poisoning. Brain Res 1987; 409:380–385.

Acker H, Lubbers DW. Relationship between local flow, tissue P_{O_2} and total flow of the cat carotid body. In: Acker H, Fidone S, Pallot D, Eyzaguirre C, Lübbers, DW, Torrance RW, eds. Chemoreception in the Carotid Body. Berlin: Springer-Verlag, 1977a: 271–276.

Acker H, Lubbers DW. The kinetics of local tissue P_{O_2} decrease after perfusion stop within the carotid body of the cat in vivo and in vitro. Pflüger's Arch 1977b; 369:135–140.

Acker H, Lubbers DW. The meaning of the tissue P_{O_2} of the carotid body for the chemoreceptive process. In: Purves MJ, ed. The Peripheral Arterial Chemoreceptors. London: Cambridge University Press, 1975:325–343.

Acker H, O'Regan RG. The effects of stimulation of autonomic nerves on carotid body blood flow in the cat. J Physiol (Lond) 1981; 315:99–110.

Acker H, Delpiano M, Degner M. The meaning of the P_{O_2} field in the carotid body for the chemoreceptive process. In: Acker H, O'Regan RG, eds. Physiology of the Peripheral Arterial Chemoreceptors. Amsterdam, The Netherlands: Elsevier, 1983: 89–115.

Almaraz L, Fidone S. Carotid sinus nerve C-fibers release catecholamines from the cat carotid body. Neurosci Lett 1986; 67:153–158.

Almaraz L, Gonzalez C, Obeso A. Effects of high potassium on the release of ³H-dopamine from the cat carotid body in vitro. J Physiol (Lond) 1986; 379:293–307.

Almaraz L, Perez-Garcia MT, Gonzalez C. Presence of D1 receptors in the rabbit carotid body. Neurosci Lett 1991; 132:259–262.

Almaraz L, Rigual R, Obeso A, Evrard Y, Gonzalez C. Effects of almitrine on the release of catecholamines from the rabbit carotid body in vitro. Br J Pharmacol 1992; 106: 697–702.

Aminoff MJ, Jaffe RA, Sampson SR, Vidruk EH. Effects of droperidol on activity of carotid body chemoreceptors in cat. Br J Pharmacol 1978; 63:245–250.

Anichkov SV, Belenki'i ML. Pharmacology of the Carotid Body Chemoreceptors. New York: Macmillan, 1963.

Aronson PS. Kinetic properties of the plasma membrane Na⁺-H⁺ exchanger. Annu Rev Physiol 1985; 47:545–560.

Avenet P, Hofman F, Lindeman B. Transduction in taste receptor cells requires cAMP-dependent protein kinase. Nature 1988; 331:351–356.

Bacopoulos NG, Bhatnagar RK. Correlation between tyrosine hydroxylase activity and catecholamine concentration or turnover in brain regions. J Neurochem 1977; 29: 639–643.

Bakhit C, Gibb JW. In vitro effects of pH and phosphorylation on neostriatal tyrosine hydroxylase from control and haloperidol-treated rats. Life Sci 1979; 25:1389–1396.

Barnett S, Mulligan E, Wagerle LC, Lahiri S. Measurement of carotid body blood flow in cats by use of radioactive microspheres. J Appl Physiol 1988; 65:2484–2489.

Baron M, Eyzaguirre C. Effects of temperature on some membrane characteristics of carotid body cells. Am J Physiol 1977; 233:C35–C46.

Bartfai T, Iverfeldt K, Fisone G. Regulation of the release of coexisting neurotransmitters. Annu Rev Pharmacol Toxicol 1988; 28:385–310.

Belmonte C, Gonzalez C, Garcia AG. Dopamine β-hydroxylase activity in the cat carotid body. In: Acker H, Fidone S, Pallot D, Eyzaguirre C, Lübbers DW, Torrance RW. Chemoreception in the Carotid Body. Berlin: Springer-Verlag, 1977:99–105.

Benot A, Lopez-Barneo J. Feedback inhibition of Ca²⁺ currents by dopamine in glomus cells of the carotid body. Eur J Neurosci 1990; 2:809–812.

Bernon R, Leitner LM, Roumy M, Verna A. Effects of ion-containing liposomes upon the chemoafferent activity of the rabbit carotid body superfused in vitro. Neurosci Lett 1983; 35:289–295.

Biscoe TJ. Carotid body: structure and function. Physiol Rev 1971; 51:437–495.

Biscoe TJ, Duchen MR. Electrophysiological responses of dissociated type I cells of the rabbit carotid body to cyanide. J Physiol (Lond) 1989; 413:447–468.

Biscoe TJ, Duchen MR. Responses of type I cells dissociated from the rabbit carotid body to hypoxia. J Physiol (Lond) 1990a; 428:39–59.

Biscoe TJ, Duchen MR. Cellular basis of transduction in carotid chemoreceptors. Am J Physiol 1990b; 258:L271–L278.

Biscoe TJ, Duchen MR. Monitoring Po₂ by the carotid chemoreceptor. News Physiol Sci 1990c; 5:229–233.

Biscoe TJ, Purves MJ, Sampson SR. The frequency of nerve impulses in single carotid body chemoreceptor afferent fibres recorded in vivo with intact circulation. J Physiol (Lond) 1970; 208:121–131.

Biscoe TJ, Duchen MR, Eisner DA, O'Neill SC, Valdeolmillos M. Measurements of intracellular Ca^{2+} in dissociated type I cells of the rabbit carotid body. J Physiol (Lond) 1989; 416:421–434.

Bisgard GE, Mitchell RA, Herbert DA. Effects of dopamine, norepinephrine and 5-hydroxytryptamine on the carotid body of the dog. Respir Physiol 1979; 37:61–80.

Black AM, Comroe JHJ, Jacobs L. Species difference in carotid body response of cat and dog to dopamine and serotonin. Am J Physiol 1972; 223:1097–1102.

Blaustein MP. Calcium transport and buffering in neurons. Trends Neurosci 1988; 11: 438–443.

Bock P. Adenine nucleotides in the carotid body. Cell Tissue Res 1980a; 206:279–290.

Bock P. Histochemical demonstration of adenine nucleotides in carotid body type I cells. Adv Biochem Psychopharmacol 1980b; 25:235–239.

Bolme P, Fuxe K, Hokfelt T, Goldstein M. Studies on the role of dopamine in cardiovascular and respiratory control: central versus peripheral mechanisms. Adv Biochem Psychopharmacol 1977; 16:281–290.

Boron WF. Intracellular pH regulation. In: Andreoli TE, Hoffman JF, Fanestil DD, Schultz SG, eds. Physiology of Membrane Disorders. New York: Plenum Press, 1986: 423–435.

Boron WF, Knakal RC. Na^+-dependent $Cl-HCO_3$ exchange in the squid axon. J Gen Physiol 1992; 99:817–837.

Boron WF, Boyarsky G, Ganz M. Regulation of intracellular pH in renal mesangial cells. Ann NY Acad Sci 1989; 574:321–332.

Bountra C, Vaughan-Jones RD. Effect of intracellular and extracellular pH on contraction in isolated, mammalian cardiac muscle. J Physiol (Lond) 1989; 418:163–187.

Brokaw JJ, Hansen JT, Christie DS. The effects of hypoxia on catecholamine dynamics in the rat carotid body. J Auton Nerv Syst 1985; 13:35–47.

Brown RH, Noble D. Displacement of activation thresholds in cardiac muscle by protons and calcium ions. J Physiol (Lond) 1978; 282:333–343.

Buckler KJ, Vaughan-Jones RD. Raising P_{CO_2} elevates $[Ca^{2+}]_i$ in neonatal rat carotid body glomus cells. J Physiol (Lond) 1992; 452:228P.

Buckler KJ, Vaughan-Jones RD, Peers C, Nye PC. Intracellular pH and its regulation in isolated type I carotid body cells of the neonatal rat. J Physiol (Lond) 1991a; 436:107–129.

Buckler KJ, Vaughan-Jones RD, Peers C, Lagadic-Gossmann D, Nye PCG. Effects of extracellular pH, P_{CO_2} and HCO_3^- on intracellular pH in isolated type I cells of the neonatal rat. J Physiol (Lond) 1991b; 444:703–721.

Buerk DG, Nair PK, Whalen WJ. Evidence for second metabolic pathway for O_2 from Pti_{O_2} measurements in denervated cat carotid body. J Appl Physiol 1989a; 67:1578–1584.

Buerk DG, Nair PK, Whalen WJ. Two-cytochrome metabolic model for carotid body Pti_{O_2} and chemosensitivity changes after hemorrhage. J Appl Physiol 1989b; 67:60–68.

Campbell G. Cotransmission. Annu Rev Pharmacol Toxicol 1987; 27:51–70.

Carbonetto ST, Fambrough DM, Muller KJ. Nonequivalence of α-bungarotoxin receptors and acetylcholine receptors in chick sympathetic neurons. Proc Natl Acad Sci USA 1978; 75:1016–1020.

Chen IL, Yates RD. Two types of glomus cell in the rat carotid body as revealed by α-bungarotoxin binding. J Neurocytol 1984; 13:281–302.

Chen IL, Hansen JT, Yates RD. Dopamine β-hydroxylase-like immunoreactivity in the rat and cat carotid body: a light and electron microscopic study. J Neurocytol 1985; 14:131–144.

Chiocchio SR, Biscardi AM, Tramezzani JH. 5-Hydroxytryptamine in the carotid body of the cat. Science 1967; 158:790–791.

Chiocchio SR, Barrio-Rendo ME, Tramezzani JH. Increased norepinephrine and dopamine content of the rat carotid body after chronic hypoxia. In: Belmonte C, Pallot DJ, Acker H, Fidone SJ, eds. Arterial Chemoreceptors. Leicester, UK: Leicester University Press, 1981:237–244.

Chiocchio SR, Hilton SM, Tramezzani JH, Willshaw P. Loss of peripheral chemoreflexes to hypoxia after carotid body removal in the rat. Respir Physiol 1984; 57:235–246.

Clark JD, Limbird LE. Na⁺-H⁺ exchanger subtypes: a predictive review. Am J Physiol 1991; 261:C945–C953.

Coburn RF, Forman HJ. Carbon monoxide toxicity. In: Fishman AP, ed. Handbook of Physiology. The Respiratory System. Bethesda, MD: American Physiological Society, 1987:439–456.

Coxon RV. Regulation of biochemical reactions by oxygen and carbon dioxide. In: Torrance RW, ed. Arterial Chemoreceptors. Oxford, UK: Blackwell Scientific Publications, 1968:91–102.

Cross AR, Henderson L, Jones OT, Delpiano MA, Hentschel J, Acker H. Involvement of an NAD(P)H oxidase as a Po_2 sensor protein in the rat carotid body. Biochem. J. 1990; 272:743–747.

Cuello AC. Peptides as neuromodulators in primary sensory neurons. Neuropharmacology 1987; 26:971–979.

Czyzyk-Krzeska MF, Bayliss DA, Lawson EE, Millhorn DE. Regulation of tyrosine hydroxylase in the rat carotid body by hypoxia. J Neurochem 1992; 58:1538–1546.

Daly M de B., Lambertsen CJ, Schweitzer A. Observations on the volume of blood flow and oxygen utilization of the carotid body in the cat. J Physiol (Lond) 1954; 125:67–89.

Dashwood MR, McQueen DS, de Burgh Daly M, Spyer KM, Evrard Y. Autoradiographic studies on the effects of chronic unilateral sectioning of a carotid sinus nerve on 5-HT and SP binding sites in the carotid body and NTS. In: Acker H, Trzebski A, O'Regan RG, eds. Chemoreceptors and Chemoreceptor Reflexes. New York: Plenum Press, 1990:305–309.

De Castro F. Sur la structure et l'innervation de la glande intercarotidienne (glomus caroticum) de l'homme et des mammifères, et sur un nouveau système d'innervation autonome du nerf glossopharyngien. Trab Lab Invest Biol Univ Madrid 1926; 24: 365–432.

De Castro F. Sur la structure et l'innervation du sinus carotidien de l'homme et des mammifères: Nouveaux faits sur l'innervation et la fonction du glomus caroticum. Trab Lab Invest Biol Univ Madrid 1928; 25:330–380.

De Castro F. Nuevas observaciones sobre la inervación de la región carotidea. Los quimio y presorreceptores. Trab Lab Invest Biol Univ Madrid 1940; 32:297–384.

De Castro F. Sur la structure de la synapse dans les chemorecepteurs: leur mécanisme d'excitation et rôle dans la circulation sanguine locale. Acta Physiol Scand 1951; 22:14–43.

De Castro F, Rubio M. The anatomy and innervation of the blood vessels of the carotid body and the role of chemoreceptive reactions in the autoregulation of the blood flow. In: Torrance RW, ed. Arterial Chemoreceptors. Oxford, UK: Blackwell Scientific Publications, 1968:267–277.

Dearnaley DP, Fillenz M, Woods RI. The identification of dopamine in the rabbit's carotid body. Proc R. Soc Lond Biol 1968; 170:195–203.

Degner F, Acker H. Mathematical analysis of Po_2 and local flow distribution in the carotid body. Adv Exp Med Biol 1985; 191:719–726.

Degner F, Acker H. Mathematical analysis of tissue Po_2 distribution in the cat carotid body. Pflüger's Arch 1986; 407:305–311.

De Kock LL. History of the carotid body. Nature 1951; 167:611–612.

De Kock LL. The intra-glomerular tissues of the carotid body. Acta Anat 1954; 21: 101–116.

Delpiano MA, Acker H. Extracellular pH changes in the superfused cat carotid body during hypoxia and hypercapnia. Brain Res 1985; 342:273–280.

Delpiano MA, Acker H. Hypoxia increases the cyclic AMP content of the cat carotid body in vitro. J Neurochem 1991; 57:291–297.

Delpiano MA, Hescheler J. Evidence for a Po_2-sensitive K^+ channel in the type-I cell of the rabbit carotid body. FEBS Lett 1989; 249:195–198.

Delpiano MA, Hescheler J. Does an inward-rectifying K channel regulate. In: Acker H, Trzebski A, O'Regan RG, eds. Chemoreceptors and Chemoreceptor Reflexes. New York: Plenum Press, 1990:15–19.

Delpiano MA, Starlinger H, Fischer M, Acker H. The c-AMP content of the cat carotid body in vivo and in vitro under normoxia and after stimulation by hypoxia. In: Pallot DJ, ed. The Peripheral Arterial Chemoreceptors. London: Croom Helm, 1984:401–408.

Dinger B, Gonzalez C, Yoshizaki K, Fidone S. Localization and function of cat carotid body nicotinic receptors. Brain Res 1985; 339:295–304.

Dinger BG, Hirano T, Fidone SJ. Autoradiographic localization of muscarinic receptors in rabbit carotid body. Brain Res 1986; 367:328–331.

Dinger B, Hirano T, Gonzalez C, Yoshizaki K, Gomez-Nino A, Fidone S. Muscarinic receptor localization and function in rabbit carotid body. Brain Res 1991; 562: 190–198.

Docherty RJ, McQueen DS. Inhibitory action of dopamine on cat carotid chemoreceptors. J Physiol (Lond) 1978; 279:425–436.

Docherty RJ, McQueen DS. The effects of acetylcholine and dopamine on carotid chemosensory activity in the rabbit. J Physiol (Lond) 1979; 288:411–423.

Donnelly DF, Kholwadwala D. Hypoxia decreases intracellular calcium in adult rat carotid body glomus cells. J Neurophysiol 1992; 67:1543–1551.

Donnelly DF, Smith EJ, Dutton RE. Neural response of carotid chemoreceptors following dopamine blockade. J Appl Physiol 1981; 50:172–177.

Duchen MR, Biscoe TJ. Relative mitochondrial membrane potential and $[Ca^{2+}]_i$ in type I cells isolated from the rabbit carotid body. J Physiol (Lond) 1992a; 450:33–61.

Duchen MR, Biscoe TJ. Mitochondrial function in type I cells isolated from rabbit arterial chemoreceptors. J Physiol 1992b; 450:13–31.

Duchen MR, Biscoe TJ. Relative mitochondrial membrane potential and $[Ca^{2+}]_i$ in type I cells isolated from the rabbit carotid body. J Physiol 1992c; 450:33–61.

Duchen MR, Caddy KW, Kirby GC, Patterson DL, Ponte J, Biscoe TJ. Biophysical studies of the cellular elements of the rabbit carotid body. Neuroscience 1988; 26:291–311.

Eldridge FL, Gill-Kumar P. Mechanisms of hyperpnea induced by isoproterenol. Respir Physiol 1980; 40:349–363.

Erecinska M, Dagani F. Relationships between the neuronal sodium/potassium pump and energy metabolism. J Gen Physiol 1990; 95:591–616.

Erecinska M, Silver IA. ATP and brain function. J Cereb Blood Flow Metab 1989; 9:2–19.

Erecinska M, Wilson DF. Regulation of cellular energy metabolism. J Memb Biol 1982; 70:1–14.

Eyzaguirre C, Koyano H. Effects of hypoxia, hypercapnia and pH on the chemoreceptor activity of the carotid body in vitro. J Physiol (Lond) 1965; 178:385–409.

Eyzaguirre C, Zapata P. Transmitter substance release from carotid body chemoreceptors. Actual Neurophysiol Paris 1968a; 8:73–88.

Eyzaguirre C, Zapata P. The release of acetylcholine from carotid body tissues. Further study on the effects of acetylcholine and cholinergic blocking agents on the chemosensory discharge. J Physiol (Lond) 1968b; 195:589–607.

Eyzaguirre C, Zapata P. A discussion of possible transmitter or generator substances in carotid body chemoreceptors. In: Torrance RW, ed. Arterial Chemoreceptors. Oxford, UK: Blackwell Scientific Publications, 1968c:213–251.

Eyzaguirre C, Koyano H, Taylor JR. Presence of acetylcholine and transmitter release from carotid body chemoreceptors. J Physiol (Lond) 1965; 178:463–476.

Eyzaguirre C, Fidone S, Nishi K. Recent studies on the generation of chemoreceptor impulses. In: Purves MJ, ed. The Peripheral Arterial Chemoreceptors. London: Cambridge University Press, 1975:175–194.

Eyzaguirre C, Monti-Bloch L, Hayashida Y, Baron M. Biophysics of the carotid body receptor complex. In: Acker H, O'Regan RG, eds. Physiology of the Peripheral Arterial Chemoreceptors. Amsterdam: Elsevier Science Publishers, 1983:59–87.

Eyzaguirre C, Monti-Bloch L, Baron M, Hayashida Y, Woodbury JW. Changes in glomus cell membrane properties in response to stimulants and depressants of carotid nerve discharge. Brain Res 1989; 477:265–279.

Eyzaguirre C, Monti-Bloch L, Woodbury JW. Effects of putative neurotransmitters of the carotid body on its own glomus cells. Eur J Neurosci 1990; 2:77–88.

Fidone SJ, Gonzalez C. Catecholamine synthesis in rabbit carotid body in vitro. J Physiol (Lond) 1982; 333:69–79.

Fidone SJ, Gonzalez C. Initiation and control of chemoreceptor activity in the carotid body. In: Fishman AP, ed. Handbook of Physiology. The Respiratory System. Bethesda, MD: American Physiological Society, 1986:247–312.

Fidone SJ, Sato A. A study of chemoreceptor and baroreceptor A and C-fibres in the cat carotid nerve. J Physiol (Lond) 1969; 205:527–548.

Fidone SJ, Weintraub ST, Stavinoha WB. Acetylcholine content of normal and denervated cat carotid bodies measured by pyrolysis gas chromatography/mass fragmentometry. J Neurochem 1976; 26:1047–1049.

Fidone S, Weintraub S, Stavinoha W, Stirling C, Jones L. Endogenous acetylcholine levels in cat carotid body and the autoradiographic localization of a high affinity component of choline uptake. In: Acker H, Fidone S, Pallot D, Eyzaguirre C, Lübbers DW, Torrance RW, eds. Chemoreception in the Carotid Body. Berlin: Springer-Verlag, 1977:106–113.

Fidone SJ, Gonzalez C, Yoshizaki K. Putative neurotransmitters in the carotid body: the case for dopamine. Fed Proc 1980; 39:2636–2640.

Fidone S, Gonzalez C, Yoshizaki K. A study of the relationship between dopamine release and chemosensory discharge from the rabbit carotid body in vitro: preliminary findings. In: Belmonte C, Pallot DJ, Acker H, Fidone S. Arterial Chemoreceptors. Leicester, UK: Leicester University Press, 1981:209–219.

Fidone S, Gonzalez C, Yoshizaki K. Effects of low oxygen on the release of dopamine from the rabbit carotid body in vitro. J Physiol (Lond) 1982a; 333:93–110.

Fidone S, Gonzalez C, Yoshizaki K. Effects of hypoxia on catecholamine synthesis in rabbit carotid body in vitro. J Physiol (Lond) 1982b; 333:81–91.

Fidone SJ, Gonzalez C, Dinger BG, Hanson GR. Mechanisms of chemotransmission in the mammalian carotid body. Prog Brain Res 1988; 74:169–179.

Fidone S, Gonzalez C, Dinger B, Stensaas L. Transmitter dynamics in the carotid body. In: Acker H, Trzebski A, O'Regan RG. Chemoreceptors and Chemoreceptor Reflexes. New York: Plenum Press, 1990a:3–14.

Fidone SJ, Gonzalez C, Obeso A, Gomez-Niño A, Dinger B. Biogenic amine and neuropeptide transmitters in carotid body chemotransmission. Experimental findings and perspectives. In: Sutton JR, Coates G, Remmers JE, eds. Hypoxia. The Adaptations. Philadelphia: BC Decker, 1990b:116–126.

Fidone S, Gonzalez C, Dinger B, Gomez-Niño A, Obeso A, Yoshizaki K. Cellular aspects of peripheral chemoreceptor function. In: Crystal RG, West JB, eds. The Lung. Scientific Foundations. New York: Raven Press, 1991:1319–1332.

Fishman MC, Greene WL, Platika D. Oxygen chemoreception by carotid body cells in culture. Proc Natl Acad Sci USA 1985; 82:1448–1450.

Fitzgerald RS, Parks DC. Effect of hypoxia on carotid chemoreceptor response to carbon dioxide in cats. Respir Physiol 1971; 12:218–229.

Fitzgerald RS, Rogus EM, Dehghani A. Catecholamines and 3',5' cyclic AMP in carotid body chemoreception in the cat. Adv Exp Med Biol 1977; 78:245–258.

Fitzgerald RS, Raff H, Garger P, Fletcher L, Anand A, Said S. Vasoactive intestinal polypeptide (VIP) and the carotid body. In: Belmonte C, Pallot DJ, Acker H, Fidone S, eds. Arterial Chemoreceptors. Leicester, UK: Leicester University Press, 1981:289–298.

Fitzgerald RS, Garger P, Hauer MC, Raff H, Fechter L. Effect of hypoxia and hypercapnia on catecholamine content in cat carotid body. J Appl Physiol 1983; 54:1408–1413.

Folgering H, Ponte J, Sadig T. Adrenergic mechanisms and chemoreception in the carotid body of the cat and rabbit. J Physiol (Lond) 1982; 325:1–21.

Forster RE. The diffusion of gases in the carotid body. In: Torrance RW, ed. Arterial Chemoreceptors. Oxford, UK: Blackwell Scientific Publications, 1968:115–132.

Fried G., Meister B, Wikstrom M, Terenius L, Goldstein M. Galanin-, neuropeptide Y- and enkephalin-like immunoreactivities in catecholamine-storing paraganglia of the fetal guinea pig and newborn pig. Cell Tissue Res 1989; 255:495–504.

Fuortes MGF. Generation of responses in receptor. In: Loewenstein WR, ed. Handbook of Sensory Physiology. Vol I, Principles of Receptor Physiology. Berlin: Springer-Verlag, 1971:243–268.

Gallman EA, Millhorn DE. Two long-lasting central respiratory responses following acute hypoxia in glomectomized cats. J Physiol (Lond) 1988; 395:333–347.

Ganfornina MD, Lopez-Barneo J. Single K^+ channels in membrane patches of arterial chemoreceptor cells are modulated by O_2 tension. Proc Natl Acad Sci USA 1991; 88:2927–2930.

Ganfornina MD, Lopez-Barneo J. Potassium channel types in arterial chemoreceptor cells and their selective modulation by oxygen. J Gen Physiol 1992a; 100:401–426.

Ganfornina MD, Lopez-Barneo J. Gating of O_2-sensitive K^+ channels of arterial chemo-receptor cells and kinetic modulation induced by low Po_2. J Gen Physiol 1992b; 100:427–455.

Ganz MB, Boyarsky G, Sterzel RB, Boron WF. Arginine vasopressin enhances pHi regulation in the presence of HCO_3^- by stimulating three acid-based transport systems. Nature 1989; 337:648–651.

Goldberg M, Dunning SP, Bunn HF. Regulation of the erythropoietin gene: evidence that the oxygen sensor is a heme protein. Science 1988; 242:1412–1415.

Gomez-Niño A. Liberación diferencial de catecolaminas por las células quimiorreceptoras del cuerpo carotídeo. Regulación por autorreceptores. Doctoral thesis, University of Vallodolid, 1989.

Gomez-Niño A, Dinger B, Gonzalez C, Fidone SJ. Differential stimulus coupling to dopamine and norepinephrine stores in rabbit carotid body type I cells. Brain Res 1990; 525:160–164.

Gomez-Niño A, Almaraz L, Gonzalez C. Potentiation by cyclooxygenase inhibitors of the release of catecholamines from the rabbit carotid body and its reversal by prostaglandin E_2. Neurosci Lett 1992; 140:1–4.

Gonsalves SF, Smith EJ, Nolan WF, Dutton RE. Beta-adrenoceptor blockade spares chemoreceptor responsiveness to hypoxia. Brain Res 1984; 324:349–353.

Gonzalez C, Fidone S. Increased release of ³H-dopamine during low O_2 stimulation of rabbit carotid body in vitro. Neurosci Lett 1977; 6:95–99.

Gonzalez C, Kwok Y, Gibb J, Fidone S. Effects of hypoxia on tyrosine hydroxylase activity in rat carotid body. J Neurochem 1979a; 33:713–719.

Gonzalez C, Kwok Y, Gibb JW, Fidone SJ. Reciprocal modulation of tyrosine hydroxylase activity in rat carotid body. Brain Res 1979b; 172:572–576.

Gonzalez C, Obeso A, Fidone S. Tris buffer: effects on catecholamine synthesis. J Neurochem 1979c; 32:1143–1145.

Gonzalez C, Kwok Y, Gibb J, Fidone S. Physiological and pharmacologic effects on TH activity in rabbit and cat carotid body. Am J Physiol 1981a; 240:R38–R43.

Gonzalez C, Kwok Y, Gibb J, Fidone S. Regulation of tyrosine hydroxylase activities in carotid body, superior cervical ganglion and adrenal gland of rat, rabbit and cat. In: Belmonte C, Pallot DJ, Acker H, Fidone S, eds. Arterial Chemoreceptors. Leicester, UK: Leicester University Press, 1981b:187–197.

Gonzalez E, Rigual R, Fidone SJ, Gonzalez C. Mechanisms for termination of the action of dopamine in carotid body chemoreceptors. J Auton Nerv Syst 1987; 18: 249–259.

Gonzalez C, Rocher A, Obeso A, Lopez-Lopez JR, Lopez-Barneo J, Herreros B. Ionic mechanisms of the chemoreception process in type I cells of the carotid body. In: Eyzaguirre C, Fidone SJ, Fitzgerald RS, Lahiri S, McDonald DM, eds. Arterial Chemoreception. New York: Springer-Verlag, 1990:44–57.

Gonzalez C, Perez-Garcia MT, Mintenig GM, Gual A. Transmisión sináptica por neuro-transmisores múltiples. Cotransmisión en el cuerpo carotídeo. In: Esquerda JE, Gallego R, Gual A, Ramirez G, Rubia F. Neurotransmisión y Plasticidad Sinaptica. Barcelona: Expaxs, 1991:109–128.

Gonzalez C, Almaraz L, Obeso A, Rigual R. Oxygen and acid chemoreception in the carotid body chemoreceptors. Trends Neurosci 1992; 15:146–153.

Gonzalez C, Almaraz L, Obeso A, Rigual R. Carotid body chemoreceptors: from natural stimuli to sensory discharges. Physiol Rev (in press).

Gonzalez-Guerrero PR, Rigual R, Gonzalez C. Catecholamine and opioid peptides in the rabbit carotid body. Adaptative changes in chronic hypoxia. J Neurochem 1993a; 60:1769–1776.

Gonzalez-Guerrero PR, Rigual R, Gonzalez C. Co-utilization and interactions of cate-cholamine and opioid peptides in the carotid body chemoreceptors. J Neurochem 1993b; 60;1762–1768.

Gray BA. Response of the perfused carotid body to changes in pH and P_{CO_2}. Respir Physiol 1968; 4:229–245.

Griffiths TL, Warren SJ, Chant AD, Holgate ST. Ventilatory effects of hypoxia and adenosine infusion in patients after bilateral carotid endarterectomy. Clin Sci 1990; 78:25–31.

Grinstein S, Cohen S. Cytoplasmic $[Ca^{2+}]$ and intracellular pH in lymphocytes. Role of membrane potential and volume-activated Na^+/H^+ exchange. J Gen Physiol 1987; 89:185–213.

Grinstein S, Furuya W. Characterization of the amiloride-sensitive Na^+-H^+ antiport of human neutrophils. Am J Physiol 1986; 250:C283–C291.

Grinstein S, Rothstein A. Mechanisms of regulation of the Na^+/H^+ exchanger. J Memb Biol 1986; 90:1–12.

Grönblad M, Liesi P, Rechardt L. Serotonin-like immunoreactivity in rat carotid body. Brain Res 1983; 276:348–350.

Grundfest H. The electrophysiology of input membrane in electrogenic excitable cells. In: Loewenstein WR, ed. Handbook of Sensory Physiology. Principles of Receptor Physiology. New York: Springer-Verlag, 1971:135–165.

Gual A, Marsal J. Application of the chemiluminiscent method to carotid body for detecting choline and acetylcholine. In: Ribeiro JA, Pallot DJ, eds. Chemoreceptors in Respiratory Control. London: Croom Helm, 1987:108–113.

Hagiwara S, Miyazaki S, Moody W, Patlak J. Blocking effects of barium and hydrogen ions on the potassium current during anomalous rectification in the starfish egg. J Physiol (Lond) 1978; 279:167–185.

Hanbauer I. Molecular biology of chemoreceptor function: induction of tyrosine hydroxylase in the rat carotid body elicited by hypoxia. In: Acker H, Fidone S, Pallot D, Eyzaguirre C, Lübbers DW, Torrance RW, eds. Chemoreception in the Carotid Body. Berlin: Springer-Verlag, 1977:114–121.

Hanbauer I, Hellstrom S. The regulation of dopamine and noradrenaline in the rat carotid body and its modification by denervation and by hypoxia. J Physiol (Lond) 1978; 282:21–34.

Hanbauer I, Lovenberg W, Costa E. Induction of tyrosine 3-monooxygenase in carotid body of rats exposed to hypoxic conditions. Neuropharmacology 1977; 16:277–282.

Hanbauer I, Karoum F, Hellstrom S, Lahiri S. Effects of hypoxia lasting up to one month on the catecholamine content in rat carotid body. Neuroscience 1981; 6:81–86.

Hansen JT. Ultrastructure of the primate carotid body: a morphometric study of the glomus cells and nerve endings in the monkey (*Macaca fascicularis*). J Neurocytol 1985; 14:13–32.

Hansen J, Ord T. Effects of 6-hydroxydopamine on rat carotid body chief cells. Experientia 1978; 34:1357–1358.

Hansen JT, Brokaw J, Christie D, Karasek M. Localization of enkephalin-like immunoreactivity in the cat carotid and aortic body chemoreceptors. Anat Rec 1982; 203: 405–410.

Hanson MA, Nye PCG, Torrance RW. The exodus of an extracellular bicarbonate theory of chemoreception and the genesis of an intracellular one. In: Belmonte C, Pallot DJ, Acker H, Fidone S, eds. Arterial Chemoreceptors. Leicester, UK: Leicester University Press, 1981:403–416.

Hanson GR, Jones JF, Fidone S. Physiological chemoreceptor stimulation decreases enkephalin and substance P in the carotid body. Peptides 1986; 7:767–769.

Hayashida Y, Eyzaguirre C. Voltage noise of carotid body type I cells. Brain Res 1979; 167:189–194.

He SF, Wei JY, Eyzaguirre C. Intracellular pH of cultured carotid body cells. In: Eyzaguirre C, Fidone SJ, Fitzgerald RS, Lahiri S, McDonald DM, eds. Arterial Chemoreception. New York: Springer-Verlag, 1990:18–23.

He SF, Wei JY, Eyzaguirre C. Effects of relative hypoxia and hypercapnia on intracellular pH and membrane potential of cultured carotid body glomus cells. Brain Res 1992; 556:333–338.

Heistad DD, Wheeler RC, Mark AL, Schmid PG, Abboud FM. Effects of adrenergic stimulation on ventilation in man. J Clin Invest 1972; 51:1469–1475.

Hellstrom S. Morphometric studies of dense-cored vesicles in type I cells of rat carotid body. J Neurocytol 1975; 4:77–86.

Hellstrom S. Putative neurotransmitters in the carotid body. Mass fragmentographic studies. Adv Biochem Psychopharmacol 1977; 16:257–263.

Hellstrom S, Koslow SH. Biogenic amines in carotid body of adult and infant rats. A gas chromatographic-mass spectrometric assay. Acta Physiol Scand 1975; 93:540–547.

Hellstrom S, Hanbauer I, Costa E. Selective decrease of dopamine content in rat carotid body during exposure to hypoxic conditions. Brain Res 1976; 118:352–355.

Hellstrom S, Pequignot JM, Dahlqvist A. Catecholamines in the carotid body are unaffected by hypercapnia. Neurosci Lett 1989; 97:280–284.

Hescheler J, Delpiano MA. Ionic currents on carotid body type I cells and the effects of hypoxia and NaCN. In: Eyzaguirre C, Fidone SJ, Fitzgerald RS, Lahiri S, McDonald DM. Arterial Chemoreception. New York: Springer-Verlag, 1990:58–62.

Hescheler J, Delpiano MA, Acker H, Pietruschka F. Ionic currents on type-I cells of the rabbit carotid body measured by voltage-clamp experiments and the effect of hypoxia. Brain Res 1989; 486:79–88.

Hess A. The effects of 6-hydroxydopamine on the appearance of granulated vesicles in glomus cells of the rat carotid body. Tissue Cell 1976; 8:381–387.

Heym C, Kummer W. Immunohistochemical distribution and co-localization of regulatory peptides in the carotid body. J Electron Microsc Tech 1989; 12:331–342.

Hille B. Ionic Channels of Excitable Membranes. Sunderland, MA: Sinauer Associates, 1984.

Hirano T, Dinger B, Yoshizaki K, Gonzalez C, Fidone S. Nicotinic versus muscarinic binding sites in cat and rabbit carotid bodies. Biol Signals 1992; 1:143–149.

Hornbein TF. The relation between stimulus to chemoreceptors and their response. In: Torrance RW, ed. Arterial Chemoreceptors. Oxford, UK: Blackwell Scientific Publications, 1968:65–78.

Hornbein TF. Hypoxia and the brain. In: Crystal RG, West JB, eds. The Lung Scientific Foundations. New York: Raven Press, 1991:1535–1543.

Horowitz, Larrabee. Ref 13 in Obeso et al., 1993.

Hudgel DW, Kressin NA, Nielsen AM, Bisgard GE. Role of β-adrenergic receptors in carotid body function of the goat. Respir Physiol 1986; 64:203–221.

Iturriaga R, Lahiri S, Mokashi A. Carbonic anhydrase and chemoreception in the cat carotid body. Am J Physiol 1991; 261:C565–C573.

Jacobs L, Comroe JHJ. Stimulation of the carotid chemoreceptors of the dog by dopamine. Proc Natl Acad Sci USA 1968; 59:1187–1193.

Joels N, Neil E. The idea of a sensory transmitter. In: Torrance RW, ed. Arterial Chemoreceptors. Oxford, UK: Blackwell Scientific Publications, 1968:153–178.

Jones JV. Localization and quantitation of the carotid body enzymes: their relevance to the cholinergic transmitter hypothesis. In: Purves MJ, ed. The Peripheral Arterial Chemoreceptors. London: Cambridge University Press, 1975:143–162.

Kanno M, Dunning BB, Mochne X. Calcium dependence of acetylcholine induced conductance changes. Life Sci 1976; 18:3111–3118.

Kato E, Narahashi T. Characteristics of the electrical response to dopamine in neuroblastoma cells. J Physiol (Lond) 1982; 333:213–236.

Keller HP, Lubbers DW. Flow measurement in the carotid body of the cat by the hydrogen clearance method. Pflüger's Arch 1972; 336:217–224.

Kety SS. Cerebral circulation and its measurement by inert diffusible tracers In: Adelman G, ed. Encyclopedia of Neuroscience. Boston: Birkhäuser, 1987:206–208.

Kinnamon SC. Taste transduction: a diversity of mechanisms. Trends Neurosci 1988; 11: 492–496.

Kirby GC, McQueen DS. Effects of the antagonists MDL 72222 and ketanserin on responses of cat carotid body chemoreceptors to 5-hydroxytryptamine. Br J Pharmacol 1984; 83:259–269.

Kirby GC, McQueen DS. Characterization of opioid receptors in the cat carotid body involved in chemosensory depression in vivo. Br J Pharmacol 1986; 88:889–898.

Kobayashi S. Comparative cytological studies of the carotid body. 1. Demonstration of monoamine-storing cells by correlated chromaffin reaction and fluorescence histochemistry. Arch Histol Jpn 1971a; 33:319–339.

Kobayashi S. Comparative cytological studies of the carotid body. 2. Ultrastructure of the synapses on the chief cell. Arch Histol Jpn 1971b; 33:397–420.

Kobayashi S, Uchida T, Ohashi T, Fujita T, Nakao K, Yoshimasa T, Imura H, Mochizuki T, Yanaihara C, Yanaihara N, et al. Immunocytochemical demonstration of the co-storage of noradrenaline with met-enkephalin-Arg6-Phe7 and met-enkephalin-Arg6-Gly7-Leu8 in the carotid body chief cells of the dog. Arch Histol Jpn 1983; 46: 713–722.

Kohn A. Ueber den Bau und die Entwicklung der sog. Carotisdrüse. Arch Mikrosk Anat 1900; 56:81–148.

Kondo H, Iwanaga T, Nakajima T. Immunocytochemical study on the localization of neuron-specific enolase and S-100 protein in the carotid body of rats. Cell Tissue Res 1982; 227:291–295.

Kondo H, Kuramoto H, Fujita T. Neuropeptide tyrosine-like immunoreactive nerve fibers in the carotid body chemoreceptor of rats. Brain Res 1986; 372:353–356.

Kou YR, Ernsberger P, Cragg PA, Cherniack NS, Prabhakar NR. Role of α_2-adrenergic receptors in the carotid body response to isocapnic hypoxia. Respir Physiol 1991; 83:353–364.

Krafte DS, Kass RS. Hydrogen ion modulation of Ca channel current in cardiac ventricular cells. J Gen Physiol 1988; 91:641–657.

Kummer W. Three types of neurochemically defined autonomic fibres innervate the carotid baroreceptor and chemoreceptor regions in the guinea pig. Anat Embryol Berl 1990; 181:477–489.

Kupfermann I. Functional studies of cotransmission. Physiol Rev 1991; 71:683–732.

Lackovic Z, Neff NH. Evidence that dopamine is a neurotransmitter in peripheral tissues. Life Sci 1983; 32:1665–1674.

Lagercrantz H, Milerad J, Walker D. Control of ventilation in the neonate. In: Crystal RG, West JB, eds. The Lung. Scientific Foundations. New York: Raven Press, 1991: 1711–1722.

Lahiri S. Introductory remarks: oxygen linked response of carotid chemoreceptors. Adv Exp Med Biol 1977; 78:185–202.

Lahiri S. Chemical modification of carotid body chemoreception by sulfhydryls. Science 1981; 212:1065–1066.

Lahiri S, Delaney RG. The nature of response of single chemoreceptor fibers of carotid body to changes in arterial PO_2 and PCO_2-H^+. In: Paintal AS, ed. Morphology and Mechanisms of Chemoreceptors. Delhi, India: Vallabhbhai Patel Chest Institute, 1976:18–26.

Lahiri S, Nishino T. Inhibitory and excitatory effects of dopamine on carotid chemoreceptors. Neurosci Lett 1980; 20:313–318.

Lahiri S, Pokorski M, Davies RO. Augmentation of carotid body chemoreceptor responses by isoproterenol in the cat. Respir Physiol 1981; 44:351–364.

Lee FL. The relation between norepinephrine content and response to sympathetic nerve stimulation of various organs of cats pretreated with reserpine. J Pharmacol Exp Ther 1967; 156:137–141.

Leitner LM, Roumy M. Effects of dopamine superfusion on the activity of rabbit carotid chemoreceptors in vitro. Neuroscience 1985; 16:431–438.

Leitner LM, Roumy M. Chemoreceptor response to hypoxia and hypercapnia in catecholamine depleted rabbit and cat carotid bodies in vitro. Pflüger's Arch 1986; 406:419–423.

Leitner LM, Roumy M, Verna A. In vitro recording of chemoreceptor activity in catecholamine-depleted rabbit carotid bodies. Neuroscience 1983; 10:883–891.

Leitner LM, Roumy M, Ruckenbusch M, Sutra JF. Monoamines and their catabolites in the rabbit carotid body. Effects of reserpine, sympathectomy and carotid sinus nerve section. Pflüger's Arch 1986; 406:552–556.

Leitner LM, Roumy M, Ruckenbusch M, Sutra JF. Monoamine content and metabolism in the rabbit carotid body. In: Ribeiro JA, Pallot DJ, eds. Chemoreceptors in Respiratory Control. London: Croom Helm, 1987:114–123.

Lever JD, Boyd JD. Osmiophile granules in glomus cells of the rabbit carotid body. Nature (Lond) 1957; 179:1082–1083.

Livett BG. Peptide modulation of adrenal chromaffin cell secretion. In: Rosenheck K, Lelkes PI, eds. Stimulus-Secretion Coupling in Chromaffin Cells. Boca Raton, FL: CRC Press, 1987:117–150.

Llados F, Zapata P. Effects of dopamine analogues and antagonists on carotid body chemosensors in situ. J Physiol (Lond) 1978a; 274:487–499.

Llados F, Zapata P. Effects of adrenoceptor stimulating and blocking agents on carotid body chemosensory inhibition. J Physiol (Lond) 1978b; 274:501–509.

Lloyd BB, Cunningham DJC, Goode RC. Depression of hypoxic hyperventilation in man by sudden inspiration of carbon monoxide. In: Torrance RW, ed. Arterial Chemoreceptors. Oxford, UK: Blackwell Scientific Publications, 1968:145–148.

Lopez-Barneo J, Lopez-Lopez JR, Ureña J, Gonzalez C. Chemotransduction in the carotid body: K^+ current modulated by Po_2 in type I chemoreceptor cells. Science 1988; 241:580–582.

Lopez-Lopez JR, Gonzalez C. Time course of K^+ current inhibition by low oxygen in chemoreceptor cells of adult rabbit carotid body: effects of carbon monoxide. FEBS Lett 1992; 299:251–254.

Lopez-Lopez J, Gonzalez C, Ureña J, Lopez-Barneo J. Low Po_2 selectively inhibits K^+ channel activity in chemoreceptor cells of the mammalian carotid body. J Gen Physiol 1989; 93:1001–1015.

Lopez-Lopez JR, De Luis DA, Gonzalez C. Properties of a transient K^+ current in chemoreceptor cells of rabbit carotid body. J Physiol (Lond) 1993; 460:15–32.

Lundberg JM, Hökfelt T. Coexistence of peptides and classical neurotransmitters. In: Bousfield D, ed. Neurotransmitters in Action. Amsterdam: Elsevier Biomedical Press, 1985:104–118.

Lundberg JM, Hokfelt T, Fahrenkrug J, Nilsson G, Terenius L. Peptides in the cat carotid body (glomus caroticum): VIP-, enkephalin-, and substance P-like immunoreactivity. Acta Physiol Scand 1979; 107:279–281.

Lundberg JM, Rudehill A, Sollevi A, Theodorsson-Hornehim E, Hamberger B. Frequency and reserpine-dependent chemical coding of sympathetic transmission: differential release of noradrenaline and neuropeptide from pig spleen. Neurosci Lett 1986; 63: 96–100.

Mata M, Fink DJ, Gainer H, Smith CB, Davidsen L, Savaki H, Schwartz WJ, Sokoloff L. Activity-dependent energy metabolism in rat posterior pituitary reflects sodium pump activity. J Neurochem 1980; 34:213–215.

Matsumoto S, Nakajima T, Uchida T, Ozawa H, Ushiyama J. Effects of sodium cyanide, dopamine and acetylcholine on the resting membrane potential of glomus cells in the rabbit. Brain Res 1982; 239:674–678.

Mayer ML, Vyklicky L Jr, Clements J. Regulation of NMDA receptor desensitization in mouse hippocampal neurons by glycine. Nature 1989; 338:425–427.

McCormack JG, Halestrap AP, Demtom RM. Role of calcium ions in regulation of intramitochondrial metabolism. Physiol Rev 1990; 70:391–425.

McDonald DM. Regulation of chemoreceptor sensitivity in the carotid body: the role of presynaptic sensory nerves. Fed Proc 1980; 39:2627–2635.

McDonald DM. Peripheral chemoreceptors. Structure-function relationships of the carotid body. In: Hornbein TF, ed. Regulation of Breathing, Part I. New York: Marcel Dekker, 1981:105–319.

McDonald DM, Haskell A. Morphology of connections between arterioles and capillaries in the rat carotid body analysed by reconstructing serial sections. In: Pallot DJ, ed. The Peripheral Arterial Chemoreceptors. London: Croom Helm, 1984:195–206.

McDonald DM, Lurue DT. The ultrastructure and connections of blood vessels supplying the rat carotid body and carotid sinus. J Neurocytol 1983; 12:117–153.

McDonald DM, Mitchell RA. The innervation of glomus cells, ganglion cells and blood vessels in the rat carotid body: a quantitative ultrastructural analysis. J Neurocytol 1975; 4:177–230.

McLennan H. Synaptic Transmission. Philadelphia: Saunders, 1963.

McQueen DS. Pharmacological aspects of putative transmitters in the carotid body. In: Acker H, O'Regan RG, eds. Physiology of the Peripheral Arterial Chemoreceptors. Amsterdam: Elsevier Science Publishers, 1983:149–195.

McQueen DS. Effects of selective dopamine receptor agonists and antagonists on carotid body chemoreceptors activity. In: Pallot DJ, ed. The Peripheral Arterial Chemoreceptors. London: Croom Helm, 1984:325–333.

McQueen DS. Does adenosine stimulate rat carotid body chemoreceptors? In: Data PG, Acker H, Lahiri S, eds. Neurobiology and Cell Physiology of Chemoreception. Advances in Experimental Medicine and Biology, Vol 337. New York: Plenum Press, 1993:289–294.

McQueen DS, Evrard Y. Use of selective antagonists for studying the role of putative transmitters in chemoreception. In: Eyzaguirre C, Fidone SJ, Fitzgerald RS, Lahiri S, McDonald DM, eds. Arterial Chemoreception. New York: Springer-Verlag, 1990: 168–173.

McQueen DS, Ribeiro JA. Effects of β-endorphin, vasoactive intestinal polypeptide and cholecystokinin octapeptide on cat carotid chemoreceptor activity. Q J Exp Physiol 1981; 66:273–284.

McQueen DS, Ribeiro JA. On the specificity and type of receptor involved in carotid body chemoreceptor activation by adenosine in the cat. Br J Pharmacol 1983; 80:347–354.

McQueen DS, Mir AK, Brash HM, Nahorski SR. Increased sensitivity of rabbit carotid body chemoreceptors to dopamine after chronic treatment with domperidone. Eur J Pharmacol 1984; 104:39–46.

McQueen DS, Ritchie IM, Birrell GJ. Arterial chemoreceptor involvement in salicylate-induced hyperventilation in rats. Br J Pharmacol 1989; 98:413–424.

Mefford IN, Foutz A, Noyce N. Distribution of norepinephrine, epinephrine, dopamine, serotonin, 3,4-dihidroxyphenylacetic acid, homovanilic acid and 5-hydroxyndole-3-acetic acid in dog brain. Brain Res 1982; 236:339–349.

Meszaros K, Bagby GJ, Lang CH, Spitzer JJ. Increased uptake and phosphorylation of 2-deoxyglucose by skeletal muscles in endotoxin-treated rats. Am J Physiol 1987; 253:E33–E39.

Millhorn DE, Eldridge FL, Kiley JP, Waldrop TG. Prolonged inhibition of respiration following acute hypoxia in glomectomized cats. Respir Physiol 1984; 57:331–340.

Mills E. Spectrophotometric and fluorometric studies on the mechanism of chemoreception in the carotid body. Fed Proc 1972; 31:1394–1398.

Mills E. Metabolic aspects of chemoreceptor function. In: Purves MJ, ed. The Peripheral Arterial Chemoreceptors. London: Cambridge University Press, 1975:373–385.

Mills E, Jobsis FF. Mitochondrial respiratory chain of carotid body and chemoreceptor response to changes in oxygen tension. J Neurophysiol 1972; 35:405–428.

Milsom WK, Sadig T. Interaction between norepinephrine and hypoxia on carotid body chemoreception in rabbits. J Appl Physiol 1983; 55:1893–1898.

Mir AK, Al Neamy K, Pallot DJ, Nahorski SR. Catecholamines in the carotid body of several mammalian species: effects of surgical and chemical sympathectomy. Brain Res 1982; 252:335–342.

Mir AK, Pallot DJ, Nahorski SR. Biogenic amine-stimulated cyclic adenosine-3',5'-monophosphate formation in the rat carotid body. J Neurochem 1983; 41:663–669.

Mir AK, McQueen DS, Pallot DJ, Nahorski SR. Direct biochemical and neuropharmacological identification of dopamine D2-receptors in the rabbit carotid body. Brain Res 1984a; 291:273–282.

Mir AK, Pallot DJ, Nahorski SR. Catecholamines; their receptors and cyclic AMP generating systems in the carotid body. In: Pallot DJ, ed. The Peripheral Arterial Chemoreceptors. London: Croom Helm, 1984b:311–323.

Monteiro EC, Ribeiro JA. Ventilatory effects of adenosine mediated by carotid body chemoreceptors in the rat. Naunyn Schmiedeberg's Arch Pharmacol 1987; 335: 143–148.

Monteiro EC, Ribeiro JA. Inhibition by 1,3-dipropyl-8(p-sulfophenyl)xanthine of the respiratory stimulation induced by common carotid occlusion in rats. Life Sci 1989a; 45:939–945.

Monteiro EC, Ribeiro JA. Adenosine deaminase and adenosine uptake inhibitions facilitate ventilation in rats. Naunyn Schmiedeberg's Arch Pharmacol 1989b; 340:230–238.

Monteiro EC, Ribeiro JA. Respiratory responses to common carotid occlusion in the rat: evidence for involvement of adenosine. In: Acker H, Trzebski A, O'Regan RG, eds. Chemoreceptors and Chemoreceptor Reflexes. New York: Plenum Press, 1990:49–56.

Monti-Bloch L, Abudara V, Eyzaguirre C. Electrical communication between glomus cells of the rat carotid body. Brain Res 1993; 622:119–131.

Monti-Bloch L, Eyzaguirre C. A comparative physiological and pharmacological study of cat and rabbit carotid body chemoreceptors. Brain Res 1980; 193:449–470.

Monti-Bloch L, Eyzaguirre C. Effects of methionine-enkephalin and substance P on the chemosensory discharge of the cat carotid body. Brain Res 1985; 338:297–307.

Monti-Bloch L, Eyzaguirre C. Effects of different stimuli and transmitters on glomus cell membranes and intercellular communications. In: Eyzaguirre C, Fidone SJ, Fitzgerald RS, Lahiri S, McDonald DM, eds. Arterial Chemoreception. New York: Springer-Verlag, 1990:157–167.

Morgado E, Llados F, Zapata P. Dopamine-β-hydroxylase activity in normal and sympathectomized carotid bodies. Neurosci Lett 1976; 3:139–143.

Mulligan E, Lahiri S. Separation of carotid body chemoreceptor responses to O_2 and CO_2 by oligomycin and by antimycin A. Am J Physiol 1982; 242:C200–C206.

Mulligan E, Lahiri S, Storey BT. Carotid body O_2 chemoreception and mitochondrial oxidative phosphorylation. J Appl Physiol 1981; 51:438–446.

Mulligan E, Lahiri S, Mokashi A, Matsumoto S, McGregor KH. Adrenergic mechanism in oxygen chemoreception in the cat aortic body. Respir Physiol 1986; 63:375–382.

Mullins LJ. An electrogenic saga: consequences of sodium-calcium exchange in cardiac muscle. In: Blaustein MP, Lieberman M, eds. Electrogenic Transport. Fundamental Principles and Physiological Implications. New York: Raven Press, 1984:161–179.

Nair PK, Buerk DG, Whalen WJ. Cat carotid body oxygen metabolism and chemoreception described by a two-cytochrome model. Am J Physiol 1986; 250:H202–H207.

Nishi K. The action of 5-hydroxytryptamine on chemoreceptor discharges of the cat's carotid body. Br J Pharmacol 1975; 55:27–40.

Nishi K. A pharmacologic study on a possible inhibitory role of dopamine in the cat carotid body chemoreceptor. In: Acker H, Fidone S, Pallot D, Eyzaguirre C, Lübbers DW, Torrance RW, eds. Chemoreception in the Carotid Body. Berlin: Springer-Verlag, 1977:145–151.

Nolan WF, Donnelly DF, Smith EJ, Dutton RE. Haloperidol-induced suppression of carotid chemoreception in vitro. J Appl Physiol 1985; 59:814–820.

Nurse CA. Localization of acetylcholinesterase in dissociated cell cultures of the carotid body of the rat. Cell Tissue Res 1987; 250:21–27.

Obeso A, Almaraz L, Gonzalez C. Effects of 2-deoxy-D-glucose on in vitro cat carotid body. Brain Res 1986; 371:25–36.

Obeso A, Fidone S, Gonzalez C. Pathways for calcium entry into type I cells: significance for the secretory response. Ribeiro JA, Pallot DJ, eds. Chemoreceptors in Respiratory Control. London: Croom Helm, 1987:91–98.

Obeso A, Almaraz L, Gonzalez C. Effects of cyanide and uncouplers on chemoreceptor activity and ATP content of the cat carotid body. Brain Res 1989a; 481:250–257.

Obeso A, Gonzalez C, Dinger B, Fidone S. Metabolic activation of carotid body glomus cells by hypoxia. J Appl Physiol 1989b; 67:484–487.

Obeso A, Rocher A, Fidone S, Gonzalez C. The role of dihydropyridine-sensitive Ca^{2+} channels in stimulus-evoked catecholamine release from chemoreceptor cells of the carotid body. Neuroscience 1992; 47:463–472.

Obeso A, Gonzalez C, Rigual R, Dinger B, Fidone S. The effect of low-oxygen on glucose uptake in rabbit carotid body. J Appl Physiol 1993; 74:2387–2393.

Okajima Y, Nishi K. Analysis of inhibitory and excitatory actions of dopamine on chemoreceptor discharges of carotid body of cat in vivo. Jpn J Physiol 1981; 31:396–704.

O'Regan RG. Responses of carotid body chemosensory activity and blood flow to stimulation of sympathetic nerves in the cat. J Physiol (Lond) 1981; 315:81–98.

Paintal AS. Further evidence that acetylcholine is not a transmitter at chemoreceptors. J Physiol (Lond) 1969; 204:94P–95P.

Paintal AS. Cardiovascular receptors. In: Neil E, ed. Handbook of Sensory Physiology Enteroceptors. Berlin: Springer-Verlag, 1972:1–45.

Paiva ACM, Paiva TB. A model of angiotensin receptors in smooth muscle cells. In: Rocha e Silve M, Suarez-Kurtz G, eds. Concepts for Membranes in Regulation and Excitation. New York: Raven Press, 1975:145–154.

Pallot DJ. The mammalian carotid body. Adv Anat Embryol Cell Biol 1987; 102:1–91.

Pallot DJ, Al Neamy KW. The effects of hypoxia, hypercapnia and almitrine bismesylate on carotid body catecholamines. Eur J Respir Dis 1983; 126(Suppl):203–207.

Pang L, Eyzaguirre C. Different effects of hypoxia on the membrane potential and input resistance of isolated and clustered carotid body glomus cells. Brain Res 1992; 575: 167–173.

Patrick JM, Pearson SB. β-Adrenoceptor blockage and ventilation in man. Br J Clin Pharmacol 1980; 10:624–625.

Peers C. Hypoxic suppression of K^+ currents in type I carotid body cells: selective effect on the Ca^{2+}-activated K^+ current. Neurosci Lett 1990; 119:253–256.

Peers C. Effect of lowered extracellular pH on Ca^{2+}-dependent K^+ currents in type I cells from the neonatal rat carotid body. J Physiol (Lond) 1990a; 422:381–395.

Peers C. Effects of D600 on hypoxic suppression of K^+ currents in isolated type I carotid body cells of the neonatal rat. FEBS Lett 1990b; 271:37–40.

Peers C. Selective effect of reduced extracellular pH. In: Acker H, Trzebski A, O'Regan RG, eds. Chemoreceptors and Chemoreceptor Reflexes. New York: Plenum Press, 1990c:21–27.

Peers C, Green FK. Inhibition of Ca^{2+}-activated K^+ currents by intracellular acidosis in isolated type I cells of the neonatal rat carotid body. J Physiol (Lond) 1991; 437: 589–601.

Peers C, O'Donnell J. Potassium currents recorded in type I carotid body cells from the neonatal rat and their modulation by chemoexcitatory agents. Brain Res 1990a; 522: 259–266.

Peers C, O'Donnell J. Effects of chemoexcitatory agents on K^+ currents of isolated type I cells from neonatal rat carotid body. In: Eyzaguirre C, Fidone SJ, Fitzgerald RS, Lahiri S, McDonald DM, eds. Arterial Chemoreception. New York: Springer-Verlag, 1990b:63–69.

Pequignot JM, Hellstrom S, Johansson C. Intact and sympathectomized carotid bodies of long-term hypoxic rats: a morphometric ultrastructural study. J Neurocytol 1984; 13:481–493.

Pequignot JM, Cottet-Emard JM, Dalmaz Y, De Haut De Sigy M, Peyrin L. Biochemical evidence for norepinephrine stores outside the sympathetic nerves in rat carotid body. Brain Res 1986; 367:238–243.

Pequignot JM, Cottet-Emard JM, Dalmaz Y, Peyrin L. Dopamine and norepinephrine dynamics in rat carotid body during long-term hypoxia. J Auton Nerv Syst 1987a; 21:9–14.

Pequignot JM, Tavitian E, Boudet C, Evrard Y, Claustre J, Peyrin L. Inhibitory effect of almitrine on dopaminergic activity of rat carotid body. J Appl Physiol 1987b; 63:746–751.

Pequignot JM, Hellström S, Hertzberg T. Long-term hypoxia and hypercapnia in the carotid body: a review. In: Eyzaguirre C, Fidone SJ, Fitzgerald RS, Lahiri S, McDonald DM, eds. Arterial Chemoreception. New York: Springer-Verlag, 1990:100–114.

Perez-Garcia MT, Almaraz L, Gonzalez C. Participation of cAMP in low Po$_2$ chemotransduction. In: Acker H, Trzebski A, O'Regan RG, eds. Chemoreceptors and Chemoreceptor Reflexes. New York: Plenum Press, 1990a:57–65.

Perez-Garcia MT, Almaraz L, Gonzalez C. Effects of different types of stimulation on cyclic AMP content in the rabbit carotid body: functional significance. J Neurochem 1990b; 55:1287–1293.

Perez-Garcia MT, Almaraz L, Gonzalez C. Cyclic AMP modulates differentially the release of dopamine induced by hypoxia and other stimuli and increases dopamine synthesis in the rabbit carotid body. J Neurochem 1991; 57:1992–2000.

Perez-Garcia MT, Obeso A, Lopez-Lopez JR, Herreros B, Gonzalez C. Characterization of chemoreceptor cells in primary culture isolated from adult rabbit carotid body. Am J Physiol 1992; 263:C1152–C1159.

Perez-Garcia MT, Gomez-Niño A, Almaraz L, Gonzalez C. Neurotransmitters and second messenger systems in the carotid body. In: Data PG, Acker H, Lahiri S, eds. Neurobiology and Cell Physiology of Chemoreception. Advances in Experimental Medicine and Biology, Vol 337. New York: Plenum Press, 1993:279–288.

Perrin DG, Chan W, Cutz E, Madapallimattam A, Sole MJ. Serotonin in the human infant carotid body. Experientia 1986; 42:562–564.

Perrin DG, Chan W, Newman C, Cutz E. Serotonin in the human infant carotid body: normal and pathological states. In: Eyzaguirre C, Fidone SJ, Fitzgerald RS, Lahiri S, McDonald DM, eds. Arterial Chemoreception. New York: Springer-Verlag, 1990: 374–387.

Pizarro J, Warner MM, Ryan M, Mitchell GS, Gisgard GE. Intracarotid norepinephrine infusions inhibit ventilation in goats. Respir Physiol 1992; 90:299–310.

Pokorski M, Lahiri S. Effects of naloxone on carotid body chemoreception and ventilation in the cat. J Appl Physiol 1981; 51:1533–1538.

Ponte J, Purves MJ. Frequency response of carotid body chemoreceptors in the cat to changes of Paco$_2$, Pao$_2$ and pHa. J Appl Physiol 1974; 37:635–647.

Ponte J, Sadler CL. Interactions between hypoxia, acetylcholine and dopamine in the carotid body of rabbit and cat. J Physiol (Lond) 1989; 410:395–410.

Potter DD, Furshpan EJ, Landis SC. Multiple-transmitter status and "Dale's principle." Neurosci Commun 1981; 1:1–9.

Potter EK, McCloskey DI. Excitation of carotid body chemoreceptors by neuropeptide-Y. Respir Physiol 1987; 67:357–365.

Prabhakar NR, Kou YR. Inhibitory influence of sympathetic innervation on the carotid body response to sustained hypoxia; role of α-adrenergic receptors. Respir Physiol 1993 (in press).

Prabhakar NR, Runold M, Yamamoto Y, Lagercrantz H, Von Euler C. Effect of substance P antagonist on the hypoxia-induced carotid chemoreceptor activity. Acta Physiol Scand 1984; 121:301–303.

Prabhakar NR, Mitra J, Cherniack NS. Role of substance P in hypercapnic excitation of carotid chemoreceptors. J Appl Physiol 1987; 63:2418–2425.

Prabhakar NR, Landis SC, Kumar GK, Mullikin-Kilpatrick D, Cherniack NS, Leeman S. Substance P and neurokinin A in the cat carotid body: localization, exogenous effects and changes in content in response to arterial Po_2. Brain Res 1989; 481:205–214.

Prabhakar NR, Gauda E, Cherniack NS. The mechanism of action of tachykinins in the carotid body. In: Eyzaguirre C, Fidone SJ, Fitzgerald RS, Lahiri S, McDonald DM, eds. Arterial Chemoreception. New York: Springer-Verlag, 1990a:192–198.

Prabhakar NR, Kou YR, Runold M. Chemoreceptor responses to substance P, physalaemin and eledoisin: evidence for neurokinin-1 receptors in the cat carotid body. Neurosci Lett 1990b; 120:183–186.

Purves MJ. The effect of hypoxia, hypercapnia and hypotension upon carotid body blood flow and oxygen consumption in the cat. J Physiol (Lond) 1970a; 209:395–416.

Purves MJ. The role of the cervical sympathetic nerve in the regulation of oxygen consumption of the carotid body of the cat. J Physiol (Lond) 1970b; 209:417–431.

Reese TS. Synapse, active zone. In: Adelman G, ed. Encyclopedia of Neuroscience. Boston: Birkhäuser, 1987:1158.

Reid PG, Watt AH, Penny WJ, Newby AC, Smith AP, Routledge PA. Plasma adenosine concentrations during adenosine-induced respiratory stimulation in man. Eur J Clin Pharmacol 1991; 40:175–180.

Rigual R, Gonzalez E, Fidone S, Gonzalez C. Effects of low pH on synthesis and release of catecholamines in the cat carotid body in vitro. Brain Res 1984; 309:178–181.

Rigual R, Iñiguez C, Carreres J, Gonzalez C. Carbonic anhydrase in the carotid body and the carotid sinus nerve. Histochemistry 1985; 82:577–580.

Rigual R, Gonzalez E, Gonzalez C, Fidone S. Synthesis and release of catecholamines by the cat carotid in vitro: effects of hypoxic stimulation. Brain Res 1986; 374:101–109.

Rigual R, Gonzalez E, Gonzalez C, Jones L, Fidone S. A comparative study of the metabolism of catecholamines in the rabbit and cat carotid body. In: Ribeiro JA, Pallot DJ, eds. Chemoreceptors in Respiratory Control. London: Croom Helm, 1987:124–134.

Rigual RJ, Diliberto EJ, Sigafoos J, Gonzalez-Guerrero PR, Gonzalez, C, Viveros OH. Proenkephalin-derived peptides in the carotid body. In: Eyzaguirre C, Fidone SJ, Fitzgerald RS, Lahiri S, McDonald DM, eds. Arterial Chemoreception. New York: Springer-Verlag, 1990:143–147.

Rigual R, Lopez-Lopez JR, Gonzalez C. Release of dopamine and chemoreceptor discharge induced by low pH and high Pco_2 stimulation of the cat carotid body. J Physiol (Lond) 1991; 433:519–531.

Riley DJ, Legawiec BA, Santiago TV, Edelman NH. Ventilatory responses to hypercapnia and hypoxia during continuous aspirin ingestion. J Appl Physiol 1977; 43:971–976.

Rocher A, Obeso A, Herreros B, Gonzalez C. Activation of the release of dopamine in the carotid body by veratridine. Evidence for the presence of voltage-dependent Na^+ channels in type I cells. Neurosci Lett 1988; 94:274–278.

Rocher A, Obeso A, Herreros B, Gonzalez C. Involvement of Na^+:H^+ and Na^+:Ca^{2+} antiporters in the chemotransduction of acidic stimuli. In: Acker H, Trzebski A, O'Regan RG, eds. Chemoreceptors and Chemoreceptor Reflexes. New York: Plenum Press, 1990:35–41.

Rocher A, Obeso A, Gonzalez C, Herreros B. Ionic mechanisms for the transduction of acidic stimuli in rabbit carotid body glomus cells. J Physiol (Lond) 1991; 433:533–548.

Roos A, Boron WF. Intracellular pH. Physiol Rev 1981; 61:296–434.

Roumy M, Leitner LM. Role of calcium ions in the mechanism of arterial chemoreceptor excitation. In: Acker H, Fidone S, Pallot D, Eyzaguirre C, Lübbers DW, Torrance RW, eds. Chemoreception in the Carotid Body. Berlin: Springer-Verlag, 1977:257–263.

Roumy M, Ruckebusch M, Sutra JF, Leitner LM. Rate of dopamine metabolism in the rabbit carotid body in vivo. Pflüger's Arch 1986; 407:575–576.

Rubin RP. Calcium and Cellular Secretion. New York: Plenum Press, 1982.

Rudy B. Diversity and ubiquity of K^+ channels. Neuroscience 1988; 25:729–749.

Rumsey WL, Iturriaga R, Spergel D, Lahiri S, Wilson DF. Optical measurements of the dependence of chemoreception on oxygen pressure in the cat carotid body. Am J Physiol 1991; 261:C614–C622.

Runold M, Cherniack NS, Prabhakar NR. Effect of adenosine on isolated and superfused cat carotid body activity. Neurosci Lett 1990; 113:111–114.

Samet P, Fierer EM, Bernstein WH. Effect of salicylates on the ventilatory response to inhaled carbon dioxide in normal subjects. J Appl Physiol 1960; 15:826–828.

Sampson SR. Mechanism of efferent inhibition of carotid body chemoreceptors in the cat. Brain Res 1972; 45:266–270.

Sampson SR, Aminoff MJ, Jaffe RA, Vidruk EH. A pharmacological analysis of neurally induced inhibition of carotid body chemoreceptor activity in cats. J Pharmacol Exp Ther 1976a; 197:119–125.

Sampson SR, Aminoff MJ, Jaffe RA, Vidruk EH. Analysis of inhibitory effect of dopamine on carotid body chemoreceptors in cats. Am J Physiol 1976b; 230:1494–1498.

Sapru HN, Krieger AJ. Effect of 5-hydroxytryptamine on the peripheral chemoreceptors in the rat. Res Commun Chem Pathol Pharmacol 1977; 16:245–250.

Sato M, Yoshizaki K, Koyano H. Veratridine stimulation of sodium influx in carotid body cells from newborn rabbits in primary culture. Brain Res 1989; 504:132–135.

Sato M, Ikeda K, Yoshizaki K, Koyano H. Response of cytosolic calcium to anoxia and cyanide in cultured glomus cells of newborn rabbit carotid body. Brain Res 1991; 551:327–330.

Sato M, Yoshizaki K, Koyano H. Elevation of cytosolic calcium induced by pH changes in cultured carotid body glomus cells. In: Data PG, Acker H, Lahiri S, eds. Neurobiology and Cell Physiology of Chemoreception, Advances in Experimental Medicine and Biology, Vol 337. New York: Plenum Press, 1993:205–212.

Schamel A, Verna A. Norepinephrine-containing glomus cells in the rabbit carotid body. I. Autoradiographic and morphometric study after tritiated norepinephrine uptake. J Neurocytol 1992a; 21:341–352.

Schamel A, Verna A. Norepinephrine-containing cells in the rabbit carotid body. II. Immunocytochemical evidence of dopamine-β-hydroxylase and norepinephrine. J Neurocytol 1992b; 21:352–362.

Schamel A, Verna A. Localization of dopamine D2 receptor mRNA in the rabbit carotid body and petrosal ganglion by in situ hybridization. In: Data PG, Acker H, Lahiri S, eds. Neurobiology and Cell Physiology of Chemoreception, Advances in Experimental Medicine and Biology, Vol 337. New York: Plenum Press, 1993:85–92.

Shaw K, Montague W, Pallot DJ. Biochemical studies on the release of catecholamines from the rat carotid body in vitro. Biochim Biophys Acta 1989; 1013:42–46.

Shaw K, Montague W, Pallot DJ. Biochemical studies on the release of catecholamines from the rat carotid body in vitro. In: Eyzaguirre C, Fidone SJ, Fitzgerald RS, Lahiri S, McDonald DM, eds. Arterial Chemoreception. New York: Springer-Verlag, 1990: 87–91.

Scheibner T, Read DJ, Sullivan CE. Distribution of substance P–immunoreactive structures in the developing cat carotid body. Brain Res 1988; 453:72–78.

Schweitzer A, Wright S. Action of prostigmine and acetylcholine on respiration. Q J Exp Physiol 1938; 28:33–47.

Shirahata M. Effects of substance P on the carotid chemoreceptor responses to natural stimuli. In: Lahiri S, Forster RE, Davies RO, Pack AI, eds. Chemoreceptors and Reflexes in Breathing. New York: Oxford University Press, 1989:139–145.

Shirahata M, Andronikou S, Lahiri S. Differential effects of oligomycin on carotid chemoreceptor responses to O_2 and CO_2 in the cat. J Appl Physiol 1987; 63:2083–2092.

Shirahata M, Fitzgerald RS. Dependency of hypoxic chemotransduction in cat carotid body on voltage-gated calcium channels. J Appl Physiol 1991; 71:1062–1069.

Siggins GR. Monoamines and message transduction in central neurons. In: Magistretti PJ, Morrison JH, Reisine TD, eds. Transduction of Neuronal Signals. Geneva: FESN, 1986:61–68.

Smith P, Gosney J, Heath D, Burnett H. The occurrence and distribution of certain polypeptides within the human carotid body. Cell Tissue Res 1990; 261:565–571.

Smith PG, Mills E. Physiological and ultrastructural observations on regenerated carotid sinus nerves after removal of the carotid bodies in cats. Neuroscience 1979; 4:2009–2020.

Sokoloff L. The radioactive deoxyglucose method: theory, procedure, and applications for the measurement of local glucose utilization in the central nervous system. In: Agranoff BW, Aprison MH, eds. Advances in Neurochemistry, vol. 4. New York: Plenum Press, 1982:1–82.

Starlinger H. Enzymes and inhibitors of the catecholamine metabolism in the cat carotid body. In: Acker H, Fidone S, Pallot D, Eyzaguirre C, Lübbers DW, Torrance RW, eds. Chemoreception in the Carotid Body. Berlin: Springer-Verlag, 1977:136–141.

Starlinger H. Activity of dopamine β-monooxygenase in the tissue of the cat's carotid body. Hoppe Seyler's Z Physiol Chem 1979; 360:103–106.

Starlinger H. Tyrosine 3-monooxygenase activity in the cat carotid body tissue. Hoppe Seyler's Z Physiol Chem 1980; 361:1457–1460.

Starlinger H, Acker H. The norepinephrine and dopamine content of the cat carotid body in vivo under normoxic and hypoxic conditions. Neurosci Lett 1986; 64:65–68.

Starlinger H, Lubbers DW. Oxygen consumption of the isolated carotid body tissue (cat). Pflüger's Arch 1976; 366:61–66.

Starlinger H, Acker H, Heinrich R. Dopamine β-hydroxylase activity of the cat carotid body under different arterial O_2 and CO_2 conditions. J Neurochem 1983; 41:1533–1537.

Stea A, Nurse CA. Whole-cell and perforated-patch recordings from O_2-sensitive rat carotid body cells grown in short- and long-term culture. Pflüger's Arch 1991; 418: 93–101.

Stea A, Alexander SA, Nurse CA. Effects of pHi and pHe on membrane currents recorded with the perforated-patch method from cultured chemoreceptors of the rat carotid body. Brain Res 1991; 567:83–90.

Stea A, Jackson A, Nurse CA. Hypoxia and $N^6,O^{2'}$-digutyryladenosine $3',5'$-cyclic monophosphate, but not nerve growth factor, induce Na^+ channels and hypertrophy in chromaffin-like arterial chemoreceptors. Proc Natl Acad Sci USA 1992; 82:9469–9473.

Stensaas LJ, Stensas SS, Gonzalez C, Fidone SJ. Analytical electron microscopy of granular vesicles in the carotid body of the normal and reserpinized cat. In: Belmonte C, Pallot DJ, Acker H, Fidone SJ, eds. Arterial Chemoreceptors. Leicester, UK: Leicester University Press, 1981:176–186.

Thomas RC. Review Lecture: Experimental displacement of intracellular pH and the mechanism of its subsequent recovery. J Physiol (Lond) 1984; 354:3–22.

Tonosaki K, Funokoshi M. Cyclic nucleotides may mediate taste transduction. Nature 1988; 331:354–356.

Torrance RW. Arterial chemoreceptors. In: Widdicombe JG, ed. Respiratory Physiology. Baltimore: University Park Press, 1974:247–271.

Torrance RW. Manipulation of bicarbonate in the carotid body. In: Acker H, Fidone S, Pallot D, Eyzaguirre C, Lübbers DW, Torrance RW, eds. Chemoreception in the Carotid Body. Berlin: Springer-Verlag, 1977:286–293.

Ureña J, Lopez-Lopez J, Gonzalez C, Lopez-Barneo J. Ionic currents in dispersed chemoreceptor cells of the mammalian carotid body. J Gen Physiol 1989; 93:979–999.

Van Buskirk R, Dowling JE. Calcium alters the sensitivity of intact horizontal cells to dopamine antagonist. Proc Natl Acad Sci USA 1982; 79:3350–3354.

Varndell IM, Tapia FJ, De Mey J, Rush RA, Bloom SR, Polak JM. Electron immunocytochemical localization of enkephalin-like material in catecholamine-containing cells of the carotid body, the adrenal medulla, and in pheochromocytomas of man and other mammals. J Histochem Cytochem 1982; 30:682–690.

Vega Saenz De Miera E, Rudy B. Modulation of K^+ channels by hydrogen peroxide. Biochem Biophys Res Commun 1992; 186:1681–1687.

Verna A, Contribution a l'étude du glomus carotidien du lapin. Recherches cytologiques, cytochimiques et expérimentales. Doctoral thesis, University of Bordeaux, 1975.

Verna A. Ultrastructure of the carotid body in the mammals. Int Rev Cytol 1979; 100: 13–23.

Verna A. The carotid body blood supply: evidence against plasma skimming. In: Belmonte C, Pallot DJ, Acker H, Fidone S, eds. Arterial Chemoreceptors. Leicester, UK: Leicester University Press, 1981:336–343.

Verna A, Roumy M, Leitner LM. Loss of chemoreceptive properties of the rabbit carotid body after destruction of the glomus cells. Brain Res 1975; 100:13–23.

Verna A, Barets A, Salat C. Distribution of sympathetic nerve endings within the rabbit carotid body: a histochemical and ultrastructural study. J Neurocytol 1984; 13: 849–865.

Wakade AR, Kruz J. Effect of reserpine, phenoxybenzamine and cocaine on neuromuscular transmission in the vas deferens of the guinea pig. J Pharmacol Exp Ther 1972; 181:310–317.

Wakade AR, Wakade TD. Absence of catecholamines uptake mechanism in the isolated perfused adrenal gland of the rat. Neurosci Lett 1984; 50:139–143.

Wang WJ, Cheng GF, Dinger BG, Fidone SJ. Effects of hypoxia on cyclic nucleotide formation in rabbit carotid body in vitro. Neurosci Lett 1989; 105:164–168.

Wang WJ, Cheng GF, Yoshizaki K, Dinger B, Fidone S. The role of cyclic AMP in chemoreception in the rabbit carotid body. Brain Res 1991; 540:96–104.

Wang ZZ, Stensaas LJ, Dinger B, Fidone SJ. Immunocytochemical localization of choline acetyltransferase in the carotid body of the cat and rabbit. Brain Res 1989; 498: 131–134.

Wang ZZ, He L, Stensaas LJ, Dinger BG, Fidone SJ. Localization and in vitro actions of atrial natriuretic peptide in the cat carotid body. J Appl Physiol 1991a; 70:942–946.

Wang ZZ, Stensaas LJ, Dinger B, Fidone SJ. Co-existence of tyrosine hydroxylase and dopamine β-hydroxylase immunoreactivity in glomus cells of the cat carotid body. J Auton Nerv Syst 1991b; 32:259–264.

Wang ZZ, Stensaas LJ, Dinger B, Fidone SJ. The co-existence of biogenic amines and neuropeptides in the type I cells of the cat carotid body. Neuroscience 1992a; 47: 473–480.

Wang ZZ, Stensaas LJ, Wang WJ, Dinger B, De Vente J, Fidone SJ. Atrial natriuretic peptide increases cyclic guanosine monophosphate immunoreactivity in the carotid body. Neuroscience 1992b; 49:479–486.

Wang ZZ, He L, Cheng B, Dinger BG, Fidone SJ. Mechanisms underlying chemoreceptor inhibition induced by atrial natriuretic peptide in the rabbit carotid body. J Physiol 1993; 460:427–441.

Ward DS. Stimulation of hypoxic ventilatory drive by droperidol. Anesth Analg 1984; 63:106–110.

Watt AH, Reid PG, Stephens MR, Routledge PA. Adenosine-induced respiratory stimulation in man depends on site of infusion. Evidence for an action on the carotid body? Br J Clin Pharmacol 1987; 23:486–490.

Weil JV. Ventilatory control at high altitude. In: Fishman AP, ed. Handbook of Physiology. The Respiratory System. Bethesda: American Physiological Society, 1986:703–727.

West JB. High altitude. In: Crystal RG, West JB, eds. The Lung Scientific Foundations. New York: Raven Press, 1991:2093–2104.

Whalen WJ, Nair P. Some factors affecting tissue P_{O_2} in the carotid body. J Appl Physiol 1975; 39:562–566.

Whalen WJ, Nair P. P_{O_2} in the carotid body perfused and/or superfused with cell-free media. J Appl Physiol 1976; 41:180–184.

Whalen WJ, Nair P. "Hypoxic" discharge of chemoreceptors in the carotid body. Microvasc Res 1977a; 13:371–376.

Whalen WJ, Nair P. Functional correlates of tissue P_{O_2} in the carotid body. In: Reivich M,

Coburn R, Lahiri S, Chance C, eds. Tissue Hypoxia and Ischemia. New York: Plenum Press, 1977b:545–550.

Whalen WJ, Nair P. Factors affecting O_2 consumption of the cat carotid body. In: Acker H, Fidone S, Pallot D, Eyzaguirre C, Lübbers DW, Torrance RW, eds. Chemoreception in the Carotid Body. Berlin: Springer-Verlag, 1977c:233–239.

Whalen WJ, Nair P. Oxidative metabolism and tissue Po_2 of the carotid body. In: Physiology of the Peripheral Arterial Chemoreceptors. Amsterdam, The Netherlands: Elsevier, 1983:117–132.

Whalen WJ, Nair P, Sidebotham T, Spande J, Lacerna M. Cat carotid body: oxygen consumption and other parameters. J Appl Physiol 1981; 50:129–133.

Wharton J, Polak JM, Pearse AG, McGregor GP, Bryant MG, Bloom SR, Emson PC, Bisgard GE, Will JA. Enkephalin-, VIP- and substance P–like immunoreactivity in the carotid body. Nature 1980; 284:269–271.

Wilding TJ, Cheng B, Ross A. pH regulation in adult rat carotid body glomus cells. J Gen Physiol 1992; 100:593–608.

Wilson DF, Rumsey WL, Green TJ, Vanderkooi JM. The oxygen dependence of mitochondrial oxidative phosphorylation measured by a new optical method for measuring oxygen concentration. J Biol Chem 1988; 263:2712–2718.

Wray S. Smooth muscle intracellular pH: measurement, regulation and function. Am J Physiol 1988; 254:C213–C225.

Yarowsky P, Ingvar OH. Neuronal activity and energy metabolism. Fed Proc 1981; 40:2353–2362.

Yoshioka M. Effect of a novel 5-hydroxytryptamine 3-antagonist, GR38032F, on the 5-hydroxytryptamine-induced increase in carotid sinus nerve activity in rats. J Pharmacol Exp Ther 1989; 250:637–641.

Zapata P. Effects of dopamine on carotid chemo- and baroreceptors in vitro. J Physiol (Lond) 1975; 244:235–251.

Zapata P, Llados F. Blockade of carotid body chemosensory inhibition. In: Acker H, Fidone S, Pallot D, Eyzaguirre C, Lübbers DW, Torrance RW, eds. Chemoreception in the Carotid Body. Berlin: Springer-Verlag, 1977:152–159.

Zapata P, Torrealba F. Blockade of dopamine-induced chemosensory inhibition of domperidone. Neurosci Lett 1984; 51:359–364.

Zapata P, Stensaas LJ, Eyzaguirre C. Axon regeneration following a lesion of the carotid nerve: electrophysiological and ultrastructural observations. Brain Res 1976; 113: 235–253.

Zapata P, Serani A, Lavados M. Inhibition in carotid body chemoreceptors mediated by D-2 dopaminoceptors: antagonism by benzamides. Neurosci Lett 1983; 42:179–184.

Zapata P, Serani A, Cardenas H, Lavados M. Characterization of dopaminoceptors in carotid body chemoreceptors. In: Pallot DJ, ed. The Peripheral Arterial Chemoreceptors. London; Croom Helm, 1984:335–344.

Zuazo A, Zapata P. Effects of 6-hydroxy-dopamine on carotid body chemosensory activity. Neurosci Lett 1978; 9:323–328.

10

Central Chemoreception

EUGENE E. NATTIE

Dartmouth Medical School
Lebanon, New Hampshire

I. Introduction

The perfusion of acidic fluids in the cerebral ventricles of anesthetized dogs (1) and conscious goats (2,3) stimulates breathing, as does systemic hypercapnia or the intravenous infusion of acidic solutions in animals without peripheral chemoreceptors (4). These and similar results clearly indicate the presence of central chemoreceptors and have led to the hypothesis that central chemoreceptors could account for most, if not all, of the ventilatory response to acidic stimuli (3).

A series of studies have placed the location of these central chemoreceptors at or within a few hundred micrometers of the ventral surface of the medulla. Initially, acid infusions via the cerebral ventricles were found to be particularly effective when made at the lateral recesses of the fourth ventricle (5), which would preferentially affect the composition of the fluid coming into contact with the ventral medullary surface. Then Mitchell et al. produced large effects on ventilation by bathing the subarachnoid region of the ventrolateral medulla (VLM) directly with acidic solutions (6). Subsequent work utilized the direct application of acidic or basic artificial cerebrospinal fluid to specific locations on the VLM surface using small cotton pledgets or a superperfusion apparatus. A rostral chemosensitive area, referred to as Mitchell's area (M), and a caudal chemosensi-

473

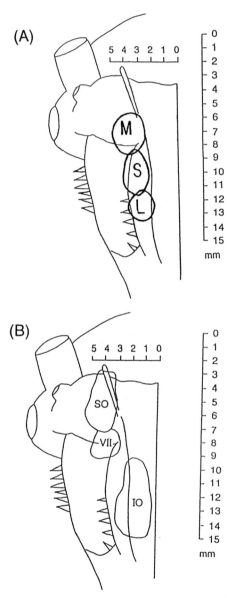

Figure 1 Schematic representations of the topographical anatomy of the traditional central chemoreceptor locations on the ventrolateral medulla (A), the ventral surface projection of some anatomical structures (B), and sagittal (C) and cross-sectional (D) depictions of the medulla. (A) Topographical representation of the rostral chemosensitive area (Mitchell's area; M), the caudal chemosensitive area (Loeschcke's area; L), and the

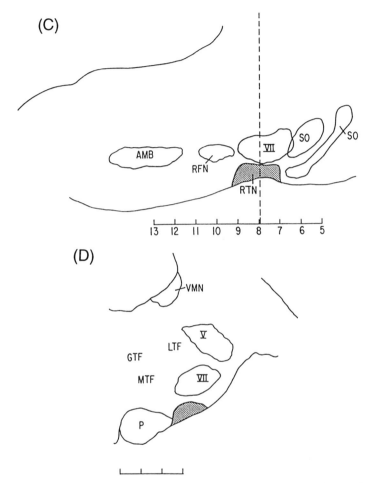

intermediate area (Schlaefke's area; S). The scale marking the lateral distance from the midline is in millimeters in this and the other panels. The vertical scale marks the distance in millimeters caudal from the interaural plane. (B) Same as A but with the topographical projection of three anatomical structures used as landmarks: the superior olive (SO), the inferior olive (IO), and the facial nucleus (VII). (C) Saggital section 3.7 mm lateral to the midline. Scale at the bottom marks the distance caudal from the interaural plane. The vertical dotted line marks the plane of the cross-section shown in D. The shaded area in C and D represents the retrotrapezoid nucleus. AMB, nucleus ambiguus; VII, facial nucleus; GTF, gigantocellular tegmental field; IO, inferior olive; LTF, lateral tegmental field; MTF, magnocellular tegmental field; RFN, retrofacial nucleus; RTN, retrotrapezoid nucleus; SO, superior olive; V, trigeminal nucleus; VMN, medial vestibular nucleus; P, pyramidal tracts. (C and D modified from Ref. 163.)

tive area, referred to as Loeschcke's area (L), were described (7,8) (see Fig. 1). A surface area lying between the M and L areas, referred to as the intermediate area (IMA; Schlaefke's area; S), was also described. The IMA was not thought to be chemosensitive but was still of some importance (9) as cooling of this area produced depression of ventilation and of chemosensitivity (10–12).

This location for central chemoreceptors, at or within a few hundred micrometers of the VLM surface at rostral and caudal locations, has received widespread acceptance, but it is not without its critics. In rats, for example, some have found ventilatory responses to VLM acid application (13) and others not (14). Lipscomb and Boyarski proposed that substances applied to the VLM surface actually are transported deeper within the medulla by the numerous blood vessels that penetrate from the ventral surface and affect neurons at these locations (15). Both large (16) and small (17–19) radiolabeled molecules applied to the VLM surface have been shown to penetrate to a depth of up to 2 mm, an observation that supports this hypothesis. The precise location of central chemoreceptors cannot be accurately deduced from surface application studies.

Many recent reviews cover in depth the introductory material outlined above (8,20–24). This chapter will focus on four topics: (1) recent evidence for the location of central chemoreceptors at or within 800 μm of the VLM surface as well as at more widespread sites deeper within the medulla, (2) possible molecular mechanisms for sensing CO_2/H^+ related to the alphastat hypothesis and to the enzyme carbonic anhydrase, (3) new experimental models for the study of central chemoreception, and (4) the anatomical substrates of the IMA and the functions of neurons within these sites.

Initially, we shall refer to the chemoreceptor stimulus as CO_2/H^+, acknowledging that we do not know its precise chemical nature; later, we shall focus on H^+ as the putative stimulus.

II. Widespread Locations of Central Chemoreceptors

A. Evidence of Single Units Responsive to Changes of CO_2/H^+

A number of studies have asked whether the activity of neurons recorded by extracellular or intracellular electrodes changes with local or systemic changes in CO_2 or H^+. All of these studies suffer from the weakness that the observed changes in neural activity may or may not reflect central respiratory chemoreceptor activity. Cells or molecules sensitive to pH are not necessarily ventilatory chemoreceptors.

In Vivo Studies

A large proportion of medullary single units with discharge patterns that vary with the respiratory cycle (respiratory-modulated) increase their firing rate with increased CO_2. Cohen (25) showed that the majority of 167 units recorded in dorsal medullary locations and within the pons in decerebrate and anesthetized cats retained their discharge pattern and increased their firing rate with systemic hypercapnia. St. John and Wang (26) reported similar findings. We have observed, in a study of a region of the cat VLM lying at the border of the IMA and the rostral chemosensitive area, that 8/17 respiratory-modulated units increased their firing rate with systemic hypercapnia (27).

Medullary single units with discharge patterns that are tonic (i.e., they do not vary with the respiratory cycle) have also been shown to increase firing with increased CO_2. Lipscomb and Boyarski (15) perfused the surface of the VLM with acidic fluid and recorded from 68 units just dorsal to the rostral chemosensitive area. Figure 1 in their paper shows that four to eight units increased their firing rate. Similar studies found 9/44 responsive units at the rostral area (28), a smaller number of units just dorsal to the caudal area and the IMA (29), and no responsive cells within the ventral respiratory group (VRG; nucleus ambiguus and retroambiguus) (30). We found that 11/29 tonic units recorded at the border of the IMA and the rostral chemosensitive area increased their discharge rate in hypercapnia (27).

Using a slightly different approach, Arita and colleagues injected CO_2-laden saline in a vertebral artery to produce brief, transient stimulation of central chemoreceptors within the medulla (31,32). They found 18/46 tonic units deep to the caudal chemosensitive area and the IMA that were responsive only to increased medullary CO_2 (unresponsive to carotid body or nociceptive stimulation). The responses of these units occurred temporally just prior to the transient increase in ventilation that followed the injection, suggesting that they were causally related to ventilation. These units were located (1) near the VLM surface, (2) near the rostral aspect of the VRG, and (3) ventral to the nucleus tractus solitarius (dorsal respiratory group, DRG). Local acidic microinjections made within these regions containing responsive units showed 16/164 that were sensitive to local pH changes Of these 16 units, 10 were also excited upon injection of CO_2-laden saline into the vertebral artery, this excitation having a time course similar to that for the increase in ventilation. These 10 units, located within 2 mm of the VLM surface at the level of the caudal chemosensitive area and more dorsally, just ventral to the nucleus tractus solitarius, were thought to be ventilatory chemoreceptors (33).

These in vivo studies show that both respiratory-modulated and tonic units at many locations within the brainstem increase their firing rate with increased CO_2-H^+ produced both locally and systemically. In many (? most) cases the increase in unit discharge may merely reflect the response of the control system; i.e., the unit is part of the respiratory control system responding to the chemoreceptor stimulation; it is not a chemosensitive neuron. The presence in many studies of tonic units that respond to CO_2 and the findings of Arita and colleagues suggest that chemosensitive neurons are not necessarily respiratory-modulated and that their location may be deeper within the medulla than deduced from earlier studies.

In Vitro Studies

The use of the whole-cell patch-clamp technique on neurons in regions of rat medullary slices with known high densities of respiratory-modulated cells and at other regions has shown a variety of responses to changes in pH (34). In similar studies, cells responsive to acidic perfusates have been found in brain slices at such sites as the IMA and the caudal chemosensitive regions (35–38). Perfusion with a low-Ca^{2+}/high-Mg^{2+} solution, which interferes with synaptic transmission, failed to block the stimulation, suggesting that the sensing mechanism is nonsynaptic. In slices including the rostral chemosensitive area (39), 136 of 316 neurons were found to be responsive to changes in local tissue pH produced by changes in perfusate pH. In this study, synaptic blockade reduced the response, suggesting that a synaptic mechanism is involved. Cells responsive to acidic stimulation have also been found at more dorsal locations near the nucleus tractus solitarius (37,38) as well as in parts of the slice not usually associated with respiratory control (38).

Dean et al. (40,41) recorded with both intra- and extracellular electrodes in the rat medullary slice and found that cells in the VRG were unresponsive to hypercapnia. More dorsally near the nucleus tractus solitarius, in a slice with the ventral half removed to eliminate input from putative VLM chemoreceptors, 35% of the neurons depolarized with increased CO_2 (41). These neurons remained responsive in the presence of low-Ca^{2+}/high-Mg^{2+} medium, suggesting the CO_2 effect did not require synaptic input.

These studies using brain slices indicate that many neurons within the brainstem are excited by CO_2/H^+. These neurons are located near the VLM surface as well as more dorsally both at sites associated with respiratory-modulated neurons and at other sites. There is evidence to support both synaptic and nonsynaptic mechanisms for the CO_2/H^+ sensing process. Whether any of these responses represent ventilatory chemoreception is unknown since no measure of ventilatory output could be included.

B. Phrenic Nerve Responses to Focal Increases in CO_2/H^+ at Widespread Brainstem Sites

We applied acetazolamide (AZ) to the surface of the VLM in anesthetized cats with end-tidal P_{CO_2} held constant to examine the effect of carbonic anhydrase inhibition in the medulla on central chemoreception (42). On average, phrenic nerve activity increased and the medullary tissue pH measured within 1–2 mm of the VLM surface decreased. The time course of the average tissue pH change was similar to that of the average increase in phrenic activity, although in individual cats there was not always a correlation. The increase in phrenic activity in response to a step increase in P_{CO_2} was slower after AZ treatment but the steady-state response was not diminished. The results suggest that carbonic anhydrase inhibition locally in the VLM produced a tissue acidosis that resulted in an increase in phrenic activity via local chemoreceptor stimulation. These data provide support for the VLM as a site for central chemoreception. But the experiments are subject to the criticisms of all surface application studies; i.e., the depth of penetration of the AZ and the size of the resultant region of acidosis are unknown. We also made microinjections (10–100 nl) of AZ unilaterally at putative VLM chemoreceptor sites and were surprised that they also brought about large increases in phrenic activity. These responses were presumed to result from local regions of decreased pH, produced by the AZ microinjections, which were smaller in size than those produced by AZ application to the surface of the VLM.

To determine the size of the region of tissue acidosis produced by AZ microinjections, we made 1 nl AZ (10^{-5} M or 5×10^{-6} M) injections in anesthetized rats and measured pH at varying distances from the AZ injection center using pH-sensitive glass microelectrodes (43). Figure 2 shows the change

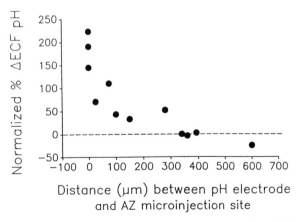

Distance (μm) between pH electrode
and AZ microinjection site

Figure 2 Relationship of the change in medullary tissue extracellular fluid pH produced by 1-nl injections of acetazolamide and the distance between the acetazolamide injection center and the pH electrode. The change in tissue pH is normalized as a percent of the pH change measured in each rat in response to a 20 mmHg increase in end-tidal P_{CO_2}. Each point is from an individual rat. Note that at distances >350 μm from the center of the acetazolamide injection no pH changes are detectable. (From Ref. 43, with permission of the *Journal of Applied Physiology*.)

(decrease) in measured tissue pH produced by AZ injections as a function of distance between the injection center and the pH electrode. The measured pH change following AZ injection is normalized to that produced in each animal by a 20 mmHg increase in end-tidal P_{CO_2}. At the center of the AZ injection, the tissue pH change was equivalent to that produced by a 36 mmHg increase in end-tidal P_{CO_2}. The pH change produced by AZ rapidly decreased with radial distance away from the injection center such that at distances greater than 350 μm, tissue pH was unaffected. With this knowledge of the size of the region of tissue acidosis produced, we then used this injection volume with these AZ concentrations as a probe to search for the locations of central chemoreceptor sites.

In anesthetized cats and rats, we made such 1-nl AZ injections to produce focal brainstem regions of decreased pH and we measured phrenic nerve responses, an index of the whole respiratory control system response to the local pH change. Figure 3 shows a typical response. At lower right the AZ injection site is marked anatomically, in this case in the region dorsal to the caudal chemosensitive area. The nondiffusible fluorescent microbeads included with each injection mark the injection site shown on the figure. The prior measured tissue pH changes indicate that the entire region affected by the combination of the subsequent AZ diffusion from the injection site and the AZ effects on tissue pH lies within 350 μm of the injection center. While many neurons could be affected, the region of decreased tissue pH is small enough to allow the use of this approach to probe the brainstem for the location of central chemoreceptor sites.

Figure 3A shows the time course of the increase in phrenic nerve activity, measured with constant end-tidal P_{CO_2}, which resulted from this injection. The response to increased systemic P_{CO_2} shown at lower left indicates the maximum response to stimulation of all central chemoreceptors in this cat. Note that at 60 min following the AZ injection, which stimulated only the chemoreceptors within the region of decreased pH produced by the injection, the phrenic nerve activity has increased to be a large fraction of the maximum observed with systemic CO_2. Overall in these experiments, 26 of 57 (46%) injections in 30 cats produced a significant increase in phrenic activity, which returned to baseline within 120 min. For these 26 positive injections, on average the normalized phrenic activity increased from 35% of maximum to 56% of maximum following the AZ injection. The sites of these positive injections are shown in Figure 4. They can be grouped into three regions: first, sites within 800 μm of the VLM surface at the rostral and caudal chemosensitive areas and at the IMA; second, sites near the nucleus tractus solitarius; and third, sites more rostrally located in the vicinity of the locus coeruleus. Similar findings were obtained in rats.

The use of 1-nl AZ injections to produce focal regions of decreased pH apparently results in the stimulation of a sufficient population of chemoreceptors to result in a measurable whole control system output. This fortunate outcome allows us to know that the AZ injection did stimulate a ventilatory chemoreceptor site; it did not merely excite a group of medullary neurons of unknown function. The

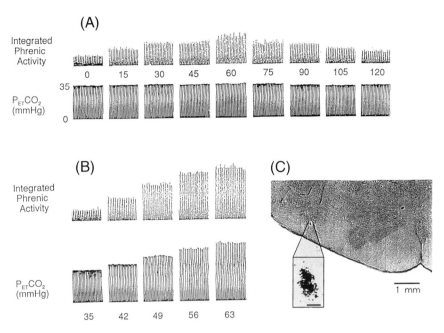

Figure 3 Phrenic nerve response to an injection of 1 nl of acetazolamide at a putative central chemoreceptor site. (A) Integrated phrenic nerve response at various times (shown as numbers) over 120 min following the injection and the corresponding values for end-tidal P_{CO_2}. Each segment shows 1 min of data. (B) Response of phrenic nerve activity to increased end-tidal CO_2. The numbers at the bottom represent the P_{CO_2} values in mmHg. (C) Quadrant of a medullary cross-section showing the acetazolamide injection site lateral to the inferior olivary nucleus. The section was stained with cresyl violet and computer-enhanced. (Inset) Magnified view of the fluorescent beads used as an injection marker. Bar in the inset = 100 μm. (From Ref. 43, with permission of the *Journal of Applied Physiology.*)

results indicate that central chemoreception is located at widespread sites within the brainstem. In fact, there may well be other sites. For example, hypercapnia excites neurons in hypothalamic slices (44), and the approach of the AZ micro-injection probe can be used to ask if local acidosis within the hypothalamus results in ventilatory stimulation. The only caveat in the interpretation of these studies is that the AZ could possibly have an effect independent from the local pH change. The presence of many ineffective injection sites and the absence of any response to injections of an inactive analog are helpful controls for the specificity of the AZ injection. The absence of any inhibitory effect on the steady-state CO_2 response of larger amounts of AZ applied on the surface of the VLM indicates that carbonic anhydrase inhibition does not affect the CO_2/H^+ transduction process (42).

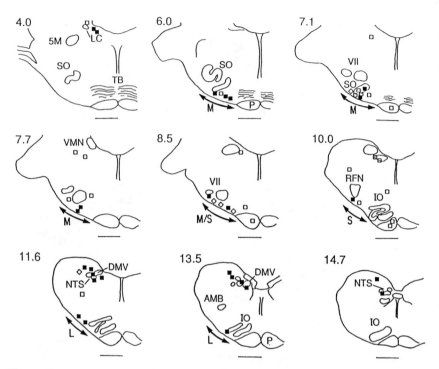

Figure 4 Central chemoreception sites within the brainstem of the cat identified by 1-nl injections of acetazolamide. These injections produced localized regions of decreased pH within the brainstem. The region of decreased pH had a radius of <350 μm from the injection center. Positive injections, those that produced a significant increase in integrated phrenic nerve activity, are shown by solid squares. Open squares denote injection sites associated with no effect on phrenic activity. Open diamonds indicate sites of injection of an inactive analog of acetazolamide. Cross-sections are labeled in millimeters caudal to the interaural plane (see Fig. 1, A and B). Bars at the bottom of each section = 2 mm. Location at the ventral surface of the M, S, and L areas is drawn at the bottom of the appropriate cross-sections with bidirectional arrows. 5M, trigeminal nucleus; LC, locus coeruleus; TB, trapezoid body; P, pyramidal tract; DMV, dorsal motor nucleus of the vagus; NTS, nucleus of the solitary tract. (Modified from Ref. 43, with permission of the *Journal of Applied Physiology*.)

C. Medullary Sites of Decreased pH Induced by Systemic Hypercapnia

It seems reasonable that with systemic hypercapnia tissue pH would decrease to a similar extent within the entire medulla; i.e., there would be a homogeneous distribution of low pH sites within the tissue. This is not the case. As shown by measurement of tissue pH profiles during hypercapnia induced by injection of CO_2-laden saline into the vertebral artery, tissue pH changes vary by location (45). Surprisingly, at many sites dorsal to the caudal chemosensitive area and the IMA, the pH did not decrease. Sites at which the pH did decrease are shown in Figure 5, and Arita et al. propose that central chemoreceptors are located at such sites. Thus, according to their view, Figure 5 shows a potential distribution of central chemoreceptor locations. Note that the sites are distributed throughout the caudal medulla and that the locations overlap with those of the 10 single units, discussed above (33), which are responsive to both local acidosis and systemic hypercapnia and whose activity increases just prior to that of the phrenic following systemic hypercapnia. The location of some sites at which pH decreased in response to injection of high CO_2 solutions into the vertebral artery, i.e., within 800 μm of the VLM surface and in the vicinity of the nucleus tractus solitarius, agree well with some 1-nl AZ injection sites associated with phrenic responses. There are also a number of sites of decreased pH within the VRG, a location not thoroughly

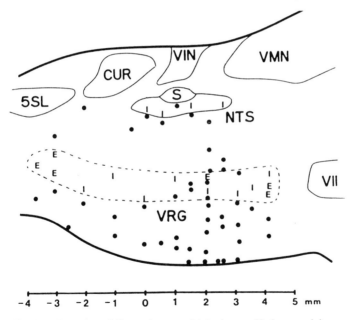

Figure 5 Location of medullary sites at which tissue pH decreased in response to vertebral artery injection of CO_2-laden saline (solid circles). At many other sites, pH was unchanged by the hypercapnic injection. (I and E) Sites of unit recordings of inspiratory and expiratory neurons. Plane of the sagittal section is 3 mm lateral to the midline. 5SL, laminar spinal trigeminal nucleus; CUR, cuneate nucleus, rostral division; S, solitary nucleus; VIN, inferior vestibular nucleus. (From Ref. 45, with permission of Elsevier Medical Publishers.)

evaluated in the initial AZ injection study, raising the possibility of central chemoreceptors being located there as well. Tissue pH responses were not evaluated at more rostral areas.

D. Brain Sites of Increased Neuronal Activity Induced by Systemic Hypercapnia

c-fos

There are methods to localize neurons within the central nervous system with increased activity in response to external stimuli. The localization by immuno-histochemistry of the *fos* protein product of the c-*fos* oncogene is one such approach, and it has been applied to the brainstem of rats exposed to 13–15% CO_2 for 1 hr (46). *fos*-like immunoreactivity was found at sites within 150 μm of the VLM surface from 1.5 mm caudal to the obex to 2.5 mm rostral to the obex, locations that match the rostral and caudal chemosensitive areas of the VLM as well as the IMA. *fos*-like immunoreactivity was also observed near the nucleus tractus solitarius. While the CO_2 levels used were quite high, the sites of *fos*-like immunoreactivity observed match some of the positive sites of the 1-nl AZ injection study and, interestingly, include the IMA, as did that study. In a similar study (47) also using 15% CO_2, *fos*-like immunoreactivity was found in the re-gion of the locus coeruleus, also a chemoreceptor site in the 1-nl AZ study. Part, but not all, of this *fos*-like immunoreactivity in the locus coeruleus was attributed to a pathway involving the VLM as lidocaine block of the VLM decreased but did not entirely eliminate it. A weakness of the c-*fos* approach is that it identifies only neurons, activated by the hypercapnia, which can express *fos*-like immunoreac-tivity. Conceivably, other neurons could be excited by CO_2 which do not express *fos*-like immunoreactivity. Also, expression of *fos*-like immunoreactivity does not prove that the neuron is chemosensitive but only that it is activated by hypercapnia; i.e., the neuron could be in any part of the respiratory control network involved in the CO_2 response. Nevertheless, these observations support those cited above indicating that central chemoreceptors have a widespread distribution within the brainstem.

2-Deoxyglucose

An alternative approach to determine the location of neurons with increased activity in hypercapnia is to measure the uptake of the nonmetabolizable glucose analog 2-deoxyglucose (48). In peripherally chemodenervated rats exposed to 10% CO_2 for 45 min, cerebral autoradiographs of 2-deoxyglucose uptake indicate that in much of the brain neuronal activity was depressed. Sites with increased neuronal activity included: (1) the lateral parabrachial region, (2) the region ventrolateral to the nucleus tractus solitarius, (3) the region of the nucleus retroambiguus, (4) a region of the ventrolateral medullary reticular formation, (5) the region of the ventral nucleus raphe pallidus, and (6) regions of the hypothalamus. Many of these sites are common to those identified by 1-nl AZ injections. As with the expression of c-*fos*, this approach only indicates neurons with increased activity in hypercapnia and does not give any specific indication of central chemoreceptive sites. The fact that the 2-deoxyglucose technique identifies many structures with increased activity in hypercapnia while the c-*fos* technique identifies only some of these adds to the difficulty of interpreting these data. However, in the context of the other data presented above, the c-*fos* and 2-deoxyglucose results do provide support for the proposal that central chemoreceptor sites have a widespread distribution.

III. Mechanism(s) of Central Chemosensitivity

A. CO_2 Versus H^+

So far we have referred to the chemoreceptor stimulus as CO_2/H^+, an admission that the exact chemical stimulus is uncertain. In general, CO_2 hyperpolarizes mammalian cortical neurons and depresses monosynaptic reflexes (49). In studies related to respiratory control, three groups of investigators have examined the relationship of ventilatory output to pH measured on the surface of the VLM in response to increased CO_2 and to intravenous infusion of metabolic acid (50–52). The pH measurement in extracellular fluid at the medullary surface is used as an index of the pH at the chemoreceptor site. All studies found that ventilatory output expressed per unit change in the extracellular pH measured at the surface of the VLM is greater following increased CO_2. It was concluded (50) that either CO_2 and H^+ have separate, independent effects that stimulate ventilation, or the chemoreceptor site is in a location that is more easily accessible to an increase in CO_2 than to an increase in extracellular H^+; e.g., the location is intracellular. Given the regional heterogeneity of medullary pH responses to hypercapnia discussed above (45), it is also possible that the pH electrode on the surface of the VLM may not have detected pH values like those at the exact chemoreceptor site(s). These results do not prove the identity of the chemoreceptor stimulus but do indicate the difficulty in measuring it.

Results of in vitro studies have also indicated differences in neuronal responses to CO_2 versus H^+. In rat medullary slices (53) and in the neonatal rat brainstem (54), exposure to solutions with the same pH but differing P_{CO_2} and HCO_3^- result in different effects. And in medullary cells grown in tissue culture (55), the neurons responsive to hypercapnia have no response to decreased pH produced under isocapnic conditions by decreasing the HCO_3^- concentration. Again, the interpretation is that either separate sensing mechanisms exist or the chemoreceptor site is more easily accessible to CO_2; i.e., the site is intracellular (55).

It is important to remember in this context the careful studies of Pappenheimer et al. (2) and Fencl et al. (3) in conscious goats. In steady-state conditions of acid-base disorders and in hypercapnia, they found that ventilation was a unique function of an estimated pH lying at a fixed distance between the [H^+] of cerebral ventricle and capillary blood. These data provide persuasive support for the hypothesis that H^+ is the chemoreceptor stimulus. In the mechanistic discussion below we shall focus on H^+ as the chemoreceptor stimulus.

B. The Alphastat Hypothesis

Homeotherms maintain pH at a constant, normal value by means of a number of physiological systems one of which involves the use of ventilatory chemoreceptors. Yet, vertebrate ectotherms, e.g., turtles (56) and toads (57,58), also have ventilatory chemoreceptors, as do invertebrate ectotherms, e.g., the pulmonate snail, *Helix aspersa* and *pomatia* (59,59a,60). In ectotherms, extracellular fluid pH varies inversely with temperature, the coefficient being approximately 0.015 pH unit/degree centigrade. This occurs without apparent effect on ventilation (61), suggesting that pH per se is unlikely to be the unique molecular stimulus for chemoreception among both the homeotherms and ectotherms. How can this be so, given the powerful effects of small pH changes in homeotherms? A solution for this paradox lies in the alphastat hypothesis (see Ref. 67).

Reeves (62,63) noted that the coefficient for the variation of ectotherm extracellular pH with temperature is similar to the coefficient for the variation of the pK' of imidazole with temperature. This means that as temperature changes the fractional dissociation of imidazole (called alpha-imidazole) remains constant. Further, any protein with imidazole groups in locations that determine function would have constant charge state and thereby be functionally unaffected by changes in temperature. But the function of this same protein could be quite sensitive to changes in pH in isothermal conditions. The exact coefficient for the change in imidazole pK' with temperature may vary depending on the histidine site within the protein and the effects of neighboring amino acids (64,65). The closer this coefficient is to that for the variation of pH with temperature in that species and at that site, the more constant would be the fractional dissociation of imidazole. The alpha-stat hypothesis has general biological significance for all pH-sensitive proteins (64–67) and it has particular relevance for the issue of central ventilatory chemoreception (67).

There is evidence for the involvement of imidazole-histidine in central chemoreception. Hitzig (61) measured ventilation in unanesthetized turtles during ventriculocisternal perfusion with solutions of differing pH at different temperatures. He found ventilation to be a unique function of calculated cerebrospinal fluid alpha-imidazole, not pH. In contrast, in anesthetized cats, Kiley et al. (68) found that phrenic nerve activity measured in conditions of varying CO_2 and temperature does not correlate uniquely with medullary alpha-imidazole in this case, using measured VLM surface pH for the calculation. In both cases the estimate of alpha-imidazole is crucially dependent on the assumed value for the variation of imidazole pK' with temperature. As Burton pointed out (64), by making slightly different assumptions the alpha-imidazole values estimated from the data of the Kiley et al. study could actually support the alpha-stat hypothesis. Nevertheless, these studies cannot be considered conclusive given the requirement in the calculation of alpha-imidazole for an estimate of a crucial variable, the value for the change in pK' imidazole with temperature for the key imidazole site(s) of the protein(s) in question.

In my laboratory (69–71) we have examined the possible role of imidazole histidine in central chemoreception by the use of a substance that is thought to be relatively specific for binding to imidazole histidine, diethylpyrocarbonate (DEPC). The pH optimum for DEPC binding to imidazole-histidine is 7.0, and the resultant carbethoxy derivative is stable for hours allowing time for physiological measurements. Unbound DEPC is rapidly hydrolyzed to ethanol and CO_2. Infusion of DEPC in the cisterna magna of conscious, awake rabbits depresses ventilation and the ventilatory responses both to hypercapnia and to the infusion of acidic mock cerebrospinal fluid in the cisterna magna. Direct application of DEPC on the rostral chemosensitive area of the VLM in anesthetized, peripherally denervated, paralyzed, and ventilated cats decreases baseline phrenic nerve activity, the response to hypercapnia, and the response to intravenous infusion of acidic solutions. These results support the hypothesis that an imidazole-histidine is involved in central chemoreception at sites accessible via VLM surface application.

Other studies have shown effects of DEPC on physiological functions attributed to its binding to imidazole-histidine. For example, the effect of external pH on an inward current induced by stimulation of excitatory amino acid receptors in catfish retinal cone cells is blocked by DEPC (71), and the pH-dependent chloride efflux from frog skeletal muscle is inhibited by DEPC (73).

C. Proteins Possibly Involved in
Chemoreception via Imidazole-Histidine

To identify proteins that might be involved in central chemoreception, we used the following strategy. First, we deduced from the alpha-state hypothesis that imidazole-histidine is a likely pH sensor molecule. Second, we utilized information concerning the molecular structure of proteins derived from cloning studies to identify proteins with histidines in locations that could affect function. In most cases, we have used the data from initial reports of cDNAs that describe the sequence of a protein subunit or of the first of a series of proteins subsequently described as a family. For example, there appear to be multiple glutamate receptor subtypes and multiple potassium channels. The proteins chosen for discussion are meant to be representative of the categories outlined below, and this selection is by no means all-inclusive. We chose proteins that could possibly be involved in sensing pH, examined their amino acid sequence for the presence of histidines, and located these histidine sites on proposed molecular models of the protein structure. When possible, evidence of pH sensitivity in regard to function has been included. We categorized the proteins into four groups: (1) membrane receptors, (2) enzymes that affect neurotransmitters, (3) ion transport proteins that can alter neuronal function, and (4) ion channels.

Receptors

Figure 6 shows, in cartoon form, the estimated molecular structures for a combined M1 and M3 subtype of the cholinergic muscarinic receptor (74) and for a subunit of the glutamate receptor (75) together with the location of all of the histidines for these molecules. In both cases the predominant histidine location

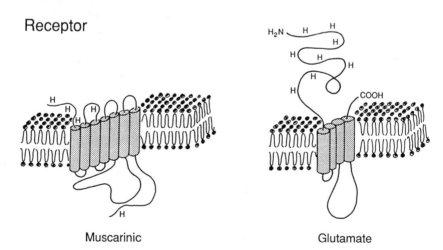

Figure 6 Molecular models for two receptors, the muscarinic cholinergic receptor and the glutamate receptor, are shown together with the location of the histidine residues on the model. These were determined from sequence analysis of the receptor structure. Similar models can be constructed for the gamma-aminobutyric acid receptor, the membrane ion channels for sodium, potassium, calcium, and chloride, and the transmembrane ion exchange proteins for sodium/potassium, chloride/bicarbonate, and sodium/proton (see text). (Data from Ref. 74 and Ref. 75.)

in the molecular model is on the outside of the cell membrane. In respect to glutamate receptors, in catfish retinal neurons (72), rat cerebellar neurons (76), and mouse (77) and rat (78) hippocampal cells, extracellular acidosis inhibits depolarizing currents induced by glutamate probably by reducing the open time of the ion channel associated with the receptor. In one case (72), this effect is inhibited by treatment at the external surface with DEPC, the imidazole-histidine blocker. Could this known pH effect on glutamate receptors be involved in central chemoreception? Inhibition of the postsynaptic effect of an excitatory amino acid by acidosis would diminish excitation. Unless the effect of the neuron excited by glutamate (the hypothetical chemoreceptor) was itself inhibitory to the respiratory control system, acidosis would presumably decrease chemosensitivity. In vivo studies have shown that microinjections of glutamate at VLM chemosensitive areas excite phrenic activity (79) and microinjections of glutamate receptor antagonists at the caudal aspect of the rostral chemosensitive area decrease phrenic activity and the response to hypercapnia (80). From this analysis, it seems unlikely that a pH effect on the glutamate receptor is the mechanism for respiratory chemosensitivity but it appears that functional glutamate receptors in the region of the VLM are required for expression of central ventilatory chemosensitivity.

For the muscarinic receptors, the M1 and M3 subtypes have a greater number of extracellular histidines than does the M2 subtype (74), and binding of muscarinic agonists to rat brainstem (81) and corpus striatum (82) membranes is inhibited by low pH. In respect to respiratory control, ventriculocisternal perfusion with acetylcholine in anesthetized dogs stimulates ventilation while atropine inhibits the response to perfusion of cerebrospinal fluid made acidic by increased CO_2 or by decreased HCO_3^- (83). A cholinergic mechanism for central chemosensitivity has long been a popular hypothesis (84,85), and recent studies have shown that application to the VLM surface of both atropine in low doses and the M1 receptor subtype antagonist pirenzepine inhibits chemosensitivity (86). Microinjections into the rostral chemosensitive region of pirenzepine and the M3 receptor subtype antagonist, 4-diphenylacetoxy-*N*-methylpiperidine (DAMP) have the same effect (87). Normal muscarinic cholinergic receptor function in the region of the VLM appears to be necessary to obtain a normal ventilatory response to hypercapnia, but the pH-sensing mechanism does not appear to be via a pH effect on cholinergic receptor binding as judged by the inhibition by low pH of agonist binding to muscarinic receptors.

The receptor for the inhibitory amino acid neurotransmitter gamma-aminobutyric acid (GABA) also has a large number (7) of histidines located at the outside of the cell membrane (88). A decreased pH is known to potentiate GABA effects in crayfish muscle (89,90) and cat dorsal root ganglion (91). One would predict from these observations that decreased pH would enhance any existing GABA-induced inhibition. Infusion of GABA into the cerebral ventricles depresses ventilation and the hypercapnic ventilatory response (92). Thus it seems unlikely that the pH-sensing mechanism for central chemoreception involves the GABA receptor.

At present it is difficult to reconcile the known effects of glutaminergic, cholinergic muscarinic, and GABAergic agonists and antagonists on ventilation and CO_2 sensitivity in vivo with the known pH effects on their respective receptors studied in vitro. In each case the pH effect in vitro seems to be in the opposite direction from that expected were that receptor involved in chemoreception. Glutamate and acetylcholine, which have excitatory effects at the VLM on breathing, are, in vitro, less excitatory at their postsynaptic receptor in acidosis. GABA, which has an inhibitory effect at the VLM on breathing, has, in vitro, its inhibitory postsynaptic effect enhanced by acidosis. However, it remains possible that these receptors are involved in sensing pH via a pH effect on receptor function that differs from those cited above or via a net neurotransmitter effect on ventilation that differs from those cited above. In any case, the normal ventilatory control system response to central chemoreceptor stimulation requires intact, functional glutamate and acetylcholine receptors in the VLM.

Enzymes that Affect Neurotransmitters

Chemoreception could result from a pH effect, not on a neurotransmitter receptor, but on an enzyme involved in transmitter production or degradation. For example, acetylcholinesterase is pH sensitive and could provide a means for pH-sensitive physiological regulation (84). DEPC inhibits acetylcholinesterase activity (93,94), suggesting that the active site of this pH-sensitive enzyme involves a histidine. We can hypothesize that low pH would inhibit the enzyme via its effect on the imidazole-histidine resulting in less acetylcholine degradation and enhanced stimulation of the postsynaptic receptor and of ventilation as well. In respect to the alpha-stat hypothesis and acetylcholinesterase, the prediction would be that the pH optima for the enzyme activity would vary inversely with temperature, as does ectotherm extracellular fluid pH and the pK' of imidazole. Thus with temperature-induced changes in pH, the enzyme optimum would remain constant. We found experimentally that the pH optima varied directly with temperature, not inversely as predicted (94). Nevertheless, pH effects on acetylcholinesterase remain a viable mechanism for central chemoreception.

Ion Transport

The cloned alpha subunit of rat brain sodium/potassium ATPase has 14 histidines located on the proposed intracellular portion of the membrane-spanning molecule (95). Ouabain-sensitive sodium flux is inhibited by a decrease in intracellular pH well within the physiological range (96), and frog skin sodium/potassium ATPase, when tested for pH optima at different temperatures, behaves according to the alpha-stat prediction (97). The effects of DEPC appear to be untested. Intracellular acidosis could, via inhibition of this ion transporter, result in cell swelling, decreased intracellular potassium, and changes in cell excitability.

The amiloride-sensitive sodium/proton antiporter involved in cell pH regulation and in the secretory function of specialized epithelium increases acid extrusion with intracellular acidosis (98). A cDNA clone of this protein has 16 of a total of 29 histidines located on the proposed intracellular aspect of the molecule (99). In rabbit renal cortical cells, this antiporter is inactivated by DEPC and it is no longer responsive to changes in pH (100), suggesting a role for histidine in its pH-sensitive function. Infusion of amiloride, which inhibits the sodium/proton antiporter, into the cisterna magna of conscious rabbits inhibits the normal regulation of cerebrospinal fluid pH in hypercapnia but has no effect on the ventilatory response to hypercapnia (101).

The chloride/bicarbonate antiporter is also involved with intracellular pH regulation and secretory epithelial function. A cDNA clone of this protein (102) shows 9 of 13 histidines located on the proposed intracellular aspect of the molecule. These presumably sense changes in intracellular pH and activate chloride extrusion, which increases intracellular bicarbonate and pH. The function of this antiporter is inhibited by 4,4'-diisothiocyanostilbene-2,2'-disulfonic acid (DIDS). Infusion of DIDS via the cisterna magna in conscious rabbits inhibits cerebrospinal fluid acid-base regulation in hypercapnia (103), but in this case the ventilatory response to hypercapnia is actually enhanced.

One interpretation of these data related to the sodium/proton and chloride/bicarbonate antiporters is that the infusion into the cisterna magna of the inhibitor of amiloride or DIDS interferes with the choroid plexus and blood-brain barrier secretory processes that regulate cerebrospinal fluid pH in hypercapnia. Thus, in both cases the usual cerebrospinal fluid pH regulation in hypercapnia is inhibited. But, only one inhibitor, DIDS, has an effect on the ventilatory response to hypercapnia. The presumed effect of amiloride or DIDS on accessible neurons would be to inhibit intracellular pH regulation in hypercapnia, resulting in a greater, more prolonged intracellular acidosis. The enhanced ventilatory response to hypercapnia after DIDS treatment suggests that (1) central chemoreceptor cells sense intracellular pH, and (2) these cells utilize a DIDS-inhibitable process for intracellular pH regulation.

Ion Channels

A cloned sodium channel (104) has eight and three histidines located on the intra- and extracellular aspects, respectively, of the membrane-spanning molecule, and extracellular acidosis inhibits sodium conductance in squid axon (105). It is not known whether the histidines are involved in this effect, which would presumably decrease cell excitability.

A cloned potassium channel has five histidines located inside and two outside the cell (106) on the proposed molecular structure, and intracellular acidosis inhibits potassium conductance (107,108) via histidines that could increase cell excitability.

A cloned skeletal muscle dihydropyridine-sensitive calcium channel (109) has five intracellular and eight extracellular histidines. Extracellular acidosis results in a greater frequency of transitions between high- and low-conductance states of a dihydropyridine-sensitive calcium channel via a histidine site in PC-12 cells and ventricular myocytes (110), and intracellular acidosis decreases calcium current in myocytes (111).

A chloride channel cloned from *Torpedo* (112) has seven intracellular histidines, but there appear to be no functional studies involving pH effects and histidine.

It is possible that any ion channel could be a site for the mechanism of sensing pH involved in ventilatory chemosensitivity.

Proteins and pH

This evaluation of proteins that might be involved in chemoreception is selective and by no means all-inclusive. It is easy to think of other possibilities, e.g., second-messenger systems. Still, the ubiquitous presence of histidines in the proteins chosen for evaluation, often in locations that would be predicted to be pH-sensitive based on the function of the protein, provides general support for the alpha-stat hypothesis. Does it help in thinking of possible mechanisms for central chemoreception? I believe it does. Although no specific mechanism can be proven from these data, they do indicate that a large number of possible mechanisms exist for a cell to sense pH and raise the possibility that ventilatory chemosensitivity may involve more than one mechanism.

In a growing number of examples, cells have been shown to use pH-sensitive proteins for physiological regulatory function. The pH-sensitive ion transport proteins are, in many cases, involved in intracellular pH regulation, and as shown above, these proteins have many histidines located at intracellular sites. Changes in pH influence fertilization via effects on potassium conductance brought about via pH effects on a calcium pump (113). Aldosterone promotes potassium secretion via a pH effect that results from aldosterone stimulation of the sodium/proton antiporter (114). A recently proposed model for the carotid body pH-sensing mechanism (115) involves many steps. Intracellular acidosis stimulates the sodium/proton antiporter and a sodium-coupled chloride/bicarbonate exchange, which increase cell sodium. The sodium drives calcium into the cell via a sodium/calcium antiporter, which activates secretion of dopamine and increases afferent nerve activity. These observations raise the possibility that central chemoreception also might be a multistep process at the cellular level initiated by pH sensitivity of one or more protein(s).

Finally, Chesler and Kaila (116) have recently reviewed pH regulation within the nervous system. They emphasize some new concepts that involve changes in pH locally within and around neurons at the synaptic level, which occur as a result of neuronal activity. They propose that these activity-dependent pH changes may modulate neuronal excitability via affects on pH-sensitive proteins. For example, the ion currents induced by glutamate at its postsynaptic receptor also produce changes in intra- and extracellular pH. These could then affect the pH-sensitive glutamate receptor and modulate subsequent glutamate effects at that receptor. Central chemoreception could conceivably involve an influence of systemic or regional acidosis on this activity-dependent modulation brought about via local pH changes at the synaptic level.

D. Carbonic Anhydrase

The enzyme carbonic anhydrase deserves mention in the consideration of mechanisms for central chemoreception. Carbonic anhydrase is located in cells within the VLM chemosensitive areas (117) and in neurons cultured from the medulla (118) many of which can be excited by hypercapnia (55). Inhibition of brain carbonic anhydrase using acetazolamide administered systemically (119) and via local application on, or microinjection into, the VLM (42,43) increases ventilatory output and decreases medullary tissue pH. In response to increased CO_2, the phrenic output at any level of CO_2, is increased; i.e., the response is shifted upward. This reflects the additive effects of the greater baseline levels of ventilatory output produced by AZ injection and the stimulation of the hypercapnia (42,119). The slope of the steady-state phrenic nerve response to hypercapnic stimulation is unaffected, and responses to step increases in PCO2 are delayed in reaching the steady state (42,120,121). One interpretation for these observations is that intracellular pH is sensed by the chemoreceptor mechanism and that carbonic anhydrase within neurons speeds the response to hypercapnia. However, with the inhibition of carbonic anhydrase increased CO_2 still results in intracellular acidosis, but with a slower time course via the uncatalyzed CO_2 hydration reaction.

Recent in vitro evidence also points to an important role for carbonic anhydrase in pH-mediated events. Dean et al. used intracellular micropipettes to measure neuronal activity and described CO_2-sensitive neurons located dorsally in medullary slices near the nucleus tractus solitarius and the dorsal motor nucleus of the vagus (41). But when using a whole-cell patch-clamp technique, Dean found that this CO_2 sensitivity had disappeared (122). It was restored by addition of carbonic anhydrase to the pipette, suggesting that in this preparation carbonic anhydrase is necessary for the neuron to respond to hypercapnia. In their review Chesler and Kaila (116) evaluated the role of carbonic anhydrase in the activity-dependent changes in extra- and intracellular pH in the nervous system. For example, in crayfish, the use of carbonic anhydrase inhibitors with varying ability to penetrate into the cells has shown that the GABA-induced increase in extracellular pH and decrease in intracellular pH are dependent on the presence of carbonic anhydrase in both compartments (123). They have proposed that carbonic anhydrase is necessary for these activity-dependent pH changes to occur.

Thus, carbonic anhydrase appears to be required for some single neurons to be excited by hypercapnia in vitro and for activity-dependent pH changes to take place at the synaptic level. In contrast, the steady-state ventilatory response to hypercapnic stimulation of central chemoreceptors measured in vivo does not appear to require the presence of this enzyme. It seems that nature has evolved a plethora of pH-sensing mechanisms many of which can alter neuronal excitability at the synaptic or nonsynaptic level. Which one participates in central chemoreception remains to be seen. Could there be more than one?

IV. Other Experimental Approaches to Central Chemosensitive Mechanisms

Three intriguing and novel approaches that have promise in the evaluation of central chemoreceptive mechanisms have been described recently.

A. Cells in Culture

Neubauer (55,118,124) has used two in vitro approaches to study medullary cells possibly involved in chemoreception. Tissue explant cultures, prepared from 1-day-old neonatal rats, with time produce layers of a few cells in thickness. Cells from both the dorsal and ventral medulla have been identified which are excited by decreased pH produced under hypercapnic or under isocapnic conditions via decreased bicarbonate. Neubauer has further studied isolated neurons in dissociated cell cultures again from 1- to 2-day-old rats. These cells can also be excited by hypercapnia, and using an immunocytochemical approach, their content of carbonic anhydrase has been identified. This approach provides single mammalian medullary neurons for study of potential cellular mechanisms for central chemosensitivity. The problem, as for the use of brain slices to approach this question, is to show which cells studied in vitro might actually be involved in ventilatory control.

B. Neonatal Rat Brainstem

Issa and Remmers (125) have used the isolated neonatal rat brainstem preparation (126,127) to evaluate central chemosensitivity. This preparation has a distinct advantage over an in vivo approach; the effects of cerebral blood flow are avoided. For example, in my laboratory we have had great difficulty in producing stable, reproducible ventilatory responses to changes in medullary pH produced by tissue injection of acidic fluid or of CO_2-loaded fluid or by microdialysis of the medulla with CO_2-loaded dialysate. We feel that this is predominantly due to the large blood flow of the medulla, which can quickly remove or dilute the relatively small and transient changes produced by such techniques. Issa and Remmers used a specially designed pipette to ensure delivery of an injection with an increased CO_2. In the absence of medullary blood flow, the changes in tissue P_{CO_2} and their distribution produced by the injection are determined in their preparation only by diffusion and local buffer mechanisms. They found a number of sites within 500 μm of the VLM surface, shown on Figure 7, at which the respiratory frequency was stimulated by the local hypercapnic injection. These sites agree well with some of those reported in other mammalian studies (see Figs. 1, 4). However, recent reports suggest that the core of this preparation actually has quite low tissue oxygen levels (128), and this may limit its utility for studies of central chemoreceptors in other locations.

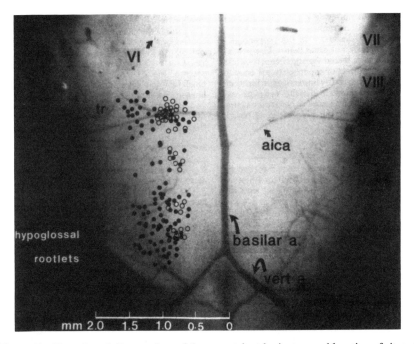

Figure 7 Ventral medullary surface of the neonatal rat brainstem and location of sites at which the injection of CO_2-enriched saline either stimulated (open circles) or had no effect on (solid circles) the frequency of ventilatory output, measured as the activity of the C-3 rootlet. aica, anterior inferior cerebellar artery. (From Ref. 125, with permission of the *Journal of Applied Physiology*.)

C. Invertebrate Models

The terrestrial gastropod *Helix aspersa* exchanges gas via a diffusion lung called the mantle, which has an opening to the environment, the pneumostome. The size of the pneumostome is sensitive to CO_2, dilating in hypercapnia. Erlichman and Leiter (59,59a) have shown that in this model of ventilatory chemoreception the CO_2 is sensed at a specific site within the central nervous system, in the visceral ganglion. In this case they were able to stimulate small groups of neurons focally, using a specially designed CO_2 perfusion pipette, and to observe changes in respiratory control system output, namely the size of the pneumostome. When they blocked synaptic transmission in the brain, they found that the pneumostome response disappeared and concluded that the entire response requires polysynaptic transmission. The use of ammonia to alkalinize the cells and DIDS pretreatment provided evidence of an intracellular site for the pH-sensing mechanism (59). In *Helix pomatia* (60) they were able to repeat these findings and to make intracellular recordings from neurons within these CO_2-sensitive regions. They found neurons that (1) are excited by local CO_2 and (2) when electrically stimulated cause pneumostome opening. Elimination of synaptic input does not affect the response of these neurons to hypercapnia. This appears to be a promising model to examine possible nonsynaptic mechanisms for sensing CO_2 in cells with known respiratory control output. It has a number of advantages. The absence of blood flow minimizes the dispersion of injected substances. Small groups of neurons and single neurons are accessible and can be examined while the investigator simultaneously monitors ventilatory chemosensitive output at the pneumostome.

V. The Intermediate Area: Anatomical Substrates and Function

A. The Intermediate Area

Studies of the ventral medullary surface, which originally described the rostral and caudal chemosensitive areas, also described an area lying between them that was labeled the intermediate area or Schlaefke's area after Marianne Schlaefke (6–9). The approximate topographical location of the IMA was 3–4 mm lateral to the midline and rostral to the rootlets of the 12th cranial nerve (Fig. 1). This medullary region is remarkable in that surface cooling using temperatures that blocked neuronal function but not that of passing axons results in apnea (10,11). The use of a cooling probe at the IMA and, just rostrally, at the level of the caudal aspect of the rostral chemosensitive area also results in apnea and in decreased CO_2 sensitivity (12). Initially the IMA was proposed to be an integrative site not directly involved in chemoreception (129).

The use of 1-nl injections of acetazolamide to probe for central chemoreceptive locations (43; see above) showed that chemoreception is present at regions all along the VLM including the IMA (Fig. 4). However, this does not detract from the significance of the effects of IMA cooling on ventilatory output; it suggests that neurons within this medullary region may have many respiratory control functions. Below I shall review data from recent studies that delineate the probable anatomical substrates of the IMA. I believe that the IMA cooling experiments were affecting respiratory neurons in the retrotrapezoid nucleus, the retrofacial nucleus, the subretrofacial region, the nucleus paragigantocellularis lateralis, and perhaps aspects of the rostral VRG, including the Bötzinger and pre-Bötzinger regions.

B. Retrotrapezoid Nucleus

Initial attempts in my laboratory to ask if neuronal cell bodies, not axons of passage, lying near to the VLM surface were involved in chemoreception involved the use of the excitatory amino acid analog and neurotoxin kainic acid. Kainic acid application to the VLM surface at the level of the rostral aspect of the IMA and caudal aspect of area M (130) and, subsequently, kainic acid microinjection within 800 μm of the VLM surface specifically at one anatomical location (131) results in decreased phrenic activity, often to apnea, and an absent response to hypercapnia. These effects last for many hours. The specific site of greatest effect (Fig. 1) lies just ventral and ventromedial to the facial nucleus, a location that appears to be beneath the topographical border of area M and the rostral aspect of the IMA. Electrolytic as well as chemical lesions produced in decerebrate as well as anesthetized cats have similar effects (132).

Following injection of retrograde tracers into the DRG and VRG, Smith et al. (133) described labeling in this same region indicating the presence of monosynaptic anatomical connections between DRG and VRG and this new location for respiratory neurons. They labeled this site lying ventral and ventromedial to the facial nucleus the retrotrapezoid nucleus. Studies have now shown the presence of respiratory-modulated single units in the retrotrapezoid nucleus of the cat (134) and rat (135) some of which increase their firing rate with hypercapnia (27). The fact that rather small amounts of destruction produced unilaterally at this location can result in long-lasting apnea and absent chemosensitivity suggests an important role for these respiratory neurons.

C. Retrofacial Nucleus and Subretrofacial
Region

Large, bilateral electrolytic and chemical lesions within the retrofacial nucleus of the cat (136) and blockade of the same region by large procaine injections in the rabbit (137) result in decreased phrenic nerve activity, sometimes to apnea, and in decreased sensitivity to hypercapnia. Smaller unilateral lesions in the cat (138) having similar effects were located approximately 5 mm rostral to the obex, 3.0–

4.2 mm lateral to the midline, and within 2.5 mm of the VLM surface, a region that included the subretrofacial region. Respiratory units recorded in the cat (139) and rat (140) retrofacial and subretrofacial region are of a variety of types, some with projections that reach to the VLM surface. In the rat, these respiratory units do not stain for the presence of catecholamines.

D.   More Caudal VRG Sites

At sites 3.0 mm rostral to the obex, 4 mm lateral to the midline, and 1.5 mm deep to the VLM surface, bilateral injections of glutamate receptor antagonists produce apnea in anesthetized cats (141,142) and rats (143,144). McCrimmon et al. (145), using small (0.2–10 nl) injections of excitatory amino acids at low concentrations (e.g., 1–100 mM for glutamate), described a heterogeneity of responses to injections within the VRG. They also found specific locations within the VRG associated with phrenic inhibition and excitation. These were in the dorsomedial and ventrolateral VRG, respectively, lying from the level of the obex to 2.5 mm rostral to the obex.

E.   Nucleus Paragigantocellularis Lateralis (PGCL)

This structure in the cat (149) and rat (150) lies between the nucleus ambiguus and the VLM surface extending rostrally from the lateral reticular nucleus to the region medial to the caudal aspect of the facial nucleus. It is lateral to the inferior olive and medial to the trigeminal nucleus (Fig. 1). It lies essentially just dorsal to the center of the IMA. Anatomical studies of retrograde transport of wheat germ agglutinin-conjugated horseradish peroxidase or Fluoro-Gold injected into the PGCL proper have shown that afferent inputs converge there from a variety of sites, including: spinal cord, caudal lateral medulla, contralateral PGCL, the nucleus of the solitary tract, the A1 area, the lateral parabrachial nucleus, the Kölliker-Fuse nucleus, the periaqueductal gray, and the supraoculomotor nucleus (151). More specific studies have focused on the retrograde transport of injections limited to the rostral pole of PGCL, the juxtafacial portion, which lies lateral to the pyramids and medial to the facial nucleus just dorsal to the VLM surface (152). A different, but also diverse, pattern of afferent sources was described, including: dorsal column nucleii, inferior colliculus, the paralemniscus, paramedian reticular formation, paraolivary reticular formation, retrofacial PGCL, caudal medullary reticular formation, and dorsal periaqueductal gray. These workers propose that the PGCL is the source of convergence of many afferent inputs involved in pain, analgesia, cardiovascular control, respiratory control, exteroceptive sensation, and arousal. A major source of efferents from the PGCL is the locus coeruleus, which itself has widespread inputs to the higher nervous system and is thought to be primarily involved in arousal and vigilance (153).

F. The IMA and Evidence for the Site of Respiratory Rhythmogenesis

Using the in vitro neonatal rat brainstem preparation, Onimaru et al. (146) have reported the presence of neurons, called pre-I neurons, which have an onset of firing just prior to that of the phrenic. These neurons are located within a small region of the VLM just medial to the caudal aspect of the facial nucleus and close to the surface of the VLM. These workers have hypothesized that this is the site of respiratory rhythm generation, at least in this preparation. Smith et al. (147) systematically sectioned the neonatal rat brainstem from rostral and caudal directions to locate the crucial region necessary to maintain a rhythmic respiratory output. They found this region to be in the VLM just caudal to the level of the retrofacial nucleus and labeled it the pre-Bötzinger region. In slices of this region, pacemaker-like activity of neurons has also been identified (147,148). The relative importance and functional roles of neurons in these two locations found in the in vitro neonatal rat brainstem are not quite clear. It is a difficult preparation in that it has a clearly demarked hypoxic central core of tissue with the viable outside ring of medullary tissue being of the order of 800 μm in thickness (128). Yet, it is striking that both these proposed regions for respiratory rhythmogenesis lie approximately within those anatomical regions discussed above as possible substrates for the IMA in adult mammals and that cooling or lesioning at sites within these regions in adult mammals has dramatic effects on ventilatory control.

G. Nonrespiratory Functions in the Regions Dorsal to the IMA

The anatomical studies reviewed above indicate that neurons accessible from the IMA are very important in the control of breathing but are also involved in many physiological functions. While the focus of this chapter is on chemoreception, it is important to realize that neurons important in other physiological control systems lie close to and are, at some sites, probably intermingled with those whose primary purpose is in the control of breathing. For example, the subretrofacial pressor region (154), also called the C-1 region (155), includes a large portion of the PGCL. This pressor region has known efferent projections to the intermediolateral column of the spinal cord, has many catecholamine-containing neurons, and is thought to be important in the origin and maintenance of sympathetic tone to the cardiovascular system. Analogous to the respiratory system, conditional pacemaker neurons thought to be cardiovascular in function have been reported here (156), and the important link between respiratory and cardiovascular sympathetic output apparently occurs here (80,157). In this link, a large portion of cardiovascular sympathetic tone is phasically related to phrenic nerve output. The neurons in this rostral pressor region lie just caudal and dorsal to the retrotrapezoid nucleus, within the region ventral to the retrofacial nucleus.

These neurons are accessible to surface manipulations at the IMA, and such studies often had blood pressure as well as respiratory effects. Hypercapnia increases cardiovascular sympathetic tone and blood pressure (80,157) as well as ventilation. The role of central chemoreceptors in these changes is unknown.

H. Physiological Importance of This Medullary Region

The studies cited above that used surface cooling and lesions to examine the role of the IMA and the more specific anatomical sites beneath the IMA were performed in anesthetized or decerebrate animals. Studies in conscious animals provide further support for the importance of this region. Schlaefke et al. (158,159) coagulated the IMA bilaterally in cats and demonstrated a chronic loss of chemosensitivity in these animals as well as resting hypoventilation. They related these findings to Ondine's curse and to the sudden infant death syndrome and have begun efforts to train the nervous system both in lesioned animals and in human patients to attempt to overcome the chronic deficits in these situations (160). Forster and colleagues (162) have begun studies with cooling of the IMA in conscious goats. They have found severe depression of ventilation at rest, in response to hypercapnia, and in exercise during IMA cooling (H. V. Forster, personal communication). In conscious dogs, Dormer (161) has reported periods of cluster breathing after unilateral lesioning of the retrotrapezoid region by kainic acid injections. In my laboratory we have found it difficult to keep rats alive after lesioning the retrotrapezoid nucleus bilaterally, an experience shared by Dormer (161) and Forster (personal communication) in their experiments. These studies suggest an important role for this region of the VLM in the control of breathing, which is demonstrable in the more physiological conditions of a chronic, conscious animal preparation.

VI. Summary and Conclusions

1. Central chemoreceptors exist and appear to be very important in respiratory control.

2. Central chemoreceptors have widespread brainstem locations. They appear to be located at or just dorsal to the ventral medullary surface at the previously described rostral, caudal, and intermediate areas and at deeper sites near the nucleus tractus solitarius and more rostrally in the vicinity of the locus coeruleus.

3. Focal stimulation of central chemoreceptors at any one of these locations increases whole respiratory control system output. This suggests

that central chemoreceptors are involved in the regulation of regional brainstem pH via a ventilatory feedback loop.

4. The mechanism(s) of CO_2/H^+ sensing appear(s) to involve the enzyme carbonic anhydrase, but the steady-state ventilatory response does not require it.

5. Use of the alpha-stat hypothesis to identify proteins with histidines at potentially functional sites results in a large number of chemoreceptor candidates, including ion channels, ion transport proteins, enzymes, and receptors. Histidine block in vivo inhibits CO_2 sensitivity.

6. There is evidence from a number of approaches to support the hypothesis that intracellular pH is sensed.

7. Elucidation of chemoreceptor mechanism(s) will require both mammalian studies to ensure that the proposed mechanism does in fact affect ventilation and studies in more reduced preparations that allow cellular and molecular approaches.

Acknowledgments

The author is supported by National Institutes of Health Grant RO1 HL 28066. The assistance of Elizabeth Burnside in the search for and evaluation of protein amino acid sequences is gratefully acknowledged.

References

1. Leusen IR. Chemosensitivity of the respiratory center. Influence of CO_2 in the cerebral ventricles on respiration. Am J Physiol 1954; 176:39–44.

2. Pappenheimer JR, Fencl V, Heisey SR, Held D. Role of cerebral fluids in control of respiration as studied in unanesthetized goats. Am J Physiol 1965; 208:436–450.

3. Fencl V, Miller TB, Pappenheimer JR. Studies on the respiratory response to disturbances of acid-base balance, with deductions concerning the ionic composition of cerebral interstitial fluid. Am J Physiol 1966; 210:459–472.

4. Nattie EE. Ventilation during acute HCl infusion in intact and chemodenervated conscious rabbits. Respir Physiol 1983; 54:97–107.

5. Loeschcke HH, Koepchen HP, Gertz KH. Über den einfluss von wasserstoffionenkonzentration und CO_2-druck im liquor cerebrospinalis auf die atmung. Pflüger's Arch 1958; 266:565–585.

6. Mitchell RA, Loeschcke HH, Massion WH, Severinghaus JW. Respiratory responses mediated through superficial chemosensitive areas on the medulla. J Appl Physiol 1963; 18:523–533.

7. Mitchell RA, Loeschcke HH, Severinghaus JL, Richardson BW, Massion WH. Regions of respiratory chemosensitivity on the surface of the medulla. Ann NY Acad Sci 1963; 109:661–681.

8. Loeschcke HH. Central chemosensitivity and the reaction theory. J Physiol (Lond) 1982; 332:1–24.

9. Schlaefke ME, See WR, Loeschcke HH. Ventilatory response to alterations of H+ ion concentration in small areas of the ventral medullary surface. Respir Physiol 1970; 10:198–212.

10. Cherniack NS, von Euler C, Homma I, Kao FF. Graded changes in central chemoreceptor input by local temperature changes on the ventral surface of the medulla. J Physiol (Lond) 1979; 287:191–211.

11. Millhorn DE, Eldridge FL, Waldrop TG. Effects of medullary area I(S) cooling on respiratory response to chemoreceptor inputs. Respir Physiol 1982; 49:23–39.

12. Budzinska K, von Euler C, Kao FF, Pantaleo T, Yamamoto Y. Effects of graded focal cold block in rostral areas of the medulla. Acta Physiol Scand 1985; 124:329–340.

13. Hori T, Roth GI, Yamamoto WS. Respiratory sensitivity of rat brainstem surface to chemical stimuli. J Appl Physiol 1970; 28:721–724.

14. Malcolm JL, Sarelius IH, Sinclair JD. The respiratory role of the ventral surface of the medulla studied in the anesthetized rat. J Physiol (Lond) 1980; 307:503–515.

15. Lipscomb WT, Boyarski LL. Neurophysiological investigations of medullary chemosensitive areas of respiration. Respir Physiol 1972; 16:362–376.

16. Borison HL, Borison R, McCarthy LE. Brain stem penetration by horseradish peroxidase from the cerebrospinal fluid spaces in the cat. Exp Neurol 1980; 69: 271–289.

17. Keeler JR, Shults CW, Chase TN, Helke CJ. The ventral surface of the medulla in the rat: pharmacological and autoradiographical localization of GABA-induced cardiovascular effects. Brain Res 1984; 297:217–224.

18. Nattie EE, Mills JW, Ou LC, St. John WM. Kainic acid on the rostral ventrolateral medulla inhibits phrenic output and CO_2 sensitivity. J Appl Physiol 1988; 65:1525–1534.

19. Yamada KA, McAllen RM, Loewy AD. GABA antagonists applied to the ventral surface of the medulla oblongata block the baroreceptor reflex. Brain Res 1984; 297:175–180.

20. Bledsoe SW, Hornbein TF. Central chemosensors and the regulation of their environment. In: Hornbein TF, ed. Regulation of Breathing, Part I. New York: Marcel Dekker, 1981;347–428.

21. Feldman JL. Neurophysiology of breathing in mammals. In: Mountcastle VB, Bloom FE, Geiger SR, eds. Handbook of Physiology. The Nervous System. Intrinsic Regulatory Systems of the Brain. Bethesda, MD: American Physiological Society, 1986:463–524.

22. Millhorn DE, Eldridge FL. Role of ventrolateral medulla in regulation of respiratory and cardiovascular systems. J Appl Physiol 1986; 61:1249–1263.

23. Bruce EN, Cherniack NS. Central chemoreceptors (brief review). J Appl Physiol 1987; 62:389–402.

24. Nattie EE. Central respiratory chemoreceptors. In: Haddad GG, Farber JP, eds.

Developmental Neurobiology of Breathing. New York: Marcel Dekker, 1991: 341–371.

25. Cohen MI. Discharge patterns of brainstem respiratory neurons in relation to carbon dioxide tension. J Neurophysiol 1968; 31:142–165.

26. St John WM, Wang SC. Response of medullary respiratory neurons to hypercapnia and isocapnic hypoxia. J Appl Physiol 1977; 43:812–821.

27. Nattie EE, Fung ML, Li A, St John WM. Responses of respiratory modulated and tonic units in the retrotrapezoid nucleus to CO_2. Respir Physiol 1993; 94:35–50.

28. Pokorski M. Neurophysiological studies on central chemosensor in medullary areas. Am J Physiol 1976; 230:1288–1295.

29. Euler C von, Soderberg U. Medullary chemosensitive receptors. J Physiol (Lond) 1952; 118:545–554.

30. Mitchell RA, and Hebert DA. The effect of carbon dioxide on the membrane potential of medullary respiratory neurons. Brain Res 1974; 75:345–349.

31. Arita H, Kogo N, Ichikawa K. Rapid and transient excitation of respiration mediated by central chemoreceptor. J Appl Physiol 1988; 64:1369–1375.

32. Arita H, Kogo N, Ichikawa K. Locations of medullary neurons with non-phasic discharges excited by stimulation of central and/or peripheral chemoreceptors and by activation of nociceptors in cat. Brain Res 1988; 442:1–10.

33. Kogo N, Arita H. In vivo study on medullary H^+-sensitive neurons. J Appl Physiol 1990; 69:1408–1412.

34. Richerson GB. Electrophysiologic effects of changes in P_{CO_2} on rat medullary neurons in vitro. Soc Neurosci Abstr 1992; 18:828.

35. Fukuda Y, Honda Y. pH-sensitive cells at ventro-lateral surface of rat medulla oblongata. Nature 1975; 256:317–318.

36. Fukuda Y, Honda Y. pH sensitivity of cells located at the ventrolateral surface of the cat medulla oblongata in vitro. Pflüger's Arch 1976; 364:243–247.

37. Fukuda Y, Loeschcke HH. Effect of H^+ on spontaneous neuronal activity in the surface layer of the rat medulla oblongata in vitro. Pflüger's Arch 1977; 371:125–134.

38. Miles R. Does low pH stimulate central chemoreceptors located near the ventral medullary surface? Brain Res 1983; 271:349–353.

39. Jarolimek W, Misgeld U, Lux HD. Neurons sensitive to pH in slices of the rat ventral medulla oblongata. Pflüger's Arch 1990; 416:247–253.

40. Dean JB, Lawing WL, Millhorn DE. CO_2 decreases membrane conductance and depolarizes neurons in the nucleus tractus solitarii. Exp Brain Res 1989; 76:656–661.

41. Dean JB, Bayliss DA, Erickson JT, Lawing WL, Millhorn DE. Depolarization and stimulation of neurons in nucleus tractus solitarii by carbon dioxide does not require chemical synaptic input. Neuroscience 1990; 36:207–216.

42. Coates EL, Li A, Nattie EE. Acetazolamide on the ventral medulla of the cat increases phrenic output and delays the ventilatory response to CO_2. J Physiol (Lond) 1991; 441:433–451.

43. Coates EL, Li A, Nattie EE. Widespread sites of brainstem ventilatory chemoreceptors. J Appl Physiol 1993; 75:5–14.

44. Dillon GH, Waldrop TG. Intracellular and extracellular recordings of posterior hypothalamic neurons in vitro: response to hypoxia and hypercapnia. Soc Neurosci Abstr 1991; 17:200.

45. Arita H, Ichikawa K, Kuwana S, Kogo N. Possible locations of pH-dependent central chemoreceptors: intramedullary regions with acidic shift of extracellular fluid pH during hypercapnia. Brain Res 1989; 485:285–293.

46. Sato M, Severinghaus JW, Basbaum A. Medullary CO_2 chemoreceptor neuron identification by c-*fos* immunocytochemistry. J Appl Physiol 1992; 73:96–100.

47. Haxhiu MA, Erokwu B, Prabhakar NR, Cherniack NS, Strohl KP. Locus coeruleus neurons express c-*fos* immunoreactivity upon stimulation of central chemosensory system. Soc Neurosci Abstr 1992; 18:828.

48. Ciriello J, Rohlicek CV, Polosa C. 2-Deoxyglucose uptake in the central nervous system during systemic hypercapnia in the peripherally chemodenervated rat. Exp Neurol 1985; 88:673–687.

49. Carpenter DO, Hubbard JH, Humphrey DR, Thompson HK, Marshall WH. Carbon dioxide effects on nerve cell function. In: Nahas G, Schaefer KE, eds. Carbon Dioxide and Metabolic Regulations. New York: Springer-Verlag, 1974:49–62.

50. Eldridge FL, Kiley JP, Millhorn DE. Respiratory responses to medullary hydrogen ion changes in cats: different effects of respiratory and metabolic acidoses. J Physiol (Lond) 1985; 358:285–297.

51. Teppema LJ, Barts PWJA, Folgering H Th, Evers JAM. Effects of respiratory and (isocapnic) metabolic acid-base disturbances on medullary extracellular fluid pH and ventilation in cats. Respir Physiol 1983; 53:379–395.

52. Shams H. Differential effects of CO_2 and H+ as central stimuli of respiration in the cat. J Appl Physiol 1985; 58:357–364.

53. Fukuda Y. Difference between actions of high PCO_2 and low [HCO_3] on neurons in the rat medullary chemosensitive areas in vitro. Pflüger's Arch 1983; 398:324–330.

54. Harada Y, Kuno M, Wang YZ. Differential effects of carbon dioxide and pH on central chemoreceptors in the rat in vitro. J Physiol (Lond) 1985; 368:679–693.

55. Neubauer JA, Gonsalves SF, Chou W, Geller HM, Edelman NH. Chemosensitivity of medullary neurons in explant tissue cultures. Neuroscience 1991; 45:701–708.

56. Hitzig BM, Jackson DC. Central chemical control of ventilation in the unanesthetized turtle. Am J Physiol 1978; 235:R257–R264.

57. Smatresk NJ, Smits AW. Effects of central and peripheral chemoreceptor stimulation on ventilation in the marine toad, *Bufo marinus*. Respir Physiol 1991; 83:223–238.

58. Branco LGS, Glass ML, Hoffman A. Central chemoreceptor drive to breathing in unanesthetized toads, *Bufo paracnemis*. Respir Physiol 1991; 87:195–204.

59. Erlichman JS, Leiter JC. Central chemoreceptor stimulus in the terrestrial pulmonate snail, *Helix aspersa*. Respir Physiol 1994; 95:209–226.

59a. Erlichman JS, Leiter JC. CO_2 reception in the pulmonate snail, *Helix aspersa*. Respir Physiol 1993; 93:347–363.

60. Erlichman JS, Leiter JC. CO_2 chemoreceptor cells in the pulmonate snail, *Helix pomatia*. Exp Biol Abstr 1993; 7(3):A458.

61. Hitzig BM. Temperature induced changes in turtle CSF pH and central chemical control of ventilation. Respir Physiol 1982; 49:205–222.

62. Reeves RB. An imidazole alphastat hypothesis for vertebrate acid-base regulation: tissue carbon dioxide content and body temperature in bullfrogs. Respir Physiol 1972; 14:219–236.

63. Reeves RB. The interaction of body temperature and acid-base balance in ectothermic vertebrates. Annu Rev Physiol 1977; 39:559–586.

64. Burton RF. The role of imidazole ionization in the control of breathing. Comp Biochem Physiol A Comp Physiol 1986; 83:333–336.

65. Cameron JN. Acid-base homeostasis: past and present perspectives. Physiol Zool 1989; 62:845–865.

66. Hochachka PW, Guppy M. Metabolic Arrest and the Control of Time. Cambridge, MA: Harvard University Press, 1987:63–64, 75–76.

67. Nattie EE. The alphastat hypothesis in respiratory control and acid-base balance (brief review). J Appl Physiol 1990; 69:1201–1207.

68. Kiley JP, Eldridge FL, Millhorn DE. The effect of hypothermia on central neural control of respiration. Respir Physiol 1984; 58:295–312.

69. Nattie EE. Intracisternal diethylpyrocarbonate inhibits central chemosensitivity in conscious rabbits. Respir Physiol 1986; 64:1161–176.

70. Nattie EE. Diethylpyrocarbonate (an imidazole binding substance) inhibits rostral VLM CO_2 sensitivity. J Appl Physiol 1986; 61:843–850.

71. Nattie EE. Diethyl pyrocarbonate inhibits rostral ventrolateral medullary H+ sensitivity. J Appl Physiol 1988; 64:1600–1609.

72. Christensen BN, Hida E. Protonation of histidine groups inhibits gating of the quisqualate/kainate channel protein in isolated catfish cone horizontal cells. Neuron 1990; 5:471–478.

73. Spalding BC, Taber P, Swift JG, Horowicz P. Response of chloride efflux from skeletal muscle of *Rana pipiens* to changes of temperature and membrane potential and diethylpyrocarbonate treatment. J Memb Biol 1991; 123:223–233.

74. Bonner TI, Buckley NJ, Young AC, Brann MR. Identification of a family of muscarinic acetylcholine receptor genes. Science 1987; 237:527–532.

75. Hollman M, O'Shea-Greenfield A, Rogers SW, Heineman S. Cloning by functional expression of a member of the glutamate receptor family. Nature 1989; 342:643–648.

76. Traynelis SF, Cull-Candy SG. Proton inhibition of N-methyl-D-aspartate receptor in cerebellar neurons. Nature 1990; 345:347–350.

77. Viklicky Jr L, Vlachová V, Krusek J. The effect of external pH changes on responses to excitatory amino acids in mouse hippocampal neurones. J Physiol (Lond) 1990; 430:497–517.

78. Tang C, Dichter M, Morad M. Modulation of the N-methyl-D-aspartate channel by extracellular H^+. Proc Natl Acad Sci USA 1990; 87:6445–6449.

79. McAllen RM. Location of neurons with cardiovascular and respiratory function, at the ventral surface of the cat's medulla. Neuroscience 1986; 18:43–49.

80. Nattie EE, Gdovin M, Li A. Retrotrapezoid nucleus glutamate receptors: control of CO_2 sensitive phrenic and sympathetic output. J Appl Physiol 1993; 74:2958–2968.

81. Anthony BL, Aronstam RS. Effect of pH on muscarinic acetylcholine receptors from rat brainstem. J Neurochem 1986; 46:556–561.

82. Ehlert FJ, Delen FM. Influence of pH on the binding of scopolamine to muscarinic receptors in the corpus striatum and heart of rats. Mol Pharm 1990; 38:143–147.
83. Burton MD, Johnson DC, Kazemi H. CSF acidosis augments ventilation through cholinergic mechanisms. J Appl Physiol 1989; 66:2565–2572.
84. Gesell R, Hansen ET. Anticholinesterase activity of acid as a biological instrument of nervous integration. Am J Physiol 1945; 144:126–163.
85. Dev NB, Loeschcke HH. A cholinergic mechanism involved in the respiratory chemosensitivity of the medulla oblongata in the cat. Pflüger's Arch 1979; 379: 29–36.
86. Nattie EE, Wood J, Mega A, Goritski W. Rostral ventrolateral medulla muscarinic receptor involvement in central ventilatory chemosensitivity. J Appl Physiol 1989; 66:1462–1470.
87. Nattie EE, Li A. Ventral medulla sites of muscarinic receptor subtypes involved in cardiorespiratory control. J Appl Physiol 1990; 69:33–41.
88. Schofield PR, Darlison MG, Fujita N, Burt DR, Stephenson FA, Rodriguez H, Rhee LM, Ramachandran J, Reale V, Glencorse TA, Seeburg PH, Barnard EA. Sequence and functional expression of the $GABA_A$ receptor shows a ligand-gated receptor super-family. Nature 1987; 328:221–227.
89. Takeuchi A, Takeuchi N. Anion permeability of the inhibitory post-synaptic membrane of the crayfish neuromuscular junction. J Physiol (Lond) 1967; 191:575–590.
90. Pasternack M, Bountra C, Voipio J, Kaila K. Dependence of GABA-gated Cl^- conductance on extracellular and intracellular pH in crayfish muscle fibers. Acta Physiol Scand 1989; 136(suppl 582):78.
91. Gallagher JP, Nakamura J, Shinnick-Gallagher P. The effects of temperature, pH and Cl^- pump inhibitors on GABA responses recorded from cat dorsal root ganglia. Brain Res 1983; 267:249–259.
92. Hedner J, Hedner T, Wessberg P, Jonason J. An analysis of the mechanism by which gamma-aminobutyric acid depresses ventilation in the rat. J Appl Physiol 1984; 56: 849–856.
93. Roskoski R. Choline acetyltransferase and acetylcholinesterase: evidence for essential histidyl residues. Biochemistry 1974; 13:5141–5144.
94. Klimek K, Nattie EE. (unpublished observations).
95. Shull GE, Greeb J, Lingrel JB. Molecular cloning of three distinct forms of the Na^+,K^+-ATPase alpha-subunit from rat brain. Biochemistry 1986; 25:8125–8132.
96. Eaton DC, Hamilton KL, Johnson KE. Intracellular acidosis blocks the basolateral Na-K pump in rabbit urinary bladder. Am J Physiol 1984; 247 (Renal Fluid Electrolyte Physiol 16):F946–F954.
97. Park YS, Hong SK. Properties of toad skin Na-K-ATPase with special reference to effects of temperature. Am J Physiol 1976; 231:1356–1363.
98. Tolkovsky AM, Richards CD. Na^+/H^+ exchange is the major mechanism of pH regulation in cultured sympathetic neurons measured in single cell bodies and neurites using a fluorescent pH indicator. Neuroscience 1987; 22:1093–1102.
99. Sardet M, Franchi A, Pouyssegur J. Molecular cloning, primary structure, and expression of the human growth factor activatable Na^+/H^+ antiporter. Cell 1989; 56:271–280.

100. Grillo FG, Aronson PA. Inactivation of the renal microvillus membrane Na^+-H^+ exchange by histidine-specific reagents. J Biol Chem 1986; 261:1120–1125.

101. Nattie EE, Giddings B. Effects of amiloride and diethylpyrocarbonate on CSF HCO_3 and ventilation in hypercapnia. J Appl Physiol 1988; 65:242–248.

102. Kopita RR, Lodish HF. Primary structure and transmembrane orientation of the murine anion exchange protein. Nature 1988; 316:234–238.

103. Nattie EE, Adams JM. DIDS decreases CSF HCO_3 and increases breathing in response to CO_2 in awake rabbits. J Appl Physiol 1988; 64:397–403.

104. Noda M, Ikeda T, Kanyano T, Suzuki H, Takashima H, Takahashi H, Kuno M, Numa S. Expression of functional sodium channels from cloned cDNA. Nature 1986; 322:826–828.

105. Begenisich T, Danko M. Hydrogen ion block of the sodium pore in squid giant axons. J Gen Physiol 1983; 82:599–618.

106. Hartman HA, Kirsch GE, Drewe JA, Taglialatela M, Joho RH, Brown AM. Exchange of conduction pathways between two related K^+ channels. Science 1989; 251:942–944.

107. Moody Jr W. Effects of intracellular H^+ on the electrical properties of excitable cells. Annu Rev Neurosci 1984; 7:257–278.

108. Wanke E, Carbone E, Teste PL. K^+ conductance modified by a titratable group accessible to protons from the intracellular side of the squid axon membrane. J Biophys Soc 1979; 26:319–324.

109. Tanaba T, Takeshima H, Mikamia A, Flockerzi V, Takahashi H, Kangawa K, Kojima M, Matsuo H, Hirose T, Numa S. Primary structure of the receptor for calcium channel blockers from skeletal muscle. Nature 1987; 328:315–318.

110. Prod'hom B, Pietrobon D, Hess P. Interactions of protons with single open L-type calcium channels. J Gen Physiol 1989; 94:23–42.

111. Kaibara M, Kameyama M. Inhibition of the calcium channel by intracellular protons in single ventricular myocytes of guinea pig. J Physiol (Lond) 1988; 403:621–640.

112. Jentsch TJ, Steinmeyer K, Schwarz G. Primary structure of *Torpedo marmorata* chloride channel isolated by expression cloning in *Xenopus* oocytes. Nature 1990; 348:510–514.

113. Georgiu P, House CR, McNiven AI, Yoshida S. On the mechanism of a pH-induced rise in membrane potassium conductance in hamster eggs. J Physiol (Lond) 1988; 402:121–138.

114. Oberleithner H, Kersting U, Hunter M. Cytoplasmic pH determines K^+ conductance in fused renal epithelial cells. Proc Natl Acad Sci USA 1988; 85:8345–8349.

115. Rocher A, Obeso A, Gonsalez C, Herreros B. Ionic mechanisms for the transduction of acidic stimuli in rabbit carotid body glomus cells. J Physiol (Lond) 1991; 433:533–548.

116. Chesler M, Kaila K. Modulation of pH by neuronal activity. Trends Neurosci 1992; 15:396–402.

117. Ridderstråle, Y, Hanson M. Histochemical study of the distribution of carbonic anhydrase in the cat brain. Acta Physiol Scand 1985; 124:557–564.

118. Neubauer J. Carbonic anhydrase and sensory function in the central nervous system.

In: Dodgson SJ, ed. The Carbonic Anhydrases: Cellular Physiology and Molecular Genetics. New York: Plenum Press, 1991.

119. Teppema LJ, Rochette F, Demedts M. Effects of acetazolamide on medullary extracellular pH and P_{CO_2} and on ventilation in peripherally chemodenervated cats. Pflüger's Arch 1990; 415:519–525.

120. Hanson MA, Nye PCG, Torrance RW. The location of carbonic anhydrase in relation to the blood-brain barrier at the medullary chemoreceptors of the cat. J Physiol (Lond) 1981; 320:113–125.

121. Toyjimia H, Kuriyama T, Fukuda Y. Delayed ventilatory response to CO_2 after carbonic anhydrase inhibition with acetazolamide administration in the anesthetized rat. Jpn J Physiol 1988; 38:55–65.

122. Dean JB. Brainstem whole-cell responses to CO_2 after intracellular dialysis with carbonic anhydrase II. Exp Biol Abstr 1993; 7(3):A403.

123. Kaila K, Saarikoski J, Voipio J. Mechanism of action of GABA on intracellular pH and on surface pH in crayfish muscle fibers. J Physiol (Lond) 1990; 427:241–260.

124. Neubauer JA, Chou W, Gonsalves S, Sterbenz G, Geller HM, Edelman NH. Chemosensitivity of medullary neurons in tissue cultures. Adv Biosci 1991; 79: 19–25.

125. Issa FG, Remmers JE. Identification of a subsurface area in the ventral medulla sensitive to local changes in P_{CO_2}. J Appl Physiol 1992; 72:439–446.

126. Onimaru H, Homma I. Respiratory rhythm generator neurons in medulla of brain stem–spinal cord preparation from newborn rat. Brain Res 1987; 403:380–384.

127. Smith JC, Feldman JL. In-vitro brain stem-spinal cord preparations for study of motor systems for mammalian respiration and locomotion. J Neurosci Meth 1987; 21:321–333.

128. Brockhaus J, Ballanyi K, Smith JC, Richter DW. Microenvironment of respiratory neurons in the in vitro brainstem-spinal cord of neonatal rats. J Physiol (Lond) 1993; 462:421–445.

129. Schlaefke ME. Central chemosensitivity: a respiratory drive. Rev Physiol Biochem Pharm 1981; 90:171–172.

130. Nattie EE, Mills JW, Ou LC, St. John WM. Kainic acid on the rostral ventrolateral medulla inhibits phrenic output and CO_2 sensitivity. J Appl Physiol 1988; 65:1525–1534.

131. Nattie EE, Li A. Fluorescence location of RVLM kainate microinjections that alter the control of breathing. J Appl Physiol 1990; 68:1157–1166.

132. Nattie EE, Li A, St. John WM. Lesions in retrotrapezoid nucleus decrease ventilatory output in anesthetized or decerebrate cats. J Appl Physiol 1991; 71:1364–1375.

133. Smith JC, Morrison DE, Ellenberger HH, Otto MR, Feldman JL. Brainstem projections to the major respiratory neuron populations in the medulla of the cat. J Comp Neurol 1989; 281:69–96.

134. Connelly CA, Ellenberger HH, Feldman JL. Respiratory activity in retrotrapezoid nucleus in cat. Am J Physiol (Lung Cell Mol Physiol) 1990; 258:L33–L44.

135. Pearce RA, Stornetta RL, Guyenet PG. Retrotrapezoid nucleus in the rat. Neurosci Lett 1989; 101:138–142.

136. St. John WM, Hwang Q, Nattie EE, Zhou D. Functions of the retrofacial nucleus in chemosensitivity and ventilatory neurogenesis. Respir Physiol 1989; 76:159–172.

137. Zhang F, Wu Z, Li Y. Effect of blocking medial area of nucleus retrofacialis on respiratory rhythm. Respir Physiol 1991; 85:73–81.

138. Nattie EE, Blanchford C, Li A. Retrofacial lesions: effects on CO_2-sensitive phrenic and sympathetic activity. J Appl Physiol 1992; 73:1317–1325.

139. Bianchi AL, Grélot L, Iscoe S, Remmers JE. Electrophysiological properties of rostral medullary respiratory neurones in the cat: an intracellular study. J Physiol (Lond) 1988; 407:293–310.

140. Pilowsky PM, Jiang C, Lipski J. An intracellular study of respiratory neurons in the rostral ventrolateral medulla of the rat and their relationship to catecholamine-containing neurons. J Comp Neurol 1990; 301:604–617.

141. Abrahams TP, Hornby PJ, Walton DP, Taveira DaSilva AM, Gillis RA. An excitatory amino acid(s) in the ventrolateral medulla is (are) required for breathing to occur in the anesthetized cat. J Exp Pharm Ther 1991; 259:1388–1395.

142. McManigle JE, Panico WH, Pineo S, Da Silva AMT, Dretchen KL, Gillis RA. Evidence for a role for tonic release of an excitatory amino acid at the caudal-subretrofacial area in the control of ventilation. Soc Neurosci Abstr 1991; 17:201.

143. Jung R, Bruce EN, Katona PG. Cardiorespiratory responses to glutaminergic antagonists in the caudal ventrolateral medulla of rats. Brain Res 1991; 564: 286–295.

144. Dillon GH, Welsh DE, Waldrop TG. Modulation of respiratory reflexes by an excitatory amino acid mechanism in the ventrolateral medulla. Respir Physiol 1991; 85:55–72.

145. McCrimmon DR, Feldman JL, Speck DF. Respiratory motoneuron activity is altered by injections of picomoles of glutamate into cat brainstem. J Neurosci 1986; 6:2384–2392.

146. Onimaru H, Arata A, Homma I. Localization of respiratory rhythm-generating neurons in the medulla of brainstem-spinal cord preparations from newborn rats. Neurosci Lett 1987; 78:151–155.

147. Smith JC, Ellenberger HH, Ballanyi K, Richter DW, Feldman JL. Pre-Bötzinger complex: a brainstem region that may generate respiratory rhythm in mammals. Science 1991; 254:726–729.

148. Smith JC, Ballanyi K, Richter DW. Whole-cell patch-clamp recording from respiratory neurons in mammalian brainstem in vitro. Neurosci Lett 1992; 134:153–156.

149. Taber E. The cytoarchitecture of the brain stem of the cat. I. Brain stem nuclei. J Comp Neurol 1961; 116:27–70.

150. Andrezik JA, Chan-Palay V. The nucleus paragigantocellularis (PGCL): definition and afferents. Anat Rec 1977; 187:524–525.

151. Van Bockstaele EJ, Pieribone VA, Aston-Jones G. Diverse afferents converge on the nucleus paragigantocellularis in the rat ventrolateral medulla: retrograde and anterograde tracing studies. J Comp Neurol 1989; 290:561–584.

152. Van Bockstaele EJ, Akaoka H, Aston-Jones G. Brainstem afferents to the rostral (juxtafacial) nucleus paragigantocellularis: integration of exteroceptive and interoceptive sensory inputs in the ventral tegmentum. Brain Res 1993; 603:1–18.

153. Aston-Jones G, Ennis VA, Pieribone VA, Nickell WT, Shipley MT. The brain nucleus locus coeruleus: restricted afferent control of a broad efferent network. Science 1986; 234:734–737.

154. Dampney R. The subretrofacial nucleus: its pivotal role in cardiovascular regulation. News Physiol Sci 1990; 5:63–66.

155. Reis DJ, Ross C, Granata AR, Ruggiero DA. Role of C1 area of rostroventrolateral medulla in cardiovascular control. In: Buckley JP, Ferrario CM, eds. Brain Peptides and Catecholamines in Cardiovascular Regulation. New York: Raven Press, 1987:1–14.

156. Sun M-K, Young BS, Hackett JT, Guyenet PG. Reticulospinal pacemaker neurons of the rat rostral ventrolateral medulla with putative sympathoexcitatory function: an intracellular study "in vitro." Brain Res 1988; 442:229–239.

157. Guyenet P, Darnall RA, Riley TA. Rostral ventrolateral medulla and sympathorespiratory integration in the rat. Am J Physiol 1990; 259 (Regul Integrat Comp Physiol 28):R1063–R1074.

158. Schlaefke ME. Elimination of central chemosensitivity by coagulation of a bilateral area on the ventral medullary surface in awake cats. Pflüger's Arch 1979; 379: 231–241.

159. Burghardt F, Schlaefke ME. Loss of central chemosensitivity: an animal model to overcome respiratory insufficiency. J Auton Nerv Syst 1986; Suppl:105–109.

160. Schlaefke ME. Central chemosensitivity. Adv Biosci 1991; 79:27–33.

161. Dormer KJ, Bedford TG. Cardiovascular control by the rostral ventrolateral medulla in the conscious dog. In: Ciriello J, Caverson MM, Polosa E, eds. The Central Neural Organization of Cardiovascular Control, Progress Brain Research 81. Amsterdam: Elsevier, 1981:265–277.

162. Pan LG, Forster HV, Erickson BK, Lowry T. Effect of transient cooling of the ventral surface of the medulla (VLM) in awake goats. FASEB J 1991; 5:A665.

163. Berman AL. The Brainstem of the Cat. Madison: University of Wisconsin Press, 1968.

11

Role of Airway Afferents on Upper Airway Muscle Activity

OOMMEN P. MATHEW and TAPAN K. GHOSH

East Carolina University School of Medicine
Greenville, North Carolina

I. Introduction

The nose, the pharynx, the larynx, and the extrathoracic portion of the trachea constitute the upper airway, a vital part of the respiratory tract. Recognition of clinical problems such as obstructive sleep apnea has generated an immense interest in the patency of the upper airway in recent years. Activity of upper airway muscles plays a critical role in maintaining upper airway patency. The role of airway afferents in regulating upper airway muscle activity is the focus of this chapter.

II. Muscles of the Upper Airway

Dynamic changes in upper airway size and resistance occur throughout the respiratory cycle. Over 20 pairs of muscles located around the upper airway can potentially influence its size, shape, and function. Some are active during eupnea; others are recruited when respiratory drive increases. However, only a few muscles have been well studied; the role of others is far from clear. This is especially true of the interaction among the various upper airway muscles, which is complex and

511

remains largely speculative. In addition to their respiratory role, most upper airway muscles participate in nonrespiratory tasks such as mastication, deglutition, vocalization, olfaction, and airway protection.

Based on their location, upper airway muscles can be divided into nasal, palatal, pharyngeal, laryngeal, and cervical. Most of the muscle groups can modify airflow resistance through valve-like mechanisms attributable to their strategic locations. Alae nasi is innervated by the buccal branch of the facial nerve. Increase in its activity decreases the nasal resistance by as much as 29% (1). Palatal muscles are critical in determining the route of breathing. Contraction of tensor veli palatini, levator veli palatini, and musculus uvulae favors oral breathing, whereas contraction of palatopharyngeal and palatoglossal muscles favors nasal breathing. All the palatal muscles, except tensor veli palatini, are innervated by the vagus nerve through the pharyngeal plexus. The mandibular branch of the trigeminal nerve supplies tensor veli palatini.

The pharyngeal dilators are located on the lateral and ventral aspects of the pharynx. The genioglossus, an extrinsic muscle of the tongue, is the most extensively studied pharyngeal dilator. All tongue muscles with the exception of palatoglossus are innervated by the hypoglossal nerve. The pharyngeal constrictors, superior, middle, and inferior, are supplied by the pharyngeal plexus. The role of the pharyngeal constrictors during respiration is not entirely clear. A number of upper airway muscles are attached to the hyoid bone. Interaction among the supra- and infrahyoid muscles is particularly important in stabilizing this portion of the pharyngeal airway.

The posterior cricoarytenoid, lateral cricoarytenoid, transverse arytenoid, and thyroarytenoid muscles are innervated by the recurrent laryngeal nerve, whereas the cricothyroid muscle is supplied by the external branch of the superior laryngeal nerve (SLN). The posterior cricoarytenoid is the principal laryngeal abductor.

III. Upper Airway Afferents

A. Nose

The nasal cavities lie within a bony and cartilaginous skeleton and are separated by a midline septum communicating externally by means of the nostrils and posteriorly with the nasopharynx by means of the choanae. Mucous membrane of the nasal cavity is innervated by the trigeminal nerve through branches of the anterior ethmoidal nerve and the maxillary nerve. Olfaction has been the focus of research on nasal afferents; until recently, very few studies have investigated the respiratory role of nasal afferents. The main respiratory function of the upper airway that most standard textbooks discuss is inspiratory air modification (humidification, filtration, and temperature control).

No structurally differentiated sensory end-organs have been identified in the nose; nonmyelinated endings in and under the epithelium are presumed to mediate the nasal reflexes. Nasal receptors sensing airflow was first suggested by Glebovski:i and Baev (2). Tsubone (3) recently confirmed the presence of nasal flow receptors by single-fiber recording of the anterior ethmoidal nerve in rats. As for laryngeal flow receptors, the stimulus for these endings appears to be a decrease in temperature (3). Although it is difficult to envision pressure receptors in the nose, a cavity surrounded by bone, endings responding to transmural pressure changes have been identified in the ethmoidal nerve of the rat; most of these nasal pressure receptors respond to negative transmural pressure changes (4). Recently, Wallois et al. (5) investigated the respiratory-related afferent activities in three branches of trigeminal nerve (anterior ethmoidal nerve, posterior nasal nerve, and infraorbital nerve). Nearly two-thirds of the receptors exhibiting respiratory modulation during nasal breathing were classified as nondrive receptors and the remaining as drive receptors. The stimulus for the nondrive receptors was flow related; however, only two endings responding to decreases in temperature were identified. Hence, transmural pressure changes appear to be the primary stimulus for the nondrive receptors. Some of the trigeminal nerve endings are also stimulated by irritants (like cigarette smoke, ammonia); these endings are presumably responsible for the reflexes elicited by nasal irritants (6,7).

B. Pharynx

The pharyngeal airway lies in front of the cervical vertebral column and prevertebral fascia and consists of the nasopharynx, oropharynx, and laryngopharynx. Although the reflex effects originating from the pharynx have been fairly well studied, relatively little is known of the role of pharyngeal receptors in respiratory control. The glossopharyngeal nerve, through the pharyngeal branch, provides sensory innervation to the mucous membrane below the nasopharynx, whereas the maxillary nerve innervates the nasopharynx.

Nail and co-workers showed that glossopharyngeal nerve contains afferents that adapt rapidly to mechanical deformation of the pharyngeal mucosa; these endings are also excited by chemical irritants (8–10). Hwang et al. (11) documented the presence of slowly adapting receptors in the glossopharyngeal nerve that respond to transmural pressure changes in the upper airway. The role of these endings in respiratory control remains unclear.

C. Larynx

The laryngeal afferents have been extensively studied. The internal branch of the SLN provides the primary afferent innervation of the larynx (for review see 12). The external branch of the SLN and the recurrent laryngeal nerve (RLN) carry some laryngeal afferents (13), although these nerves contain primarily efferent fibers. Laryngeal receptors have been studied in several species, including the rabbit (14–16), cat (17,18), dog (19,20), guinea pig (21), and rat (22). Histologically, laryngeal endings can be classified as mucosal, articular (joint), and muscular. Earlier studies evaluating the behavior of laryngeal afferents with an open larynx have documented the responses to gentle probing, topically applied anesthetics, and selective manipulation of the articulation or stretching of the muscles so that these endings can be correlated with the histological classification (23). Recent studies, on the other hand, have focused on functional classification of laryngeal endings. Whole-nerve recording of the SLN reveals a clear respiratory modulation (Figs. 1 and 2). Responses of SLN afferents to changes in airflow, transmural pressure, and active and passive laryngeal motion (drive) were assessed by single-fiber recording. On the basis of their response to the above stimuli, respiratory-modulated laryngeal endings are classified into flow, pressure, and drive receptors (Fig. 3; 19). Subsequent studies have shown that flow receptors respond to decreases in laryngeal temperature (24). These flow/cold receptors are located superficially since lidocaine blocks their discharge within a few seconds (25). Unlike laryngeal cold receptors, pressure and drive receptors are mechanosensitive. Some of these are superficial, stimulated with gentle probing of the mucosa, and blocked rather promptly by topically applied anesthetics such as lidocaine; others are located more deeply, responding only to firm laryngeal pressure, and are either unaffected by lidocaine or blocked after a long delay (26). Earlier studies have shown that water and CO_2 can alter the discharge pattern of some laryngeal receptors (27–29). Recent studies by Anderson et al. (30,31) in spontaneously breathing dogs show that some of the endings responding to water

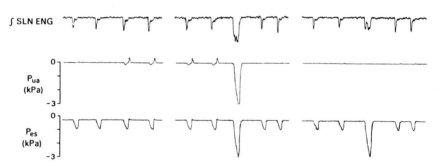

Figure 1   Effect of diversion of breathing and airway occlusion on the activity of the superior laryngeal nerve. Traces are integrated superior laryngeal neurogram, upper airway pressure, and esophageal pressure. Pressure changes in the upper airway are seen during upper airway breathing and upper airway occlusion. Note that maximal increase in inspiratory activity of the SLN occurs during upper airway occlusion. (Modified from Ref. 12, p. 210, by courtesy of Marcel Dekker, Inc.)

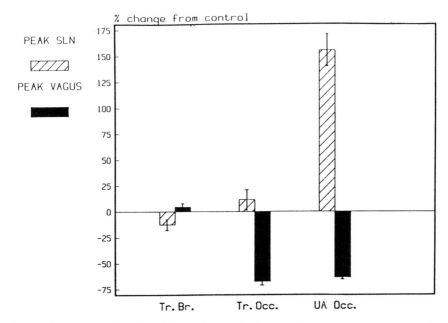

Figure 2 Changes in peak activity of the superior laryngeal and vagus nerves expressed as percent change from upper airway breathing. Note that the greatest increase in SLN activity occurs during upper airway occlusion, whereas a marked decrease in vagal activity is seen during airway occlusions. (Reprinted from Ref. 20.)

and CO_2 are indeed respiratory modulated and respond to transmural pressure changes. Other investigators have confirmed the CO_2 sensitivity of laryngeal pressure receptors in paralyzed animal models (32). Recently we have been able to demonstrate that intralaryngeal CO_2 can alter the pressure sensitivity of laryngeal endings (33). All these findings indicate that CO_2-sensitive laryngeal receptors are not specialized chemoreceptors.

D. Developmental Changes

Data on upper airway afferents during development are sparse. Morphological studies performed on the SLN in newborn kittens show that only 22% of the fibers (both afferent and efferent) are myelinated at birth; this increases to 48% at 2 months (34). In contrast, 90% of fibers are myelinated in adult cats (35). All the respiratory-modulated SLN afferents (cold, pressure, drive) in adult dogs have myelinated fibers (12). The myelinated endings constitute the majority of the fibers in the SLN of adult dogs (36). A similar morphological change has also been observed in the vagus nerve of the kitten (37). Studies in dogs show that

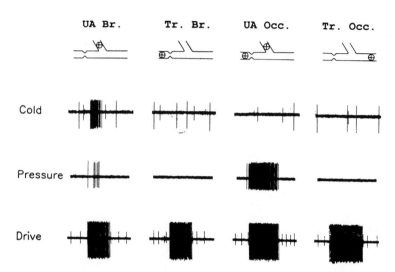

Figure 3 Behavior of respiratory modulated laryngeal receptors during upper airway breathing (UA Br.), tracheal breathing (Tr. Br.), upper airway occlusion (UA Occ.), and tracheal occlusion (Tr. Occ.). Laryngeal cold receptors are activated only when airflow-related temperature change occurs, whereas pressure receptors respond to transmural pressure changes within the larynx. In contrast, "drive" receptors, in general, reflect respiratory drive to upper airway muscles, which is increased during airway occlusions. (Reprinted from Ref. 23a, p. 226, by courtesy of Marcel Dekker, Inc.)

development of myelination and increase in nerve conduction velocity in RLN is most rapid during the first 2 months (38).

IV. Control of Upper Airway Muscle Activity: Influence of Upper Airway Afferents

A. Nasal Afferents

The nose is a source of many powerful reflexes, most of which are defensive or airway protective in nature and will be discussed separately. McBride and Whitelaw (39) reported a temperature-dependent respiratory inhibition of upper airway origin. Cold air breathing depresses the ventilatory response to CO_2 (40). These effects are presumed to be mediated by nasal afferents. Nerve endings sensitive to airflow and transmural pressure in the nose have been subsequently identified (3,4).

Negative pressure in the nasal airway augments the activity of the alae nasi and other upper airway dilator muscles such as the posterior cricoarytenoid and genioglossus (41–43). The above responses are markedly attenuated or abolished after topical anesthesia of the nasal mucosa, suggesting that trigeminal afferents mediate these reflex effects originating from the nasopharynx (44). Recently, Horner et al. (45), in a series of protocols in humans, have shown that the primary afferent pathway for activation of the genioglossus by negative pressure is carried by the superior laryngeal and trigeminal nerves.

B. Pharyngeal Afferents

The role of pharyngeal afferents in respiratory control has been much less studied than their role in defensive reflexes. Pressure-sensitive receptors have been identified in the pharynx (18). Hypoglossal nerve responses to upper airway pressure changes were augmented following glossopharyngeal nerve section, suggesting that glossopharyngeal afferents have an inhibitory influence on hypoglossal motoneurons or modulate the effect of superior laryngeal and trigeminal afferents (11). However, the role of glossopharyngeal nerve afferents in the above response in humans appears to be small, if any (45).

C. Laryngeal Afferents

Electrical stimulation of the SLN has an inhibitory effect on breathing frequency; stronger stimulation results in apnea. It also reduces the activity of thoracic inspiratory muscles such as the diaphragm. The effect of electrical stimulation on upper airway muscles is complex. The majority of studies suggest that the activity of laryngeal adductors (thyroarytenoid, interarytenoid, and cricothyroid) is increased (46–49). Both excitation and inhibition of the posterior cricoarytenoid muscle activity have been reported with SLN stimulation (43,46,49,50). Although electrical stimulation experiments have provided valuable insights into the functional role of laryngeal afferents, it is difficult to interpret the reflex responses because of simultaneous stimulation of multiple afferent types. These afferents can be activated by several stimuli such as airflow, transmural pressure, "drive," temperature, osmolarity, and chemical irritants.

Pressure changes in the upper airway alter the activity of several upper airway muscles (41,42,51). Mathew et al. (44,52) suggested that pressure-sensitive, slowly adapting receptors of the upper airway mediate these responses. The presence of such receptors in the larynx has been subsequently documented (19,53). Negative pressure in the upper airway enhances the phasic activity of the genioglossus, posterior cricoarytenoid, cricothyroid, and alae nasi muscles (Fig. 4; 42,43,54,55). These reflex changes of laryngeal origin are abolished by topical anesthesia of the laryngeal mucosa or sectioning of the SLN (44). The magnitude of the reflex response to negative pressure depends on several factors, such as stimulus strength, time of application, concurrent presence or absence of other afferent inputs, and level of consciousness. For example, as the strength of the stimulus increases, greater effects are observed. The effect of negative pressure

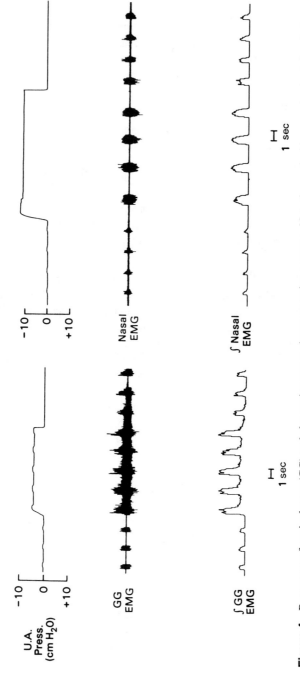

Figure 4 Responses of genioglossus (GG) and alae nasi to upper airway negative pressure. Note the marked increase in phasic inspiratory activity during the negative pressure application. (Adapted from Ref. 42.)

decreases at deeper levels of anesthesia (42). Sleep also reduces the responsiveness to upper airway negative pressure (56). Mathew and co-workers have investigated the timing of the stimuli as well as the role of other afferent inputs on the response to upper airway pressure changes (57,58). These results indicate that negative pressure applied to the upper airway during inspiration is more effective than that applied during expiration (Fig. 5); even during inspiration, early application augments the genioglossus muscle activity more than late application (57). Volume feedback from the lungs also has an effect on upper airway negative pressure reflex; in fact, negative pressure is more effective in the absence of volume feedback (Fig. 6; 58). Together these findings underscore the importance of integration of various phasic and tonic afferent inputs in determining upper airway muscle activity. The nucleus tractus solitarius is believed to be an important site where such integration occurs. We are only beginning to understand the mechanisms involved in this process. As early as 1973, the inhibitory effect of laryngeal CO_2 on breathing frequency was noted by Boushey and Richardson (59); however, the physiological significance of this finding still remains unclear. There has been a resurgence of interest in the effect of intralaryngeal CO_2 in recent years. The receptors responding to laryngeal CO_2 are fairly well characterized (27,31,60). In addition to its inhibitory effect on the phrenic nerve activity, intralaryngeal CO_2 has an excitatory effect on genioglossal muscle (hypoglossal nerve) activity (61,62). Recently Bartlett et al. (63) also examined the influence of intralaryngeal CO_2 on the respiratory activity of motor nerves to other muscles of the upper airway. Compared to the increase in activity of the nasolabial branch of the facial nerve, no consistent response was seen in the posterior cricoarytenoid branch of the recurrent laryngeal nerve; an intermittent exaggeration of the early expiratory burst was observed in the nerve to the thyroarytenoid muscle. These investigators

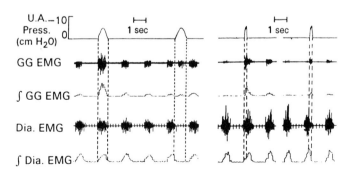

Figure 5 Time of application of upper airway pressure on genioglossus muscle response. (Left) Inspiratory versus expiratory; (right) early versus late inspiratory application. (Adapted from Ref. 57.)

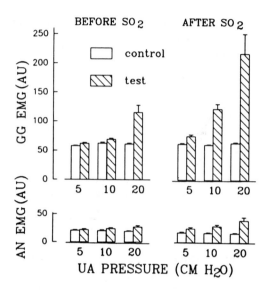

Figure 6 Role of volume feedback on the response of upper airway muscles to negative pressure changes in the upper airway. An increase in the response is seen following blockade of slowly adapting receptors with SO_2 in the rabbit. (Reprinted from Ref. 58.)

have also shown that intralaryngeal CO_2 exerted a greater effect on upper airway muscle activity following vagotomy; i.e., vagal afferents have a stabilizing influence on the effect of CO_2 (62). These findings indicate that airway CO_2 may play a greater role in upper airway maintenance during decreases in lung volume feedback.

Airflow can stimulate laryngeal receptors either by distorting the mucosal structures or by changing the laryngeal temperature. Jammes and co-workers reported that cooling of the isolated larynx produces marked increases in lower airway resistance especially when the temperature decreases below 10°C; this is associated with a reduction in laryngeal expiratory muscle activity and laryngeal resistance (64). However, only the increase in lower airway resistance is abolished by SLN section. In contrast, a small reduction in peak inspiratory activity of posterior cricoarytenoid muscle, suggesting an increase in laryngeal resistance, was observed in dogs following modest decreases in laryngeal temperature (65). Differences in experimental conditions, afferent source, and species could account for the observed discrepancy. Results of a recent study by Ukabam et al. (66) may have provided some insight into this issue. These investigators assessed the effect of upper airway cooling on hypoglossal and phrenic nerve activity in decerebrate, paralyzed, artificially ventilated adult cats. The hypoglossal response to laryngeal cooling was consistent in individual cats but varied markedly among different animals (an increase in hypoglossal nerve activity in some vs. a decrease in activity in others). These investigators speculated that two reflexes with divergent consequences are elicited by cooling. Since stimulation and inhibition of both myelinated (24,26) and nonmyelinated (67) endings have been documented with laryngeal cooling, the above hypothesis remains attractive.

The role of "drive" receptors in respiratory control, at least in anesthetized animals, appears small, if any. These receptors may play an important role in vocalization.

D. Changes During Development

Laryngeal chemoreflex has been studied extensively. Instillation of water and a number of other liquids into the larynx induces apnea in newborn lambs (68,69), kittens (70), and piglets (71), a response mediated through laryngeal afferents. The principal stimulus for this apneic reflex is the absence or reduced concentration of Cl^- or other small anions in the surface liquid of the laryngeal airway (72).

Negative pressure applied to the upper airway can produce apnea in newborn puppies (73). Airflow through the larynx has similar effects in kittens and puppies (73–75). The respiratory depressant effect of airflow is due to its cooling effect on the laryngeal mucosa (76). Laryngeal cooling stimulates cold receptors and inhibits the mechanoreceptors (24,26); however, the relative contribution of the two types of receptors in the respiratory depressant effect is unclear. Menthol, a specific laryngeal cold receptor stimulant in adult dogs (77), induces respiratory depression in puppies (78). Apnea induced by laryngeal negative pressure, cooling, and chemoreflex disappears in older puppies. Maturational changes in the central nervous system appear to underlie this age-related difference in response. Indeed, solitary tract neurons in newborn kittens are more susceptible to inhibition than those in adults (70,79).

Laryngeal abduction during hypoxic and hypercapnic stimulation decreases airway resistance less in newborn than in adult dogs (80). Laryngeal adductor response to SLN stimulation, absent immediately after birth, develops within the first few days of birth (38). A period of transient state of laryngeal adductor hyperexcitability has been observed between 50 and 70 days of life (81). Activation of the adductor muscles, like thyroarytenoid, during expiration is a prominent feature in the newborn (82,83). This is perceived as an important mechanism for slowing expiration and elevating end-expiratory volume in newborns since they have a poorly compliant lung and a highly compliant chest wall (84).

V. Lower Airway Afferents

Sensory innervation of the lower airway is provided primarily through the vagus nerve. Branches from the left side of the trachea and mainstem bronchus join the recurrent laryngeal nerve, whereas the branches on the right side join the main vagus trunk. Afferents from the extrathoracic portion of the trachea join, for the most part, the SLN or the recurrent laryngeal nerve (85). Vagal afferents can be divided into myelinated and nonmyelinated endings. A comprehensive review of vagal afferents is beyond the scope of this chapter, and the readers are referred to reviews on this subject (86,87).

Two distinct types of endings have been recognized in the myelinated category. They are termed rapidly adapting receptors (RAR) and slowly adapting receptors (SAR). Responses to a maintained stimulus and regularity of discharge form the basis of this classification. Activity of SARs and RARs has been studied in several species, including cat, rabbit, guinea pig, and dog (88–92). SARs generally exhibit a respiratory modulation consisting of an increase in frequency during inspiration (91,93–95). The majority of these endings are active at end-expiration and the rest are recruited during inspiration. In contrast, activity of SARs in the extrathoracic trachea decreases during inspiration and increases during expiration (96). Although SARs respond with a slowly adapting and regular discharge to a maintained stimulus (97), they do exhibit significant dynamic sensitivity initially (98). Light probing of mucosal surface does not activate these endings, suggesting a deeper location. Functional studies as well as electron microscopic studies suggest a location in close association with airway smooth muscle (99–102). RARs, on the other hand, reveal an irregular discharge and adapt completely to a maintained stimulus. These endings terminate as free nerve endings at the base of the tracheobronchial mucosa and respond to light mucosal stimulation with a rapidly adapting discharge pattern. One-fourth to one-half of myelinated endings are estimated to be RARs (97,103). Topically applied local anesthetics block SARs; however, higher concentration and longer time, compared to RARs, are required to block SAR activity, indicating a deeper location (104).

The vast majority of the vagal afferents are nonmyelinated. Two principal types are identified (bronchial and pulmonary C-fibers) based on the circulatory accessibility by agents such as capsaicin and phenyl-biguanide. They also respond to mechanical stimulation and certain irritants. Most nonmyelinated endings respond to intravenous administration of hypertonic saline solution into the pulmonary or bronchial circulation (105).

Vagal afferents carry information originating from the lower airway to the central nervous system during inspiration and expiration and play an important role in shaping the motor output of various respiratory muscles. However, it is not clear whether the absolute number or the pattern of discharge is the critical variable in determining the response to stimulation. At least in the apnea associated with high-frequency ventilation, the temporal pattern of afferent input from SARs appears to be more important than the absolute number (106). If one records the overall afferent activity emerging from the vagus, a clear inspiratory modulation is observed (Figs. 2 and 7). Since nonmyelinated endings do not show any clear respiratory modulation, this increase in activity originates mostly from SARs and RARs, whereas the activity during end-expiration represents SARs and C-fibers. The increase in inspiratory activity is primarily due to SARs. Although

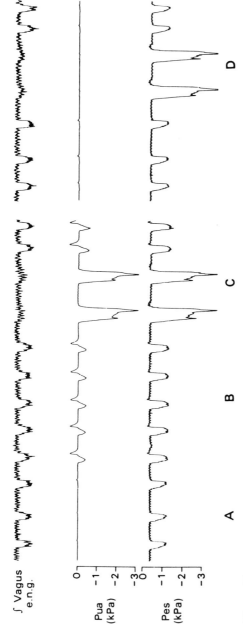

Figure 7 Activity of vagus nerve during tracheostomy breathing (A), upper airway breathing (B), upper airway occlusion (C) and tracheal occlusion (D). Although the peak inspiratory activity is markedly less during occlusions, a phasic inspiratory activity persists. (Adapted from Ref. 20.)

increase in lung volume acts as a stimulus, changes in transpulmonary pressure seem to correlate better with changes in SAR and RAR activity. The individual C-fiber shows only sparse activity; however, since the vast majority of vagal afferents fall in this category, their overall contribution to respiratory control cannot be ignored.

Cell bodies of vagal afferents are located primarily in the nodose ganglion. Central projections of vagal afferents are discussed in Chapter 5.

A. Developmental Changes

Vagal afferents innervating the tracheobronchial tree and lung show considerable difference in myelination during the newborn period (106,107). For example, only 10–20% of adult values of myelination are observed at birth in kittens (106). Although both SARs and RARs have been recognized, the relative frequency of RARs appears to be less in newborns (108,109). Similarly, discharge frequencies of SARs, at any given transpulmonary pressure, are lower in the newborn (110). No direct recording of C-fibers has been reported in the newborn.

VI. Control of Upper Airway Muscle Activity: Influence of Lower Airway Afferents

Lower airway afferents alter both respiratory timing and pattern of activation of upper airway muscles. Our attempts to selectively alter the afferent input from the lower airway have considerable limitations and should, therefore, be interpreted with caution. It must be recognized that the concept of one type of endings exclusively mediating a given response is not necessarily accurate.

A. Slowly Adapting Receptors

The role of SARs in respiratory control has been studied primarily in one of two ways: by inflating the lungs or by preventing lung expansion. Lung inflation maintains SAR activation at increased levels, whereas prevention of lung expansion by airway occlusion at end-expiration reduces the phasic increase in SAR activity. Increased SAR activation, as in lung inflation, terminates inspiration and prolongs expiration. In contrast, decreases in volume-related feedback, as in airway occlusion, prolong inspiratory duration. Generally the changes in respiratory timing observed in thoracic respiratory muscles are reflected in upper airway muscles as well. However, the changes observed during airway occlusion cannot be solely attributed to the lack of increase in SAR activity. For example, RAR activation seen near peak inflation is also eliminated during occluded breaths. In addition, afferent activity originating from the upper airway in spontaneously breathing animals increases during airway occlusion compared to unoccluded breaths (20). Although the overall activity emerging from the airway is markedly decreased during airway occlusion at end-expiration, Miserocchi et al. (95) and, recently, Iscoe and Gordon (111) showed that the activity of a significant percentage of SARs increases during airway occlusion. Nevertheless, the above conclusions about the role of SAR on respiratory timing appear justified, since qualitatively similar results have been obtained under varied experimental conditions.

The effect of volume feedback on the activity of upper airway muscles has been studied by several investigators (112–115). During tidal breathing, some upper airway muscles are either silent or display tonic activity; others exhibit phasic activity, predominantly during inspiration. Thoracic inspiratory muscles, such as the diaphragm, exhibit a ramp-like increase during inspiration; peak activity often occurs close to the end of inspiration. In contrast, upper airway muscles often exhibit a different discharge profile. Activity of upper airway muscles starts early and abruptly, reaches a peak quickly, and begins to decline well before the end of inspiration, similar to the inspiratory airflow profile. Earlier onset of changes in recurrent laryngeal and hypoglossal nerve activity during airway occlusion, compared to phrenic nerve activity, suggest that volume-related feedback on cranial motoneurons may not operate through inspiratory off-switch mechanism. Withholding lung inflation alters the discharge of these muscles (or their nerves) into a late-peaking pattern (Fig. 8). These increases in nerve activity indicate the inhibitory effect of lung volume (113,114). The volume threshold for inhibiting cranial nerve activity is not time dependent (116). Effects similar to those observed in paralyzed animals are seen during airway occlusion in spontaneously breathing animals as well. The inhibitory effect is greatest on hypoglossal nerve activity and least on phrenic nerve activity (115). Increase in the discharge frequency of phasically active motoneurons as well as recruitment of previously inactive motoneurons accounts for the incrementing pattern (113,114). When lung inflation is withheld, even the expiratory activity of hypoglossal and recurrent laryngeal nerves increases (Fig. 8). Alternatively, SAR input can be reduced by blocking SAR activity. In rabbits this can be accomplished by selectively blocking SARs with sulfur dioxide (SO_2). An increase in the duration of genioglossus muscle activity, without significant change in peak activity, was observed following SO_2 block (58,117).

These results are in sharp contrast to the results of airway occlusions in spontaneously breathing vagally intact animals and withholding lung inflation in paralyzed, artificially ventilated animals; an increase in peak genioglossus muscle or hypoglossal nerve activity is observed under these conditions. Differences in excitation of SARs and RARs could account for the observed difference. Continued RAR activation occurs during breathing in SO_2-exposed rabbits, which is not likely during airway occlusion or withholding of inflation. Incomplete block of SARs with SO_2 is another potential confounding variable. However, Hering-Breuer inflation tests indicate nearly complete blockade of SARs. A reduction in

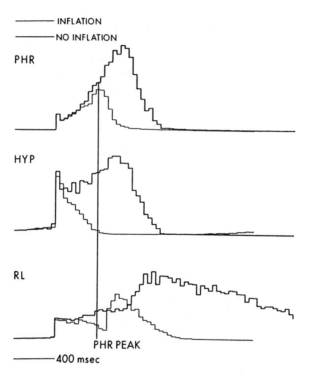

Figure 8 Effects of withholding of inflation on cranial nerve activity. Hypoglossal and recurrent laryngeal nerve activity increases indicating the inhibitory effect of volume feedback. (Reprinted from Ref. 113.)

tonic SAR activity occurs with SO_2 block, whereas it is preserved during airway occlusions. This difference in tonic discharge could account, at least in part, for the observed difference. Agostoni et al. (117) have suggested that SARs have a facilitatory input on genioglossus at end-expiratory volume but an inhibitory influence at higher lung volumes. Moreover, these investigators have suggested that the effects of tracheal and bronchial SARs on the control of breathing may not be uniform.

There is no consensus on the effect of lung inflation on upper airway muscles. Lung inflation is reported to decrease the activity of a number of upper airway muscles and cranial nerves supplying these muscles (118–120). A tonic activation of the posterior cricoarytenoid, instead of complete inhibition, was observed by Bartlett et al. (121). Inspiratory motoneurons with a low-level tonic activity may be responsible for this observation (120). The original description of the Hering-Breuer reflex suggests that lung inflation inhibits the alae nasi, since the naris is seen to narrow immediately. But this observation has not been confirmed by electromyographic (EMG) studies.

Lung deflation increases the activity of both inspiratory and expiratory upper airway muscles (120,122,123). Since reduction in lung volume from functional residual capacity (FRC) to half-lung collapse decreases primarily SAR activity (124), changes in SAR activity appear to play a major role in the above response.

B. Rapidly Adapting Receptors

The role of RARs in airway reflexes is much less clear. In part, this difficulty is due to our inability to precisely define the reflexes elicited by RAR stimulation. At present there is no chemical agent that stimulates these endings selectively. Most agents either directly or indirectly stimulate other vagal afferents as well. In addition to their role in the control of breathing, RARs are believed to play an important role in initiating cough and sigh. In a recent study, Green and Kaufman (124) used reduction in lung volume as a stimulus for RARs. Reduction in lung volume from half-lung collapse to full-lung collapse stimulated primarily RARs. In parallel studies, reflex effects of RAR stimulation were investigated; the only significant change observed was an increase in breathing frequency due to shortening of expiration. Davies et al. (125) reached similar conclusions following the block of SARs with SO_2 in rabbits. Unfortunately, upper airway muscle activity was not monitored in these experiments. RARs are presumed to mediate tracheobronchial cough; however, Sant'Ambrogio et al. (126) have shown that SAR input is important in eliciting cough reflexes. Lack of SAR facilitation of expiratory muscles is one mechanism by which SARs could affect cough responses. RARs are also believed to play a role in the genesis of augmented breaths or sighs. Increased frequency of augmented breaths is seen following airway occlusions. Although the precise mechanism is unclear, a change in lower airway afferent activity resulting from decreased compliance and FRC presumably accounts for this finding. Increased discharge of RARs seen immediately following airway occlusion is consistent with this notion (94). During augmented breaths, the activity of chest wall muscles increases. Without a proportionate increase in upper airway muscle activity, flow limitation or even airway obstruction would ensue. Van Lunteren et al. (126a) reported that activity of various upper airway muscles increases markedly during augmented breaths (Fig. 9). Hiccough, on the other hand, is an excellent example in which a disproportionate increase in diaphragmatic activity results in airway obstruction.

C. C-Fibers

The role of airway C-fiber afferents in respiratory control during eupnea is not clear. Perineural capsaicin treatment of vagus, which blocks the C-fibers selectively, does not alter the breathing pattern significantly (127), whereas stimulation of C-fibers alters the breathing pattern.

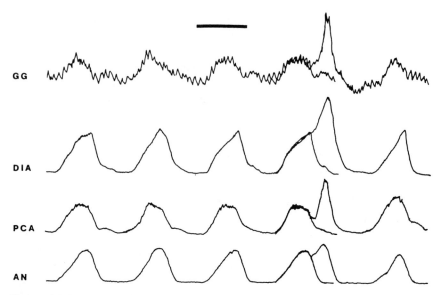

Figure 9 Discharge pattern of diaphragm and upper airway muscles during augmented breaths. (Reprinted from Ref. 126a.)

Intravenous injection of C-fiber stimulant such as capsaicin induces apnea followed by rapid, shallow breathing. Using isolated pulmonary vasculature, Schertel et al. (128) have shown that lower doses of capsaicin produce rapid shallow breathing without apnea. Haxhiu et al. (129) recorded the activity of upper airway dilators and constrictors during capsaicin administration (Fig. 10). During the period of apnea, both the thoracic inspiratory muscles and the upper airway dilating muscles are completely inhibited (129). An increase in tonic discharge appeared in upper airway dilating muscles immediately prior to the reappearance of phasic activity. Following apnea, when rapid shallow breathing ensued, the ratio of upper airway muscle activity to diaphragm activity increased markedly and remained elevated for several minutes. This increased ratio reflects, at least in part, a greater activation of upper airway muscles by chemical stimuli developed during apnea. Capsaicin increases laryngeal resistance, indicating that laryngeal adductors are activated during the period of apnea. Recently Haxhiu et al. (129) have shown that pharyngeal constrictor activity is also increased during capsaicin-induced apnea.

D. Changes During Development

The Hering-Breur reflex, mediated by SARs, is believed to be stronger in the neonate than in the adult. Since the threshold of activation of SARs is higher and

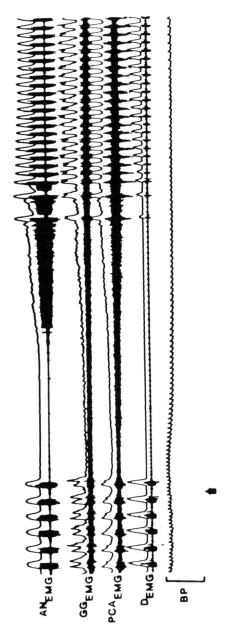

Figure 10 Effects of capsaicin administration into right atrium on alae nasi (AN), genioglossus (GG), posterior cricoarytenoid (PCA), and diaphragm (D) EMGs. (Reprinted from Ref. 129.)

SAR discharge frequency, at any given transmural pressure, is lower in the neonate than in the adult, the respiratory center in the newborn must be more responsive to volume feedback. Decrease in inhibitory influences from higher centers may account, at least in part, for the increased responsiveness. Alternatively, differences in the mechanical properties of the lungs and/or differences in rib cage afferents could account for some of the observed difference between newborns and adults.

Available data suggest that RARs are scant in the lower airway of newborns. Absent or weak cough reflex observed in the newborn is consistent with this finding. Some infants, especially preterm infants, may develop apnea in response to mechanical irritation of the airway (130). An increased incidence of augmented breaths or sighs is seen in the newborn, which may reflect the lower compliance of their lungs. It is interesting that increased lung compliance observed during growth is accompanied by a decrease in sigh frequency.

Injection of phenyl-biguanide to right heart results in a weak or absent chemoreflex response in kittens (131), suggesting a minimal role for pulmonary C-fibers in the newborn.

VII. Upper Airway Muscle Activity During Defensive Reflexes

The upper airway participates in a number of vital functions, some of which clearly interrupt tidal breathing. The general strategy is to limit further penetration of foreign materials into the tracheobronchial tree (airway protective responses) or to facilitate expulsion of foreign materials from the airway (defensive responses) through reflexes such as cough, sneeze, and swallow. The precise role of various upper airway muscles in these reflexes is yet to be determined.

The diving reflex (apnea, bradycardia, and laryngeal closure) is one of the protective reflexes originating from the nose (132,133). Increase in laryngeal adductor muscle activity appears to be an integral part of this response.

A sneeze can be induced by many mechanical and chemical stimuli (133,134). Although the activity of upper airway muscles during sneezing has not been studied, such activity can be inferred from available data on pressure and airflow. A sneeze consists of an initial deep inspiration followed by forced expiration and has several features in common with cough. Laryngeal adductor muscles probably play a critical role in developing this explosive pressure through their initial activation followed by their subsequent sudden relaxation. As in coughing, the palatal muscles play an important role in sneezing. The position of the soft palate has to be maintained such that a significant portion of the expiratory airflow occurs through the nose. Recently, Widdicombe and Tatar (135) observed a great reduction in upper airway resistance during sneezing induced by mechanical stimulation of the nasal mucosa. A significant decrease in upper airway resistance occurred even in the absence of sneezing, suggesting that the upper airway dilator response is not dependent on the sneeze response.

Aspiration and swallowing are two important reflexes that have a great impact on upper airway muscles. The aspiration reflex causes vigorous contraction of the diaphragm associated with reflex laryngeal abductions (136). Stimulation of the rapidly adapting receptors in the submucosa of the nasopharynx is presumed to mediate the response. Mechanical stimulation of the posterior wall of the nasopharynx also increases the peak activity of the expiratory pharyngeal muscles (137). The role of these expiratory pharyngeal muscles in aspiration reflex response is unclear. The developmental aspects of the aspiration reflex have been studied in animal models. In rats, this reflex is absent at birth and remains weak at 15–20 days, whereas in kittens it is present at birth and fully developed by the second day of life (134).

Several upper airway muscles that exhibit respiratory activity participate in swallowing. The magnitude of activation of these muscles during swallowing is usually greater than their respiratory activity. Swallowing can be elicited from multiple sites in the upper airway. Although receptors that initiate swallow have not been identified histologically, slowly adapting receptors that respond to water and light touch are presumed to initiate swallow. Water is the most effective stimulus from the larynx, whereas light pressure or touch is most effective from the pharynx. Anesthesia of the entire upper airway mucosa can cause difficulty in initiating a swallow. Peripheral feedback mechanisms have been shown to alter the activation of muscles during swallowing. This feedback is thought to be more important in the newborn than in the adult (138). Various upper airway muscles have to be recruited in a coordinated and sequential manner in order to propel the bolus into the esophagus. Some of these muscles are antagonistic during breathing, illustrating the complexity of this task. During swallowing, food particles are prevented from entering the respiratory tract by inhibiting the activity of posterior cricoarytenoid muscle, enhancing the activity of thyroarytenoid and lateral cricoarytenoid muscles along with repositioning of the epiglottis (83,139).

A number of irritants, such as cigarette smoke, ammonia, phenyl-biguanide, and veratridine, applied to laryngeal mucosa alter the respiratory pattern; cough is elicited less often. Data on upper airway muscle activity during airway defense responses are sparse. Szereda-Przestaszewska and Widdicombe (132) have shown that ammonia, even at concentrations that do not alter breathing frequency, increases laryngeal resistance. Glogowska et al. (140) have confirmed the excitatory effect of ammonia on expiratory activity of recurrent laryngeal nerve. In a recent study, Palecek et al. (141) observed that both ammonia and capsaicin increase laryngeal resistance (indicating increased laryngeal adductor activity) in rats but not in dogs. Since capsaicin is a selective C-fiber stimulant, a difference in C-fiber afferent innervation between the two species could account for the observed difference.

Cough, an airway defense reflex, can be elicited from the upper or lower respiratory tract (134). However, there are some distinct differences between laryngeal and tracheobronchial cough (136). The initial inspiratory component is quite variable and may even be absent in laryngeal cough. Laryngeal muscles play an integral role in cough. Increased activation of laryngeal adductors is followed by sudden relaxation, resulting in explosive expiratory airflow. Activation of abdominal expiratory muscles continues. The discharge pattern of various pharyngeal muscles during a cough has not been well studied. Since the inspiratory flow is nasal and the expiratory flow is oral, palatal muscle activation during the two phases of cough is critical.

VIII. Relevance to Humans

Relatively few studies have evaluated the role of airway afferents in humans. The role of vagal feedback in conscious humans is weak or absent, except at large inspired lung volumes. Several studies in human infants, on the other hand, have shown a clear prolongation of inspiration during end-expiratory airway occlusion. An increase in inspiratory duration accompanying end-expiratory occlusion has also been observed in anesthetized human subjects (142). Upper airway muscle activity was not monitored in the above studies. State-dependent effects of airway reflexes are discussed in greater detail in Chapter 22.

The role of sensory feedback from the upper airway on the activity of upper airway muscles in humans is still emerging. Basner et al. (143) reported an increase in phasic activity of upper airway muscles during nose breathing compared to mouth breathing in awake adults; this was independent of airway resistance and was abolished by topical anesthesia, suggesting the involvement of superficial nasal receptors. It is unclear whether these effects are mediated by cold receptors or mechanoreceptors. In a recent study, Mezzanotte et al. (144) provided supportive evidence for the presence of a neural reflex mechanism augmenting the alae nasi during inspiratory resistive loading, implicating both mucosal and nonmucosal mechanoreceptors.

Effects of upper airway negative pressure on genioglossal activity have been the focus of two recent studies (145,146). Selective activation of the genioglossal muscle by upper negative pressure during wakefulness was confirmed in both studies. Moreover, Horner et al. (45) have shown that the superior laryngeal and trigeminal nerve afferents are involved in this response. In contrast, Kuna and Smickley (147) observed no augmentation of genioglossus muscle activity attributable to upper airway negative pressure when the effects of nasal occlusions on genioglossus muscle were evaluated in sleeping subjects. Nevertheless, Kuna et al. (148) were able to show an effect of laryngeal anesthesia on flow-volume loop in awake humans. Sleep state emerged as a significant factor in the response to upper airway negative pressure from these studies. Attenuation of the reflex effects of upper airway negative pressure during sleep has been well documented in the animal model (56). The effect of sleep state on the above response was the focus of two recent investigations in humans (149,150); preliminary data from these studies reveal a state-dependent response: a marked reduction or complete elimination of the response during sleep. Unlike adults, infants exhibit an increase in submental EMG during the first occluded breath (151). Also, decreases in inspiratory airflow by upper airway negative pressure indicting a marked inhibitory effect on thoracic inspiratory muscles have been documented in sleeping infants (152). These findings suggest a greater loss or attenuation of the negative pressure response during sleep in adults, compared to children. Several questions remain unanswered. Is the attenuation of the reflex exclusively a central nervous system effect? If so, which group(s) of neurons is responsible for the state-dependent effect? Does the afferent activity emerging from the upper airway decrease with the onset of sleep? Although the upper airway may be subjected to greater transmural pressure changes during sleep, a reduction in upper airway muscle activity is associated with a reduction in the response of laryngeal afferents to negative pressure (55). Why does the loss of this compensatory neural reflex during sleep predispose the patients to upper airway obstruction? Although the answers to many of the above questions remain to be elucidated, upper airway afferents are known to play an important role in inducing arousal (153,154), which facilitates recovery from airway obstructions.

IX. Conclusions

There has been an explosion of information on upper airway muscle activity during the last decade. It is clear from these studies that airway receptors play an important role in regulating the activity of these muscles. Most of these observations were originally made in anesthetized animals; recent studies have extended these findings to wakefulness and sleep as well. Despite this wealth of information, we are only beginning to understand the role of airway afferents in the control of upper airway muscle activity in humans. Current evidence suggests that airway afferents play a greater role in respiratory control in infants than in adults.

References

1. Strohl KP, O'Cain CF, Slutsky AS. Alae nasi activation and nasal resistance in healthy subjects. J Appl Physiol 1982; 52:1432–1437.
2. Glebovski:i VD, Baev AV. Stimulation of trigeminal receptors of the nasal mucosa by respiratory airflow [Rus]. Fiziol Z Sssr Imeni I-M-Sechenova 1984; 70:1534–1541.
3. Tsubone H. Nasal "flow" receptors of the cat. Respir Physiol 1989; 75:51–64.

4. Tsubone H. Nasal "pressure" receptors. Nippon Juigaku Zasshi—Jpn J Vet Sci 1990; 52:225–232.

5. Wallois F, Macron JM, Jounieaux V, Duron B. Trigaminal nasal receptors related to respiration and to various stimuli in cats. Respir Physiol 1991; 85:111–125.

6. Dawson WW. Chemical stimulation of the peripheral trigeminal nerve. Nature 1962; 196:341–345.

7. Ulrich CE, Haddock MP, Alarie Y. Airborne chemical irritants. Role of the trigeminal nerve. Arch Environ Health 1972; 24:37–42.

8. Nail BS, Sterling GM, Widdicombe JG. Epipharyngeal receptors responding to mechanical stimulation. J Physiol 1969; 204:91–98.

9. Nail BS, Sterling GM, Widdicombe JG. Patterns of spontaneous and reflexly-induced activity in phrenic and intercostal motoneurons. Exp Brain Res 1972; 15: 318–332.

10. Nail BS. Sensitization of polymodal airway receptors. In: Hutas J, Debreczeni LA, eds. Advances in Physiological Sciences: Respiration, Vol. 10. Budapest: Akad Kido, 1981:479–448.

11. Hwang J, St. John WM, Bartlett D. Afferent pathways for hypoglossal and phrenic responses to changes in upper airway pressure. Respir Physiol 1984; 55:341–354.

12. Widdicombe JG, Sant'Ambrogio G, Mathew OP. Nerve receptors of the upper airway. In: Mathew OP, Sant'Ambrogio G, eds. Respiratory Function of the Upper Airway. New York: Marcel Dekker, 1988:193–231.

13. Sant'Ambrogio FB, Tsubone H, Mathew OP, Sant'Ambrogio G. Afferent activity in the external branch of the superior laryngeal and recurrent laryngeal nerves. Ann Otol Rhinol Laryngol 1991; 100:944–950.

14. Aldaya F. Le controle reflexe de la respiration par la sensibilite du larynx. CR Soc Biol (Paris) 1936; 123:1001–1002.

15. Mortola JP, Citterio G, Agostoni E. Sulphur dioxide block of laryngeal receptors in rabbits. Respir Physiol 1985; 62:195–202.

16. Tsubone H, Mathew OP, Sant'Ambrogio G. Respiratory activity in the superior laryngeal nerve of the rabbit. Respir Physiol 1987; 69:195–207.

17. Sumi T. Spontaneous afferent impulses of the superior laryngeal nerve of the cat. Seitai No Kagaku 1958; 9:235–240.

18. Hwang J, St. John WM, Bartlett D. Receptors responding to changes in upper airway pressure. Respir Physiol 1984; 55:355–366.

19. Sant'Ambrogio G, Mathew OP, Fisher JT, Sant'Ambrogio FB. Laryngeal receptors responding to transmural pressure, airflow and local muscle activity. Respir Physiol 1983; 54:317–330.

20. Mathew OP, Sant'Ambrogio G, Fisher JT, Sant'Ambrogio FB. Respiratory afferent activity in the superior laryngeal nerves. Respir Physiol 1984; 58:41–50.

21. Tsubone H, Sant'Ambrogio G, Anderson JW, Orani GP. Laryngeal afferent activity and reflexes in the guinea pig. Respir Physiol 1991; 86:215–231.

22. Sekizawa S, Tsubone H. The respiratory activity of the superior laryngeal nerve in the rat. Respir Physiol 1991; 86:355–368.

23. Wyke BD, Kirchner JA. Neurology of the larynx. In: Hinchcliffe R, Harrison D, eds. Scientific Foundations of Otolaryngology. London: Heinemann, 1976:546–574.

23a. Fisher JT, Mathew OP, Sant'Ambrogio G. Morphological and neurophysiological aspects of airway and pulmonary receptors. In: Haddad GG, Farber JP, eds. Developmental Neurobiology of Breathing. New York: Marcel Dekker, 1991: 219–244.

24. Sant'Ambrogio G, Mathew OP, Sant'Ambrogio FB. Laryngeal cold receptors. Respir Physiol 1985; 59:35–44.

25. Sant'Ambrogio G, Mathew OP, Sant'Ambrogio FB. Characteristics of laryngeal cold receptors. Respir Physiol 1988; 71:287–297.

26. Sant'Ambrogio G, Brambilla-Sant'Ambrogio F, Mathew OP. Effect of cold air on laryngeal mechanoreceptors in the dog. Respir Physiol 1986; 64:45–56.

27. Boushey HA, Richardson PS, Widdicombe JG, Wise JCM. The response of laryngeal afferent fibres to mechanical and chemical stimuli. J Physiol 1974; 240: 153–175.

28. Storey AT, Johnson P. Laryngeal water receptors initiating apnea in the lamb. Exp Neurol 1975; 47:42–55.

29. Harding R, Johnson P, McClelland ME. Liquid-sensitive laryngeal receptors in the developing sheep, cat and monkey. J Physiol 1978; 277:409–422.

30. Anderson JW, Sant'Ambrogio FB, Mathew OP, Sant'Ambrogio G. Water-responsive laryngeal receptors in the dog are not specialized endings. Respir Physiol 1990; 79: 33–43.

31. Anderson JW, Sant'Ambrogio FB, Orani GP, Sant'Ambrogio G, Mathew OP. Carbon dioxide-responsive laryngeal receptors in the dog. Respir Physiol 1990; 82:217–226.

32. Bradford A, Nolan P, McKeogh D, Bannon C, O'Regan RG. The responses of superior laryngeal nerve afferent fibres to laryngeal airway CO_2 concentration in the anaesthetized cat. Exp Physiol 1990; 75:267–270.

33. Ghosh TK, Mathew OP. Influence of intralaryngeal carbon dioxide on the response of laryngeal afferents to upper airway pressure. J Appl Physiol (in press).

34. Miller AJ, Dunmire CR. Characterization of the postnatal development of superior laryngeal nerve fibers in the postnatal kitten. J Neurobiol 1976; 7:483–494.

35. Miller AJ, Loizzi RF. Anatomical and functional differentiation of superior laryngeal nerve fibers affecting swallowing and respiration. Exp Neurol 1974; 42:369–387.

36. Chung K, Sant'Ambrogio F, Sant'Ambrogio G. The fiber composition of the superior laryngeal nerve of the dog. FASEB J 1993; 7:A402 (abstract).

37. Marlot D, Duron B. Postnatal maturation of phrenic, vagus, and intercostal nerves in the kitten. Biol Neonat 1979; 36:264–272.

38. Sasaki CT, Suzuki M. Horiuchi M. Postnatal development of laryngeal reflexes in the dog. Arch Otolaryngol 1977; 103:143–144.

39. McBride B, Whitelaw WA. A physiological stimulus to upper airway receptors in humans. J Appl Physiol 1981; 51:1189–1197.

40. Burgess KR, Whitelaw WA. Reducing ventilatory response to carbon dioxide by breathing cold air. Am Rev Respir Dis 1984; 129:687–690.

41. Mathew OP, Abu-Osba YK, Thach BT. Genioglossus muscle responses to upper airway pressure changes: afferent pathways. J Appl Physiol 1982; 52:445–450.

42. Mathew OP. Upper airway negative-pressure effects on respiratory activity of upper airway muscles. J Appl Physiol 1984; 56:500–505.

43. van Lunteren E, Van de Graaff WB, Parker DM, Mitra J, Haxhiu MA, Strohl KP, Cherniack NS. Nasal and laryngeal reflex responses to negative upper airway pressure. J Appl Physiol 1984; 56:746–752.

44. Mathew OP, Abu-Osba YK, Thach BT. Influence of upper airway pressure changes on genioglossus muscle respiratory activity. J Appl Physiol 1982; 52:438–444.

45. Horner RL, Innes JA, Holden HB, Guz A. Afferent pathway(s) for pharyngeal dilator reflex to negative pressure in man: a study using upper airway anaesthesia. J Physiol 1991; 436:31–44.

46. Yamashita T, Urabe K. Uber den Stimmbandtensorreflex. Z Laryng Rhinol Otol 1959; 38:759–766.

47. Martensson A. Reflex responses and recurrent discharges evoked by stimulation of laryngeal nerves. Acta Physiol Scand 1963; 57:248–269.

48. Murakami Y, Kirchner JA. Electrophysiological properties of laryngeal reflex closure. Acta Oto-Laryngol 1971; 71:416–425.

49. Sasaki CT, Suzuki M. Laryngeal reflexes in cat, dog, and man. Arch Otolaryngol 1976; 102:400–402.

50. Yamashita T, Urabe K. Glottisschlussreflex and M. cricoarytaenoid eus posterior. Arch Ohr Nas Kehlk Heilkd 1960; 177:39–44.

51. Mathew OP, Farber JP. Effect of upper airway negative pressure on respiratory timing. Respir Physiol 1983; 54:259–268.

52. Mathew OP, Abu-Osba YK, Thach BT. Influence of upper airway pressure changes on respiratory frequency. Respir Physiol 1982; 49:223–233.

53. Mathew OP, Sant'Ambrogio G, Fisher JT, Sant'Ambrogio FB. Laryngeal pressure receptors. Respir Physiol 1984; 57:113–122.

54. Sant'Ambrogio FB, Mathew OP, Clark WD, Sant'Ambrogio G. Laryngeal influences on breathing pattern and posterior cricoarytenoid muscle activity. J Appl Physiol 1985; 58:1298–1304.

55. Mathew OP, Sant'Ambrogio FB, Woodson GE, Sant'Ambrogio G. Respiratory activity of the cricothyroid muscle. Ann Otol Rhinol Laryngol 1988; 97:680–687.

56. Issa FG, Edwards P, Szeto E, Lauff D, Sullivan CE. Genioglossus response to airway occlusion in dogs: effect of sleep and route of occlusion. J Appl Physiol 1988; 64:543–549.

57. Woodall DL, Hokanson JA, Mathew OP. Time of application of negative pressure pulses and upper airway muscle activity. J Appl Physiol 1989; 67:366–370.

58. Zhang S, Mathew OP. Response of laryngeal mechanoreceptors to high-frequency pressure oscillation. J Appl Physiol 1992; 73:219–223.

59. Boushey HA, Richardson PS. The reflex effects of intralaryngeal carbon dioxide on the pattern of breathing. J Physiol 1973; 228:181–191.

60. Lee LY, Morton RF, McIntosh MJ, Turbek JA. An isolation upper airway preparation in conscious dogs. J Appl Physiol 1986; 60:2123–2127.

61. Nolan P, Bradford A, O'Regan RG, McKeogh D. The effects of changes in laryngeal airway CO_2 concentration on genioglossus muscle activity in the anaesthetized cat. Exp Physiol 1990; 75:271–274.

62. Bartlett D, Jr., Knuth SL, Leiter JC. Alteration of the ventilatory activity by intralaryngeal CO_2 in the cat. J Physiol 1992; 457:117–185.

63. Bartlett D., Jr., Knuth SL, Gdovin MJ. Influence of laryngeal CO_2 on respiratory activities of motor nerves to accessary muscles. Respir Physiol 1992; 90: 289–297.

64. Jammes Y, Barthelemy P, Delpierre S. Respiratory effects of cold air breathing in anesthetized cats. Respir Physiol 1983; 54:41–54.

65. Mathew OP, Sant'Ambrogio FB, Sant'Ambrogio G. Effects of cooling on laryngeal reflexes in the dog. Respir Physiol 1986; 66:61–70.

66. Ukabam CU, Knuth SL, Bartlett D, Jr. Phrenic and hypoglossal neural responses to cold airflow in the upper airway. Respir Physiol 1992; 87:157–164.

67. Jammes Y, Nail B, Mei N, Grimaud C. Laryngeal afferents activated by phenyldiguanide and their response to cold air or helium-oxygen. Respir Physiol 1987; 67:379–389.

68. Johnson P, Salisbury DM, Storey AT. Apnea induced by stimulation of sensory receptors in the larynx. In: Bosma JF, Showacre J, eds. Development of upper respiratory anatomy and function. Washington, DC: US Government Printing Office, 1975:160–178.

69. Kovar I, Selstam U, Catterton WZ, Stahlman MT, Sundell HW. Laryngeal chemoreflex in new born lambs: respiratory and swallowing response to salts, acids, and sugars. Pediatr Res 1979; 13:1144–1149.

70. Lucier GE, Storey AT, Sessle BJ. Effects of upper respiratory tract stimuli on neonatal respiration: reflex and single neuron analyses in the kitten. Biol Neonate 1979; 35:82–89.

71. Downing SE, Lee JC. Laryngeal chemosensitivity: a possible mechanism for sudden infant death. Pediatrics 1975; 55:640–649.

72. Boggs DF, Bartlett D. Chemical specificity of a laryngeal apneic reflex in puppies. J Appl Physiol 1982; 53:455–462.

73. Fisher JT, Mathew OP, Sant'Ambrogio FB, Sant'Ambrogio G. Reflex effects and receptor responses to upper airway pressure and flow stimuli in developing puppies. J Appl Physiol 1985; 58:258–264.

74. Al-Shway SF, Mortola JP. Respiratory effects of airflow through the upper airways in newborn kittens and puppies. J Appl Physiol 1982; 53:805–814.

75. Mortola JP, Al-Shway S, Noworaj A. Importance of upper airway airflow in the ventilatory depression of laryngeal origin. Pediatr Res 1983; 17:550–552.

76. Mathew OP, Anderson JW, Orani GP, Sant'Ambrogio FB, Sant'Ambrogio G. Cooling mediates the ventilatory depression associated with airflow through the larynx. Respir Physiol 1990; 82:359–367.

77. Sant'Ambrogio FB, Anderson JW, Sant'Ambrogio G. Effect of l-menthol on laryngeal receptors. J Appl Physiol 1991; 70:788–793.

78. Sant'Ambrogio FB, Anderson JW, Sant'Ambrogio G. Menthol in the upper airway depresses ventilation in newborn dogs. Respir Physiol 1992; 89:299–307.

79. Sessle BJ, Greenwood LF, Lund JP, Lucier GE. Effects of upper respiratory tract stimuli on respiration and single respiratory neurons in the adult cat. Exp Neurol 1978; 61:245–259.

80. Blum DJ, McCaffrey TV. Effect of maturation on the sensitivity of laryngeal

81. Sasaki CT. Development of laryngeal function: etiologic significance in the sudden infant death syndrome. Laryngoscope 1979; 89:1964–1982.

82. Farber JP. Development of pulmonary reflexes and pattern of breathing in Virginia opossum. Respir Physiol 1972; 14:278–286.

83. Harding R, Johnson P, McClelland ME. Respiratory function of the larynx in developing sheep and the influence of sleep state. Respir Physiol 1980; 40:165–179.

84. Mortola JP, Fisher JT, Smith B, Fox G, Weeks S. Dynamics of breathing in infants. J Appl Physiol 1982; 52:1209–1215.

85. Lee BP, Sant'Ambrogio G, Sant'Ambrogio F. Afferent innervation and receptors of the canine extrathoracic trachea. Respir Physiol 1992; 90:55–65.

86. Sant'Ambrogio G. Information arising from the tracheobronchial tree of mammals. Physiol Rev 1982; 62:531–569.

87. Coleridge HM, Coleridge JCG. Reflexes evoked from tracheobronchial tree and lungs. In: Cherniack NS, Widdicombe JG, eds. Handbook of Physiology, The Respiratory System, Section 3, Vol. 2. Bethesda, MD: American Physiological Society, 1986.

88. Knowlton GC, Larrabee MG. A unitary analysis of pulmonary volume receptors. Am J Physiol 1946; 147:100–114.

89. Dixon M, Jackson DM, Richards IM. The effects of histamine, acetylcholine and 5-hydroxytryptamine on lung mechanics and irritant receptors in the dog. J Physiol 1979; 287:393–403.

90. Mills J, Sellick H, Widdicombe JG. The role of lung irritant receptors in respiratory responses to multiple pulmonary embolism, anaphylaxis and histamine-induced bronchoconstriction. J Physiol 1969; 200:79P–80P.

91. Koller EA, Ferrer P. Studies on the role of the lung deflation reflex. Respir Physiol 1970; 10:172.

92. Kohl J, Koller EA. Stretch receptor activity during irritant-induced tachypnoea in the rabbit. Pflügers Arch 1980; 386:231–237.

93. Paintal AS. Re-evaluation of respiratory reflexes. Q J Exp Physiol 1966; 51:151–163.

94. Richardson PS, Sant'Ambrogio G, Mortola J, Bianconi R. The activity of lung afferent nerves during tracheal occlusion. Respir Physiol 1973; 18:273–283.

95. Miserocchi G, Sant'Ambrogio G. Responses of pulmonary stretch receptors to static pressure inflations. Respir Physiol 1974; 21:77–85.

96. Sant'Ambrogio G, Mortola JP. Behavior of slowly adapting stretch receptors in the extrathoracic trachea of the dog. Respir Physiol 1977; 31:375–385.

97. Widdicombe JG. Receptors in the trachea and bronchi of the cat. J Physiol (Lond) 1954; 123:71–104.

98. Davenport PW, Sant'Ambrogio FB, Sant'Ambrogio G. Adaptation of tracheal stretch receptors. Respir Physiol 1981; 44:339–349.

99. Bartlett D, Sant'Ambrogio G, Wise JCM. Transduction properties of tracheal stretch receptors. J Physiol 1976; 258:421–432.

100. Bradley GW, Scheurmier N. Transduction properties of tracheal stretch receptors in vitro. Respir Physiol 1977; 31:356–375.

101. von During M, Andres KH, Iravani J. The fine structure of the pulmonary stretch receptor in the rat. Z Anat Entwicklungsgesch 1974; 143:215–222.

102. Krauhs JM, Salinas NL. Structure of presumptive stretch receptors in dog trachea. Physiologist 1980; 23:21.

103. Roumy M, Leitner LM. Localization of stretch and deflation receptors in the airways of the rabbit. J Physiol (Paris) 1980; 76:67–70.

104. Camporesi EM, Mortola JP, Sant'Ambrogio F, Sant'Ambrogio G. Topical anesthesia of tracheal receptors. J Appl Physiol 1979; 47:1123–1126.

105. Pisarri TE, Jonzon A, Coleridge HM, Coleridge JC. Intravenous injection of hypertonic NaCl solution stimulates pulmonary C-fibers in dogs. Am J Physiol 1991; 260:H1522–H1530.

106. Thompson-Gorman SL, Fitzgerald RS, Mitzner W. Quantitative evaluation of pulmonary stretch receptor activity during high-frequency ventilation. J Appl Physiol 1992; 72:1101–1110.

107. De Neef KJ, Jansen JR, Versprille A. Developmental morphometry and physiology of the rabbit vagus nerve. Brain Res 1982; 256:265–274.

108. Fisher JT, Sant'Ambrogio G. Location and discharge properties of respiratory vagal afferents in the newborn dog. Respir Physiol 1982; 50:209–220.

109. Farber JP, Fisher JT, Sant'Ambrogio G. Airway receptor activity in the developing opossum. Am J Physiol 1984; 246:R753–R758.

110. Fisher JT, Sant'Ambrogio G. Airway and lung receptors and their reflex effects in the newborn. Pediatr Pulmonol 1985; 1:112–126.

111. Iscoe S, Gordon SP. Chest wall distortion and discharge of pulmonary slowly adapting receptors. J Appl Physiol 1992; 73:1619–1625.

112. Brouillette RT, Thach BT. Control of genioglossus muscle inspiratory activity. J Appl Physiol 1980; 49:801–808.

113. Sica AL, Cohen MI, Donnelly DF, Zhang H. Hypoglossal motoneuron responses to pulmonary and superior laryngeal afferent inputs. Respir Physiol 1984; 56:339–357.

114. Sica AL, Cohen MI, Donnelly DF, Zhang H. Responses of recurrent laryngeal motoneurons to changes of pulmonary afferent inputs. Respir Physiol 1985; 62:153–168.

115. van Lunteren E, Strohl KP, Parker DM, Bruce EN, Van de Graaff WB, Cherniack NS. Phasic volume-related feedback on upper airway muscle activity. J Appl Physiol 1984; 56:730–736.

116. Kuna ST. Inhibition of inspiratory upper airway motoneuron activity by phasic volume feedback. J Appl Physiol 1986; 60:1373–1379.

117. Agostoni E, Cavagna AM, Citterio G. Effects of stretch receptors of bronchi or trachea on genioglossus muscle activity. Respir Physiol 1987; 67:335–345.

118. Green JH, Neil E. The respiratory function of the laryngeal muscles. J Physiol 1955; 129:134–141.

119. Eyzaguirre C, Taylor JR. Respiratory discharge of some vagal motoneurons. J Neurophysiol 1963; 26:61–78.

120. Barillot JC, Bianchi AL. Activity of laryngeal motoneurons during the Hering-Breuer reflex. J Physiol (Paris) 1971; 63:783–792.

121. Bartlett D Jr, Remmers JE, Gautier H. Laryngeal regulation of respiratory airflow. Respir Physiol 1973; 18:194–204.

122. Sherrey JH, Megirian D. Analysis of the respiratory role of intrinsic laryngeal motoneurons of cat. Exp Neurol 1975; 49:456–465.

123. Mann DG, Sasaki CT, Fukuda H, Suzuki M, Hernandez JR. Dilator naris muscle. Ann Otol Rhinol Laryngol 1977; 86:362–370.

124. Green JF, Kaufman MP. Pulmonary afferent control of breathing as end-expiratory lung volume decreases. J Appl Physiol 1990; 68:2186–2194.

125. Davies A, Dixon M, Callanan D, Huszczuk A, Widdicombe JG, Wise JCM. Lung reflexes in rabbits during pulmonary stretch receptor block by sulphur dioxide. Respir Physiol 1978; 34:83–101.

126. Sant'Ambrogio G, Sant'Ambrogio FB, Davies A. Airway receptors in cough. Bull Eur Physiopathol Respir 1984; 20:43–47.

126a. van Lunteren E, Van de Graff WR, Parker DM, Strohl KP, Mitra J, Salamone J, Cherniack NS. Activity of upper airway muscles during augmented breaths. Respir Physiol 1983; 53:87–98.

127. Lee BP, Morton RF, Lee LY. Acute effects of acrolein on breathing: role of vagal bronchopulmonary afferents. J Appl Physiol 1992; 72:1050–1056.

128. Schertel ER, Adams L, Schneider DA, Smith KS, Green JF. Rapid shallow breathing evoked by capsaicin from isolated pulmonary circulation. J Appl Physiol 1986; 61: 1237–1240.

129. Haxhiu MA, van Lunteren E, Deal EC, Cherniack NS. Effect of stimulation of pulmonary C-fiber receptors on canine respiratory muscles. J Appl Physiol 1988; 65:1087–1092.

130. Fleming PJ. Functional immaturity of pulmonary irritant receptors and apnoea in newborn preterm infants. Pediatrics 1978; 61:515–518.

131. Kalia M. Visceral and somatic reflexes produced by J pulmonary receptors in newborn kittens. J Appl Physiol 1976; 41:1–6.

132. Szereda-Przestaszewska M, Widdicombe JG. Reflex effects of chemical irritation of the upper airways on the laryngeal lumen in cats. Respir Physiol 1973; 18: 107–115.

133. Widdicombe JG. Reflexes from the upper respiratory tract. In: Cherniack NS, Widdicombe JG, eds. Handbook of Physiology. Section 3, The Respiratory System. Vol II, Control of Breathing. Bethesda, MD: American Physiological Society, 1986:363–394.

134. Korpas J, Tomori Z. Cough and Other Respiratory Reflexes. Basel: Karger, 1979.

135. Widdicombe JG, Tatar M. Upper airway reflex control. Ann NY Acad Sci 1988; 533:252–261.

136. Tomori Z, Widdicombe JG. Muscular, bronchomotor and cardiovascular reflexes elicited by mechanical stimulation of the respiratory tract. J Physiol 1969; 200:25–49.

137. Miyaoka Y, Takahashi Y, Sato S, Shimada K. Autonomic nervous reflexes in respiration elicited by mechanical stimulation of the velopharyngeal region in rabbits. J Autonom Nerv Syst 1989; 26:177–180.

138. Sumi T. The nature and postnatal development of reflex deglutition in the kitten. Jpn J Physiol 1967; 17:200–210.

139. Harding R, Titchen DA. Oesophageal and diaphragmatic activity during suckling in lambs. J Physiol 1981; 321:317–329.

140. Glogowska M, Stransky A, Widdicombe JG. Reflex control of discharge in motor fibres to the larynx. J Physiol 1974; 239:365–379.

141. Palecek F, Sant'Ambrogio G, Sant'Ambrogio FB, Mathew OP. Reflex responses to capsaicin: intravenous, aerosol, and intratracheal administration. J Appl Physiol 1989; 67:1428–1437.

142. Polacheck J, Strong R, Arens J, Davies C, Metcalf I, Younes M. Phasic vagal influence on inspiratory motor output in anesthetized human subjects. J Appl Physiol 1980; 49:609–619.

143. Basner RC, Simon PM, Schwartzstein RM, Weinberger SE, Weiss JW. Breathing route influences upper airway muscle activity in awake normal adults. J Appl Physiol 1989; 66:1766–1771.

144. Mezzanotte WS, Tangel DJ, White DP. Mechanisms of control of alae nasi muscle activity. J Appl Physiol 1992; 72:925–933.

145. Leiter JC, Daubenspeck JA. Selective reflex activation of the genioglossus in humans. J Appl Physiol 1990; 68:2581–2587.

146. Horner RL, Innes JA, Murphy K, Guz A. Evidence for reflex upper airway dilator muscle activation by sudden negative airway pressure in man. J Physiol 1991; 436: 15–29.

147. Kuna ST, Smickley J. Response to genioglossus muscle activity to nasal occlusion in normal sleeping adults. J Appl Physiol 1988; 64:347–353.

148. Kuna ST, Woodson GE, Sant'Ambrogio G. Effect of laryngeal anesthesia on pulmonary function testing in normal subjects. Am Rev Respir Dis 1988; 137:656–661.

149. Horner RL, Innes JA, Morrel M, Shea SA, Guz A. Effect of sleep on reflex pharyngeal dilator muscle activation by negative airway pressure stimuli in man. Am Rev Respir Dis 1992; 145:A212 (abstract).

150. Wheatley JR, Mezzanotte WS, Tangel DJ, White DP. Influence of sleep on genioglossus muscle activation by negative pressure in normal men. Am Rev Respir Dis 1993; 148:597–605.

151. Carlo WA, Miller MJ, Martin RJ. Differential response of respiratory muscles to airway occlusion in infants. J Appl Physiol 1985; 59:847–852.

152. Thach BT, Menon AP, Schefft GL. Effects of negative upper airway pressure on pattern of breathing in sleeping infants. J Appl Physiol 1989; 66:1599–1605.

153. Issa FG, McNamara SG, Sullivan CE. Arousal responses to airway occlusion in sleeping dogs: comparison of nasal and tracheal occlusion. J Appl Physiol 1987; 62:1832–1836.

154. Basner RC, Ringler J, Garpestad E, Schwartzstein RM, Sparrow D, Winberger SE, Lilly J, Weiss JW. Upper airway anaesthesia delays arousal from airway occlusion induced during human NREM sleep. J Appl Physiol 1992; 73:642–648.

12

Respiratory Control by Diaphragmatic and Respiratory Muscle Afferents

YVES JAMMES

Jean Roche Institute Faculty of Medicine
Marseilles, France

DEXTER F. SPECK

University of Kentucky
Lexington, Kentucky

I. Introduction

Although the vagal pulmonary stretch receptors and the arterial chemoreceptors are generally considered to be the primary respiratory receptors, many other types of receptors can and do affect respiratory control mechanisms. Much of the research on these receptors has been based on more general information obtained from the study of skeletal muscles. This chapter summarizes the available information pertaining to the mechanoreceptors and chemoreceptors of the respiratory musculature, with special emphasis on the diaphragm and intercostal muscles. Attention is focused on the functional roles played by respiratory muscle afferents in daily life and also pathophysiological circumstances, including diaphragmatic fatigue.

II. Respiratory Muscle Afferent Pathways

A. Receptor Types and Physiological Stimuli

General Considerations

Identification of Receptor Types

Recordings of afferent nerve activity are often performed from the distal extremity of a cut nerve trunk, which suppresses any reflex loop. Alternatively, recordings can be made from nerve filaments dissected from an entire nerve trunk, thereby leaving most of reflex loops intact. A more rarely used procedure, which leaves the reflex paths intact, uses glass or tungsten microelectrodes to make extracellular recordings of sensory neurons in the spinal cord ganglia. In all cases, strictly single afferent unit activity is rarely recorded, and the use of window discriminators allows separate analysis of one or two action potentials of different amplitudes. Quantitative analysis involves counting nerve impulses for consecutive fixed epochs of time or computing interspike histograms. When single afferent activity is obtained, subsequent identification of the receptor type is generally based on two successive steps: (1) measurement of conduction velocity in afferent nerve fibers by stimulating the nerve distal to the electrophysiological recording; this allows identification of the afferent fiber as a large or thin myelinated or unmyelinated fiber; (2) classification of afferent units into mechano-, chemo-, or thermoreceptors.

The receptive field of mechanoreceptors is determined by probing the muscle with a blunt rod to ensure that the discharge recorded was initiated in the muscle group studied. However, this test cannot serve to identify selective chemo- or thermosensitive afferents. The spontaneous discharge of mechanoreceptors in respiratory muscles can be easily recorded in phase with the respiratory movements; this is an interesting situation, not easy to reproduce for the study of limb muscle afferents in anesthetized animals. A more specific technique commonly used to activate muscle spindles in limb (Burke et al., 1976; Jammes et al., 1981) or intercostal muscles (Homma et al., 1984) involves the application of high-frequency mechanical vibrations on muscle tendons. The identification of muscle spindles is based on their high frequency of activation (Fig. 1A) and also on recordings of the reflex tonic contractile response of the vibrated muscle, which results from activation of the facilitatory gamma reflex loop.

Identification of chemosensory nerve endings in a muscle is based on the activation of afferent units by endogenous or exogenous chemicals injected into the arterial blood supplying the muscle group studied. Different test agents are well known to activate chemosensory nerve endings in skeletal or respiratory muscles including the diaphragm: there are endogenous substances such as lactic acid solution (Fig. 1B), hyperosmolar NaCl or KCl solutions, and other noxious substances, like bradykinin or serotonin, released during severe muscle contraction, or exogenous chemicals, such as phenyldiguanide (PDG) or capsaicin, an extract from the plant *Capsicum* (Serratrice et al., 1978; Mense, 1986; Jammes et al., 1986a; Graham et al., 1986; Kaufman et al., 1987; Hussain et al., 1990). PDG and capsaicin are commonly used to activate unmyelinated afferent fibers in visceral or somatic tissues, and they have no effect on the activity of muscular proprioceptors. Muscle ischemia is also a potent stimulus for the chemoreceptor activation in limb muscles (Kaufman et al., 1984; Lagier-Tessonnier et al., 1993) or the diaphragm (Graham et al., 1986) (Fig. 1C).

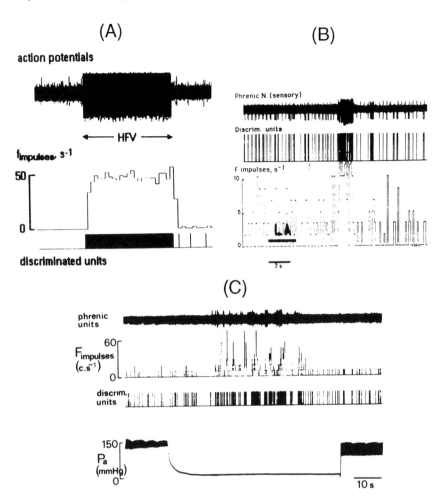

Figure 1 Some test agents used to activate skeletal or respiratory muscle afferents in animals. (A) Response of muscle spindles to high-frequency mechanical vibrations applied to the tendon (raw action potentials, discriminated units, and their counting with a frequency meter); (B) intra-arterial injection of lactic acid solution (LA) markedly activates groups III and mostly IV muscle afferents; (C) thin-fiber muscle afferents are also stimulated by metabolic changes produced by local ischemia.

Warm- or cold-sensitive afferent units are identified in limb muscles from their activation by local temperature variations at the muscle surface.

Functional Categories of Muscle Receptors

Two main functional categories of receptors are described in limb muscles: there are mechanoreceptors or proprioceptors, which are length or force receptors, and chemoreceptors, called metaboreceptors by Kaufman (Kaufman and Rybicki, 1987). The first category includes encapsulated structures, represented by primary (group Ia afferent fibers) and secondary (group II fibers) muscle spindles that detect the magnitude and velocity of change in muscle length and Golgi tendon organs (group Ib fibers) acting as force receptors. All these proprioceptors are slowly adapting receptors, connected to myelinated fibers ranging in diameter between 2 and 20 μm (group I: 12–20 μm; group II: 2–16 μm). The second functional category of muscle receptors includes free nerve endings that terminate in various locations in the muscle, including the interstitium between intrafusal and extrafusal muscle fibers, the arterioles and venules, and also the tendon tissues and capsules of Golgi tendon organs (Stacey, 1969). The afferent supply of these receptors consists of thin myelinated (group III: 1–6 μm) or unmyelinated fibers (group IV: diameter <2 μm). The physiological stimuli of groups III and IV afferents have been extensively studied in limb muscles. Both types of thin-fiber afferents can be activated by a variety of mechanical, chemical, and thermal stimuli, and thus, they act as polymodal receptors (for review, see Mense, 1986). However, group III fibers are mostly activated by local touch, pressure applied locally to muscles, or muscular contraction or stretching, whereas group IV afferents mostly increase their spontaneous discharge rate in response to the aforementioned pain-producing substances and also under the circumstances of reduced muscular oxygen supply (ischemia or hypoxemia), leading to the accumulation of lactic acid in muscle tissue (Kaufman et al., 1984; Mense, 1986; Lagier-Tessonnier et al., 1993). Thus, metaboreceptors detect the changes in glycolytic metabolic path associated with high levels of dynamic or static exercise. Numerous animal studies have also revealed that hypertonic KCl solutions injected into the muscle arteries constitute a potent stimulus for the activation of limb muscle metaboreceptors (Serratrice et al., 1978; Mense, 1986). A gross dysfunction of voltage-operated membrane channels in the muscle sarcolemma, responsible for the outflow of intracellular potassium, may be the consequence of falling intramuscular pH. Some of these test agents that constitute potent stimuli for the activation of thin-fiber limb muscle afferents (lactic acid, ischemia, hypoxemia) are also responsible for a markedly depressed activity of muscle proprioceptors (Matthews, 1972; Lagier-Tessonnier et al., 1993). Groups III and IV muscle afferents are also sensitive to temperature changes in muscle tissues. Mense (1986) describes both warm- and cold-sensitive units in hindlimb muscles.

    With the introduction of electron microscopy it is generally agreed that the number of unmyelinated (group IV) fibers in the sensory component of nerves supplying limb muscles is almost two-fold higher than large myelinated fibers (groups I and II). The small myelinated fibers (group III) constitute a relatively small contingent of muscle afferents (Stacey, 1969).

Respiratory Muscle Innervation

Diaphragmatic Innervation

This has been detailed in a recent well-documented review by Hussain and Roussos (1994). The existence of a sensory diaphragmatic innervation was detected from clinical observations as early as 1800. The identification of both afferent and efferent fibers in the cat phrenic nerve was performed by Fergusson in 1891, and numerous studies have been devoted to the analysis of phrenic fiber composition in cats, dogs, rats, rabbits, and humans. In most of the studied species, including humans, the phrenic nerve contains two populations of myelinated fibers (bimodal distribution); the majority of them (around 84%) have diameters ranging from 9 to 12 μm, whereas less than 16% of the myelinated fibers have diameters less than 6 μM (Duron, 1981). A large number of unmyelinated fibers have been reported in the cat phrenic nerve by Duron and Condamin (1970), who used electron microscopy. In their studies more than 70% of the nerve fibers were unmyelinated, with diameters ranging between 0.1 and 1.4 μm. However, in the aforementioned observations, myelinated as well as unmyelinated fibers may be sensory or motor. Only the studies by Hinsey et al. (1939) in the cat phrenic nerve and by Langford and Schmidt (1983) in the rat phrenic nerve have estimated, after degeneration of the motor component, that unmyelinated fibers constituted more than 50% of the afferent fibers traveling through the dorsal roots. Hinsey and co-workers also reported that the myelinated sensory component amounts to about 10% of the total myelinated population. Also in cats, when phrenic nerves were examined 35–40 days after excision of the 3rd to 6th spinal cervical ganglia and compared to entire nerve samples, Duron (1981) estimated that 20–30% of total myelinated fibers appear to be sensory and that most of their axons have diameters between 2 and 6 μm. The recent study by Rose et al. (1990) used retrograde labeling of dorsal root ganglia with horseradish peroxidase to estimate that unmyelinated fibers constitute 67% of the phrenic afferents.

Histological identification of diaphragmatic receptors has been performed in cats and humans. In cats, Hinsey (1939) could not identify any muscle spindle in the diaphragm, and Duron (1981) counted a few muscle spindles, exclusively located in the crural portion. However, many more spindles are probably present in the human diaphragm (Winckler and Delaloye, 1957). Golgi tendon organs, which consist of a fascia of tendinous fibers attached at one end to a large number of muscle fibers, are located at the junction of the muscle and its tendon. Their afferent fibers seem to constitute the major component of the large myelinated sensory phrenic fibers, with a conduction velocity ranging between 10 and 60 m/sec (Jammes et al., 1986a; Jammes and Balzamo, 1992). The diaphragm also contains pacinian and paciniform corpuscules, which consist of a nerve ending surrounded by a lamellated capsula. They are located adjacent to the Golgi tendon organs and distributed throughout the diaphragm. These mechanoreceptors are rapidly adapting receptors (Corda et al., 1965), and they may be connected to group III afferent fibers. A particular type of receptors with characteristic terminal arborization has been described by Dogiel (1902) in the diaphragm, but the stimuli as well as the functional importance of Dogiel's corpuscules has not been yet identified. Finally, the diaphragm of cats contains numerous metaboreceptors connected to groups III and IV fibers. The conduction velocity of group III phrenic fibers ranges between 2 and 11 m/sec (Speck and Revelette, 1987; Jammes and Balzamo, 1992) and that of group IV phrenic afferents between 0.5 and 1.3 m/sec (Jammes et al., 1986a; Jammes and Balzamo, 1992).

The stimuli and circumstances for activation of these afferents are the same as those previously described for limb muscle afferents. In addition, it has been demonstrated in cats that electrically induced diaphragm fatigue elicits a marked increase in the spontaneous activity of metaboreceptors, which develops in parallel to depressed proprioceptor discharge (Jammes and Balzamo, 1992). Other test agents used to activate thin-fiber phrenic afferents, such as intra-arterial lactic acid injection or diaphragmatic ischemia, also markedly decrease the activity of proprioceptive phrenic afferents activated by the spontaneous diaphragmatic contractions (Graham et al., 1986; Jammes and Balzamo, 1992). The decreased firing rate of diaphragmatic mechanoreceptors in these situations may result simply from reduced changes in muscle tension due to the reflex inhibition of phrenic motor drive. However, depressed proprioceptor activity persisted when the motor drive to the diaphragm (Graham et al., 1986) or hindlimb muscles (Zimmerman and Grossie, 1963; Matthews, 1972; Lagier-Tessonnier et al., 1993) was unchanged or absent. The mechanisms of the inhibitory effects on muscle mechanoreceptors exerted by physiological stimulation of metaboreceptors are yet unknown. In a first approximation, one may speculate that the common denominator is the fall in muscle pH, produced by lactic acid injection and associated with muscle fatigue or reduced oxygen supply to a contracting muscle. However, the opposite effects elicited by muscle ischemia or hypoxemia on mechano- and metaboreceptors are also reported in noncontracting hindlimb muscles (Lagier-Tessonnier et al., 1993), i.e., under the circumstances where phosphorus nuclear magnetic resonance studies were unable to demonstrate any significant change in muscle pH (Sahlin and Katz, 1989). Unpublished personal observations on changes in limb muscle blood flow associated with lactic acid injection or general hypoxemia suggest that the mechanisms for reduced mechanoreceptor activity could be the fall in arterial blood pressure and thus in interstitial pressure in muscle tissues.

Sensory Innervation of Intercostal Muscles

The sensory innervation of the intercostal musculature includes most, if not all, of the receptor types associated with the limb muscles. The various receptors and their specific activation have been reviewed extensively by Duron (1981) and Shannon (1986). Histologically, the mechanoreceptors include both primary and secondary muscle spindles, Golgi tendon organs, and costovertebral joint receptors. In the cat the secondary muscle spindle endings are the most plentiful (Barker, 1962), with the density of these receptors being greatest in the external intercostal muscles (Jung Caillol and Duron, 1976). The distribution of spindles within the respiratory muscles decreases markedly in the caudal interspaces (Duron, 1981). This distribution is inversely correlated with the degree of phasic respiratory activity in these muscles, suggesting that the receptors may be more important in postural reflexes than in respiratory ones.

The reflexes associated with the individual receptor types have been studied by using "physiological" stimuli such as mechanical stimulation, chest compression, rib vibration, lung inflation, and loading (see review by Shannon, 1986). Because of the complexity of the respiratory pump and the extensive interactions between the movements of the different muscle groups, it has been difficult to determine the specific receptors implicated in the reflexes initiated by these manipulations. Many studies have utilized dorsal root sections and/or spinal transections to ascertain the origin of the afferents. Several studies indicate that removal of the intercostal afferents by thoracic dorsal rhizotomies may have little (Shannon, 1977) or no (Speck and Webber, 1979) effect on respiratory pattern. However, since supraspinal reflexes are easily suppressed by anesthesia (Speck and Webber, 1981), these studies may not be applicable to the conscious animal.

Most studies of the intercostal afferents have relied on direct electrical stimulation of the intercostal nerves to demonstrate the potential reflexes that can be evoked. These reflexes can be initiated by low-threshold stimulation, suggesting that they are mediated primarily through large myelinated afferents. However, there are many unmyelinated fibers (0.2–1.5 μm diameter) in the intercostal nerve. These fibers have been reported to be associated with free nerve endings in the muscle, skin, and pleura (Duron, 1981).

Sensory Supply to the Abdominal Muscles

Information concerning the sensory innervation of abdominal muscles is sparse. The knowledge of proprioceptors, namely muscle spindles, in these muscles is based on the recordings of a tonic contraction, i.e., electromyographic (EMG) activation, in rectus abdominis muscle in response to high-frequency mechanical stimulation applied to the linea alba (Jammes et al., 1983a), a procedure commonly used to activate muscle spindles in limb muscles and the chest wall. The identification of metaboreceptors in abdominal muscles, based on their specific activation by endogenous or exogenous chemicals, has not yet been performed.

However, it is amazing that this category of receptors, found in all skeletal muscles studied, was absent in abdominal muscle groups.

B. Central Projections and Reflex Actions

The respiratory muscle afferents project to the spinal cord and different supraspinal structures such as the brainstem, the cerebellum, and the cerebral sensory cortex. Numerous studies have been devoted to these anatomical projections. For more details see the general reviews by Duron (1981), Shannon (1986), and Hussain and Roussos (1994). Most data were deduced from the responses of central neurons to single or repetitive electrical stimuli applied to the central end of the intercostal, abdominal, or phrenic nerves. Thus, the assessment of spinal and supraspinal projections of respiratory muscle afferent was based either on intra- and mostly extracellular recordings of evoked neuronal activities or, more simply, on the analysis of phrenic motor output changes in response to peripheral nerve stimulation; any changes in the ventilatory timing [inspiratory (T_I) and/or expiratory (T_E) duration and duty cycle, i.e., the T_I/T_{tot} ratio] were then related to the influences of muscle afferents on the central structures governing the breathing rhythm. In some instances, the use of mechanical or chemical test agents, well known to activate a specific category of muscular receptors, allows examination of the role of a particular type of sensory ending in the observed response.

Phrenic Afferents

In the cat the phrenic afferents ascend and also descend in the dorsal spinal cord column at the level of the 4th and 5th cervical segments before terminating in laminae I–IV of the dorsal horns (Duron, 1981) where they influence the activity of ipsi- and contralateral phrenic motoneurons (Gill and Kuno, 1963). However, this afferent path concerns probably only that of large myelinated sensory fibers (proprioceptive afferents), and there is some evidence that the group I and II afferent fibers project through the dorsal columns (Marlot et al., 1985). Indeed, thin fibers carrying noxious and local metabolic informations from skeletal muscles ascend in the lateral and ventrolateral columns in the spinal cord. In addition to the main entry of thin-fiber phrenic afferents in the spinal cord through the dorsal roots, Langford et al. (1983) have shown that few unmyelinated phrenic fibers enter the spinal cord through the ventral roots. The functional study by Revelette et al. (1988) in dogs has also confirmed that ventral roots may be one route of spinal cord entry for the responses to thin-fiber phrenic afferent stimulation. A small number of large-fiber phrenic afferents may enter the cervical spinal cord through the ventral roots (Duron, 1981). Phrenic afferents project also to supraspinal structures such as brainstem respiratory neurons in the dorsal and ventral respiratory groups (Macron et al., 1985, 1986; Speck and Revelette, 1987).

Based on the latencies of respiratory neuron activation in response to single shock stimulation of the phrenic nerve, Speck (1987) has proposed that group III and perhaps also IV phrenic afferents project contralaterally on phrenic motoneurons through brainstem relays. Additional brainstem projection sites include the lateral reticular nucleus (Macron et al., 1985), the external cuneate nucleus (Marlot et al., 1985), and the Bötzinger complex (Speck, 1989). Projections of phrenic afferents on the cerebellum are also described (Marlot et al., 1984), but the persistence of the phrenic motor response to contralateral stimulation of phrenic afferents after decerebration and decerebellation suggests that the cerebellum is of negligible importance in this reflex (Speck and Revelette, 1987). Phrenic afferent projections to the sensorimotor cortex have also been demonstrated (Davenport et al., 1985; Balzamo et al., 1992).

Gill and Kuno (1963) first recorded inhibitory postsynaptic potentials in phrenic motoneurons in response to dorsal root stimulation in cats. Speck (1987) has elegantly demonstrated in decerebrated or C-2 spinalized cats that the inhibitory ipsilateral phrenic response is due to spinal cord circuits (short latency: 5 msec), whereas the contralateral inhibitory phrenic response is abolished after C-2 spinal section, thus involving supraspinal connections (long latency: 20 msec) (Fig. 2). Speck (1989) has also shown that pathways important in producing the phrenic-to-phrenic inhibitory reflex pass through the region of the Bötzinger complex, although there does not seem to be a synaptic connection in this area. In the above studies the stimuli were single or double electric pulses. When repetitive phrenic nerve stimulation was applied for a few consecutive inspiratory discharges or for 1-min, the ventilatory effects of phrenic afferent fiber stimulation were more complex. A triggering inspiratory effect ("on-switch" mechanism) by phrenic afferents is shown when brief (2 sec), repetitive (80 Hz) phrenic nerve stimulation is delivered early in the expiratory period (Marlot et al., 1987; Jammes, 1988a) (Fig. 3). A 30-sec train of rectangular shocks delivered to one or both phrenic nerves induced immediate changes in breathing pattern, characterized by tachypnea, a marked shortening in the firing time of motor phrenic discharge (T_{phr}) with concomitant decline in the T_{phr}/T_{tot} ratio, and reduction in the peak firing rate of motoneurons (Jammes et al., 1986a). When repetitive stimulation of the phrenic nerve was maintained for 1 min, Marlot et al. (1987) reported a diphasic response: a short-term inhibitory response for a few breaths, which was suppressed in animals pretreated with bicuculline (an antagonist of $GABA_A$ neurotransmission), followed by a long-term excitation beginning after 15–20 sec of nerve stimulation. The aforementioned data concern nonselective electrical activation of all phrenic afferents, including the thin-fiber ones.

Some authors have tried to preferentially activate group III and IV fibers using either appropriate parameters for electric shocks, high-voltage stimulation under cold block of conduction in large myelinated fibers, or the chemical activation of metaboreceptors by specific test agents. Road et al. (1987) and Ward

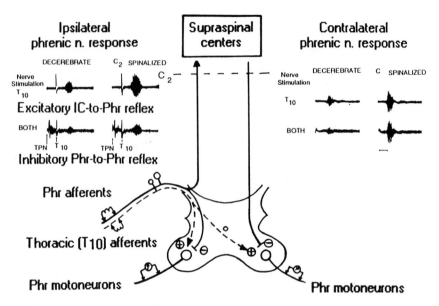

Figure 2 Synaptic connections between thoracic (T-10) and phrenic afferents and the phrenic motoneurons deduced from data obtained by Speck (1987) in decerebrate or C-2 spinalized cats. Excitatory intercostal-to-phrenic responses are found ipsilaterally and contralaterally. Since these responses are exaggerated in C-2 spinalized animals, supraspinal synaptic connections are not obligatory. However, ipsilateral and contralateral inhibitory phrenic-to-phrenic responses involve the participation of supraspinal centers because they are attenuated or abolished after C-2 spinal cord section. The persistence of some ipsilateral phrenic-to-phrenic inhibition suggests that a segmental pathway may be involved in this reflex.

et al. (1992a,b) found an excitatory effect on the rate and depth of breathing, whereas Jammes et al. (1986a) observed a tachypnea with reduced firing rate of phrenic motoneurons. These discrepancies possibly could be attributed to the difficulty in achieving selective electrical stimulation of thin fibers, since the simultaneous activation of both categories of muscle receptors (proprio- and metaboreceptors) could exert some antagonistic central influences. However, most of these observations, including ours, may be irrelevant. Indeed, repetitive high-intensity electrical stimulation of any somatic nerve, including phrenic, intercostal, limb muscle, and cutaneous nerves (personal observations), elicits hyperventilation, which may be attributed to nonspecific painful stimuli. Revelette et al. (1988) have reported that capsaicin injection into the phrenic artery of dogs induced tonic diaphragmatic contractions within 1 or 2 sec. This response, interpreted as an excitatory effect on phrenic motoneurons exerted by the activation of group III and/or IV phrenic sensory fibers, was abolished after surgical

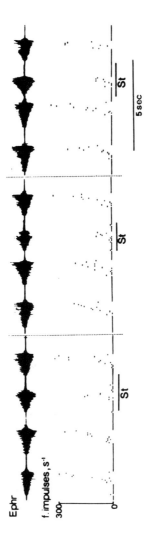

Figure 3 Repetitive electrical stimulation of phrenic afferents reduces the contralateral motor phrenic activity (decreased impulse rate) but also triggers inspiration. Marked triggering effect is observed when the stimulation begins early during the expiratory period.

destruction of the cervical spinal cord but persisted after cervical dorsal rhizotomy or C-2 spinal cord transection. However, there is a marked contradiction between the very short latency of the capsaicin-induced diaphragmatic response and the minimal 5-sec delay needed to activate free muscle endings in the diaphragm (Graham et al., 1986; Jammes et al., 1986a; Jammes and Balzamo, 1992). Hussain et al. (1990) reported a 7-sec latency to increased peak EMG in different respiratory muscles, including the diaphragm, after capsaicin injection into the phrenic artery of an in situ isolated and innervated hemidiaphragm. These facilitatory phrenic-to-phrenic and phrenic-to-intercostal reflexes associated with a weak shortening of inspiratory and expiratory durations could be attributed to the chemical activation of diaphragmatic metaboreceptors. However, increased discharge frequency of these receptors with diaphragmatic fatigue, a more realistic circumstance, does not increase, but reduces, the breathing rhythm (see Section III.D).

Chest Wall Muscle Afferents

Afferents of primary muscle spindle endings in inspiratory and expiratory intercostal muscles monosynaptically excite the homonymous motoneurons of the same spinal segment and also of adjacent segments (Sears, 1964; Kirkwood and Sears, 1982). Unlike group Ia afferents of antagonistic limb muscles, afferents from intercostal muscles do not inhibit the heteronymous motoneurons (Shannon, 1986). Instead, the intercostal afferents can evoke phrenic excitation in the spinal cat (Downman, 1955; Decima and von Euler, 1969; Remmers, 1973). Golgi tendon organ afferents (group Ib fibers) from intercostal muscles exert an inhibitory effect on their respective homonymous motoneurons of the same thoracic segment. The effects of intercostal muscle proprioceptive afferents on medullary inspiratory and expiratory neurons are more controversial. Two recent studies in cats by Shannon and colleagues (Bolser et al., 1987; Shannon et al., 1987) demonstrate that intercostal muscle spindle endings have no direct influence on medullary neurons, while external and internal intercostal tendon organs exert an inhibitory effect on all inspiratory neurons and a population of expiratory neurons driving intercostal and abdominal muscles, constituting the arm of an intercostal-to-abdominal reflex loop.

Intercostal-to-phrenic reflexes include both spinal facilitatory and supraspinal inhibitory effects. Afferents of secondary muscle spindle endings (group II fibers) and Golgi tendon organs in intercostal muscles of the caudal thoracic segments (T-9 to T-12) project to phrenic motoneurons. These proprioceptive afferents are involved in a facilitatory intercostal-to-phrenic reflex. Some studies reviewed by Shannon (1986) have also suggested the existence of an inhibitory intercostal-to-phrenic reflex elicited by electrical stimulation of the intercostal nerves, chest compression in vagotomized animals, or sustained high-frequency mechanical vibrations in the lower thoracic regions. However, in a recent work

Bolser et al. (1988) have shown that costovertebral joint mechanoreceptors mostly contribute to the inspiratory inhibitory effect of intercostal muscle/rib vibration. The presence and involvement of thoracic interneurons within these reflexes has recently been reviewed (Monteau and Hilaire, 1991). These interneurons are located primarily dorsal to the intercostal motor nuclei (Kirkwood et al., 1988) and appear to receive appreciable input from both respiratory and nonrespiratory sources. In addition to central respiratory drive, many of these neurons respond to segmental and supraspinal afferent input linked to respiration, posture, and proprioception (Monteau and Hilaire, 1991).

There is limited information concerning the central projections of the intercostal afferents. Afferent activity in phase with breathing has been recorded in the dorsal columns of the cat (Yamamoto et al., 1960). This finding is supported by the observation that lesioning of the dorsal columns abolishes the inspiratory inhibitory effects of intercostal nerve stimulation (Remmers and Tsiaras, 1973). At supraspinal levels, the intercostal afferents are known to provide input to the cerebellum (Coffee et al., 1971; Baker et al., 1993), the external cuneate nucleus, the Bötzinger complex (Shannon et al., 1983), and the dorsal, ventral, and pontine respiratory groups (Shannon et al., 1987; Shannon, 1986). These influences have been demonstrated primarily with extracellular recording techniques, which have not determined whether these are direct or multisynaptic projections. Despite the presence of a strong intercostal input to the cerebellum, the inhibitory effects of these afferents on inspiratory activity persist in animals that are decerebrated and decerebellated (Speck and Webber, 1982). Similarly, ablation studies have demonstrated that the cuneate nuclei are not essential for the inhibitory intercostal-to-phrenic reflex (Shannon et al., 1982). Although intercostal nerve stimulation can influence the discharge of pontine respiratory-modulated neurons, the long latency for their activation suggests that they are not part of the circuitry involved in the inhibitory reflex (Shannon and Lindsey, 1983). This conclusion is supported by the persistence of the intercostal-to-phrenic inhibition after lesions of the pontine respiratory group (Remmers and Marttila, 1975; Karius et al., 1991).

Abdominal Muscle Afferents

As for the chest wall muscles, afferents from the abdominal muscle groups enter the spinal cord through the dorsal roots at lower thoracic segments (T-9 to T-12) (Shannon, 1986). Proprioceptive afferents project onto homonymous alpha motoneurons, as assessed by the facilitatory stretch reflex elicited in abdominal muscles of rabbits and dogs (Bishop, 1964; Jammes et al., 1983a). However, data concerning abdominal-to-phrenic reflexes and supraspinal influences are contradictory. Compression of the abdominal wall in vagotomized mammals does not induce changes in the ventilatory timing (D'Angelo et al., 1976). Shannon (1980) and then Shannon and Freeman (1981) reported that stimulation of afferent fibers from abdominal muscles reflexly facilitates phrenic motor activity via spinal and supraspinal pathways. On the other hand, other authors observed that electrical stimulation of group I afferent fibers in the muscle branch of the lateral intercostal nerve, which innervates the external oblique muscle (Sears, 1964), or intense mechanical activation of abdominal muscle mechanoreceptors with tetanic contraction (Jammes et al., 1983a) reduced the phrenic motor discharge and the activity of inspiratory neurons of dorsal and ventral respiratory groups. It was tempting to attribute these inhibitory influences to the activation of Golgi tendon organs in the abdominal wall. However, an inspiratory depression was also recorded during the selective mechanical activation of muscle spindles in the rectus abdominis (Jammes et al., 1983a). Group I afferent fibers from abdominal muscles inhibit the activity of brainstem expiratory neurones (Shannon, 1986), and this results in shortening of the expiratory period, also observed with high-frequency mechanical stimulation of muscle spindles (Jammes et al., 1983a).

The neurotransmitters and neurochemical modulators associated with respiratory muscle sensory pathways are widely documented in Chapter 4.

C. Spontaneous Activities in Respiratory Muscle Afferents

Phrenic Afferents

Diaphragmatic proprioceptors have high-frequency spontaneous discharge. Their afferent impulses are in phase with respiration; phasic phrenic afferent activities during the inspiratory phase of the breathing cycle have the highest firing frequency, which may reach 150 impulses per second (Duron, 1981; Jammes and Balzamo, 1992; Balzamo et al., 1992); i.e., it was in the range of that measured for limb muscle spindles and Golgi tendon organs (Matthews, 1972). There are some "active" spindles, which receive gamma motor drive parallel to the alpha motor command to extrafusal muscle fibers (Corda et al., 1965; Duron and Jung-Caillol, 1973), and mostly low-excitation threshold Golgi receptors, activated by the tendon stretching accompanying each diaphragmatic contraction (Jammes et al., 1986a; Revelette et al., 1992). However, the peak discharge rate of Golgi receptors is less than that of spindles (Jammes et al., 1986a) (Fig. 4). These afferent units discharging in phase with diaphragmatic contraction constitute the main phasically active sensory component: Corda et al. (1965): 54/85 afferent units; Jammes et al. (1986a): 42/50; Graham et al. (1986): 19/25. Phrenic afferent units with peak discharge during the expiratory phase, i.e., diaphragmatic relaxation, have lower firing frequency (around 50 impulses/sec) (Duron and Jung-Caillol, 1973; Jammes and Balzamo, 1992). They most likely correspond to "passive" muscle spindles, which do not depend on the gamma motor control (Corda et al., 1965; Duron, 1981). They are less numerous than high-frequency units activated during inspiration: Corda et al. (1965): 10/85; Jammes et al. (1986a): 8/50; Graham et al. (1986): 6/25.

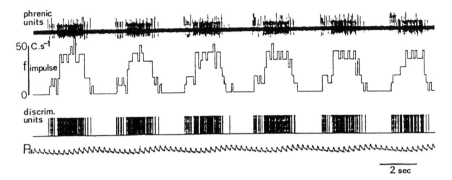

Figure 4 Typical recording of phasically active phrenic afferent units. These units are strictly activated during diaphragmatic contractions (inspiration). Because their peak firing rate is less than that measured for muscle spindles and because of their strong activation with end-expiratory tracheal occlusion, these afferent activities are probably those of Golgi tendon organs (unpublished data).

In contrast to the high-frequency, phasically active diaphragmatic proprioceptors, the thin-fiber afferents (groups III and IV) have low-frequency, erratic discharge patterns. However, the value of their tonic firing rate depends on the experimental circumstances: a very low rate, i.e., in the range of 1–3 impulses/sec, was measured in cats artificially ventilated with open chest (Jammes et al., 1986a; Jammes and Balzamo, 1992), while it was significantly higher (14 ± 3 impulses/sec) when cats breathed spontaneously (Graham et al., 1986). Such marked quantitative differences within the spontaneous discharge rate of diaphragmatic metaboreceptors are reminiscent of the observations on the changes in the spontaneous tonic activity of vagal bronchopulmonary C-fibers. Indeed, the firing rate of these polymodal receptors in the airways and alveoli is multiplied by 5 when the physiological conditions of expired CO_2 content, temperature, and tidal volume are restored (Delpierre et al., 1981), explaining the major role played by these vagal afferents in the control of the bronchoconstrictor vagal tone (Jammes and Mei, 1979). Thus, it is tempting to speculate that in daily life tonically active diaphragmatic metaboreceptors may participate in the control of ventilation and other associated functions such as the bronchomotor tone regulation (see Section III.A).

Intercostal Afferents

Recordings of afferent discharges from dorsal root filaments have indicated the presence of Golgi tendon organs and both primary and secondary muscle spindle afferents (Critchlow and Euler, 1963; Euler and Peretti, 1966). The discharges of these receptors are usually modulated by the respiratory activity, although they can have a significant tonic component with baseline discharge rates in excess of 30 impulses/sec. Based on these activity patterns and the inverse correlation between spindle distribution and respiratory activity, Duron (1973) has suggested that the major role for these afferents is in postural control, with very little influence on eupneic respiratory activity. Maximal discharge of intercostal muscle spindles occurs during the active phase of respiration; therefore, the receptors in the external intercostals generally reach their maxima during inspiration while the internal intercostal receptors are at their lowest level of activity. In addition to respiratory modulations, some variability in discharge pattern is correlated with heart rate in the muscle spindles located more ventrally (Critchlow and Euler, 1963). Tracheal occlusion leads to an initial increase in the firing of muscle spindles in the inspiratory muscles. This initial increase is followed by a marked decrease, which may be due a mismatch of the alpha and gamma motor drives to these muscles (Critchlow and Euler, 1963).

Abdominal Muscle Afferents

Abdominal respiratory muscles are not ordinarily active during eupnea, especially in anesthetized supine animals. Thus the role played by their proprioceptive afferents in the control of the eupneic ventilation seems doubtful. Since some of these afferents do involve pathways similar to the intercostal nerve afferents and send collaterals to the dorsal and ventral respiratory groups (Shannon et al., 1982), it is conceivable that they may play a more important role as ventilation increases.

III. Functional Roles of Respiratory Muscle Afferents

A. Control of Eupneic Breathing in Daily Life

Eupneic breathing results from two related functions: the ventilatory control (amplitude and timing of tidal breaths) and the control of bronchomotor tone, which governs the airway caliber and the distribution of alveolar gases. Respiratory muscle afferents, especially diaphragmatic afferents, influence these two motor drives.

Phrenic Afferents

In 1960, Nathan and Sears described the development of diaphragmatic paresis in patients who had undergone therapeutic section of the cervical dorsal roots, i.e., after diaphragmatic deafferentation. These observations suggest a major role for phrenic afferents in the eupneic breathing control of humans. Since then, few animal studies have been devoted to the functional role played by the spontaneous activity of diaphragmatic afferents. In rabbits, Dolivo (1952) reported that selective anodal blockade of conduction in myelinated phrenic fibers lengthened the inspiratory time. This was studied in spontaneously breathing animals, and it was found that the consequences of diaphragmatic paralysis on chest wall mechanics and respiratory gas exchange may influence the ventilatory control. However, we reported similar observations in cats under artificial ventilation and constant blood gases (Jammes et al., 1986a; Jammes and Balzamo, 1992). These animals presented spontaneous diaphragmatic contractions with the chest largely open, and their spinal cord was sectioned at C-8 level to suppress thoracic and abdominal muscle afferents. Then, cold block at 6°C of large phrenic fibers (Jammes et al., 1986a) or bilateral phrenic nerve section (diaphragmatic deafferentation) (Jammes and Balzamo, 1992) significantly prolonged the motor phrenic discharge, reduced the respiratory frequency, and also markedly modified the recruitment strategy of phrenic motoneurons, enhancing high-frequency power toward the end of inspiration. Compared to the effects of cold block of large phrenic fibers, procaine block of thin phrenic fibers had no effect (Fig. 5). In a recent study, Teitelbaum et al. (1993) corroborated these observations in an in situ vascularly isolated and innervated left diaphragm in dogs. They showed that selective paralysis of the left hemidiaphragm by injection of a neuromuscular junction blocker increased the peak integrated EMG activity in the right hemidiaphragm as well as in parasternal and alae nasi muscles. This was associated with significant increase in breathing frequency. The response to left hemidiaphragmatic paralysis disappeared after section of the left phrenic nerve and also after the left isolated diaphragm was placed in a flaccid position to suppress the spontaneous rhythmic discharge of muscle spindles and mostly Golgi tendon organs, numerous in the diaphragm. Based on these observations, it is tempting to speculate that the spontaneous high-frequency phasic discharge of diaphragmatic proprioceptors, active during eupneic breathing, is responsible for a phrenic-to-phrenic reflex loop, which informs the phrenic motoneurons and also the respiratory centers on the length-tension relationship in the diaphragm. These reflex influences are inhibitory.

In addition, thin-fiber phrenic afferents exert inhibitory influences on the vagal motor control of the airway smooth muscle in dogs (McCallister et al., 1986). This was observed in dogs where repetitive high-voltage electrical stimulation of all phrenic afferents decreased lung resistance, but low-voltage stimulation of large myelinated phrenic fibers had little effect. This bronchomotor effect was abolished by atropine, and thus, it was interpreted as a withdrawal of the tonic cholinergic vagal motor drive to the airways. Similar observations have been reported by Wilson et al. (1992) in the same species. The group IV unmyelinated phrenic afferents influence the neural networks involved in bronchomotor control just like the vagal C-fibers from the lungs and airways (see review by Jammes, 1988b). It has already been mentioned that their activation by metabolic changes in

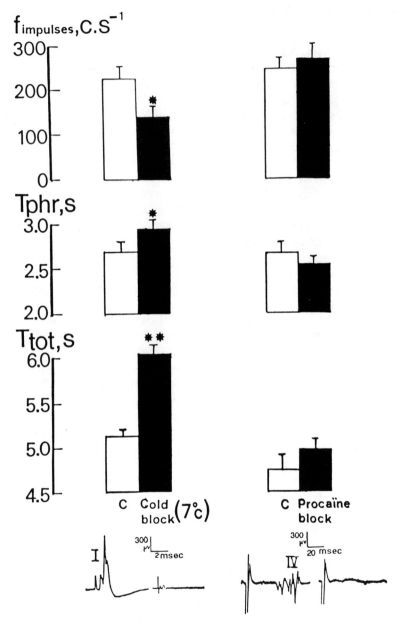

Figure 5 Changes in spontaneous control motor phrenic activity (impulse rate, phrenic discharge time, and total respiratory period) induced by distal cold block at 7°C of large myelinated phrenic fibers (group I) or procaine block of thin fibers (group IV) in cats under artificial ventilation. In either case, selective suppression of nervous conduction was assessed on electrically evoked potentials. (Redrawn from data reported by Jammes et al., 1986a.)

muscle tissues also influences the respiratory neuronal discharge. One may postulate that the tonic discharge of thin-fiber phrenic afferents may balance the facilitatory influences on the bronchoconstrictor vagal tone exerted by bronchopulmonary vagal afferents. This central interaction may be present in daily life and mostly during increased respiratory muscle work in response to loaded ventilation with asthmatic attack. Then, enhanced tonic discharge of groups III and IV phrenic afferents may constitute a protective mechanism that holds back the bronchoconstriction. Observations by Hussain et al. (1990, 1991) in dogs demonstrate that the chemical activation of groups III and IV phrenic afferents by intra-arterial injection of capsaicin in an isolated innervated diaphragm increases the systemic arterial pressure with associated tachycardia and also reduces the phrenic blood flow. In addition, activation of thin-fiber phrenic afferents redistributes blood flow away from the intestinal and renal vascular beds toward the carotid vascular bed, i.e., the brain circulation (Hussain et al., 1991). However, these data were obtained in anesthetized animals, and thus, the redistribution of thoracic blood flow toward exercising limb muscles could not be assessed. This "pressor" reflex is similar to that attributed to the activation of groups III and IV limb muscle afferents during static exercise performed at high levels of force (Kaufman et al., 1988), but Hussain et al. (1991) have reported that cardiovascular reflex from thin-fiber phrenic afferents seems less potent than that from limb muscle afferents.

Chest Wall and Abdominal Muscle Afferents

The role of thoracic wall afferents in the control of respiration has been examined by comparing the respiratory pattern before and after section of the thoracic dorsal roots. Interpretation of these experiments is often difficult because many different types of afferents are eliminated by the rhizotomies. Data concerning the role played by the rib cage afferents during quiet breathing are often contradictory. Results from several laboratories show a slight decrease in tidal volume and an increase in frequency (Gautier, 1973; Shannon, 1977), whereas others report increased integrated diaphragmatic activity with no change in ventilatory timing (Jammes et al., 1986b). Other studies have reported no change in respiratory pattern after thoracic dorsal rhizotomy (Speck and Webber, 1979; Stella, 1938). All these studies support the conclusion that thoracic afferents play little role in regulating the breathing pattern in the anesthetized cat. Discrepancies between data obtained in the different animal species and protocols may result from the fact that central integration of somatic reflexes depends on the depth and type of anesthesia (Speck and Webber, 1981). Thus, the ventilatory effects of C-8 spinal cord section were found negligible in cats under pentobarbital sodium anesthesia, a powerful depressor of spinal reflexes, whereas they were very pronounced under chloralose-ethyl carbamate, which facilitates reflex actions (Jammes et al., 1986b). In the latter case, the recruitment of phrenic motoneurons is facilitated after C-8 spinal cord section. This unmasks inhibitory influences exerted by abdominal and more probably thoracic afferents on phrenic motoneurons and perhaps also central respiratory neurons. Another important point is that chest wall and vagal afferents exert interdependent influences on the recruitment and firing rate of phrenic motoneurons; indeed, C-8 spinal section induces reverse changes in the amplitude of breathing depending on whether vagal afferents are present or suppressed (Jammes et al., 1986b).

The overall conclusion drawn from the results on spinal cord section or thoracic dorsal rhizotomies is that chest wall information is not a major factor determining the eupneic breathing pattern in anesthetized animals. However, this does not eliminate a role for these somatic afferents in the control of eupnea in conscious and mostly upright standing individuals where postural adaptations may prevail. Based on the results of thoracic dorsal rhizotomies in conscious goats, Mitchell (1990) has proposed that these afferents may also be very important in influencing the gain of ventilatory adaptations to exercise. It has been postulated that the increased ventilatory drive in exercise is associated with the coactivation of alpha and gamma motoneurons, which in turn leads to an increased proprioceptor feedback from muscle spindles. Activation of these receptors could depolarize the intercostal motoneurons and thereby increase the effectiveness of the descending respiratory command signal.

B. Role in Compensation for Posture Changes

Changes in the operating length of the respiratory muscles, namely the diaphragm, occur during the transition from decubitus to sitting to upright posture in humans and also quadrupeds. Consequently, the muscle fiber resting length must be shorter, and thus, the pressure-generating ability of the muscle should decrease. If there is no compensatory reflex increase in neural drive to the respiratory muscles, the amplitude of breathing will fall. In fact, two strategies can potentially compensate for a reduced efficacy of the diaphragm in the sitting or upright posture: one strategy is to increase the neural drive to inspiratory muscles, and the other strategy involves an activation of abdominal muscles, maximizing the diaphragmatic end-expiratory length (Banzett and Mead, 1985). Since the princeps work by Fleisch et al. (1946), numerous studies have been devoted to the description of proprioceptive reflex loops within the diaphragm and intercostal or abdominal muscles. These elementary reflex actions have already been described, and the following sections will be focused on their possible intervention with postural changes in daily life.

Postural Adaptations of Diaphragmatic Contraction

The existence of a diaphragmatic autogenic load compensation reflex has been controversial for some time. Animal studies by Sant'Ambrogio et al. (1962), Sant'Ambrogio and Widdicombe (1965), Corda et al. (1965), von Euler (1966), and Brancatisano et al. (1989) have reported no reflex change in motor phrenic activity in response to diaphragmatic distension. Experiments performed in anesthetized cats by Cheeseman and Revelette (1990) have even shown a reduction in integrated peak EMG diaphragmatic activity when the diaphragmatic length was increased, except after cervical dorsal rhizotomy. Such data favor the existence of an inhibitory phrenic-to-phrenic reflex mechanism for controlling diaphragmatic length changes. By contrast, other animal studies demonstrate an operational length compensation characterized by increased and prolonged diaphragmatic EMG activity in response to the inflation of an abdominal balloon (Cuenod, 1961), the application of lower-body negative pressure in C-7 spinalized and vagotomized cats (Fryman and Frazier, 1987), or postural changes (Lunteren et al., 1985). Increased inspiratory drive was also reported in upright conscious humans who were healthy (Druz and Sharp, 1981) or had chronic obstructive pulmonary disease (Druz and Sharp, 1981).

The Role of Chest Wall Afferents

As documented above, it is now well established that afferents of primary muscle spindles in both the internal and external intercostal muscles monosynaptically excite the homonymous motoneurones of the same and adjacent spinal segments. Afferents of secondary muscle spindles and Golgi tendon organs in intercostal muscles in the caudal thoracic segments also exert facilitatory influences on phrenic motoneurons (see the review by Shannon, 1986). Such facilitatory intercostal-to-intercostal and intercostal-to-phrenic reflexes may play a role in ventilatory compensation for posture changes. However, recent research developments reinforce the claim that proprioceptive afferents from intercostal muscles do not exert direct facilitatory influence on medullary respiratory neurons (Bolser et al., 1987). Costovertebral joint receptors do not participate in the compensatory reflex increase in ventilatory neural drive in response to postural changes, but their afferent paths are involved in the inhibitory intercostal-to-phrenic reflex (Bolser et al., 1988).

The Participation of Abdominal Muscle Afferents

The knowledge of a facilitatory abdominal-to-abdominal stretch reflex results from electrophysiological recordings in lumbar motoneurons (Bishop, 1964) or the abdominal muscles themselves (Jammes et al., 1983a). This suggests that proprioceptive information from the abdominal wall may participate in the compensatory response to postural changes. However, the existence of a facilitatory long reflex loop between abdominal muscles and phrenic motoneurons is controversial. Indeed, the activation of abdominal muscle afferents in anesthetized cats and dogs reduces the phrenic motoneuron discharge (Jammes et al., 1983a; Shannon, 1986). In addition, Fitting et al. (1989) reported in conscious chronically instrumented dogs that, with posture changes from decubitus to sitting or standing, the end-expiratory length of costal and crural diaphragm did not vary and even weakly fell when compared with the decubitus position. This was associated with phasic expiratory contractions of abdominal muscles in sitting or standing dogs.

Thus, the main compensatory mechanism for changes in diaphragmatic operational length in conscious quadrupeds is not an increase in diaphragmatic activity, but rather phasic expiratory contractions of the abdominal muscles. Due to the chronic animal preparation, it is impossible to attribute the origin of phasic expiratory activities in abdominal muscles to either the triggering action of vagal pulmonary stretch receptors on brainstem expiratory neurones (Bishop, 1964; Jammes et al., 1983a), the conscious reactions present in the unanesthetized state (Davies et al., 1980), or the intervention of proprioceptive segmental reflex loops in the abdominal wall. The latter mechanism should be mostly responsible for enhanced tonic abdominal muscle contraction rather than the phasic expiratory activities.

C. Role in Ventilatory Adaptations to Loaded Breathing

Mechanical ventilatory loading may be produced by the addition of external resistive or elastic loads, chest compression, tracheal occlusion, or internal loads such as passive hyperinflation or deflation of the lungs, high-density gas breathing, and mostly, drug- or antigen-induced bronchospasm. With external mechanical loading, single-breath loading can be performed and the immediate (first-breath) ventilatory effect studied. Then, the ventilatory response to the sole activation of mechanosensitive respiratory afferents (vagal and/or respiratory muscle afferents) can be studied, because arterial blood gases are not so rapidly altered and the chemoreflex drive is not activated. This pure condition is not found during multiple breaths or steady-state ventilatory loading, a condition where proper data analysis would require maintenance of constant arterial blood gases. Load-induced changes in ventilatory activity must be considered in intact and then vagotomized animals, to differentiate the specific influences of vagal afferents. Also, the response to loads may be studied after suppression of chest wall and abdominal muscle afferents (spinal section at C-7 or C-8 level) and/or of any reflex feedback from the diaphragm (section of C-3 to C-7 cervical dorsal roots).

External Loading

Decreased End-Expiratory Lung Volume

This situation is produced by chest compression, breathing against external inspiratory loads (resistive or elastic), or tracheal occlusion (TO) at end-expiration, which elicits an infinite inspiratory load. Prolongation of inspiratory activity leading to a near-tonic discharge in phrenic and intercostal motoneurons is commonly reported in response to TO or prolonged inspiratory resistive loading in anesthetized cats and rabbits (Siafakas et al., 1981; Seaman et al, 1983; Shannon et al., 1985; Jammes et al., 1986b; Badier et al., 1989). This facilitatory influence is also present, but reduced, when cats breathe against an inspiratory resistor and only the first or second loaded breath is considered (Mathiot et al., 1987). In any case, TO and inspiratory resistive loading never modify the time course of integrated phrenic motor discharge (Trippenbach and Milic-Emili, 1977; Siafakas et al., 1981; Jammes et al., 1986b). This suggests that the recruitment of phrenic motoneurons is not influenced by the activation of pulmonary and/or inspiratory muscle afferents. The role of chest wall and/or diaphragmatic afferents in this response to loads is controversial. Some authors report observations that bivagotomy totally suppresses the changes in inspiratory duration (Trippenbach and Milic-Emili, 1977; Siafakas et al., 1981). However, in the study by Shannon et al. (1985) in vagotomized cats, the effects of loads disappeared only after cervical plus thoracic dorsal rhizotomies. In the same species, we demonstrated that C-8 spinal cord section markedly reduced the inspiratory prolongation with TO, the response being abolished after further bivagotomy (Jammes et al., 1986b). The use of anesthetic agents such as chloralose and ethyl carbamate, which facilitate spinal reflexes, accentuates the ventilatory response to TO or inspiratory resistance (Jammes et al., 1986b; Mathiot et al., 1987). This may be interpreted as a facilitation of respiratory muscle afferent pathways. The diaphragmatic afferents are suspected to be involved in the response to TO. Indeed, TO induces no change in the inspiratory duration but a marked depression of integrated motor phrenic activity in vagotomized, C-8 spinalized cats (Jammes et al., 1986a; Jammes, 1988a). This inhibitory effect is attributed to the activation of diaphragmatic Golgi tendon organs with TO (Corda et al., 1965; Jammes et al., 1986a). However, such an inhibitory phrenic-to-phrenic reflex is only activated with very strong diaphragmatic contraction since it is never observed in the same experimental conditions when cats breathe through inspiratory resistors (Mathiot et al., 1987).

Elevated End-Expiratory Lung Volume

Increased thoracic gas volume is produced by expiratory threshold load breathing (ETL), i.e., positive expiratory pressure breathing, addition of an external resistor or elastance on the expiratory line, or application of lower-body negative pressure. An increase in phrenic efferent activity or in integrated diaphragmatic EMG is commonly reported in animals (Kelsen et al., 1981; Jammes et al., 1983a,b; Finkler and Iscoe, 1984; van Lunteren et al., 1985; Newman et al., 1986) and also humans (Banzett et al., 1981; Druz and Sharp, 1981; Alex et al., 1987). The increased inspiratory activity compensates for the decreased inspiratory muscle force due to shorter lengths in intercostal muscles and an increased radius of curvature of the diaphragm. Enhanced strength of diaphragmatic contractions is associated with a slight prolongation of inspiratory duration and, mostly, a lengthening of expiratory period due to evoked expiratory activities in internal intercostal and abdominal muscles (Jammes et al., 1983a,b; Russel and Bishop,

1976; Iscoe, 1989). This was also observed in dogs under cardiopulmonary bypass, where the chemoreflex drive of breathing was held constant (Jammes et al., 1983a,b). The compensatory response requires several loaded respiratory cycles to be complete; indeed, we recorded very weak changes in inspiratory activity for the first or even second loaded breath (Mathiot et al., 1987). The ventilatory compensation of reduced inspiratory muscle force appears to be complete in conscious humans, because alveolar CO_2 partial pressure does not change (Green et al., 1978), but not in anesthetized cats (Finkler and Iscoe, 1984; Iscoe, 1989) where the arterial or alveolar P_{CO_2} increases. Also the type of anesthesia influences the response to elevated end-expiratory lung volume, which was minimal when barbiturates were used (Jammes et al., 1986; Mathiot et al., 1987). Some observations in animals and humans suggest that the compensatory mechanism for elevated end-expiratory lung volume is mediated by phrenic and/or vagal afferents, but not the chest wall or abdominal muscle afferents. Indeed, Banzett et al. (1981) reported that the response to lower-body negative pressure persisted in quadriplegic men (low cervical cord section), and the study by Kenneth (1984) revealed that the ventilatory adjustments to elastic or resistive loads, including the changes in timing, were qualitatively the same in quadriplegic men as those found in healthy subjects. Phrenic afferents were not implicated in this response in pentobarbital-anesthetized cats (Iscoe, 1989).

Pulmonary vagal afferents play the major role in the ventilatory response to lung volume changes (increased or decreased end-expiratory volume) in anesthetized cats. Indeed, increased phrenic motor activity in response to single-breath inspiratory or expiratory resistive loading is markedly enhanced after cervical bivagotomy or procaine block of conduction in thin vagal fibers (Mathiot et al., 1987). Thus, inhibitory influences exerted by pulmonary vagal afferents, including thin-fiber afferents, seem to counterbalance the facilitatory effects of respiratory muscle afferents. The role of vagal afferents is also essential in triggering expiratory activities in intercostal and abdominal muscles during prolonged expiratory-threshold load breathing (Russel and Bishop, 1976; Jammes et al., 1983a). Elastic loading increases the respiratory frequency in vagotomized dogs and cats, but this does not occur when the chemical drive is held constant (Shannon, 1986). Thus, respiratory muscle afferents do not participate significantly in this response.

Internal Loading
Passive Lung Inflation or Deflation

Passive lung inflation in vagotomized animals exerts various and often opposite effects. Duron (1973) reports an inhibition of the EMG activity in the diaphragm and external intercostal and interchondral muscles in cats. He attributes this inhibition to increased activity of muscle spindle endings in the antagonistic muscles (stretching of internal intercostal muscles with the thoracic distension). However, in the same species Bainton et al. (1978) observed the opposite effects, and Bianchi and Barillot (1975) reported no change in the central inspiratory activity during passive expansion of the thorax in vagotomized animals. Lung deflation produces a tachypnea with evoked tonic activity in external intercostal muscles and the diaphragm; this response is no longer found after bivagotomy or procaine block of vagal C-fibers (Badier et al., 1989).

Dense Gas Breathing

Hyperbaric studies at pressure up to 91 absolute atmospheres (ATA), i.e., 900 meters of sea water (gas density = 20 g/L), in conscious cats have shown a marked increase in the tonic diaphragmatic activity with prolonged inspiratory discharge (review by Jammes and Roussos, 1994). Also, the recruitment strategy of diaphragmatic motor units is severely modified under hyperbaric conditions. Thus, EMG recordings of the spontaneous diaphragmatic activity in human volunteers compressed at pressure up to 46 ATA (gas density = 8 to 11 g/L) (Lenoir et al., 1990) and in cats studied at 101 ATA (gas density = 25 g/L) (Burnet et al., 1992) revealed a marked recruitment of diaphragmatic motor units in parallel to the increased amplitude of tidal breaths with elevated pressure. Changes in EMG power spectrum characterized by reduced centroid frequency were also observed, but they were not proportional to the elevated pressure at 31 ATA in cats. The experimental conditions did not allow determination of the role of reflex paths in these EMG changes. However, the absence of EMG power changes in skeletal muscles and in other respiratory muscles that did not participate in resting ventilation at depth (Lenoir et al., 1990; Derrien et al., 1990; Burnet et al., 1992) suggests the existence of reflex influences activated by the enhanced strength of inspiratory muscle contractions with dense gas breathing. Normobaric experiments in anesthetized cats breathing a dense gas mixture of SF_6 and O_2 (gas density: 6.6 g/L) have revealed significant lengthening in both inspiratory and expiratory periods. This effect persisted after C-8 spinal cord section but disappeared after bivagotomy (Barriere et al., 1993).

Bronchospasm

The ventilatory response to an increase in the respiratory system impedance produced by histamine-, carbachol- or antigen-induced bronchospasm is characterized by tachypnea plus marked tonic activity in inspiratory muscles. The same tonic response was described in normal humans or asthmatic subjects (Muller et al., 1980; Martin et al., 1980, 1983) as in anesthetized dogs (Kelsen et al., 1981) or rabbits (Badier et al., 1989). This was not a consistent response in cats (Barriere et al., 1993). Cervical vagotomy or selective conduction block of thin vagal fibers abolished the bronchospasm-induced tonic inspiratory activity in rabbits (Badier et al., 1989) but had no consistent effect in cats (Barriere et al., 1993). In the latter species, enhanced tonic diaphragmatic activity in response to induced broncho-spasm was absent after C-8 spinal cord section. Thus, the role played by respiratory muscle afferents from the chest and/or abdominal wall in this response depends on the animal species. However the most potent afferent path involves the activation of bronchopulmonary vagal endings by increased intra-airway pressure, smooth muscle contraction, and in some instances the direct stimulating effect of inhaled or injected chemicals.

Comparisons between the responses to external and internal loads have been performed in conscious humans (Kelsen et al., 1981) and in anesthetized rabbits (Badier et al., 1989) or cats (Barriere et al., 1993). In humans, Kelsen and co-workers have shown that facilitatory influences on inspiratory muscles, as well as the sense of effort, were more pronounced during induced bronchospasm than when subjects breathed against external resistive loads. These authors concluded that increased sensory inputs from the lungs and airways may explain the different responses. However, another explanation may be that the tonic activity in the inspiratory muscles, mostly found under the circumstances of internal loading, is responsible for enhanced afferent muscle paths, which in turn accentuate the dyspneic sensation.

In summary, despite the existence of well-known segmental and pluri-segmental spinal reflexes between the respiratory muscle groups that may play a role in the adaptations to posture changes, the ventilatory effects elicited by infra-maximal mechanical loading of the respiratory system involve a weak participa-tion of thoracic respiratory muscle afferents. This indicates that sensory inputs from the lungs and airways are sufficient to mediate normal patterns of ventilatory adjustments during loaded breathing.

D. Reflex Effects Associated with Respiratory Muscle Fatigue

Fragmentary observations concern the role of respiratory muscle afferents during muscle fatigue or metabolic changes resulting from reduced oxygen supply to muscles. Both circumstances can activate the muscle metaboreceptors via the local acidosis associated with extracellular fluid hyperosmolarity due to the outflow of intracellular potassium. In humans, it has been suggested by Roussos (1984) and also Gallagher et al. (1985) that respiratory muscle fatigue results in a pattern of rapid, shallow breathing. This response is also observed when high-intensity exercise is employed to further increase the strength of respiratory muscle contractions (Mador and Acevedo, 1991a), but the changes in breathing pattern are not found in resting individuals after induction of respiratory muscle fatigue with large inspiratory resistive loading (Mador and Acevedo, 1991b). In anesthetized dogs, Aubier et al. (1981) reported an initial tachypnea followed by bradypnea during the response to breathing against a fatiguing load or in a state of reduced diaphragmatic blood flow such as shock. Because this response was not affected by vagotomy or cross-perfusion of the head, which eliminated the activation of arterial and central chemoreceptors, it was tempting to speculate that the activation of diaphragmatic metaboreceptors may play a role in the observed delayed bradypnea. In conscious cats breathing a very dense gas mixture (gas density around 25 g/L) for several days, the occurrence of EMG signs of diaphragmatic fatigue (leftward shift in EMG power spectrum and also decreased M-wave amplitude) was associated with a progressive bradypnea (Burnet et al., 1992).

Opposite observations were reported by Supinski et al. (1989), who have shown in anesthetized dogs that fatigue of in situ muscle strips from the left diaphragm elicited a slight increase in respiratory frequency. Teitelbaum et al. (1992) also found that inspiratory motor drive and breathing frequency increased when diaphragmatic blood flow was selectively reduced in dogs. However, in all the aforementioned observations there were never simultaneous recordings of the changes in the ventilatory pattern and the phrenic sensory pathways during a fatigue run. This was recently performed in artificially ventilated cats, where diaphragm fatigue was produced by direct electrical stimulation of the two cupolae with trains of pulses (Jammes and Balzamo, 1992). Before any change in transdiaphragmatic pressure twitches and diaphragmatic EMG power spectrum could be detected, marked modifications in the motor phrenic activity were measured. These early motor phrenic changes were characterized by reduced high-frequency discharge of phrenic motoneurones. When muscle failure occurred after 10–15 min of stimulation, the firing rate of diaphragmatic metaboreceptors markedly increased. This was associated with a progressive lengthening in inspiratory and total breath durations and a persistence of altered motor phrenic electroneurogram. After diaphragmatic denervation, all fatigue-induced changes in the motor phrenic activity as well as in ventilatory timing during fatigue were abolished. This suggests that the successive activation of the different categories of diaphragmatic receptors (proprioceptors and then group III and mostly IV phrenic afferents) exerts specific influences on the phrenic motoneurons and also the supraspinal structures, which govern the recruitment of phrenic motoneurons and the respiratory frequency. The latter component seems to be mostly influenced by the peripheral inputs from diaphragmatic metaboreceptors. However, diaphragm (Jammes and Balzamo, 1992) and limb muscle studies in cats (Lagier-Tessonnier et al., 1993) have demonstrated that enhanced anaerobic metabolic paths produced by muscle fatigue not only activate the muscular metaboreceptors, but also depress the discharge of proprioceptors. Thus, the aforementioned reflex changes in ventilatory pattern associated with diaphragmatic fatigue may result from increased sensory pathways from metaboreceptors and/or depressed afferent phasic discharge of proprioceptors.

E. Central Interactions Between Respiratory Muscle Afferents and Other Respiratory Inputs

Electrophysiological and histological studies performed mostly in cats have shown that afferents from the chest and abdominal walls and also the diaphragm project to the dorsal respiratory group, which also integrates vagal and arterial chemoreceptor afferents (Cohen, 1979; Shannon, 1980; Ciriello et al., 1981). Hence the ventilatory response to a given stimulus must be interpreted as a central integration of agonistic and antagonistic information. The changes in breathing pattern observed after selective suppression of one group of respiratory afferents could be due to the removal of an agonistic influence or to the enhancement of other antagonistic respiratory inputs. Thus, the selective elimination of sensory fibers may induce different changes in breathing pattern. This could result from prevailing influences exerted by some respiratory afferents on the excitation threshold of brainstem neurons. In anesthetized cats, respiratory muscle and vagal afferents seem to interact centrally in the control of eupneic ventilation since marked increases in the amplitude of breath with no change in inspiratory duration occurred when a C-8 spinal cord section was performed first, whereas further spinal section in vagotomized cats decreased tidal volume and shortened the inspiratory period (Jammes et al., 1986b).

Speck and Webber (1981) have suggested that the activation of respiratory muscle proprioceptors may bypass the integrating network involved in the processing of vagal pulmonary stretch receptor input. Prolonged and severe expiratory loaded ventilation constitutes an experimental situation combining the activation of expiratory muscle afferents, the stimulation of vagal pulmonary stretch receptors (Davenport, 1981), and increased information from arterial and central chemoreceptors when respiratory gas exchanges are impeded. When one of these respiratory afferent paths is controlled, the interactions between the two others may be studied. Antagonistic influences have been shown in dogs under extracorporeal circulation, which allowed maintenance of constant arterial blood gases (Jammes et al., 1983b). Then, prolonged expiratory threshold load breathing was associated with a progressive reduction of the inhibitory ventilatory response to vagal afferent stimulation. This phenomenon was not observed in the absence of evoked contractions in internal intercostal and abdominal muscles. This reduction or even suppression of the inspiratory "off-switch" vagal mechanism occurred with either mechanical activation of the pulmonary stretch receptors (lung inflation) or electrical stimulation of the afferent vagal fibers. Thus, peripheral habituation of sensory processes could not be involved. Such an antagonistic central interaction between respiratory muscle and vagal afferents began after at least 10 min of loaded ventilation and persisted for 15 min during the recovery period. These relatively long delays suggest the participation of central neurotransmitters and/or neuromodulators. Antagonistic influences between respiratory muscle afferents and the CO_2 sensitivity have also been demonstrated in the same animal preparation (Jammes et al., 1983a). In conscious humans, the central interaction between respiratory muscle and vagal afferents has not been studied owing to the difficulties in exploring the inspiratory vagal "off-switch" mechanism in such circumstances. However, some observations reveal that the activation of chest wall proprioceptors using high-frequency oscillations alters the CO_2 sensitivity (Khoo et al., 1989). Interaction between phrenic and limb muscle afferents has been studied by Ward et al. (1992) in dogs. These authors found that repetitive electrical stimulation of the left phrenic and gastrocnemius nerves concurrently produced additive ventilatory effects.

F. Participation in Respiratory Sensations

In their original study, Campbell et al. (1961) suggested that sensory activity from the respiratory muscles gives rise to sensations associated with loaded ventilation. They proposed that additional external loads created an inappropriate muscle length-tension relationship, which was detected by muscle spindles abundant in intercostal muscles. In addition, Homma et al. (1984) have reported that vibration of the chest wall worsened breathlessness. Several new lines of study provided results consistent with the concept that diaphragmatic afferents may also play a role in respiratory sensation. In normal human subjects, Zechman et al. (1985) have shown that the latency for detecting added inspiratory resistive loads was inversely proportional to the magnitude of transdiaphragmatic pressure changes with increasing load intensity. Eisele et al. (1968) have also shown that spinal anesthesia at the level of T-1 did not affect elastic load detection, although chest wall and abdominal wall sensory activity, but not phrenic afferents, was suppressed in these circumstances. Similarly, in C-4 to C-7 quadriplegic patients with intact diaphragmatic innervation, the ability to detect added resistive load (Zechman et al., 1967) and the sensation of inspired volume (DiMarco et al., 1982) were normal. Human studies have revealed that the sensation of respiratory force is shaped by afferent signals from muscle receptors that gauge respiratory muscle tension (Gottfried et al., 1984). It was also shown that the sense of respiratory effort depends on the corollary enhanced neuromuscular command, increased motor output being required to achieve a given tension in weakened respiratory muscles (Campbell et al., 1980; Killian and Jones, 1988). Heightened expiratory as well as inspiratory motor output causes comparable increases in the sensation of difficulty in breathing (Chonan et al., 1990). The most recent observations also indicate that absolute sensation intensity during resistive and elastic loading was significantly reduced after strength training (Redline et al., 1991). Thus, the close connections between the sensory and motor cortex, well documented for the control of limb movements, also exist for scaling of ventilatory motion. Experi-

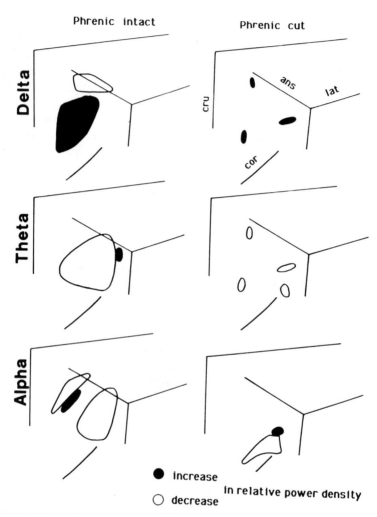

Figure 6 Schematic representation of the posterior sigmoid gyrus (cortical sensorimotor area) collecting the changes in relative power density of the three EEG frequency bands during electrically induced diaphragmatic fatigue in cats. Denervation of the diaphragm reduced or abolished quantitative EEG changes. (From Balzamo et al., 1992, by permission of *Respiration Physiology*.)

ments in cats suggest that phrenic afferents carry sensory information to the cortex when the strength of diaphragmatic contraction is enhanced. Thus, Marquez and Barillot (cited in Bassal and Bianchi, 1981), then Davenport et al. (1985), and more recently Balzamo et al. (1992) have shown that the electrical stimulation of phrenic nerve afferents evokes potentials in the sensorimotor cortex. These experimental data support the fact that, in humans, inspiratory occlusion evokes respiratory-related cortical potentials in the somatosensory cortex (Davenport et al., 1986; Revelette and Davenport, 1990).

The aforementioned influences of respiratory muscle afferents on the highest integration of sensory processes concern only those exerted by force or length receptors, but not by metaboreceptors. In humans, opposite results are reported on the interaction between respiratory muscle fatigue and the sensation of breathing. Gandevia et al. (1981) observed that the perception of added inspiratory load magnitude was elevated during inspiratory muscle fatigue, whereas Bradley et al. (1986) found that the sensation of inspiratory effort was independent of the presence of a fatiguing diaphragmatic motor pattern. The interpretation of these observations may be based on the corollary increase in afferent and efferent pathways to the fatigued respiratory muscles (central hypothesis), but also on electrophysiological data that reveal that phasically active proprioceptor discharge decreases in parallel to enhanced metaboreceptor activity when diaphragmatic fatigue occurs (peripheral hypothesis) (Jammes and Balzamo, 1992; Balzamo et al., 1992). Whatever the case, diaphragmatic fatigue is associated with alterations in the transmission of phrenic sensory activity to the cortex and also marked changes in spontaneous cortical activity (Balzamo et al., 1992). Progressive lengthening in onset and peak latencies of cortical phrenic evoked potentials recorded in the sensorimotor area were correlated with the development of electrically induced diaphragm fatigue in cats. This was associated with decreased energy in the theta frequency band of the electroencephalogram (EEG) and increased energy in the delta band. As shown in Fig. 6, denervation of the diaphragm suppressed the EEG changes during the fatigue run. Both phenomena, i.e., lengthening of cortical phrenic evoked potential latency and depression of the EEG activity, may correspond to either a central habituation or central inhibitory processes elicited by the enhanced firing rate of diaphragmatic metaboreceptors. Since part of the cortical effects persisted during the recovery after a fatigue trial, it was tempting to speculate that the central delivery of inhibitory neurotransmitters could be involved.

IV. Summary

Recent studies have greatly expanded our knowledge of the receptors, stimuli pathways, and reflexes that can be associated with the mechanoreceptor afferents from the respiratory musculature In addition to the mechanoreceptors, there is a wide variety of metaboreceptors in the respiratory muscles, which have only recently received much attention. Most of these recent research developments concern the sensory innervation of the diaphragm. Despite these advances, the actual roles and importance of these afferent systems are still being debated. Many fundamental questions remain concerning the influence of these muscle receptors in the automatic control of ventilation, postural as well as load compensatory mechanisms, perception of breathing, and behavioral responses. One of the most striking points is the knowledge of potent central interactions between respiratory afferents, including those from the respiratory musculature, a phenomenon accentuated under severe mechanical ventilatory loading. This realization further complicates the interpretation of breathing pattern changes associated with chronic respiratory insufficiency and acute ventilatory failure.

References

Alex CG, Aronson RM, Onal E, Lopata M. Effects of continuous positive airway pressure on upper airway and respiratory muscle activity. J Appl Physiol 1987; 62:2026–2030.

Aubier M, Trippenbach T, Roussos Ch. Respiratory muscle fatigue during cardiogenic shock. J Appl Physiol 1981; 51:499–508.

Badier M, Jammes Y, Romero-Colomer P, Lemerre Ch. Tonic activity in inspiratory muscles and phrenic motoneurons by stimulation of vagal afferents. J Appl Physiol 1989; 66:1613–1619.

Bainton CR, Kirkwood PA, Sears TA. On the transmission of the stimulating effects of carbon dioxide to the muscles of respiration. J Physiol (Lond) 1978; 280:249–272.

Baker S, Seers C, Sears TA. Respiratory modulation of afferent transmission to the cerebellum. In: Speck et al., ed. Respiratory Control: Central and Peripheral Mechanisms. Lexington: University of Kentucky Press, 1993:95–99.

Balzamo E, Lagier-Tessonnier F, Jammes Y. Fatigue-induced changes in diaphragmatic afferents and cortical activity in the cat. Respir Physiol 1992; 90:213–226.

Banzett RB, Ingbar GF, Brown R, Goldman M, Rossier A, Mead J. Diaphragm electrical activity during negative lower torso pressure in quadriplegic men. J Appl Physiol 1981; 51:654–659.

Banzett RB, Mead J. Reflex compensation for changes in operational length of inspiratory muscles. In: Roussos Ch, Macklem PT, eds. The Thorax, Part A. New York: Marcel Dekker, 1985:595–605.

Barker D. The structure and distribution of muscle receptors. In: Barker D, ed. Symposium on Muscle Receptors. Hong Kong: Hong Kong University Press, 1962:227–240.

Barrière JR, Delpierre S, Del Volgo MJ, Jammes Y. Comparison between external resistive loading, drug-induced bronchospasm and dense gas breathing in cats: roles of vagal and spinal afferents. Lung 1993; 171:123–136.

Bassal M, Bianchi AL. Effets de la stimulation des structures nerveuses centrales sur les activités respiratoires efférentes chez le chat. I. Reponses à la stimulation corticale. J Physiol (Paris) 1981; 77:741–757.

Bianchi AL, Barillot JC. Activity of medullary respiratory neurons during reflexes from the lungs in cats. Respir Physiol 1975; 25:335–352.

Bishop B. Reflex control of abdominal muscles during positive-pressure breathing. J Appl Physiol 1964; 19:224–232.

Bolser DC, Lindsey BG, Shannon R. Medullary inspiratory activity: influence of intercostal tendon organs and muscle spindle endings. J Appl Physiol 1987; 62:1046–1056.

Bolser DC, Lindsay BG, Shannon R. Respiratory pattern changes produced by intercostal muscle/rib vibration. J Appl Physiol 1988; 64:2458–2462.

Bradley TD, Chartrand DA, Fitting JW, Killian KJ, Grassino A. The relation of inspiratory effort sensation to fatiguing patterns of the diaphragm. Am Rev Respir Dis 1986; 134:1119–1124.

Brancatisano A, Kelly SM, Tully A, Loring SH, Engel LA. Postural changes in spontaneous and evoked regional diaphragmatic activity in dogs. J Appl Physiol 1989; 66: 1699–1705.

Burke D, Hagbarth KE, Lofstedt L, Wallin G. The response of human muscle spindle endings to vibrations of noncontracting muscles. J Physiol (Lond) 1976; 261:673–693.

Burnet H, Lenoir P, Jammes Y. Changes in respiratory muscle activity in conscious cats during experimental dives at 101 ATA. J Appl Physiol 1992; 73:465–472.

Campbell EJM, Freedman S, Smith PS, Taylor ME. The ability of man to detect added elestic loads to breathing. Clin Sci 1961; 20:223–231.

Campbell EJM, Gandevia SC, Killian KJ, Mahutte CK, Rigg JRA. Changes in the perception of inspiratory resistive loads during partial curarization. J Physiol (Lond) 1980; 309:93–100.

Cheeseman M, Revelette WR. Phrenic afferent contribution to reflexes elicited by changes in diaphragm length. J Appl Physiol 1990; 69:640–647.

Chonan T, Altose MD, Cherniack NS. Effects of expiratory resistive loading on the sensation of dyspnea. J Appl Physiol 1990; 69:91–95.

Ciriello J, Hrycyshyn AW, Calaresu FR. Glossopharyngeal and vagal afferent projections to the brain stem of the cat: a horseradish peroxidase study. J Auton Nerv Syst 1981; 4:63–79.

Coffey GL, Godwin-Austen RB, Macgillivray BB, Sears TA. The form and distribution of the surface evoked responses in cerebellar cortex from intercostal nerves in the cat. J Physiol (Lond) 1971; 212:129–145.

Cohen MI. Neurogenesis of respiratory rhythm in the mammals. Physiol Rev 1979; 59: 1105–1173.

Corda M, Euler C von, Lennerstrand G. Proprioceptive innervation of the diaphragm. J Physiol (Lond) 1965; 178:161–178.

Critchlow V, Euler C Von. Intercostal muscle spindle activity and its gamma motor control. J Physiol (Lond) 1963; 168:820–847.

Cuenod M. Reflexes proprioceptifs du diaphragme chez le lapin. Helv Physiol Acta 1961; 19:360–372.

D'Angelo E, Miserocchi G, Agostoni E. Effect of rib cage or abdomen compression at iso-lung volume on breathing patterns. Respir Physiol 1976; 28:161–177.

Davenport PW, Frazier DT, Zechman FW. The effect of the resistive loading of inspiration and expiration on pulmonary stretch receptor discharge. Respir Physiol 1981; 43: 299–314.

Davenport PW, Thompson FJ, Reep RL, Freed AN. Projection of phrenic nerve afferents to the cat sensorimotor cortex. Brain Res 1985; 328:150–153.

Davenport PW, Friedman WA, Thompson FJ, Franzen O. Respiratory-related cortical potentials evoked by inspiratory occlusion in humans. J Appl Physiol 1986; 60: 1843–1848.

Davies A, Sant'Ambrogio FG, Sant'Ambrogio G. Control of postural changes of end expiratory volume by airways slowly adapting mechanoreceptors. Respir Physiol 1980; 41:211–216.

Decima EE, Euler C von. Intercostal and cerebellar influences on efferent phrenic activity in the decerebrate cat. Acta Physiol Scand 1969; 76:148–158.

Decima EE, Euler C von, Thoden U. Intercostal-to-phrenic reflexes in the spinal cat. Acta Physiol Scand 1969; 75:568–579.

Delpierre S, Grimaud Ch., Jammes Y, Mei N. Changes in activity of vagal bronchopulmonary C-fibres by chemical and physical stimuli in the cat. J Physiol (Lond) 1981; 316: 61–74.

Derrien I, Lenoir P, Jammes Y. Etude comparative des muscles diaphragme et adducteur du pouce lors de contractions statiques fatigantes à 25 ATA. Arch Intern Physiol Biochem 1990; 98:A424.

DiMarco AF, Wolfson DA, Gottfried SB, Altose MD. Sensation of inspired volume in normal subject and in quadriplegic patients. J Appl Physiol 1982; 53:1481–1486.

Dogiel AS. Die Nervenendigungen in Bauchfell in den Sehnen der Muskelspindels und dem Centrum Tendineum des Diaphragms beim Menschen und bei Saugethieren. Arch Mikroskop Anat Entwicklungsmed 1902; 59:1–31.

Dolivo M. Effet de l'interruption de la conduction nerveuse dans le nerf phrénique sur la fréquence respiratoire. Helv Physiol Acta 1952; 10:366–371.

Downman CRB. Skeletal muscle reflexes of splanchnic and intercostal nerve origin in acute spinal and decerebrate cats. J Neurophysiol 1955; 18:217–235.

Druz WS, Sharp JT. Activity of respiratory muscles in upright and recumbent humans. J Appl Physiol 1981; 51:1552–1561.

Duron B. Postural and ventilatory function of intercostal muscles. Acta Neurobiol Exp 1973; 33:355–380.

Duron B. Intercostal and diaphragmatic muscle endings and afferents. In: Hornbein TF, ed. Regulation of Breathing, Part I, New York: Marcel Dekker, 1981:473–540.

Duron B, Condamin M. Etude au microscope électronique de la composition amyélinique du nerf phrénique du chat. CR Soc Biol 1970; 164:577–585.

Duron B, Jung-Caillol MC. Investigation of afferent activity in the intact phrenic nerve with bipolar electrodes. Acta Neurobiol Exp 1973; 33:427–432.

Eisele J, Trenchard D, Burki N, Guz A. The effect of chest wall block on respiratory sensation and control in man. Clin Sci 1968; 35:23–33.

Euler C von. The control of respiratory movements. In: Howell JBL, Campbell EJM, eds. Breathlessness. Oxford, UK: Blackwell, 1966:19–32.

Euler C von, Peretti G. Dynamic and static contributions to the rhythmic gamma-activation of primary and secondary spindle endings in external intercostal muscle. J Physiol (Lond) 1966; 187:501–516.

Fergusson J. The phrenic nerve. Brain 1891; 14:282–283.

Finkler J, Iscoe S. Control of breathing at elevated lung volumes in anesthetized cats. J Appl Physiol 1984; 53:839–844.

Fitting JW, Easton PA, Arnoux R, Guerraty A, Grassino A. Diaphragm length adjustments with body position changes in the awake dog. J Appl Physiol 1989; 66:870–875.

Fleisch A, Tripod J. Die afferente Komponente der Atmungssteurerung. Pflüger's Arch Ges Physiol Mensch Tiere 1938; 240:676–679.

Fleisch A, Grandjean E, Crusaz R. Contribution à l'étude de la fonction des fibres afférentes du phrénique. Physiol Pharmacol Acta 1946; 4:127–134.

Fryman DL, Frazier DT. Diaphragm afferent modulation of phrenic motor drive. J Appl Physiol 1987; 62:2436–2441.

Gallagher CG, Im Hof V, Younes M. Effect of inspiratory muscle fatigue on breathing pattern. J Appl Physiol 1985; 59:1152–1158.

Gandevia SC, Killian KJ, Campbell EJM. The effect of respiratory muscle fatigue on respiratory sensations. Clin Sci (Lond) 1981; 60:463–466.

Gautier H. Respiratory responses of the anesthetized rabbit to vagotomy and thoracic dorsal rhizotomy. Respir Physiol 1973; 17:238–247.

Gill PK, Kuno M. Excitatory and inhibitory actions on phrenic motoneurones. J Physiol (Lond) 1963; 168:274–289.

Gottfried SB, Leech I, DiMarco AF, Zaccardelli W, Altose MD. Sensation of respiratory muscle force following low cervical spine transection. J Appl Physiol 1984; 57: 989–994.

Graham R, Jammes Y, Delpierre S, Grimaud Ch., Roussos Ch. The effects of ischemia, lactic acid and hypertonic sodium chloride on phrenic afferent discharge during spontaneous diaphragmatic contractions. Neurosci Lett 1986; 67:257–262.

Green M, Mead J, Sears TA. Muscle activity during chest wall restriction and positive pressure breathing in man. Respir Physiol 1978; 35:283–300.

Hinsey JC, Hare K, Philips RA. Sensory components of the phrenic nerve of the cat. Proc Soc Exp Biol NY 1939; 41:411–414.

Homma I, Obata T, Sibuya M, Uchida M. Gate mechanism in breathlessness caused by chest wall vibrations in humans. J Appl Physiol 1984; 56:8–11.

Hussain S, Magder S, Chatillon A, Roussos Ch. Chemical activation of thin-fibre phrenic afferents. 1. Respiratory response. J Appl Physiol 1990; 69:1002–1011.

Hussain S, Chatillon A, Comtois A, Roussos Ch, Magder S. Chemical activation of thin-fiber phrenic afferents. 2. Cardiovascular responses. J Appl Physiol 1991; 70:77–86.

Hussain S, Roussos Ch. Thin-fiber phrenic afferents. In: Roussos Ch, Macklem PT, eds, The Thorax, 2nd ed. New York: Marcel Dekker, 1994 (in press).

Iscoe S. Phrenic afferents and ventilatory control at increased end-expiratory lung volumes in cats. J Appl Physiol 1989; 66:1297–1303.

Jammes Y. Chest wall and diaphragmatic afferents: their role during external mechanical loading and respiratory muscle ischemia. In: Grassino A, ed. Respiratory Muscles in Chronic Obstructive Pulmonary Disease. London: Springer Verlag, 1988a:49–57.

Jammes Y. Tonic sensory pathways of the respiratory system. Eur Respir J 1988b; 1:176–183.

Jammes Y, Balzamo E. Changes in afferent and efferent phrenic activities with electrically-induced diaphragmatic fatigue. J Appl Physiol 1992; 73:894–902.

Jammes Y, Mei N. Assessment of the pulmonary origin of bronchoconstrictor vagal tone. J Physiol (Lond) 1979; 291:305–316.

Jammes Y, Mathiot MJ, Roll JP, Prefaut C, Berthelin F, Grimaud Ch., Milic-Emili J. Ventilatory responses to muscular vibrations in healthy humans. J Appl Physiol 1981; 51:262–269.

Jammes Y, Bye PTP, Pardy RL, Katsardis C, Esau S, Roussos Ch. Expiratory threshold load under extracorporeal circulation: effects of vagal afferents. J Appl Physiol 1983a; 55:307–315.

Jammes Y, Bye PTP, Pardy RL, Roussos Ch. Vagal feedback with expiratory threshold load under extracorporeal circulation. J Appl Physiol 1983b; 55:316–322.

Jammes Y, Buchler B, Delpierre S, Rasidakis A, Grimaud Ch., Roussos Ch. Phrenic afferents and their role in inspiratory control. J Appl Physiol 1986a; 60:854–860.

Jammes Y, Mathiot MJ, Delpierre S, Grimaud Ch. Role of vagal and spinal sensory pathways on eupneic diaphragmatic activity. J Appl Physiol 1986b; 60:479–485.

Jammes Y, Roussos Ch. Diving. In: Roussos Ch., Macklem PT, eds. The Thorax, 2nd ed. New York: Marcel Dekker, 1994 (in press).

Jung-Caillol MC, Duron B. Number of neuromuscular spindles and electrical activity of the respiratory muscles. In: Duron B, ed. Colloque INSERM. Respiratory Centres and Afferent Systems. Paris: INSERM, 1976:165–173.

Karius DR, Ling L, Speck DF. Lesions of the rostral dorsolateral pons have no effect on afferent-evoked inhibition of inspiration. Brain Res 1991; 559:22–28.

Kaufman MP, Rybicki KJ. Discharge properties of group III and IV muscle afferents: their response to mechanical and metabolic stimuli. Circ Res 1987; 61:160–165.

Kaufman MP, Rybicki KJ, Waldrop TG, Ordway GA. Effects of ischemia on response of group III and IV afferents to contraction. J Appl Physiol 1984; 57:644–650.

Kaufman MP, Rotto DM, Rybicki KJ. Pressor reflex response to static muscular contraction: its afferent arm and possible neurotransmitters. Am J Cardiol 1988; 62:58E–62E.

Kelsen SG, Prestel TF, Cherniack NS, Chester EH, Deal EC. Comparison of the respiratory responses to external resistive loading and bronchoconstriction. J Clin Invest 1981; 67:1761–1768.

Kenneth A. Adaptations of quadriplegic men to consecutively loaded breaths. J Appl Physiol 1984; 56:1099–1103.

Khoo MCK, Gelmont D, Howell S, Johnson R, Yang F, Chang HK. Effects of high-frequency chest wall oscillations on respiratory control in humans. Am Rev Respir Dis 1989; 139:1223–1230.

Killian KJ, Jones NL. Respiratory muscles and dyspnea. In: Belman MJ, ed. Clinics in Chest Medicine. Respiratory Muscles: Function in Health and Disease. Philadelphia: Saunders, 1988:237–247.

Kirkwood PA, Sears TA. Excitatory post-synaptic potentials from single muscle spindle afferents in external intercostal motoneurones of the cat. J Physiol (Lond) 1982; 322:287–314.

Kirkwood PA, Munson JB, Sears TA, Westgaard RH. Respiratory interneurones in the thoracic spinal cord of the cat. J Physiol (Lond) 1988; 395:161–192.

Lagier-Tessonnier F, Balzamo E, Jammes Y. Comparative effects of ischemia and acute hypoxemia on muscle afferents from tibialis anterior in cats. Muscle Nerve 1993; 16:135–141.

Langford A, Schmidt RF. An electron microscopic analysis of the left phrenic nerve in the rat. Anat Rec 1983; 205:207–213.

Lenoir P, Jammes Y, Giry P, Rostain JC, Burnet H, Tomei Ch., Roussos Ch. Electromyographic study of respiratory muscles during human dive at 46 ATA. Undersea Biomed Res 1990; 17:121–137.

Lunteren van E, Haxhiu MA, Cherniack NS, Goldman MD. Differential costal and crural diaphragm compensation for posture changes. J Appl Physiol 1985; 58:1895–1900.

Macron JM, Marlot D, Duron B. Phrenic afferent input to the lateral medullary reticular formation of the cat. Respir Physiol 1985; 59:155–167.

Macron JM, Marlot D, Duron B. Effects of stimulation of phrenic afferent fibers on medullary respiratory neurons in cat. Neurosci Lett 1986; 63:231–236.

Mador MJ, Acevedo FA. Effect of respiratory muscle fatigue on breathing pattern during incremental exercise. Am Rev Respir Dis 1991a; 143:462–468.

Mador MJ, Acevedo FA. Effect of inspiratory muscle fatigue on breathing pattern during inspiratory resistive loading. J Appl Physiol 1991b; 70:1627–1632.

Marlot D, Macron JM, Duron B. Projections of phrenic afferents to the cat cerebellar cortex. Neurosci Lett 1984; 44:95–98.

Marlot D, Macron JM, Duron B. Projection of phrenic afferents to the external cuneate nucleus in the cat. Brain Res 1985; 327:328–330.

Marlot D, Macron JM, Duron B. Inhibitory and excitatory effects on respiration by phrenic nerve afferent stimulation in cats. Respir Physiol 1987; 69:321–333.

Martin JG, Habib M, Engel LA. Inspiratory muscle activity during induced hyperinflation. Respir Physiol 1980a; 39:303–313.

Martin JG, Powell Z, Shore S, Einrich J, Engel LA. The role of respiratory muscles in the hyperinflation of bronchial asthma. Am Rev Respir Dis 1980b; 121:441–447.

Mathiot MJ, Jammes Y, Grimaud Ch. Role of vagal and spinal sensory pathways in diaphragmatic response to resistive loading. Neurosci Lett 1987; 74:131–136.

Matthews PBC. Mammalian muscle receptors and their central actions. In: Dawson H, Greenfield ADN, Whitemann R, Brindley GS, eds. Monography of Physiology Society. London: Arnold, 1972:630.

McCallister LW, McCoy KW, Connelly JC, Kaufman MP. Stimulation of group III and IV phrenic afferents reflexly decreases total lung resistance in dogs. J Appl Physiol 1986; 61:1346–1351.

Mense S. Slowly conducting afferent fibres from deep tissues: neurobiological properties and central nervous actions. In: Ottoson D, ed. Progress in Sensory Physiology 6. Berlin: Springer Verlag, 1986:149–219.

Mitchell GS. Ventilatory control during exercise with increased respiratory dead space in goats. J Appl Physiol 1990; 69:718–727.

Monteau R, Hilaire G. Spinal respiratory motoneurons. Prog Neurobiol 1991; 37: 83–144.

Muller N, Bryan AC, Zamel N. Tonic inspiratory muscle activity as a cause of hyperinflation in histamine-induced asthma. J Appl Physiol 1980; 49:869–874.

Nathan PW, Sears TA. Effects of posterior root section on the activity of some muscles in man. J Neurol Neurosurg Psychiatry 1960; 23:10–22.

Newman SL, Road JD, Grassino A. In vivo length and shortening of canine diaphragm with body postural change. J Appl Physiol 1986; 60:661–669.

Redline S, Gottfried SB, Altose MD. Effects of changes in inspiratory muscle strength on the sensation of respiratory force. J Appl Physiol 1991; 70:240–245.

Remmers JE. Extra-segmental reflexes derived from intercostal afferents: phrenic and laryngeal responses. J Physiol (Lond) 1973; 233:45–62.

Remmers JE, Marttila I. Action of intercostal muscle afferents on the respiratory rhythm of anesthetized cats. Respir Physiol 1975; 24:31–41.

Remmers JE, Tsiaras WG. Effect of lateral cervical cord lesions on the respiratory rhythm of anesthetized decerebrate cats after vagotomy. J Physiol (Lond) 1973; 233:63–74.

Revelette WR, Davenport PW. Effects of timing on inspiratory occlusion on cerebral evoked potentials in humans. J Appl Physiol 1990; 68:282–288.

Revelette WR, Jewell LA, Frazier DT. Effect of diaphragm small fibre afferent stimulation on ventilation in dogs. J Appl Physiol 1988; 65:2097–2106.

Revelette R, Reynolds S, Brown D, Taylor R. Effects of abdominal compression on diaphragmatic tendon organ activity. J Appl Physiol 1992; 72:288–292.

Road JD, West NH, Van Vilet BN. Ventilatory effects of stimulation of phrenic afferents. J Appl Physiol 1987; 63:1063–1069.

Rose D, Larnicol N, Duron B. The cat cervical dorsal root ganglia: generalized cell-size characteristics and comparative study of neck muscle, neck cutaneous and phrenic afferents. Neurosci Res 1990; 7:341–357.

Roussos Ch. Ventilatory muscle fatigue governs breathing frequency. Clin Respir Physiol 1984; 20:445–451.

Russel JA, Bishop B. Vagal afferents essential for abdominal muscle activity during lung inflation in cats. J Appl Physiol 1976; 41:310–315.

Sahlin K, Katz A. Hypoxemia increases the accumulation of inosine monophosphate (IMP) in human skeletal muscle during submaximal exercise. Acta Physiol Scand 1989; 136:199–203.

Sant'Ambrogio G, Widdicombe JG. Respiratory reflexes acting on the diaphragm and inspiratory intercostal muscles of the rabbit. J Physiol (Lond) 1965; 180:766–779.

Sant'Ambrogio G, Wilson MF, Frazier DT. Somatic afferent activity in reflex regulation of diaphragmatic function in the cat. J Appl Physiol 1962; 17:829–832.

Seaman RG, Zechman FD, Frazier DT. Response of ventral inspiratory group neurons to mechanical loading. J Appl Physiol 1983; 54:254–261.

Sears TA. Some properties and reflex connections of respiratory motoneurones of the cat's thoracic spinal cord. J Physiol (Lond) 1964; 175:386–403.

Serratrice G, Mei N, Pelissier JF, Cros D. Cutaneous, muscular and visceral unmyelinated afferent fibres: comparative study. In: Carrera N, Pozza G, eds. Peripheral Neuropathies. Amsterdam: Elsevier, 1978:67–82.

Shannon R. Effects of thoracic dorsal rhizotomies on the respiratory pattern in anesthetized cats. J Appl Physiol 1977; 43:20–26.

Shannon R. Intercostal and abdominal muscle afferent influence on medullary dorsal respiratory group neurons. Respir Physiol 1980; 39:73–94.

Shannon R. Reflexes from respiratory muscles and costo-vertebral joints. In: Fishman AP, ed. Handbook of Physiology. The Respiratory System II. Bethesda, MD: American Physiology Society, 1986:431–447.

Shannon R, Freeman DL. Nucleus retroambigualis respiratory neurons: response to intercostal and abdominal muscle afferents. Respir Physiol 1981; 45:357–375.

Shannon R, Lindsey BG. Intercostal and abdominal muscle afferent influence on pneumotaxic center respiratory neurons. Respir Physiol 1983; 52:85–98.

Shannon R, Saporta S, Lindsey BG. Transmission of intercostal muscle proprioceptor afferent information to medullary respiratory areas. Exp Neurol 1982; 78:222–225.

Shannon R, Shear WT, Mercak AR, Bolser DC, Lindsay BG. Non vagal reflex effects on medullary inspiratory neurons during inspiratory loading. Respir Physiol 1985; 60:193–204.

Shannon R, Bolser DC, Lindsay BG. Medullary expiratory activity: influence of intercostal tendon organs and muscle spindle endings. J Appl Physiol 1987; 62:1057–1062.

Shannon R, Bolser DC, Lindsey BG. Medullary neurons mediating the inhibition of inspiration by intercostal muscle tendon organs. J Appl Physiol 1988; 65:2498–2505.

Siafakas NM, Chang HK, Bonora M, Gautier H, Milic-Emili J, Duron B. Time course of phrenic activity and respiratory pressure during airway occlusion in cats. J Appl Physiol 1981; 51:99–108.

Speck DF. Supraspinal involvement in the phrenic-to-phrenic inhibitory reflex. Brain Res 1987; 414:169–172.

Speck DF. Bötzinger complex region role in phrenic-to-phrenic inhibitory reflex of cat. J Appl Physiol 1989; 67:1364–1370.

Speck DF, Revelette WR. Excitation of dorsal and ventral respiratory group neurons by phrenic nerve afferents. J Appl Physiol 1987; 62:946–951.

Speck DF, Webber CL. Thoracic dorsal rhizotomy in the anesthetized cats: maintenance of eupnoeic breathing. Respir Physiol 1979; 38:347–357.

Speck DF, Webber CL. Time course of intercostal afferent termination of the inspiratory process. Respir Physiol 1981; 43:133–145.

Speck DF, Webber CL. Cerebellar influence on the termination of inspiration by intercostal nerve stimulation. Respir Physiol 1982; 47:231–238.

Stacey MJ. Free nerve endings in skeletal muscle of the cat. J Anat 1969; 105:231–254.

Stella G. On the mechanisms of production and the physiological significance of "apneusis." J Physiol (Lond) 1938; 93:10–23.

Supinski GS, Di Marco AF, Hussein F, Altose MD. Alterations in respiratory muscle activation in the ischemic fatigued canine diaphragm. J Appl Physiol 1989; 67: 720–729.

Teitelbaum J, Magder S, Roussos Ch, Hussain S. Effects of diaphragmatic ischemia on the inspiratory motor drive. J Appl Physiol 1992; 72:447–454.

Teitelbaum J, Borel C, Magder S, Traystman R, Hussain S. Effect of selective diaphragmatic paralysis on the inspiratory motor drive. J Appl Physiol 1993 (in press).

Trippenbach T, Milic-Emili J. Vagal contribution to the inspiratory "off-switch" mechanism. Fed Proc 1977; 36:2395–2399.

Ward M, Deschamps A, Roussos Ch., Hussain S. Effect of phrenic afferent stimulation on pattern of respiratory muscle activation. J Appl Physiol 1992a; 73:563–570.

Ward M, Vanelli G, Hashefi M, Hussain S. Ventilatory effects of the interaction between phrenic and limb muscle afferents. Respir Physiol 1992b; 88:63–76.

Wilson C, Gottfried S, Hussain S. Influence of phrenic afferents on tracheal tension in dogs. FASEB J 1992; 6:A1805.

Winckler G, Delaloye B. A propos de la présence de fuseaux neuromusculaires dans le diaphragme humain. Acta Anat 1957; 29:114–116.

Yamamoto S, Miyajima M, Urabe M. Respiratory neuronal activities in spinal afferents of cat. Jpn J Physiol 1960; 10:509–517.

Zechman FW, O'Neill R, Shannon R. Effect of low cervical cord lesions on detection of increased airflow resistance in man. Physiologist 1967; 10:356.

Zechman FW, Muza SR, Davenport PW, Wiley RL, Shelton R. Relationship of transdiaphragmatic pressure and latencies for detecting added inspiratory loads. J Appl Physiol 1985; 58:236–243.

Zimmerman GW, Grossie J. Sensitivity and behaviour of muscle spindles to systemic arterial hypoxia. Proc Soc Exp Biol Med 1963; 132:1114–1118.

13

Afferents from Limb Skeletal Muscle

MARC P. KAUFMAN

University of California—Davis
Davis, California

I. Introduction

Stimulation of sensory nerves with endings in hindlimb skeletal muscles is well known to have marked reflex effects on the respiratory system of anesthetized animals. Some of these reflex effects include increases in tidal volume, increases in the frequency of breathing, and increases in airway caliber. The purpose of this chapter is to define the reflex arc arising from contracting hindlimb skeletal muscle that functions to increase breathing and to dilate the airways. This reflex arc also has important effects on the cardiovascular system. These include vasoconstriction as well as increases in cardiac rate and contractility.

The reflex arc arising from contracting skeletal muscle is comprised of three components, namely the sensory nerves, the central neural pathways, and the motor nerves to the effector organs. Particular attention will be paid to the discharge properties of the sensory nerves that are responsible for evoking these reflex effects. Discussion of these components will be preceded by a description of the types of sensory nerves that supply hindlimb skeletal muscle.

II. Sensory Innervation of Skeletal Muscle

There is widespread agreement that hindlimb as well as forelimb skeletal muscle is innervated by five types of sensory nerves. These have been labeled groups I–IV, with the first group having two subtypes, Ia and Ib. This classification scheme is based on both the diameter and the degree of myelination of the afferent fibers. Both factors are important determinants of axonal conduction velocity (1,2).

Group Ia and Ib muscle afferents are thickly myelinated and conduct impulses between 72 and 120 m/sec. The receptors of group Ia afferents are primary muscle spindles and those of group Ib afferents are Golgi tendon organs. Primary spindle afferents (i.e., group Ia) are believed to be situated "in parallel" with the skeletal muscle fibers that they innervate. Simply put, this is another way of saying that the discharge of primary spindle afferents is stimulated by stretch (i.e., lengthening) of the muscle and is inhibited by contraction (i.e., shortening). Golgi tendon organs, on the other hand, are believed to be situated "in series" with the muscle fibers they innervate because these afferents are stimulated by both muscle stretch and contraction.

Group II afferents, also known as secondary spindles, conduct impulses between 31 and 71 m/sec. The receptors of these afferents (i.e., the spindles), like their group Ia counterparts, are situated in parallel with the muscle fibers that they innervate. Although secondary spindle afferents (i.e., group II) are stimulated by muscle stretch, they are unable to signal the rate at which this occurs. On the other hand, primary spindle afferents (i.e., group Ia) do signal the rate of stretch and consequently are said to be "dynamically sensitive."

Group III afferents are thinly myelinated and conduct impulses between 2.5 and 30 m/sec. Their receptors are free, unencapsulated nerve endings. Group IV afferents are unmyelinated and conduct impulses at less than 2.5 m/sec. Like their group III counterparts, the receptors of group IV afferents are free nerve endings. Group III afferents are also known as "A δ fibers," whereas group IV afferents are also known as "C-fibers."

Recently, von Düring and Andres (3) have described the ultrastructural anatomy of the free nerve endings of group III and IV afferents innervating the triceps surae muscles of cats. Electron microscopy revealed three locations for these free nerve endings within the muscle. The first location was in the adventitia of arteries (group III), arterioles (group IV), precapillary segments (group IV), as well as veins and lymphatic vessels (groups III and IV). The second location was in the endoneurium of the muscle nerves (group IV), and the third location was in connective tissue of the perimysium (group IV).

Similarly, Andres et al. (4) have described the ultrastructural anatomy of group III and IV endings within the Achilles (i.e., calcaneal) tendon. Group III endings were found in four locations: venules, lymph vessels, the connective tissue surrounding vessels and nerves, and the endoneurium of small nerve bundles. Group IV endings were found in the walls of both blood and lymph vessels supplying the Achilles tendon. In addition, group IV, but not group III, endings contain granulated vesicles, the content of which is not known (4). It would be interesting to know whether these granulated vesicles contained neuropeptides whose release via the "axon reflex" evokes vasodilation. In both the triceps surae muscles and the Achilles tendon, the diameters of the group III endings were found to be larger than those of the group IV endings (3,4). Finally, group III endings have more mitochondria and have a more distinct receptor matrix than do group IV endings (3).

III. Reflex Responses

Three types of stimuli have been used to investigate the reflex respiratory responses to activation of sensory nerves supplying hindlimb skeletal muscle. The three stimuli are electrical current applied to the hindlimb nerves, injection of algesic (i.e., painful) chemicals into the arterial supply of the hindlimb muscles, and contraction of hindlimb muscles. The use of each of the three types of stimuli presents difficulties and limitations in the interpretation of the findings; each of these will be discussed. Despite these difficulties and limitations, important information has been obtained from the use of each type of stimulus. This information has led consistently to the conclusion that stimulation of group III (i.e., thinly myelinated) and group IV (i.e., unmyelinated) muscle afferents reflexly increases tidal volume, increases breathing frequency, and dilates the airways, whereas stimulation of group I and II afferents has, at best, only small effects on some of these variables and none on others.

A. Electrical Stimulation

Electrical stimulation of sensory nerves supplying hindlimb skeletal muscle is well known to increase ventilation by a reflex mechanism. The utility of electrical stimulation of muscle nerves is that it provides an easily quantifiable stimulus whose timing is precisely controlled. In addition, measurement of the compound action potential allows one to reach some conclusions about the fiber populations recruited by the electrical pulses. Nevertheless, the use of electrical stimulation has severe drawbacks. These include the fact that applying electrical pulses to a nerve does not simulate the discharge pattern of afferent fibers stimulated by physiological conditions. Moreover, the frequency of the electrical pulses applied to a nerve often exceeds the frequency of the action potentials generated by physiological or pathophysiological stimuli. Finally, compound action potential measurements, which indicate the synchronous activation of many fibers by an electrical pulse, may not reveal the activation of a small number of other fibers, which in fact may be the initiators of any reflex effect that was observed.

Although there is widespread agreement that ventilation is increased reflexly by electrical stimulation of muscle nerves at current intensities that recruit group III and IV afferents, there is considerable controversy over whether ventilation is also increased by electrical stimulation of group I and II afferents. Several investigators have reported that stimulation of group I and II muscle afferents reflexly increases ventilation in anesthetized cats and dogs (5–9). In contrast, other investigators have reported that stimulation of these thick-fiber afferents had no effect on ventilation in anesthetized cats, dogs, and rabbits (10–12).

This controversy might be resolved by a detailed examination of the types of afferent fibers recruited by the electrical pulses applied to the muscle nerves. Two methods of identifying the fiber types recruited by the electrical pulses were used in the studies reporting that activation of group I and II afferents reflexly increased ventilation. These were the measurement of compound action potentials from the whole nerve and measurement of the stimulus current as a multiple of the threshold current needed to evoke a muscle twitch (i.e., motor threshold). One might offer the speculation that neither method was capable of revealing that the axons of a small number of group III afferents were recruited by electrical pulses that were thought to activate only the axons of group I and II afferents. On the other hand, it is entirely possible that stimulation of group I and II muscle afferents reflexly stimulates ventilation, although the increase is most probably modest compared to that reflexly evoked by stimulation of group III and IV afferents.

Electrical stimulation of sensory nerves supplying hindlimb skeletal muscle has been shown to relax reflexly airway smooth muscle in both anesthetized dogs (Figs. 1 and 2) (13,14) and cats (15). In addition, electrical stimulation of

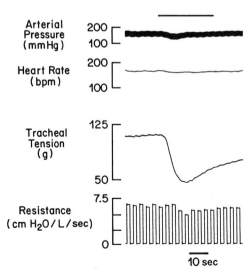

Figure 1 Bilateral electrical stimulation of the gracilis nerves at 20 Hz and 20 times motor threshold, which recruited groups I–III afferents, decreased arterial pressure, tracheal tension, and total pulmonary resistance. Stimulation period is signaled by the bar. Note that the dog was paralyzed with gallamine triethiodide. (Reprinted from Ref. 13 with permission.)

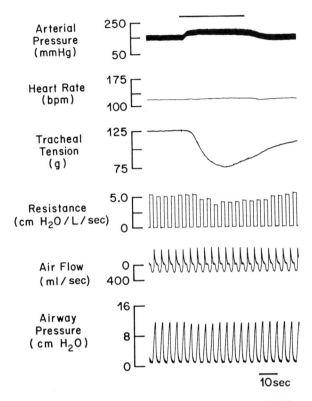

Figure 2 Bilateral electrical stimulation of the gracilis nerves at 20 Hz and 200 times motor threshold, which recruited groups I–IV afferents, increased arterial pressure, but decreased tracheal tension and total pulmonary resistance. Stimulation period is signaled by the bar. Note that results in Figure 1 and this figure are from different dogs, although both were paralyzed with gallamine. (Reprinted from Ref. 13 with permission.)

hindlimb sensory nerves has been shown to increase reflexly the activity of upper airway dilating muscles in these species (15). The afferent arm of the reflex arc evoking airway dilation was comprised of group III and IV fibers innervating the hindlimb. No evidence could be found that electrical stimulation of group I and II afferents reflexly evoked this effect (Fig. 3) (13,16). In addition, the efferent arm of this reflex arc in dogs was comprised of a withdrawal of cholinergic tone to airway smooth muscle. Excitation of beta-adrenergic pathways was shown to play no role in evoking this reflex (13). The efferent arm of the reflex airway dilation evoked by group III and IV afferents in species other than dogs is unknown. One candidate is the nonadrenergic, noncholinergic dilator pathway, which is found in cats, monkeys, and humans, but not in dogs (17).

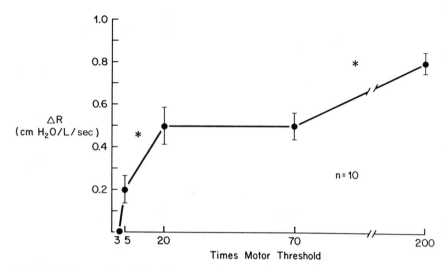

Figure 3   Decrease in total pulmonary resistance is dependent on the stimulus intensity. Bilateral electrical stimulation (20 Hz) of the gracilis nerves at 3 times motor threshold, which recruited groups I and II afferents, had no effect on resistance. Increasing the current intensity to either 5, 20, 70, or 200 times motor threshold evoked, for the most part, progressively greater decreases in resistance. Five times motor threshold is the minimum current intensity needed to recruit group III afferents. Likewise, 70 times motor threshold is the minimum needed to recruit group IV afferents. Asterisks indicate significant differences between adjacent means ($p < 0.05$). (Reprinted from Ref. 13 with permission.)

B. Algesic Chemicals

Injection of algesic chemicals into the arterial supply of hindlimb skeletal muscle of anesthetized animals has reflex effects on the respiratory system that are highly similar to those evoked by electrical stimulation of hindlimb muscle nerves. These reflex effects include increases in tidal volume, breathing frequency, and relaxation of airway smooth muscle. The algesic substances used to evoke these increases included potassium (18–21), capsaicin (22–24), bradykinin (20,21), sodium citrate (21), acid sodium phosphate (NaH_2PO_4) (21), and lactic acid (25). Moreover, these reflex increases in breathing and decreases in airway smooth muscle tone have been obtained in several species, including dogs, cats, and rabbits; because injection of these substances is quite painful, it is not possible to perform these experiments without benefit of anesthesia or decerebration. It is interesting to note that in rabbits injection of other substances, such as adenosine, serotonin, nicotine, vasopressin, and oxytocin, has been found to have no reflex respiratory effects (20).

It is useful to point out that the algesic substances capable of evoking reflex respiratory effects from hindlimb skeletal muscle are potent stimulants of group III and IV afferents. Moreover, these substances have little direct effect on the discharge of group I and II afferents, although they can increase the activity of these thick fiber afferents indirectly by reflex activation of gamma motoneurons (see below). Succinylcholine, which has proved to stimulate muscle spindles and to a lesser extent Golgi tendon organs, had no effect on breathing when injected into the arterial supply of hindlimb muscle in anesthetized cats (26). Moreover, succinylcholine had no effect on the discharge of group III and IV muscle afferents provided the muscles were not allowed to fasciculate in response to injection (26). In addition, tendon vibration, a maneuver that stimulates selectively group Ia and II muscle spindles, had no effect on ventilation (27,28).

C. Muscular Contraction

Contraction is the third stimulus used to investigate the respiratory responses to activation of hindlimb skeletal muscle afferents. Frequently, contraction of hindlimb muscle is induced in anesthetized animals by electrical stimulation of the peripheral cut ends of the lumbar and sacral ventral roots, which contain alpha and gamma motoneurons. There is substantial evidence that maintained tetanic contraction (often called static contraction), intermittent tetanic contraction, or repetitive twitch contraction at 5 Hz reflexly increases minute volume of ventilation and relaxes airway smooth muscle, effects that have been reported in both cats (29–31) and dogs (Fig. 4) (32–35). In addition, intermittent tetanic contraction of the gastrocnemius muscles of anesthetized dogs has been shown to increase reflexly the activity of upper airway dilator muscles (36). There is also evidence that static and intermittent tetanic contraction of hindlimb muscles in rabbits increases minute volume of ventilation (37). The reflex effect of muscular contraction on airway caliber in rabbits has not been investigated.

The use of three types of neural blockade has led to the conclusion that group III and IV muscle afferents comprise the afferent arm of reflex respiratory responses to contraction. Lidocaine applied topically to the dorsal roots of anesthetized cats was the first type of neural blockade to be used. When Mc-Closkey and Mitchell (30) applied this local anesthetic in concentrations that blocked impulse conduction in group III and IV afferents but not in group I and II afferents, they found that the ventilatory and pressor responses to contraction were greatly reduced. Moreover, when the lidocaine was washed away, the responses to contraction were restored to their original magnitude.

Anodal blockade applied to the dorsal roots of anesthetized cats was the second type of neural blockade used. When McCloskey and Mitchell (30) used this technique to block impulse conduction in group I and II afferents, but not in group III and IV afferents, they found that the ventilatory and pressor responses to contraction were no different than those to contraction before anodal blockade. The third technique to be used was the application of cold to the hindlimb muscle nerves of anesthetized dogs (32). Cooling the sciatic nerves to 4–8°C, a tempera-

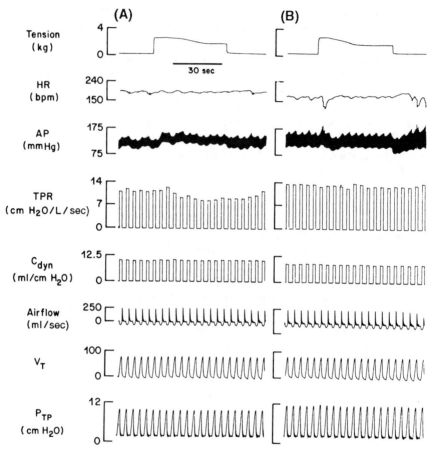

Figure 4 Static contraction of hindlimb muscles reflexly decreases total pulmonary resistance (TPR). (A) Static contraction induced by stimulating L-6 to L-7 ventral roots at 50 Hz decreased TPR. (B) S-3 to L-4 dorsal and ventral roots were cut and hindlimb muscles statically contracted again. Note that TPR did not change. Also note that baseline transpulmonary pressure (P_{TP}), TPR, and arterial pressure (AP) increased, presumably owing to a decrease in level of anesthesia. HR, heart rate; C_{dyn}, dynamic compliance; V_T, tidal volume. (Reprinted from Ref. 33 with permission.)

ture that blocks impulse conduction in groups I and II fibers, had only a small attenuating effect on the ventilatory, pressor, and cardiac responses to intermittent tetanic contraction of the hindlimb muscles in barbiturate-anesthetized dogs (32). At 4–8°C impulse frequency across the cooled portion of nerve is slowed but it is not blocked in group III and IV fibers. On the other hand, cooling the sciatic nerves to 1°C, a temperature that blocks impulse conduction in all afferent fibers, almost abolished the respiratory and cardiovascular responses to contraction (32). The direction of the ventilatory response to stimulation of hindlimb muscle afferents has been shown to depend on whether the neuraxis is intact or sectioned at the cervical spinal level. Stimulation of these afferents by stretching the gastrocnemius muscle or by electrically stimulating the tibial nerve at high current intensities in intact paralyzed, anesthetized cats reflexly increased phrenic nerve activity, although a short-lasting early inhibition of this activity was usually observed as well. When the spinal cord was sectioned between C-1 and C-2 and phrenic nerve discharge was evoked by electrical stimulation of intercostal nerves, both stretch and electrical stimulation reflexly decreased phrenic nerve activity (38), an inhibition that was both rapid in onset and long-lasting. Eldridge et al. (38) concluded that stimulation of muscle afferents evoked a reflex inhibition of breathing that was expressed over spinal pathways. Eldridge et al. (38) further concluded that supraspinal pathways are required for the expression of the ventilatory increase evoked by stimulation of thin-fiber muscle afferents. One might speculate that supraspinal pathways are required no matter what the method used to stimulate muscle afferents. For example, ventilation is sometimes inhibited immediately after the onset of static muscular contraction, only to increase progressively as the contraction period continues. Most likely, this initial inhibition of ventilation is a spinal reflex.

Stimulation of sensory nerves with endings in hindlimb skeletal muscle has important reflex cardiovascular consequences, which can only be described briefly in this chapter. These reflex cardiovascular effects occur concomitantly with the respiratory ones described above. Regardless of whether muscle afferents are activated by electrical stimulation, by injection of algesic substances, or by static contraction, the reflex cardiovascular effects almost always include increases in cardiac rate, cardiac contractility, mean arterial pressure, and peripheral vascular resistance (30,32,34,39,40).

There is some evidence that rhythmic contraction of hindlimb muscles in anesthetized dogs and rabbits reflexly decreases mean arterial pressure and heart rate (11,12,41,42). This does not, however, appear to be the case in cats that were either decerebrated or anesthetized. In either feline preparation, any repetitive twitch contraction of the hindlimb muscles that decreased mean arterial pressure (43,44) remained after section of the dorsal roots innervating the hindlimb and was therefore attributed to a metabolic vasodilation.

IV. Discharge Properties of Thin-Fiber Muscle Afferents

The evidence that group III and IV afferents are responsible for the large majority of the reflex respiratory and cardiovascular responses to stimulation of sensory endings in hindlimb skeletal muscle is overwhelming. This section, therefore, will focus on the discharge properties of these thin-fiber (i.e., group III and IV) muscle afferents. While muscle spindles and Golgi tendon organs (i.e., group I and II afferents) may play important roles in regulating skeletal muscle function in the hindlimb, these thick-fiber afferents have at best only small reflex effects on both the respiratory and cardiovascular system. Muscle spindles and Golgi tendon organs supplying respiratory muscles such as the diaphragm and the intercostals may reflexly affect the respiratory system, but that is because these afferents are regulating the function of muscles that cause the lungs to be ventilated.

A. Sensitivity to Mechanical Stimuli

Sensitivity to mechanical stimuli is one important discharge property of group III and IV afferents. The most frequently used mechanical stimuli include tendon stretch (usually the calcaneal) as well as probing the receptive field of the afferent. This latter maneuver consists of punctate probing with a blunted instrument such as a von Frey hair, lightly stroking the receptive field with a painter's brush, and nonnoxious squeezing with a blunted forceps. When applied to the forearm of an investigator, none of these maneuvers are perceived as noxious. The findings of many studies have led to the conclusion that group III muscle afferents are much more sensitive to mechanical stimuli than are group IV afferents.

Paintal (45) was one of the first to investigate the mechanical sensitivity of group III afferents located in the hindlimb muscles of anesthetized dogs. He found that these thinly myelinated afferents responded to nonnoxious stimulation of their receptive fields. Since Paintal's report, several independent laboratories have reached a similar conclusion, namely that these afferents, which are almost always silent when the muscles are at rest, can be discharged by nonnoxious probing of their receptive fields (46–52). This nonnoxious probing is usually more forceful than the probing used to stimulate the receptive fields of Golgi tendon organs and muscle spindles. Moreover, not every group III afferent responds to nonnoxious probing of its receptive field; a minority require noxious squeezing of the muscle to stimulate them.

Tendon stretch is another maneuver that has been used to assess the mechanical sensitivity of group III afferents. Paintal (45) found that tendon stretch was not a particularly effective stimulus to group III afferents, with only a few responding to it. Other investigators have found that tendon stretch stimulated about half of the group III afferents tested (49,51), and still others have found that tendon stretch stimulated the great majority of the afferents tested (52).

Group IV afferents are much less sensitive to mechanical stimulation than are group III afferents. Nonnoxious probing of the receptive fields of group IV afferents has been shown to stimulate very few of them (49–51). In contrast, nonnoxious probing of the receptive fields of group III afferents stimulated at least half, if not more, of these myelinated fibers (see above). When probing receptive fields, one must frequently apply noxious pressure to the muscle to discharge group IV afferents (49–51). Indeed, some of these unmyelinated afferents are so insensitive to probing that when one vigorously pinches their receptive fields, they discharge only a few impulses. This vigorous pinching maneuver, by comparison, would elicit an explosive burst of impulses from many group III muscle afferents.

Group IV afferents are also much less sensitive to stretching the calcaneal (i.e., Achilles) tendon than are group III afferents. In fact, only a few group IV afferents were stimulated by tendon stretch in the physiological range (49–51,53). In contrast, at least half of the group III afferents tested are stimulated by tendon stretch within the physiological range (49,51,52).

B. Sensitivity to Chemical Stimuli

Sensitivity to chemical stimuli is a second discharge property of group III and IV muscle afferents. To assess this sensitivity, investigators have recorded the discharge of an individual group III or IV afferent before, during, and for several minutes after intra-arterial injection of the substance under examination. One such substance is bradykinin, which is known to be algesic (54) and which has been shown to be a potent stimulus to group III and IV muscle afferents (47,51,55–57). Roughly equal percentages of group III and IV afferents have been shown to be stimulated by bradykinin, and these percentages are always at least 50%, a finding that has been confirmed by several independent laboratories in both anesthetized dogs and cats.

Bradykinin has been shown to be released by contraction of the triceps surae muscles in anesthetized cats (58). This finding has raised the possibility that this substance plays a role in stimulating group III and IV afferents during exercise. However, one must keep in mind that the relationship between the concentration of bradykinin found in the interstitial space of contracting muscle and the concentration of this substance when it is injected intra-arterially is unclear. Dose-response studies in cats have revealed that the smallest effective dose, injected close arterially, was usually 2.6 μg (56), and sometimes 10 times that dose was needed to stimulate them.

Because both painful chemical agents such as bradykinin and nonnoxious mechanical stimuli such as probing of receptive fields have both been shown to stimulate many of the same group III and IV muscle afferents, Kumazawa and Mizumura (47) have proposed that they are polymodal. In contrast, others have proposed that these thin-fiber afferents display a high degree of specificity, responding either to algesic chemical stimuli or to nonnoxious ones, but not both (45,46,56). Mense and Meyer (53) stated that the controversy over specificity versus polymodality might be due to the use of algesic chemicals, such as bradykinin, that are "strong inadequate stimuli." One might interpret that statement to mean that the doses of bradykinin used by previous authors created concentrations of this substance in the hindlimb muscles that exceeded those produced by tissue inflammation and damage. Although neither concentration has been measured owing to limited technology, it is reasonable to speculate that Mense and Meyer's (53) point is correct. Mense and Meyer (53) concluded that thin-fiber afferents innervating hindlimb skeletal muscle and tendons of cats are not polymodal, but rather display discharge properties specific to different functions, such as thermoception, nociception, mechanoreception, and ergoreception.

Group III and IV muscle afferents are also stimulated by intra-arterial injection of several other substances, many of which are produced by hindlimb muscle during either contraction or tissue inflammation. For example, potassium (50,59,60), lactic acid (61–63), arachidonic acid (62), and PGE_2 (64,65) have been shown to stimulate these thin-fiber afferents. Each of these substances stimulates equal percentages of group III and IV afferents, with potassium being the most frequently effective stimulus and PGE_2 appearing to be the least effective.

Using an ion-selective electrode placed on the surface of the gracilis muscle, Rybicki et al. (60) found that bolus intra-arterial injections of KCl solution evoked increases in potassium activities in the muscle that lasted 3–4 min, but that the afferents' responses to injection lasted less than 30 sec. In addition, Rybicki et al. (60) found that infusions of KCl solution, lasting 10 min, only transiently stimulated the group III and IV afferents. These findings led Rybicki et al. (60) to suggest that increases in potassium activity, induced by hindlimb muscle contraction, were capable of initiating autonomic reflexes, but that these increases were not capable of maintaining these reflexes.

Capsaicin, an extract of jalapeño pepper, has been shown to stimulate about 75% of the group IV afferents tested but only 25% of the group III afferents tested (51,57). Capsaicin, therefore, is a potent pharmacological tool that is useful for stimulating thin-fiber afferents, most of which belong to the group IV category. Nevertheless, capsaicin is a bizarre, foreign compound that discharges group IV afferents at much higher frequencies than do "natural" stimuli. Its use needs to be considered carefully.

Several other substances, each of which is naturally produced by skeletal muscle, have been shown to have only small effects on the discharge of group III and IV afferents. Both serotonin and histamine, injected intra-arterially, have been shown to stimulate only a few afferents in cats. This is the case even when high doses of either substance are injected (56). In addition, lactate at a neutral pH, phosphate at a neutral pH, and adenosine have been shown to stimulate only a small percentage of group III and IV afferents (50,62).

C. Sensitivity to Muscular Contraction

Sensitivity to muscular contraction is a third important discharge property of group III and IV afferents. To test this sensitivity, investigators usually have contracted hindlimb muscles by applying electrical pulses to either the ventral roots or the muscle nerves themselves. The advantages of the former method over the latter is that the ventral roots contain few afferent fibers; therefore, one does not need to be concerned about attributing an afferent's response to contraction when in fact it was caused by electrical stimulation of afferent fibers. Regardless of whether the hindlimb muscles were contracted in an intermittent tetanic fashion (49) or in a maintained tetanic fashion (51,52,66,67), neither type of contraction is representative of an alpha motoneuron discharge pattern and recruitment order similar to that evoked by static or dynamic exercise. In fact, electrical stimulation of ventral roots and muscle nerves recruits alpha motoneurons in the opposite order of that recruited during exercise (68).

Despite the fact that electrical stimulation of ventral roots does not cause hindlimb skeletal muscle to contract in the same manner as that seen during either static or dynamic exercise as performed by a behaving, intact animal, studies using electrical stimulation of ventral roots or muscle nerves have provided some valuable insights into the discharge properties of group III and IV muscle afferents. For example, several groups of investigators have reported that some group III afferents respond quite rapidly at the onset of contraction (Fig. 5). Sometimes this rapid response occurs within 100 msec of the onset of ventral root or muscle nerve stimulation and is expressed as an explosive burst of impulses that decrease in frequency as the contracting muscle fatigues (51,52). Sometimes, group III afferents display during contraction a second increase in activity, an effect that occurs usually 30 sec after the start of ventral root stimulation (Fig. 5) (51). One might speculate that this second increase in activity by group III afferents during static (i.e., maintained tetanic) contraction is caused by a metabolic by-product released by the working muscle.

Not all group III afferents respond vigorously at the start of contraction. Some (about 35–50%) do not respond at all and others respond only weakly at the start of contraction, but then discharge as the contraction period progresses. These diverse responses to contraction strongly suggest that group III afferents possess discharge properties that fall along a continuum, with one end being mechanosensitivity and the other end being chemical (i.e., metabolic) sensitivity. With respect to the mechanosensitive group III afferents, many will synchronize their discharge to rhythmic (oscillating) contractions of the triceps surae muscles of cats (49,66). In addition, the more forceful the contraction, the greater their discharge (49,51,52).

Group IV afferents, in contrast to group III afferents, rarely discharge an explosive burst of impulses at the onset of a static contraction (Figs. 5 and 6). Nevertheless, these unmyelinated afferents may discharge an impulse or two at the onset of contraction, especially if it is forceful. Frequently, their discharge in response to the first 5–10 sec of static contraction will be sparse, after which impulse activity will increase provided the static contraction is maintained. Moreover, group IV afferents usually do not synchronize their discharge to

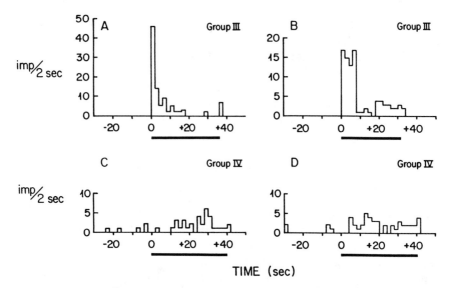

Figure 5 Discharge patterns of four thin-fiber muscle afferents that responded to static contraction. Contraction period depicted by black bar. (A) Group III fiber (conduction velocity 17.8 m/sec) discharged vigorously at onset of contraction, but then its firing rate decreased even though muscle continued to contraction. (B) Group III fiber (conduction velocity 9.6 m/sec) discharged vigorously at start of contraction, adapted, and then fired again during contraction. (C) Group IV fiber (conduction velocity 1.3 m/sec) started to fire 10 sec after onset of contraction and then gradually increased its firing rate during contraction period. Note that firing of fiber slowed even though muscle continued to contract. (D) Group IV fiber (conduction velocity 1.1 m/sec) fired irregularly 4 sec after onset of static contraction. (Reprinted from Ref. 51 with permission.)

rhythmic contractions and usually do not increase their discharge frequency as the force of contraction increases.

The different discharge patterns displayed by group III and IV afferents responsive to muscular contraction have led to the hypothesis that group III afferents are stimulated, at least in part, by mechanical distortion of their receptive fields, whereas group IV afferents are stimulated by the metabolic by-products of contraction. A partial test of this hypothesis has been performed. This test has compared an afferent's response to contraction while the triceps surae muscles were freely perfused with the afferent's response to contraction while the triceps surae muscles were ischemic. The reasoning underlying this test is that ischemia will increase the levels of metabolic by-products in the contracting muscle because it will cause a mismatch between blood supply and demand. The results have shown that few group III afferents respond more to "ischemic contractions" than

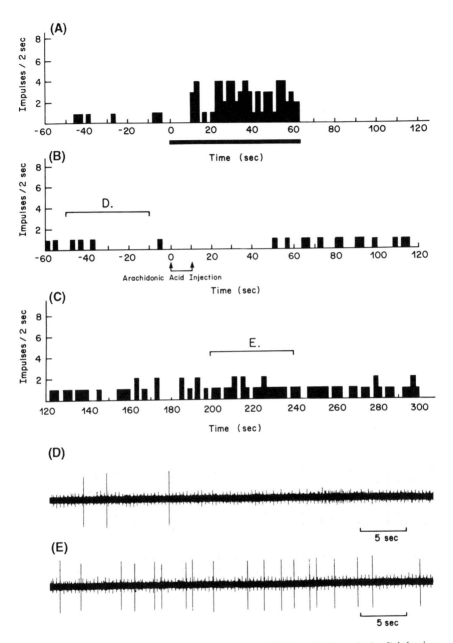

Figure 6 Effects of static contraction (A) and arachidonic acid (1 mg in 1 ml) injection into femoral artery (B and C) on discharge of a group IV afferent (conduction velocity = 1.1 m/sec). ■, Contraction period in A. Note that B and C are continuous in time. (D) Recording of the impulse activity of afferent during period of time depicted by bracket with D over it in B. (E) Recording of impulse activity of afferent during period of time depicted by the bracket with E over it in C. (Reprinted from Ref. 62 with permission.)

to "freely perfused contractions," whereas many group IV afferents respond more to the former type of contraction than respond to the latter (49,67,69). Specifically, only 12% of the group III afferents tested responded more to static contraction when the triceps surae muscles were ischemic than when they were freely perfused (67). In contrast, 47% of the group IV afferents responded more to static contraction when these muscles were ischemic than when they were freely perfused. The difference between these percentages was found to be statistically significant ($p < 0.05$).

As yet, the metabolic by-product that signals a mismatch between blood supply and demand in contracting skeletal muscle while it is ischemic is unknown. Some candidates include lactic acid, bradykinin, and cyclooxygenase products of arachidonic acid (see above; Fig. 6). Exogenous injection of each of these candidates, however, appears to stimulate equal percentages of group III and IV afferents (47,56,62), whereas ischemia increases the responses to contraction of many more group IV than group III afferents (49,67). This difficulty remains to be resolved. It may be that none of these substances (i.e., bradykinin, arachidonic acid, and lactic acid) function as the ischemic metabolite.

The hypothesis that an ischemic metabolite signals a mismatch between blood supply and demand in the working muscle is based on one of three circumstances. The first is that metabolites accumulate in the muscle owing to insufficient washout. The second is that the mismatch causes the production of a metabolite that is not produced when there is not a mismatch. The third is that the mismatch might be signaled by hypoxia in the working muscle. The evidence, so far, does not offer strong support for hypoxia to be the signal. For example, with hindlimb muscles at rest, ventilation of the lungs for 3–4 min with 5% oxygen in nitrogen, a maneuver that decreased the mean arterial Po_2 to about 22 mmHg, had only a modest stimulatory effect on the discharge of group IV afferents and had no effect on the discharge of group III afferents (70). In addition, hypoxic ventilation of the lungs for the above period of time had no effect on femoral venous lactate or hydrogen ion concentrations. Moreover, static contraction during hypoxic ventilation of the lungs did not stimulate most group III and IV afferents to a greater extent than did static contraction during normoxic ventilation (70).

The sensitivity of group III and IV afferents to contraction has been shown to be changed by alterations in the chemical environment of the muscle. For example, intra-arterial injection of bradykinin has been shown to increase the responses to intermittent tetanic contraction of both group III and IV afferents innervating the triceps surae muscles (53). Similarly, intra-arterial injections of arachidonic acid has been shown to increase the responses of group III, but not the responses of group IV, afferents to static contraction (65,71). Decreasing the concentrations of various chemicals in the muscle's environment has been shown to alter the responses of these afferents to contraction. Thus, both indomethacin and aspirin, substances that decreased the muscles' ability to synthesize prostaglandins and thromboxanes, decreased both group III and IV afferents' responses to static contraction (65,71). In addition, sodium dichloroacetate, which decreases the concentration of lactic acid in the muscles, decreased the responses of group III afferents to static contraction (63). In particular, the decrease in sensitivity to contraction by dichloroacetate occurred during the first 10 sec of the contraction period, which was interpreted to mean that lactic acid concentrations in skeletal muscle can affect the mechanical sensitivity of group III afferents (63). The effect of dichloroacetate on the responses of group IV afferents to contraction is not known.

The finding that the concentration of various substances in skeletal muscle affects the responses of group III and IV afferents to contraction has an important implication. Inflammation and injury are both likely to increase the concentrations of bradykinin and cyclooxygenase metabolites in skeletal muscle. Both substances have been shown to increase the sensitivity of group III and IV afferents to contraction. Therefore, inflammation and injury may markedly increase the magnitude of any reflex autonomic responses to contraction of hindlimb skeletal muscle. Consequently, one needs to consider the degree of inflammation and injury to skeletal muscle when interpreting data. This might be especially important in preparations that have undergone extensive surgery or have been manipulated manually to stimulate the receptive fields of thin fiber afferents.

V. The Dorsal Horn—Site of the First Synapse

Group III and IV hindlimb muscle afferents enter the spinal cord by the dorsal roots and synapse in the dorsal horn of the gray matter. A few group IV afferents, however, project their axons into the ventral roots, which some may interpret as an exception to the Law of Bell and Magendie. This Law states that the ventral roots contain only motor fibers, whereas the dorsal roots contain only sensory fibers. Convincing evidence has been presented that these unmyelinated ventral root afferents make a U-turn and enter the spinal cord via the dorsal root (72,73). Furthermore, most of these ventral root afferents appear to innervate the viscera and skin (74).

Light and Perl (75) were among the first investigators to use horseradish peroxidase (HRP) to trace the termination of thin-fiber afferents in the dorsal horn of the spinal cord. Using light microscopy, they found terminal labeling from small myelinated afferents in Rexed's lamina I (i.e., the marginal zone) and the inner portion of lamina II (i..e, the substantia gelatinosa). Furthermore, terminal labeling of the endings of presumed unmyelinated afferents was found in both the inner and outer portions of lamina II. The terminal labeling described by Light and Perl (75) arose from the application of HRP to the cut central ends of the cervical, lumbar, and sacral dorsal roots of cats, rats, and monkeys. This labeling, therefore, represented the termination of afferent fibers supplying a variety of structures, including muscle, skin, joints, and bone.

Subsequently, Craig and Mense (76) and Mense and Craig (77) applied wheat germ agglutin conjugated to HRP (WGA-HRP) to the gastrocnemius and soleus nerves of cats. The application of WGA-HRP to these nerves was an attempt to restrict transport of this substance and, therefore, terminal labeling to only muscle afferents. Using light microscopy, these investigators reported terminal labeling in laminas I and V; they did not find significant amounts of labeling in laminas II–IV. The terminal labeling in laminas I and V was attributed to group III and IV muscle afferents, because WGA-HRP is believed to label predominantly C-fiber (i.e., group IV) terminals in the dorsal horn (78).

These findings have been supplemented by studies in which the cell bodies of group III gastrocnemius afferents were impaled and filled with HRP. Terminal labeling in these filled dorsal root ganglion cells was found in laminas I and V (79). Impaling and filling small cells such as those supplying the axons of group III and IV afferents is extremely difficult, and consequently it has not been done for the cell bodies of group IV afferents.

Electrophysiological studies have also provided some useful information about the location of the synapses made by group III and IV afferents. Thus, group III afferents, when stimulated electrically, were shown to excite cells in laminas I, II, V, and VI (80,81). In addition, group III and IV muscle afferents, when stimulated by algesic substances, were shown to excite spinothalamic cells, whose dendrites were located in laminas II–VI, but were not located in lamina I (82). Electrophysiological information, although valuable, must be interpreted carefully because of the difficulty involved in determining the number of synapses between the stimulus and the dorsal horn cell responsive to it. This is especially true when dealing with slowly conducting afferents.

Electrophysiological studies have also provided two other important findings. The first is that cold block of descending input from central structures above the lumbar spinal cord increased the number of receptive fields of dorsal horn cells receiving hindlimb input. The second is that cold block increased the mechanical responsiveness of these cells to a given stimulus (81). One interpretation of these findings is that the dorsal horn receives from higher central structures a tonic inhibitory input that functions to gate or dampen group III and IV afferent input.

VI. Neurotransmitters and Neuromodulators Released in the Dorsal Horn

A. Release by Thin-Fiber Muscle Afferents

Group III and IV muscle afferents are believed to release onto dorsal horn cells a fast-acting chemical messenger, referred to as a neurotransmitter, and a slow-acting chemical messenger, referred to as a neuromodulator. The nature of the neurotransmitter is unknown, although glutamate is one candidate that is frequently mentioned. The neuromodulator might be substance P, although others such as somatostatin and calcitonin gene-related peptide (CGRP) may also function in this role.

Glutamate is well known to be contained by primary afferents synapsing in the dorsal horn (83,84). Moreover, glutamate is released when these afferents are activated (85) and is a powerful stimulant of spinal neurons (86). These findings provide strong support for glutamate to serve as the fast-acting neurotransmitter for the first synapse in the reflex arc arising from hindlimb skeletal muscle that functions to activate the autonomic nervous system. Unfortunately, there is no hard experimental evidence that this is in fact the case. Thus, the effects of glutamate receptor blockade on the reflex autonomic responses to stimulation of group III and IV muscle afferents are unknown.

Two reports shed some light on the role of glutamate in the spinal transmission of afferent input from hindlimb muscles. First, Schneider and Perl (87), using a hamster spinal cord preparation in vitro, reported that L-glutamate or L-aspartate excited less than a third of the dorsal horn cells tested. These cells were located in laminas I–V and many received input from dorsal root afferent C-fibers. Second, Yoshimura and Jessell (88), using a rat spinal cord preparation in vitro, reported that CNQX was much more effective than APV in decreasing the amplitude of EPSPs evoked in the substantia gelatinosa (i.e., lamina II) by electrical stimulation of Aδ (i.e., group III) and C (i.e., group IV) fibers in the dorsal roots. Because CNQX blocks non-NMDA receptors and APV blocks NMDA receptors, these investigators concluded that the former play an important role in the fast neurotransmission in the spinal cord. In addition, Yoshimura and Jessell (88) showed that both AMPA and kainate, which are not substrates for the high-affinity L-glutamate uptake system, markedly depolarized glutamate-insensitive cells in the substantia gelatinosa. Moreover, both the AMPA- and kainate-induced depolarizations were reduced by CNQX. These latter findings were interpreted to mean that a lack of sensitivity of cells to glutamate, such as that shown by Schneider and Perl (87), might be attributable to rapid reuptake of this excitatory amino acid.

There is considerable evidence that substance P functions as a slow transmitter (i.e., neuromodulator) in the first synapse of the reflex arc arising from hindlimb skeletal muscle that increases autonomic output. For example, electrical stimulation of Aδ- and C-fiber afferents in the sciatic nerve releases substance P in the dorsal horn (89). In addition, static contraction of hindlimb muscle releases substance P as well as neurokinin A in the dorsal horn (90,91). The release of substance P is greatly attenuated by dorsal root section (91). In addition, substance P has been localized in the terminals of thin-caliber axons traveling in the dorsal roots (92–94). Finally, substance P has been shown to evoke a slow depolarization of dorsal horn cells (95).

Support for the hypothesis that substance P functions as a neuromodulator in the reflex arc arising from skeletal muscle has come from studies on anesthetized cats. These studies have shown that intrathecal injections of either a peptide antagonist to substance P or an antibody to this peptide decreased by half the reflex pressor response to static contraction of the hindlimb muscles (96,97). Subsequently, microinjection of this peptide antagonist into the gray matter of the spinal cord has been shown to attenuate the reflex pressor response to static contraction, but to have no effect on the reflex pressor response to stretching the calcaneal (i.e., Achilles) tendon (98).

The peptide antagonist to substance P (i.e., D-Pro^2, D-Phe^7, D-Trp^9-substance P) used in the above studies (96,98) has been shown to antagonize two of the three neurokinin receptors found in the spinal cord. Recently, specific antagonists to the two receptors, NK-1 and NK-2, have been developed. Using these two specific receptor antagonists, Hill et al. (99) showed that blockade of the NK-1 receptor with CP-96345 attenuated both reflex ventilatory and pressor responses to static contraction, but that blockade of the NK-2 receptor had no effect on these reflex responses. Hill et al. (99) concluded that although both substance P and neurokinin A are released in the dorsal horn by the group III and IV afferents activated by muscular contraction, the two neuropeptides exert their reflex effects on autonomic function by stimulating NK-1 receptors.

Although considerable evidence exists in support of substance P as a neuromodulator in the first synapse of the reflex arc arising from hindlimb skeletal muscle, a note of caution should be raised. Microinjection of substance P into the lumbosacral dorsal horn does not increase either arterial blood pressure or heart rate (98). This is a disturbing finding because it is reasonable to expect that exogenous administration of substance P into its purported site of action in the dorsal horn should evoke similar cardiovascular responses as those arising reflexly from stimulation of group III and IV afferents. One possible explanation for this discrepancy might be that substance P, a slow-acting neuromodulator, must be coreleased, with a fast-acting neurotransmitter in the dorsal horn to evoke autonomic effects.

Somatostatin is another neuromodulator candidate in the dorsal horn. This peptide has been localized in the terminals of thin-fiber afferents of the dorsal roots. Hökfelt et al. (92) reported that somatostatin was located in different terminals than those in which substance P was located. In contrast, Cameron et al. (93) found somatostatin and substance P to be located in the same terminals. In the rat, somatostatin is rarely found in muscle afferents, whereas it is frequently found in skin afferents (94). Contraction of hindlimb skeletal muscle in rats does not evoke reflex pressor effects (100), whereas it does evoke this effect in many other species. It would be of interest to ascertain whether muscle afferents contain somatostatin in these other species.

As with substance P, evidence exists that somatostatin functions as a neuromodulator in the dorsal horn. Intrathecal injection or microinjection of a peptide antagonist to somatostatin has been shown to attenuate the reflex pressor response to static contraction of the hindlimb muscles in anesthetized cats (98,101). Moreover, microinjection of the somatostatin antagonist had no effect on the pressor response to tendon stretch (98). Microinjection of somatostatin into the lumbosacral dorsal horn had no effect on arterial pressure or heart rate (98), a finding that raises some doubt about its neuromodulator function. Although studies using receptor blockade or immunoneutralization of substance P and somatostatin have provided some valuable insights into neurotransmission in the dorsal horn, they do not offer any information that attenuation of the reflex responses to muscular contraction occurred at the first synapse of this reflex arc.

CGRP is also believed to be released in the dorsal horn by the terminals of group IV (102) muscle afferents. In addition, CGRP has been colocalized with substance P in the spinal terminals of these afferents (94,103). The role of CGRP in the spinal transmission of reflex autonomic responses arising from the stimulation of limb thin-fiber muscle afferents is not known.

B. Release by Interneurons

Norepinephrine (104), metenkephalin (105), and serotonin (106) are found in the dorsal horn of the spinal cord. Both norepinephrine and met-enkephalin are believed to be released by axon terminals whose cell bodies are located in the dorsal horn, whereas serotonin is believed to be released by terminals whose cell bodies are located in the medullary and pontine raphé. Intrathecal injections of opioid, alpha-adrenergic, or serotonergic agonists (done one at a time and not in combination) greatly attenuated the reflex pressor and ventilatory responses to static contraction in anesthetized cats. However, intrathecal injections of antagonists to these substances did not potentiate the reflex responses to contraction (107–109). The simplest interpretation of these latter findings is that endogenous release of norepinephrine, met-enkephalin, and serotonin plays little if any role in buffering the reflex pressor response to contraction.

Vasopressin has also been found in the dorsal horn of the spinal cord. The source of this peptide is both the dorsal root ganglia (i.e., primary afferents) and the terminals of axons whose cell bodies are located in the paraventricular nucleus of the hypothalamus (110,111). Intrathecal injection of vasopressin has been shown to attenuate the reflex pressor response to static contraction, whereas intrathecal injection of a receptor antagonist to vasopressin has been shown to potentiate this reflex response (112). These findings suggest that the release of vasopressin in the dorsal horn by axon terminals projecting from the paraventricular nucleus has a tonic inhibitory role in the reflex autonomic responses to contraction.

VII. The Ventrolateral Medulla

An intact caudal ventrolateral medulla appears to be needed for the full expression of the reflex airway dilation arising from the stimulation of group III and IV hindlimb muscle afferents. In anesthetized dogs, Padrid et al. (14) showed that microinjection of either ibotenic acid or cobalt chloride into the caudal ventrolateral medulla attenuated the reflex airway dilation evoked by either electrical stimulation of C-fiber afferents in the sciatic nerve or by static contraction of the gastrocnemius muscles. The attenuation by ibotenic acid, which destroys cell bodies but not axons of passage, was not reversible, whereas the attenuation by cobalt chloride, which by blocking calcium channels prevented neurotransmitter release, was reversible. In anesthetized cats, Strohl et al. (15) showed that topical application of lidocaine to the ventrolateral medullary surface abolished the reflex tracheal dilation evoked by electrical stimulation of the sciatic nerve.

The ventrolateral medullary site inactivated by Padrid et al. (14) in dogs appeared to be anatomically and functionally different than the site inactivated by Strohl et al. (15) in cats. Anatomically, the site inactivated by Padrid et al. (14) was in the substance of the caudal ventrolateral medulla and was near, but not in, the lateral reticular nucleus. In contrast, the site inactivated by Strohl et al. (15) was on the surface of the ventrolateral medulla and corresponded to the intermediate area described by Schlaefke and Loeschcke (113). Functionally, stimulation of the substance of the caudal ventrolateral medulla with DL-homocysteic acid dilated the airways in dogs (114), whereas stimulation of the ventrolateral medullary surface with N-methyl D-aspartic acid constricted the airways and stimulated phrenic nerve discharge in cats (115). In addition, blockade of the ventrolateral medullary surface with either lidocaine or cooling attenuated the reflex tracheal constriction evoked by mechanical stimulation of pulmonary vagal afferents in cats (116).

There is also electrophysiological evidence that stimulation of group III and IV hindlimb muscle afferents relays their input to the ventrolateral medulla. Iwamoto and Kaufman (117) reported that capsaicin, injected into the arterial supply of the hindlimb, stimulated cells in the caudal ventrolateral medulla of anesthetized cats. Capsaicin has been shown to excite most group IV muscle afferents, a few group III afferents, but almost no group I and II afferents (51,57). Iwamoto and Kaufman (117) also showed that static contraction of the triceps surae muscles stimulate many of the same caudal ventrolateral medullary cells as those stimulated by capsaicin. These findings were confirmed and extended by Bauer et al. (118), who showed that ventrolateral medullary neurons responded to hindlimb muscular contraction in anesthetized cats. In addition, Bauer et al. (118) showed that many of these ventrolateral medullary neurons discharged in synchrony with sympathetic nerve activity and projected axons to the intermediolateral cell column. The cells described by Bauer et al. (118) were probably involved in controlling sympathetic outflow and appeared to be somewhat more rostrally located than some of those described by Iwamoto and Kaufman (117). Other central neural structures in and rostral to the medulla have been examined for their participation in the reflex arc arising from hindlimb skeletal muscle that causes autonomic effects. For example, bilateral electrolytic lesions of the subthalamic locomotor region, which is in or near the fields of Forel of the hypothalamus, potentiated both the ventilatory frequency and heart rate increases reflexly evoked by static contraction of the hindlimb muscles in anesthetized cats (119). These lesions, however, had no effect on the increases in mean arterial pressure and minute ventilation that were evoked by contraction. At this point, the best available evidence suggests that central neural structures rostral to the inferior colliculus of the midbrain play only a small role in expressing the autonomic responses to contraction of hindlimb muscles in animals (44). Finally, bilateral electrolytic lesions of the nucleus reticularis gigantocellularis, which is located near the pontomedullary border, have been shown to have no effect on the reflex ventilatory and cardiovascular responses to hindlimb muscle contraction in anesthetized cats (120).

VIII. Final Common Path

There are many reflex autonomic responses to stimulation of hindlimb muscle afferents. This portion of the chapter, however, will be concerned only with the final common pathway to airway smooth muscle that causes it to relax when group III and IV afferents with endings in hindlimb skeletal muscle are stimulated. The best available evidence to date strongly suggests that this reflex relaxation is caused by vagal withdrawal and not by $beta_2$-adrenergic excitation regardless of whether group III and IV afferents are stimulated by algesic substances (121) or by muscle contraction (33). Likewise, the relaxation of airway smooth muscle evoked by chemical stimulation of the caudal ventrolateral medulla is also caused by vagal withdrawal and not by $beta_2$-adrenergic excitation (114,122). These conclusions are based on data from chloralose-anesthetized dogs, and it is not clear that they can be extended to other species or to conscious preparations. One must remember that dogs do not have a nonadrenergic, noncholinergic pathway to airway smooth muscle (17), whereas other species, including cats, monkeys, and humans, do have this pathway.

There is evidence that the nucleus ambiguus contains the cells of origin of the vagal efferent fibers whose activation causes constriction of airway smooth muscle. In an electrophysiological study, McAllen and Spyer (123) showed that cells in the nucleus ambiguus of cats could be antidromically invaded from the pulmonary branches of the vagus nerves. Subsequently, Ford et al. (124) showed that cells in the dorsal motor nucleus could also be antidromically invaded from the pulmonary vagus nerve. The vagal motoneurons activated by McAllen and Spyer (123) were innervated by axons conducting in the B-fiber range, whereas the vagal motoneurons activated by Ford et al. (124) conducted in the C-fiber range. Because the cells by Ford et al. (124) had unmyelinated axons, these investigators concluded that vagal motoneurons in the dorsal motor nucleus were not bronchomotor in function (see below).

Widdicombe (125) reported that vagal preganglionic fibers innervating the lungs conducted impulses in the B-fiber range (i.e., 10 m/sec) and discharged spontaneously with an inspiratory rhythm. These findings were confirmed and extended by McAllen and Spyer (123), who reported that the cells of origin of these vagal preganglionic fibers were in the nucleus ambiguus of cats. Widdicombe (125) and McAllen and Spyer (123) speculated that excitation of these vagal preganglionic fibers displaying an inspiratory rhythm caused airway smooth muscle to constrict.

Subsequently, Mitchell et al. (126) recorded intracellular potentials from parasympathetic postganglionic cell bodies lying on the trachea of chloralose-anesthetized cats. These investigators found two distinct populations of tracheal ganglion cells. The first discharged spontaneously with an expiratory rhythm and were reflexly excited by lung hyperinflation. When Mitchell et al. (126) injected these cells with Lucifer yellow dye they traced their postganglionic axons into the intercartilaginous spaces near the mucous glands.

The second population of tracheal ganglion cells found by Mitchell et al. (126) discharged spontaneously with an inspiratory rhythm and were reflexly activated by stimulation of the carotid chemoreceptors. In contrast to the first population of the tracheal ganglion cells, the spontaneous discharge of the second population of cells was reflexly inhibited by lung hyperinflation. Intracellular injections of Lucifer yellow dye revealed that the postganglionic axons of these ganglion cells projected to tracheal smooth muscle. In addition, the axonal projections of two distinct populations of tracheal ganglion cells in ferrets (127) have been shown to parallel the axonal projections of the two populations of ganglion cells found in cats (126).

Anatomical studies have shown that both the nucleus ambiguus and dorsal motor nucleus contain the cells of origins for vagal preganglionic fibers innervating the airways. For example, Bennett et al. (128) reported that application of HRP to the intrapulmonary branches of the vagus nerve in dogs resulted in cell body labeling in both medullary nuclei. These findings have been confirmed and extended to the extrapulmonary airways as well (129). A limitation of these anatomical studies is that they do not distinguish between cell bodies that cause airway smooth muscle constriction and those that cause airway mucous secretion. Nevertheless, they have provided valuable information and have advanced our understanding about the control of airway caliber.

Previous evidence strongly suggests that muscular contraction reflexly dilates the airways by decreasing the spontaneous activity of vagal preganglionic neurons, whose stimulation causes airway constriction. Although some progress has been made in this area (e.g., the caudal ventrolateral medulla), the central integrating mechanisms and neural pathways contributing to this reflex airway dilation are poorly understood. The elucidation of these mechanisms and pathways remains to be accomplished. Likewise, the ability of the vagal postganglionic cell bodies to integrate inputs from both sensory nerves and central neural structures remains to be determined. The possibility exists that these postganglionic cell bodies have an important integratory role, as do their preganglionic counterparts in the medulla.

IX. Relevance to Humans Performing Exercise

The contribution of the muscle reflex to the respiratory responses to exercise is unclear. Whereas the role of the muscle reflex in the human cardiovascular responses to exercise has received considerable attention, the role of this reflex in the human airway response to exercise has been almost ignored. For example, although exercise is known to dilate human airways by withdrawing cholinergic tone (130,131), the neural mechanisms causing this effect have not been determined.

The few attempts made to elucidate the mechanisms causing the human ventilatory responses to exercise have been inconclusive. For example, occlusion of the blood flow to the legs while subjects exercised on a bicycle has been shown to increase minute volume of ventilation (132,133). As has been pointed out by the authors of these reports, the ventilatory increase in response to circulatory occlusion while exercising can be attributed to either a muscle chemoreflex induced by ischemia or an increase in central command induced by a weakening of the skeletal muscles.

Consequently, postexercise circulatory occlusion has been used to examine the role of the muscle chemoreflex in the ventilatory responses to exercise. This technique has been used since the time of Alam and Smirk (134) to show that part of the pressor response to exercise remains if metabolic by-products are trapped in resting muscles that were previously contracting. Rowell et al. (135) found that postexercise circulatory occlusion caused arterial blood pressure but not ventilation to remain above preexercise level. These findings led Rowell et al. (135) to conclude that the muscle chemoreflex had no effect on ventilation in humans.

Using another experimental method, Galbo et al. (136) reached a conclusion about the role of the muscle reflex in the ventilatory response to exercise that might be viewed as different from that reached by Rowell et al. (135). Galbo et al.

(136) examined the ventilatory response to bicycle exercise before and during partial paralysis with curare. They reported that at a given oxygen uptake, ventilation was higher in partly paralyzed subjects than in unparalyzed subjects. This finding was interpreted as support for a role for central command in causing the ventilatory responses to exercise. However, Galbo et al. (136) also reported that when central command was held near maximal, increasing the oxygen uptake, which occurred as the effect of the curare wore off, led to large increases in ventilation. This latter finding was interpreted as support for a large role for peripheral factors, such as the muscle reflex, in causing the ventilatory response to exercise in humans.

One important caveat must be kept in mind when considering the above findings. While exercising, humans have more than one peripheral factor capable of increasing ventilation. In addition to the muscle reflex, these factors include a reflex arising from the carotid body as well as a reflex arising from the lungs. The carotid body reflex, which is well known to increase ventilation, is believed to be evoked by increases in plasma potassium concentrations, which in turn arise from the extrusion of this ion from the exercising muscles. The lung reflex, which can also increase ventilation, may arise from an increase in pulmonary arterial P_{CO_2} and may have a vagal afferent pathway (137). The relative contribution of each of these three peripheral factors, as well as central command, in causing the ventilatory responses to exercise remains to be clarified.

References

1. Hunt CC: Relation of function to diameter in afferent fibers of muscle nerves. J Gen Physiol 1954; 38:117–131.
2. Boyd IA, Davy MR: Composition of Peripheral Nerves. Edinbugh: Livingston, 1968.
3. von Düring M, Andres KH: Topography and ultrastructure of group III and IV nerve terminals of cat's gastrocnemius-soleus muscle. In: Zenker W, Neuhuber WL, eds. The Primary Afferent Neuron: A Survey of Recent Morpho-functional Aspects. New York: Plenum Press, 1990.
4. Andres KH, von Düring M, Schmidt RF: Sensory innervation of the Achilles tendon by group III and IV afferent fibers. Anat Histol Embryol 1985; 172:145–156.
5. Bessou P, Dejours P, LaPorte Y: Effets ventilatoires réflexes de la stimulation de fibres afférentes de grand diamètre, d'origine musculaire, chez le chat. CR Soc Biol (Paris) 1959; 153:477–481.
6. Koizumi K, Ushiyama J, Brooks CMcC: Muscle afferents and activity of respiratory neurons. Am J Physiol 1961; 200:679–684.
7. Senapati JM: Effect of stimulation of muscle afferents on ventilation of dogs. J Appl Physiol 1966; 21:242–246.
8. Carcassi AM, Concu A, Decandia M, Onnis M, Orani GP, Piras MB: Respiratory

responses to stimulation of large fibers afferent from muscle receptors in cats. Pflüger's Arch 1983; 399:309–314.

9. Orani GP, Decandia M: Group I afferent fibers: effects on cardiorespiratory system. J Appl Physiol 1990; 68:932–937.

10. Matthews PBC: Mammalian Muscle Receptors and Their Central Actions. London: Arnold, 1972.

11. Tallarida G, Baldoni F, Peruzzi G, Raimondi G, Massaro M, Sangiorgi M: Cardiovascular and respiratory reflexes from muscles during dynamic and static exercise. J Appl Physiol 1981; 50:784–791.

12. Tallarida G, Baldoni F, Peruzzi G, Raimondi G, Di Nardo P, Massaro M, Visigalli G, Franconi G, Sangiorgi M: Cardiorespiratory reflexes from muscles during dynamic and static exercise in the dog. J Appl Physiol 1985; 58:844–852.

13. Rybicki KJ, Kaufman MP: Stimulation of group III and IV muscle afferents reflexly decreases total pulmonary resistance in dogs. Respir Physiol 1985; 59:185–195.

14. Padrid PA, Haselton JR, Kaufman MP: Role of caudal ventrolateral medulla in reflex and central control of airway caliber. J Appl Physiol 1991; 71:2274–2282.

15. Strohl KP, Norcia MP, Wolin AD, Haxhiu MA, VanLunteren E, Deal EC Jr: Nasal and tracheal responses to chemical and somatic afferent stimulation in anesthetized cats. J Appl Physiol 1988; 65:870–877.

16. Haxhiu MA, Van Lunteren E, Mitra J, Cherniack NS, Strohl KP: Comparison of the responses of the diaphragm and upper airway muscles to central stimulation of the sciatic nerve. Respir Physiol 1984; 58:65–76.

17. Russell JA: Noradrenergic inhibitory innervation of canine airways. J Appl Physiol 1980; 48:16–22.

18. Liu CT, Huggins RA, Hoff HE: Mechanisms of intra-arterial K^+-induced cardiovascular and respiratory responses. Am J Physiol 1969; 217:969–973.

19. Wildenthal K, Mierzwiak DS, Skinner NS Jr, Mitchell JH: Potassium-induced cardiovascular and ventilatory reflexes from the dog hindlimb. Am J Physiol 1968; 215:542–548.

20. Tallarida G, Baldoni F, Peruzzi G, Brindisi F, Raimondi G, Sangiorgi M: Cardiovascular and respiratory chemoreflexes from the hindlimb sensory receptors evoked by intra-arterial injection of bradykinin and other chemical agents in the rabbit. J Pharmacol Exp Ther 1979; 208:319–329.

21. Tallarida G, Baldoni F, Peruzzi G, Raimondi G, Massaro M, Abate A, Sangiorgi M: Different patterns of respiratory responses to chemical stimulation of muscle receptors in the rabbit. J Pharmacol Exp Ther 1982; 223:552–559.

22. Crayton CS, Mitchell JH, Payne FC III: Reflex cardiovascular response during the injection of capsaicin into skeletal muscle. Am J Physiol 1981; 240:H315–H319.

23. Coleridge JCG, Coleridge HM, Roberts AM, Kaufman MP, Baker DG: Tracheal contraction and relaxation initiated by lung and somatic afferents in dogs. J Appl Physiol 1982; 52:984–990.

24. Baker DG, Don H: Reversal of the relation between respiratory drive and airway tone in cats. Respir Physiol 1988; 73:21–30.

25. Rotto DM, Stebbins CL, Kaufman MP: Reflex cardiovascular and ventilatory

responses to increasing H⁺ activity in cat hindlimb muscle. J Appl Physiol 1989; 67:256–263.

26. Waldrop TG, Rybicki KJ, Kaufman MP: Chemical activation of group I and II muscle afferents has no cardiorespiratory effects. J Appl Physiol 1984; 56:1223–1228.

27. Hodgson HJF, Matthews PBC: The ineffectiveness of excitation of the primary endings of the muscle spindle by vibration as a respiratory stimulate in the decerebrate cat. J Physiol 1968; 194:555–563.

28. McCloskey DI, Matthews PBC, Mitchell JH: Absence of appreciable cardiovascular and respiratory responses to muscle vibration. J Appl Physiol 1972; 33:623–626.

29. Coote JH, Hilton SM, Perez-Gonzalez JF: The reflex nature of the pressor response to muscular exercise. J Physiol 1971; 215:789–804.

30. McCloskey DI, Mitchell JH: Reflex cardiovascular and respiratory responses originating in exercising muscle. J Physiol 1972; 224:173–186.

31. Longhurst JC: Static contraction of hind limb muscles in cats reflexly relaxes tracheal smooth muscle. J Appl Physiol 1984; 57:380–387.

32. Tibes U: Reflex inputs to the cardiovascular and respiratory centers from dynamically working canine muscles: some evidence for involvement of group III or IV nerve fibers. Circ Res 1977; 41:332–341.

33. Kaufman MP, Rybicki KJ, Mitchell JH: Hindlimb muscular contraction reflexly decreases total pulmonary resistance. J Appl Physiol 1985; 59:1521–1526.

34. Fisher ML, Nutter DO: Cardiovascular reflex adjustments to static muscular contraction in the canine hindlimb. Am J Physiol 1974; 226:648–655.

35. Kaufman MP, Rybicki KJ: Muscular contraction reflexly relaxes tracheal smooth muscle in dogs. Respir Physiol 1984; 56:61–72.

36. Sakurai M, Hiba W, Chonan T, Kikuchi Y, Takishima T: Responses of upper airway muscles to gastrocnemius muscle contraction in dogs. Respir Physiol 1991; 84: 311–321.

37. Tallarida G, Baldoni F, Peruzzi G, Raimondi G, Massaro M, Abate A, Sangiorgi M: Different patterns of respiratory reflexes originating in exercising muscle. Am J Physiol 1983; 55:84–91.

38. Eldridge FL, Gill-Kumar P, Millhorn DE, Waldrop TG: Spinal inhibition of phrenic motoneurons by stimulation of afferents from peripheral muscles. J Physiol 1981; 311:67–79.

39. Mitchell JH, Mierzwiak DS, Wildenthal K, Willis WD Jr, Smith AM: Effect on left ventricular performance of stimulation of an afferent nerve from muscle. Circ Res 1968; 22:507–516.

40. Clement DL, Pannier JL: Cardiac output distribution during induced static muscular contractions in the dog. Eur J Appl Physiol 1980; 45:199–207.

41. Clement DL: Neurogenic influences on blood pressure and vascular tone from peripheral receptors during muscular contraction. Cardiology 1976; 61 (Suppl 1): 65–68.

42. Clement DL, Pelletier CL, Shepherd JT: Role of muscular contraction in the reflex vascular responses to stimulation of muscle afferents in the dog. Circ Res 1973; 33:386–392.

43. Kaufman MP, Rybicki KJ, Waldrop TG, Mitchell JH: Effect on arterial pressure of

rhythmically contracting the hindlimb of cats. J Appl Physiol 1984; 56:1265–1271.

44. Iwamoto GA, Waldrop TG, Kaufman MP, Botterman BR, Rybicki KJ, Mitchell JH: Pressor reflex evoked by muscular contraction: contributions by neuraxis levels. J Appl Physiol 1985; 59:459–467.

45. Paintal AS: Functional analysis of group III afferent fibres of mammalian muscles. J Physiol 1960; 152:250–270.

46. Bessou P, LaPorte Y: Étude des récepteurs musculaires innervés par les fibres afférentes du group III (fibres myéllinisées fines) chez le chat. Arch Ital Biol 1961; 99:293–321.

47. Kumazawa TN, Mizumura K: Thin-fibre receptors responding to mechanical, chemical and thermal stimulation in the skeletal muscle of the dog. J Physiol 1977; 273:179–194.

48. Ellaway PH, Murphy PR, Tripathi A: Closely coupled excitation of gamma-motoneurons by group III muscle afferents with low mechanical threshold in a cat. J Physiol 1982; 331:481–498.

49. Mense S, Stahnke M: Responses in muscle afferent fibers of slow conduction velocity to contractions and ischemia in the cat. J Physiol 1983; 342:383–397.

50. Kniffki K-D, Mense S, Schmidt RF: Responses of group IV afferent units from skeletal muscle to stretch, contraction and chemical stimuli. Exp Brain Res 1978; 31:511–522.

51. Kaufman MP, Longhurst JC, Rybicki KJ, Wallach JH, Mitchell JH: Effects of static muscular contraction on impulse activity of groups III and IV afferents in cats. J Appl Physiol 1983; 55:105–112.

52. Hayward L, Wesselmann U, Rymer WZ: Effects of muscle fatigue on mechanically sensitive afferents of slow conduction velocity in the cat triceps surae. J Neurophysiol 1991; 65:360–370.

53. Mense S, Meyer H: Bradykinin-induced modulation of the response behaviour of different types of feline group III and IV muscle receptors. J Physiol 1988; 398:49–63.

54. Guzman F, Braun C, Lim RKS, Potter GD, Rodgers DW: Visceral pain and the pseudaffective response to intra-arterial injection of bradykinin and other algesic agents. Arch Int Pharmacodyn Ther 1964; 149:571–588.

55. Mense S, Schmidt RF: Activation of group IV afferent units from muscle by algesic agents. Brain Res 1974; 72:305–310.

56. Mense S: Nervous outflow from skeletal muscle following chemical noxious stimulation. J Physiol 1977; 267:75–88.

57. Kaufman MP, Iwamoto GA, Longhurst JC, Mitchell JH: Effects of capsaicin and bradykinin on afferent fibers with endings in skeletal muscle. Circ Res 1982; 50:133–139.

58. Stebbins CL, Carretero OA, Mindroiu T, Longhurst JC: Bradykinin release from contracting skeletal muscle of the cat. J Appl Physiol 1990; 69:1225–1230.

59. Hnik P, Hudlická O, Kucera J, Payne R: Activation of muscle afferents by non-proprioceptive stimuli. Am J Physiol 1969; 217:1451–1458.

60. Rybicki KJ, Waldrop TG, Kaufman MP: Increasing gracilis interstitial potassium

concentrations stimulates group III and IV afferents. J Appl Physiol 1985; 58: 936–941.

61. Thimm F, Baum K: Response of chemosensitive nerve fibers of group III and IV to metabolic changes in rat muscles. Pflüger's Arch 1987; 410:143–152.

62. Rotto DM, Kaufman MP: Effects of metabolic products of muscular contraction on the discharge of group III and IV afferents. J Appl Physiol 1988; 64:2306–2313.

63. Sinoway LI, Hill JM, Pickar JG, Kaufman MP: Effects of contraction and lactic acid on the discharge of group III muscle afferents in cats. J Neurophysiol 1993; 69: 1053–1059.

64. Mense S: Sensitization of group IV muscle receptors to bradykinin by 5-hydroxy-tryptamine and prostaglandin E-2. Brain Res 1981; 225:95–105.

65. Rotto DM, Hill JM, Schultz HD, Kaufman MP: Cyclooxygenase blockade attenuates the responses of group IV muscle afferents to static contraction. Am J Physiol 1990; 259:H745–H750.

66. Kaufman MP, Rybicki KJ, Waldrop TG, Ordway GA, Mitchell JH: Effects of static and rhythmic twitch contractions on the discharge of group III and IV muscle afferents. Cardiovasc Res 1984; 18:663–668.

67. Kaufman MP, Rybicki KJ, Waldrop TG, Ordway GA: Effect of ischemia on responses of group III and IV afferents to contraction. J Appl Physiol 1984; 57: 644–650.

68. Henneman E, Somjen G, Carpenter DO: Functional significance of cell size in spinal motoneurons. J Neurophysiol 1965; 28:560–580.

69. Iggo A: Non-myelinated afferent fibers from mammalian skeletal muscle. J Physiol 1961; 155:52–53P.

70. Hill JM, Pickar JG, Parrish M, Kaufman MP: Effects of hypoxia on the discharge on group III and IV muscle afferents in cats. J Appl Physiol 1992; 73:2524–2529.

71. Rotto DM, Schultz HD, Longhurst JC, Kaufman MP: Sensitization of group III muscle afferents to static contraction by products of arachidonic acid metabolism. J Appl Physiol 1990; 68:861–867.

72. Risling M, Dalsgaard C-J, Cukierman A, Cuello AC: Electron microscopic and immunohistochemical evidence that unmyelinated ventral root axons make u-turns or enter the spinal pia mater. J Comp Neurol 1984; 225:53–63.

73. Azerad J, Hunt CC, LaPorte Y, Pollin B, Thiesson D: Afferent fibres in cat ventral roots: electrophysiological and histological evidence. J Physiol 1986; 379:229–243.

74. Coggeshall RE, Ito H: Sensory fibres in ventral roots L7 and S1 in the cat. J Physiol 1977; 267:215–235.

75. Light AR, Perl ER: Reexamination of the dorsal root projection to the spinal dorsal horn including observations on the differential termination of coarse and fine fibers. J Comp Neurol 1979; 186:117–131.

76. Craig AD, Mense S: The distribution of afferent fibers from the gastrocnemius-soleus muscle in the dorsal horn of the cat as revealed by the transport of horseradish peroxidase. Neurosci Lett 1983; 41:233–238.

77. Mense S, Craig ADIII: Spinal and supraspinal terminations of primary afferent fibers from the gastrocnemius-soleus muscle in the cat. Neuroscience 1988; 26:1023–1035.

78. Swett J, Woolf CJ: The somatotopic organization of primary afferent terminals in the superficial laminae of the dorsal horn of the rat spinal cord. J Comp Neurol 1985; 231:66–77.

79. Mense S, Prabhakar NR: Spinal termination of nociceptive afferent fibres from deep tissues in the cat. Neurosci Lett 1986; 66:169–174.

80. Pomeranz B, Wall PD, Weber WV: Cord cells responding to fine myelinated afferents from viscera, muscle, and skin. J Physiol 1968; 199:511–532.

81. Hoheisel U, Mense S: Response behaviour of cat dorsal horn neurons receiving input from skeletal muscle and other deep somatic tissues. J Physiol 1990; 426:265–280.

82. Foreman RD, Schmidt RF, Willis WD: Effects of mechanical and chemical stimulation of fine muscle afferents upon primate spinothalamic tract cells. J Physiol 1979; 286:215–231.

83. Johnson JL, Aprison MH: The distribution of glutamic acid, a transmitter candidate, and other amino acids in the dorsal sensory neuron of the cat. Brain Res 1970; 24: 285–292.

84. Graham LT, Shank RP, Werman R, Aprison MH: Distribution of some synaptic transmitter suspects in cat spinal cord. J Neurochem 1967; 14:465–472.

85. Roberts PJ: The release of amino acids with proposed neurotransmitter function from the cuneate and gracile nuclei of the rat in vivo. Brain Res 1974; 67:419–428.

86. Curtis DR, Johnston GAR: The chemical excitation of spinal neurones by certain acidic amino acids. J Physiol 1960; 150:656–682.

87. Schneider SP, Perl ER: Comparison of primary afferent and glutamate excitation of neurons in the mammalian spinal dorsal horn. J Neurosci 1988; 8:2062–2073.

88. Yoshimura M, Jessell T: Amino acid-mediated EPSPs at primary afferent synapses with substantia gelatinosa neurones in the rat spinal cord. J Physiol 1990; 430:315–335.

89. Go VLW, Yaksh TL: Release of substance P from the cat spinal cord. J Physiol 1987; 391:141–167.

90. Duggan AW, Hope PJ, Lang CW, Williams CA: Sustained isometric contraction of skeletal muscle results in release of immunoreactive neurokinins in the spinal cord of the anaesthetized cat. Neurosci Lett 1991; 122:191–194.

91. Wilson LB, Fuchs IE, Matsukawa K, Mitchell JH, Wall PT: Substance P release in the spinal cord during the exercise pressor reflex in anaesthetized cats. J Physiol 1993; 460:79–90.

92. Hökfelt T, Elde R, Johansson O, Luft R, Nilsson G, Arimura A: Immunohistochemical evidence for separate populations of somatostatin-containing and substance P-containing primary afferent neurons in the rat. Neuroscience 1976; 1:131–136.

93. Cameron AA, Leah JD, Snow PJ: The coexistence of neuropeptides in feline sensory neurons. Neuroscience 1988; 81:969–979.

94. O'Brien C, Woolf CJ, Fitzgerald M, Lindsay RM, Molander C: Differences in the chemical expression of rat primary afferent neurons which innervate skin, muscle or joint. Neuroscience 1989; 32:493–502.

95. Murase K, Randic M: Actions of substance P on rat spinal dorsal horn neurones. J Physiol 1984; 346:203–217.

96. Kaufman MP, Kozlowski GP, Rybicki KJ: Attenuation of the reflex pressor response to muscular contraction by a substance P antagonist. Brain Res 1985; 333:182–184.

97. Kaufman MP, Rybicki KJ, Kozlowski GP, Iwamoto GA: Immunoneutralization of substance P attenuates the reflex pressor response to muscular contraction. Brain Res 1986; 377:199–203.

98. Wilson LB, Wall PT, Matsukawa K, Mitchell JH: The effect of spinal microinjections of an antagonist to substance P or somatostatin on the exercise pressor reflex. Circ Res 1992; 70:213–222.

99. Hill JM, Pickar JG, Kaufman MP: Attenuation of reflex pressor and ventilatory responses to static contraction by an NK-1 receptor antagonist. J Appl Physiol 1992; 73:1389–1395.

100. Overton JM, Stremel RW: Hindlimb muscle contraction elicits depressor responses in anesthetized rats. Physiologist 1992; 35:238.

101. McCoy KW, Rotto DM, Rybicki KJ, Kaufman MP: Attenuation of the reflex pressor response to muscular contraction by an antagonist to somatostatin. Circ Res 1988; 62:18–24.

102. Klein CM, Coggeshall RE, Carlton SM, Westlund KN, Sorkin LS: Changes in calcitonin gene-related peptide immunoreactivity in the rat dorsal horn following electrical stimulation of the sciatic nerve. Neurosci Lett 1990; 115:149–154.

103. Wiesenfeld-Hallin Z, Hökfelt T, Lundberg JM, Forssmann WG, Reinecke M, Tschopp FA, Fischer JA: Immunoreactive calcitonin gene-related peptide and substance P coexist in sensory neurons to the spinal cord and interact in spinal behavioral responses of the rat. Neurosci Lett 1984; 52:199–204.

104. Dahlstrom A, Fuxe K: Evidence for the existence of monoamine neurons in the central nervous. II. Experimentally-induced changes in interneuronal amine levels of bulbospinal neurone systems. Acta Physiol Scand 1964; 64 (Suppl):247.

105. Miller KE, Seybold VS: Comparison of met-enkephalin, dynorphin A- and neurotension-immunoreactive neurons in the cat and rat spinal cords. I. Lumbar cord. J Comp Neurol 1984; 255:293–304.

106. Kagerberg GS, Bjorklund A: Topographic principles in the spinal projections of serotonergic and non-serotonergic brainstem neurons in the rat. Neuroscience 1985; 15:445–480.

107. Hill JM, Kaufman MP: Attenuation of reflex pressor and ventilatory responses to static muscular contraction by intrathecal opioids. J Appl Physiol 1990; 68:2466–2472.

108. Hill JM, Kaufman MP: Attenuating effects of intrathecal clonidine on the exercise pressor reflex. J Appl Physiol 1991; 70:516–522.

109. Hill JM, Kaufman MP: Intrathecal serotonin attenuates the pressor response to static contraction. Brain Res 1991; 550:157–160.

110. Kai-Kai MM, Anderton BH, Keen P: A quantitative analysis of the interrelationships between subpopulations of rat sensory neurons containing arginine vasopressin or oxytocin and those containing substance P, fluoride-resistant acid phosphatase or neurofilament protein. Neuroscience 1986; 18:475–486.

111. Millan MJ, Millan MH, Czlonkowski A, Herz A: Vasopressin and oxytocin in the rat spinal cord: Distribution and origins in comparison to metenkephalin, dynorphin, and related opioids and their irresponsiveness to stimuli modulating neurohypophyseal secretion. Neuroscience 1984; 13:179–187.

112. Stebbins CL: Reflex cardiovascular response to exercise is modulated by circulating vasopressin. Am J Physiol 1992; 263:R1104–R1109.

113. Schaefke ME, Loeschcke HH: Lokalisation eines an der Regulation von Atmung und Kreislauf beteiligten Gebietes an der ventralen Oberfläche der Medulla oblongata Pflüger's Arch 1967; 297:201–220.

114. Connelly JC, McCallister LW, Kaufman MP: Stimulation of the caudal ventrolateral medulla decreases total lung resistance in dogs. J Appl Physiol 1987; 63:912–917.

115. Haxhiu MA, Deal EC, Jr, Norcia MP, VanLunteren E, Cherniack NS: Effect of N-methyl-D-aspartate applied to the ventral surface of the medulla on the trachea. J Appl Physiol 1987; 63:1268–1274.

116. Haxhiu MA, Deal EC, Norcia MP, Van Lunteren E, Mitra J, Cherniack NS: Influence of ventrolateral surface of medulla on reflex tracheal constriction. J Appl Physiol 1986; 61:791–796.

117. Iwamoto GA, Kaufman MP: Caudal ventrolateral medullary cells responsive to static muscular contraction. J Appl Physiol 1987; 62:149–157.

118. Bauer RM, Waldrop TG, Iwamoto GA, Holzwarth MA: Properties of ventrolateral medullary neurons that respond to muscular contraction. Brain Res Bull 1992; 28:167–178.

119. Waldrop TG, Mullins DC, Henderson MC: Effects of hypothalamic lesions on the cardiorespiratory responses to muscular contraction. Respir Physiol 1986; 66: 215–224.

120. Richard CA, Waldrop TG, Bauer RM, Mitchell JH, Stremel RW: The nucleus reticularis gigantocellularis modulates the cardiopulmonary responses to central and peripheral drives related to exercise. Brain Res 1989; 482:49–56.

121. Rybicki KJ, Kaufman MP: Atropine prevents the reflex tracheal relaxation arising from the stimulation of intestinal and skeletal muscle afferents in dogs. Brain Res 1983; 270:159–161.

122. Haselton JR, Padrid PA, Kaufman MP: Activation of neurons in the rostral ventrolateral medulla increases bronchomotor tone in dogs. J Appl Physiol 1991; 71: 210–216.

123. McAllen RM, Spyer KM: Two types of vagal preganglionic motoneurons projecting to the heart and lungs. J Physiol 1978; 282:353–364.

124. Ford TW, Bennett JA, Kidd C, McWilliam PN: Neurones in the dorsal motor vagal nucleus of the cat with non-myelinated axons projecting to the heart and lungs. Exp Physiol 1990; 75:459–473.

125. Widdicombe JG: Action potentials in parasympathetic and sympathetic efferent fibres to trachea and lungs of dogs and cats. J Physiol 1966; 186:56–88.

126. Mitchell RA, Herbert DA, Richardson CA: Neurohumoral regulation of airway smooth muscle: role of tracheal ganglia. In: Lahiri S, Forster RE III, et al, eds. Chemoreceptors and Reflexes in Breathing: Cellular and Molecular Aspects. New York: Oxford University Press, 1989:299–309.

127. Baker DG, McDonald DM, Basbaum CB, Mitchell RA: The architecture of nerves and ganglia of the ferrett trachea as revealed by acetylcholinesterase histochemistry. J Comp Neurol 1986; 246:513–526.

128. Bennett JA, Kidd C, Latif AB, McWilliam PN: A horseradish peroxidase study of

vagal motoneurons with axons in cardiac and pulmonary branches of the cat and dog. Q J Exp Physiol 1981; 66:145–154.

129. Wallach JH, Rybicki KJ, Kaufman MP: Anatomical localization of the cells of origin of efferent fibers in the superior laryngeal and recurrent laryngeal nerves of dogs. Brain Res 1983; 261:307–311.

130. Kagawa J, Kerr HD: Effects of brief graded exercise on specific airway conductance in normal subjects. J App Physiol 1970; 28:138–144.

131. Warren JB, Jennings SJ, Clark TJH: Effect of adrenergic and vagal blockade on the normal human airway response to exercise. Clin Sci 1984; 66:79–85.

132. Asmussen E, Nielsen M: Experiments on nervous factors controlling respiration and circulation during exercise employing blocking of the blood flow. Acta Physiol Scand 1964; 60:103–111.

133. Stanley WC, Lee WR, Brooks GA: Ventilation studied with circulatory occlusion during two intensities of exercise. Eur J Appl Physiol 1985; 54:269–277.

134. Alam M, Smirk FH: Observation in man upon a blood pressure raising reflex arising from the voluntary muscles. J Physiol 1937; 89:372–383.

135. Rowell LB, Hermansen L, Blackmon JR: Human cardiovascular and respiratory responses to grades muscle ischemia. J Appl Physiol 1976; 41:693–701.

136. Galbo H, Kjaer M, Secher NJ: Cardiovascular ventilatory and catecholamine responses to maximal dynamic exercise in partially curarized man. J Physiol 1987; 389:557–568.

137. Sheldon MI, Green JF: Evidence for pulmonary CO_2 chemosensitivity: effects on ventilation. J Appl Physiol 1982; 52:1192–1197.

14

Peripheral and Central Effects of Hypoxia

GERALD E. BISGARD

University of Wisconsin
Madison, Wisconsin

JUDITH A. NEUBAUER

UMDNJ–Robert Wood Johnson Medical
School
New Brunswick, New Jersey

I. Introduction

Responses and adaptation of humans and animals to environmental hypoxia have long been the subject of intense interest to physiologists. The respiratory effects of hypoxia have received more extensive attention as it became obvious that the ventilatory response to hypoxia is more complex than earlier thought. It is now well known that the acute response to hypoxia is dramatically modified depending on the severity and duration of hypoxic exposure. Initially, hypoxia produces a rapid increase in ventilation. In adult humans and some animals, this initial ventilatory increase is not sustained and declines during the first 30 min of hypoxic exposure (1,2). This biphasic response is generally referred to as roll-off or hypoxic ventilatory decline (HVD). More prolonged exposure (hours to several days) produces a secondary increase in breathing, a phenomenon that has been termed ventilatory acclimatization to hypoxia. Finally, long life at high altitude (years) has a moderating effect on respiration by reducing the amount of hyperventilation found during acclimatization (3–5).

From these observations it is apparent that there are both excitatory and inhibitory effects of hypoxia on ventilation and that there are important time-dependent influences on mechanisms controlling ventilation during hypoxia.

Some time-dependent influences on the ventilatory response to hypoxia require only minutes to be seen; others require hours, days, or years to manifest themselves. In addition to time dependency, it is also now being recognized that hypoxia can have varying effects on different central nervous system (CNS) structures, and these effects may also change with maturation, or during different states such as anesthesia or sleep. Various conditioning stimuli may also modify the ventilatory response to hypoxia. For example, repeated hypoxic stimuli (vs. sustained hypoxia), may produce a prolonged augmentation of breathing (6).

Our goal in this chapter is to review the current state of knowledge of the effects of hypoxia on the respiratory control system. We will first discuss the peripheral arterial chemoreceptor response to hypoxia, for it is these receptors that are primarily responsible for the ventilatory stimulation produced by hypoxia. Second, we will discuss the effects of hypoxia on the CNS and how this modulates ventilatory responses. Finally, we will discuss the integrated ventilatory responses under acute and chronic hypoxic conditions.

II. Peripheral Chemoreceptors

The basic effects of hypoxia on the peripheral chemoreceptors and the consequent reflex effects are very well known. There have been excellent reviews on the subject (7–9). Therefore, we will only briefly review the response to hypoxia of the peripheral chemoreceptors. Putative modulators of carotid body function will be discussed in Section IV, as they pertain to ventilatory responses to hypoxia. Detailed review of the transduction and modulation of arterial chemoreceptor function is provided in Chapter 9.

In humans and, under most conditions, in nonhuman mammals, the peripheral chemoreceptors, carotid and aortic bodies, are considered the only source for reflex ventilatory stimulation with hypoxia. However, ventilatory stimulation has been observed in animal studies as a result of CNS hypoxia (see below). It is well accepted that the carotid bodies are the most important of the two sets of peripheral chemoreceptors with regard to ventilatory stimulation during hypoxia. Both carotid and aortic bodies are stimulated by a fall in Pao_2, although the response of the aortic body is much smaller than the response of the carotid body (10). Unlike the carotid body, the aortic body is stimulated by reductions in arterial O_2 content, e.g., carboxyhemoglobinemia and anemia (11,12), as well as by hypotension. These observations have led to the conclusion that the aortic body is much more sensitive to total O_2 flow or delivery (13) whereas the carotid body is exquisitely sensitive to Pao_2. The contribution of the aortic chemoreceptor stimulation to the overall ventilatory response to hypoxia was recently examined in a study of anesthetized dogs (14). Chemical stimulation of the aortic chemoreceptors produced clear effects on phase timing, reducing both T_I and T_E, with no change in phrenic amplitude, and, overall, had only very minimal effects on ventilation. This is in contrast to carotid body stimulation, which produces significant increases in ventilation by affecting timing as well as phrenic amplitude (or V_T) (see below). In any case, hypoxia produced by a reduction in Pao_2 causes an increase in ventilation by an intense stimulation of the carotid chemoreceptors and relatively little or no stimulation of ventilation via the aortic chemoreceptors [cf. Fitzgerald and Lahiri (9)].

In animals, progressive isocapnic hypoxic hypoxia (lowered Pao_2) carotid body stimulation produces an hyperbolic-life afferent discharge pattern (15–17) (Fig. 1). There is no true threshold for carotid body afferent activity because even under hyperoxic conditions ($Pao_2 > 500$ torr) discharge is not completely inhibited (16,18). In the cat the Pao_2 where an increase in discharge frequency is

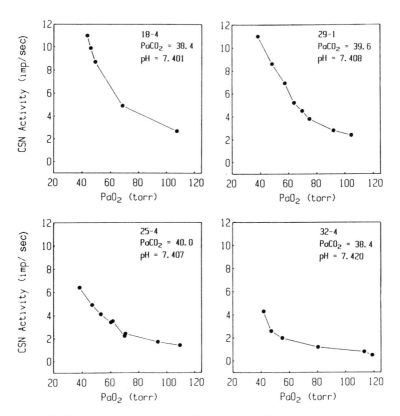

Figure 1 Single carotid chemoreceptor fiber discharge frequency obtained from four chloralose anesthetized goats illustrating the curvilinear response to a change in Pao_2 during maintained isocapnia. (From Ref. 17.)

detected has been shown to be in the range of 140–400 torr (mean = 190 torr) (16). However, the rapid increase in afferent activity is produced only after Pa_{O_2} falls below 100 torr (16,17).

There is no evidence of time-dependent adaptation (reduced discharge frequency) in the afferent activity of the carotid chemoreceptor fibers during up to 1 hr of steady-state hypoxia recorded from adult cats and goats (17,19). However, in adult rabbits, after 1 hr of hypoxia afferent discharge frequency decreased to a mean of 72% of the initial hypoxic response (20). Similarly, in 1-week-old kittens it has been reported that after a brief period of excitation lasting less than 1 min, a reduction in firing frequency occurs (21,22). The observation that the responsiveness of the carotid body to hypoxia is weaker in the neonate than in the adult has been made in several species, including the newborn rat, cat, pig, and sheep (21–25). In very prolonged hypoxia (hours to days), recent evidence has shown an increased sensitivity to hypoxic stimulation, and in at least one adult animal, the goat, firing frequency is increased in a time-dependent manner after 1 hr of steady-state hypoxia (17). The importance of these observations will be discussed more thoroughly in Section IV.

III. Effects of CNS Hypoxia on Ventilation

While reflex stimulation of respiration during hypoxia is ascribed to the arterial chemoreceptors, the effects of hypoxia on the CNS are believed to primarily promote respiratory depression. The carotid chemoreceptors respond to hypoxia and stimulate respiration within a few seconds (26). In contrast, the time constant of the depressant response to central hypoxia is 80–150 sec (27,28). Thus, the physiological influence of hypoxic respiratory depression in the intact animal becomes apparent when the temporal profile of the responses to hypoxia is examined. The slow depressant effect of central hypoxia has been observed in the awake subject in several situations. The ventilatory response of human subjects to transient hypoxia is 18% greater than the ventilatory response to an equivalent magnitude of steady-state hypoxia (29). For any given level of alveolar Po_2, ventilation is greater during production of hypoxia than during recovery from hypoxia (30). The central depressant effects of hypoxia have been proposed to explain the biphasic nature of the respiratory response to hypoxia in both the neonatal and adult mammal (2,31–37). In neonatal and adult humans and animals, the initial increase in ventilation is followed within minutes by a decline in ventilation (HVD), although the decline is more pronounced and has faster dynamics in the neonate. There is considerable experimental evidence that this decline in ventilatory response to hypoxia reflects the effects of CNS hypoxia (see Section IV.C).

Early studies in awake chemodenervated dogs and humans found that hypoxia caused a transient ventilatory depression (38–41). More recent studies in awake chemodenervated animals have found that CNS hypoxia may not cause hypoventilation (42–47). In some cases there is evidence of stimulation of ventilation. For example, in awake goats, when sustained or severe CNS hypoxia is produced either by inhalation of CO or by inhalation of hypoxic gas mixtures while the isolated carotid bodies are simultaneously perfused with normoxic blood, there is an increase in respiratory frequency and an increase in V_T resulting in a moderate hyperventilation (48–52). And in awake chemodenervated cats CNS hypoxia causes a pronounced tachypnea (53,54). In contrast, hypoxic respiratory depression is observed consistently in chemodenervated animals during states associated with low respiratory drive such as anesthesia, sleep, or hypocapnia (55–62). The state dependence of the responses to hypoxia in chemodenervated animals suggests that the level of CNS arousal modulates the hypoxic vulnerability of the neural structures involved in generating the respiratory pattern.

Graded hypoxia in anesthetized, peripherally chemodenervated animals results in a stereotypical sequence of patterning changes of the phrenic neurogram characterized by an initial decline in the peak amplitude, followed by a reduction in frequency, with apnea generally occurring when the arterial oxygen content is reduced by 50–60% (57,61,62). If the hypoxia is made more severe (Cao_2 reduced by 80–85%), respiratory activity reappears in the form of high-amplitude, short-duration bursts (gasping). This later event is associated with increases in extracellular [K^+] (57) and probably represents a hyperexcitable state in the transition from hyperpolarization and energy conservation to depolarization, membrane instability, and the events that, if not reversed quickly, could ultimately result in cell death. This respiratory pattern is a very effective autoresuscitation mechanism producing rapid reoxygenation (63,64). Survival from severe hypoxic exposures appears to be critically dependent on this response since failure to gasp or the inability to sustain gasping during reoxygenation is predictive of animals that will not recover (65,66).

The net effect of central hypoxia on respiration reflects the fundamental response of central neurons to reductions in available oxygen, i.e., decreases in neuronal excitability (67–72). However, depending on the configuration of the neural network and whether there is any selective vulnerability of individual neurons within the network, the net effect of this generalized depression of neuronal excitability may manifest as either a reduction or an excitation of the integrated output. This phenomenon of dynamic reconfiguration due to temporal and spatial modulation of excitatory and inhibitory connections in a neural network has been proposed as a mechanism for stabilizing neural activity in a particular state or level of activity (73). Thus the net respiratory response to generalized neuronal depression in peripherally chemodenervated animals (hypoxic depression in anesthetized animals and ventilatory stimulation in some unanesthetized animal models) may provide important information regarding the relative contributions and sources of both excitatory and inhibitory elements that shape the final respiratory output. In the future it will be important to correlate the contribution of individual excitatory and inhibitory components of the respiratory neural network with the integrated respiratory output to determine how the hypoxic responses of these components are modulated by the state of the system.

Several salient features of hypoxic depression of central neurons have been observed both in vivo (74) and in vitro (68,70,75–80). In response to a reduction in oxygen, the sequence of events can be summarized as a transient initial modest intracellular alkalinization that is rapidly followed by an intracellular acidosis (74), an initial small rise in intracellular $[Ca^{2+}]$ (74,81–84), an increase in potassium conductance (gK$^+$) (70,72,74,77–79,85) membrane hyperpolarization (68,70,72,74,77–79,85), and a reduction in cell excitability (68,70,72,74,77–79). These initial events are readily reversible if oxygen is reinstituted and have been proposed by many to subserve a protective function for the neuron by reducing the utilization of energy substrates when oxygen is limited. In contrast, if the hypoxia is severe and sustained, and intracellular acidosis becomes severe (74), there is progressive membrane depolarization (68,70,72,74,77–79,85) with substantial influx of Ca^{2+} and Na^+ and efflux of K^+ potentially resulting in cell death (74,78,81,82,84,86). However, these changes can still be reversed as long as activation of proteolytic processes that result in cell damage does not occur (87). Thus, while the initial events occurring with modest to moderate hypoxia probably reflect the physiological response to CNS hypoxia, the later events are more closely associated with ischemic cell death.

The mechanisms responsible for the events that lead to reductions in neuronal excitability can be broadly classified into presynaptic and postsynaptic effects. Presynaptic reductions in neurotransmitter release, reuptake, or synthesis act to reduce the net excitatory input required to reach the threshold for neuronal activation (76,89–95). Postsynaptic increases in gK$^+$ (70,72,74,77–79,85) and Na$^+$ channel kinetics (67) also promote hyperpolarization and reduced excitability. In addition, reductions in oxygen availability promote the metabolic production of adenosine (96) and lactic acid (90,97), which act as neuromodulators to reduce the excitability of CNS neurons. Taken together, and depending on the severity of the CNS hypoxia, these events promoting a reduction in neuronal excitability can result in a spectrum of responses ranging from impairment of function to complete silencing of neurons.

The initial transient alkalinization has been observed to occur in the ventral medulla during mild isocapnic hypoxia and to be associated with a small reduction in respiratory output in anesthetized peripherally chemodenervated animals presumably by reducing the amount of acid stimulation of the central chemoreceptors (58,98). Since brain blood flow increases in response to hypoxia, one potential explanation for the transient alkalosis is a secondary washout of CO_2 secondary to an overperfusion (58). An alternative explanation for the transient alkalosis is that an initial cellular response to reductions in oxygen availability is to utilize the limited stores of creatine phosphate as an energy source (74,99). Hydrolysis of CrP would reduce free protons as well as act to maintain ATP levels constant. This initial response could probably maintain neuronal excitability as long as cellular ATP levels do not decline. However, this ability is probably relatively limited since evidence of decreases in cellular [ATP] is quickly demonstrable. The initial small increase in intracellular Ca^{2+} without a change in membrane potential or changes in extracellular Ca^{2+} reflects a decreased intracellular ability to sequester cytosolic Ca^{2+}, a process which is ATP-dependent (100,101). Likewise, there is evidence that the voltage-independent increase gK^+ is due to the opening of the ATP-sensitive K^+ channel the closure of which is ATP-dependent (85,102–104), although the small rise in intracellular calcium may also contribute to changes in the calcium-dependent potassium channel. These changes in gK^+ have been used to explain the initial hyperpolarization of the cell membrane and may account at least in part for the reduction in neuronal excitability. Changes in potassium conductance may not be the only ion change responsible for reductions in neuronal excitability during hypoxia. Recently Cummins et al. (67) have also attributed a large negative shift in the ATP-dependent inactivation of the voltage-dependent sodium current as a mechanism for reductions in neuronal excitability during hypoxia. Thus, these mechanisms permit reductions in cellular excitability and metabolism to occur with only small reductions in [ATP]. This reduction in metabolism should contribute to neuronal survival during hypoxic stress.

Presynaptic events and neuromodulators reinforce the reduction of neuronal excitability. For example, acidosis promotes membrane stabilization by hyperpolarization via an action on channels (105–108). In addition, acidosis may also reduce excitability by inhibition of glutamergic activation of NMDA receptors (109). There is evidence suggesting that hypoxia reduces calcium-mediated release of neurotransmitters from presynaptic terminals (94,110). This effect of hypoxia would not influence the inhibitory action of adenosine since adenosine release is not calcium dependent (69,111). Failure of certain reuptake systems, such as those for GABA, has been used to explain the increase in extracellular concentrations of this inhibitory neurotransmitters (112) and may explain why GABA antagonists are so effective in reversing respiratory depression (113).

The effect of CNS hypoxia on most individual neurons is to reduce excitability (68,70,72,74,77–79). However, the net effect of hypoxia on the discharge rate of that individual neuron will reflect the net result of hypoxia on its presynaptic inputs and the summation of effects of both inhibitory and excitatory processes within the network. In general, CNS hypoxia depresses both inspiratory and expiratory neurons (114–116). Intracellular recordings from respiratory neurons have demonstrated a loss of both EPSPs and IPSPs, suggesting that both excitatory and inhibitory presynaptic input are depressed by CNS hypoxia (117). Since respiratory rhythmogenesis is largely determined by reciprocal inhibition, this loss of both excitation and inhibition on the firing pattern of individual neurons within the network produces major changes in respiratory pattern (117). For example, while the firing frequency of late inspiratory neurons declines progressively with increasing hypoxia (due to loss of excitability), these late inspiratory neurons begin to fire earlier and earlier in the inspiratory cycle (due to loss of inhibition) (118). This modification of the circuitry may provide an advantage by synchronizing the firing of both early and late inspiratory units especially at a time when there may be fewer units reaching threshold and those that are firing have a slower discharge rate.

Another important consideration in describing the effects of CNS hypoxia is the heterogeneity of hypoxic vulnerability within the neuraxis, which may explain the apparently paradoxical tachypneic response to hypoxia in the unanesthetized, awake, peripherally chemodenervated animal (53,54). Based on studies done in unanesthetized decorticate and decerebrate animals, Tenney and his colleagues (119,120) proposed that this tachypneic response was mediated by hypoxic effects on suprapontine structures, specifically, that tachypnea was due to a disinhibition of the diencephalic rate-facilitating centers. Under euoxic conditions, the diencephalon is modulated by inhibitory input from the cerebral cortex. During hypoxia in the awake state, there is a rostral-to-caudal hierarchy of vulnerability along the neuraxis, a phenomenon that has been well described in humans, especially in regard to impairment of higher cortical functions (121,122). Thus, during hypoxia, depression of cortical function should result in a loss of cortical inhibition, a disinhibition of the diencephalon, and an increase in respiratory frequency. Anesthesia results in a general depression of the neuraxis and thus abolishes selective hypoxic vulnerability and eliminates the tachypneic response. Instead, in anesthetized states there is as generalized depression of respiratory activity.

There is also some evidence that there may be unique sites within the brain that are directly stimulated by hypoxia to elicit excitatory and inhibitory effects on ventilation. Dillon and Waldrop (123), using whole-cell patch recordings in tissue slices of the caudal hypothalamus, found that neurons depolarized and increased their firing rates when exposed to hypoxia. Direct stimulation of this region of the hypothalamus has been shown to result in increases in respiratory frequency (124). Based on these observations, these investigators have suggested that a direct hypoxic stimulation of these neurons may mediate the tachypneic response in awake chemodenervated animals. Additionally, there is evidence suggesting that brain hypoxia may directly stimulate neurons in higher brain centers, which then act to depress respiration. These studies in neonates (125–127) have demonstrated that hypoxic depression of breathing is attenuated in fetal and newborn lambs and rabbits after a site in the upper lateral pons is transected. Thus, although the general neuronal response to hypoxia is a reduction in excitability, there may be a subpopulation of neurons located within specific brain regions that are excited by hypoxia. The mechanism by which these neurons are directly excited is unresolved. Whether these neurons are acting as oxygen "chemosensors" excited via cellular responses similar to those in carotid chemosensitive cells or whether they are simply more vulnerable to hypoxia and rapidly depolarize in response to hypoxia, as has been suggested for hypoglossal neurons (128,129), is yet to be determined.

To summarize, the effect of hypoxia on the brain is to cause a generalized reduction in neuronal excitability through mechanisms that should conserve energy during the stress of reduced availability of oxygen. This reduction in neuronal excitability can manifest as either decrease or increase in net respiratory output, depending on the selective vulnerability of the excitatory and inhibitory components of the central respiratory network and the level of respiratory drive. The physiological and clinical relevance of reduced neuronal excitability is also important. The key to surviving the detrimental effects of hypoxia is critically linked to an ability to maintain the integrity of transmembrane ionic gradients (130). Neuronal survival is facilitated by metabolic mechanisms that promote membrane hyperpolarization, reduce ionic conductance, and minimize neuronal activity. These mechanisms may represent a remnant adaptation to fetal life. In utero a respiratory response to hypoxia would be counterproductive and a reduction in neuronal activity would not only preserve neuronal integrity, but would also limit motor activity and preserve O_2 stores in the whole organism.

IV. Integrated Effects of Hypoxia on Ventilatory Control

A. Normoxia

Our main goal in this chapter is to discuss the ventilatory responses to hypoxia. However, since peripheral chemoreceptor activity during "control" normoxic conditions provides a tonic input that contributes to normoxic respiratory drive, it is an important consideration when assessing the changes that ensue upon transition to hypoxia.

The neural mechanisms that generate the rhythm and pattern of breathing are modulated by several afferent inputs that integrate to set central respiratory drive. During eupnea under normoxic conditions, a primary determinant of respiratory drive is thought to come from the central chemoreceptors. In the awake subject, another important determinant of respiratory drive during normoxia comes from neural mechanisms associated with wakefulness (131). In eupneic normoxia, although most of the chemical drive to breathe originates from the $[H^+]/CO_2$ stimulation of the medullary chemoreceptors (3), the peripheral chemoreceptors also provide a varying amount of chemical drive in normoxia. Evidence that the peripheral chemoreceptors are partly responsible for setting respiratory drive comes from the observation that there is an elevation in resting $Paco_2$ in animals that have been subjected to carotid body denervation. The approximate mean elevation of $Paco_2$ ranges from 20 torr in calves (45), 10–15 torr in ponies (46), 11 torr in sheep (132), 5–8 torr in goats (44,133), 8 torr in rats (134) and cats (135), to 6 torr in human subjects (41). In awake goats subjected to isolated carotid body perfusion, carotid body hypocapnia, a reduction in $Pcbco_2$ from 37 to 26 torr during normoxia, increased mean systemic $Paco_2$ 6 torr and decreased minute ventilation 24%, further indicating that some resting chemical drive may also be the result of CO_2 chemosensitive stimulation of the normoxic carotid body (136). In addition to a resting drive from CO_2 stimulation, inhalation of a few breaths of O_2 also results in an acute reduction in ventilation during normoxia in intact animals (137–140) and humans (141,142), suggesting that there is also an O_2-related drive from the normoxic carotid body.

B. Ventilatory Responses to Acute Hypoxia

In awake humans (143) and animals (144) the hyperbolic increase in carotid chemoreceptor afferent activity induced by progressive isocapnic hypoxia produces an increase in ventilation that also has a hyperbolic shape (Fig. 2), although the two are not precisely parallel (145). The increase in ventilation occurs because of an increase in both tidal volume (V_T) and respiratory frequency in animals, whereas in human subjects acute hypoxia produces primarily a rise in V_T and only a small increase in frequency (146–148). For example, in anesthetized dogs carotid sinus nerve stimulation or isolated carotid body simulation reduces T_E and also increases phrenic neurogram amplitude, thus having effects on both phase timing and drive to breathe (14). In cats both aortic and carotid chemoreceptor stimulation produce increases in V_T and respiratory frequency (149,150); however, in the dog isolated hypoxic aortic body stimulation shortens T_I and T_E with no effect on V_T (14). Engwall et al. (151) observed the effect of 5 min of isolated carotid body hypoxia in awake goats with systemic arterial blood maintained normoxic and isocapnic. In these studies carotid body hypoxia ($Pcbo_2$ 40 torr) produces an increase in V_T, V_T/T_I, and reduced T_E. Thus, in animal studies there is clear evidence that hypoxic stimulation of the carotid body can affect both the amplitude and timing of ventilation. Furthermore, these changes occur in the presence or absence of coexistent CNS hypoxia.

Modulators of the Ventilatory Response to Acute Hypoxia

Important modulators of the ventilatory response to hypoxia include Pco_2, state of consciousness, CNS hypoxia (as discussed above), and neurochemical modulation of peripheral chemoreceptor function. Other influences that affect the hypoxic response include sex hormones, genetics, state of maturity, and level of metabolic

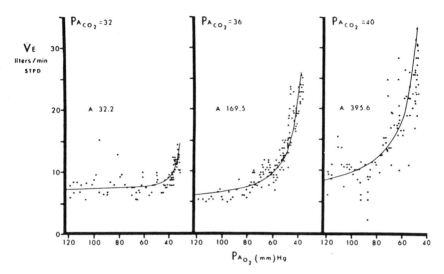

Figure 2 Acute ventilatory response to hypoxia in a single subject with ventilation plotted against alveolar P_{O_2} at three levels of maintained isocapnia. "A" Values determine the shape of the curve and are an index of the strength of the hypoxic response. (From Ref. 143.)

activity. These may be touched on briefly, but they are covered in more detail elsewhere in this book.

Modulation of the Hypoxic Ventilatory Response by CO_2

In the absence of maintained systemic arterial isocapnia, the ventilatory response to acute hypoxia is severely attenuated by the hypocapnia associated with the hyperventilation (Fig. 2). This attenuation of ventilation is due to an effect on the carotid body as well as to reduced drive from the central chemoreceptors. The effect of hypocapnia on the carotid body is greater than would be predicted by the reduction in Pa_{CO_2} alone because there is a strong hyperadditive interaction between Pa_{O_2} and Pa_{CO_2} at the carotid body. This has been well documented by recordings of afferent carotid sinus nerve chemoreceptor activity (152–154). In addition, this interaction at the carotid body has been shown to alter the ventilatory response of awake goats subjected to isolated carotid body stimulation (155). Hypocapnia greatly diminishes carotid body hypoxic stimulation (153). Hypocapnic alkalosis also diminishes the afferent activity arising from the central chemoreceptors, further reducing respiratory drive. Thus, poikilocapnic hypoxia (allowing Pa_{CO_2} to fall during hypoxic hyperventilation) provides a markedly attenuated ventilatory stimulation as compared to isocapnic hypoxia (156,157).

Adrenergic Neurochemical Modulation of the Carotid Body

Because of the emphasis and interest of clinicians and researchers on the effects of catecholamines on the carotid body, a brief review of their role in modulating ventilatory responses, especially the hypoxic response, is warranted.

Dopamine is found in significant quantity in carotid body type I cells (see Chapter 9). It is released from the carotid body during hypoxia (158,159), and intravenous or intracarotid infusions of dopamine produce a depression of ventilation and a reduction in the ventilatory response to hypoxia in a variety of animals (133,160–163) and in humans (164–166). One exception to this is in the dog, where high doses of exogenous dopamine stimulate the carotid body briefly followed by an inhibition (160,167). However, more physiological doses of dopamine are inhibitory to the carotid body and ventilation in the dog (160).

Blockade of carotid body inhibitory D_2 dopamine receptors with domperidone, an agent that does not cross the blood-brain barrier, increases the ventilatory response to acute hypoxia in humans (168–170). Domperidone does not change resting ventilation in human subjects, indicating that there is no significant endogenous release of carotid body dopamine in the normoxic human or that any increase in carotid body activity attendant on a small endogenous release is insufficient to increase normoxic breathing. By contrast, ventilation in both normoxic and hypoxic awake goats is increased significantly by an increase in carotid body activity after domperidone administration (171). Similar ventilatory findings were reported for anesthetized rabbits after domperidone administration (172). In another study, afferent carotid body activity was shown to be augmented by domperidone in the rabbit in normoxia and acute hypoxia, but this increased level of carotid body stimulation was not sustained during a 1-hr period of hypoxia (20). These data taken together indicate that dopamine provides inhibitory modulation of the ventilatory response to hypoxia by an effect on the carotid body.

The carotid sinus nerve contains efferents that originate primarily from cells in the rostral nucleus ambiguus (173–175). These efferents are inhibitory to the carotid body, as cutting the carotid sinus nerve increases the carotid body afferent response to hypoxia (176,177). The inhibition is thought to be via release of dopamine (178). The significance of these efferents has been questioned because of the relatively small numbers of efferent fibers in the carotid sinus nerve (173). However, they may provide a pathway by which the ventilatory response to acute or prolonged hypoxia may be modulated.

A second carotid body catecholamine is norepinephrine, and there is a considerable body of work attempting to understand the role of carotid body norepinephrine as well as sympathetically released and circulating norepinephrine on the carotid body and consequently on ventilation. Norepinephrine is found in both the carotid body type I cells and sympathetic nerve terminals on vessels in the carotid body (7). Thus, at least two sources of norepinephrine potentially interact with hypoxia at the level of the carotid body, the sympathetic nerve terminals and the carotid body type I cells. Circulating norepinephrine could also influence the carotid body, but it has not been consistently found to be elevated by acute hypoxia in resting humans or animals (179–182). However, during prolonged hypoxia (21 days at 4300 m) in human subjects resting plasma norepinephrine was significantly elevated above sea level values (180). Exogenously infused norepinephrine has been found to be primarily excitatory on the rabbit (183) and cat carotid body (184,185) while primarily inhibitory to the dog (160) and goat carotid body (186). Biphasic effects of norepinephrine, inhibition followed by excitation, have been described in the cat and dog (160,184), with the excitatory effect being ascribed to vasoconstriction in the CB (7,184). Excitatory effects of norepinephrine on the CB have also been attributed to adrenergic β_2-receptor stimulation (183). In humans, intravenous administration of norepinephrine stimulates breathing, an effect potentiated in hypoxia, attenuated by hyperoxia, and blocked by propranolol (187–189). This effect is thought to be mediated by the carotid body (187).

Recent studies in cats have shown the presence of carotid body α_2-adrenergic receptors that are inhibitory to the function of the carotid body (190). Specific α_2-adrenergic antagonists increased the response of the cat carotid body to hypoxia. An inhibitory effect of norepinephrine on the carotid body and ventilation has also been demonstrated recently in awake goats (186). This effect was inhibited by a nonspecific alpha-adrenergic antagonist, phenoxybenzamine, and also by domperidone, suggesting that both adrenergic and dopaminergic effects produced the inhibitory effect of norepinephrine.

The above brief review of the effects of norepinephrine indicates excitatory, inhibitory, and/or mixed effects on the carotid body of different species. Therefore, the potential is present for a modulating role of norepinephrine in the ventilatory response to hypoxia, but the effects vary with species. It is quite possible that giving exogenous adrenergic agents to the carotid body does not reflect the function of these agents released either from type I cells or from sympathetic nerve terminals within the carotid body.

The carotid body receives a significant sympathetic innervation from the superior cervical ganglion via one or more ganglioglomerular nerves. This innervation is distributed primarily to the vasculature of the carotid body, but some is also distributed in close proximity to type I and type II cells (191). There has been a series of studies on the function of the sympathetic innervation of the carotid body (cf. Ref. 177). Several observers found that electrical stimulation of the sympathetic innervation of the carotid body causes a stimulation of carotid chemoreceptor afferent activity (177,192–196). One careful study revealed that about 50% of pre- or postganglionic stimulations had no effect on carotid sinus nerve activity. Of the half responding, 82% were excitatory and 12% were inhibitory (195). Some of the stimulatory effect was attributed to a reduction in blood flow, but increased activity in the absence of a change in tissue P_{O_2} supports the view that some nonvascular mechanism can cause stimulation of the carotid

body during sympathetic stimulation (197). Studies after carotid body sympathectomy have provided little evidence of an important functional role of carotid body
sympathetic innervation in ventilatory control. Matsumoto et al. (198) have shown
that chemoreceptor afferent discharge frequency is not significantly changed
during either hypoxic or hypercapnic stimulation of the carotid body after section
of its ganglioglomerular nerve. This was true even though these stimuli can
increase ganglioglomerular efferent activity (198,199). In awake cats studied
before and after the sympathetic innervation to the carotid bifurcation was cut,
there were no changes in mean normoxic ventilation, but a tendency for V_T to
increase and respiratory frequency to decrease was noted (200). In anesthetized
cats the ventilatory response to isolated hypoxic stimulation of the carotid bodies
was unchanged after sympathectomy by removal of the superior cervical ganglion
(201). It was shown recently that the ventilatory response to acute isocapnic
hypoxia in awake goats is not altered after section of the ganglioglomerular
nerve (202).

Thus, the general conclusion is that while effects of sympathetic activity
may mildly modulate carotid body function, these effects are not powerful enough
to have a particularly important effect on hypoxic ventilation. Norepinephrine
effects are variable and species dependent, but dopamine appears to have a
consistent inhibitory role in modulating the carotid body and ventilatory responses
of hypoxia.

Other Intrinsic Neuromodulators Within the Carotid Body

There are additional putative neuromodulators/neurotransmitters in the carotid
body. These include acetylcholine, 5-hydroxytryptamine, adenosine, nitric oxide,
and peptides such as substance P, atrial natriuretic factor, and enkephalins.
Chapter 9 includes specific information on these agents.

Effects of Plasma Potassium on Ventilation

Elevated plasma potassium is a potent stimulus for the carotid body (203). This
may play an important role in the hyperpnea of exercise, particularly in hypoxia
(cf. Ref. 204). However, this hypothesis was not supported by a recent study in
awake goats showing that artificial elevation of plasma [K$^+$] produced only mild
hyperventilation, which did not differ between normoxic and hypoxic conditions (205).

C. Ventilatory Responses to Sustained Hypoxia: Hypoxic Ventilatory Decline

In adult human subjects if steady-state isocapnic hypoxia is maintained for a
period of up to 60 min, a biphasic change in ventilation occurs; the initial acute
response, reaching a peak in about 3–5 min, is followed by a decrease to a new,
lower steady state (2,35,36,206–211) (Fig. 3). An example of the change in

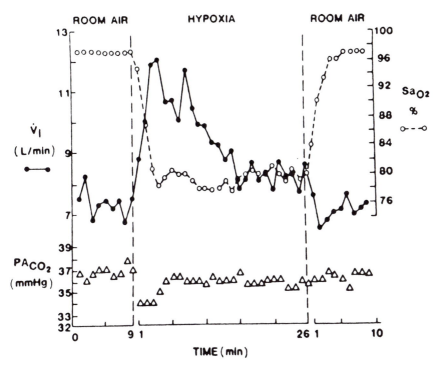

Figure 3 Ventilatory response to sustained hypoxia in an adult human subject. Mean ventilation (closed circles), mean SaO_2 (open circles), and mean PA_{CO_2} (triangles). (From Ref. 2.)

ventilation is demonstrated by the work of Easton et al., who found that when maintaining SaO_2 at 80% the initial mean increase in ventilation was about 40–60% above normoxic ventilation, whereas after 25 min of hypoxia mean ventilation had declined to a value that was 11–20% above control ventilation and remained stable at that level for 1 hr (206). This time-dependent fall in ventilation has been termed roll-off or hypoxic ventilatory decline (HVD).

In neonatal humans and several animal species, a biphasic response to hypoxia is well known, but it varies from the adult response in that the initial peak response is lower, the decline occurs more rapidly, and ventilation is frequently reduced to levels below the initial room air control values (31,34,212–217). A biphasic effect of sustained hypoxia on ventilation has not been consistently reported in adult animals with the exception of cats, in which it has been demonstrated in both awake and anesthetized state (1,201,218). A recent report specifically studying HVD indicated that there is no biphasic hypoxic response in conscious adult dogs (219).

Mechanisms of Hypoxic Ventilatory Decline

The mechanism of HVD is not thoroughly understood; however, several hypotheses have been tested and there is both negative and positive support for these mechanisms. These include declining carotid chemoreceptor activity, carotid body–mediated depression of central respiratory drive, reduced stimulation of central chemoreceptors, and CNS hypoxic depression of ventilation.

Carotid Chemoreceptor Activity

There has been considerable controversy regarding the possibility that a time-dependent decline in chemoreceptor activity could be responsible for the biphasic ventilatory response to hypoxia in newborn animals. As mentioned earlier in this chapter, carotid chemoreceptor activity has recently been demonstrated to decline during sustained hypoxia in kittens less than 10 days old (21,22). This appears to be a developmental characteristic because the hypoxic decline in discharge activity diminished with age and was eliminated in kittens by 8 weeks of age (22). Furthermore, adult cats do not exhibit a time-dependent decline in the carotid body response to hypoxia (1,19,218). These findings provide evidence that in the newborn kitten there may be a component of the hypoxic decline brought about by immaturity of the carotid chemoreceptor response to hypoxia. However, this may be species dependent as newborn 1-day- and 6-day-old piglets do not exhibit ventilatory decline during sustained hypoxia (220,221). This finding suggests adequately functioning carotid chemoreceptors in piglets. Anesthetized piglets do have a biphasic hypoxic response, indicating that anesthesia plays a role in this species (34). A CNS mechanism for decline in the hypoxic ventilatory response in anesthetized piglets has been postulated (34).

As indicated for the adult cat, there is less evidence for a time-dependent change in chemoreceptor activity in adult animals with the possible exception of the rabbit, which exhibits a diminished activity during a 1-hr period of steady-state isocapnic hypoxia (20). There is no reduction in carotid chemoreceptor afferent activity during the first hour of hypoxia in goats (17), but awake goats show little, if any, evidence of HVD in this time frame (222). In adult humans, Bascom et al. (223) assessed ventilatory response to brief pulses of additional hypoxia or hypercapnia during 23 min of sustained hypoxia and found that the responses to hypoxic pulses late in the period of hypoxia (after 17 min) were attenuated compared to the first response (after 2 min), and responses to hypercapnic pulses during the hypoxic period were little changed. They interpreted this to mean that the peripheral chemoreceptors themselves mediated the HVD. This hypothesis was not supported by Berkenbosch et al., who found no significant change in peripheral chemoreceptor sensitivity after 25 min of hypoxia using the fast component of the response to CO_2 as an index of the function of the peripheral chemoreceptors (224). They suggested the possibility that central modulation of the input from peripheral chemoreceptors could be altered to produce HVD. A similar conclusion was reached in studies done to determine the interaction of the specific peripheral chemoreceptor stimulant almitrine (225). Oral pretreatment of subjects with almitrine greatly increased the initial peak hypoxic ventilatory response and the subsequent decline of ventilation. These results were interpreted as suggesting that peripheral chemoreceptor input not only reflexively stimulates breathing, but also activates a central modulating mechanism that could be responsible for the ventilatory decline. This is compatible with previous data showing that the degree of HVD is correlated with the magnitude of the initial ventilatory stimulation (2). However, Bascom et al., contrary to the effects with almitrine, found that the peripheral dopamine D_2 antagonist domperidone increased the acute initial response to hypoxia but did not attenuate HVD, supporting their view that the cause of HVD is in the peripheral chemoreceptor itself (168). Thus, there remains a controversy as to whether HVD is mediated by mechanisms acting primarily at the peripheral chemoreceptor or primarily within the CNS.

The hypothesis that HVD is initiated by peripheral chemoreceptor stimulation is supported by studies in awake cats in which HVD occurs in carotid-body-intact cats whereas no change in ventilation occurs in carotid-body denervated cats during sustained hypoxia (47). In a similar experiment performed in anesthetized adult rabbits (226), it was found that dopamine was released in the nucleus tractus solitarius by hypoxic stimulation of the carotid body, and it was suggested that this mechanism could be responsible for HVD. Tatsumi et al. found that haloperidol, a dopamine antagonist that crosses the blood-brain barrier, blocks the HVD in cats, further supporting a role for a carotid-body-mediated inhibition of ventilation by release of dopamine in the CNS (218).

In summary, there is little evidence to support a role for a decline in chemoreceptor discharge as a cause for HVD in adult animals; however, there is substantial support for a CNS mechanism that is activated by peripheral chemoreceptor stimulation. This mechanism may be mediated by dopamine release in the nucleus tractus solitarius. In this regard, it is interesting to note that, in both awake cats and humans, domperidone, which does not cross the blood-brain barrier, increases the initial acute response to hypoxia, but does not attenuate HVD (168), while haloperidol blocks HVD in awake cats (218). The same mechanism may contribute to HVD in the newborn, but carotid chemoreceptor immaturity may contribute to the decline as well in some species.

CNS Mechanisms of HVD

The possibility that there is a change in CNS chemical neuromodulators or neurotransmitters during sustained hypoxia, from the direct effects of brain hypoxia and/or from peripheral chemoreceptor stimulation, is strongly suggested by the slow recovery process of the ventilatory response to acute hypoxia after return to normoxic conditions. Full recovery of the acute response to hypoxia following sustained hypoxia requires 30–60 min on normoxia, a process that can be accelerated by inhalation of 100% oxygen (206,210). Several candidates for inhibitory neuromodulators/transmitters have been proposed to account for HVD. Dopamine has been mentioned above; in addition, adenosine, GABA, serotonin, and opioids have been proposed or tested as possible candidates.

Adenosine is known to increase in the brain during hypoxia (96) and has been shown to depress ventilation (227,228). The possibility that adenosine is contributory to HVD has been tested by giving the adenosine antagonist aminophylline (209,211). Hypoxic ventilatory decline was attenuated by aminophylline, suggesting a contribution of adenosine to the mechanism, but because there remains some HVD, particularly the V_T component (209), and because of the other possible respiratory effects of aminophylline, it is not likely the sole mechanism of HVD.

The extracellular concentration of GABA is also increased in the brain during hypoxia in both adult and neonatal animals (229– 231) and may also be a possible cause of hypoxic ventilatory decline. It has been shown that administration of GABA or its agonist muscimol produces ventilatory and cardiovascular depression when placed in the fourth ventricle or on the ventral surface of the medulla of anesthetized cats (232,233) or dogs (234). These actions were prevented by the GABA antagonist bicuculline (232,233). This has not been directly tested on HVD in awake humans. It is known that benzodiazepines potentiate GABA effects, and the finding that one such drug, midazolam, increased HVD in adult human subjects is compatible with a role for GABA in HVD (235). Thus, CNS neurotransmitters/modulators, such as GABA, adenosine, and dopamine, may contribute to HVD.

Hypoxia is also associated with a cerebral lactic acidosis. While an acidosis would be expected to increase ventilation by stimulation of the chemoreceptors rather than depress respiration, recent data show that prevention of brain acidosis abolishes the depression of respiration during progressive modest to moderate hypoxia (97). To test whether lactic acidosis could be the mediator of HVD in awake humans, dichloroacetate, which inhibits lactate production, was given to subjects before hypoxic exposure (236). This treatment, however, failed to attenuate HVD, suggesting that lactic acidosis probably does not mediate HVD.

Other CNS neuromodulator/transmitter mechanisms have been tested for an effect on HVD in adults and have not been found to have a role in the mechanism of the reduced hypoxic ventilation. These include serotonin (207) and opioids (35). However, since opioid antagonists have been shown to reverse hypoxic depression in the newborn (32,237), it remains possible that opioids have a role in the biphasic response to hypoxia in the neonate.

Role of Central Chemoreceptors in HVD

A reduction in stimulus level at the central chemoreceptor has also been postulated to mediate HVD. This could be mediated by a washout of brain CO_2 due to the initial hypoxic hyperventilation or by an hypoxia-induced increase in cerebral blood flow. While the location and stimulus parameters for the central chemo-receptors remain controversial (3), monitoring of the ventral medullary extracellular fluid (ECF) has been used to represent the most proximal stimulus of the central chemoreceptors. Hypoxia has been shown to be associated with increases in the pH of ventral medullary ECF, although with sustained or more severe hypoxia this initial alkalosis is replaced with a reduction in pH (58,97,238). Although hypoxia is associated with an initial alkalosis, there is no evidence that diminished central chemoreceptor stimulation is responsible for HVD. In fact, there is lack of change in cerebral venous (internal jugular vein) P_{CO_2} during HVD, which should reflect brain tissue P_{CO_2} during sustained hypoxia (239). In addition, it seems unlikely that a change in brain blood flow and central alkalosis would persist for the prolonged period necessary to account for the decline in ventilatory response (>15 min) and for the posthypoxic suppression of ventilation that remains on return to normoxic conditions after HVD (206,240). Finally, in adult human subjects it has been shown that the ventilatory response to CO_2 is unaffected after 25 min of hypoxia while the response to hypoxia is selectively depressed (240).

Exercise and HVD

There is some evidence that exercise may attenuate HVD. In a study by Ward and Nguyen (241), exercise during mild hypoxia eliminated the decline in ventilation. However, ventilation was maintained because of an increase in respiratory frequency while VT still exhibited a progressive decline. A similar study by Pandit and Robbins (242) also reported that ventilation changed minimally during hypoxic exercise, but a control study in the same subjects showed that ventilation progressively increased during normoxic exercise. The results of these two studies suggest that some elements of HVD, perhaps the V_T component, remain during sustained hypoxic exercise, but that, overall, HVD may be attenuated by exercise compared to resting HVD. These findings do little to sort out the mechanisms of HVD, but suggest that the CNS mechanisms do not impair the ability to maintain ventilation during the stress of hypoxic exercise.

In summary, studies in adult animals provide good evidence for a CNS mechanism of HVD that is initiated by hypoxic peripheral chemoreceptor stimulation. In addition, there is evidence that the CNS mediator released by carotid body stimulation in HVD is dopamine. Other cellular or CNS neurochemical mediators of hypoxic brain depression may also be involved as outlined in Section III. While these mechanisms may be responsible for HVD in awake adult human subjects, there remains controversial evidence that the primary source of declining ventilatory drive may be at the peripheral chemoreceptors. Newborn animals show a more exaggerated HVD, which may involve immaturity of peripheral chemoreceptor input and centrally mediated mechanisms including opioids, adenosine, GABA, and so forth. In addition, the newborn may have neuromechanical components that contribute (216,217) as well as a decrease in metabolic rate in hypoxia (243,244).

D. Ventilatory Acclimatization to Short-Term Hypoxia

We have discussed the ventilatory responses to acute and sustained hypoxia. These are effects that we consider to have a time course of up to about 1 hr in duration. Beyond 1 hr there are two other distinct phases of response to hypoxia. The next phase is the response in sea-level or low-altitude residents that occurs over time on ascent to altitude from low elevations. In humans this phase requires days to reach completion and then ventilation may remain stable for years. This is termed ventilatory acclimatization to short-term hypoxia (ASTH). ASTH is characterized by a time-dependent increase in ventilation, which becomes stable at a value greater than the ventilatory response to acute hypoxia. The last phase, termed acclimatization to long-term hypoxia (ALTH), is characteristic of natives or very long-term residents of altitude in which ventilation is reduced somewhat from that in ASTH. We will discuss ALTH in the next section.

The time course of ASTH varies with species and altitude. In humans, acclimatization to an altitude of 2900 m requires 4 days (245), to 4300 m requires approximately 10 days (246), and to the greatest terrestrial heights (>8000 m), more than 30 days (247). Generally, animals have a shorter time course of ASTH. Acclimatization to 4300 m in ponies is significant after 6 hr and is complete in 24 hr (43). In goats, acclimatization to the same altitude is complete in 4–6 hr (42,44). Dogs also acclimatize rapidly (3 hr at 3550 m) (248), and rats have time course similar to that of human subjects (249). The time course in cats has not been studied in detail, but it is known that significant acclimatization is apparent after 2 days at 4570 m (250). The finding of HVD (as described above) in human subjects has made the sequence of events interesting and may be one reason that ASTH requires a longer time course in humans than in most animals. Factors responsible for HVD combined with hypocapnia delay ASTH, but these tend to diminish over approximately the first 5 days of hypoxia at 4300 m (Fig. 4) (156,251).

The degree of hyperventilation is illustrated by the arterial or alveolar P_{CO_2} recorded in human subjects after completion of ASTH at several different altitudes: 2900 m, $P_{ACO_2} = 30.9$ torr (245); 3100 m, $Pa_{CO_2} = 32.3$ torr (252); and 4300 m, $Pa_{CO_2} = 25.2$ torr (246). At extreme altitude on Mt. Everest the mean Pa_{CO_2} at 8050 m was 11.0 torr and on the summit at 8848 m the P_{ACO_2} was 7.5 torr (253). These hyperventilatory responses defend Pa_{O_2}, and this is probably the most important physiological response that improves O_2 transport after ascent to high altitude (254).

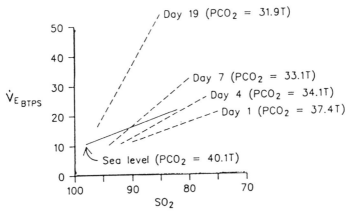

Figure 4   Mean ventilatory responses to acute hypoxia from six subjects measured at sea level and after variable durations of sojourn at 4300 m. The depressed ventilatory response early in the sojourn is likely due to the same mechanism causing HVD. Later responses indicate an increased response to acute hypoxia in the acclimatized subjects. (From Ref. 251.)

Mechanisms Responsible for Short-Term Acclimatization

Several mechanisms have been investigated historically, and we will mention them only briefly as they have been thoroughly reviewed (3–5).

Central Chemoreceptors in ASTH

Historically, a widely held theory of acclimatization was that proposed by Severinghaus et al. (255). These workers concluded that the pH of the cerebral fluid surrounding the central chemoreceptors was at first alkaline from hyperventilation owing to stimulation of the peripheral chemoreceptors, but with time this pH was corrected and allowed the full expression of the peripheral chemoreceptor input and the time-dependent hyperventilation characteristic of ASTH. A major part of this conclusion was based on the assumption that measurement of acid-base balance in cerebrospinal fluid (CSF) would reflect the acid-base status at the central chemoreceptor. In their studies they found that CSF pH was normalized in four subjects during ASTH (255). However, this could not be confirmed by numerous other investigators who found that CSF consistently remained alkaline during ASTH in either human or animal subjects (43,246,252,256–259).

Further animal studies attempted to determine whether pH near the putative central chemoreceptor (and therefore not reflected in bulk CSF pH) might be responsible for increasing ventilatory drive in ASTH. Some support for this theory was obtained by Davies using anesthetized dogs in which he calculated that cerebral interstitial pH was acidified in the region of putative central chemorecep-tors, while bulk CSF remained alkaline (260). Fencl et al. used ventriculocisternal perfusion in awake goats following 5 days of hypoxic exposure. They found that the cerebral interstitial fluid was not in equilibrium with the CSF and estimated that interstitial fluid was acidified by a lactic acidosis in the area of the central chemoreceptors, thus causing hyperventilation typical of ASTH (261). A theory based on hypoxia-induced acidification of central chemoreceptor pH is not consistent with the finding that ASTH is attenuated significantly in animals with peripheral chemoreceptor denervation (42–44,248). These animals would be expected to have at least the same degree of central chemoreceptor acidification and should also hyperventilate. That they do not during prolonged hypoxia is evidence against the central acidification hypothesis.

Recent studies in anesthetized cats (262) and awake goats (263) found greater acidification over putative ventral medullary surface chemoreceptors during acute hypoxia. The workers concluded that since this acidification did not stimulate breathing, central chemoreceptors may not respond to ECF [H$^+$], but may respond to transmembrane [H$^+$] gradient. Further, these studies provide more evidence that acidification of cerebral ECF per se does not play a role in ASTH.

In a study of CSF acid-base compensation and ventilation after controlled hyperventilation during either normoxia or hypoxia, Dempsey et al. (264) found independent effects of hypoxia on ventilation as compared to normoxia that could not be explained by CSF compensation. These studies provided further evidence against local regulation of CSF acid-base balance as a cause of ASTH. Taking this to the cellular level, studies of cerebral acid-base balance in rats exposed to hypoxia failed to provide a correlation between cerebral acidosis and the time course of ventilatory acclimatization (265).

Two attempts were made to determine whether maintaining eucapnia during acclimatization in human studies (preventing the fall in Pa$_{CO_2}$ that occurs with hyperventilation in ASTH) could also prevent acclimatization (266,267). The hypothesis was based on the premise that compensation for hypocapnic alkalosis was essential in production of acclimatization. Because of technical limitations, e.g., measuring only alveolar gases, and data that could not be fully interpreted, these studies were unable to conclusively support the hypothesis.

Similar studies of eucapnic hypoxia have been completed in awake goats in which ASTH can be completed in a period of only 4 hr of hypoxia (222). In goats it is possible to frequently sample and measure arterial blood gases to more accurately maintain arterial isocapnic conditions. The results of these studies indicate significant time-dependent increases in ventilation that are indicative of ASTH (Fig. 5) (268), illustrating that maintaining isocapnic hypoxia does not prevent acclimatization in the goat. In addition, studies with isolated carotid body perfusion in awake goats provide further evidence against central chemoreceptors as the primary site of ASTH (discussed more fully below). Thus, current evidence

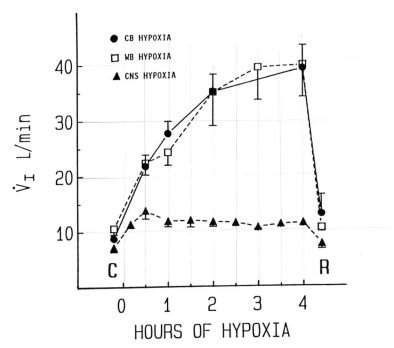

Figure 5 Mean ventilatory responses in three groups of goats subjected to either whole-animal hypoxia (open squares), isolated carotid body hypoxia (closed circles), or CNS (systemic arterial) hypoxia with isolated carotid body remaining normoxic (closed triangles). In all cases steady-state isocapnic hypoxia was sustained with arterial or carotid body hypoxia near 40 torr P_{O_2}. The data indicate time-dependent hyperventilation with either whole-body or isolated carotid body hypoxia (acclimatization or ASTH) whereas CNS hypoxia produced mild hyperventilation but no acclimatization. (From Ref. 268.)

is against a primary role for central chemoreceptors in ASTH; however, it is not possible to completely rule out some contribution from central chemoreceptors in acclimatization until one can precisely localize them and directly measure their stimuli during ASTH.

Other Possible CNS Mechanisms of ASTH

CNS Hyperexcitability. A general increase in CNS excitability was postulated to contribute to ASTH by Forster and Dempsey (4). This was based on studies in cats by Tenney et al. and Ou et al., who provided evidence of cortical facilitation of ventilation during prolonged hypoxia (120,269). Forster, Dempsey, and co-workers found additional evidence to support their view based on exaggerated ventilatory responses to hypoxia, hypercapnia, exercise, and IV doxapram as well as changes in electroencephalographic tracings in human subjects during or after ASTH (3,43,270–274).

Changes in brain monoamine metabolism have been postulated to cause increased ventilatory drive during ASTH (275–277). Olson et al. measured monoamine metabolism in rats exposed for up to 7 days of hypoxia (275). These investigators found reductions in serotonin and dopamine turnover, but norepinephrine turnover did not change. However, it was not possible to directly link these changes in monoamines to the mechanism of ASTH.

Millhorn et al. found that repeated stimulation of the carotid sinus nerve or carotid body produced a long-term elevation in ventilation in anesthetized or decerebrate cats that could be blocked by serotonin antagonists (277,278). This novel observation was the discovery of a neural long-term facilitation mechanism involved in control of ventilation that was postulated to contribute to ASTH. Recently, awake dogs were shown to hyperventilate for more than 30 min on return to normoxic conditions after 6–13 repeated hypoxia exposures (6).

Gallman and Millhorn also discovered a form of long-term facilitation of ventilation persisting for more than 1 hr after a 10-min period of hypoxia in peripheral chemoreceptor-denervated anesthetized cats (56). In brain-sectioning experiments, they found that the source for this facilitation was the diencephalic region and postulated that this facilitation could contribute to ASTH. This mechanism would be compatible with the hypothesis of Forster and Dempsey of increased CNS excitability during acclimatization (4). However, studies in goats do not support a long-term-facilitation mechanism of ASTH, from either carotid body stimulation or a diencephalic facilitation. This is based on the finding that if isocapnia is maintained during the hypoxic exposure, then goats do not hyperventilate after return to normoxic conditions following ASTH; i.e., there is no long-term facilitation (222,279). Furthermore, isolated carotid body hypoxia produces acclimatization whereas isolated carotid body hypercapnia does not in awake systemically normoxic goats (280) (see below). A mechanism involving long-term facilitation would require that any mode of carotid body stimulus would induce ASTH. Finally, Olson found that serotonergic antagonists do not modify ASTH in rats, not supporting involvement of a serotonergic long-term-facilitation mechanism of ASTH (276).

The Peripheral Chemoreceptors in ASTH

Carotid Body Denervation. Animals exposed to hypoxia without intact carotid bodies have much lower Pa_{O_2} at any given altitude or FI_{O_2} (43,44,134). Furthermore, acclimatization as assessed by time-dependent fall in Pa_{CO_2} is reported to be significantly attenuated in the goat (42,44,281), pony (43), cat (282), rat (134), and dog (248). Contrary to these findings one group of investigators found that carotid-body-denervated goats exhibited a significant fall in Pa_{CO_2} after 3 days of hypoxia (283). There is no obvious explanation for this discrepancy, but recent studies using carotid body perfusion in awake goats showed that systemic hypoxia (including the CNS) did not induce ASTH when the carotid body was maintained normoxic (51). Taken together, these studies indicate that carotid bodies are an essential element in ASTH.

   Carotid Body Perfusion Studies. Isolated perfusion of the carotid body of awake goats has allowed a greater understanding of acclimatization (51,279,280, 284). In this preparation one carotid body is perfused with blood from an extracorporeal circuit and this blood is prevented from circulating to the brain by previous vascular ligations (284). The system allows independent control of blood perfusing the carotid body from that in the systemic circulation (and brain). Using this preparation, it was first demonstrated that the goat underwent ASTH as assessed by time-dependent fall in Pa_{CO_2} during hypoxic perfusion of the carotid body while the systemic arterial blood (including the CNS) now normoxic; i.e., brain hypoxia was not required for acclimatization to occur (Fig. 6) (284). In addition, acclimatization also occurred in the absence of hypocapnic alkalosis in the carotid body perfusion model, indicating that acclimatization was not depen-

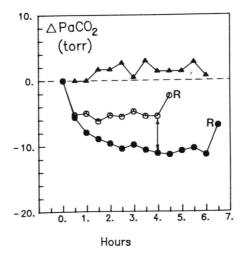

Hours

Figure 6   Mean changes in systemic arterial P_{CO_2} during isolated carotid body perfusion in awake goats. Initial value at time 0 is control with normoxic carotid body perfusate. Closed circles indicate isolated carotid body hypoxia (Pcb_{O_2} = 40 torr), open circles indicate isolated carotid body normoxic-hypercapnia (Pcb_{CO_2} = 78 torr), closed triangles indicate normoxic-normocapnic control carotid body perfusion. In all cases systemic arterial normoxia was maintained. These data indicate that isolated carotid body hypoxia produces typical time-dependent hyperventilation (acclimatization or ASTH), whereas isolated carotid body hypercapnia produces sustained hyperventilation, but with no time-dependent increasing hyperventilation (no acclimatization). (From Ref. 280.)

dent on the development of cerebral hypocapnic alkalosis (Fig. 5) (279). It was further shown that systemic arterial (including brain) hypoxia did not produce acclimatization when the isolated carotid body was maintained normoxic although brain hypoxia produced mild hyperventilation (Fig. 5) (280). All these studies were done using a steady-state hypoxic blood stimulus level near 40 torr Po_2 and in some cases with isocapnia maintained. It is appreciated that neither constant Pao_2 nor constant $Paco_2$ is present in natural acclimatization; however, in some cases it was necessary to control these conditions in order to answer the question at hand, and it was believed that the fundamental mechanism of acclimatization would not be affected by these conditions.

The above studies suggested that carotid body input was key in eliciting ASTH in goats. A further question was asked: is carotid body stimulus mode, e.g., hypoxia versus hypercapnia, critical to induction of ASTH? To answer this question, the isolated carotid body was stimulated with hypercapnic-normoxic blood (280). Care was taken to provide the same initial level of stimulation that was present when the carotid body was stimulated by hypoxic blood (a mean $Pcbco_2$ of 78 torr). This level of steady-state stimulation produced a brisk hyperventilation in the goats, but no further time-dependent hyperventilation, i.e., no acclimatization (Fig. 6) (280). These findings indicated that ASTH requires that the carotid body be hypoxic, and that steady-state carotid body input to the CNS does not result in some time-dependent change in the central respiratory controller to produce ASTH. These results strongly suggested that the carotid body was the primary locus of ASTH in the goat.

Carotid Sinus Nerve Recording Studies. Support for the above conclusions was obtained by recording carotid body afferent activity in anesthetized goats over periods of up to 4 hr during either steady-state hypoxia (17) or normoxic hypercapnia (285). The results of these studies were compatible with the above findings using carotid body perfusion; i.e., hypoxia produced time-dependent increasing afferent activity and hypercapnia produced a steady-state stimulation of afferent activity. These findings are supported by studies in cats by Vizek et al. (250), who showed that carotid sinus nerve afferent and ventilatory response to acute hypoxia are increased after 48 hr of hypoxia. In a related study, Barnard et al. found that up to 3 hr of hypoxia did not increase carotid body afferent activity in cats (286). However, this is likely related to a longer time course of acclimatization in cats. This group found that after 4 weeks of hypoxia cats had an exaggerated carotid body response to hypoxia (286).

Ventilatory Response to Acute Hypoxia in ASTH. The carotid body as a primary location for the mechanism of ASTH is supported by the finding of increased ventilatory response to acute hypoxia in both animal (222,250,287–290) and human studies (271,291–295) either during or after ASTH (Fig. 4). This is a relatively recent observation as the response to acute hypoxia was not consistently found to be changed in most earlier studies (cf. Ref. 271). The increased ventilatory response to acute hypoxia has been found to be present after as long as 1 year in residence at high altitude in human subjects (295).

Mechanisms of Increased Carotid Body Response to Hypoxia in ASTH

The mechanism(s) responsible for increased carotid body response to hypoxia during ASTH are not fully understood. Possible intrinsic carotid body mechanisms could involve increased activity of excitatory neuromodulators, inhibition or down-regulation of inhibitory neuromodulators, or some fundamental change in expression of the transduction mechanism. It is also possible that extrinsic influences via carotid sinus nerve or sympathetic efferent innervation of the carotid body could change the response to hypoxia. Circulating factors conceivably could affect carotid body function during prolonged hypoxia, but none have been proposed or tested. Similarly, no studies of the transduction mechanism have been carried out during or after ASTH.

Dopamine and Carotid Sinus Nerve Afferents. As indicated above, there is strong evidence that dopamine is an important inhibitory neuromodulator in the carotid body. It has been postulated that diminishing dopaminergic inhibition may be responsible for increasing carotid body activity during ASTH (288,296). This could occur by depletion of carotid body dopamine or a down-regulation of the dopamine receptors in the carotid body. Goats were given dopamine infusions intravenously or directly into the common carotid arteries before and after ASTH, and there was no change in the carotid-body-mediated reduction in ventilation, strongly suggesting no change in dopamine receptor effectiveness after ASTH (222,297). Additional studies were done in goats to determine whether dopamine blockade initiated before hypoxic exposure and maintained throughout for up to 28 hr of hypoxia could modify ASTH (296). A dopamine antagonist was used that does not readily cross the blood-brain-barrier, domperidone (298). The time course of acclimatization was hypothesized to significantly shorten with dopamine blockade, if dopamine was depleted or not released from carotid body type I cells. The findings indicated a partial acceleration of ASTH, but the results were not clear enough to strongly support the hypothesis. More recent studies in cats by Tatsumi et al. (288) have found that the maximal acute response to hypoxia after domperidone treatment could not be further augmented after ASTH in cats, suggesting that decreased carotid body dopaminergic activity was playing an important role in ASTH. In summary, the above studies together are compatible with a decrease in dopamine release but not a change in dopamine receptor sensitivity as a possible mechanism for increased hypoxic sensitivity of the carotid body during ASTH.

As described above, the carotid sinus nerve contains inhibitory efferents that originate primarily from cells in the rostral nucleus ambiguus (173–177). The inhibition via these efferents is thought to be via release of dopamine (178).

Elevated hypoxic sensitivity recorded from carotid body afferents was not changed by section of the carotid sinus nerve in acclimatized cats after 48 hr of hypoxia (250). This suggests that efferents are not involved in ASTH. Unlike this result, previous studies found increased carotid body efferent inhibition in cats after 3–7 weeks of hypoxia (178,299). The disagreement between these studies is likely due to the longer duration of hypoxia in the second set of studies (178,299) and may reflect changes occurring in acclimatization to more prolonged hypoxia (see below). Carotid sinus nerve efferents were not found necessary for time-dependent increased carotid body afferent neural discharge frequency during prolonged hypoxia in goats (17). Thus, the balance of evidence suggests carotid sinus nerve efferents do not appear to play an important role in ASTH.

After a few hours of hypoxia, carotid body dopamine content is decreased in rats (158,159,275). However, after days or weeks of hypoxia the carotid body contains a greatly increased level of dopamine (275,300,301), dopamine turnover is increased (301), and this increased dopaminergic activity is partially under the control of sympathetic innervation (302). All of these changes taken together are intriguing and hint of important role(s) for carotid body dopamine during prolonged hypoxic exposure. These putative dopaminergic mechanisms that may mediate or modulate changes in carotid body responses to hypoxia in ASTH remain to be more completely elucidated.

Noradrenergic/Sympathetic Efferent Mechanisms. Carotid body norepinephrine contents and turnover rate, like dopamine, are increased during chronic hypoxia, but the changes are smaller and are slower to occur (275,301). And, as outlined above, there are at least three possible sources of norepinephrine influence on the carotid body: the type I cells of the carotid body, sympathetic nerve terminals in the carotid body, and circulating norepinephrine. The finding of inhibitory α_2-adrenergic receptors in the cat carotid body (190) followed by the demonstration that this inhibition disappeared after 24 hr of hypoxia (303) suggested that down-regulation of another inhibitory catecholaminergic mechanism could be contributing to increased carotid body hypoxic sensitivity in the cat during ASTH. Pizarro et al., using intracarotid infusions, recently demonstrated that norepinephrine was inhibitory to the goat carotid body (186). To further examine the possibility that noradrenergic sensitivity could be reduced in ASTH, the responses to intracarotid norepinephrine infusion were determined in awake goats during and after ASTH (297). No change in the carotid-body-induced inhibition of ventilation by norepinephrine was detected, providing no evidence for a change in noradrenergic sensitivity in goats during ASTH. In related studies, the magnitude and time course of ASTH were determined before and after sympathetic denervation of the carotid body in goats (202). These studies revealed no change in ASTH after sympathetic denervation. Thus, in the goat there is no evidence that carotid body noradrenergic activity or sympathetic innervation plays a significant role in ASTH.

One study has examined the role of β-adrenergic receptors in human subjects on ASTH and metabolic rate during hypoxic acclimitization (304). These workers found that propranolol inhibited the metabolic rate increase but had no effect on ventilatory acclimatization to an altitude of 4300 m, indicating that β-adrenergic receptors in the carotid body or elsewhere were unlikely to be involved in the mechanism of ASTH.

The above-described studies indicate a potential role for carotid body dopaminergic but no noradrenergic mechanisms having a role in ASTH. As stated earlier, the carotid body contains many other putative neuromodulators/transmitters that could play a role in ASTH. None of these agents have been tested for their potential role in ASTH. The findings from peripheral chemoreceptor denervation and isolated perfusion studies in animals and more direct assessment of peripheral arterial chemoreceptor function as outlined above point to the peripheral arterial chemoreceptors as the initiators of ASTH rather than a primary role for hypoxia-induced brain mechanisms in ASTH. Nevertheless, there are data suggesting both CNS excitation and inhibition due to hypoxia in animals. Thus, CNS mechanisms have the potential to modify ASTH depending on the balance of CNS modulation of ventilatory drive. This brings up the distinct possibility of species differences in ASTH. For example, the goat and cat seem to be primarily dependent on peripheral chemoreceptor input during ASTH whereas humans may have a peripheral chemoreceptor component along with CNS component(s). We could further speculate that strength and importance of both peripheral chemoreceptor and CNS components could vary according to the severity of hypoxia.

Deacclimatization After Short-Term Acclimatization

Upon return to normoxic conditions following ASTH at an altitude of 4300 m, a period of hyperventilation is present for more than 13 hr in human subjects (257). This continued hyperventilation is termed *deacclimatization* (3). Few studies have been carried out on deacclimatization and its mechanism remains unknown. In one systematic study in humans and ponies, no correlations could be found between arterial and CSF acid-base changes and the rising Pa_{CO_2}; thus, the cause for continued hyperventilation was not determined (257). Acid-base changes were the main theme of this study, and the stimulus level of central chemoreceptors remains uncertain; thus, their contribution to deacclimatization cannot be determined.

The assumption held for many years is that the same mechanism is responsible for acclimatization and deacclimatization. This assumption has been questioned recently as more emphasis has been placed on the carotid body rather than the central chemoreceptor as the main locus of the mechanism of ASTH. Indeed, it has been shown that if eucapnic conditions are maintained during acclimatization in awake goats during either whole-body hypoxia (222,297) or isolated carotid body hypoxia (279), then the animals do not hyperventilate after return to normoxia. Goats in which Pa_{CO_2} is allowed to fall, as in natural acclimatization, do hyperventilate in the classic way after return to normoxia (42,44,222,284). This finding indicates that there are probably different mechanisms for acclimatization and deacclimatization and further suggests that hypocapnic alkalosis is required for deacclimatization. Vizek et al. found that carotid bodies were primarily responsible for acclimatization in cats with little evidence for a CNS contribution; nevertheless, acclimatized cats continued to hyperventilate after the carotid sinus nerves are cut, suggesting the possibility that CNS mechanisms are responsible for deacclimatization (250). A study in anesthetized goats found no evidence of increased carotid body afferent activity after return to normoxia following prolonged hypoxia (305), indicating that the carotid bodies do not contribute to deacclimatization.

E. Ventilatory Acclimatization to Long-Term Hypoxia

Very long-term altitude residents who have moved from low elevations and native altitude residents have changed ventilatory characteristics compared to those after ASTH even though ASTH can be maintained for a period of years in humans (3,5). We term this ventilatory acclimatization to long-term hypoxia (ALTH). For the most part, there are no differences between long-term residents and long-term natives; therefore, they are considered as a single group termed *highlanders* (see exception below regarding Tibetans). Highlanders differ in that they have a resting Pa_{CO_2} indicative of hyperventilation relative to sea level residents but not as low as the Pa_{CO_2} characteristic of ASTH (3,306–311). The decreased ventilation is accompanied by a significant reduction (blunting) of the ventilatory response to acute hypoxia (Fig. 7) (3,306–311). However, in most highlanders there is no change in the ventilatory response to acute hypercapnia (271,308,310,312). Reduced transient ventilatory responses to CO_2, 100% O_2, or N_2 are consistent with a diminished peripheral chemoreceptor reflex (308,313). Steady-state administration of O_2 is reported to cause hyperventilation in highlanders (306,308,314). This could be due to relief of central hypoxic depression or to CNS stimulation effects of hyperoxia (315).

Reduced or total absence of hypoxic sensitivity is the most striking finding in highlanders (Fig. 7). This blunting of the hypoxic response is apparently an acquired characteristic as children born and resident at high altitude do not have blunted responses to hypoxia (316,317). And the degree of blunting is correlated with years in residence at altitude (271,311) and may also be associated not only with time in residence (years), but also proportional to the altitude (km) (314). Blunting has generally been considered to be a permanent change in the ventilatory control system (306,318), but some exceptions have been reported (319). One exception has recently been described to the above description of

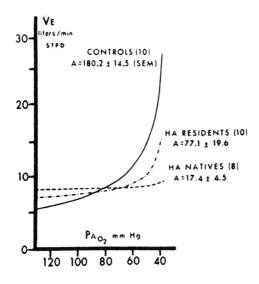

Figure 7 Average ventilatory responses from lowlander controls, highlanders (long-term residents of high altitude (HA), and natives of high altitude (Leadville, CO, 3100 m). The data illustrate the blunted ventilatory response to acute hypoxia in highlanders. (From Ref. 311.)

highlanders (320). This exception has been found in life-long adult Tibetan residents ($n = 27$) of the Lhasa region of Tibet (3650 m). This group was compared to age-, body size-, and activity-matched residents of the same region who had emigrated from lowland China (Han) 1–20 years earlier ($n = 30$). It was found that the lifelong Tibetans did not have the expected blunted ventilatory response to acute hypoxia compared to the short-term acclimatized Han subjects, who behaved as Andeans or North Americans would have who had emigrated from low altitude; i.e., they had ventilatory response that were becoming blunted over time. In addition, the Tibetans maintained the same PET_{CO_2} as the Han, as would be expected after ASTH. Thus, not all natives of altitude have the characteristics classically attributed to highlanders as described above. Reasons for the differences are not clear, but Tibetans are the longest-residing high-altitude population, suggesting the possibility of a natural adaptation or selection process that has developed over many generations.

Mechanisms of ALTH in Highlanders (Non-Tibetans)

Investigators examining changes in ventilatory control in highlanders have focused on the hypoxic chemoreflex. CNS translation of peripheral chemoreceptor input and function of the arterial chemoreceptors themselves are the two components of the system receiving the most attention. The carotid body has logically been the focus of attention not only because of the failed ventilatory response to hypoxia, but because of the significant changes in the biochemistry and morphology of the carotid body in highlander animals and humans. The carotid bodies are markedly enlarged in chronically hypoxic animals and humans whether from altitude residence or disease (321–326). There is hypertrophy of type I cells (321,325,326) as well as an increase in vascular volume (321,325). We have previously mentioned the increased dopamine and norepinephrine content and turnover in rats exposed to prolonged hypoxia (275,300–302). There have been few studies, but biochemical and morphological changes have not correlated well with function of the chemoreflex (327), thus leaving the functional implications of hypoxia-induced carotid body changes unsettled.

There are no natural animal models of blunting of the acute ventilatory response as native or resident animals of high altitude do not exhibit the reduced hypoxic ventilatory response (328–332). However, cats exposed to a barometric pressure simulating 5500 m for 3–4 weeks exhibit a diminished hypoxic ventilatory response (333,334). This model has been used to examine the mechanisms of the blunted hypoxic response, but unlike humans, the cat quickly recovers the normal ventilatory response to hypoxia (318,334). Tenney and Ou originally described this model and showed that midcollicular decerebration induced recovery of the normal hypoxic response, suggesting cortical inhibition was responsible for blunting (334). This cat model was also used by Tatsumi et al. (333), who found that both the ventilatory and carotid body responses to hypoxia were blunted after the animals were exposed to 5500 m for 4 weeks. Their data suggested that CNS translation of carotid body input was depressed, implicating a CNS involvement in blunting. They further found that cutting the carotid sinus nerve increased the carotid body response to acute hypoxia, suggesting that descending inhibitory efferent activity was increased. The same investigators have found that the dopamine antagonist domperidone restored the blunted response to hypoxia (335). Since this agent does not effectively cross the blood-brain barrier, these findings indicate a dopaminergic carotid body inhibition contributes to blunting. The data on the cat model taken together are compatible with a CNS mechanism and a carotid body dopaminergic inhibition in blunting of the hypoxic ventilatory response.

While blunting of the acute hypoxic response is not found in altitude native or resident animals, resting ventilation is attenuated as in humans; i.e., more moderate hyperventilation continues but not at the same level as seen in ASTH. This has been observed in dogs (256), cats (330,334), goats (336,337), and ponies (258) and requires a shorter time to develop, a matter of a few weeks, rather than many years as in human subjects. This phenomenon in animals may provide a valid model to examine mechanisms of hyperventilation in long-term residents of altitude. One study has examined the role of opiate receptors in awake goats during long-term acclimatization; however, these investigators did not confirm a role for opiate mechanisms as the full hyperventilation was not restored with naloxone (334). Mechanisms similar to those suggested to explain hypoxic blunting in the cat, e.g., a combination of cortical inhibition, CNS modulation of carotid body activation, and excessive carotid body dopaminergic inhibitory activity, as described above, may be operating during resting ventilation. It would be relatively easy to examine dopaminergic activity in human subjects and other animal models, but more creative investigation will be needed to discover specific mechanisms controlling ventilation in long-term hypoxia.

V. Summary

We have attempted, in this chapter, to briefly review the increasing knowledge of the complexity of hypoxic effects on ventilation.

A large effort has been put into the understanding of roll-off or HVD as it may have important clinical implications, for example, in recovery from anesthesia. Much data point to hypoxic CNS depression as a cause for HVD, but a few investigators believe the carotid body itself may be the cause for falling ventilation. Animal studies suggest that CNS dopaminergic inhibition may be responsible for HVD and this may be dependent on carotid sinus nerve input. This needs to be further elucidated and, if confirmed, extended to human subjects. It is likely that HVD is delaying the onset of acclimatization in those species such as humans and cats who exhibit HVD. Once the mechanisms of HVD are better defined, its influence on acclimatization to hypoxia can be better assessed.

Most evidence indicates that CNS hypoxia produces decreased neuronal excitability and that, within limitations, the mechanisms responsible for this reduction are also providing some protection of neuronal integrity. The net effect on ventilation is inhibition, but this is state-dependent and may also depend on the presence of peripheral chemoreceptors. There is increasing evidence for selective CNS neuronal stimulation by hypoxia, and much needs to be done to further our understanding of the neuroanatomical and neurophysiological significance of these findings and their potential effects on respiratory control.

Long-term potentiation of ventilation was briefly mentioned. The evidence to date does not support its having an important role in acclimatization to short-term hypoxia in goats and cats. However, further studies need to be done to characterize this phenomenon and determine whether it has a physiological role in ventilatory control.

A brief review of the mechanisms of ASTH supports the view that central chemoreceptors are not the primary locus of the mechanism of ASTH. However, time-dependent changes in CNS excitability may play a role in delaying the onset of ASTH in humans due to HVD and may, at a later time, increasing ventilatory drive. However, most recent data suggest that there is increased sensitivity of the carotid body to hypoxia during acclimatization and that this may be the primary initiating factor of ASTH. There is evidence that carotid body dopaminergic mechanisms play a role in this increased carotid body response to hypoxia. This needs to be further explored and additional studies directed toward the mechanisms increasing the time-dependent carotid response to hypoxia. The increased hypoxic sensitivity that has been documented on the cat and goat carotid body after relatively short periods (4 hr in goats and 48 hr in cats) raises interesting questions about plasticity of the function of the carotid body. This phenomenon has both physiological and clinical implications and deserves further study. Carotid body plasticity may also play a role in ALTH. While there is evidence of an increase in carotid body dopaminergic activity during ALTH in cats, further animal studies and investigation in human subjects are warranted.

Significant progress has been made in understanding mechanisms and effects of hypoxia on the ventilatory control system. However, in addition to the specific areas mentioned above regarding effects of hypoxia on the control of breathing, work must continue to broaden our knowledge in fundamental areas, including: (1) the basic cellular transduction mechanism in peripheral chemoreceptor cells during hypoxia and how these are modulated by intrinsic and extrinsic factors; (2) the cellular and biophysical responses of respiratory neurons to different levels of brain hypoxia; (3) the structure and function of the neural circuitry mediating the CNS responses to hypoxia; (4) the effect of these components on ventilation and homeostasis during conditions of acute and chronic hypoxia; and (5) the reasons for the marked time dependency of ventilatory responses to hypoxia.

References

1. Vizek M, Pickett CK, Weil JV. Biphasic ventilatory response of adult cats to sustained hypoxia has central origin. J Appl Physiol 1987; 63:1658–1664.
2. Easton PA, Slykerman LJ, Anthonisen NR. Ventilatory response to sustained hypoxia in normal adults. J Appl Physiol 1986; 61:906–911.
3. Dempsey JA, Forster HV. Mediation of ventilatory adaptations. Physiol Rev 1982; 62:262–346.
4. Forster HV, Dempsey JA. Ventilatory adaptations. In: Hornbein T, ed. Lung Biology in Health and Disease. Regulation of Breathing. New York: Marcel Dekker, 1981:845–904.
5. Weil JV. Ventilatory control at high altitude. In: Cherniack NS, Widdicombe JG, eds. Handbook of Physiology. Section 3: The Respiratory System. Vol II: Control of Breathing. Part 2. Bethesda, MD: American Physiological Society, 1986:703.
6. Cao K-Y, Zwillich CW, Berthon-Jones M, Sullivan CE. Increased normoxic ventilation induced by repetitive hypoxia in conscious dogs. J Appl Physiol 1992; 73:2083–2088.
7. Eyzaguirre C, Zapata P. Perspectives in carotid body research. J Appl Physiol 1984; 57:931–957.
8. Fidone SJ, Gonzales C. Initiation and control of chemoreceptor activity in the carotid body. In: Cherniack NS, Widdicombe JG, eds. Handbook of Physiology. Section 3:

The Respiratory System. Vol II: Control of Breathing, Part 1. Bethesda, MD: American Physiological Society, 1986:247–312.

9. Fitzgerald RS, Lahiri S. Reflex response to chemoreceptor stimulation. In: Cherniack NS, Widdicombe JG, eds. Handbook of Physiology. Section 3: The Respiratory System. Vol II: Control of Breathing, Part 1. Bethesda, MD: American Physiological Society, 1986:313–362.

10. Lahiri S, Nishino A, Mulligan E, Nishino T. Comparison of aortic and carotid chemoreceptor response to hypercapnia and hypoxia. J Appl Physiol 1981; 51: 55–61.

11. Lahiri S. Role of arterial O_2 flow in peripheral chemoreceptor excitation. Fed Proc 1980; 39:2648–2652.

12. Lahiri S, Nishino T, Mulligan E, Mokashi A. Relative latency of responses of chemoreceptor afferents from aortic and carotid bodies. J Appl Physiol 1980; 48: 262–269.

13. Lahiri S. Oxygen biology of peripheral chemoreceptors. In: Lahiri S, Cherniack NS, Fitzgerald RS, eds. Response and Adaptation to Hypoxia. Bethesda, MD: American Physiological Society, 1991:95–106.

14. Hopp FA, Seagard JL, Bajic J, Zuperku EJ. Respiratory responses to aortic and carotid chemoreceptor activation in the dog. J Appl Physiol 1991; 70:2539–2550.

15. Biscoe TJ, Bradley GW, Purves MJ. The relation between carotid body chemoreceptor discharge, carotid sinus pressure and carotid body venous flow. J Physiol (Lond) 1970; 208:99–120.

16. Biscoe TJ, Purves MJ, Sampson SR. The frequency of nerve impulses in single carotid body chemoreceptor afferent fibres recorded in vivo with intact circulation. J Physiol (Lond) 1970; 208:121–131.

17. Nielsen AM, Bisgard GE, Vidruk EH. Carotid chemoreceptor activity during acute and sustained hypoxia in goats. J Appl Physiol 1988; 65:1796–1802.

18. Eyzaguirre C, Koyano H. Effects of hypoxia, hypercapnia, and pH on the chemoreceptor activity of the carotid body in vitro. J Physiol (Lond) 1965; 178:385–409.

19. Andronikou S, Shirahata M, Mokashi A, Lahiri S. Carotid body chemoreceptor and ventilatory responses to sustained hypoxia and hypercapnia in the cat. Respir Physiol 1988; 72:361–374.

20. Li K, Ponte JL, Sadler CL. Carotid body chemoreceptor response to prolonged hypoxia in the rabbit: effects of domperidone and propranolol. J Physiol (Lond) 1990; 430:1–11.

21. Marchal F, Bairam A, Haouzi P, et al. Carotid chemoreceptor response to natural stimuli in the newborn kitten. Respir Physiol 1992; 87:183–193.

22. Carroll JL, Bamford OS, Fitzgerald RS. Postnatal maturation of carotid chemoreceptor responses O_2 and CO_2 in the cat. J Appl Physiol 1993; 75:2383–2391.

23. Kholwadwala D, Donnelly DF. Maturation of carotid chemoreceptor sensitivity to hypoxia: in vitro studies in the newborn rat. J Physiol (Lond) 1992; 453:461–473.

24. Blanco CE, Dawes GS, Hanson MA, McCooke HB. The response to hypoxia of arterial chemoreceptors in fetal sheep and new-born lambs. J Physiol 1984; 351: 25–37.

25. Mulligan EM. Discharge properties of carotid bodies: developmental aspects. In:

Haddad GG, Farber JP, eds. Developmental Neurobiology of Breathing. New York: Marcel Dekker, 1991:321–340.

26. Dutton RE, Smith EJ, Ghatak PK, Davies DG. Dynamics of the respiratory controller during carotid body hypoxia. J Appl Physiol 1973; 35:844–850.

27. Ward DS, Berkenbosch A, DeGoede J, Olievier CN. Dynamics of the ventilatory response to central hypoxia in cats. J Appl Physiol 1990; 68:1107–1113.

28. Yu GP, Melton JE, Li JK-J, Neubauer JA, Edelman NH. The response of the phrenic neurogram to sinusoidal brain hypoxia. FASEB J 1991:A665.

29. Edelman NH, Epstein PE, Lahiri S, Cherniack NS. Ventilatory responses to transient hypoxia and hypercapnia in man. Respir Physiol 1973; 17:302–314.

30. Weiskopf RB, Gabel RA. Depression of ventilation during hypoxia in man. J Appl Physiol 1975; 39:911–915.

31. Blanco CE, Hanson MA, Johnson P, Rigatto H. Breathing pattern of kittens during hypoxia. J Appl Physiol 1984; 56:12–17.

32. Grunstein MM, Hazinski TA, Schleuter MA. Respiratory control during hypoxia in newborn rabbits: implied action of endorphins. J Appl Physiol 1981; 51:122–130.

33. Haddad GG, Mellins RB. Hypoxia and respiratory control in early life. Annu Rev Physiol 1984; 46:629–643.

34. Lawson EE, Long WW. Central origin of biphasic breathing pattern during hypoxia in newborns. J Appl Physiol 1983; 55:483–488.

35. Kagawa S, Stafford MJ, Waggener TB, Severinghaus JW. No effect of naloxone on hypoxia-induced ventilatory depression in adults. J Appl Physiol 1982; 52:1030–1034.

36. Weil JV, Zwillich CW. Assessment of ventilatory response to hypoxia: methods and interpretation. Chest 1976; 70 (Suppl):124S–128S.

37. Woodrum DF, Standaert TA, Maycock DE, Guthrie RD. Hypoxic ventilatory response in the newborn monkey. Pediatr Res 1981; 5:1278–1286.

38. Watt JG, Dumke PR, Comroe JH Jr. Effects of inhalation of 100 percent and 14 percent oxygen upon respiration of unanesthetized dogs before and after chemoreceptor denervation. Am J Physiol 1943; 138:610–617.

39. Davenport HW, Brewer G, Chambers AH, Goldschmidt S. The respiratory responses to anoxemia of unanesthetized dogs with chronically denervated aortic and carotid chemoreceptors and their causes. Am J Physiol 1947; 148:406–417.

40. Holton P, Wood JB. The effects of bilateral removal of the carotid bodies and denervation of the carotid sinuses in two human subjects. J Physiol (Lond) 1965; 181:365–378.

41. Wade JG, Larson CP, Jr., Hickey RF, Ehrenfeld WK, Severinghaus JW. Effect of carotid endarterectomy on carotid chemoreceptor and baroreceptor function in man. N Engl J Med 1970; 282:823–829.

42. Forster HV, Bisgard GE, Klein JP. Effect of peripheral chemoreceptor denervation on acclimatization of goats during hypoxia. J Appl Physiol 1981; 50:392–398.

43. Forster HV, Bisgard GE, Rasmussen B, Orr JA, Buss DD, Manohar M. Ventilatory control in peripheral chemoreceptor-denervated ponies during chronic hypoxemia. J Appl Physiol 1976; 41:878–885.

44. Smith CA, Bisgard GE, Nielsen AM, et al. Carotid bodies are required for ventilatory acclimatization to chronic hypoxia. J Appl Physiol 1986; 60:1003–1010.

45. Bisgard GE, Vogel JHK. Hypoventilation and pulmonary hypertension after carotid body excision. J Appl Physiol 1971; 31:431–437.
46. Bisgard GE, Forster HV, Orr JA, Buss DD, Rawlings CA, Rasmussen B. Hypoventilation in ponies after carotid body denervation. J Appl Physiol 1976; 40:184–190.
47. Long WQ, Giesbrecht GG, Anthonisen NR. Ventilatory response to moderate hypoxia in awake chemodenervated cats. J Appl Physiol 1993; 74:805–810.
48. Santiago TV, Edelman NH. Mechanisms of the ventilatory response to carbon monoxide. J Clin Invest 1976; 57:977–986.
49. Smith CA, Engwall MJA, Dempsey JA, Bisgard GE. Effects of specific carotid body and brain hypoxia on respiratory muscle control in the awake goat. J Physiol (Lond) 1993; 460:623–640.
50. Chapman RW, Santiago TV, Edelman NH. Brain hypoxia and control of breathing: role of the vagi. J Appl Physiol 1982; 53:212–217.
51. Weizhen N, Engwall MJA, Daristotle L, Pizarro J, Bisgard GE. Ventilatory effects of prolonged systemic (CNS) hypoxia in awake goats. Respir Physiol 1992; 87: 37–48.
52. Daristotle L, Engwall MJA, Niu WZ, Bisgard GE. Ventilatory effects and interactions with change in Pa_{O_2} in awake goats. J Appl Physiol 1991; 71:1254–1260.
53. Miller M, Tenney SM. Hypoxia-induced tachypnea in carotid-deafferented cats. Respir Physiol 1975; 23:31–39.
54. Gautier H, Bonora M. Possible alterations in brain monoamine metabolism during hypoxia-induced tachypnea in cats. J Appl Physiol 1980; 49:769–777.
55. Chin K, Motoharu O, Masashi H, Takanobu K, Yanosuke S, Kenshi K. Breathing during sleep with mild hypoxia. J Appl Physiol 1989; 67:1198–1207.
56. Gallman EA, Millhorn DE. Two long-lasting central respiratory responses following acute hypoxia in glomectomized cats. J Physiol (Lond) 1988; 395:333–347.
57. Melton JE, Oyer Chae LO, Neubauer JA, Edelman NH. Extracellular potassium homeostasis in the cat medulla during progressive brain hypoxia. J Appl Physiol 1991; 70:1477–1482.
58. Neubauer JA, Santiago TV, Posner MA, Edelman NH. Ventral medullary pH and ventilatory responses to hyperfusion and hypoxia. J Appl Physiol 1985; 58:1659–1668.
59. Neubauer JA, Melton JE, Edelman NM. Modulation of respiration during brain hypoxia. J Appl Physiol 1990; 68(2):441–451.
60. Mitra J, Dev NB, Romaniuk JR, Trivedi R, Prabhakar NR, Cherniack NS. Cardiorespiratory changes induced by vertebral artery injection of sodium cyanide in cats. Respir Physiol 1992; 87:49–61.
61. Melton JE, Neubauer JA, Edelman NH. CO2 sensitivity of cat phrenic neurogram during hypoxic respiratory depression. J Appl Physiol 1988; 65:736–743.
62. Wasicko MJ, Melton JE, Neubauer JA, Krawciw N, Edelman NH. Cervical sympathetic and phrenic nerve responses to progressive brain hypoxia. J Appl Physiol 1990; 68:53–58.
63. Guntheroth WG, Kawabori I. Hypoxic apnea and gasping. J Clin Invest 1975; 56: 1371–1377.
64. Sanocka UM, Donnelly DF, Haddad GG. Autoresuscitation: a survival mechanism in piglets. J Appl Physiol 1992; 73:749–753.

65. Jacobi MS, Gershan WM, Thach BT. Mechanism of failure of recovery from hypoxic apnea by gasping in 17-23-day-old mice. J Appl Physiol 1991; 71:1098–1105.

66. Jacobi MS, Thach BT. Effect of maturation on spontaneous recovery from hypoxic apnea by gasping. J Appl Physiol 1989; 66:2384–2390.

67. Cummins TR, Jiang C, Haddad GG. Human neocortical excitability is decreased during anoxia via sodium channel modulation. J Clin Invest 1993; 91:608–615.

68. Doll CJ, Hochachka PW, Reiner PB. Effects of anoxia and metabolic arrest on turtle and rat cortical neurons. Am J Physiol 1991; 260:R747–R755.

69. Fowler JC. Adenosine antagonists delay hypoxia-induced depression of neuronal activity in hippocampal brain slice. Brain Res 1989; 490:378–384.

70. Fujiwara N, Higashi H, Shimoji K, Yoshimura M. Effects of hypoxia on rat hippocampal neurones in vitro. J Physiol (Lond) 1987; 384:131–151.

71. Hansen AJ. Effect of anoxia on ion distribution in the brain. Physiol Rev 1985; 65:101–148.

72. Hansen AJ, Hounsgaard J, Jahnsen H. Anoxia increases potassium conductance in hippocampal nerve cells. Acta Physiol Scand 1982; 115:301–310.

73. Lindsey BG, Hernandez YM, Morris KF, Shannon R, Gerstein GL. Dynamic reconfiguration of brain stem neural assemblies: respiratory phase-dependent vs modulation of firing rates. J Neurophysiol 1992; 67:923–930.

74. Silver IA, Erecinska M. Intracellular and extracellular changes of $[Ca^{2+}]$ in hypoxia and ischemia in rat brian in vivo. J Gen Physiol 1990; 95:837–866.

75. Clark GD, Rothman SM. Blockade of excitatory amino acid receptors protects anoxic hippocampal slices. Neuroscience 1987; 21:665–671.

76. Davis AK, Janigro D, Schwartzkoin PA. Effect of tissue preincubation and hypoxia on CA3 hippocampal neurons in the in vitro slice. Brain Res 1986; 370:44–53.

77. Cummins TR, Donnely DF, Haddad GG. Effect of metabolic inhibition on the excitability of isolated hippocampal CA1 neurons: developmental aspects. J Neurophysiol 1991; 66:1471–1482.

78. Leblond J, Krnjevic K. Hypoxic changes in hippocampal neurons. J Neurophysiol 1989; 62:1–14.

79. Misgeld U, Frotscher M. Dependence of the viability of neurons in hippocampal slices on oxygen supply. Brain Res Bull 1982; 8:95–100.

80. Sick TJ, Rosenthal M, LaManna JC, Lutz PL. Brain potassium ion homeostasis, anoxia, and metabolic inhibition in turtles and rats. Am J Physiol 1982; 243:R281–R288.

81. Dubinsky JM, Rothman SM. Intracellular calcium concentrations during chemical hypoxia and excitotoxic neuronal injury. J Neurosci 1991; 11:2545–2551.

82. Duchen MR, Valdeomillos M, O'Neill SC, Eisner DA. Effects of metabolic blockade on the regulation of intracellular calcium in dissociated mouse sensory neurones. J Physiol (Lond) 1990; 424:411–426.

83. Kass IS, Lipton P. Calcium and long-term transmission damage following anoxia in dentate gyrus and CA1 regions of the rat hippocampal slice. J Physiol (Lond) 1986; 38:313–334.

84. Uematsu D, Greenberg JH, Reivich M, Kobayashi S, Karp A. In vitro fluorometric measurement of changes in cytosolic free calcium from the cat cortex during anoxia. J Cereb Blood Flow Metab 1988; 380:367–374.

85. Murphy KPSJ, Greenfield SA. Neuronal selectivity of ATP-sensitive potassium channels in guinea pig substatia nigra revealed by response to anoxia. J Physiol (Lond) 1992; 453:167–183.

86. Choi DW. Glutamate neurotoxicity and diseases of the nervous system. Neuron 1988; 1:623–634.

87. Choi DW, Rothman SM. The role of glutamate neurotoxicity in hypoxic-ischemic neuronal death. Annu Rev Neurosci 1990; 13:171–182.

88. Davis JN, Carlsson A. Effect of hypoxia on monoamine synthesis, levels and metabolism in rat brain. J Neurochem 1973; 21:783–790.

89. Brown RM, Snider SR, Carlsson A. Changes in biogenic amine synthesis and turnover induced by hypoxia and/or foot shock stress. II. The central nervous system. J Neurol Trans 1974; 35:293–305.

90. Duffy TE, Nelson SR, Lowry OH. Cerebral carbohydrate metabolism during acute hypoxia and recovery. J Neurochem 1972; 19:959–977.

91. Erecinska M, Nelson D, Wilson DF, Silver IA. Neurotransmitter amino acids in the CNS. I. Regional changes in amino acid levels in rat brain during ischemia and reperfusion. Brain Res 1984; 304:9–22.

92. Wood JD, Watson WJ, Drucker AJ. The effect of hypoxia on brain gamma-aminobutyric acid levels. J Neurochem 1968; 15:603–608.

93. Gibson GE, Shimada M, Blass JP. Alterations in acetylcholine synthesis and in cyclic nucleotides in mild cerebral hypoxia. J Neurochem 1978; 31:757–760.

94. Young JN, Somjen GG. Suppression of presynaptic calcium currents by hypoxia in hippocampal tissue slices. Brain Res 1992; 573:70–76.

95. Rader RK, Lanthorn THE, Lipton P. Effects of hypoxia on responses to acidic amino acids in the in vitro hippocampal slice. Soc Neurosci Abstr 1987; 13:1495.

96. Winn HR, Rubio R, Berne RM. Brain adenosine concentration during hypoxia in rats. Am J Physiol 1981; 241:H235–H242.

97. Neubauer JA, Simone A, Edelman NH. Role of brain lactic acidosis in hypoxic depression of respiration. J Appl Physiol 1988; 65:1324–1331.

98. Brown DL, Lawson EE. Brain stem extracellular fluid pH and respiratory drive during hypoxia in newborn pigs. J Appl Physiol 1988; 64:1055–1059.

99. Lawson JWR, Veech RL. Effects of pH and free Mg++ on the Keq of the creatine kinase reaction and other phosphate hydrolyses and phosphate transfer reactions. J Biol Chem 1979; 254:6528–6534.

100. Blaustein MP. Calcium transport and buffering in neurons. Trends Neurosci 1988; 11:438–443.

101. DiPolo R, Beauge L. Ca^{2+} transport in nerve fibers. Biochim Biophys Acta 1988; 947:549–569.

102. Lipton P, Whittingham TS. Reduced ATP concentration as a basis for synaptic transmission failure during hypoxia in the in vitro guinea-pig hippocampus. J Physiol 1982; 325:51–65.

103. Grigg JJ, Anderson EG. Glucose and sulfonylureas modify different phases of the membrane potential change during hypoxia in rat hippocampal slices. Brain Res 1989; 489:302–310.

104. Zhang L, Krnjevic K. Whole-cell recording of anoxic effects on hippocampal neuronal slices. J Neurophysiol 1993; 69:118–127.

105. Gifford RG, Monyer H, Cristine CW, Choi DW. Acidosis reduces NMDA receptor activation, glutamate neurotoxicity and oxygen-glucose deprivation neuronal injury in cortical neurons. Brain Res 1990; 506:339–342.

106. Gifford RG, Weiss JH, Choi DW. Extracellular alkalinity exacerbates injury of cultured cortical neurons. Stroke 1992; 23:1817–1821.

107. Traynelis SF, Cull-Candy SG. Proton inhibition of N- methyl-D-aspartate receptors in cerebellar neurons. Nature 1990; 345:347–350.

108. Vylicky L, Jr., Viktorie V, Krusek J. The effect of external pH changes on responses to excitatory amino acids in mouse hippocampal neurons. J Physiol (Lond) 1990; 430:497–517.

109. Tang CM, Dichter M, Morad M. Modulation of the N-methyl-D-aspartate channel by extracellular H^+. Proc Natl Acad Soc USA 1990; 87:6445–6449.

110. Czeh G, Somjen GG. Hypoxic failure of synaptic transmission in the isolated spinal cord and the effects of divalent cations. Brain Res 1990; 527:224–233.

111. Fowler JC. Modulation of neuronal excitability by endogenous adenosine in the absence of synaptic transmission. Brain Res 1988; 463:368–373.

112. Hagberg H, Lehmann A, Sandberg M, Nystrom B, Jacobson I, Hamberger A. Ischemia-induced shift of inhibitory and excitatory amino acids from intra- to extracellular compartments. J Cereb Blood Flow Metab 1985; 5:413–419.

113. Melton JE, Neubauer JA, Edelman NH. GABA antagonism reverses hypoxic respiratory depression in the cat. J Appl Physiol 1990; 69:1296–1301.

114. Bianchi AL, St. John WM. Changes in antidromic latencies of medullary respiratory neurons in hypercapnia and hypoxia. J Appl Physiol 1985; 59:1208–1213.

115. St. John WM, Bianchi AL. Responses of bulbospinal and laryngeal respiratory neurons to hypercapnia and hypoxia. J Appl Physiol 1985; 59:1201–1207.

116. St. John WM, Wang SC. Response of medullary respiratory neurons to hypercapnia and isocapnic hypoxia. J Appl Physiol 1977; 43:812–821.

117. Richter DW, Bischoff A, Anders K, Bellingham M, Windhorst U. Response of the medullary respiratory network of the cat to hypoxia. J Physiol (Lond) 1991; 443: 231–256.

118. Melton JE, England SJ, Duffin J, Neubauer JA. Activity of respiratory neurons during hypoxia in chemodenervated cats. Soc Neurosci 1992; 18:826.

119. Tenney SM, Ou LC. Ventilatory response of decorticate and decerebrate cats to hypoxia and CO_2. Respir Physiol 1976; 29:81–92.

120. Tenney SM, Scotio P, Ou LC, Bartlett D Jr, Remmers JE. Suprapontine influences on hypoxia ventilatory control. In: Porter R, Knight J, eds. High Altitude Physiology: Cardiac and Respiratory Effects. London: Churchill Livingstone, 1971:89–102.

121. Mayevskey A, Chance B. Metabolic responses of the awake cerebral cortex to anoxic hypoxia, spreading depression and epileptiform activity. Brain Res 1975; 98: 149–165.

122. Siesjo BK, Johannsson H, Ljunggren B, Norberg K. Brain dysfunction in cerebral hypoxia and ischemia. In: Plum F, ed. Brain Dysfunction in Metabolic Disorders. New York: Raven Press, 1974; 75–112.

123. Dillon GH, Waldrop TG. In vitro responses of caudal hypothalamic neurons to hypoxia and hypercapnia. Neuroscience 1992; 51:941–950.

124. Waldrop TG, Bauer RM, Iwamoto GA. Microinjection of GABA antagonists into the posterior hypothalamus elicits locomotor activity and cardiorespiratory activation. Brain Res 1988; 444:84–94.

125. Dawes GS, Gardner WN, Johnston BM, Walker DW. Breathing in fetal lambs: the effect of brainstem section. J Physiol (Lond) 1983; 335:535–553.

126. Gluckman PD, Johnston BM. Lesions in the upper-lateral pons abolish the hypoxic depression of breathing in unanesthetized fetal lambs in utero. J Physiol (Lond) 1987; 382:373–383.

127. Martin-Body RL, Johnston BM. Central origin of the hypoxic depression of breathing in the newborn. Respir Physiol 1988; 71:25–32.

128. Haddad GG, Donnelly DF. O2 deprivation induces a major depolarization in brain stem neurons in the adult but not in the neonatal rat. J Physiol (Lond) 1990; 429:411–428.

129. Jiang C, Haddad GG. Effect of Anoxia on intracellular and extracellular potassium activity in hypoglossal neurons in vitro. J Neurophysiol 1991; 66:103–111.

130. Hochachka PW. Defense strategies against hypoxia and hypothermia. Science (Washington DC) 1986; 231:234–241.

131. Von Euler C. Brian stem mechanisms for generation and control of breathing pattern. In: Cherniack NS, Widdicombe JG, eds. Handbook of Physiology. Section 3: The Respiratory System. Vol. II: Control of Breathing, Part 1. Bethesda, MD: American Physiological Society, 1986:1–67.

132. Hales JRS, Dampney RAL, Bennett JW. Influences of Chronic denervation of the carotid bifurcation regions on panting in the sheep. Pflüger's Arch 1975; 360:243–253.

133. Bisgard GE, Forster HV, Klein J, Manohar M, Bullard VA. Depression of ventilation by dopamine in goats—effects of carotid body excision. Respir Physiol 1980; 41:379–392.

134. Olson EB, Jr., Vidruk EH, Dempsey JA. Carotid body excision significantly changes ventilatory control in awake rats. J Appl Physiol 1988; 64:666–671.

135. Gautier H, Bonora M. Effects of carotid body denervation on respiratory pattern of awake cats. J Appl Physiol 1979; 46:1127–1131.

136. Daristotle L, Berssenbrugge A, Engwall MJA, Bisgard GE. The effects of carotid body hypocapnia on ventilation in goats. Respir Physiol 1990; 79:123–136.

137. Bouverot P, Candas V, Libert JP. Role of the arterial chemoreceptors in ventilatory adaptation to hypoxia of awake dogs and rabbits. Respir Physiol 1973; 17:209–217.

138. Bouverot P, Flandrois R, Puccinelli R, Dejours P. Etude du role des chemorecepteurs arteriels dans la regulation de la respiration pulmonaire chez le chien eveille. Arch Int Pharmacodyn Ther 1965; 157:253–271.

139. Bouverot P, Sebert P. O2-chemoreflex drive of ventilation in awake birds at rest. Respir Physiol 1979; 37:201–218.

140. Engwall MJ, Daristotle L, Zuba M, Bisgard GE. Ventilatory response to Dejours O_2 test during hypoxia in the awake goat. FASEB J 1988; 2:A1294.

141. Dejours P. Chemoreflexes in breathing. Physiol Rev 1962; 42:335–358.

142. Downs JJ, Lambertsen CJ. Dynamic characteristics of ventilatory depression in man on abrupt administration of O_2. J Appl Physiol 1966; 21:447–453.

143. Weil JV, Byrne-Quinn E, Sodal IE, et al. Hypoxic ventilatory drive in normal man. J Clin Invest 1970; 49:1061–1071.

144. Bisgard GE, Ruiz AV, Grover RF, Will JA. Ventilatory control in the Hereford calf. J Appl Physiol 1973; 35:220–226.

145. Lahiri S, DeLaney RG. Relationship between carotid chemoreceptor activity and ventilation in the cat. Respir Physiol 1975; 24:267–286.

146. Bender PR, Weil JV, Reeves JT, Moore LG. Breathing pattern in hypoxic exposures of varying duration. J Appl Physiol 1987; 62:640–645.

147. Mahutte CK, Woodley WE, Rebuck AS. A comparison of the effects of steady-state and progressive hypoxia on the ventilatory and frequency response. Adv Exp Med Biol 1978; 99:315–324.

148. Reynolds WJ, Milhorn HT Jr. Transient ventilatory response to hypoxia with and without controlled alveolar P_{CO_2}. J Appl Physiol 1973; 35:187–196.

149. Comroe JH. Location and function of the chemoreceptors of the aorta. Am J Physiol 1939; 127:176–190.

150. Marek W, Prabhakar NR, Loeschcke HH. Electrical stimulation of arterial and central chemosensory afferents at different times in the respiratory cycle. Pflüger's Arch 1985; 403:415–421.

151. Engwall MJA, Daristotle L, Niu WZ, Dempsey JA, Bisgard GE. Ventilatory afterdischarge in the awake goat. J Appl Physiol 1991; 71:1511–1517.

152. Fitzgerald RS, Parks DC. Effect of hypoxia on carotid chemoreceptor response to carbon dioxide in cats. Respir Physiol 1971; 12:218–229.

153. Lahiri S, DeLaney RG. Stimulus interaction in the responses of carotid body chemoreceptor single afferent fibers. Respir Physiol 1975; 24:249–266.

154. Fitzgerald RS, Dehghani GA. Neural responses of the cat carotid and aortic bodies to hypercapnia and hypoxia. J Appl Physiol 1982; 52:596–601.

155. Daristotle L, Berssenbrugge AD, Bisgard GE. Hypoxic-hypercapnic interaction at the carotid body of awake goats. Respir Physiol 1987; 70:63–72.

156. Huang SY, Alexander JK, Grover R, et al. Hypocapnia and sustained hypoxia blunt ventilation on arrival at high altitude. J Appl Physiol 1984; 56:602–606.

157. Moore LG, Huang SY, McCullough RE, et al. Variable inhibition by falling CO_2 of hypoxic ventilatory response in humans. J Appl Physiol 1984; 56:207–210.

158. Hellstrom S, Hanbauer I, Costa E. Selective decrease of dopamine content in rat carotid body during exposure to hypoxic conditions. Brain Res 1976; 118: 352–355.

159. Hanbauer I, Hellstrom S. The regulation of dopamine and noradrenaline in the rat carotid body and its modification by denervation and by hypoxia. J Physiol (Lond) 1978; 282:21–34.

160. Bisgard GE, Mitchell RA, Herbert DA. Effects of dopamine, norepinephrine and 5-hydroxytryptamine on the carotid body of the dog. Respir Physiol 1979; 37: 61–80.

161. Docherty RJ, McQueen DS. Inhibitory action of dopamine on cat carotid chemoreceptors. J Physiol (Lond) 1978; 279:425–436.

162. Zapata P. Modulatory role of dopamine on arterial chemoreceptors. Adv Biochem Psychopharmacol 1977; 16:291–298.

163. Zapata P. Effects of dopamine on carotid chemo- and baroreceptors in vitro. J Physiol (Lond) 1975; 224:235–251.

164. Henson LC, Ward DS, Whipp BJ. Effect of dopamine on ventilatory response to incremental exercise in man. Respir Physiol 1992; 89:209–224.

165. Ward DS, Bellville JW. Reduction of hypoxic ventilatory drive by dopamine. Anesth Analg 1982; 61:333–337.

166. Welsh MJ, Heistad DD, Abboud FM. Depression of ventilation by dopamine in man. J Clin Invest 1978; 61:708–713.

167. Black AMS, Comroe JHJ, Jacobs L. Species difference in carotid body response of cat and dog to dopamine and serotonin. Am J Physiol 1972; 223:1097–1102.

168. Bascom DA, Clement ID, Dorrington KL, Robbins PA. Effects of dopamine and domperidone on ventilation during isocapnic hypoxia in humans. Respir Physiol 1991; 85:319–328.

169. Javaheri S, Guerra LF. Effects of domperidone and medroxyprogesterone acetate on ventilation in man. Respir Physiol 1990; 81:359–370.

170. Delpierre S, Fornaris M, Guillot C, Grimaud C. Increased ventilatory chemosensitivity induced by domperidone, a dopamine antagonist, in healthy humans. Bull Eur Physiopathol Respir 1987; 23:31–35.

171. Kressin NA, Nielsen AM, Laravuso R, Bisgard GE. Domperidone induced potentiation of ventilatory responses in awake goats. Respir Physiol 1986; 65: 169–180.

172. Delpierre S, Peyrot J, Guillot C, Grimaud C. Ventilatory effects of domperidone, a new dopamine antagonist, in anaesthetized rabbits. Arch Int Pharmacodyn 1985; 275:47–57.

173. Berger AJ. The distribution of the cat's carotid sinus nerve afferent and the efferent cell bodies using the horseradish peroxidase technique. Brain Res 1980; 190: 309–320.

174. Davies RO, Kalia M. Carotid sinus nerve projections to the brain stem in the cat. Brain Res. 1981; 6:531–541.

175. DeGroat WC, Nadelhaft I, Morgan C, Schauble T. The central origin of efferent pathways in the carotid sinus nerve of the cat. Science 1979; 205:1017–1018.

176. Neil E, O'Regan RG. Efferent and Afferent impulse activity recorded from few-fibre preparations of otherwise intact sinus and aortic nerves. J Physiol (Lond) 1971; 215:33–47.

177. O'Regan RG, Majcherczyk S. Control of peripheral chemoreceptors by efferent nerves. In: Acker H, O'Regan R, eds. Physiology of the Peripheral Arterial Chemoreceptors, 1983:257–298.

178. Lahiri S, Smatresk N, Pokorski M, Barnard P, Mokashi A, McGregor KH. Dopaminergic efferent inhibition of carotid body chemoreceptors in chronically hypoxic cats. Am J Physiol 1984; 247:R24–R28.

179. Luenberger U, Gleeson K, Wroblewski K, et al. Norepinephrine clearance is increased during acute hypoxemia in humans. Am J Physiol 1991; 261:H1659–H1664.

180. Mazzeo RS, Bender RP, Brooks GA, et al. Arterial catecholamine responses during exercise with acute and chronic high-altitude exposure. Am J Physiol 1991; 24: E419–E424.

181. Rose CE, Althaus JA, Kaiser DL, Miller ED, Carey RM. Acute hypoxia and hypercapnia: increase in plasma catecholamines in conscious dogs. Am J Physiol 1983; 245:H924–H929.

182. Warner MM, Mitchell GS. Role of catecholamines and B-receptors in ventilatory response during hypoxic exercise. Respir Physiol 1991; 85:41–53.

183. Milsom WK, Sadig T. Interaction between norepinephrine and hypoxia on carotid body chemoreception in rabbits. J Appl Physiol 1983; 55:1893–1898.

184. Llados F, Zapata P. Effects of adrenoreceptors stimulating and blocking agents on carotid body chemosensory inhibition. J Physiol (Lond) 1978; 274:501–509.

185. Joels N, White H. The contribution of the arterial chemoreceptors to the stimulation of respiration by adrenaline and noradrenaline in the cat. J Physiol (Lond) 1968; 197:1–23.

186. Pizarro J, Warner MM, Ryan ML, Mitchell GS, Bisgard GE. Intracarotid norepinephrine infusions inhibit ventilation in goats. Respir Physiol 1992; 90:299–310.

187. Heistad DD, Wheeler RC, Mark AL, Schmid PG, Abboud FM. Effects of adrenergic stimulation on ventilation in man. J Clin Invest 1972; 51:1469–1475.

188. Dempsey JA, Gledhill N, Reddan WG, Forster HV, Hanson P, Claremont AD. Pulmonary adaptation to exercise: effects of exercise type and duration, chronic hypoxia and physical training. Ann NY Acad Sci 1977; 301:243–261.

189. Patrick JM, Pearson SB. Beta-adrenergic blockade and ventilation in man. Br J Clin Pharmacol 1980; 10:624–625.

190. Kou YR, Ernsberger P, Cragg PA, Cherniack NS, Prabhakar NR. Role of alpha-2 adrenergic receptors in the carotid body response to isocapnic hypoxia. Respir Physiol 1991; 83:353–364.

191. Verna A, Barets A, Salat C. Distribution of sympathetic nerve endings within the rabbit carotid body: A histochemical and ultrastructural study. J Neurocytol 1984; 13:849–865.

192. Eyzaguirre C, Lewin J. The effect of sympathetic stimulation on carotid nerve activity. J Physiol 1961; 159:251–267.

193. Floyd WF, Neil E. The influence of the sympathetic innervation of the carotid bifurcation on chemoreceptor and baroreceptor activity in the cat. Arch Int Pharmacodyn Ther 1952; 91:230–239.

194. McClosky DI. Mechanisms of autonomic control of carotid chemoreceptor activity. Respir Physiol 1975; 25:53–61.

195. O'Regan RG. Responses of carotid body chemosensory activity and blood flow to stimulation of sympathetic nerves in the cat. J Physiol (Lond) 1981; 315:81–98.

196. O'Regan RG. Carotid chemoreceptor responses to sympathetic excitation. J Physiol (Lond) 1976; 263:267P–268P.

197. Acker H, O'Regan RG. The effects of stimulation of autonomic nerves on carotid body blood flow in the cat. J Physiol (Lond) 1981; 315:99–110.

198. Matsumoto S, Mokashi A, Lahiri S. Influence of ganglioglomerular nerve on carotid chemoreceptor activity in the cat. J Auton Nervous Sys 1986; 15:7–20.

199. Lahiri S, Matsumoto S, Mokashi A. Responses of ganglioglomerular nerve activity to respiratory stimuli in the cat. J Appl Physiol 1986; 60:391–397.

200. Szlyk PC, Jennings DB. Respiration in awake cats: sympathectomy and deafferentation of carotid bifurcations. J Appl Physiol 1987; 62:932–940.

201. Carmody JJ, Scott MJ. Respiratory and cardiovascular responses to prolonged stimulation of the carotid body chemoreceptors in the cat. Aust J Exp Biol Med Sci 1974; 52:271–283.

202. Ryan ML, Hedrick MS, Pizarro J, Li Q, Bisgard GE. Ventilatory acclimatization to hypoxia does not require sympathetic innervation to the carotid body in awake goats. FASEB J 1993; 7:A396.

203. Burger RE, Estavillo JA, Nye PCG, Paterson DJ. Effects of potassium, oxygen and carbon dioxide on the steady-state discharge of cat carotid body chemoreceptors. J Physiol (Lond) 1988; 401:519–531.

204. Paterson DJ. Potassium and ventilation in exercise. J Appl Physiol 1992; 72: 811–820.

205. Warner MM, Mitchell GS. Ventilatory responses to hyperkalemia and exercise in normoxic and hypoxic goats. Respir Physiol 1990; 82:239–250.

206. Easton PA, Slykerman LJ, Anthonisen NR. Recovery of the ventilatory response to hypoxia in normal adults. J Appl Physiol 1988; 64:521–528.

207. Long GR, Filuk R, Balakumar M, Easton PA, Anthonisen NR. Ventilatory response to sustained hypoxia: effect of methysergide and verapamil. Respir Physiol 1989; 75:173–182.

208. Easton PA, Anthonisen NR. Carbon dioxide effects on the ventilatory response to sustained hypoxia. J Appl Physiol 1988; 64:1451–1456.

209. Easton PA, Anthonisen NR. Ventilatory response to sustained hypoxia after pretreatment with aminophylline. J Appl Physiol 1988; 64:1445–1450.

210. Holtby SG, Berezanski DJ, Anthonisen NR. Effect of 100% O_2 on hypoxic eucapnic ventilation. J Appl Physiol 1988; 65:1157–1162.

211. Georgopoulos D, Holtby SG, Berezanski D, Anthonisen NR. Aminophylline effects on ventilatory response to hypoxia and hyperoxia in normal adults. J Appl Physiol 1989; 67:1150–1156.

212. Bonora M, Marlot D, Gautier H, Duron B. Effects of hypoxia on ventilation during postnatal development in conscious kittens. J Appl Physiol 1984; 56:1464–1471.

213. Bureau MA, Cote A, Blanchard PW, Hobbs S, Foulon P, Dalle D. Exponential and diphasic ventilatory response to hypoxia in conscious lambs. J Appl Physiol 1986; 61:836–842.

214. Bureau MA, Zinman R, Foulon P, Begin R. Diphasic ventilatory response to hypoxia in the newborn lamb. J Appl Physiol 1984; 56:84–90.

215. Rigatto H, Wiebe C, Rigatto C, Lee DS, Cates D. Ventilatory response to hypoxia in unanesthetized newborn kittens. J Appl Physiol 1988; 64:2544–2551.

216. LaFramboise WA, Guthrie RD, Standaert TA, Woodrum DE. Pulmonary mechanics during the ventilatory response to hypoxemia in the newborn monkey. J Appl Physiol 1983; 55:1008–1014.

217. LaFramboise WA, Woodrum DE. Elevated diaphragm electromyogram during neonatal hypoxic ventilatory depression. J Appl Physiol 1985; 59:1040–1045.

218. Tatsumi K, Pickett CK, Weil JV. Effects of haloperidol and domperidone on

ventilatory roll off during sustained hypoxia in cats. J Appl Physiol 1992; 72:1945–1952.

219. Cao K, Zwillich CW, Berthon-Jones M, Sullivan CE. Ventilatory response to sustained eucapnic hypoxia in the adult conscious dog. Respir Physiol 1992; 89:65–73.

220. Davis GM, Bureau MA, Gaultier C. The sustained ventilatory response to hypoxic challenge in the awake newborn piglet with an intact upper airway. Respir Physiol 1988; 71:307–314.

221. Rosen CL, Schecter WS, Mellins RB, Haddad GG. Effect of acute hypoxia on metabolism and ventilation in awake piglets. Respir Physiol 1993; 91:307–319.

222. Engwall MJA, Bisgard GE. Ventilatory responses to chemoreceptor stimulation after hypoxic acclimatization in awake goats. J Appl Physiol 1990; 69:1236–1243.

223. Bascom DA, Clement ID, Cunningham DA, Painter R, Robbins PA. Changes in peripheral chemoreflex sensitivity during sustained, isocapnic hypoxia. Respir Physiol 1990; 82:161–176.

224. Berkenbosch A, Dahan A, DeGoede J, Olievier ICW. The ventilatory response to CO_2 of the peripheral and central chemoreflex loop before and after sustained hypoxia in man. J Physiol (Lond) 1992; 456:71–83.

225. Georgopoulos D, Walker S, Anthonisen NR. Increased chemoreceptor output and ventilatory response to sustained hypoxia. J Appl Physiol 1989; 67:1157–1163.

226. Goiny M, Lagercrantz H, Srinivasan M, Ungerstedt U, Yamamoto H. Hypoxia-mediated in vivo release of dopamine in nucleus tractus solitarii of rabbits. J Appl Physiol 1991; 70:2395–2400

227. Eldridge FL, Millhorn DE, Kiley JP. Respiratory effects of a long-acting analog of adenosine. Brain Res 1984; 301:273–280.

228. Eldridge FL, Millhorn DE, Kiley JP. Antagonism by theophylline of respiratory inhibition induced by adenosine. J Appl Physiol 1985; 59:1428–1433.

229. Iversen K, Hedner T, Lundborg P. GABA concentrations and turn-over in neonatal rat brain during asphyxia and recovery. Acta Physiol Scand 1983; 118:91–94.

230. Weyne J, VanLeuven F, Leusen I. Brain amino acids in conscious rats in chronic normocapnic and hypocapnic hypoxemia. Respir Physiol 1977; 31:231–239.

231. Wood JB, Watson WJ, Drucker AJ. The effect of hypoxia on brain gamma-aminobutyric acid levels. J Neurochem 1968; 15:603–608.

232. Yamada KA, Hamosh P, Gillis RA. Respiratory depression produced by activation of GABA receptors in hind-brain of cat. J Appl Physiol 1981; 51:1278–1286.

233. Yamada KA, Norman WP, Hamosh P, Gillis RA. Medullary ventral surface GABA receptors affect respiratory and cardiovascular function. Brain Res 1982; 248:71–78.

234. Kneussl MP, Pappagianopoulos P, Hoop B, Kazemi H. Reversible depression of ventilation and cardiovascular function by ventriculo-cisternal perfusion with gamma-aminobutyric acid in dogs. Am Rev Respir Dis 1986; 133:1024–1028.

235. Dahan A, Ward DS. Effect of i.v. midazolam on the ventilatory response to sustained hypoxia in man. Br J Anaesth 1991; 66:454–457.

236. Georgopoulos D, Berezanski D, Anthonisen NR. Effect of dichloroacetate on ventilatory response to sustained hypoxia in normal adults. Respir Physiol 1990; 82:115–122.

237. Chernick V, Craig RJ. Naloxone reverses neonatal depression caused by fetal asphyxia. Science (Washington DC) 1982; 216:1252–1253.

238. Javaheri S, Teppema LJ, Evers JA. Effects of aminophylline on hypoxemia-induced ventilatory depression in the cat. J Appl Physiol 1988; 64:1837–1843.

239. Suzuki A, Nishimura M, Yamamoto H, Miyamoto K, Kishi F, Kowakami Y. No effect of brain blood flow on ventilatory depression during stained hypoxia. J Appl Physiol 1989; 66:1674–1678.

240. Georgopoulos D, Walker S, Anthonisen NR. Effect of sustained hypoxia on ventilatory response to CO2 in normal adults. J Appl Physiol 1990; 68:891–896.

241. Ward DS, Nguyen TT. Ventilatory response to sustained hypoxia during exercise. Med Sci Sports Exer 1991; 23:719–626.

242. Pandit JJ, Robbins PA. The ventilatory effects of sustained isocapnic hypoxia during exercise in humans. Respir Physiol 1991; 86:393–404.

243. Mortola JP, Rezzonico R, Lanthier C. Ventilation and oxygen consumption during acute hypoxia in newborn mammals: a comparative analysis. Respir Physiol 1989; 78:31–43.

244. Mortola JP, Rezzonico R. Metabolic and ventilatory rates in newborn kittens during acute hypoxia. Respir Physiol 1988; 73:55–68.

245. Rahn H, Otis AB. Man's respiratory response during and after acclimatization to high altitude. Am J Physiol 1949; 157:445–462.

246. Forster HV, Dempsey JA, Chosy LW. Incomplete compensation of CSF [H+] in man during acclimatization to high altitude (4,300 m). J Appl Physiol 1975; 38:1067–1072.

247. West JB. Rate of Acclimatization to extreme altitude. Respir Physiol 1988; 74:323–333.

248. Bouverot P, Bureau M. Ventilatory acclimatization and CSF acid-base balance on carotid chemodenervated dogs at 3,550 m. Pflüger's Arch 1975; 361:17–23.

249. Olson EB, Jr., Dempsey J. Rat as a model for human-like ventilatory adaptation to chronic hypoxia. J Appl Physiol 1978; 44:763–769.

250. Vizek M, Pickett CK, Weil JV. Increased carotid body hypoxic sensitivity during acclimatization to hypobaric hypoxia. J Appl Physiol 1987; 63:2403–2410.

251. Weil JV. Control of ventilation in chronic hypoxia: role of peripheral chemoreceptors. In: Lahiri S, Cherniack NS, Fitzgerald RS, eds. Response and Adaptation to Hypoxia. New York: Oxford University Press, 1991:122–132.

252. Dempsey JA, Forster HV, DoPico GA. Ventilatory acclimatization to moderate hypoxemia in man. The role of spinal fluid [H+]. J Clin Invest 1974; 53:1091–1100.

253. West JB, Hackett PH, Maret KH, et al. Pulmonary gas exchange on the summit of Mount Everest. J Appl Physiol 1983; 55:678–687.

254. West JB. Acclimatization and Adaptation: Organ to Cell. Response and Adaptation to Hypoxia organ to organelle. In: Lahiri S, Cherniack NS, Fitzgerald RS, eds. Response and Adaptation to Hypoxia. New York: Oxford University Press, 1991:177–190.

255. Severinghaus JW, Mitchell RA, Richardson BW, Singer MM. Respiratory control at high altitude suggesting active transport regulation of CSF pH. J Appl Physiol 1963; 18:1155–1166.

256. Bureau M, Bouverot P. Blood and CSF acid-base changes, and rate of ventilatory acclimatization of awake dogs to 3550m. Respir Physiol 1975; 24:203–216.

257. Dempsey JA, Forster HV, Bisgard GE, et al. Role of cerebrospinal fluid [H+] in ventilatory deacclimatization from chronic hypoxia. J Clin Invest 1979; 64:199–205.

258. Orr JA, Bisgard GE, Forster HV, Buss DD, Dempsey JA, Will JA. Cerebrospinal fluid alkalosis during high-altitude sojourn in unanesthetized ponies. Respir Physiol 1975; 25:23–37.

259. Weiskopf RB, Gabel RA, Fencl V. Alkaline shift in lumbar and intracranial CSF in man after 5 days at high altitude. J Appl Physiol 1976; 41:93–97.

260. Davies DG. Evidence for cerebral extracellular fluid [H+] as a stimulus during acclimatization to hypoxia. Respir Physiol 1978; 32:167–182.

261. Fencl V, Gabel RA, Wolfe D. Composition of cerebral fluids in goats adapted to high altitude. J Appl Physiol 1979; 47:508–513.

262. Xu F, Sato M, Spellman MJ, Jr., Mitchell RA, Severinghaus JW. Topography of cat medullary ventral surface hypoxic acidification. J Appl Physiol 1992; 73:2631–2637.

263. Xu FD, Spellman MJ, Jr., Sato M, Baumgartner JE, Ciricillo SF, Severinghaus JW. Anomalous hypoxic acidification of medullary ventral surface. J Appl Physiol 1991; 71:2211–2217.

264. Dempsey JA, Forster HV, Gledhill N, DoPico GA. Effects of moderate hypoxemia and hypocapnia on CSF [H+] and ventilation in man. J Appl Physiol 1975; 38: 665–674.

265. Musch TI, Dempsey JA, Smith CA, Mitchell GS, Bateman NT. Metabolic acids and [H+] regulation in brain tissue during acclimatization to chronic hypoxia. J Appl Physiol 1983; 55:1486–1495.

266. Cruz JC, Reeves JT, Grover RF, et al. Ventilatory acclimatization to high altitude is prevented by CO2 breathing. Respiration 1980; 39:121–130.

267. Eger EI, II, Kellogg RH, Mines AH, Lima-Ostos M, Morrill CG, Kent DW. Influence of CO2 on ventilatory acclimatization to altitude. J Appl Physiol 1968; 24:607–615.

268. Bisgard GE, Engwall MJA, Niu WZ, Daristotle L, Pizarro J. Respiratory responses to prolonged central or peripheral hypoxia. In: Speck DF, Dekin MS, Revlette WR, Frazier DT, eds. Respiratory Control, Central and Peripheral Mechanisms. Lexington: University of Kentucky, 1993:191–194.

269. Ou LC, St. John WM, Tenney SM. The contribution of central mechanisms rostral to the pons in high altitude ventilatory acclimatization. Respir Physiol 1983; 54: 343–351.

270. Dempsey JA, Forster HV, Birnbaum ML, et al. Control of exercise hyperpnea under varying durations of exposure to moderate hypoxia. Respir Physiol 1972; 16: 213–231.

271. Forster HV, Dempsey JA, Birnbaum ML, et al. Effect of chronic exposure to hypoxia on ventilatory response to CO2 and hypoxia. J Appl Physiol 1971; 31:586–592.

272. Forster HV, Dempsey JA, Vidruk E, DoPico GA. Evidence of altered regulation of ventilation during exposure to hypoxia. Respir Physiol 1974; 20:379–392.

273. Forster HV, Soto RJ, Dempsey JA, Hosko MJ. Effect of sojourn at 4,300 m altitude

on electroencephalogram and visual evoked response. J Appl Physiol 1975; 39: 109–113.

274. Schmeling WT, Forster HV, Hosko MJ. Effect of sojourn at 3200 m altitude on spinal reflexes in young adult males. Aviat Space Environ Med 1977; 48:1039–1045.

275. Olson EB, Jr., Vidruk EH, McCrimmon DR, Dempsey JA. Monoamine neuro-transmitter metabolism during acclimatization to hypoxia in rats. Respir Physiol 1983; 54:79–96.

276. Olson EB, Jr. Ventilatory adaptation to hypoxia occurs in serotonin-depleted rats. Respir Physiol 1987; 69:227–235.

277. Millhorn DE, Eldridge FL, Waldrop TG. Prolonged stimulation of respiration by endogenous central serotonin. Respir Physiol 1980; 42:171–188.

278. Millhorn DE, Eldridge FL, Waldrop TG. Prolonged stimulation of respiration by a new central neural mechanism. Respir Physiol 1980; 41:87–103.

279. Bisgard GE, Busch MA, Forster HV. Ventilatory acclimatization to hypoxia is not dependent on cerebral hypocapnic alkalosis. J Appl Physiol 1986; 60:1011–1015.

280. Bisgard GE, Busch MA, Daristotle L, Berssenbrugge A, Forster HV. Carotid body hypercapnia does not elicit ventilatory acclimatization in goats. Respir Physiol 1986; 65:113–125.

281. Lahiri S, Edelman NH, Cherniack NS, Fishman AP. Role of carotid chemoreflex in respiratory acclimatization to hypoxemia in goat and sheep. Respir Physiol 1981; 46:367–382.

282. Fordyce WE, Tenney SM. Role of the carotid bodies in ventilatory acclimation to chronic hypoxia by the awake cat. Respir Physiol 1984; 58:207–221.

283. Steinbrook RA, Donovan JC, Gabel RA, Leith DE, Fencl V. Acclimatization to high altitude in goats with ablated carotid bodies. J Appl Physiol 1983; 55:16–21.

284. Busch MA, Bisgard GE, Forster HV. Ventilatory acclimatization to hypoxia is not dependent on arterial hypoxemia. J Appl Physiol 1985; 58:1874–1880.

285. Engwall MJA, Vidruk EH, Nielsen AM, Bisgard GE. Response of the goat carotid body to acute and prolonged hypercapnia. Respir Physiol 1988; 74:335–344.

286. Barnard P, Andronikou S, Pokorski M, Smatresk N, Mokashi A, Lahiri S. Time-dependent effect of hypoxia on carotid body chemosensory function. J Appl Physiol 1987; 63:685–691.

287. Ou LC, Chen J, Fiore E, et al. Ventilatory and hematopoietic responses to chronic hypoxia in two rat strains. J Appl Physiol 1992; 72:2354–2363.

288. Tatsumi K, Pickett CK, Weil JV. Possible role of dopamine in ventilatory acclimati-zation to high altitude. Am Rev Respir Dis 1992; 145:A677.

289. Mathew L, Gopinath PM, Purkayastha SS, Sen Gupta J, Nayar HS. Chemoreceptor sensitivity in adaptation to high altitude. Aviat Spac Environ Med 1983; 54: 121–126.

290. Aaron EA, Powell FL. Effect of chronic hypoxia on hypoxic ventilatory response in awake rats. J Appl Physiol 1993; 74:1635–1640.

291. Goldberg SV, Schoene RB, Haynor D, et al. Brain tissue pH and ventilatory acclimatization to high altitude. J Appl Physiol 1992; 72:58–63.

292. Sato M, Severinghaus JW, Powell FL, Xu F-D, Spellman MJ, Jr. Augmented hypoxic ventilatory response in men at altitude. J Appl Physiol 1992; 73:101–107.

293. Schoene RB, Roach RC, Hackett PH, Sutton JR, Cymerman A, Houston CS. Operation everest II: ventilatory adaptation during gradual decompression to extreme altitude. Med Sci Sports Exer 1990; 22:804–810.

294. White DP, Gleeson K, Pickett CK, Rannels AM, Cymerman A, Weil JV. Altitude acclimatization: influence on periodic breathing and chemoresponsiveness during sleep. J Appl Physiol 1987; 63:401–412.

295. Serebrovskaya TV, Ivashkevich AA. Effects of a 1-yr stay at altitude on ventilation, metabolism, and work capacity. J Appl Physiol 1992; 73:1749–1755.

296. Bisgard GE, Kressin NA, Nielsen AM, Daristotle L, Smith CA, Forster HV. Dopamine blockade alters ventilatory acclimatization to hypoxia in goats. Respir Physiol 1987; 69:245–255.

297. Ryan ML, Hedrick MS, Pizarro J, Bisgard GE. Carotid body noradrenergic sensitivity in ventilatory acclimatization to hypoxia. Respir Physiol 1993; 92:77–90.

298. Laduron PM, Leysen JE. Domperidone, a specific in vitro dopamine antagonist, devoid of in vivo central dopaminergic activity. Biochem Pharmacol 1979; 28:2161–2165.

299. Lahiri S, Smatresk N, Pokorski M, Barnard P, Mokashi A. Efferent inhibition of carotid body chemoreception in chronically hypoxic cats. Am J Physiol 1983; 245: R678–R683.

300. Hanbauer I, Karoum F, Hellstrom S, Lahiri S. Effects of hypoxia lasting up to one month on the catecholamine content in rat carotid body. Neuroscience 1981; 6: 81–86.

301. Pequignot JM, Cottet-Emard JM, Dalmaz Y, Peyrin L. Dopamine and norepinephrine dynamics in rat carotid body during long-term hypoxia. J Auton Nervous Sys 1987; 21:9–14.

302. Pequignot JM, Dalmaz Y, Claustre J, Cottet-Emard JM, Borghini N, Peyrin L. Preganglionic sympathetic fibres modulate dopamine turnover in rat carotid body during long-term hypoxia. J Auton Nervous Sys 1991; 32:243–250.

303. Cao H, Kou YR, Prabhakar NR. Absence of chemoreceptor inhibition by alpha-2 adrenergic receptor agonist in cats exposed to low Po_2. FASEB J 1991; 5:A1118.

304. Moore LG, Cymerman A, Huang SY, et al. Propranolol blocks metabolic rate increase but not ventilatory acclimatization to 4300 m. Respir Physiol 1987; 70: 195–204.

305. Bisgard GE, Engwall MJA, Weizhen N, Nielsen AM, Vidruk E. The effect of prolonged stimulation on afferent activity of the goat carotid body. In: Acker H, Trzebski A, O'Regan R, eds. Chemoreceptors and Chemoreceptor Reflexes. New York: Plenum Press, 1990:165–170.

306. Lahiri S, Kao FF, Velasquez TM, Martinez C, Pezzia W. Irreversible blunted respiratory sensitivity to hypoxia in high altitude natives. Respir Physiol 1969; 6:360–374.

307. Lefrancois R, Gautier H, Pasquis P. Ventilatory oxygen drive in acute and chronic hypoxia. Respir Physiol 1968; 4:217–228.

308. Milledge JS, Lahiri S. Respiratory control in lowlanders and Sherpa highlanders at altitude. Respir Physiol 1967; 2:310–322.

309. Severinghaus JW. Hypoxic respiratory drive and its loss during chronic hypoxia. Clin Physiol 1972; 2:57–79.

310. Severinghuas JW, Bainton CR, Carcelen A. Respiratory insensitivity to hypoxia in chronically hypoxic man. Respir Physiol 1966; 1:308–334.

311. Weil JV, Byrne-Quinn E, Sodal IE, Filley GF, Grover RF. Acquired attenuation of chemoreceptor function in chronically hypoxic man at high altitude. J Clin Invest 1971; 50:186–195.

312. Chiodi H. Respiratory adaptation to chronic high altitude hypoxia. J Appl Physiol 1957; 10:81–87.

313. Sorensen SC, Cruz JC. Ventilatory response to a single breath of CO_2 in O_2 in normal man at sea level and high altitude. J Appl Physiol 1969; 27:186–190.

314. Hackett PH, Reeves JT, Reeves CD, Grover RF, Rennie D. Control of breathing in Sherpas at low and high altitude. J Appl Physiol 1980; 49:374–379.

315. Daristotle L, Engwall MJA, Weizhen N, Bisgard G. Ventilatory effects and interactions with change in Pao_2 in awake goats. J Appl Physiol 1991; 71:1254–1260.

316. Byrne-Quinn E, Sodal IE, Weil JV. Hypoxic and hypercapnic ventilatory drives in children native to high altitude. J Appl Physiol 1972; 32:44–46.

317. Lahiri S. Respiratory control in Andean and Himalayan high-altitude natives. In: West JB, Lahiri S, eds. High Altitude and Man. Bethesda, MD: American Physiological Society, 1984:147–162.

318. Sorensen SC, Severinghaus JW. Irreversible respiratory insensitivity to acute hypoxia in man born at high altitude. J Appl Physiol 1968; 25:217–220.

319. Lahiri S. Adaptive respiratory regulation-lessons from high altitudes. In: Horvath SM, Yousef MK, eds. Environmental Physiology: Aging, Heat and Altitude. Amsterdam: Elsevier/North Holland, 1980:341–347.

320. Zhuang J, Droma T, Sun S, et al. Hypoxic ventilatory responsiveness in Tibetan compared with Han residents of 3,658 m. J Appl Physiol 1993; 74:303–311.

321. Dhillon DP, Barer GR, Walsh M. The enlarged carotid body of the chronically hypoxic and chronically hypoxic and hypercapnic rat: a morphometric analysis. Q J Exp Physiol 1984; 69:301–317.

322. Heath D, Smith P, Fitch R. Comparative pathology of the enlarged carotid body. J Comp Pathol 1985; 95:259–271.

323. Laidler P, Kay JM. A quantitative morphological study of the carotid bodies of rats living at a simulated altitude of 4300 metres. J Pathol 1975; 117:183–191.

324. Laidler P, Kay JM. Ultrastructure of carotid body in rats living at a simulated altitude of 4300 metres. J Pathol 1978; 124:27–33.

325. McGregor KH, Gil J, Lahiri S. A morphometric study of the carotid body in chronically hypoxic rats. J Appl Physiol 1984; 57:1430–1438.

326. Pequignot JM, Hellstrom S, Johannsson H. Intact and sympathectomized carotid bodies of long-term hypoxic rats: a morphometric ultrastructural study. J Neurocytol 1984; 13:481–493.

327. Barer GR, Edwards CW, Jolly AI. Short communication. Changes in the carotid body and the ventilatory response to hypoxia in chronically hypoxic rats. Clin Sci Mol Med 1976; 50:311–313.

328. Bisgard GE, Ruiz AV, Grover RF, Will JA. Ventilatory acclimatization to 3,400 meters altitude in the Hereford calf. Respir Physiol 1974; 21:271–296.

329. Brooks JG, III, Tenney SM. Ventilatory response of llama to hypoxia at sea level and high altitude. Respir Physiol 1968; 5:269–278.

330. Hornbein TF, Sorensen SC. Ventilatory response to hypoxia and hypercapnia in cats living at high altitude. J Appl Physiol 1969; 27:834–836.
331. Lahiri S. Unattenuated ventilatory hypoxic drive in ovine and bovine species native to high altitude. J Appl Physiol 1972; 32:95–102.
332. Lahiri S. Ventilatory response to hypoxia in intact cats living at 3850 m. J Appl Physiol 1977; 43:114–120.
333. Tatsumi K, Pickett CK, Weil JV. Attenuated carotid body hypoxic sensitivity after prolonged hypoxic exposure. J Appl Physiol 1991; 70:748–755.
334. Tenney SM, Ou LC. Hypoxic ventilatory response of cats at high altitude: an interpretation of "blunting." Respir Physiol 1977; 30:185–199.
335. Tatsumi K, Pickett CK, Weil JV. Effects of a dopamine antagonist on decreased carotid body and ventilatory hypoxic sensitivity in chronically hypoxic cats. Am Rev Respir Dis 1991; 143:A189.
336. Lahiri S, Cherniack NS, Edelman NH, Fishman AP. Regulation of respiration in goat and its adaptation to chronic and life-long hypoxia. Respir Physiol 1971; 12: 388–403.
337. Weinberger SE, Steinbrook RA, Carr DB, et al. Endogenous opioids and ventilatory adaptation to prolonged hypoxia in goats. Life Sci 1987; 40:605–613.

15

Respiratory Sinus Arrhythmia and Other Human Cardiovascular Neural Periodicities

DWAIN L. ECKBERG

Hunter Holmes McGuire Department of Veterans Affairs Medical Center
and Medical College of Virginia
Richmond, Virginia

I. Introduction

Generations of preeminent physiologists and physicians have studied respiratory periodicities present in measures of cardiovascular function. In general, these rhythms have been regarded as curiosities, worthy of attention more because they are interesting than because they have practical importance. Investigation of respiratory-cardiovascular periodicities continues as pure science; however, increasing numbers of research workers are studying these rhythms because they convey information about other physiological or pathophysiological processes. For example, in healthy (1), diabetic (2), and postmyocardial infarction (3) subjects, respiration-related fluctuations of R-R intervals (respiratory sinus arrhythmia) predict the gain of vagal baroreceptor-cardiac reflex responses (1), acute reductions of fetal respiratory sinus arrhythmia during labor portend fetal death (4), and chronic reductions of heart rate fluctuations after myocardial infarctions portend sudden cardiac death (5).

The most important reason for the burgeoning (6) literature dealing with sinus arrhythmia may be that study of respiration-related rhythms opens windows on otherwise elusive human central neural integrative mechanisms. Such research is made possible by an array of well-validated, non- or minimally invasive methods that characterize autonomic periodicities with precision. Changes (if not absolute levels) of vagal-cardiac nerve traffic can be estimated with confidence; in anesthetized dogs, changes of R-R intervals measured from surface electrocardiograms reflect linearly changes of vagal-cardiac nerve activity over a wide range of vagal traffic (7,8). Sympathetic nerve traffic to skin and muscle vascular beds can be measured directly in humans (9,10) with safety (11). Beat-by-beat systolic and diastolic arterial pressures can be estimated with surprising accuracy with a finger photoplethysmograph invented by Penáz (12), refined by Wesseling (13), validated by Imholz (14) and Parati (15) and their co-workers, and manufactured by Ohmeda (Englewood, CO) and Ueda (Tokyo, Japan). Moreover, powerful frequency-domain methods of analysis are now readily available. These provide indexes of R-R interval fluctuations that correlate closely with traditional time-domain measures, such as R-R interval means and standard deviations (16,17). More important, frequency-domain methods also permit study of interrelations between rhythms and, thus, speculation regarding mechanisms.

In this research, human subjects have unique advantages over other species. Foremost of these is that humans can cooperate—they can hold their breath; they can breathe slowly or rapidly, and deeply or shallowly; and they can even breathe without interrupting their cadence during brief neck suction (18,19) or pressure (20). Implicit in the use of controlled breathing in human research is the notion that voluntary control exerts no independent influence on the rhythms being studied. Although this is controversial (see below), most of the limited data published suggest that voluntary control of respiration does not alter vagal or sympathetic neural efferent cardiovascular traffic.

In contrast, use of anesthetized animals to study cardiovascular rhythms brings great complexity to the subject; the directness that comes with actual recordings of neural traffic carries a price. It seems likely that intubation, use of muscle relaxants, and mechanical ventilation distort respiration-related neural periodicities. General anesthesia provokes quantitative and even qualitative changes of the variables being measured. Chief among the quantitative changes is that most general anesthetic agents suppress vagal firing. Kunze (21) found that in anesthetized cats, vagal-cardiac motoneuron activity was not present until mean arterial pressure had been raised to over 150 mmHg. Other workers have found it necessary to iontophorese excitant amino acids, such as DL-homocysteic acid or glutamate, directly onto vagal-cardiac motoneurons to elicit firing in the presence of general anesthesia.

General anesthesia may also lead to qualitative changes of autonomic neural rhythms. Low-frequency (centered at about 0.1 Hz) blood pressure waves typically are absent in anesthetized animals and can be brought out only by unusual measures, such as hemorrhage or bilateral carotid artery occlusion (22). Low-frequency rhythms are not only present in conscious humans, they may be dominant (23). In some studies, the choice of anesthetic agent determines whether a rhythm (such as the 10-Hz sympathetic rhythm found in cats) will be present or absent (24). In other studies, *quantitative* changes of the depth of anesthesia provoke *qualitative* changes of results; Koizumi et al. (25) reported that small additions of chloralose change the amount and timing of vagal-cardiac nerve traffic within the respiratory cycle.

Difficulties involved with study of autonomic rhythms in anesthetized animals render use of conscious cooperative human subjects attractive indeed. However, this chapter suggests that the elegant methods available for human research yield results whose complexities are not well appreciated. The chapter discusses the physiological bases underlying respiratory influences on cardiovascular neural outputs. It indicates that attempts to use these respiratory influences to quantitate autonomic neural outflow suffer from want of a gold standard and from a frequent failure of investigators to recognize the importance of breathing parameters to the estimates of nerve traffic. Finally, this chapter indicates that use of measures of respiratory sinus arrhythmia as practical tools may have entered the mainstream in clinical medicine without having been evaluated sufficiently.

II. History

The famous experiment published by Stephen Hales in 1733 (26) is depicted in Figure 1. This technologically advanced study marked the first demonstration and direct observation of rhythmic changes of arterial pressure. Hales describes fluctuations of the level of blood in a glass pipe connected to the crural artery of a mare "tied down alive on her back."

> When it was its full height, it would rise and fall at and after each pulse two, three, or four Inches; and sometimes it would fall twelve or fourteen Inches, and have there for a time the same vibrations up and down at and after each pulse, as it had, when it was at its full height; to which it would rise again, after forty or fifty pulses.

Hales did not relate blood pressure waves to respiratory activity. Clearly, Hales describes the existence in this conscious mare of low-frequency blood pressure waves.

In 1847, the famous physiologist and teacher of physiologists Carl Ludwig recorded (on smoked drums) physiological signals from dogs and horses and documented respiration-related fluctuations of arterial pressure (27). He suggested that the respiratory periodicity seen in blood pressure recordings results simply from mechanical imposition of changes of intrathoracic pressure on blood vessels. This explanation soon became untenable when quantitative measurements of arterial and intrathoracic pressure changes became possible; arterial pressure fluctuations were found to be much larger than intrathoracic pressure changes and,

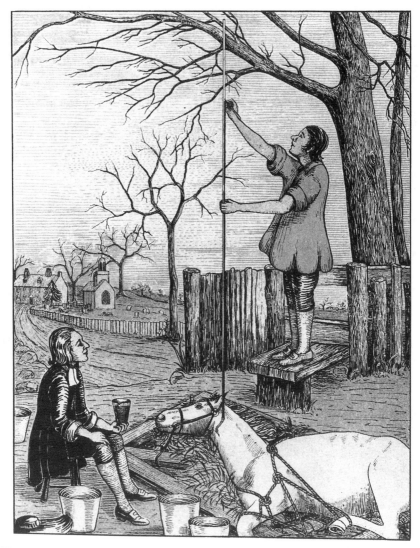

Figure 1 Stephen Hales and assistant measuring arterial pressure in a mare.

therefore, could not result simply from the mechanical influences of intrathoracic pressure on arteries.

Subsequent studies of rhythmic blood pressure waves by Traube, Hering, and Mayer were given the names of the scientists who described them. Traube (28) documented the occurrence of rhythmic blood pressure waves in mechanically ventilated curarized dogs, at times when the ventilator was turned off. Hering (29) reported similar blood pressure waves in animals who exerted feeble respiratory efforts, in the presence of partial curarization and suggested that such waves had their origin in respiration. He also showed that blood pressure waves resulted from vasomotion, since they persisted after exclusion of the heart from the circulation. Although Mayer (30) reported blood pressure waves whose periods were longer than those of respiration, he ascribed such waves to respiration. [Cyon described slow blood pressure waves in 1874 (31), 3 years before Mayer, but was not awarded the eponymic designation.] In 1882, Fredericq (32) recommended that Mayer waves be distinguished from Traube-Hering waves on the basis that Traube-Hering waves are respiration-related, but that Mayer waves are slower than respiration. [A similar suggestion was made by Schweitzer in 1945 (33).]

Koepchen has reviewed the early, largely German literature dealing with blood pressure waves authoritatively (34). He points out that a thread that is woven throughout this literature is that all blood pressure waves betray an influence of respiration. He iterates (and helps to restore some order to current thinking) the view that Traube-Hering waves occur at respiratory rates, and that Mayer waves occur at rates slower than respiration. Implicit in this reduction is the notion that "respiratory" and "low" periodicities are distinct from each other, as they usually are, and that more rapid Traube-Hering waves do not influence less rapid Mayer waves. As discussed below, human respiratory periodicity is not fixed, and slow respiratory and autonomic neural rhythms influence each other, in poorly defined ways.

Another thread that runs through the literature on respiratory sinus arrhythmia is the either/or question: Are respiratory influences on autonomic neural outflow mediated by central neural mechanisms (28,32) or by afferent input coming to the brain from slowly adapting pulmonary and thoracic stretch receptors (35,36)? This question has been difficult to sort out in humans; however, Seals and co-workers (37) joined the issue by studying patients (who, therefore, can cooperate) with denervated, surgically transplanted lungs (which presumably have intact thoracic stretch receptors). (Seals et al. concluded that afferent lung inputs modulate muscle sympathetic nerve activity, but only at supranormal tidal volumes.)

Human research into respiratory sinus arrhythmia has been pushed forward in other less spectacular, but nevertheless important ways. A variety of inputs to the central nervous system, known to influence sinus arrhythmia, have been controlled experimentally; these include those from chemoreceptors (38), baroreceptors (18–20), and trigeminal receptors (39). Respiratory rate and depth have been controlled (40–42) [but by a small minority of workers (6)]. Sympathetic nerve traffic has been measured directly (9). Importantly, results have been subjected to sophisticated mathematical analyses. Clynes (43) and, subsequently, Angelone and Coulter (44) analyzed respiratory sinus arrhythmia with mathematical techniques drawn from control systems theory. More recently, frequency-domain methods have been applied to neural outputs, including vagal-cardiac, as reflected by heart rate or R-R intervals (23,45,46) and muscle sympathetic nerve activity (20). The above litany suggests that powerful tools can be marshaled to investigate and understand respiration-related autonomic neural periodicities in humans.

III. Study of Human Autonomic Neural Periodicities

The general inaccessibility of human autonomic nerves imposes a need for compromise. Some of the constraints involved with such human research and the means taken to circumvent them are discussed below. This critical treatment of methodology is included to provide the perspective that is necessary to understand data on physiological mechanisms discussed later in the chapter. This review focuses on *physiological* mechanisms in *humans*. It takes its place as a new entry in what has become an ongoing review of this important topic (47–51).

A. Neural Recordings

Vagal-cardiac nerve traffic has not been measured directly in humans. Therefore, all quantitation of human vagal activity is indirect. All the approaches used currently are based on a measure of the interval between heart beats (usually R-R intervals) and the assumption that interbeat intervals in some way sample the underlying neural traffic that shapes them. This usage is supported by research conducted in animals and humans. The most important support is that changes of R-R intervals are linear functions of changes of vagal-cardiac nerve traffic. This was shown convincingly by Katona and co-workers (52), who used a linear model to predict changes of R-R intervals from changes of vagal-cardiac nerve activity during moderate arterial pressure changes in anesthetized dogs. Linearity between R-R intervals and vagal traffic also was proven indirectly by Parker et al. (8), who showed that in anesthetized dogs, R-R intervals are linear functions of the frequency of electrical vagus nerve stimulation.

A second assumption (which usually is not owned) is that the sinoatrial node translates changes of vagal (and sympathetic) traffic faithfully in time. Vagal-cardiac nerve traffic fluctuates on a heartbeat-by-heartbeat basis (53,54). Surges of vagal traffic are followed by release of acetylcholine, slowing of the rate of sinoatrial node diastolic depolarization, and dissipation of the effects of acetylcholine. The human sinoatrial node tracks changes of vagus nerve traffic well, but not perfectly; the response to a square wave reflex input, if such could be applied in humans, is not a square wave output. There are minimum latencies, of about 0.25 sec, from an abrupt increase of baroreceptor input until a prolongation of the R-R interval (55), and there is a decay, lasting about 2 sec, of R-R interval responses after abrupt cessation of baroreceptor stimulation (56). The implication of these observations is that the human sinoatrial node can follow rapid changes of vagus nerve traffic [such as those associated with breathing at usual rates (57)], but that the kinetics of sinoatrial node responses to acetylcholine modify and distort such rhythms.

A third assumption involved with estimates of human vagal-cardiac nerve traffic is that *changes* of R-R intervals (and, therefore, changes of vagal-cardiac traffic) can be used to predict *absolute levels* of vagus traffic to the heart. This usage is supported by the study of Katona and Jih (7), which showed that in anesthetized dogs, vagal-cardiac neurons fall silent during inspiration and fire during expiration, in proportion to the level of (baroreceptor) stimulation. In this study, the amount of vagal firing during expiration was proportional to total vagal-cardiac nerve activity. This study led to the use of human peak minus valley R-R intervals (or some mathematical derivation thereof) as surrogates for steady-state vagal-cardiac nerve traffic.

Sympathetic-cardiac nerve traffic also has not been measured directly in humans. Therefore, as with studies of vagal mechanisms, studies of sympathetic-cardiac mechanisms are based on indirect methods. The most prevalent of these is to extract information regarding sympathetic activity from periodicities present in surface electrocardiograms. In my view, the assumptions underlying this genre of research are not nearly as well validated as assumption underlying research into vagal mechanisms.

Sympathetic, as well as vagal nerve, activity fluctuates on a heartbeat-by-heartbeat basis (58). However, there are major differences between the time constants of effector responses to the two neural outflows. First, there is a substantial delay, averaging about 5 sec, between the occurrence of a (muscle) sympathetic burst and the peak heart rate and arterial pressure changes, and even longer delays in the decays of those changes (59). Thus, human sympathetic-cardiac responses are sluggish and begin and dissipate more slowly than vagal responses. The sinoatrial node functions as a low-pass filter, whose responses to rapidly changing sympathetic neural inputs, such as those related to respiration, are small [but not absent altogether (60,61)]. In part because of sympathetic-cardiac time constants, the assumption is made that sympathetic can be distinguished from vagal rhythms on the basis of their frequencies. According to this usage (23), R-R interval fluctuations occurring at the respiratory frequency are purely vagal, and R-R interval fluctuations occurring at slower frequency are mainly sympathetic.

A second assumption invoked to justify indirect measures of sympathetic-cardiac nerve traffic is that sympathetic can be distinguished from vagal rhythms by the use of autonomic blocking drugs. This assumption is not supported adequately by experimental data. First, beta-adrenergic blocking drugs, in poorly understood ways, seem to increase vagal periodicities (62–64). Second, again in poorly understood ways, large doses of cholinergic blocking drugs such as atropine sulfate abolish nearly all cardiac periodicities (1,65).

Sympathetic traffic to skin and muscle vascular beds has been measured directly in humans, with needles inserted percutaneously into mixed peripheral nerves. This method, developed in Sweden by Vallbo and Hagbarth (66), has been described in explicit detail recently (67). Two groups (20,37,68) have studied the effects of respiration on directly recorded muscle sympathetic nerve traffic. This genre of research provides clear insights into how respiration influences sympathetic neural outflow. However, use of sympathetic-*muscle* nerve recordings to derive information about sympathetic-*cardiac* mechanisms (69) involves a major assumption, that sympathetic rhythms to muscle and cardiac vascular beds are (qualitatively, if not quantitatively) similar. Although I suspect that this is true, I am aware of no direct data that bear on the possibility. It is known that there is a statistically significant correlation between average levels of human muscle sympathetic nerve activity and an indirect index of cardiac sympathetic nerve traffic, myocardial norepinephrine spillover (70). However, some studies in animals indicate that respiration-related patterns of sympathetic traffic may be different in different sympathetic outflows (71,72).

B. Data Treatment

The simplest way to study human autonomic rhythms is to regard them as series of events occurring in time. Before such time series can be analyzed, however, certain of the recorded signals must be modified. Systolic and diastolic pressures can be registered simply at their times of occurrence. Sympathetic neurograms must be changed in at least two ways. First, sympathetic bursts must be normalized, so that they can be compared across subjects. (Signal-to-noise ratios of these recordings depend on factors that cannot be controlled.) One way to do this is to measure burst heights during a control period, assign some numerical value to the highest burst or bursts, and then normalize bursts in the remainder of the record according to this standard (73). Second, sympathetic bursts must be shifted in time. Human sympathetic traffic is carried from ganglia near the spinal cord to mixed nerve peripheral recording sites over slowly conducting, unmyelinated C-fibers. If the timing of sympathetic bursts is to be correlated with the timing of other events, bursts must be advanced on the time axis. The value for this shift (which averages about 1.3 sec to the peroneal nerve) can be calculated by inserting subjects' heights into empirical formulas, such as one derived from data published by Fagius and Wallin [0.0038 × height in cm + 0.687 (74)]. Alternatively, the value for this shift can be determined experimentally, from the delay from an R wave until the peak of a burst in the next complete cardiac cycle.

R-R intervals (used as substitutes for P-P intervals) also must be manipulated before they can be analyzed. Several authors discuss issues involved in transformations of R-R intervals into suitable time series (75–79). Figure 2 illustrates several ways to treat R-R interval data. The left panels show an individual data sweep triggered on inspiration. Figure 2C shows a simple R-R interval plot; in this panel, the value of each R-R interval is plotted at the R wave that ended each interval. One problem with this real-time plot is that measured R-R intervals are delayed by one heartbeat. Another is that each R-R interval is weighted as though it persisted throughout the next R-R interval.

Figure 2D–F depict ways (not real-time) for correcting problems arising from the one-beat phase lag of actual R-R interval signals. In D, R-R intervals were plotted at the times they actually occurred. In E and F, the points on C were shifted to the left by one beat and connected with straight lines (E) or with lines derived with spline regression (F). The right panels of Figure 2 show average (± SEM) measurements made during 10 breaths; tracings shown in H–K represent simply averages derived from the methods illustrated in C–F. The main difference between the average shown in H and those shown in I–K is that there is a one heartbeat phase shift; changes shown in H appeared later than they actually occurred. [There is also a small (between 0.12 and 0.20 sec) phase shift produced by use of R-R, instead of P-P, intervals; the phase lag that results from use of R-R instead of P-P intervals is almost always ignored.]

After the data are transformed into satisfactory time series, they can be analyzed with time-domain methods (such as the one illustrated in Fig. 2) or with *frequency-domain methods*. There are at least two rationales for preferring frequency- to time-domain analyses of R-R intervals. First, simple averages of R-R intervals provide highly ambiguous information regarding underlying autonomic nerve traffic. A study by Inoue and Zipes (80) underscores complexities involved with use of average R-R intervals to understand underlying changes of autonomic input. They stimulated sympathetic- and vagal-cardiac nerves electrically in anesthetized dogs and measured R-R and A-H (atrioventricular node conduction time) intervals. They identified several combinations of stimulus frequencies that yielded identical R-R intervals, but highly disparate A-H intervals. Other animal studies show that inputs from one autonomic division modulate sinoatrial node responses to inputs from the other division importantly [through both pre- and postganglionic mechanisms (81)]. (However, the practical importance of such autonomic interactions has not been defined well in humans.)

Second, measures of R-R interval fluctuations based on respiration, including peak minus valley R-R interval changes during individual breaths and power spectra at respiratory frequencies, may fail to identify periodicities different from respiration. For example, frequency-domain methods may delineate Mayer waves—blood pressure rhythms with center frequencies at about 0.1 Hz, whose frequency is, by definition, less than that of respiration (see Section II). If these waves exist entirely independent of respiration [as the power spectral analyses of Saul and co-workers (61)], they will occur at all times in the breathing

678 Eckberg

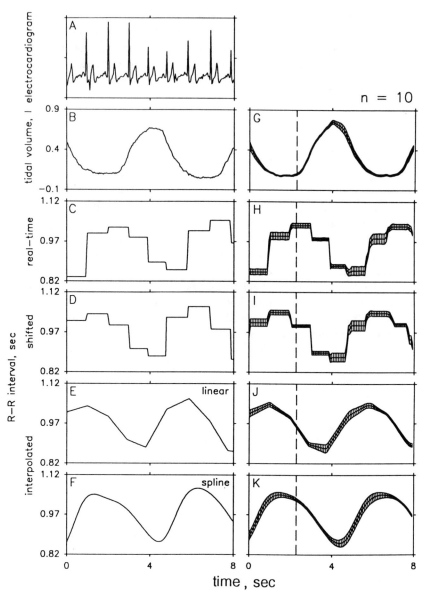

Figure 2 Methods for preparing R-R intervals for analysis. (G–K) Mean ± SEM values for 10 data sweeps.

cycle and will, therefore, be filtered out in data sweeps triggered by respiration.

Frequency-domain methods hold several important advantages over time-domain methods. First, since net human autonomic rhythms reflect interplays among several oscillations, methods that characterize all rhythms are preferable to methods that delineate only one rhythm. Second, with frequency-domain methods, information derived from different signals (such as arterial pressure, respiration, cardiac activity, and temperature) can be correlated to obtain insights into mechanisms. For example, if it is shown that increases of blood pressure precede increases of R-R intervals, the inference may be drawn that a baroreflex mechanism is operative. Also, if two signals change together at a given frequency (in the same direction or opposite directions), this fact will be noted by high (>0.5) coherence values. The presence of high degrees of coherence suggests that one rhythm drives the other, or that both rhythms are driven by a third oscillation.

Finally, frequency-domain methods yield results that can reduce bewilderingly complex waveforms into tight, economical graphical representations. Such graphs (as shown below) comprise snapshots; they indicate what the rhythms were at the time they were recorded. In the rapidly growing literature involving frequency-domain methods, much is made of the need for *stationarity* of the analyzed signals. If a series of events occurring in time is to be reduced to a single frequency-domain characterization, such as a power spectrum, all segments of the record should have stationary statistical properties, including mean, probability distribution, and covariance.

Human physiological signals are not mathematically stationary, however. It may be that investigators who use frequency-domain methods have borrowed the language of mathematicians without fully grasping its limited relevance to human research. A power spectrum (for example) does no more than characterize a subject at the time the recording was made. The characterization will be different if the subject's situation is different. At the onset of intense exercise, the R-R interval shortens within 1 sec (82), and the power spectrum changes accordingly. Requirements that signals be stationary are not peculiar to frequency-domain methods; all attempts to reduce complex waveforms to concise mathematical expressions are influenced by nonstationarities. Simple R-R interval standard deviations increase with the length of recordings, because of unavoidable nonstationarities. Moreover, it is unlikely that one method, such as autoregressive power spectra, is immune to concerns about stationarity, and another, such as fast-Fourier transform power spectra, is not. It is good science to require that experimental data represent subjects at the time recordings are made. In this connection, it may be worthwhile to examine experimental records for stationarity (83,84). If trends are not found, or if sequential segments are statistically similar, results can be considered representative of the subject at the time recordings were made. [However, Grossman argues persuasively, from experimental data, that lack of stationarity does not influence measures of respiratory sinus arrhythmia importantly (85).]

Finally, to assure stationarity, the length of recordings can be shortened; the shorter the record, the less likely nonstationarities will be present. However, the length of recordings determines in part the results obtained. There are trade-offs involved in the selection of the length of recordings. If recordings are long, the resolution of separate rhythms will be better, and it will be possible to define low-frequency rhythms. Short recordings yield data that are more likely to be stationary. There are also practical considerations that enter into decisions regarding the lengths of recordings. Human subjects can control their breathing frequencies exquisitely and their tidal volumes well; however, even the most dedicated volunteers eventually lapse, and yawn, sigh, or fall asleep. Also, there are limits to the length of experiments conscious human subjects can tolerate. If experiments involve many interventions, the length of recordings made during each intervention cannot be too long. Thus, for a variety of reasons, researchers choose shorter rather than longer recording times (typically 128 or 256 heartbeats). In limiting the lengths of recordings, they preclude study of slow rhythms. In part because of this, there is little research on very slow (0–0.02 sec) human autonomic periodicities (which are thought to reflect thermoregulation).

Several types of frequency-domain methods are used to explore respiration-related autonomic neural periodicities. The most widely used are based on fast-Fourier transform (41,45,86) or autoregressive approaches (23). Examples of these are included in the subsequent discussion. The technical merits of each approach are ably discussed by Kay and Marple (87). The autoregressive method yields graphs that are aesthetically more pleasing and have several other advantages over graphs obtained with fast-Fourier transform methods. Autoregressive methods yield better resolution of components with close frequencies. They calculate center frequencies and powers of component spectra automatically. (In fast-Fourier transforms, the investigator arbitrarily defines a region for scrutiny.) They calculate very low-frequency power (DC, or $1/f^x$ noise) as individual components. (In fast-Fourier transforms, low-frequency power is mixed with other components and increases their power.) These advantages are mathematical; it is less clear that autoregressive methods characterize autonomic nerve traffic better than other approaches. Figure 3, left (J Koh, TE Brown, LA Beightol, and DL Eckberg, unpublished), depicts an R-R interval time series obtained from one supine patient with an incomplete cervical spinal cord transection, during infusion of saline (upper panel) or phenylephrine (lower panel), during controlled breathing. The right panels show power spectra derived with fast-Fourier transform and autoregressive methods.

In addition, there are methods designed specifically to characterize periodicities that are nonstationary. These include complex demodulation (46,88) and wavelets (89). The technique of complex demodulation (46) involves iterative computation of phase and frequency components in a window that is moved

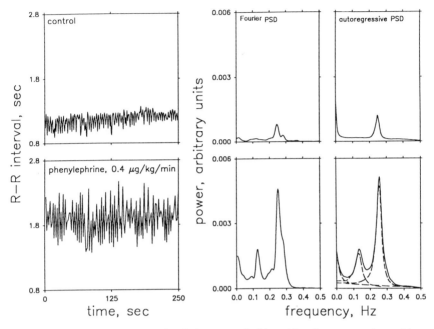

Figure 3 R-R interval time series during controlled breathing from one patient with an incomplete cervical spinal cord injury, during saline (control) and phenylephrine infusions. (J Koh, TE Brown, LA Beightol, and DL Eckberg, unpublished.)

progressively through the record. Figure 4, top panel (JA Taylor, AR Patwardhan, J Hayano, and DL Eckberg, unpublished) shows an R-R interval time series made during successive, 5-min applications of 0 (control), 5, 10, 15, 20, and 40 mmHg suction to the lower body, during controlled breathing at a rate of 15 breaths/min. The lower two panels show complex demodulations of the signal at 0.25 Hz (the frequency of breathing) and 0.1 Hz (the average center frequency of Mayer waves). Figure 5 shows a wavelet analysis of the same time series shown in Figure 4. The wavelet approach, which is not yet widely used in human physiology, has the advantage that it depicts changes over all frequencies; complex demodulation depicts changes at only one frequency per analysis. [Another type of wavelet analysis, the Wigner distribution (90), was used to derive the time/frequency plots of respiratory periodicities shown in Fig. 37.]

The remainder of this review deals with several questions: What is the temporal relation between breathing and other human autonomic rhythms? What underlying changes of autonomic efferent activity are responsible for such rhythms? How do changes of breathing affect efferent autonomic cardiovascular outflow? What are the practical implications of respiratory modulation of autonomic cardiovascular outflow?

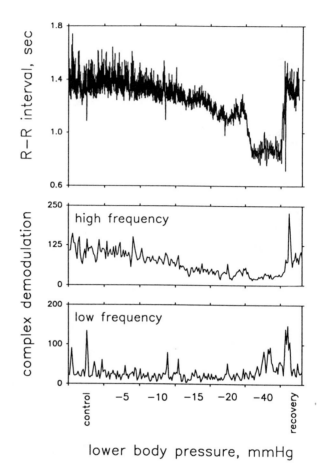

Figure 4   Time series from one healthy supine subject before, during, and after a series of
5-min applications of lower-body suction. (JA Taylor, AR Patwardhan, J Hayano, and DL
Eckberg, unpublished.)

IV.   Relations Between Respiration and
   Other Autonomic Rhythms

Figure 6 (20) illustrates the ebb and flow of arterial pressure, muscle sympathetic
nerve activity, respiration (inspiration is denoted by an upgoing signal), and vagal
activity (heart period) in one subject who was breathing spontaneously. This
recording was obtained from a healthy young woman who was lying supine. This
record says nothing about mechanisms; however, it does indicate that during quiet
breathing, vagal and sympathetic outflows, arterial pressure, and respiratory
rhythms may be synchronized closely. [Although R-R interval fluctuations at
respiratory frequencies are thought to be mediated entirely by changes of *vagal-*

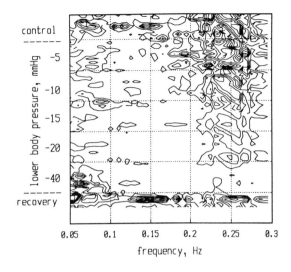

Figure 5 Wavelet analysis of the same time series shown in Figure 4. (JA Taylor, AR Patwardhan, J Hayano, and DL Eckberg, unpublished.)

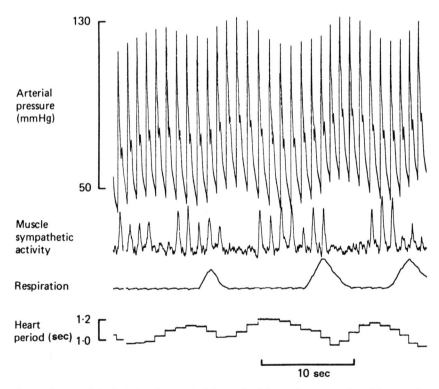

Figure 6 Physiological signals recorded from a healthy supine woman breathing spontaneously. In this subject, all four signals fluctuated in a 1:1 relation. (Reproduced with permission from Ref. 20.)

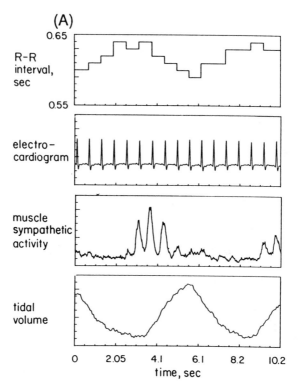

Figure 7 Data obtained from one healthy supine subject during controlled respiration. The three lower panels on the right depict data obtained from 10 data sweeps triggered on early inspiration. (Reproduced with permission from Ref. 91.)

cardiac nerve traffic (65), muscle *sympathetic* nerve activity also fluctuates with a strong respiratory periodicity.]

Data shown in Figure 7 (91), left, are similar to those shown in Figure 6 (but without arterial pressure). These data were recorded during fixed-rate breathing, at a rate of 12 breaths/min. The right panels show data sweeps begun after an early inspiratory threshold crossing. From above downward, these panels show sympathetic traffic from the same breath shown on the left, sympathetic traffic from 10 superimposed sweeps of data triggered by 10 inspirations, average (± SEM) sympathetic traffic during those 10 breaths, and average tidal volumes. In this subject, sympathetic firing began in midexpiration and peaked in late inspiration. The average sympathetic neurogram indicates that under these experimental circumstances, sympathetic firing occurred systematically during a breath, in an almost deterministic fashion.

Figure 8 (20) provides a clear indication of the interrelations that exist

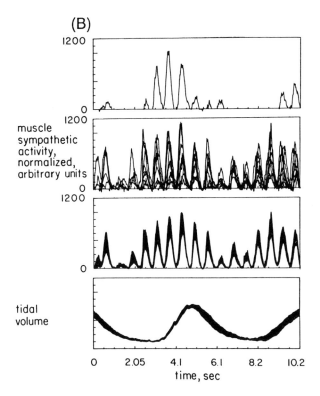

Figure 7 (Continued)

among breathing, intra-arterial pressure, and vagal and sympathetic neural out-flows, across subjects. This figure depicts average (+ SEM) inspiratory-triggered measurements obtained from nine healthy supine subjects who were breathing spontaneously. The results show that during a breath (0% marks the beginning of inspiration), muscle sympathetic nerve activity declines as arterial pressure rises (in these subjects, by an extremely small amount), and that vagal activity changes directly, not reciprocally with sympathetic activity. Possible explanations for the apparent coactivation of vagal and sympathetic motoneurons are given below. The data in Figure 8 are descriptive and do not necessarily define mechanisms. Moreover, these data in no way indicate that the periodicities shown *always* occur in the same way. [Several groups (22,92,93) have reported that in anesthetized animals, changes of breathing patterns may change the timing of sympathetic activity within breaths.]

Figure 6 illustrates a very simple relation among autonomic and respiratory periodicities: during this recording, all rhythms tended to vary with respiration, in a simple 1:1 ratio. The recording shown in Figure 9, left, introduces new com-

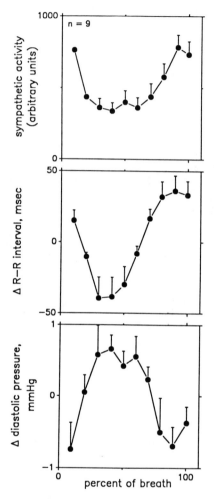

Figure 8 Signal-averaged (± SEM) muscle sympathetic nerve activity, R-R interval, and diastolic pressure from nine healthy supine subjects who were breathing spontaneously. (Reproduced with permission from Ref. 20.)

plexities. These data were obtained from a healthy supine young woman who was breathing at a constant tidal volume and a controlled rate of 15 breaths/min. Although this volunteer breathed about eight times during this recording, she had only five major volleys of sympathetic bursts and changes of diastolic pressure waves. Systolic pressures and R-R intervals varied with periods different from diastolic pressures and sympathetic activity. This tracing underscores the inade-

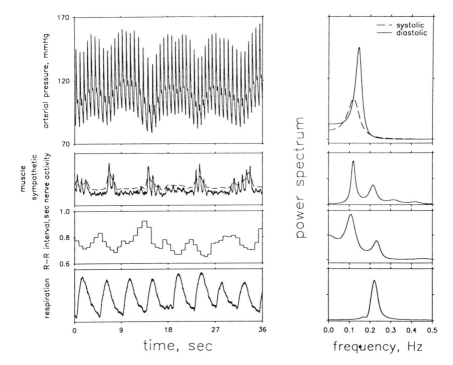

Figure 9 Time series from one supine subject who was breathing spontaneously. Data on right were obtained with autoregressive power spectral analysis. In this subject, respiratory frequency was much greater than that of other signals; the primary efferent sympathetic and R-R interval rhythms were centered at about 0.1 Hz.

quacy of time-domain methods, such as the simple strip-chart recordings or postevent triggered averages shown in Figures 6–9 (left), as guides to understanding human autonomic periodicities.

The autoregressive power spectrum shown in Figure 9, right, second panel from the top shows unambiguously that resting humans have low- as well as respiratory-frequency efferent sympathetic rhythms, which (presumably) are responsible for low-frequency blood pressure waves. These muscle sympathetic neurograms, however, provide no direct information about efferent sympathetic rhythms to the *heart*. Sympathetic traffic to the human heart has not been measured. In the absence of direct recordings, investigators have attempted to discern human sympathetic-cardiac rhythms in R-R interval fluctuations.

Human R-R interval fluctuations are mediated almost entirely by fluctuations of neural input to the heart. This assertion is proven most convincingly by recordings obtained from heart transplant patients, each of whom has atrial remnants that include innervated and denervated sinoatrial nodes. In such patients, the rhythm of the denervated sinoatrial node is nearly monotonic (94). Figure 10 shows respiration, and P-P intervals calculated from innervated and denervated atrial electrograms, measured in a patient with a transplanted heart. Fluctuations of rhythm in the innervated sinoatrial node (left middle panel) were substantial, and fluctuations of rhythm in the denervated sinoatrial node (left bottom panel) were small. Autoregressive power spectral analysis of respiration and the two atria are shown on the right. Respiratory periodicities were unmistakable in both innervated and denervated atria (right middle and bottom panels). However, the amplitudes of these fluctuations were decidedly different; power was approximately 250 times greater in the innervated than the denervated atrium. The most likely explanation for respiratory periodicity in the denervated atrium is that it is nonautonomic and secondary to rhythmic stretching (95,96) caused by inspiratory augmentation of venous return to the right heart.

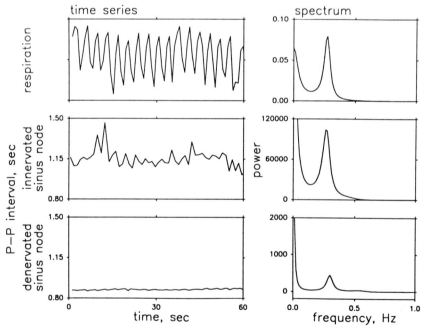

Figure 10   Respiration and P-P interval during controlled breathing in a patient with an orthotopic heart transplant. Spectral analyses were made with autoregressive techniques. Note that the gain of the power spectrum for the denervated atrial electrogram signal (right bottom panel) is about one-sixtieth that of the innervated atrial electrogram signal (right middle panel).

V. Mechanisms Responsible for Interrelations Between Respiration and Autonomic Outflow

A. Sympathetic Firing

Data depicted in Figure 8 suggest that firing does not occur simply because sympathetic motoneurons are stimulated by *inspiratory* neurons (97); sympathetic firing reaches its nadir in late inspiration (after about 40% of the breath), when phrenic motoneuron activity is greatest (98). A more likely explanation is that sympathetic firing falls steadily as inspiration progresses, because of steadily increasing levels of slowly adapting pulmonary and thoracic stretch receptor activity (99). Others also have remarked that human muscle sympathetic bursts occur more often in *expiration* than inspiration (9,68).

The question of whether inspiratory or expiratory neurons are responsible assumes that respiration-related sympathetic periodicities are secondary to breathing, rather than to other rhythms also related to breathing. One candidate for a respiration-related rhythm is arterial pressure. The fall and rise of sympathetic traffic during the breath shown in Figure 8 can be explained entirely on the basis of an arterial *baroreflex* mechanism, since human muscle sympathetic neuronal firing occurs reciprocally with changes of arterial pressure (100,101). Such an interpretation, however, probably is simplistic. Preiss and Polosa (22) showed in cats that some rhythmic changes of sympathetic nerve activity related reciprocally to arterial pressure persist after blood pressure changes are buffered mechanically or prevented pharmacologically by administration of ganglionic blocking drugs. Their observations suggest that respiratory activity itself is sufficient to explain the sympathetic periodicities depicted in Figures 6–8.

The notion that within-breath modulation of sympathetic nerve activity is due simply to arterial pressure changes occurring within the breath was discredited also by Seals and co-workers (68), who measured peroneal nerve muscle sympathetic activity during low-level ("nonhypotensive") lower-body suction. They showed that when sympathetic bursts occurring after similar diastolic pressures were compared, bursts were always greater in expiration than inspiration. [Seals et al. did not indicate whether the reference pressure was preceded by a higher or lower pressure. This detail may be important, because Sundlöf and Wallin (102) showed that sympathetic bursts are more likely to occur when pressure is falling than when it is rising.]

In a second study (37), Seals and associates devised an ingenious strategy to alter aortic baroreceptor firing in opposite directions, with application of inspiratory resistance or positive pressure. Resistance breathing increases negative intrathoracic pressure, the pressure gradient across the aortic wall, aortic dimensions (103), and probably aortic baroreceptor firing (104). Positive pressure breathing produces opposite changes. The results of Seals's study, shown in Figure 11, indicate that respiratory modulation of sympathetic outflow is similar when aortic distending pressure is increased by inspiratory resistance or decreased by positive pressure breathing.

Does this mean that respiration-related changes of sympathetic outflow occur independent of baroreceptor input? It does not, because input from baroreceptors (and other sensory receptors, including chemoreceptors) determines the amount of sympathetic activity upon which respiratory influences act. The effect of ambient arterial pressure on respiration-related peroneal nerve muscle sympathetic traffic is shown in Figures 12 and 13 (91). Figure 12 shows signal-averaged muscle sympathetic nerve activity (± SEM) at four levels of diastolic pressure, during intravenous infusions of phenylephrine (top panel), saline (second panel), and graded nitroprusside (third and fourth panels) in one subject. At the highest pressure (uppermost panel), muscle sympathetic bursts were few and appeared mainly at the peak of inspiration. At lower arterial pressures, the number of bursts increased, and bursts occurred progressively earlier in the breath. At the lowest pressure (fourth panel), sympathetic firing began in mid-expiration, and peaked in late expiration. These results suggest that when sympathetic firing is suppressed by high levels of baroreceptor input, respiration exerts little effect on sympathetic outflow. Sympathetic activity must be present for respiration to modulate it. Conversely, when baroreceptor inhibition of sympathetic firing is minor and sympathetic firing levels are high, respiration exerts strong modulatory effects on sympathetic outflow.

Figure 13 depicts integrated inspiratory and expiratory sympathetic activity in 10 subjects during pharmacological alterations of arterial pressure. This figure

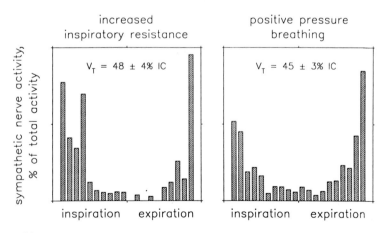

Figure 11   Average respiratory distribution of muscle sympathetic nerve activity in six subjects during two conditions chosen to alter aortic transmural pressure in opposite directions (see text). (Reproduced with permission from Ref. 37.)

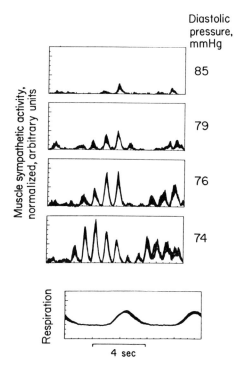

Figure 12 Inspiratory signal-averaged muscle sympathetic nerve activity and respiration from one supine subject during controlled breathing. Changes of diastolic pressure were produced by infusions of phenylephrine (top panel), saline (second panel), and two doses of nitroprusside (third and fourth panels). (Reproduced with permission from Ref. 91.)

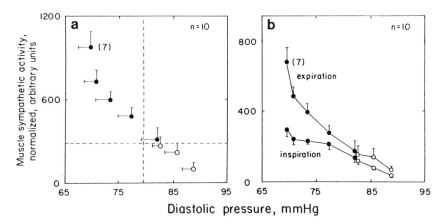

Figure 13 Average (± SEM) muscle sympathetic nerve activity measured in nine supine subjects during controlled breathing. (Reproduced with permission from Ref 91.)

shows that (as expected) sympathetic firing is related inversely to arterial pressure, and that the greatest disparities between inspiratory and expiratory levels of sympathetic firing occur when sympathetic activity is greatest. Differences between inspiratory and expiratory sympathetic firing are minimal when sympathetic activity is minimal (as it is when arterial pressure is high).

The data shown in Figures 12 and 13 document parallel increases of sympathetic activity and respiration-related fluctuations of sympathetic activity, as arterial pressure falls. In this study, average diastolic pressure was lowered only to 70 mmHg; therefore, these data provide little information on how breathing modulates sympathetic activity at low arterial pressures. However, an animal study and a human case report provide clues regarding respiration modulation of sympathetic activity at very low pressures.

McAllen (105) recorded activity of subretrofacial nucleus units in anesthetized, paralyzed, and artificially ventilated cats. [This medullary recording site was chosen because cells in this region provide the primary stimulus for spinal sympathetic motoneurons to fire (106). When connections between the medulla and the spinal cord are severed, as they are in patients with clinically complete cervical spinal cord injuries, (muscle) sympathetic nerve activity is sparse (107).] Figure 14 underscores several of McAllen's observations. The top tracings depict firing of a unit in the subretrofacial nucleus (second and third tracings) and phrenic nerve activity (which was unrelated to the rate of artificial ventilation, reflected in the CO_2 tracing). The lower panels illustrate frequency histograms of the medullary unit and concurrent activity of a multifiber postganglionic cervical sympathetic nerve, triggered by (inspiratory) phrenic nerve threshold crossings. These data were recorded with one carotid sinus nerve and both vagus nerves cut. The left portion of Figure 14 shows data obtained with the remaining, innervated carotid artery open to pulsatile flow, and the right portion shows data obtained with that carotid artery clamped. These results indicate that respiration imposes an "imprint" on the medullary neuron pool that drives spinal sympathetic motoneurons, and that this imprint is translated into fluctuations of postganglionic sympathetic nerve activity (as shown in the lowest tracings). Although McAllen did not comment on it, these data show also that when sympathetic activity is increased to high levels, as it is when there is no baroreceptor inhibition, respiratory modulation is reduced.

A case report included in a review of human vasovagal reactions (108) may provide clues about what happens to respiratory modulation of human sympathetic outflow when pressure is reduced profoundly. Figure 15 shows muscle sympathetic nerve activity in a subject who developed a vasovagal reaction during a graded infusion of sodium nitroprusside. (This record is one of four published human sympathetic recordings obtained during vasovagal reactions.) Respiratory modulation of sympathetic activity is obvious during saline infusion (first panel), and during infusion of nitroprusside at the lower rate (second panel). During

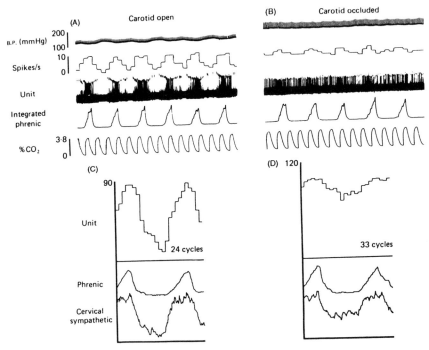

Figure 14 Subretrofacial nucleus unit and phrenic and cervical sympathetic nerve firings in an anesthetized cat. The bottom graphs represent signal-averaged activity, triggered on phrenic nerve activity. When the remaining baroreceptive artery was open to the circulation (left) there was striking modulation of the medullary unit and cervical sympathetic activity. When that carotid was occluded (and baroreceptor input was effectively reduced to zero, right), medullary unit firing was greater, but the respiratory variation was less. (Reproduced with permission from Ref. 105.)

infusion of nitroprusside at the higher rate (third panel), sympathetic activity was augmented greatly, but respiratory modulation was not apparent. Finally, during the full-blown vasovagal reaction (which developed *after* the nitroprusside infusion had been stopped), sympathetic activity was less than during infusion of the higher nitroprusside dose, and again, respiratory modulation of sympathetic outflow was not apparent. These data suggest that the ability of respiration to modulate human sympathetic outflow can be overridden by intense stimulatory drive of sympathetic motoneurons, or by the apparent disengagement of baroreflex control of sympathetic activity that occurs during vasovagal reactions.

There are few published data regarding biochemical mechanisms responsible for the respiratory periodicities found in efferent sympathetic neurograms.

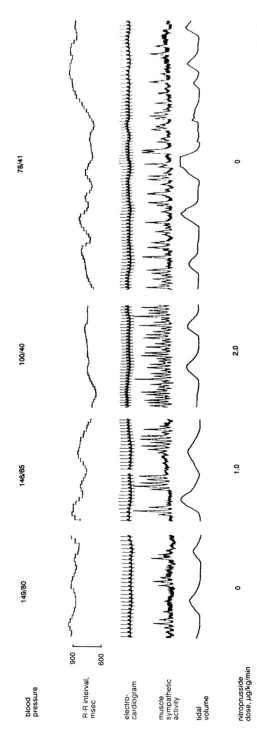

Figure 15 Development of a vasovagal reaction in healthy supine subject breathing spontaneously. Respiratory modeling of muscle sympathetic nerve activity was not apparent during infusion of the higher dose of nitroprusside or during the vasovagal reaction that followed it. (Reproduced with permission from Ref. 108.)

Sundlöf and co-workers (109) showed that acute intravenous injections of metoprolol, a lipophilic beta-adrenergic blocking drug that crosses the blood-brain barrier readily, increase muscle sympathetic nerve activity. Sundlöf et al. speculated that this effect was due to hemodynamic effects, including bradycardia and prolongation of diastolic run-off; he did not attribute it to a central action of metoprolol. Porter and co-workers (110) showed that sequential (small, as well as large) doses of the muscarinic cholinergic blocking drug atropine sulfate, which also crosses the blood-brain barrier, do not influence human muscle sympathetic nerve activity.

Others have suggested that respiratory activity modulates the ability of arterial baroreceptors to influence sympathetic (and vagal) firing. Results adapted from a study published by Seller and associates (111) are shown in Figure 16. This analysis depicts the persistence of renal sympathetic nerve inhibition after electrical carotid sinus nerve stimuli delivered at different times during the respiratory cycle. (Such electrical stimuli excite afferent chemoreceptor as well as baroreceptor neurons.) Seller's results show clearly that carotid sinus nerve stimuli provoke longer-lasting sympathetic inhibition when they are delivered during expiration than inspiration.

Eckberg et al. (20) performed a related study in humans. They applied abrupt, brief (about one cardiac cycle) pressure pulses to the neck at different times in the respiratory cycle. [Such pressure pulses reduce carotid dimensions (112) and trigger increases of sympathetic activity (73).] Eckberg's results are summarized in Figure 17. Abrupt reductions of carotid dimensions were much more likely to increase sympathetic activity when they were applied during expiration than inspiration. Although these findings indicate clearly that respiration modulates sympathetic responsiveness to baroreceptor influences, they do not

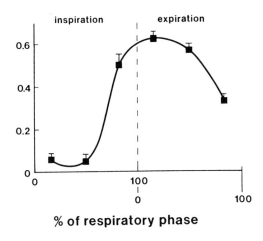

% of respiratory phase

Figure 16 Duration of sympathetic inhibition after electric carotid sinus nerve stimuli delivered at various times in the cardiac cycle. (Adapted with permission from Ref. 111.)

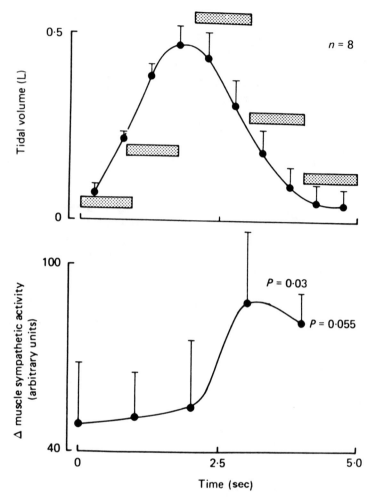

Figure 17 Average increases of muscle sympathetic nerve activity provoked by brief neck pressure, in eight healthy subjects. Changes of nerve traffic were plotted at the time in the breathing cycle that the neck pressure was delivered, as shown in the upper graph. (Reproduced with permission from Ref. 20.)

exclude the possibility that respiration influences sympathetic firing through central mechanisms that are independent of baroreceptor inputs. Bainton and co-workers (113) showed that some respiratory modulation of cardiac and renal sympathetic activity persists after sinoaortic baroreceptor denervation.

B. Vagal Firing

The reduction of vagal restraint (shortening of R-R intervals) that occurs during inspiration (Fig. 8, left) cannot be explained on the basis of a baroreflex mechanism; over a wide arterial pressure range, vagal firing is proportionally, not reciprocally, related to arterial pressure (114). Moreover, Koepchen and Thurau (115) showed that respiratory periodicity of vagally mediated heart rate changes is preserved when arterial pressure is varied artificially, out of phase with respiration. Thus, both changes of sympathetic and vagal outflow during quiet breathing may be due more to respiration itself than to arterial pressure changes coincident with respiration.

In a series of articles (18,19,91), Eckberg and his colleagues explored the relation between breathing phase and responsiveness of vagal-cardiac motoneurons to baroreceptor stimulation. The results of one of these studies (19) are summarized in Figure 18. The upper panel of this figure shows the average tidal

tidal volume, L

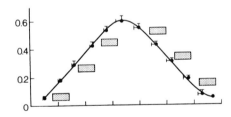

△P-P interval, sec

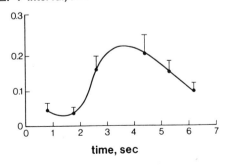

time, sec

Figure 18   Average P-P ($\pm$ SEM) interval changes after delivery of moderate neck suction at different times in the respiratory cycle. Responses were plotted at the time stimuli were begun, as shown in upper panel. (Reproduced with permission from Ref. 19.)

volume of six volunteers and the times and durations (0.6 sec) of carotid baroreceptor stimulation with neck suction (30 mmHg). The lower panel depicts integrated P-P interval changes occurring after stimuli, plotted at the time in the respiratory cycle that each stimulus was delivered. These results illustrate how respiration modulates the ability of baroreceptor inputs to stimulate vagal-cardiac motoneurons, and they complement animal research published much earlier by Koepchen et al. (116). They belie the notion that respiratory sinus arrhythmia reflects simply inspiratory suppression and expiratory facilitation of vagal firing; rather, the data illustrate an ongoing, almost sinusoidal process wherein vagal responsiveness to baroreceptor input may be large in late inspiration and small in late expiration.

Electrophysiological mechanisms responsible for the human observations shown in Figure 18 were published in a study of anesthetized, spontaneously breathing dogs by Davidson et al. (117). Figure 19 shows activity of a single vagal-cardiac efferent neuron to brief, large pressure pulses delivered to a carotid sinus. The stimulus delivered during expiration (left) provoked an intense barrage of vagal activity; the stimulus delivered during inspiration (right) elicited no vagal response.

Eckberg and Orshan (18) applied brief (0.6 sec) negative pressure pulses to a neck chamber (118) during different phases of respiration. Their findings are summarized in Figure 20. Moderate (30 mmHg) neck suction provoked greater R-R interval prolongation when it was delivered in expiration than inspiration. Intense (60 mmHg) neck suction, however, provoked similar R-R interval lengthening in expiration and inspiration. These results suggest that inspiration interferes with the ability of baroreceptors to stimulate vagal motoneurons. They also

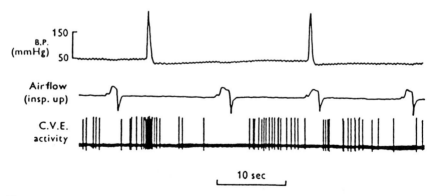

Figure 19   Effect of carotid pressure pulses delivered at different times in the cardiac cycle, on a single cardiac vagal unit (C.V.E.) in an anesthetized dog. (Reproduced with permission from Ref. 117.)

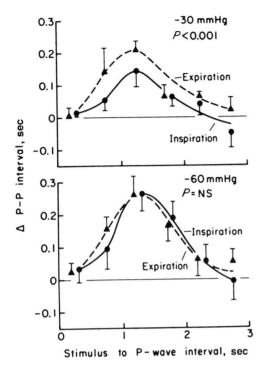

Figure 20 Average P-P interval prolongation caused by brief neck suction delivered at different times in the breathing cycle in six subjects. (Reproduced with permission from Ref. 18.)

indicate that this influence is finite; intense baroreceptor stimuli can override inspiratory inhibition of vagal firing.

The results shown in Figure 20 are related closely to those published much earlier by Anrep et al. (36). In their classic work, which was begun in Cambridge, finished in Cairo, and published in 1936, they measured inspiratory and expiratory R-R intervals during pressure elevations produced by infusions of epinephrine (the methods are not described explicitly). Anrep's data are adapted in Figure 21. At low arterial pressures, inspiratory and expiratory R-R intervals were equal, and sinus arrhythmia was absent. At higher pressures, inspiratory R-R intervals remained constant, but expiratory R-R intervals and, consequently, sinus arrhythmia increased. At the highest arterial pressures studied, inspiratory and expiratory R-R intervals were equal, and again, sinus arrhythmia was absent. These results document the importance of baroreceptor stimulation in generation of sinus arrhythmia, and they indicate that the ability of inspiration to prevent baroreceptor stimulation of vagal-cardiac motoneurons is limited. This conclusion supports the one drawn by Eckberg and Orshan (18) from their data obtained with human subjects and intense neck suction (Fig. 20).

One of the advantages of the neck suction technique is that very large

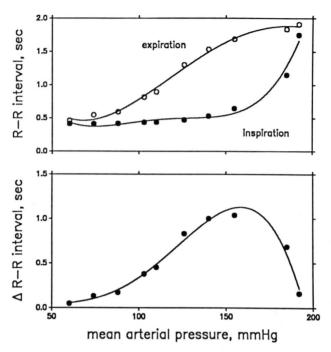

Figure 21 Inspiratory and expiratory R-R intervals during pharmacological arterial pressure changes in anesthetized dogs. (Adapted with permission from Ref. 36.)

pressure changes can be delivered. Unpublished data (D.L. Eckberg) suggest that it may be impossible to raise arterial pressure to high levels with pressor infusions, in healthy young subjects. However, the effects of lesser pressure changes can be studied in humans. Eckberg and co-workers (91) lowered and raised arterial pressure by modest levels with graded infusions of nitroprusside and phenyl-ephrine. Figure 22 depicts peak minus valley R-R interval changes as functions of mean R-R intervals during frequency-controlled breathing in nine healthy supine subjects. These data are very similar to the results of Anrep, shown in the left portion of the lower panel in Figure 21. They indicate that respiratory sinus arrhythmia is small with low levels of baroreceptor stimulation, and that sinus arrhythmia increases asymptotically with higher levels of baroreceptor stimulation. In this study, the range of average diastolic pressures achieved with drug infusions was only 70–89 mmHg; presumably, if pressures had been raised to higher levels, peak minus valley R-R interval changes would have declined, as they did in Anrep's study (Fig. 21).

There is a large published literature from animals and humans on central

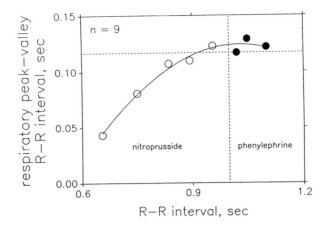

Figure 22 Average respiratory R-R interval changes during graded infusions of vasoactive drugs in nine subjects during controlled breathing. (Reproduced with permission from Ref. 91.)

biochemical mechanisms responsible for respiration-related fluctuations of vagal-cardiac efferent nerve activity. The following is a summary of some of the more important points.

First, vagal-cardiac motoneurons discharge with cardiac rhythms. Figure 23 shows an arterial pulse-triggered histogram of a cardiac vagal neuron in an aortic-nerve-denervated cat (119). Both carotids were open to flow in A, one was closed in B and C, and both were closed in D. These results indicate clearly that vagal-cardiac motoneurons receive information from baroreceptors. This observation led

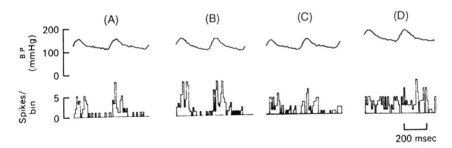

Figure 23 Femoral pulse-triggered histogram of cardiac vagal motoneuron firing in an aortic denervated, anesthetized cat. (A) Both carotids open to the circulation; (B and C) contralateral and ipsilateral carotid arteries occluded; (D) bilateral carotid artery occlusion. (Reproduced with permission from Ref. 119.)

McAllen and Spyer to speculate that imposition of respiratory rhythm on vagal firing occurs importantly at the membrane of vagal-cardiac motoneurons.

Second, firing of vagal-cardiac motoneurons is modulated by muscarinic cholinergic mechanisms. Figure 24 shows integrated phrenic nerve activity and respiration-triggered histograms of a single vagal motoneuron whose level of firing had been increased by iontophoresis of the excitant amino acid DL-homocysteic acid (120). Figure 24B shows that iontophoresis of acetylcholine

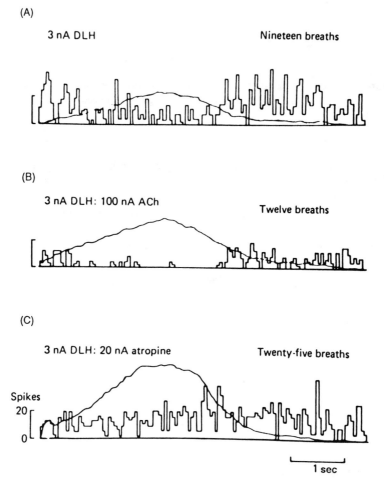

Figure 24   Cardiac vagal neuronal firing histogram in anesthetized cat during iontophoresis of DL homocysteic acid (DLH), acetylcholine (ACh), and atropine sulfate in one anesthetized cat. (Reproduced with permission from Ref. 120.)

reduced firing levels, in a way that provoked a clear respiratory periodicity (with nearly complete suppression of firing in late inspiration and early expiration). Figure 24C shows that iontophoresis of atropine nearly abolished respiration-related differences in firing levels. On the basis of these data, Gilbey and associates proposed that respiratory influences are imprinted on vagal firing at the membrane of the vagal-cardiac motoneuron, and that this influence is mediated by inhibitory cholinergic receptors.

Third, others have shown that intravenous atropine increases vagal-cardiac neuronal firing and R-R intervals. It has long been recognized that low atropine doses paradoxically slow the heart rate in humans (121). The study of Katona et al. (122) in anesthetized dogs showed that small atropine doses increase vagal activity and prolong R-R intervals. Large atropine doses further increase vagal-cardiac activity but, owing to their peripheral muscarinic blocking action, shorten R-R intervals. Raczkowska et al. (1) studied the effects of very low intravenous atropine doses in healthy subjects who controlled their tidal volumes and breathing frequencies. Their results are summarized in Figure 25. Atropine increased both

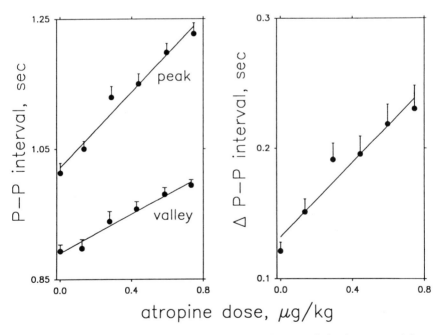

atropine dose, μg/kg

Figure 25 Average respiratory P-P interval changes after cumulative intravenous injections of atropine sulfate in six subjects during controlled breathing. (Reproduced with permission from Ref. 1.)

peak and valley P-P intervals (left) and increased respiratory sinus arrhythmia (right). A similar conclusion was reached by Alcalay and co-workers, who gauged the effects of low atropine doses on R-R interval changes with frequency-domain methods (123). These changes of P-P intervals are nearly identical to the peak-and-valley changes of vagal firing reported by Katona and co-workers (122). They suggest that atropine sulfate, which freely crosses the blood-brain barrier, occupies inhibitory cholinergic receptors and thereby increases vagal firing rates. [They do not exclude other mechanisms; low-dose atropine also may inhibit sino-atrial node firing by raising arterial pressure (a baroreflex mechanism) (122) or by augmenting responsiveness of the sinoatrial node to neuronally released acetylcholine (124).]

Raczkowska's results, obtained from cooperative human subjects, tend to discredit the proposal of Gilbey and associates (120) that respiratory modulation of vagal firing results from cholinergic inhibition restricted primarily to *inspiration*. If this were the case in humans, low atropine doses should increase inspiratory, and not change expiratory, vagal firing and, thus, reduce, not increase, respiratory sinus arrhythmia. Rather, these results suggest that vagal-cardiac motoneuron activity is inhibited by cholinergic mechanisms throughout the breathing cycle. When cholinergic receptors are occupied by atropine, their level of firing is increased in all phases of the respiratory cycle, but more in expiration (peak) than inspiration (valley).

C. Low-Frequency Rhythms

The right panels of Figure 9 depict the results of autoregressive power spectral analyses of the time series shown in the left panel. These data support a notion gained from visual inspection that in this subject, respiration occurred much more frequently than other periodicities. Particularly noteworthy is the low-frequency (0.1 Hz, or one every 10 sec) periodicity in arterial pressure, sympathetic, and R-R interval tracings. In anesthetized animals, low-frequency arterial pressure waves result from low-frequency firing of spinal sympathetic motoneurons (22,125). Low-frequency R-R interval fluctuations are thought to represent, in part, baroreflex-mediated changes of efferent sympathetic (60) and vagal-cardiac nerve traffic (25).

The autonomic mediation of low-frequency human R-R interval rhythms is controversial. Cholinergic blockade with large doses of atropine sulfate nearly abolishes all R-R interval fluctuations in supine subjects, including those at respiratory and lower frequencies (1,65,126), and beta-adrenergic blockade with propranolol reduces (but does not abolish) R-R interval fluctuations centered at about 0.1 Hz (23). Some workers consider low-frequency R-R interval fluctuations to be mediated almost *exclusively* by changes of sympathetic outflow (23,127). Others, however, consider that the great reduction of low-frequency R-R interval fluctuations after large doses of atropine point toward an important vagal contribution to these rhythms (65,126).

Koh and associates (126) recently explored this issue in an unusual human model: patients with clinically complete cervical spinal cord transections. Although such patients have intact spinal sympathetic motoneurons and peripheral sympathetic pathways, they lack connections between spinal sympathetic motoneurons and the medullary neurons that supply most of their stimulatory drive (128). Koh measured the influence of arterial pressure on fast-Fourier transform R-R interval power spectra in supine tetraplegic and age-matched healthy subjects, during frequency and tidal volume controlled breathing. The main results are summarized in the insets of Figure 26. Low-frequency R-R interval power varied *directly* with arterial pressure in tetraplegic subjects (inset, upper panel). Had these fluctuations resulted in some way from a baroreflex mechanism (I am aware of no spinal baroreflex mechanism that exists independent of medullary influences), sympathetic-cardiac traffic should have varied *inversely*, not directly, with arterial pressure. Low-frequency R-R interval power did not vary appreciably in the healthy subjects (inset, lower panel). Further proof that in tetraplegic patients, low-frequency R-R interval fluctuations result from the ebb and flow of vagal traffic comes from their disappearance after large doses of atropine, as shown in the inserts of Figure 27.

VI. Influence of Breathing Parameters on Autonomic Neural Outflow

Figures 6–9 document certain temporal relations between breathing (spontaneous or voluntarily controlled) and efferent autonomic neural outflow. As mentioned, these records do not necessarily indicate that the relations between breathing and autonomic traffic are fixed, or that the patterns of autonomic outflow shown are caused by breathing. Before the influence of breathing parameters on autonomic outflow is discussed, some attention will be paid to how *absence of breathing* or *absence of control of breathing* affects autonomic outflow.

Figure 28 depicts average autonomic activities of one subject during held expiration, in data sweeps triggered by late expiratory threshold crossings. These data (129) document a progressive augmentation of muscle sympathetic nerve activity and arterial pressure, and a nearly constant R-R interval, in the absence of breathing. In an article published earlier (55), constant R-R intervals during held expiration were taken to reflect constant levels of efferent vagal-cardiac nerve traffic. The data in Figure 28, however, suggest that since arterial pressure rises during held expiration (presumably as a consequence of increasing sympathetic traffic), vagal-cardiac activity must also rise. This record does not indicate why, in the absence of breathing, muscle sympathetic nerve activity and blood pressure

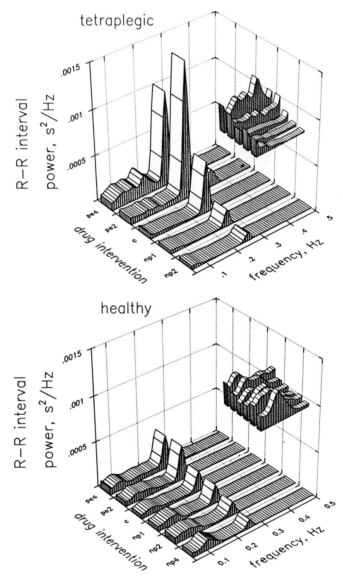

Figure 26 Average fast-Fourier transform R-R interval power spectra in eight patients with clinically complete cervical spinal cord transections and 10 age-matched healthy subjects at different arterial pressures during controlled breathing. pe4 and pe2 = phenyl-ephrine infusion at rates of 0.4 and 0.2 μg/kg/min, respectively; c = control; np1, np2, and np4 = nitroprusside infusion at rates of 0.1, 0.2, and 0.4 μg/kg/min, respectively. (Insets) R-R interval spectral power between 0.05 and 0.15 Hz, displayed at the same gain. (Reproduced with permission from Ref. 126.)

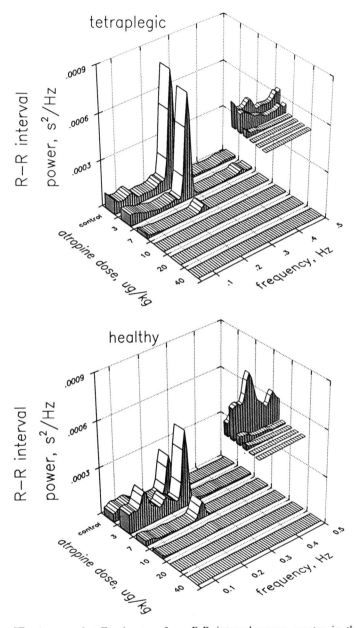

Figure 27 Average fast-Fourier transform R-R interval power spectra in the same subjects as Figure 25, during graded intravenous infusions of atropine sulfate. Insets show low-frequency power at the same gain as in Figure 25. (Reproduced with permission from Ref. 126.)

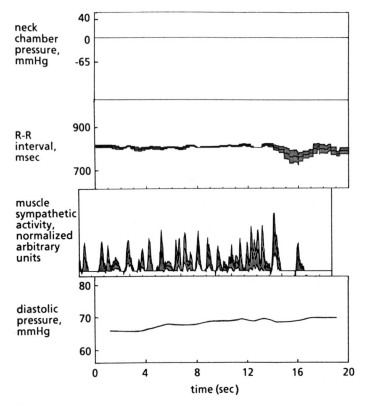

Figure 28 Muscle sympathetic nerve activity in one subject during held expiration. Data sweeps were triggered at the end of expiration (time zero). (Reproduced with permission from Ref. 129.)

rise. This record also does not indicate what rhythmic changes might have occurred, had held expiration been maintained. According to the much more comprehensive analysis published by Penáz and Burianek (130), the data shown in Figure 28 comprise only part of a rhythm that was truncated by the end of data collection.

The question of whether voluntary control of respiration influences autonomic neural outflow has not been answered definitively. The most careful study of this issue was published by Hirsch and Bishop (40). These authors (whose main results are depicted in Figure 34) compared respiratory R-R interval fluctuations during controlled and spontaneous breathing at similar rates. They concluded that voluntary control of breathing frequency and tidal volume do not alter respiratory peak minus valley R-R interval fluctuations. This conclusion was challenged by

Pagani et al. (23), who made the case (on the basis of much more limited data) that voluntary control of respiration increases R-R interval power at the respiratory-frequency and decreases R-R interval power at low frequencies. This conclusion was based on autoregressive analyses of R-R interval power in 16 young subjects at spontaneous and controlled breathing rates of about 19.8 and 15.6 breaths/min. Tidal volume was measured (but not controlled) in seven of these subjects. In this study, voluntary control of breathing led to small reductions of tidal volume and transcutaneous P_{CO_2}.

The profound influence of breathing control on autoregressive respiratory and R-R interval power in one subject is shown in Figure 29 (JA Taylor, JR Halliwill, J Hayano, and DL Eckberg, unpublished). In this subject whose breathing was highly variable, energy in both respiratory and R-R interval power was distributed over a range from 0 to 0.5 Hz. The extremely narrow band of respiratory power (right upper panel) illustrates how exquisitely human volunteers can control respiratory frequency.

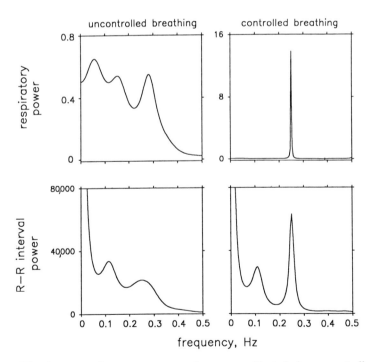

Figure 29 Autoregressive power spectra from one subject during uncontrolled and controlled (at 15 breaths/min) breathing in one subject. (JA Taylor, JR Halliwill, J Hayano, and DL Eckberg, unpublished.)

Data published by Eckberg et al. (20), shown in Figure 30, complement those reported by Hirsch and Bishop and provide some indication regarding how voluntary control of breathing influences muscle *sympathetic* nerve activity. (In this record obtained from eight healthy supine subjects, inspiration began at time zero.) These limited data, and the more comprehensive data published by Hirsch and Bishop (40), suggest that voluntary control of respiratory frequency and tidal volume do not modify human vagal and sympathetic nerve activity importantly. Clearly, however, as the study of Pagani and co-workers (23) suggests, this question deserves further study.

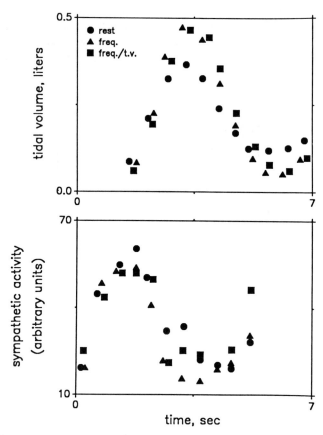

Figure 30   Average tidal volume and peroneal muscle sympathetic nerve activity from eight healthy supine subjects during uncontrolled breathing (rest), frequency-controlled (freq.), and frequency- and tidal volume-controlled breathing (freq./t.v.). (Reproduced with permission from Ref. 20.)

Figures 31–35 address the simple question, How does respiratory rate influence R-R (or P-P) intervals? Figure 31 (TE Brown, LA Beightol, J Koh, and DL Eckberg, unpublished) shows inspiratory volume, R-R intervals, and R-R interval probability distributions measured in one supine subject at three respiratory rates. These data document an inverse relation between R-R interval fluctuations and breathing rate. At very slow breathing rates (left), R-R interval (and presumably vagal-cardiac neural traffic) fluctuations were much greater than at rapid breathing rates (right). Probability distributions (lowest panels) show that during slow breathing, there was a preponderance of short R-R intervals, and during rapid breathing, there was a preponderance of long R-R intervals. This shift of frequency distributions suggests that as breathing rate increases, vagal withdrawal becomes progressively less complete. [These data do not indicate why vagal withdrawal is incomplete at rapid breathing rates; the observation may indicate that vagal-cardiac firing lasts longer than the breathing interval, or (more likely) that decay of vagal effects extends over more than one breath because of the time constants of hydrolysis of acetylcholine.] Figure 32 (42) depicts average

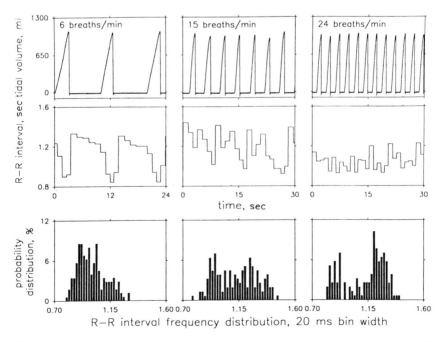

Figure 31 Inspiratory volume (measured with an ultrasonic transit-time analyzer), R-R interval, and R-R interval probability distribution in nine subjects at three rates of controlled breathing. (TE Brown, LA Beightol, J Koh, and DL Eckberg, unpublished.)

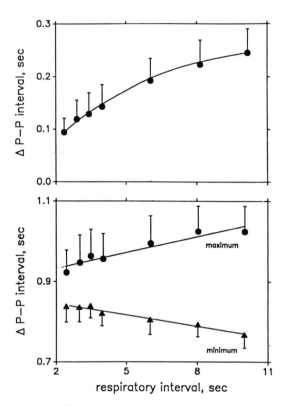

Figure 32 Average (± SEM) respiratory peak and valley P-P intervals at different breathing intervals and a constant tidal volume in six healthy supine subjects. (Reproduced with permission from Ref. 42.)

measurements obtained from six healthy supine subjects during tidal volume controlled breathing. The top panel shows that respiration-related (peak minus valley) P-P interval fluctuations increase directly (and asymptotically) as breathing interval increases (as breathing rate slows). The bottom panel indicates that respiratory sinus arrhythmia increased at lower breathing intervals because maximum P-P intervals increased and minimum P-P intervals shortened.

The main responses of the single subject reported in the early study of Angelone and Coulter (44) are shown in Figure 33. This seated volunteer breathed at rates between about 1 and 40 breaths/min. Although tidal volume, estimated from changes of thoracic circumference, was controlled, P_{CO_2} and P_{O_2} were not measured. It is apparent from this early study, that at very rapid breathing rates (extreme right), heart rate is almost monotonic, and that at slower breathing rates

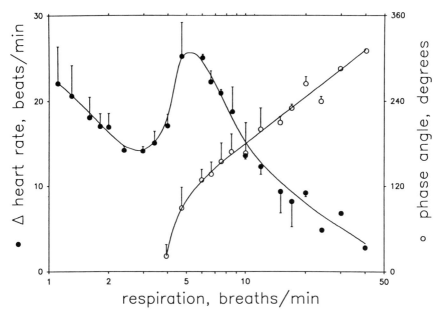

respiration, breaths/min

Figure 33 Average (± SEM) respiratory changes of heart rate and breathing frequency in one subject. For phase angle, 0 degrees indicates that heart rate speeding began at the beginning of expiration. (Reproduced with permission from Ref. 44.)

(middle), heart rate is widely variable. Angelone and Coulter suggested that the peak heart rate fluctuations that occurred at about 5 breaths/min represented "system resonance." The reasons for the reductions of heart rate changes at breathing rates below 5 breaths/min are not clear from this study. It seems likely that respiratory gases changed importantly as this subject's breathing rate approached 1 breath/min. The change of phase angle (open circles) is discussed below.

Hirsch and Bishop (40) published a comprehensive analysis of the influence of both respiratory rate and tidal volume on respiratory peak minus valley R-R interval changes, in 17 subjects, and published their subjects' responses as Bode plots (logs of both respiratory frequency and heart rate changes). Their results are summarized in Figure 34. As in the study of Angelone and Coulter (Fig. 33), peak heart rate changes occurred at a respiratory rate of about 5 breaths/min, and progressively smaller heart rate changes occurred at faster breathing frequencies. The data in Figure 34 indicate that tidal volume contributes importantly to respiratory sinus arrhythmia; when tidal volume was increased from 0.5 to 1.0 liters, peak heart rate fluctuations nearly doubled.

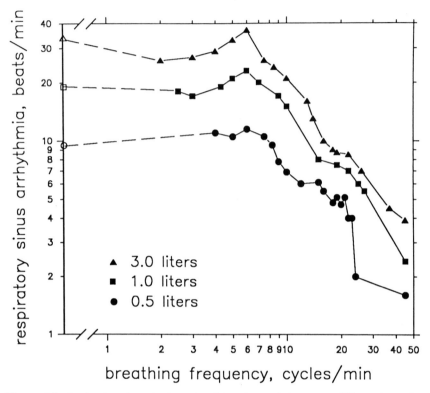

Figure 34   Bode plot of respiration-related R-R interval changes at different breathing frequencies and tidal volumes. (Adapted with permission from Ref. 40.)

Figure 35 shows fast Fourier transform R-R interval power spectral densities (6) from nine healthy supine subjects who breathed at a constant tidal volume (about 1000 ml). This frequency-domain analysis yielded data qualitatively similar to the time-domain analyses shown in Figures 33 and 34. It indicates that R-R interval fluctuations are large at slow breathing rates and are small at fast (more than 10 breaths/min) breathing rates. [This record also illustrates an aspect of R-R interval rhythms that time-domain methods cannot show: as respiratory rate slows, respiratory-frequency R-R interval fluctuations merge with low-frequency fluctuations (at about 0.1 Hz).] Figure 36 depicts average R-R intervals for the subjects whose power spectra are shown in Figure 35. (This figure also shows average R-R intervals measured when subjects were breathing with tidal volumes of about 1500 ml.) Brown and co-workers concluded from these data that

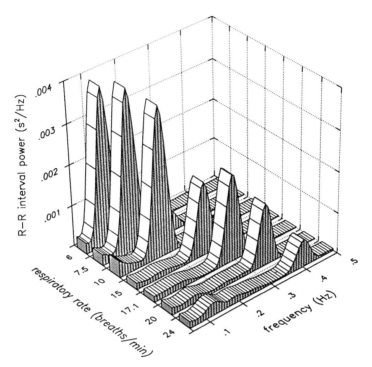

Figure 35 Fast-fourier transform R-R interval power spectra from nine supine healthy subjects breathing at different rates and a constant tidal volume. (Reproduced with permission from Ref. 6.)

changes of breathing rate distribute vagal firing within breaths, but do not alter mean levels of vagal firing.

The important influence of respiratory frequency on R-R intervals and systolic and diastolic pressures is also illustrated by the exquisite Wigner distributions published by Novak and her colleagues (90), shown in Figure 37. These results, obtained during programmed breathing at rates between about 3 and 28 breaths/min, document inverse relations between all signals and breathing frequency. [As the Wigner distribution of respiration (top, left) indicates, tidal volume was not controlled; therefore, these data provide no information on the contributions of tidal volume to the changes registered.]

The open circles in Figure 33 (44) depict phase angle changes between heart rate and respiration at different breathing rates. According to the scheme used by Angelone and Coulter, there was a 0 phase angle when heart rate began to increase at the beginning of expiration. Thus, the phase angle of about 180 degrees found

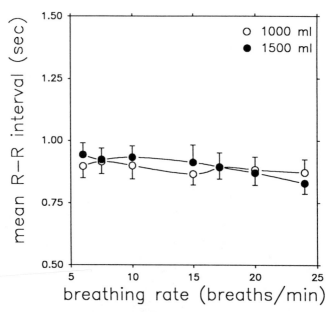

Figure 36   Average R-R intervals (± SEM) for the same subjects whose power spectra are depicted in Figure 35, during breathing at two different tidal volumes. (Reproduced with permission from Ref. 6.)

at a breathing rate of about 10 breaths/min indicated that at this breathing rate, heart rate began to speed at the beginning of inspiration. Angelone and Coulter considered that different phase angles at different breathing rates prove that respiratory sinus arrhythmia is frequency-dependent. They did not speculate about what mechanisms are responsible for this frequency-dependent relation.

Eckberg (42) depicted temporal relations between respiration and P-P interval changes as Lissajous figures. Figure 38 shows average responses of six subjects who controlled their tidal volumes and breathed at seven different rates. This figure indicates that at breathing intervals of 6 sec or more (10 breaths/ min or less), P-P intervals shorten during inspiration and lengthen during expiration. However, at the shortest breathing interval, 2.5 sec (24 breaths/min), P-P intervals lengthen during inspiration and shorten during expiration. A plot of phase angle as a function of respiratory interval (not shown) yielded data that were qualitatively (if not quantitatively) similar to those of Angelone and Coulter, shown in Figure 33; P-P interval shortening began in expiration at very slow breathing rates, and at the beginning of inspiration at a breathing rate of about 10 breaths/min. Eckberg speculated that reductions of vagal-cardiac motoneuron firing always begin in

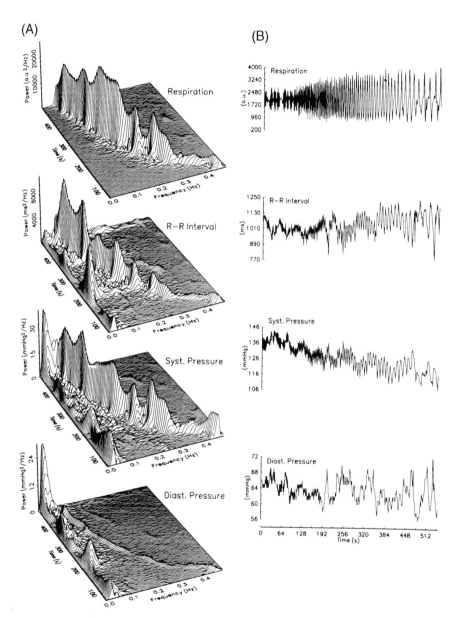

Figure 37 Wigner distributions of signals from one subject during ramped, frequency controlled breathing. (Reproduced with permission from Ref. 90.)

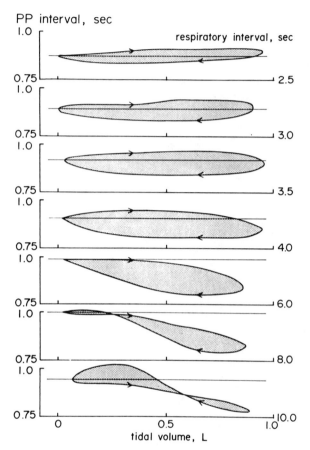

Figure 38   P-P interval changes of six subjects at different breathing intervals, plotted as Lissajous figures. (Reproduced with permission from Ref. 42.)

expiration, but that the timing of these reductions moves progressively earlier in expiration as breathing rate slows. These findings were duplicated by Saul and co-workers (61), who measured heart rate fluctuations in subjects whose respiratory rates and tidal volumes varied randomly [as "white noise" (131)]. These authors concurred with Eckberg's speculation that changes of breathing frequency alter the timing of vagal-cardiac motoneuron firing.

Saul and co-workers published a subsequent study (132) that ingeniously explored mechanisms responsible for respiration-related heart rate periodicities. As in the earlier study (61), respiratory frequencies and (derivatively) tidal volumes were varied randomly by subjects, who followed computer-generated cues, and heart rate (not R-R interval) was measured. Saul studied 14 healthy subjects in supine and standing positions before and after large doses of autonomic blocking drugs. They [and Pagani et al. (23) before them] reasoned that contributions from sympathetic mechanisms might be increased (and, therefore, recognized more easily) in the standing position (which would also reduce vagal contributions). Lying and standing measurements were repeated after administration of blocking doses of propranolol, atropine, or both. Saul characterized supine subjects after propranolol as being "purely vagal" and standing subjects after atropine as being "purely sympathetic."

Saul's principal findings are summarized in Figures 39 and 40. Figure 39 shows the average transfer function, expressed as heart rate change per liter tidal volume, in the upper panels, and the average transfer phase in the lower panels. (Saul designated zero phase as occurring when heart rate speeding coincided with the onset of inspiration.) In the purely *vagal* state (left panels), gain of the transfer function was high, and a peak occurred at a breathing rate of about 0.12 Hz (about 7 breaths/min). There was a modest reduction of transfer function gain at more rapid breathing rates. The phase angle in the vagal state was positive [probably indicating that heart rate speeding began during expiration (52)] and nearly constant over breathing ranges greater than about 2 breaths/min. In the purely

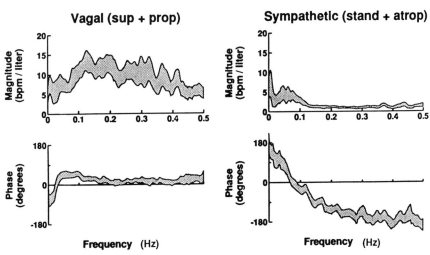

Figure 39 Average (± SEM) inspiratory lung volume–heart rate transfer function gain and phase during white noise breathing in 14 healthy subjects in supine and standing positions, without autonomic blockade. bpm = beats/min; sup = supine; prop = propranolol; atrop = atropine sulfate. See text for discussion. (Reproduced with permission from Ref. 132.)

sympathetic state (right panels), gain of the transfer function was much smaller and was nearly zero at breathing frequencies above about 0.15 Hz. The great decline of transfer function gain after about 0.1 Hz emphasizes the fact that the sinoatrial node functions as a low-pass filter in response to fluctuations of neuronally released norepinephrine. The phase angle in the sympathetic state approached 180 degrees at very slow breathing rates and declined steadily, to almost −180 degrees, at faster breathing rates. Thus, in the sympathetic state at very slow breathing rates, (presumably) heart rate speeds with inspiration, but with a 3–5 sec delay. At more rapid breathing rates, heart rate speeding begins progressively later in the respiratory cycle. These data suggest that inspiration reduces vagal- and sympathetic-cardiac neuronal firing at all breathing frequencies, and that the phase shifts that occur at different breathing rates reflect differential responsiveness of the sinoatrial node to released acetylcholine and norepinephrine.

Figure 40 shows average transfer function magnitudes and phases (without autonomic blockade) in the supine and standing positions. In this mixed (that is, physiological) autonomic state, heart rate changes at breathing frequencies above about 0.15 Hz had essentially zero phase lag and were, therefore, almost exclusively vagal. Heart rate transfer function gain was less in the standing, than in the supine, position. These data suggest that baseline levels of vagal firing were less in the standing position, but that some vagal activity remained to be modulated by respiration. Heart rate fluctuations during breathing frequencies below 0.15 Hz were nearly the same in supine and standing positions, presumably because reductions of vagal oscillations were offset by increases of sympathetic oscillations.

Figure 41 shows average transfer function and phases for instantaneous lung volume (ILV) and arterial blood pressure (ABP) and for systolic, diastolic, and

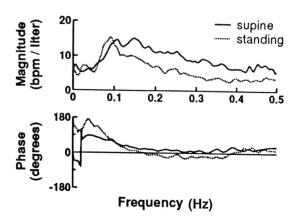

Figure 40   Data similar to those depicted in Figure 39 in supine and standing positions. (Reproduced with permission from Ref. 132.)

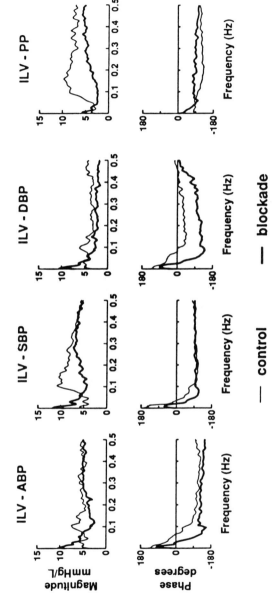

Figure 41 Average transfer function gain and phase in supine subjects before (control) and after dual autonomic blockade with propranolol, 0.2 mg/kg, and atropine, 0.03 mg/kg. ILV = inspiratory lung volume; ABP = arterial blood pressure; SBP = systolic blood pressure; DBP = diastolic blood pressure; PP = pulse pressure. (Reproduced with permission from Ref. 132.)

pulse pressures (SBP, DBP, PP). Dual autonomic blockade reduced the gain of transfer functions for systolic and pulse pressures (second and fourth panels), but only for breathing frequencies below about 0.25 Hz (15 breaths/min). The difference between control and blockade conditions represents the contribution of autonomically mediated heart rate changes to arterial pressure fluctuations. Autonomic neural contributions are important at slow breathing rates and minor at rapid breathing rates (above about 0.3 Hz, or 18 breaths/min). These data provide compelling evidence that both mechanical hemodynamic changes *and* autonomic heart rate changes related to breathing are responsible for respiration-related systolic and pulse pressure changes.

Figure 42 illustrates the average pulse pressure transfer function gain and phase in supine and standing positions. Standing greatly increased the pulse pressure transfer function gain. Several of the observations of Saul and co-workers shown above (132) confirm results published much earlier by Dornhorst et al. (133) (whom Saul does not cite). Dornhorst's study also showed (1) that the amplitude of arterial pressure changes is greater at slower than faster breathing rates, (2) that the timing of arterial pressure changes within the respiratory cycle depends on breathing rate, and (3) that blood pressure fluctuations are greater in the standing than the supine position.

Use of "white noise" breathing to study human periodicities defies predictions [that it cannot be done (134,135)] and offers the prospect that a variety of autonomic mechanisms can be characterized and understood in a new way, with efficiency and power. Clearly, white noise breathing deserves careful consideration. I have several theoretical concerns about the approach described by Berger

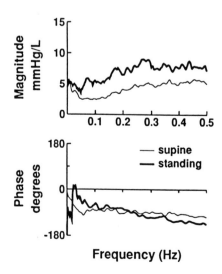

Figure 42 Average inspiratory lung volume–heart rate transfer function gain after dual autonomic blockade, in two positions. (Reproduced with permission from Ref. 132.)

and co-workers (131). First, their published time series showing the frequency and depth of breathing do not appear to be very *"white."* In some [for example, their Fig. 1 (132)], there is a preponderance of slow, deep breathing and a relative dearth of rapid breathing. (In this example, there were many breaths of about 1 liter, at a rate of about 6/min.) Moreover, it is obvious from these records that the breathing pattern is grossly unphysiological; very deep, slow breaths are succeeded by shallow, rapid breaths that are initiated before complete exhalation. Second, white noise breathing blurs distinctions between low- and respiratory-frequency power; Figure 35 shows that slow breathing leads to huge increases of low-frequency spectral power. Third, the potential contributions from chemoreceptors to autonomic patterns provoked by white noise breathing are unknown. Surely, during such slow and fast, deep and shallow breathing, chemoreceptor activity varies widely. The problem posed by chemoreceptors is not unique to protocols involving white noise breathing, and potentially confounding influences from arterial and central chemoreceptors in studies of respiratory sinus arrhythmia are often ignored. Although I did not stress it (42), I dealt with the chemoreceptor problem by obtaining measurements at different respiratory rates during *mild hypercapnia*; in my study, P_{CO_2} was measured when subjects breathed at the slowest rate and maintained when subjects breathed at more rapid rates. Finally, it is unclear why Berger, Saul, and Cohen characterize transfer functions in terms of heart rate, rather than R-R interval. Since R-R interval is a linear function of vagal-cardiac nerve traffic (8,52), heart rate (its reciprocal) manifestly is not. Since the white noise technique is used under circumstances in which baseline heart rates are systematically different (in lying and standing positions), comparisons are made on different portions of a curve. The practical importance of these objections to Berger's technique is unknown.

VII. R-R Interval Periodicities as "Probes" to Quantitate Human Autonomic Outflow

Much of the great current interest in human R-R interval (and, to a lesser extent, arterial pressure) fluctuations arises importantly from the belief that these fluctuations can be used to gauge efferent vagal- and sympathetic-cardiac nerve traffic. This usage derives from the seminal study of Katona and Jih, published in 1975 (7), which documented (in anesthetized dogs) a linear correlation between single-fiber vagal-cardiac nerve activity and respiratory peak minus valley R-R interval changes. Two conditions in Katona's study merit emphasis: respiratory rates and depths were constant (because of general anesthesia), and vagal-cardiac nerve fibers were silent during inspiration. Although many workers have based their human studies on this article, it is unlikely that either of the important conditions in the dogs Katona and Jih studied obtains in conscious humans.

First, many studies have shown that human respiration is variable. [This issue was ably reviewed by van den Aardweg and Karemaker (136).] Bendixen et al. (137) documented great variability of breathing patterns among healthy subjects (and systematic slowing of respiration during the first hour of recording). Grossman and Wientjes (138) showed that substantial percentages of breaths occur at frequencies above 20 and below 9 breaths/min. Their findings suggest that the wide-band respiratory spectral power shown in Figure 29 is not uncommon. Lenfant (139) found slow oscillations of breathing in all the subjects he studied. Figure 43 illustrates the breathing pattern of one subject in whom such fluctuations were particularly striking. Priban (140) found that breathing pattern is variable in subjects selected for the constancy of their breathing. Tobin (141) found that ventilation is variable from day to day, and Siegelová and Kopècny (156) found that ventilation is variable from year to year.

Second, certain populations have breathing patterns that are *systematically* different from those of other populations. Elderly subjects have more day-to-day variability of breathing than young subjects (141). Women have more sighs than men and breathe more deeply and slowly (137). Tetraplegic patients also have

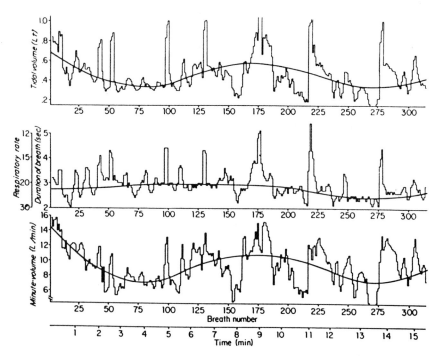

Figure 43 Respiratory parameters during quiet breathing in one subject. (Reproduced with permission from Ref 139.)

more rapid breathing than healthy subjects (142), presumably because they have impaired scalene, intercostal, and abdominal respiratory muscle function. Since breathing pattern affects R-R interval fluctuations profoundly (see above), it is likely that systematic differences of breathing patterns in different populations translate into systematic differences of R-R interval fluctuations.

Brown and co-workers (6) surveyed published literature to determine how investigators who report frequency-domain analyses of R-R intervals deal with the nettlesome influence of respiration. In many studies, including those involving ambulatory Holter monitoring, infant subjects, and psychophysiological interventions, control of respiration is impossible. However, in studies in which control of respiration was possible, only a small minority (11%) involved control of both respiratory rate and tidal volume. Brown's analysis indicates that in the great majority of published research involving frequency-domain analyses of R-R intervals, the degree to which respiration confounds the results is unknown.

Third, there is reason to believe also that in contrast with the anesthetized dogs studied by Katona and Jih (7), conscious humans have persistent vagal effects during inspiration. This was shown simply and elegantly by Kollai and Mizsei (143). They reasoned that if vagal restraint is absent during inspiration, maneuvers known to reduce vagal activity should not shorten R-R intervals to levels below those occurring during inspiration. They found that after large intravenous propranolol doses, handgrip, deep breathing, and standing all reduced R-R intervals to levels below inspiratory levels measured during quiet breathing. Moreover, they found that administration of large atropine doses (after propranolol) also reduced R-R intervals to levels much below those occurring during inspiration.

These observations raise the question, What is the gold standard for measurement of vagal-cardiac outflow in humans? In the absence of direct vagus nerve recordings, workers have relied primarily on measurements of R-R interval shortening after large atropine sulfate doses (144). [Although this measure seems to be the best available (glycopyrrolate may be better), it is not ideal; large atropine doses cause an "excess tachycardia" that cannot be explained on the basis of blockade of cholinergic muscarinic receptors (145).]

There is a small literature, comprising as few as two articles (16,146), in which different time- and frequency-domain R-R interval analysis methods have been compared. [One subheading in Grossman's article on sinus arrhythmia (RSA) is, "Quantification techniques for estimating RSA: is there a Rolls Royce of RSA or are all major estimates equally reliable Toyotas?"] Both articles indicate that R-R interval standard deviations, respiratory peak minus valley changes, and power spectra at respiratory frequencies yield similar information. This suggests that in resting humans during laboratory recording sessions, most R-R interval variability occurs at respiratory frequencies. Hayano (16) showed that all these measures of R-R interval fluctuation correlate well with the R-R interval shortening that occurs after large atropine doses. However, Hayano found no correlation between postatropine R-R interval shortening and *relative* spectral power [respiratory power divided by total power (23)].

Methods used to estimate *sympathetic*-cardiac traffic also are not free of controversy. Although sympathetic traffic to human skin and muscle vascular beds can be measured directly, sympathetic traffic to the heart cannot be (or, at least, has not been) measured. Therefore, other indexes are proposed as substitutes for direct measurements of human sympathetic-cardiac nerve activity. These include measurements of cardiac norepinephrine spillover (70) and noninvasive measurements of R-R interval spectral power at low frequencies. Since studies of myocardial norepinephrine spillover are highly invasive and require coronary sinus cannulation, most attempts to estimate sympathetic traffic to the human heart are based on analyses of R-R interval (or heart rate) fluctuations.

As mentioned, although human (muscle) sympathetic nerve traffic fluctuates on a breath-by-breath basis, sluggishness of sinoatrial node responses to released norepinephrine greatly dampens respiratory-frequency R-R interval fluctuations. Therefore, attention has focused on low (about 0.05–0.15 Hz) R-R interval fluctuations, which occur slowly enough to reflect changes of sympathetic nerve traffic. The rationale for this usage is strong in that low-frequency *arterial pressure* waves are mediated by low-frequency sympathetic nerve activity (22), and maneuvers known to increase net sympathetic traffic increase low-frequency sympathetic firing. This is illustrated very clearly by a subject studied by Burke et al. (147), whose muscle sympathetic nerve activity is depicted in Figure 44. The rationale for this usage is weak, however, in that low-frequency R-R interval fluctuations are mediated by vagal as well as sympathetic mechanisms. Some of the evidence for this assertion was discussed above. Additional evidence comes from direct recordings of vagal-cardiac nerve traffic in animals, which document the presence of low-frequency fluctuations (25,127). Figure 45 depicts the only published (autoregressive) power spectral analysis of R-R intervals and concurrent sympathetic- and vagal-cardiac nerve traffic.

In a series of articles (23,127,148,149), Malliani and co-workers have promoted use of the ratio of low- to high-frequency autoregressive R-R interval spectral power* as an index of "vagosympathetic balance." Their argument for the usefulness of this measure is based primarily on (1) the increase of the low- to high-frequency R-R interval spectral power ratio that occurs during augmentation of sympathetic (and reduction of vagal) activity by standing or pharmacological arterial pressure reductions; (2) articles published by Inoue and co-workers (150,151) which show that low-frequency arterial pressure and R-R interval waves are absent in patients with complete cervical spinal cord injuries, who lack

---

*The actual value they report is low-frequency power (if >5% of the total) divided by the sum of all peaks whose power is >5% of the total.

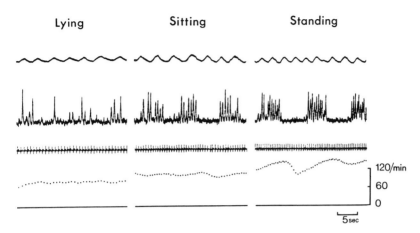

Figure 44 Respiration (top tracing), muscle sympathetic nerve activity (second tracing), electrocardiogram, and heart rate in one subject in three positions. (Reproduced with permission from Ref. 147.)

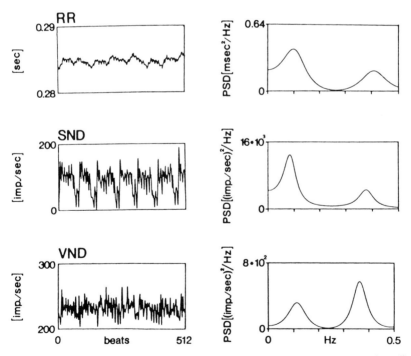

Figure 45 Time series of R-R interval (RR) and sympathetic (SND) and vagal-cardiac (VND) nerve activities and corresponding autoregressive power spectra in one ventilated decerebrate cat. (Reproduced with permission from Ref. 127.)

medullary stimulation of spinal sympathetic motoneurons; and (3) abolition of low-frequency R-R spectral interval power responses to nitroglycerin by sympathectomy in conscious dogs. In my view, Malliani's elegant new methodology has entered the mainstream of clinical research without having been critically challenged. This method has several serious, possibly fatal, flaws.

1.   Low-frequency R-R interval fluctuations cannot be taken simply as indexes of resting sympathetic traffic, because they reflect vagal, as well as sympathetic, neural changes. As mentioned, Inoue's observation that spinal patients lack low-frequency arterial pressure and R-R interval power was not replicated by Koh and co-workers (126), who found that low-frequency R-R interval power is present in tetraplegic patients. A second challenge came from a study published by Saul and co-workers (69), who reported no significant association between low-frequency R-R interval power and sympathetic traffic in healthy supine human volunteers. During infusions of saline in this study (that is, under control conditions), there was no correlation between low-frequency R-R interval power and sympathetic traffic (relative, as well as absolute). During elevations of arterial pressure produced by graded infusions of phenylephrine, sympathetic traffic declined (as expected), but low-frequency R-R interval power remained constant. This probably occurred because as pressure rose and sympathetic outflow fell, vagal outflow increased. Finally, although in some subjects, graded reductions of arterial pressure produced parallel increases of low-frequency R-R interval power and sympathetic nerve activity, in other subjects, there was no such correlation. A major weakness of Saul's study was that it involved measurements of sympathetic traffic to *skeletal muscle* rather than to the *heart*. A study published subsequently, however, provides some support for Saul's use of muscle, as a surrogate for cardiac sympathetic nerve traffic. Wallin and associates (70) showed that resting myocardial norepinephrine spillover correlates significantly with resting muscle sympathetic nerve activity, and that both measurements increase in parallel during exercise and mental arithmetic.

2.   The concept of "vagosympathetic balance" is at once attractive and vague. It is attractive in that it implies orderliness, symmetry, and balance in human cardiovascular regulation. This concept is vague, however, in that it is a construct whose existence has not been proven, and whose attributes therefore are unknown. The concept raises several questions. One is, What is the sensor that measures sympathetic and vagal activities and adjusts their levels to maintain their postulated equipoise? Another question is, Does "vagosympathetic balance" exist? I am not aware of any published evidence that documents a reciprocal relation between levels of vagal and sympathetic outflow in healthy populations. This issue was studied by Porter and colleagues (110), who estimated vagal-cardiac outflow with R-R interval standard deviations and measured (muscle) sympathetic outflow directly or estimated sympathetic outflow with antecubital vein plasma norepinephrine measurements, in supine healthy subjects and patients

with heart failure. Porter's results are summarized in Figure 46. In healthy subjects, there was no correlation between R-R interval standard deviations and either plasma norepinephrine levels or muscle sympathetic nerve activity (not shown). (However, in heart failure patients there was a strong reciprocal relation between R-R interval standard deviations and norepinephrine levels.)

A third question is, If there is no reciprocity between vagal and sympathetic outflows in healthy resting subjects, are there reciprocal *changes* in these measures in subjects during physiological interventions? This seems likely with arterial pressure changes. Most healthy resting humans lie on the "linear" portions of their arterial pressure-autonomic response relations (101), and when arterial pressure changes, vagal and sympathetic outflows usually change in opposite directions (73,101). However, not all subjects lie on the "linear" portions of their arterial pressure-autonomic response relations; champion athletes operate in the saturation range (152) and heart failure patients operate in the threshold region (110) of their carotid arterial pressure-vagal cardiac response relations. Also, reciprocal changes of sympathetic and vagal outflows do not always occur. Burke et al. (147) showed that in some subjects, both muscle sympathetic nerve activity and R-R intervals decrease when they stand. Such changes are not necessarily linear, however. For example, in some subjects, small arterial pressure increases effectively silence muscle sympathetic neurons (91), and further pressure increases are answered exclusively by increases of vagal-cardiac nerve activity. Under such circumstances, the ratio between sympathetic and vagal neural outflows should not

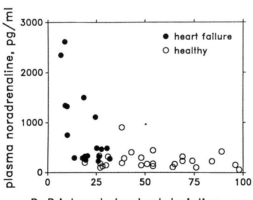

R−R interval standard deviation, msec

Figure 46 Average R-R interval standard deviations and plasma norepinephrine levels in 18 heart failure patients and 38 healthy subjects, during controlled breathing. The relation between R-R interval standard deviations and muscle sympathetic nerve activity, measured in a smaller number of subjects, was similar. (Reproduced with permission from Ref. 110.)

change linearly throughout arterial pressure increases. Moreover, there is abundant evidence from animals and humans that sympathetic and vagal cardiovascular outflows sometimes increase or decrease together. Koizumi et al. (153) documented a variety of circumstances in which sympathetic and vagal traffic covaries in anesthetized dogs. Fagius and Sundlöf (154) showed that during simulated diving (immersion of the face in cold water), sympathetic and vagal traffic increase together. Finally, Figure 8 shows that during quiet breathing, sympathetic and vagal outflows change together, not reciprocally. Thus, any measurement that is predicated on the notion that sympathetic and vagal neural outflows change reciprocally is likely to be suspect under certain circumstances.

    3.   The contribution of respiration to low- and high-frequency R-R interval ratios cannot be ignored. Figure 35 shows that small changes of respiratory frequency, between 10 and 15 breaths/min, provoke major changes of R-R interval spectral power. This figure also shows that the distinction between "low" and "high" frequencies becomes meaningless at slow breathing rates. As discussed above, healthy people breathe at slow rates (Fig. 29); therefore, they routinely contaminate their low- with respiratory-frequency R-R interval power.

    4.   It is highly unlikely that the huge differences of R-R interval spectral power caused by moderate changes of breathing frequency (as in Fig. 35) reflect differences of net vagal-cardiac nerve traffic. The minuscule changes of mean R-R interval at different breathing rates (Fig. 36) suggest that if vagal outflow changes at all, the changes must be small indeed. A similar theme was sounded by Kollai and Mizsei (143), who concluded that respiration-related changes of R-R interval fluctuations are not reliable indicators of vagal outflow *within individual subjects*. (As discussed above, however, differences of resting R-R interval fluctuations in different groups of subjects, including those with heart failure (110) and diabetes (155), probably reflect real differences of vagal-cardiac outflow.)

VIII. Summary and Conclusions

This chapter treats autonomic cardiovascular rhythms and the important influence of respiration in healthy humans. It deals with methodology at length, to call attention to pitfalls associated with use of the array of tools available for study of autonomic rhythms. Arterial pressure waves result from both the mechanical effects of respiration and related changes of sympathetic neural outflow. R-R interval rhythms result almost exclusively from changes of autonomic neural activity. Interactions between respiration and autonomic cardiovascular outflows are complex. Nevertheless, published information allows several generalizations to be made.

    Baroreceptor input is necessary for respiratory modeling of autonomic outflow. When baroreceptor activity is high and sympathetic activity is low, respiratory modeling of sympathetic activity is small; when baroreceptor activity is low and sympathetic activity is high, respiratory modeling of sympathetic activity *also* is small. When baroreceptor and vagal activities are low, respiratory modeling of vagal activity is small; when baroreceptor and vagal activities are high, respiratory modeling of vagal activity *also* is small. Thus, the largest fluctuations of both sympathetic and vagal activities appear when baroreceptor, sympathetic, and vagal activities are at moderate levels.

There is strong evidence that a primary mechanism whereby respiration modulates autonomic outflow is by interfering with the ability of baroreceptor inputs to influence autonomic motoneurons. Breathing is associated with an almost sinusoidal variability of motoneuron excitability; both sympathetic and vagal motoneurons are more susceptible to stimulation in expiration than inspiration, and both outflows are at their highest levels during expiration. This is not the only mechanism responsible for respiratory modulation of autonomic outflow, however, since some respiratory fluctuations of sympathetic activity persist when baroreceptor inputs are low or absent altogether. The biochemical mediation of respiratory effects on sympathetic motoneurons is poorly understood. The biochemical mediation of respiratory effects on vagal motoneurons is understood better. Vagal-cardiac motoneurons are inhibited by cholinergic receptors; when these are blocked with atropine sulfate, vagal firing is increased. This effect is more striking in expiration than inspiration.

Respiratory rate and depth exert important influences on the timing of autonomic motoneuronal firing within the breathing cycle. There is strong evidence that in *individual subjects*, moderate changes of breathing rate and depth alter the distribution of sympathetic and vagal firing within the breath, but do not alter the net level of either outflow. However, it is likely that in *different populations*, net vagal motoneuron activity is reflected in respiratory variations of R-R intervals. This conclusion is tentative, however, because in most published studies, respiratory rate and depth are neither measured nor controlled. Both vagal and sympathetic efferent activities contribute to low-frequency R-R interval rhythms. Therefore, in healthy subjects, R-R interval fluctuations at low frequencies cannot be taken simply as measures of sympathetic neural activity. Powerful new computerized methods available to quantitate human autonomic neural outflow hold great promise; however, these new methods require direct validation against nerve traffic itself under physiological and pathophysiological conditions, before they enter the mainstream of clinical investigation.

Acknowledgments

I thank Larry A. Beightol for his critical reading of this chapter and James Brownie for his help with the photography. Much of the research described in this chapter was supported by grants from the National Institutes of Health (HL22296), the Department of Veterans Affairs, and the National Aeronautics and Space Administration (NAS9-16046 and NAG9-412).

References

1. Raczkowska M, Eckberg DL, Ebert TJ. Muscarinic cholinergic receptors modulate vagal cardiac responses in man. J Autonom Nerv Syst 1983; 7:271–278.
2. Bennett T, Farquhar IK, Hosking DJ, Hampton JR. Assessment of methods for estimating autonomic nervous control of the heart in patients with diabetes mellitus. Diabetes 1978; 27:1167–1174.
3. Bigger JT Jr, La Rovere MT, Steinman RC, et al. Comparison of baroreflex sensitivity and heart period variability after myocardial infarction. J Am Coll Cardiol 1989; 14:1511–1518.
4. Hon EH, Lee ST. Electronic evaluation of the fetal heart rate. VIII. Patterns preceding fetal death, further observations. Am J Obstet Gynecol 1963; 87: 814–826.
5. Kleiger RE, Miller JP, Bigger JT Jr, Moss AJ, and Multicenter Post-Infarction Research Group. Decreased heart rate variability and its association with increased mortality after acute myocardial infarction. Am J Cardiol 1987; 59:256–262.
6. Brown TE, Beightol LA, Koh J, Eckberg DL. The important influence of respiration on human R-R interval power spectra is largely ignored. J Appl Physiol 1993; 75: 2310–2317.
7. Katona PG, Jih F. Respiratory sinus arrhythmia: noninvasive measure of parasympathetic cardiac control. J Appl Physiol 1975; 39:801–805.
8. Parker P, Celler BG, Potter EK, McCloskey DI. Vagal stimulation and cardiac slowing. J Autonom Nerv Syst 1984; 11:226–231.
9. Hagbarth K-E, Vallbo ÅB. Pulse and respiratory grouping of sympathetic impulses in human muscle nerves. Acta Physiol Scand 1968; 74:96–108.
10. Vallbo ÅB, Hagbarth K-E, Torebjörk HE, Wallin BG. Somatosensory, proprioceptive, and sympathetic activity in human peripheral nerves. Physiol Rev 1979; 59: 919–957.
11. Eckberg DL, Wallin BG, Fagius J, Lundberg L, Torebjörk HE. Prospective study of symptoms after human microneurography. Acta Physiol Scand 1989; 137:567–569.
12. Penáz J. Photoelectric measurement of blood pressure, volume and flow in the finger. In: Digest of the 10th International Conference on Medical and Biologic Engineering, Dresden: The Conference Committee of the X International Conference on Medical and Biological Engineering 1973:104.
13. Wesseling KH, de Wit B, Settels JJ, Klawer WH, Arntzenius AC. On the indirect registration of finger blood pressure after Peňáz. Funkt Biol Med 1982; 1:245–250.
14. Imholz BPM, van Montfrans GA, Settels JJ, van der Hoeven GMA, Karemaker JM, Wieling W. Continuous non-invasive blood pressure monitoring: reliability of Finapres device during the Valsalva manoeuvre. Cardiovasc Res 1988; 22:390–397.
15. Parati G, Casadei R, Groppelli A, di Rienzo M, Mancia G. Comparison of finger

and intra-arterial blood pressure monitoring at rest and during laboratory testing. Hypertension 1989; 13:647–655.

16. Hayano J, Sakakibara Y, Yamada A, et al. Accuracy of assessment of cardiac vagal tone by heart rate variability in normal subjects. Am J Cardiol 1991; 67: 199–204.

17. Grossman P, Karemaker J, Wieling W. Prediction of tonic parasympathetic cardiac control using respiratory sinus arrhythmia: the need for respiratory control. Psychophysiology 1991; 28:201–216.

18. Eckberg DL, Orshan CR. Respiratory and baroreceptor reflex interactions in man. J Clin Invest 1977; 59:780–785.

19. Eckberg DL, Kifle YT, Roberts VL. Phase relationship between normal human respiration and baroreflex responsiveness. J Physiol (Lond) 1980; 304:489–502.

20. Eckberg DL, Nerhed C, Wallin BG. Respiratory modulation of muscle sympathetic and vagal cardiac outflow in man. J Physiol (Lond) 1985; 365:181–196.

21. Kunze DL. Reflex discharge patterns of cardiac vagal efferent fibres. J Physiol (Lond) 1972; 222:1–15.

22. Preiss G, Polosa C. Patterns of sympathetic neuron activity associated with Mayer waves. Am J Physiol 1974; 226:724–730.

23. Pagani M, Lombardi F, Guzzetti S, et al. Power spectral analysis of heart rate and arterial pressure variabilities as a marker of sympatho-vagal interaction in man and conscious dog. Circ Res 1986; 59:178–193.

24. Barman SM, Gebber GL, Zhong S. The 10-Hz rhythm in sympathetic nerve discharge. Am J Physiol 1992; 262:R1006–R1014.

25. Koizumi K, Terui N, Kollai M. Relationships between vagal and sympathetic activities in rhythmic fluctuations. In: Miyakawa K, Koepchen HP, Polosa C, eds. Mechanisms of Blood Pressure Waves. Berlin: Springer-Verlag, 1984:43–56.

26. Hales S. Statical Essays: Containing Haemastaticks; or, An Account of some Hydraulick and Hydrostatical Experiments made on the Blood and Blood-Vessels of Animals. London: W. Innys, R. Manby, and T. Woodward, 1733.

27. Ludwig C. Beiträge zur Kenntniss des Einflusses der Respirationsbewegungen auf den Blutlauf im Aortensysteme. Muller's Arch Anat Physiol Med 1847; 242–302.

28. Traube L. Ueber periodische Thätigkeits-Aeusserungen des vasomotorischen und Hemmungs-Nervencentrums. Centralbl Med Wissenschaft 1865; 56:881–885.

29. Hering E. Über den Einfluss der Atmung auf den Kreislauf I. Über Athembewegungen des Gefässsystems. Sitzungsberichte Mathemat-Naturwissenschaft Classe Kaiserlich Akad Wissenschaft 1869; 60:829–856.

30. Mayer S. Studien zur Physiologie des Herzens und der Blutgefässe. V. Über spontane Blutdruckschwankungen. Sitzungsberichte Kaiserlich Akad Wissenschaft Mathemat-Naturwissenschaft Classe 1877; 74:281–307.

31. Cyon E. Zur Physiologie des Gefässnervencentrums. Pflüger's Arch 1874; 9: 499–513.

32. Fredericq L. De l'influence de la respiration sur la circulation. Les oscillations respiratoires de la pression artérielle chez le chien. Arch Biol (Paris) 1882; 3: 55–100.

33. Schweitzer A. Rhythmical fluctuations of the arterial blood pressure. J Physiol (Lond) 1945; 104:25P–26P.

34. Koepchen HP. History of studies and concepts of blood pressure waves. In: Miyakawa K, Koepchen HP, Polosa C, eds. Mechanisms of Blood Pressure Waves. Berlin: Springer-Verlag, 1984:3–23.

35. Hering E. Über den Einfluss der Atmung auf den Kreislauf. Zweite Mittheilung. Sitzungsberichte Akad Wissenschaft Mathemat-Naturwissenschaft Classe Abt II Wien 1871; 64:333–353.

36. Anrep GV, Pascual W, Rössler R. Respiratory variations of the heart rate. I—The reflex mechanism of the respiratory arrhythmia. Proc Roy Soc Lond B 1936; 119B: 191–217.

37. Seals DR, Suwarno O, Joyner MJ, Iber C, Copeland JG, Dempsey JA. Respiratory modulation of muscle sympathetic nerve activity in intact and lung denervated humans. Circ Res 1993; 72:440–454.

38. Eckberg DL, Bastow H, Scruby AE. Modulation of human sinus node function by systemic hypoxia. J Appl Physiol 1982; 52:570–577.

39. Eckberg DL, Mohanty SK, Raczkowska M. Trigeminal-baroreceptor reflex interactions modulate human cardiac vagal efferent activity. J Physiol Lond 1984; 347:75–83.

40. Hirsch JA, Bishop B. Respiratory sinus arrhythmia in humans: how breathing pattern modulates heart rate. Am J Physiol 1981; 241:H620–H629.

41. Selman A, McDonald A, Kitney R, Linkens D. The interaction between heart rate and respiration: Part I—Experimental studies in man. Automedica 1982; 4: 131–139.

42. Eckberg DL. Human sinus arrhythmia as an index of vagal cardiac outflow. J Appl Physiol 1983; 54:961–966.

43. Clynes M. Respiratory sinus arrhythmia: laws derived from computer simulation. J Appl Physiol 1960; 15:863–874.

44. Angelone A, Coulter NA Jr. Respiratory sinus arrhythmia: a frequency dependent phenomenon. J Appl Physiol 1964; 19:479–482.

45. Hyndman BW, Kitney RI, Sayers BMcA. Spontaneous rhythms in physiological control systems. Nature 1971; 233:339–341.

46. Hayano J, Taylor JA, Yamada A, et al. Continuous assessment of hemodynamic control by complex demodulation of cardiovascular variability. Am J Physiol 1993; 264:H1229–H1238

47. Kitney RI, Rompelman O. The Study of Heart-Rate Variability. Oxford: Clarendon Press, 1980.

48. Miyakawa K, Koepchen HP, Polosa C, Eds. Mechanisms of Blood Pressure Waves. Berlin: Springer-Verlag, 1984.

49. Porges SW. Respiratory sinus arrhythmia: physiological basis, quantitative methods, and clinical implications. In: Grossman P, Janssen KHL, Vaitl D, eds. Cardiorespiratory and Cardiosomatic Psychophysiology. New York: Plenum Press, 1986:101–115.

50. Kitney RI. Beat-by-beat interrelationships between heart rate, blood pressure, and respiration. In: Kitney RI, Rompelman O, eds. The Beat-by-beat Investigation of Cardiovascular Function. Oxford: Clarendon Press, 1987:146–178.

51. Karemaker JM. Analysis of blood pressure and heart rate variability: theoretical considerations and clinical applicability. In: Low PA, ed. Clinical Autonomic Disorders. Boston: Little, Brown, 1993:315–329.

52. Katona PG, Poitras JW, Barnett GO, Terry BS. Cardiac vagal efferent activity and heart period in the carotid sinus reflex. Am J Physiol 1970; 218:1030–1037.

53. Iriuchijima J, Kumada M. Activity of single vagal fibers efferent to the heart. Jpn J Physiol 1964; 14:479–487.

54. Jewett DL. Activity of single efferent fibres in the cervical vagus nerve of the dog, with special reference to possible cardio-inhibitory fibres. J Physiol (Lond) 1964; 175:321–357.

55. Eckberg DL. Temporal response patterns of the human sinus node to brief carotid baroreceptor stimuli. J Physiol (Lond) 1976; 258:769–782.

56. Eckberg DL, Eckberg MJ. Human sinus node responses to repetitive, ramped carotid baroreceptor stimuli. Am J Physiol 1982; 242:H638–H644.

57. Kumada M, Iriuchijima J. Cardiac output in carotid sinus reflex. Jpn J Physiol 1965; 15:397–404.

58. Ninomiya I, Nisimaru N, Irisawa H. Sympathetic nerve activity to the spleen, kidney, and heart in response to baroceptor input. Am J Physiol 1971; 221:1346–1351.

59. Wallin BG, Nerhed C. Relationship between spontaneous variations of muscle sympathetic activity and succeeding changes of blood pressure in man. J Autonom Nerv Syst 1982; 6:293–302.

60. Chess GF, Tam RMK, Calaresu FR. Influence of cardiac neural inputs on rhythmic variations of heart period in the cat. Am J Physiol 1975; 228:775–780.

61. Saul JP, Berger RD, Chen MH, Cohen RJ. Transfer function analysis of autonomic regulation. II. Respiratory sinus arrhythmia. Am J Physiol 1989; 256:H153–H161.

62. Coker R, Koziell A, Oliver C, Smith SE. Does the sympathetic nervous system influence sinus arrhythmia in man? Evidence from combined autonomic blockade. J Physiol (Lond) 1984; 356:459–464.

63. Eckberg DL. Beta-adrenergic blockade may prolong life in post-infarction patients in part by increasing vagal cardiac inhibition. Med Hypoth 1984; 15:421–432.

64. Fouad FM, Tarazi RC, Ferrario CM, Fighaly S, Alicandri C. Assessment of parasympathetic control of heart rate by a noninvasive method. Am J Physiol 1984; 246:H838–H842.

65. Pomeranz B, Macaulay RJB, Caudill MA, et al. Assessment of autonomic function in humans by heart rate spectral analysis. Am J Physiol 1985; 248:H151–H153.

66. Vallbo ÅB, Hagbarth K-E. Impulses recorded with micro-electrodes in human muscle nerves during stimulation of mechanoreceptors and voluntary contractions. Electroenceph Clin Neurophysiol 1967; 23:392.

67. Eckberg DL, Sleight P. Human Baroreflexes in Health and Disease. Oxford: Clarendon Press, 1992.

68. Seals DR, Suwarno NO, Dempsey JA. Influence of lung volume on sympathetic nerve discharge in normal humans. Circ Res 1990; 67:130–141.

69. Saul JP, Rea RF, Eckberg DL, Berger RD, Cohen RJ. Heart rate and muscle sympathetic nerve variability during reflex changes of autonomic activity. Am J Physiol 1990; 258:H713–H721.

70. Wallin BG, Esler M, Dorward P, et al. Simultaneous measurements of cardiac noradrenaline spillover and sympathetic outflow to skeletal muscle in humans. J Physiol (Lond) 1992; 453:45–58.

71. Numao Y, Koshiya N, Gilbey MP, Spyer KM. Central respiratory drive-related activity in sympathetic nerves of the rat: the regional differences. Neurosci Lett 1987; 81:279–284.

72. Boczek-Funcke A, Häbler H-J, Jänig W, Michaelis M. Respiratory modulation of the activity in sympathetic neurones supplying muscle, skin and pelvic organs in the cat. J Physiol (Lond) 1992; 449:333–361.

73. Wallin BG, Eckberg DL. Sympathetic transients caused by abrupt alterations of carotid baroreceptor activity in humans. Am J Physiol 1982; 242:H185–H190.

74. Fagius J, Wallin BG. Sympathetic reflex latencies and conduction velocities in normal man. J Neurol Sci 1980; 47:433–448.

75. Sayers BMcA. Analysis of heart rate variability. Ergonomics 1973; 16:17–32.

76. Hyndman BW, Mohn RK. A model of the cardiac pacemaker and its use in decoding the information content of cardiac intervals. Automedica 1975; 1:239–252.

77. Peňáz J. Mayer waves: history and methodology. Automedica 1978; 2:135–141.

78. de Boer RW, Karemaker JM, Strackee J. Description of heart-rate variability data in accordance with a physiological model for the genesis of heartbeats. Psychophysiology 1985; 22:147–155.

79. Kitney RI, Rompelman O. The Beat-by-beat Investigation of Cardiovascular Function. Oxford: Clarendon Press, 1987.

80. Inoue H, Zipes DP. Changes in atrial and ventricular refractoriness and in atrioventricular nodal conduction produced by combinations of vagal and sympathetic stimulation that result in a constant spontaneous sinus cycle length. Circ Res 1987; 60:942–951.

81. Levy MN. Sympathetic-parasympathetic interactions in the heart. Circ Res 1971; 29:437–445.

82. Freyschuss U. Cardiovascular adjustment to somatomotor activation. Acta Physiol Scand 1970; Suppl 342:1–63.

83. Bendat JS, Piersol AG. Random Data: Analysis and Measurement Procedures. New York: Wiley-Interscience, 1971.

84. Sugimoto H, Ishii N, Iwata A, Suzumura N. Stationarity and normality test for biomedical data. Comput Prog Biomed 1977; 7:293–304.

85. Grossman P. Breathing rhythms of the heart in a world of no steady state: a comment on Weber, Molenaar, and van der Molen. Psychophysiology 1992; 29:66–72.

86. de Boer RW, Karemaker JM, Strackee J. Relationships between short-term blood-pressure fluctuations and heart-rate variability in resting subjects. 1: A spectral analysis approach. Med Biol Eng Comput 1985; 23:352–358.

87. Kay SM, Marple SL Jr. Spectrum analysis—a modern perspective. Proc IEEE 1981; 69:1380–1419.

88. Shin S-J, Tapp WN, Reisman SS, Natelson BH. Assessment of autonomic regulation of heart rate variability by the method of complex demodulation. IEEE Trans Biomed Eng 1989; 36:274–283.

89. Rioul O, Vetterli M. Wavelets and signal processing. IEEE SP Mag 1991; 14–38.

90. Novak V, Novak P, de Champlain J, Le Blanc AR, Martin R, Nadeau R. Influence of respiration on heart rate and blood pressure fluctuations. J Appl Physiol 1993; 74:617–626.

91. Eckberg DL, Rea RF, Andersson OK, et al. Baroreflex modulation of sympathetic activity and sympathetic neurotransmitters in humans. Acta Physiol Scand 1988; 133: 221–231.

92. Cohen MI, Gootman PM. Periodicities in efferent discharge of splanchnic nerve of the cat. Am J Physiol 1970; 218:1092–1101.

93. Barman SM, Gebber GL. Basis for synchronization of sympathetic and phrenic nerve discharges. Am J Physiol 1976; 231:1601–1607.

94. Bernardi L, Keller F, Sanders M, et al. Respiratory sinus arrhythmia in the denervated human heart. J Appl Physiol 1989; 67:1447–1455.

95. Blinks JR. Positive chronotropic effect of increasing right atrial pressure in the isolated mammalian heart. Am J Physiol 1956; 186:299–303.

96. James TN. The sinus node as a servomechanism. Circ Res 1973; 32:307–313.

97. Gregor M, Jänig W, Wiprich L. Cardiac and respiratory rhythmicities in cutaneous and muscle vasoconstrictor neurones to the cat's hindlimb. Pflüger's Arch 1977; 370:299–302.

98. Eldridge FL. Relationship between phrenic nerve activity and ventilation. Am J Physiol 1971; 221:535–543.

99. Gootman PM, Cohen MI. The interrelationships between sympathetic discharge and central respiratory drive. In: Umbach W, Koepchen HP, eds. Central Rhythmic and Regulation. Circulation, Respiration, Extrapyramidal Motor System. Stuttgart: Hippokrates Verlag, 1974:195–209.

100. Sundlöf G, Wallin BG. Human muscle nerve sympathetic activity at rest. Relationship to blood pressure and age. J Physiol (Lond) 1978; 274:621–637.

101. Rea RF, Eckberg DL. Carotid baroreceptor-muscle sympathetic relation in humans. Am J Physiol 1987; 253:R929–R934.

102. Sundlöf G, Wallin BG. The variability of muscle nerve sympathetic activity in resting recumbent man. J Physiol (Lond) 1977; 272:383–397.

103. Peters J, Kindred MK, Robotham JL. Transient analysis of cardiopulmonary interactions. I. Diastolic events. J Appl Physiol 1988; 64:1506–1517.

104. Angell James JE. The effects of changes of extramural, "intrathoracic," pressure on aortic arch baroreceptors. J Physiol (Lond) 1971; 214:89–103.

105. McAllen RM. Central respiratory modulation of subretrofacial bulbospinal neurones in the cat. J Physiol (Lond) 1987; 388:533–545.

106. Guertzenstein PG, Silver A. Fall in blood pressure produced from discrete regions of the ventral surface of the medulla by glycine and lesions. J Physiol (Lond) 1974; 242:489–503.

107. Stjernberg L, Blumberg H, Wallin BG. Sympathetic activity in man after spinal cord injury. Outflow to muscle below the lesion. Brain 1986; 109:695–715.

108. van Lieshout JJ, Wieling W, Karemaker JM, Eckberg DL. The vasovagal response. Clin Sci 1991; 81:575–586.

109. Sundlöf G, Wallin BG, Strömgren E, Nerhed C. Acute effects of metoprolol on muscle sympathetic activity in hypertensive humans. Hypertension 1983; 5:749–756.

110. Porter TR, Eckberg DL, Fritsch JM, et al. Autonomic pathophysiology in heart failure patients. Sympathetic-cholinergic interrelations. J Clin Invest 1990; 85: 1362–1371.

111. Seller H, Langhorst P, Richter D, Koepchen HP. Über die Abhängigkeit der pressoreceptorischen Hemmung des Sympathicus von der Atemphase und ihre Auswirkung in der Vasomotorik. Pflügers Arch 1968; 302:300–314.

112. Kober G, Arndt JO. Die Druck-Durchmesser-Beziehung der A. carotis communis des wachen Menschen. Pflügers Arch 1970; 314:27–39.

113. Bainton CR, Richter DW, Seller H, Ballantyne D, Klein JP. Respiratory modulation of sympathetic activity. J Autonom Nerv Syst 1985; 12:77–90.

114. Koch E. Die reflektorische Selbststeuerung des Kreislaufes. In: Kisch B, ed. Dresden: Steinkopff, 1931.

115. Koepchen HP, Thurau K. Über die Entstehungsbedingungen der atemsynchronen Schwankungen des Vagustonus (Respiratorische Arrhythmie). Pflügers Arch 1959; 269:10–30.

116. Koepchen HP, Lux HD, Wagner P-H. Untersuchungen über zeitbedarf und zentrale verarbeitung des pressoreceptorischen Herzreflexes. Pflügers Arch 1961; 273:413–430.

117. Davidson NS, Goldner S, McCloskey DI. Respiratory modulation of baroreceptor and chemoreceptor reflexes affecting heart rate and cardiac vagal efferent nerve activity. J Physiol (Lond) 1976; 259:523–530.

118. Eckberg DL, Cavanaugh MS, Mark AL, Abboud FM. A simplified neck suction device for activation of carotid baroreceptors. J Lab Clin Med 1975; 85:167–173.

119. McAllen RM, Spyer KM. The baroreceptor input to cardiac vagal motoneurones. J Physiol (Lond) 1978; 282:365–374.

120. Gilbey MP, Jordan D, Richter DW, Spyer KM. Synaptic mechanisms involved in the inspiratory modulation of vagal cardio-inhibitory neurones in the cat. J Physiol (Lond) 1984; 356:65–78.

121. Morton HJV, Thomas ET. Effect of atropine on the heart-rate. Lancet 1958; 2:1313–1315.

122. Katona PG, Lipson D, Dauchot PJ. Opposing central and peripheral effects of atropine on parasympathetic cardiac control. Am J Physiol 1977; 232:H146–H151.

123. Alcalay M, Izraeli S, Wallach-Kapon R, Tochner Z, Benjamini Y, Akselrod S. Pharmacological modulation of vagal cardiac control measured by heart rate power spectrum: a possible bioequivalent probe. Neurosci Biobehav Rev 1991; 15:51–55.

124. Wellstein A, Pitschner HF. Complex dose-response curves of atropine in man explained by different functions of M_1 and M_2 cholinoceptors. Naunyn-Schmiedebergs Arch Pharmacol 1988; 338:19–27.

125. Fernandez de Molina A, Perl ER. Sympathetic activity and the systemic circulation in the spinal cat. J Physiol (Lond) 1965; 181:82–102.

126. Koh J, Brown TE, Beightol LA, Ha CY, Eckberg DL. Human autonomic rhythms: vagal-cardiac mechanisms in tetraplegic patients. J Physiol (Lond) 1994; 474: 483–495.

127. Malliani A, Pagani M, Lombardi F, Cerutti S. Cardiovascular neural regulation explored in the frequency domain. Circulation 1991; 84:482–492.

128. Haselton JR, Guyenet PG. Central respiratory modulation of medullary sympathoexcitatory neurons in rat. Am J Physiol 1989; 256:R739–R750.

129. Fritsch JM, Smith ML, Simmons DTF, Eckberg DL. Differential baroreflex modulation of human vagal and sympathetic activity. Am J Physiol 1991; 260:R635–R641.

130. Peñáz J, Buriánek P. Zeitverlauf und Dynamik der durch Atmung ausgelösten Kreislaufänderungen beim Menschen. Pflüger's Arch 1963; 276:618–635.

131. Berger RD, Saul JP, Cohen RJ. Assessment of autonomic response by broad-band respiration. IEEE Trans Biomed Eng 1989; 36:1061–1065.

132. Saul JP, Berger RD, Albrecht P, Stein SP, Chen MH, Cohen RJ. Transfer function analysis of the circulation: unique insights into cardiovascular regulation. Am J Physiol 1991; 261:H1231–H1245.

133. Dornhorst AC, Howard P, Leathart GL. Respiratory variations in blood pressure. Circulation 1952; 6:553–558.

134. Womack BF. The analysis of respiratory sinus arrhythmia using spectral analysis and digital filtering. IEEE Trans Bio-med Eng 1971; BME-18:399–409.

135. Ahmed AK, Fakhouri SY, Harness JB, Mearns AJ. Modelling of the control of heart rate by breathing using a kernel method. J Theoret Biol 1986; 119:67–79.

136. van den Aardweg JG, Karemaker JM. Respiratory variability and associated cardiovascular changes in adults at rest. Clin Physiol 1991; 11:95–118.

137. Bendixen HH, Smith GM, Mead J. Pattern of ventilation in young adults. J Appl Physiol 1964; 19:195–198.

138. Grossman P, Wientjes K. Respiratory sinus arrhythmia and parasympathetic cardiac control: some basic issues concerning quantification, applications and implications. In: Grossman P, Janssen KHL, Vaitl D, eds. Cardiorespiratory and Cardiosomatic Psychophysiology. New York: Plenum Press, 1986:117–138.

139. Lenfant C. Time-dependent variations of pulmonary gas exchange in normal man at rest. J Appl Physiol 1967; 22:675–684.

140. Priban IP. An analysis of some short-term patterns of breathing in man at rest. J Physiol (Lond) 1963; 166:425–434.

141. Tobin MJ, Mador MJ, Guenther SM, Lodato RF, Sackner MA. Variability of resting respiratory drive and timing in healthy subjects. J Appl Physiol 1988; 65:309–317.

142. Loveridge BM, Dubo HI. Breathing pattern in chronic quadriplegia. Arch Phys Med Rehabil 1990; 71:495–499.

143. Kollai M, Mizsei G. Respiratory sinus arrhythmia is a limited measure of cardiac parasympathetic control in man. J Physiol (Lond) 1990; 424:329–342.

144. Jose AD, Taylor RR. Autonomic blockade by propranolol and atropine to study intrinsic myocardial function in man. J Clin Invest 1969; 48:2019–2031.

145. Rigel DF, Lipson D, Katona PG. Excess tachycardia: heart rate after antimuscarinic agents in conscious dogs. Am J Physiol 1984; 246:H168–H173.

146. Grossman P. Respiratory and cardiac rhythms as windows to central and autonomic biobehavioral regulation: selection of window frames, keeping the panes clean and viewing the neural topography. Biol Psychol 1992; 34:131–161.

147. Burke D, Sundlöf G, Wallin BG. Postural effects on muscle nerve sympathetic activity in man. J Physiol (Lond) 1977; 272:399–414.

148. Baselli G, Cerutti S, Civardi S, et al. Heart rate variability signal processing: a quantitative approach as an aid to diagnosis in cardiovascular pathologies. Int J Bio-Med Comput 1987; 20:51–70.

149. Baselli G, Cerutti S, Civardi S, et al. Parameter extraction from heart rate and

arterial blood pressure variability signals in dogs for the validation of a physiological model. Comp Biol Med 1988; 18:1–16.

150. Inoue K, Miyake S, Kumashiro M, Ogata H, Yoshimura O. Power spectral analysis of heart rate variability in traumatic quadriplegic humans. Am J Physiol 1990; 258: H1722–H1726.

151. Inoue K, Miyake S, Kumashiro M, Ogata H, Ueta T, Akatsu T. Power spectral analysis of blood pressure variability in traumatic quadriplegic humans. Am J Physiol 1991; 260:H842–H847.

152. Levine BD, Buckey JC, Fritsch JM, et al. Physical fitness and cardiovascular regulation: mechanisms of orthostatic intolerance. J Appl Physiol 1991; 70: 112–122.

153. Koizumi K, Terui N, Kollai M. Neural control of the heart: significance of double innervation re-examined. J Autonom Nerv Syst 1983; 7:279–294.

154. Fagius J, Sundlöf G. The diving response in man: effects on sympathetic activity in muscle and skin nerve fascicles. J Physiol (Lond) 1986; 377:429–443.

155. Comi G, Sora MGN, Bianchi A, et al. Spectral analysis of short-term heart rate variability in diabetic patients. J Autonom Nerv Syst 1990; 30:S45–S50.

156. Siegelová J, Kopècny J. Spectral analysis of breathing pattern in man. Physiol Bohemoslov 1985; 34:321–331.

Part Four

DEVELOPMENTAL AND HORMONAL INFLUENCES

16

Developmental Control of Respiration: Neurobiological Basis

GABRIEL G. HADDAD, DAVID F. DONNELLY,
and ALIA R. BAZZY-ASAAD

Yale University School of Medicine
New Haven, Connecticut

I. Introduction and Overview

It is well accepted that, from an engineering viewpoint, feedback systems are generally challenged when the parameters that characterize them or when the conditions that surround them are altered. If this were the case also for the feedback system that regulates respiration, then there would be substantial reasons for this feedback system to be put to test during early postnatal development since enormous and profound changes take place in early life. Indeed, so many physiological and structural changes occur, e.g., in the lung, the respiratory musculature, central neuronal substrates and afferent systems, and their central connections in early infancy, that it is surprising, in some ways, that we do not clinically observe more pathophysiological aberrations from "normal" development. Consider, for example, a few simple facts. In the human infant, there are about 25 million alveoli at birth but about 130 million at 1 year of age. Assuming that the rate of alveolar growth is uniform in the first year of life (which is likely to be an underestimate for the first several months), then a simple calculation would reveal that there are about 290×10^3 alveoli per day and about 200 alveoli per minute that form and pop open! In contrast and of interest, studies performed by Rakic and colleagues in our institution on rhesus monkey and human brain development have shown that thousands of neuronal synapses in the neocortex are eliminated every day in early postnatal life (1). These early alterations are clearly not occurring only in the lung and brain, but also in other parts of the cardio-respiratory control system, such as in the sinus node and conduction system of the heart, in the vascular system, as well as in other organs of the body.

From the viewpoint of cardiorespiratory function, the basic physiological and structural differences between the young and the mature are expressed "phenotypically" or clinically in a number of ways. A number of studies in the past have demonstrated, for example, that the neonatal animal or human is more susceptible to respiratory pauses or apneas with airway receptor or facial trigemi-nal receptor stimulation than the more mature (2). The ventilatory response of the infant to hypoxia differs markedly from that of the adult whether during wakeful-ness or during sleep (3). The hyperoxic response of the premature has also been examined, and such studies have shown that such responses are attenuated in the neonate as compared with the older child or adult (4,5). The nature and duration of sleep states, their pattern and diurnal distribution, their neural basis and electro-physiological characterization in the infant are profoundly different from their adult counterparts (3). Temperature regulation in early life is more difficult to maintain with environmental alterations, and the metabolic rate per body weight is much higher at a stage in life when the O_2 stores are lower in the young (4). With gross differences between the immature and the adult, such as those described above, a number of major questions can be asked. For instance, what is the basis for these developmental differences in fundamental terms? How do these biolog-ical changes take place and what factors regulate the shift in structure and function? How do the interactions between the afferent components, central neurons, and efferent organs, i.e., respiratory muscles, change with maturation? How do changes in metabolism and temperature impact on the feedback system in early life as compared with the adult? These and other questions have been tackled by a large number of investigators in the past half-century, and a considerable literature is available. On the other hand, there are still major gaps in our knowledge regarding a number of these important questions, not only at the system level but also, in a major way, at the cellular and molecular levels.

Clearly, in this chapter, we will not be able to address all the questions posed above or be very comprehensive regarding the developmental neurobiology of respiration. We have therefore chosen to detail maturational aspects that are related to an important afferent system (e.g., carotid function), an efferent system (e.g., respiratory muscle structure and function) in early life, and some of the recent findings on central neurons, their synaptic connectivity, and their maturation in terms of response to stimuli. By so doing, we will give examples of how the various compartments of the respiratory feedback system function at the molecu-lar, cellular, and integrated levels. Although each of these examples will be treated separately, we will attempt to clarify how each component interacts with the rest of the feedback system.

II. Developmental Changes in Carotid Body Hypoxia Chemosensitivity

A. Peripheral Chemoreceptors and the Respiratory System in Early Life

The respiratory control system is primarily charged with providing a periodic drive to respiratory muscles such that pulmonary ventilation is appropriate for the level of O_2 consumption and CO_2 production. Normally, the level of ventilation is controlled so as to produce a gradient of 40–50 torr in O_2 and CO_2 between the outside air and alveolar gas; i.e., O_2 and CO_2 alveolar gas tensions are about 100 and 40 torr respectively, compared to ambient tensions of 150 and 0 torr, respectively. However, under conditions of reduced ambient oxygen (e.g., hypobaric conditions), it is undesirable to maintain an O_2 gradient of 40 torr because significant desaturation and loss of oxygen delivery would result. Peripheral chemoreceptors mediate this change by detecting a decrease in blood oxygen tension and increasing afferent neural activity, which increases the rate and depth of lung movements and reduces the gradient between alveolar and ambient air.

Although peripheral chemoreceptors are the primary oxygen sensors in the respiratory control system, their function is, to some extent, redundant with that of the central chemoreceptors. Central chemoreceptors, stimulated by blood or cerebral spinal fluid acidity, can alone drive the respiratory rhythm generator following peripheral denervation (6–8). Furthermore, some conditions that decrease Pa_{O_2} (for instance, central hypoventilation) also cause an increase in Pa_{CO_2}. Increased Pa_{CO_2} would increase central chemoreceptor activity and thereby increase respiratory muscle drive, thus correcting the abnormality in the absence of a hypoxia sensor. The fact that peripheral chemoreceptors are not essential for breathing, in most cases, has given rise to the postulate that peripheral chemoreceptor denervation may be a useful treatment for intractable lung conditions, such as severe asthma (9) or chronic obstructive pulmonary disease (10). The rationale for the treatment is that denervation and loss of hypoxic sensitivity would ameliorate the dyspnea caused by the chronic lung condition and thus improve the quality of life.

In comparison to the adult, peripheral chemoreceptors assume a greater role in the newborn period. Although not essential for initiation of fetal respiratory movements (11,12) or initiation of breathing at birth (12), peripheral chemoreceptor denervation in the newborn period results in several respiratory impairments. Following denervation, lambs fail to develop a mature respiratory pattern (7,8, 13,14) and, more important, have a 30% mortality rate, weeks or months following surgery. In other species, denervation also leads to lethal respiratory disturbances (15–17). For instance, denervated rats experience severe desaturation during REM sleep (16), and piglets experience periodic breathing with profound apneas during quiet sleep (15). Of particular interest is the observation that these lethal impairments occur only in a fairly narrow developmental window, and denervation before or after this window results in only relatively minor alterations in respiratory pattern (15,18). This window of vulnerability, which is opened by denervation in the newborn period, gives support to the speculation that sudden infant death syndrome (SIDS) may be due to peripheral chemoreceptor malfunction (19–21). Although no direct information is presently available to support or refute this speculation, it is intriguing that histological and neurochemical abnormalities are often present in the tissue of SIDS victims (19–21).

This heightened sensitivity to denervation in early life implies that the newborn respiratory control system is different from that of the adult. Two well-documented major differences, which pertain to chemoreceptor function, are: (1) the respiratory response to an acute change in inspired oxygen is less in the newborn than in the adult, and (2) the newborn is unable to sustain the respiratory stimulation caused by acute hypoxia (Fig. 1) (4). An acute increase in inspired oxygen rapidly inhibits arterial chemoreceptor activity, and by measuring the change in breathing before and after high oxygen exposure, the contribution of peripheral chemoreceptors to eupnea may be evaluated. By this assay, the contribution of peripheral chemoreceptors during eupnea increases in rats from 5 to 30% over the first 1–2 weeks after birth (Fig. 1) (22–24); in lambs the increase is about 10–30% in the first month (13,25). Using the opposite experimental manipulation (i.e., an acute decrease in oxygen), breathing initially increases in all ages but, in the newborn, falls back toward baseline over the next 5 min despite the continued presence of hypoxia (Fig. 1).

The reasons for the impaired response of newborns as compared to adults are incompletely understood. It is possible that elements central to the chemoreceptor have a major influence in determining the response to chemoreceptor input; i.e., ventilation may not follow the level of afferent input in a linear function. Indeed, experiments have shown that the central neural response to a constant sinus nerve stimulation train changes with time and with subject age (26), and that at least some of the ventilatory accommodation during hypoxia in the newborn is due to stimulation of descending dopaminergic projections from the hypothalamus to the brainstem (27). However, major changes also occur within the chemosensor itself, and this will be the focus of this chapter.

B. Discharge Properties of Carotid Body Afferent Nerves

As noted above, there are two differences between newborn and adult in the ventilatory response to hyperoxia or hypoxia (Fig. 1): (1) The magnitude of the decrease in ventilation with hyperoxia is less in the newborn than in the adult, and (2) the newborn fails to sustain a hyperventilation in response to hypoxia. Although these differences can be based on differences at a number of levels of respiratory control, potentially both these developmental differences may be due

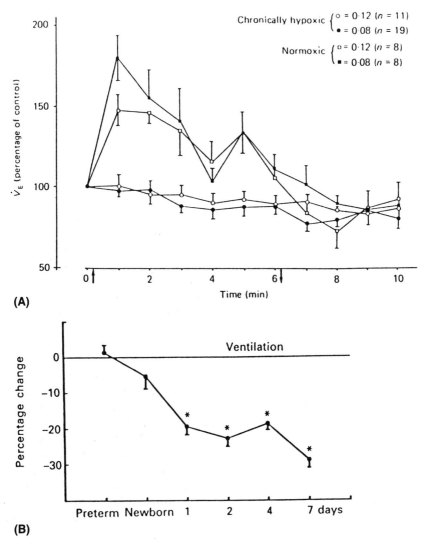

Figure 1 Ventilatory response of young rats to acute hypoxia and hyperoxia. (A) Effects on respiration of an acute reduction in $F_{I_{O_2}}$ from 0.15 to 0.12 (open circles) or to 0.08 (closed circles) for 6 min on postnatal day 5 for normal rats and rats born and maintained in chronic hypoxia. Note, in normal rats, that hypoxia increased ventilation, which was followed by adaptation despite the continued presence of hypoxia (22). (B) Percent change in ventilation in rats elicited by transient *hyperoxia* as a function of age. The effect of hyperoxia increased with age, suggesting that the contribution of peripheral chemoreceptors to eupnea increases with postnatal age.

to changes occurring at the sensor itself. The problem is to obtain a direct assay of chemoreceptor nerve activity in as close to a physiological state as can be reasonably obtained.

Classically, chemoreceptors have been recorded, in vivo, in anesthetized lambs, cats, or rabbits by surgically exposing and cutting the sinus nerve at its junction with the glossopharyngeal nerve and recording spiking activity from the cut peripheral nerve. Given that baroreceptors travel in the same nerve, the gross activity is a combination of rhythmic baroreceptor activity and tonic chemoreceptor activity unless further intervention is undertaken. Two refinements that can yield purer data on chemoreceptor activity have been (1) the crushing of nerve fibers in the sinus region to eliminate baroreceptor activity, thus yielding summated chemoreceptor activity on the sinus nerve, and (2) stranding of the sinus nerve into small axonal bundles with the hope that recording from these strands will yield activity from only one to several chemoreceptor afferent nerve fibers.

Recordings from both single fiber afferents and sinus nerve trunks have shown major differences between the fetus and newborn and between newborn and adult. Early attempts to record fetal chemoreceptor activity, in vivo, generally failed in that little, if any, definable chemoreceptor activity was present on the sinus nerve. However, the situation was greatly improved following clamping of the umbilical cord—a form of artificial birth (28). This result suggested that an increase in sympathetic outflow, which is evoked by cord clamping, is critical for initiating the chemoreceptor sensitivity to hypoxia, or alternatively, cord clamping releases some hormonal factor that establishes chemosensitivity. This latter speculation received some support by the observation that the same carotid bodies, from which no chemoreceptor activity could be recorded, in vivo, could be removed and placed in a bath of Ringer's saline, and, with this artificial perfusate, chemoreceptor activity could be readily recorded (12). Unfortunately, the hormonal or neural factors altering chemosensitivity remain undefined, but the search for them has been tempered by recent experiments that had greater success in recording chemoreceptor activity from the fetus in the absence of cord clamping.

In a seminal series of observations, Hanson and colleagues demonstrated that fetal chemoreceptor activity is present in the normal fetus and that a large increase ($5\times$) in activity may be evoked by decreasing the end-tidal oxygen to the ewe (Fig. 2) (11,29). The estimated response curve was considerably left-shifted compared to the adult such that Pao_2 values below 20 torr were required to initiate an increase in discharge (Fig. 2). As would be predicted by this left-shifted O_2 response curve, the large increase in Pao_2 at the time of birth virtually silences chemoreceptor activity in the newborn period (30). However, the left-shifted response curve does not last long and assumes a normal adult-like sensitivity by 1–2 weeks after birth (11,29,31).

Not only is the newborn chemoreceptor sensitivity to hypoxia low, but the dynamic range (or maximum discharge from a single receptor) is less in the

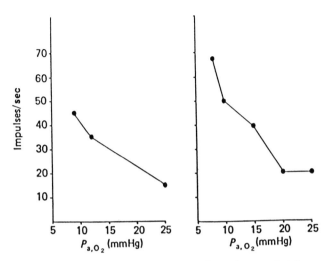

Figure 2 Chemoreceptor response to steady-state hypoxia recorded from two fetuses aged 108 days (left) and 140 days (right). The response curve is shifted to the left compared to that obtained in mature animals (29).

newborn than in the adult. Recordings from single chemoreceptor fibers in 6-day-old piglets demonstrated a dynamic range as Pao_2 was reduced from 300 to 25 torr of 0.5–6 Hz and this increased to 0.5–8 Hz in 8-day-old piglets (Fig. 3) (32). Similarly, in kittens, the discharge rate of single chemoreceptor afferent fibers at Pi_{O_2} of 55 torr (Pao_2: 31–44 torr) increased from 5.8 ± 0.6 Hz in kittens younger than 10 days to 8.8 ± 1.3 Hz in kittens older than 10 days (33). In contrast, chemoreceptors of normal adult cats increased activity from 0.5 to 15 Hz over the same Pao_2 range (34). However, a Pao_2 of 35–40 torr, which is a reasonable lower limit for experiments in vivo that do not incur severe metabolic acidosis or impaired blood pressure, does not maximally stimulate chemoreceptor discharge. The dynamic range question may, thus, be better addressed, in vitro, under conditions of constant pH and nutrient delivery. Under these conditions and using an anoxic stimulus, the maximal discharge rate obtained from rat chemoreceptors increased from about 5 Hz at 1 day of age to about 20 Hz by 15 days of age (Fig. 4) (35).

The physiological signal to initiate chemoreceptor maturation from the newborn to adult sensitivity appears to be Pao_2. Animals that are born into a hypoxic environment (Fi_{O_2} about 12%) maintain an immature respiratory response to hypoxia: a poor ventilatory response to hypoxia/hyperoxia (Fig. 1) (36–38) and a low nerve response to hypoxia (Fig. 5) (36). In the normal newborn rat, hyperoxia reduces respiratory drive by 5–8%, and this increases to 20% in the

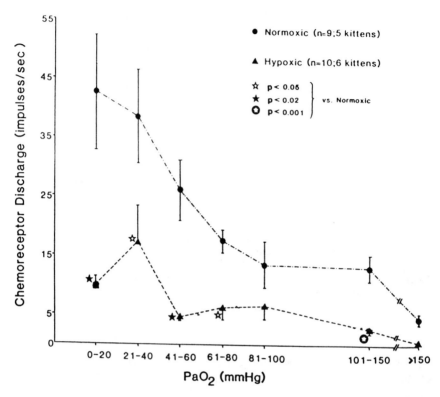

Figure 3   Effect of postnatal, chronic hypoxia on the discharge sensitivity of chemoreceptors recorded in young kittens. Note that the chemoreceptor response of the chronically
hypoxic group is less than that of the normal group. Postnatal hypoxia simarly suppressed
the respiratory response to hypoxia (see Fig. 1) (37).

normal 2-week-old rat (22). In contrast, rats born into hypoxia decrease respiration by only 5% regardless of age (36). The hyperoxic maturation signal may also
be advanced in time. Chemoreceptors of fetal lambs ventilated with oxygen for 24
hr prior to birth are right-shifted compared to chemoreceptors of lambs ventilated
with nitrogen (11).

A second major developmental change in the respiratory response to
hypoxia is the ability to sustain the hypoxia-induced hyperventilation. As mentioned above, the response of the newborn to hypoxia is characterized by a
biphasic respiratory response with an immediate increase in ventilation but then a
falloff toward baseline despite the continued presence of hypoxia (4,7,8,13,14,
30). Some of this falloff can be central in origin (26,27), but recent observations
have suggested that at least part of the falloff is due to the inability of newborn
chemoreceptor to sustain high discharge rates. A falloff in peripheral chemorecep-

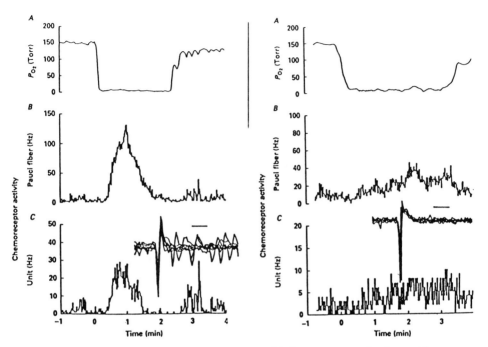

Figure 4 Increase in dynamic range of rat carotid chemoreceptors, in vitro, with age. (Left) Discharge frequency and local P_{O_2} versus time recorded from a *28-day-old* rat carotid body superfused with Ringer's saline. Anoxia evoked an increase in single-fiber activity from about 2 Hz to 24 Hz at peak. Inset, superimposed oscillographic tracings of unit activity. Scale bar is 2 msec. (Right) Discharge frequency and local P_{O_2} versus time recorded from a *1-day-old* carotid body. Anoxia caused activity to increase from about 2 Hz to 7 Hz at peak (35).

tor activity was inferred in studies of ventilatory transients in young lambs (25), and recent single fiber recordings in 6-8-day-old piglets demonstrated chemoreceptor fibers that became silent below 40 torr, despite increasing activity in the range of 100–50 torr (39). These observations were recently confirmed and extended in kittens (33) and demonstrate that some of the respiratory falloff may be due to peripheral failure. However, these are controversial observations, and some investigators see little change in peripheral chemoreceptor activity during hypoxia despite decreases in respiratory drive (30,40).

C. External Factors Dictating Maturation of Chemosensitivity

Arterial chemoreceptors are subject to external nervous and hormonal influences, which may potentially directly affect the sensor or alter tissue P_{O_2} within the

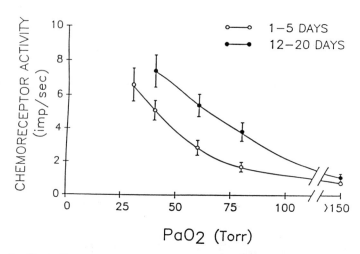

Figure 5 Single-fiber carotid chemoreceptor afferent response to isocapnic hypoxia in young (1–5 day) and older (12–20 day) piglets. The level of discharge activity was significantly elevated in older pigs at all levels of Pa_{O_2} except hyperoxia (39).

organ. In fact, measurements of tissue Po_2 in the neonatal period show a decrease over the first week after birth, and this may be an important factor in explaining the apparent increase in hypoxia sensitivity (41); however, this change in tissue oxygen tension must be due to an active change in vessel control because little or no change occurs in the characteristics of the carotid body vasculature during this period (42,43). Some of these nutritive changes may be due to nervous regulation of local blood flow; the carotid body receives a major innervation from the superior cervical ganglia (ganglioglomerular nerve) and a parasympathetic innervation from the sinus nerve (44). Stimulation of sympathetic and parasympathetic efferents causes ongoing afferent activity to increase (45) and decrease (46), respectively, and these changes are largely due to blood flow changes within the organ (41).

Blood-borne substances or neurochemicals may potentially play a major role as a modulator of chemosensitivity. This is particular true of plasma K^+ levels and endorphins, which have been implicated as modulators of chemosensitivity in the adult (47,48). A slight increase in K^+, as occurs during exercise, causes a 20–30% increase in discharge sensitivity to hypoxia (48), but its effects on the newborn are unexplored. Endorphins are documented to decrease in the newborn period, and the effect of exogenous endorphin is inhibition of chemoreceptor hypoxia sensitivity (49). Thus, part of the decreased sensitivity in the fetus and newborn may be a tonic, hormonal inhibition of chemoreceptors from circulating endorphins. Even less well understood is the effect of blood versus artificial plasma on hypoxia sensitivity. This was originally noted by Joels and Neil in 1968, who were studying chemoreceptors in vitro (50). They found that chemosensitivity decreases over time in saline until the organ is virtually unresponsive to hypoxia. However, addition of as little as 5% blood to the saline restored these "tired" chemoreceptors and prevented the decline. In the opposite sense, fetal chemoreceptor activity may be sparse in situ, but readily recorded from in the same carotid body in vitro (12). Both observations imply that blood-borne factors play a major modulatory role in determining the level of chemosensitivity, but identification of the critical substance(s) or their change in the newborn period is presently lacking.

D. Intrinsic Changes Dictating Maturation of Chemosensitivity

Even in the absence of external modulatory factors (acute hormonal or neural effects), chemosensitivity of the newborn chemoreceptor is less than in the adult. As noted above, the dynamic increase in nerve activity of rat carotid bodies, in vitro, following transition from normoxia to severe hypoxia is about fourfold greater in carotid bodies harvested from 20-day-old rats compared to 1-2-day-old rats (Fig. 4) (35). This corresponds well to the maturation pattern of respiratory response to hypoxia in the intact animal (22) and suggests that major maturational changes occur within the carotid body itself, independent of the acute effects of hormones or nerves.

Several histological, biophysical, and neurochemical changes occur with development, but the interpretation and the significance of these changes are dependent on assumptions of the internal workings of the organ. In apposition to the afferent nerve endings are glomus cells that are grouped into clusters or glomoids, and surrounding the glomoids are sustentacular or supporting cells (44). Because of the synaptic arrangement, it seems likely that hypoxia is transduced by glomus cells that elaborate an excitatory neurotransmitter that excites the afferent nerve ending. Although the nature of the synaptic transmitter remains uncertain, the number of synapses increases greatly in the newborn period. In the rat, this increase is of the order of 4–5 times between birth and 20 days of age (51), which is about the same order of increase as the respiratory response to hypoxia (22). The synthesis of some purported neurotransmitters is also developmentally linked to chemosensitivity. For instance, substance P immunocytochemical staining is sparse in fetal carotid body but rapidly appears after birth (52). Substance P has been implicated as a major mediator of the hypoxia response (53).

Catecholamines, in particular, are purported to play a major role in modulating the hypoxia response, but it is uncertain whether they act as excitatory or inhibitory modulator. Evidence for an inhibitory role of catecholamines is based on the effects of dopamine agonists or antagonists on chemoreceptor discharge rates: exogenous dopamine generally inhibits, not excites, afferent activity, and dopamine blockers generally fail to block hypoxia transduction (54,55). The low sensitivity in the newborn period may, thus, be due to high rates of tonic dopamine secretion (24,38). Indeed, this conjecture is supported by recent data on dopamine turnover rates in the newborn period, which show a large increase in the first 6 hr after birth and a gradual decrease over the next 12 hr (Fig. 6) (24). Furthermore, rats exposed to postnatal hypoxia, which delays the maturation of normal hypoxia sensitivity, show enhanced dopamine turnover rates at postnatal day 2 as compared to normoxic rats; i.e., the chronically hypoxic rats appear to maintain an immature pattern of dopamine secretion (38).

An alternative to the inhibitory modulatory function of glomus cells secretion is the postulate that enhanced glomus cell catecholamine secretion causes an increase in afferent nerve activity. An argument in support of this position is well outlined in a recent review by Gonzalez (56) and is based on the high correlation between dopamine release and afferent nerve activity (56–59). If increases in catecholamine secretion mediate the increase in nerve activity, then it would be expected that tissue catecholamine levels in the newborn carotid body would be low or the number of dopamine receptors would be low. At present, there are no data directly addressing either possibility.

The maturational increase in chemosensitivity may also, potentially, be attributed to a maturational change in the biophysical properties of glomus cells.

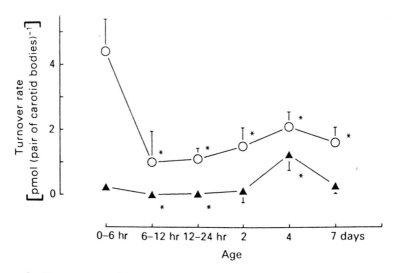

Figure 6 Turnover rates of dopamine (open circles) and norepinephrine (closed triangles) as a function of age in neonatal rats. Note high turnover rate for dopamine in the immediate newborn period. *Significantly different turnover rate compared to value obtain at 0–6 hr after birth (24).

Although no data are presently available directly addressing this postulate, comparison of results between different laboratories may give clues to the result of such a study. In adult cells, Gonzalez and colleagues proposes that molecular hypoxia directly inhibits a membrane-localized K^+ channel that is active at rest, and the resulting depolarization leads to calcium influx and enhanced secretion (56). Experimental support for this special K^+ channel has rested on recordings from cultured, adult rabbit glomus cells whose outward (or K^+ current) is apparently inhibited by hypoxia, and this may be observed in isolated membrane patches (60). In comparison, several different groups of investigators are working with glomus cells harvested from immature animals (generally rats) and report a similar decrease in whole-cell K^+ current during hypoxia as is observed in cells from the adult rabbit. However, the decrease in K^+ current is attributed to a decreased activation of a Ca^{2+}-dependent K^+ current and not a specialized K^+ channel sensitive to hypoxia (61). This is further supported by observations that intracellular calcium may actually decrease during hypoxia in some rat glomus cells (62). Thus, either the transduction mechanism for hypoxia is different between rats and rabbits or the membrane channels sensitive to hypoxia undergo a maturational change. Clearly, this is an important question that needs to be answered.

Carotid body chemoreceptors are the major sensor for early detection of hypoxia and evoke a number of reflexes that defend against further hypoxia. The primary response is an increase in neural drive of breathing, but peripheral chemoreceptor activity also leads to increase in sympathetic tone and arousal (6). These defensive maneuvers may be especially critical for the maintenance of the newborn, because denervation at early ages, as opposed to older ages, leads to an enhanced mortality in the postnatal period.

Although it is relatively well established that an increase in chemosensitivity occurs in the postnatal period and that this is triggered by the increase in Pa_{O_2} at birth, the mechanism remains unknown. However, the solution will likely be found in a better understanding of the nature of transmitters elaborated by the glomus cells or a better understanding of the biophysical changes of glomus cells. As noted above, glomus cells must be apposed to the afferent nerve endings to convey the property of chemosensitivity to the organ (63). Furthermore, glomus cells respond biophysically to hypoxia by altering intracellular calcium (62,64) and membrane currents (61,65–67). Unfortunately, although the cells often respond to the hypoxia stimulus, they appear to respond differently among laboratories. For instance, in two laboratories studying the response of mature rabbit glomus cells, one records an increase in K^+ current during chemostimulation (68), and one a decrease (65). Why glomus cells of the same species and of the same age respond in opposite directions is uncertain, but clearly needs to be resolved before synthesis of a coherent transduction scheme of the mature organ as prelude to understanding the mechanism of organ maturation.

Not only does the biophysical response of the glomus cell need to be better understood, but we need a better identification of the secretory product. Dopamine secretion, as noted above, is in direct proportion to chemoreceptor afferent activity, but instead of being an excitatory transmitter, it appears to be an inhibitory neuromodulator (54,55). Thus, other transmitters are likely involved, and there is no shortage of candidates that have been localized to the carotid body. These include, substance P, VIP, enkephalins, ACh, ANP, and neurokinin Y, to name just a few. Clearly, the first step to understanding and controlling dynamic changes in chemosensitivity is an understanding of why the nerve activity increases during hypoxia.

Ultimately, an understanding of neurotransmitter control of chemosensitivity and the (changing) biophysical properties of glomus cells will lead to questions posed at the level of transcription. An understanding of these changes is only in its nascent stage, and it has been demonstrated that the mRNA for synthesizing dopamine-β-hydroxylase in petrosal ganglion neurons changes with development and the same enzyme in glomus cells can be altered by hypoxia exposure (69). Clearly, these varied experimental approaches—neuropharmacological (transmitter and receptor identification), optical (measurement of membrane potential, calcium, pH), electrophysiological (identification of membrane currents), and genetic (protein expression)—should rapidly lead to an understanding of the determinants of hypoxia sensitivity and its change in the newborn period. This promises to lead to an improved pharmacological control of the hypoxia sensory system for the treatment of apneas and chronic lung diseases.

Some of the difficulties we encounter when we analyze the various parts of the respiratory control system during early life are due to the fact that maturational changes are occurring in all parts of the feedback system. Therefore, the properties of the glomus cells are not the only cells that are developing, but the cells in the central nervous system (CNS) that they communicate with are also maturing. In the next section, we discuss some of the interesting recent observations that characterize neurons in the brainstem and CNS and highlight their role in the overall genesis of the respiratory rhythm. In addition, we examine some of the inherent properties of such neurons that we believe are important under stressful conditions.

III. Central Neuronal Control of Respiration in Early Life

In this section, we highlight several aspects of the central nervous control of respiration in the young mammal. The first will be related to the integrated neurophysiological behavior and extracellular measurements performed in the brainstem of neonates. The second will be focused on intracellular neuronal measurements in in vitro and in vivo preparations and the new insights that these approaches are now providing. The third aspect to be emphasized is the response of central neurons to stress, their tolerance (or lack thereof) to it, and the basis for such a response. The main message in this part of our chapter is that we know now that central neurons are developing not only prenatally but also postnatally, especially in the preterm or immature infant in a number of ways, and that this maturation impacts on how respiration is controlled in early life.

In this chapter, and this is probably true for the rest of this volume, we need to consider two important tenets when we try to understand the respiratory control system in the young or in the mature organism. The first is that respiration is a *behavior* (Fig. 7) that involves, besides peripherally located organs, various regions of the brain with several neuronal groups that are intricately connected with chemical and electrical synapses. Hence, this behavior is most likely controlled by a network of nerve cells. The second tenet is that the network's output to the respiratory muscles is dependent not only on the synaptic and network properties of the neurons in that particular network, but also on the *single neuronal cellular properties*. Single neurons in a network are far from being simple "followers" of activity and are capable of modifying input/output relations (70). The importance of this tenet and of the interactions between cellular, synaptic, and network properties in initiating and shaping the final output of the system stems from inumerable studies in invertebrate model neuronal networks underlying rhythmic behavior. These models have included oscillating and rhythmic alternating muscle activation for escape swimming in the *Tritonia* (71–73), locomotion in the locust (74,75), lobster pyloric motor pattern (76), rhythmic heartbeat in the leech (77), to name a few. If we accept these two tenets, it becomes clear that experimentations at both levels are important if we wish to understand the respiratory control system (78). We believe that considering the respiratory control system as a behavior *only* will retard our progress in understanding the detailed workings of this control system. It is only when we can reduce the system, study it in its reduced form in a variety of ways, and study it also in its "native" or "in situ" form that we can make advances in this complex research area. The reason for using a reductionist approach is to be able to study (1) cell physiology and behavior and (2) the molecular mechanisms that underlie cell physiology. Unless newer technologies appear in the near future that allow us to study cell and molecular physiology in situ and understand the basis for the intricate interactions of neurons within circuits or network, we will need to reduce the system (Fig. 7). Examples abound both in vertebrates, such as the locomotion of the lamprey and the major advances made in the recent past in understanding this system, and in the invertebrate organisms mentioned above (78).

A. Neurophysiology of Respiration—In Situ Studies

The neurophysiology of respiration has fascinated a great many investigators for many centuries. However, probably the first documentation of the importance of

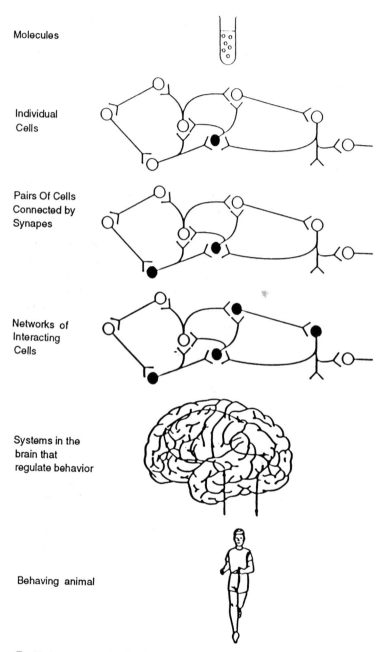

Figure 7 Various approaches for the study of a behavior in animals, i.e., from molecules to a behaving human. (Reproduced after modification from Levitan and Kaczmarek, *The Neuron*, New York: Oxford University Press, 1991.)

the brainstem in the control of respiration was made by the Frenchman LeGallois in the early 1800s in his discovery of the medullary "noeud vital" (79). Parenthetically, he attributed his interest in respiration and the brain to his clinical observation of the survival of human neonates who had sustained long periods of apneas. Subsequently this observation led him to study newborn and more mature rabbits and test their tolerance to lack of O_2 (Table 1) (79). These issues will be discussed later in this chapter. Since that time there have been many attempts to understand the neural basis for respiration. We have made a great deal of progress in the past 50 years, but we still have many unanswered questions of clinical importance.

Inspiratory and Expiratory Discharge Patterns

Although no single major animal model has been used in this research area, the cat has probably been the best-studied species for a number of reasons. However, other animals, such as the opossum, piglet, rabbit, and rat, have also been used in the study of respiratory rhythmogenesis. Therefore, the data that will be referred to are a result of experiments on these animals rather than on a single one.

One major question that investigators have examined in general is related to

Table 1 Duration of Gapings and Sensitivity of Rabbits of Different Ages (79)

Age (days)	Sensitivity (min)	Gapings (min)	Age (days)	Sensitivity (min)	Gapings (min)
After extraction of the heart					
1	14	20	20	1⅓	2⅔
5	6	9	25	1¼	1½
10	3⅓	4	30	1	1⅓
15	2⅓	2¾			
After opening of the thorax					
1	16	30	20	2¾	3½
5	12	16	25	2	2½
10	5½	7½	30	1¾	2¼
15	5¾	5½			
In asphyxia by submersion					
1	15	27	20	2¾	3¼
5	10	16	25	2	3¾
10	4⅓	5½	30	1½	2¼
15	3	4			

the location of the respiratory neurons and their distribution. The term "respiratory" is therefore reserved for those cells that fire with a phase of phrenic activity (inspiratory activity, postinspiratory activity, and expiratory silence) in a locked fashion. These studies have generated considerable knowledge and can be summarized as follows:

1. One important aspect of neuronal discharge activity in both neonatal and adult animals is that there are probably two separate functional systems in the CNS that are related to feedback control (80,81). One system is charged with the initiation of the rhythm of respiration and the other is responsible for shaping the burst of activity as it is developing. It is presumed that these two functions are fairly separate and anatomically distinct. From clinicopathological point of view, the best illustration we know of is in the infant with congenital hypoventilation syndrome (or Ondine's curse), who, typically, has an extremely low respiratory rate during sleep (8–10 breaths/min in early life) but whose tidal volume is close to normal (Table 2) (82).

2. Although recent studies in the neonatal rat in vitro (whole brainstem preparation) were not targetted at understanding the neonate in particular, these studies have shed light on basic fundamental issues pertaining to the control of respiration in the newborn (81). In fact, we know now from several such studies that the young rat (which is quite immature in the first week of life) brainstem in vitro does not need any external or peripheral drive for the oscillator in order to discharge. The inherent rate (as judged by cranial nerve output) is markedly reduced, however, and it is clear from these studies that peripheral or central (rostral to the medulla and pons) input is needed to maintain the respiratory output at a much higher frequency. These studies do not conceptually differ from

Table 2 Comparison of Tidal Volume, Mean Inspiratory Flow, and Respiratory Timing in Patient L.S. with Weight-Matched Normal Newborn Infants in REM and Quiet Sleep[a]

Ventilatory parameters	REM		Quiet	
	LS	Normal[b]	LS	Normal[b]
Vt (ml)	22	15 ± 2.2	15	15 ± 2.8
Ttot (sec)	2.8	1.4 ± 0.2	3.1	1.4 ± 0.1
Ti (sec)	0.6	0.4 ± 0.1	0.7	0.5 ± 0.1
Te (sec)	2.1	0.9 ± 0.1	2.3	0.9 ± 0.03
Vt/Ti (ml/sec)	34	33 ± 3.4	21	32 ± 8.7
Ti/Ttot	0.28	0.33 ± 0.02	0.26	0.37 ± 0.07

[a]Median values based on an entire sleep cycle.
[b]Average ± SD of four normal infants.

results obtained several years ago (4), which showed that the respiratory frequency drops to about one-tenth of normal when several peripheral inputs to the CNS are blocked. It is important to keep in mind, though, that the in vitro studies may not include all the respiratory network circuitry as claimed since O_2 diffusion may be compromised and a part of the network may not be functional. Our studies on the neuronal response to hypoxia (see below) may be relevant to this issue and in relation to the integrity of neurons bathed with very low pO_2 for more than 10–15 min, even in the neonate at low ambient temperature (83).

3. It has recently been hypothesized that the basis of the respiratory rhythm generator in the adult is a network of neurons which, by virtue of their connectivity, fire in bursts and oscillate. In the neonate, some investigators believe that the system is that of a hybrid, that is it is based on both a network and a pacemaker-type oscillator (84,85). This hypothesis stems from experiments showing that the respiratory rhythm was not abolished in the neonatal animal (brainstem preparation) when blockers of inhibitory mediators such as GABA or Cl^--free solutions were used with little disturbance of the rhythm generation (85). Such experiments led some investigators to hypothesize that it is possible that the respiratory rhythm generation is not based on inhibitory connections or synapses, and one way that this could be brought about is if the rhythm is based on pacemaker cells. Clearly this is only one hypothesis and, at present, is far from proven. Consider, for example, the following questions: Is it possible that the rhythm generation in the newborn is based on mutual excitatory connections? Is it possible that inhibitory receptor development is at the basis of this different response? Is it possible that removal of Cl^- from the medium induces changes in intracellular constituents such as pH, which, in turn, alter responsiveness?

4. In most adult animals, two groups of neurons are found to fire in synchrony with phrenic activity (80). One of them is located in the so-called dorsal respiratory group (DRG), which includes neurons in the ventral area of the nucleus of the solitary tract. The other one is ventral to this group and is called the ventral respiratory group (VRG). In the immature opossum, which was studied more than other neonatal animals, DRG and VRG neurons do not seem to be separated from each other easily (86). The piglet's units are also more diffuse (87), although it should be stated that neither the adult opossum or adult pig have been studied from this point of view. This lack of separation between DRG and VRG units can be related to age or species. In addition to young opossums and piglets, adult guinea pigs show much less concentration of units in the dorsal and ventral regions than the adult cat or the rabbit (88).

5. Since the VRG is a series of longitudinal groups of neurons, the question that has been raised is whether there is an anatomical organization within this nucleus. In the opossum, most units in the caudal or rostral areas are expiratory, but inspiratory cells are also found in the middle region. One major difference between rostral and caudal groups of neurons is that most of the caudal group projects to spinal motoneurons but most of the rostral ones do not seem to.

6. The discharge pattern of each unit seems, from extracellular recordings, to be different from that in the adult in two major ways. First, the inspiratory discharge is not ramp in shape but increases and decreases within the same breath. The second is that it is extremely brief, sometimes limited to even a few action potentials (86). The reason for this inspiratory discharge is not clear but could be related to cellular or network properties. In addition to differences in inspiratory discharge, expiratory units discharge weakly and appear often only after an expiratory load (89, 90). Adult counterparts are much more active, even at rest.

7. Since the discharge pattern of central neurons is affected by peripheral input, including input from the vagus nerve, and since this is a feedback system that can operate on a breath-by-breath basis in the adult animal, one question that has been raised on several previous occasions is whether the lack of myelination in nerve fibers that subserve feedback affects function. Indeed, this is the case not only because of the lack of myelination and the delays in signaling between feedback components, but because the inspiratory and expiratory discharges are so fast, precluding the effect of some of the information that would have impacted on the same breath. Therefore, one important issue that can be raised in this discussion is whether breath-by-breath feedback is as potent in the young as in the adult.

Synapses, Neurotransmitters, and Neonatal Responses

Our concepts regarding neurotransmitters and synaptic transmission have evolved a great deal in the past 10–20 years. There have been major changes in the way we think about transmitter content and release, the nature of storage, and the mechanisms involving neurotransmission. Besides, many neurotransmitters have been discovered, and we believe that all of them so far have been found in the brainstem. Which of those are really involved in rhythm generation versus modulation of output pattern, such as has been described for the locomotion of the lamprey, is not known at present although some information has been forthcoming (91). For example, glutamate increases and glutamate blockers decrease respiratory output in the adult animal (80, 84). Young and immature animals may respond differently to neurotransmitters, and this has been mostly documented by work on the opossum (92). Glutamate injected in various locations in the brainstem, even in large doses, induces respiratory pauses (92). Inhibitory neurotransmitters such as GABA have also been used, and these have age-dependent effects in the opossum. Indeed, Cl^--mediated inhibition is completely suppressed in the adult but not in the neonate in the isolated brainstem (80), although the pattern of each burst of activity changes. These differences in response are not quite understood at the fundamental level since there are many variables that are not controlled for in these experiments, such as the size of the extracellular space, synaptic differentiation, receptor development, ability for sensitization, and cellular properties, to name only a few.

A large number of studies have examined the effect of a variety of neuromodulators and transmitters on respiration and on pattern of neuronal activity (80). However, it is not known whether these alter the rhythm itself. For example, we do not know the full action of acetylcholine, monoamines, and other neuropeptides (which are present in the brainstem) of rhythm generation.

Intracellular Recordings and Triphasic Respiration

These are difficult measurements to make in vivo, and the little information we have on respiratory-related neurons is therefore important. Some of the problems with these measurements are that (1) they are performed under anesthesia and this may affect the functional connectivity of neurons involved in respiration, and (2) often these recordings are not optimal, indicating either injury of cells being recorded or inadequate impalement. With these caveats in mind, these studies have helped us understand further the organization of the respiratory network (80,81). For example, we know now that there are early-inspiratory and postinspiratory neurons. These two groups of neurons are probably the "primary oscillator" and are responsible for the on-switch and off-switch of the respiratory cycle. There are clearly other groups of neurons that have been characterized; these are expiratory, late-inspiratory, throughout-inspiratory, and preinspiratory. Triphasic respiration refers to the working model that inspiration is turned off by postinspiratory neurons whose activity is associated with major postsynaptic inhibitory currents in inspiratory neurons. Postinspiratory neurons seem to have inhibitory influence on early- , throughout-, and preinspiratory neurons (80).

The drive to this network of neurons is assumed to be from sources outside the network itself, but, as mentioned above, whole brainstem preparations have suggested that peripheral input (vagal, carotid, mechanoreceptors, and other peripheral receptors) are not needed in the rhythm generation (81). Indeed, in the spontaneously active brainstem slice, a respiratory rhythm, as measured by cranial nerve activity, is preserved as long as a pre-Bötzinger neuronal group is preserved in the slice (81).

Neonatal piglets also seem to show postinspiratory neuronal activity in the same general area as inspiratory neurons (93). These postinspiratory neurons, which are most likely interneurons, are hyperpolarized during inspiration and show their depolarization only immediately with a strong inhibition of inspiratory neurons. Whether this is the case with neonatal animals in general is not clear at present, keeping in mind that piglets are rather precocious at birth.

B.   Neurobiology of Respiratory Neurons: In Vitro Studies

General Properties

Major progress has been made recently in the study of cellular properties and types of ionic conductances in respiratory neurons. For DRG and VRG neurons, the intrinsic membrane currents that can shape their repetitive firing activity are impressive. These include not only the classic sodium and potassium currents responsible for the action potential, but also an A-current, two types of calcium currents, calcium-activated potassium currents, inward rectifier currents, ATP-sensitive K^+ currents, and other currents (70,94). There seems to be little disagreement about the presence of these channels in respiratory neurons since after their initial demonstration in brain slices, many of these channels were studied in identified respiratory neurons in vivo. Assignment of a role for these currents in shaping the activity of DRG neurons is still subject to study and speculation and will ultimately require their further investigation in vivo and in vitro.

A major advantage of studying the cellular properties of respiratory neurons in vitro is that is allows comparisons with other, better-characterized motor networks. Such a comparative approach could lead to new insights about how rhythmic breathing movements are controlled. An example of the apparent conservation of cellular properties among diverse types of motor networks is that based on the A-current. Some bulbospinal DRG neurons in both the guinea pig (95,96) and the rat (97) possess an A-current that, when activate, causes a long delay between the time of depolarization and the occurrence of the first action potential (Fig. 8). This is called delayed excitation and is shared by other motor systems, including *Tritonia* swimming (73) lamprey swimming (98,99), and *Aplysia* inking behavior (78). The A-current and delayed excitation have also been observed in phrenic motoneurons in the cat (70). This A-current is a fast-transient outward current that is activated by depolarization but then rapidly inactivates (95,97). In most systems, the A-current undergoes steady-state inactivation at resting membrane potential levels, and this is removed by hyperpolarization. Thus, for delayed excitation to be observed, a cell must first by hyperpolarized for its subsequent expression during depolarization unless its resting potential is not associated with A-current inactivation. For a given level of depolarizing drive, therefore, the amount of delayed excitation will depend on the preceding membrane potential level. This history-dependent expression of the A-current has particular significance for rhythmic motor networks where neurons undergo oscillations in their membrane potential between hyperpolarized and depolarized levels. Although still speculative, it has been suggested that delayed excitation may be responsible for the repetitive firing activity of "late" inspiratory neurons in the DRG (70). If this were true, it is possible that the A-current in these neurons works in conjunction with other processes such as synaptic facilitation to shape a ramp-like excitatory synaptic drive to phrenic motoneurons. Provided that individual members of this pool possessed slightly different membrane potential levels before being depolarized, they would express various amounts of delayed excitation. This would lead to a gradual recruitment of the ensemble spike activity within a pool during the course of depolarization, which, in turn, would be translated into a ramp-like excitatory synaptic drive to phrenic motoneurons.

For bulbospinal neurons in the guinea pig or rat DRG, the magnitude of delayed excitation can be modulated over a wide range of membrane potential levels. During expiration, DRG neurons receive synaptic inhibition, which hyperpolarizes their membrane potential level to between -60 and -80 mV (70,97). Over this membrane potential range, the magnitude of the delay would vary between 25 and 300 msec, respectively. These data demonstrate that, within the limits of expiratory phase membrane potential levels, the magnitude of delayed excitation can be varied by at least an order of magnitude.

With the recent data obtained about the cellular and membrane properties and synaptic efficiency of newborn neurons, differences in the integrated output between newborn and adult neural networks could be explained. For example, both active and passive cellular properties in newborn DRG cells are different from those in adults (100,101). Newborn brainstem neurons have less spike frequency adaptation, less inward rectifier currents, different afterhyperpolarization, a wider action potential waveform, and no delayed excitation (101). Such maturational changes are related to changes in a number of variables pertaining to cytosolic as well as to membrane structure and function. For example, the distribution on cells, the structural and functional nature, and the regulation and modulation of ion channels change with age in early life. Because the ramp neural drive is absent from phrenic discharge in the young rat, one hypothesis is that the phrenic discharge pattern is causally related to the lack of delayed excitation in the newborn (70). Another tenable hypothesis is that the phrenic discharge pattern in the newborn is a reflection of immature and inefficient central synapses. This immaturity is evidenced by the fact that there is a maturational decrease in the amount of current required to induce postsynaptic potentials and that these postsynaptic potentials cannot be maintained with prolonged stimulation as in the adult.

Are Neurons in the Young More or Less Tolerant to Anoxic Stress?

There are a number of reasons for trying to understand questions related to O_2 deprivation in the CNS. Some of those pertain to this chapter. For example, since the response of the cardiorespiratory and sympathetic systems depends on CNS neurons and the change in their excitability during hypoxia, the neurophysiological changes that occur in these cells become exceedingly important. In addition, since well-differentiated neurons do not "regenerate" when they are lethally injured (this dogma is at present being challenged), understanding the cascade of events that occur before irreversible damage also becomes crucial if we were to design therapies to prevent such injury.

Brainstem Neurons

Since brainstem nuclei contain neurons that are responsible for the control and regulation of vital functions such as respiration, blood pressure, and cardiac

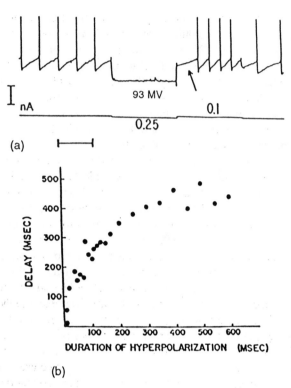

(a)

(b)

Figure 8 Delayed excitation in a neuron from the ventrolateral region of the tractus solitarius in the adult rat. (a) Arrow points to the delay that occurs at the outset of the depolarization. (b) This delay depends on the duration of the hyperpolarization that precedes the onset of the delay. (c) This delay depends also on the membrane potential reached during the prepulse hyperpolarization. (d) Firing frequency histogram showing the delay when the depolarization occurs after the prepulse (W Prepulse) (97).

micity, understanding the effect of hypoxia on these neurons and their responses has been an important topic for respiratory and cardiovascular neurobiologists and neurophysiologists. Recent studies in our laboratory on hypoglossal neurons at rest and during O_2 deprivation have shown that hypoxia produces a major depolarization in brainstem neurons of adult rats (101–104). No hyperpolarization has been observed in studies of more than 350–400 brainstem neurons to date in our laboratory. A depolarization has been observed in several cardiorespiratory neuronal groups, including hypoglossal neurons (102,103), neurons in the dorsal motor nucleus of the vagus (104,105), neurons in the nucleus of solitary tract (105), and those in the Kölliker-Fuse nucleus when exposed to hypoxia or anoxia (C Jiang and GG Haddad, unpublished observations) (Fig. 9). This depolarization starts to occur within 1 min of hypoxic exposure (Po_2 = 10–20 torr, cf. Ref. 106)

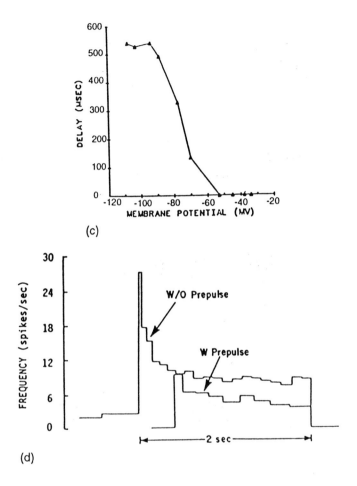

(c)

(d)

and reaches a maximum of about 30 mV in about 3–5 min (102). Anoxia ($Po_2 = 0$ torr) induces a larger a larger depolarization in even less time (103).

So far the mechanisms for this hypoxia-induced depolarization are not well understood. Blockade of action potentials and, in turn, inhibition of synaptic interactions (high Mg^{2+}, low Ca^{2+}) does not seem to affect this depolarization, suggesting that the anoxia-induced depolarization is mediated by alterations in the inherent neuronal postsynaptic membrane properties (102). Our most recent studies have shown that removal of Na^+ from ECF (extracellular fluid) blunts the depolarization (107). Furthermore, energy failure may play an important role in this depolarization since addition of ATP in the recording pipette in our studies reduces in a major way the hypoxia-induced changes in membrane currents in freshly dissociated brainstem neurons studies with patch electrodes (107) (C Jiang, TR Cummins, and GG Haddad, unpublished observations).

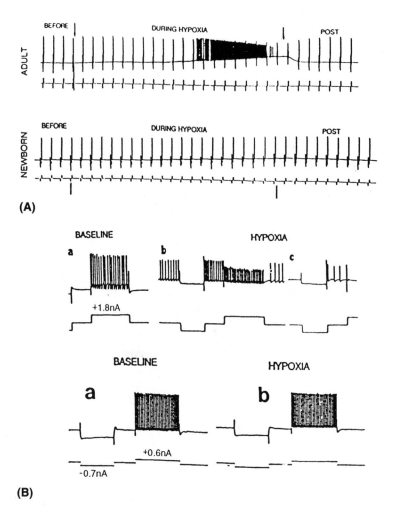

(A)

(B)

Figure 9 Hypoxia-induced depolarization is much larger in the older rat than in the neonatal rat. (A) Intracellular records from an adult hypoglossal neuron (top) and a neonatal one (bottom). Note extent of depolarization in both ages. Arrows show start and end of hypoxic period. Lower curves are current injections. (B) Higher-resolution intracellular records from the adult neuron (top, a, b, c) with current steps shown. Lower panels are obtained from a neonatal record with current injections shown below (bottom, a, b). (C) Average data at various ages representing the maximum change in V_{max} as a function of age (left) and a proportion of cells histogram showing disjoint populations between cells the first 2 weeks of life and 28 days of life (right) (102).

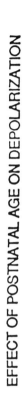

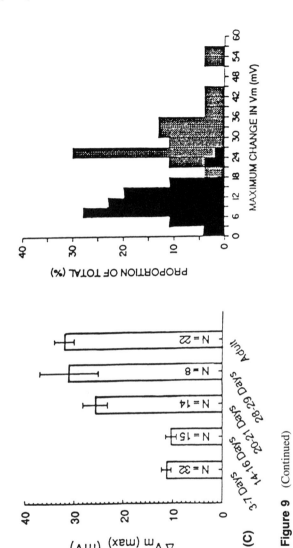

Figure 9 (Continued)

Hippocampal and Neocortical Neurons

The response and vulnerability of central neurons to O_2 deprivation varies with a number of factors, including species, age, phylum, brain region, and so forth. For example, it is well known that hippocampal CA1 neurons are exquisitely sensitive to anoxia and ischemia (108). Since other neurons in this same region (e.g., dentate gyrus) are relatively more tolerant to hypoxia (109,110), it would be advantageous to study hippocampal brain slices to learn about the differential sensitivity to hypoxia in central neurons (111). It is not surprising, therefore, that there have been numerous studies on neurons from the CA1, the CA3, and the dentate gyrus (104,112–117). Neurons in these areas may slightly hyperpolarize initially during a short period of hypoxia (2–4 min), with decreased synaptic noise and input resistance (R_N) (112,114,115). This hyperpolarization and decrease in R_N are likely mediated by activation of K^+ channels (15,112,118). With longer periods of hypoxia (5–8 min), the small hyperpolarization is followed by a depolarization, the etiology of which remains unclear (115). In contrast to brainstem neurons, a marked suppression in synaptic potentials has been found in CA1 cells (119–120). It is interesting that, although the membrane potential trajectory during hypoxia in brainstem neurons is different from that of hippocampal CA1 neurons, brainstem cells do not seem to be more resistant to O_2 deprivation than CA1 neurons. It is important also to realize that Po_2 levels in the CA1 studies were not measured and differences in response between these neurons and brainstem cells cannot be compared easily.

Rat neocortical neurons respond similarly to those in humans when challenged with hypoxia (121–123). As in the hippocampus, human and rat neocortical neurons show a small hyperpolarization (3–7 mV) at the beginning (2–4 min) of the anoxia exposure (123). In human neocortical neurons, this transient hyperpolarization is followed by return of a membrane potential (V_m) to baseline; this level is then maintained for a considerable period (5–20 min) before depolarization (123). Depolarization appears usually after several minutes have passed during anoxic exposure. Along with the early hyperpolarization, synaptic potentials are markedly suppressed, the threshold for action potential generation is significantly increased, and, in the majority of neocortical neurons studied, R_N is decreased (123). These alterations indicate that a reduction in membrane excitability occurs during anoxia in human cortical neurons. We have also shown that similar changes in V_m, R_N and rheobase occur in rat neocortical neurons (Fig. 10) (123). It is important to mention that the decrease in excitability in neocortical neurons in rats and humans is related not only to K^+ channel opening, but also to Na^+ channel inactivation, as we have subsequently shown (117,124). Indeed, one important and interesting mechanism that we have demonstrated in human and rat neocortical and CA1 neurons is that the steady-state availability of the voltage-sensitive Na^+ channels is reduced during O_2 deprivation in a major way, rendering the Na^+ current very small (Fig. 11) (124).

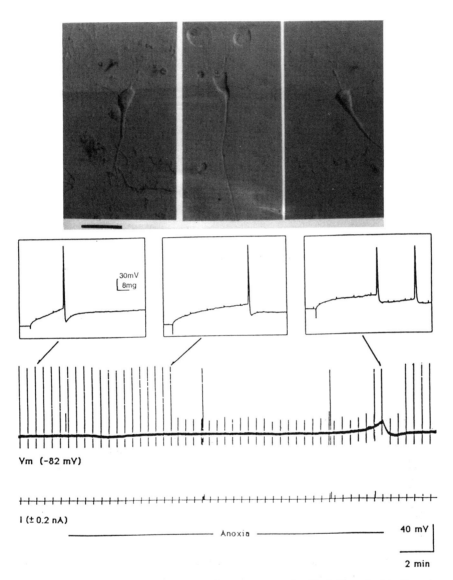

Figure 10 Human neocortical neuronal response to anoxia. (Top) Three freshly dissociated neurons from the temporal neocortex of a human. (Bottom) Intracellular records from a human neocortical cell (temporal lobe) in a slice preparation. Note that excitability decreases in time during anoxia. This is most likely due to inhibition of Na^+ channels (see text) as well as activation of K^+ channels. Window insets illustrate an increase in rheobase (note size of current injected to elicit action potential) (123).

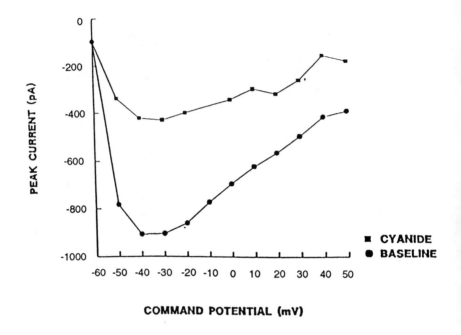

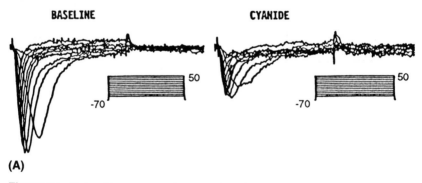

(A)

Figure 11 Rat and human central neurons inhibit their Na^+ channels during metabolic inhibition (cyanide) or during anoxia. (A) Peak voltage-sensitive Na^+ current at various command potentials during baseline and cyanide (2–4 mM) in an adult rat hippocampal neuron. Note the much decreased current induced. (Bottom) Family of curves elicited with command potentials during both conditions. (B) Similar plot (left) as in A for a human neuron exposed to anoxia. Note the similar response. (Right) Steady-state inactivation is shifted to the left during anoxia, indicating that there is inhibition of Na^+ channels during anoxia in human neurons as well. Arrows point to curves during anoxia (117,124).

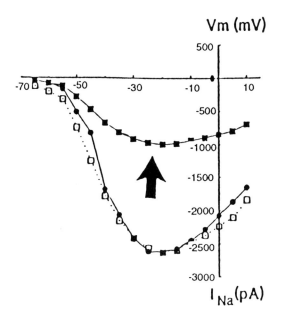

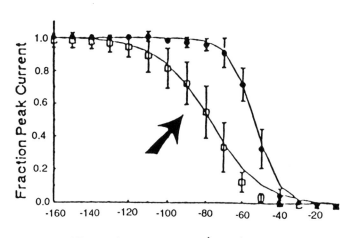

(B)

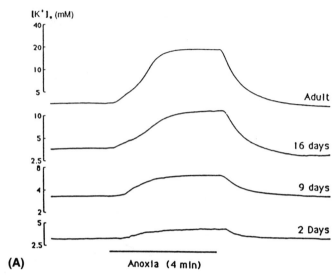

Figure 12 Extracellular K+ in slice preparation from various regions of the adult rat brain and from rats of various ages in the same region (hypoglossal, XII). (A) K+ increases as a function of age in anoxia (scales are different). (B) Dependence of extracellular K+ on region (hippocampal CA1, XII, or vagal motoneurons or DMNX) and on severity of O_2 deprivation (hypoxia = 10–15 torr, anoxia = 0 torr within 20 sec). (Bottom) K+ in neonatal slice tissue in the region of XII during anoxia along with the DC potential (104).

Neurons in the Neonate

The neonatal brain seems to be much more resistant to O_2 deprivation than that of the adult. The first documented observation related to anoxia tolerance in the newborn, made by the Frenchman Legallois in 1813 (Table 1) (79), has been confirmed since then (4,125,126). In our recent studies, neonatal brainstem hypoglossal neurons depolarize only modestly to hypoxia, and this is about one-third to one-fourth the change in their adult counterparts (102). Measurements of intracellular and extracellular ionic activities from our laboratory have also demonstrated that ionic homeostasis in the neonatal neurons is much better maintained during anoxia (Fig. 12). Also, anoxia induces only modest changes of R_N and synaptic potentials in hippocampal CA1 cells of the neonate as compared with the adult (114, 120).

The underlying mechanisms for the hypoxic tolerance in the neonatal neurons are not clear. However, it is possible that the newborn's apparent tolerance to O_2 deprivation is due to differences in metabolic pathways (127), such as the ability of the newborn to decrease its overall metabolic rate to preserve ATP levels (4,128). Supporting this idea are our recent observations that the average tissue O_2

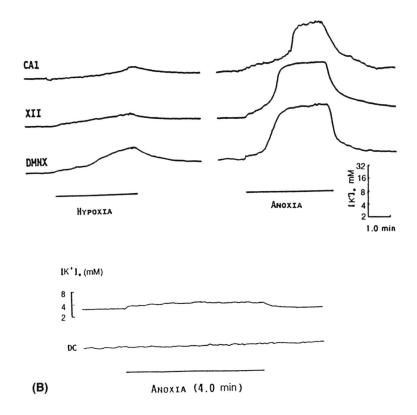

(B) ANOXIA (4.0 min)

tension in the neonatal brain slice is significantly higher than that in the adult during anoxia (106). Similarly, previous studies done in the slice have demonstrated higher ATP levels in the young than in the mature animal during and at the end of hypoxia (128).

It is clear therefore from this analysis that, although we have made tremendous strides toward the understanding of respiratory control at the central level, there are inumerable questions that are basic and fundamental to the overall integration of the cardiorespiratory control system that still do not have answers. There are also approaches now that were not available until recently, making our endeavors more exciting and more yielding.

Knowledge of afferent information and of central neuronal characteristics does not suffice for assessment of the overall respiratory function and feedback system. This is especially valid in cases of disease or conditions in which physiological homeostasis is jeopardized. For example, in cases when the ventilatory output is impaired because of mechanical abnormalities of the lung (e.g., asthma), afferent feedback and central neuronal studies are not sufficient to understand overall function. It is in these instances that detailed analysis of normal and abnormal muscle function at various levels will be invaluable.

IV. Role of Respiratory Muscles in Respiratory Control in the Young

Even in the presence of a mature and functional central nervous system and afferent input to it, the overall system can still fail because of potential immaturity or abnormalities with the pump apparatus. Therefore, we will review here the basic properties of muscle fiber physiology and biochemistry as well as their responses to loads to put in perspective the role of muscles in the overall control system, especially in the young.

A. Fatigue Resistance of the Developing Diaphragm: Structural and Metabolic Correlates

Fiber-Type Composition and Oxidative Capacity

Although many muscles constitute the respiratory musculature, the diaphragm, the major inspiratory muscle, has been studied most extensively. The literature is replete with studies showing that the respiratory muscles in the adult possess a finite tolerance to acute loading, and that increasing the intensity or the duration of the load leads to failure of the muscles to perform adequately (129–133). In comparison to the adult, fewer studies have examined the response of developing respiratory muscles to loading. In addition, data relating to the susceptibility of the newborn diaphragm to fatigue remain controversial. This controversy can probably be explained by the difference in the properties examined by various investigators. For instance, some of the earliest studies of the developing diaphragm focused on examining the muscle fiber types as identified by histochemical staining properties (134–136). This approach has been used in skeletal muscles where it has been shown that in the adult hindlimb muscle, the degree of histochemical staining of a fiber by the myosin ATPase reaction correlates with the contractile and fatigue properties of the muscle (137). For example, fibers that stain lightly with the myosin ATPase reaction, i.e., type I fibers, have a slow contraction time and half relaxation time, a low peak tension, and are resistant to fatigue when stimulated electrically using a paradigm such as the Burke protocol (trains of 40 Hz for 330 msec for a total period of 2 min) (138). These fibers usually have a high oxidative capacity as evidenced by the intensity of staining for oxidative enzymes such as succinate dehydrogenase (SDH), nicotinamide dinucleotide dehydrogenase (NADH), or cytochrome C oxidase (COX) (135,139–141). Dark-staining fibers in the myosin ATPase reaction, or type II fibers, have contractile properties that are opposite to those of type I fibers; however, these fibers may be subclassified on the basis of their fatigue resistance (139). Using this approach, Keens et al. examined the histochemical fiber types in postmortem specimens of human diaphragms from prematurity through adulthood (134). These investigators found that there was a preponderance of type II (fast, fatigable) fibers in the premature diaphragm, and that with advancing age the proportion of these fibers decreased and more type I (fatigue resistant) fibers appeared. These data suggested that the premature and newborn human diaphragm was more susceptible to fatigue than the adult. However, subsequent to this study Maxwell et al. performed a similar analysis of the developing baboon diaphragm but examined also the oxidative capacity of the muscle fibers (135). Although an increasing proportion of type I fibers was also found in the developing baboon diaphragm, these investigators identified a subgroup of type II fibers, type IIc, in the younger diaphragms, which possess oxidative properties similar to type I rather than to type II fibers. Hence they suggested that based on its oxidative capacity, the developing baboon diaphragm may be more resistant to fatigue than the mature diaphragm. To confirm this, these investigators examined the contractile properties of the baboon diaphragm in vitro and found that the immature diaphragm during prolonged electrical stimulation was much more fatigue resistant than the mature baboon diaphragm (135). However, this fatigue resistance decreased prenatally with maturation, so that the premature diaphragm was less fatigue resistant than the mature diaphragm. Sieck and co-workers have found that in other species, the rat and cat, the newborn diaphragm is more resistant to fatigue than the adult diaphragm (142,143). The fatigue resistance did not correlate with oxidative capacity of the diaphragm, as SDH activity was uniformly low at birth and increased with postnatal development (144). This led to further investigation of other structural properties that are important for energy substrate delivery to the muscle, such as capillary density. Here it was found that in the adult cat diaphragm, fatigue resistance correlated with capillary density of muscle fiber units (145). In the kitten, diaphragm capillary density correlated with SDH activity (146), but neither correlated with fatigue resistance (143).

Energy Substrate Availability

Since structural properties cannot fully explain the endurance properties of the developing diaphragm, attention has also been directed toward examining the availability of energy substrates to the muscle. This is important because it has been hypothesized that diaphragmatic fatigue develops when there is an imbalance between the energy supply and demand of the muscle (147). This hypothesis has been supported by data from the adult showing that respiratory muscle blood flow and oxygen consumption increased markedly from baseline when respiratory loads were applied (148,149). However, because of the large contractile force and the duration of the contraction associated with these loads, compression of intramuscular blood vessels may occur and blood flow to the muscle may be impeded (150). This has been examined more closely by studying the relationship between diaphragm fatigability and two indices of energy requirement, namely the force of contraction of the diaphragm (transdiaphragmatic pressure, or Pdi) and the pattern of breathing as reflected by the respiratory duty cycle (Ti/Ttot) (151). The product of these two indices is the tension time index (TTi). The results of these studies demonstrate that the endurance time of the diaphragm decreases as Pdi/Pdi_{max} and Ti/Ttot are increased (151). Also, there appears to be a strong relationship between blood flow and TTi, such that as Ti/Ttot and/or Pdi/Pdi_{max} are increased, impairment of blood flow to the diaphragm occurs and may have a detrimental effect on function (152,153). However, in recent studies in our laboratory, we have measured diaphragmatic blood flow in unanesthetized sheep subjected to inspiratory flow resistive loads and found that there was no significant decrease in blood flow at the time when Pdi decreased and respiratory failure ensued (154). This raises the question as to whether impairment of blood flow is at the basis of the development of diaphragmatic fatigue in the intact animal. Interestingly, when oxygen content and Po_2 were measured in the phrenic venous effluent of sheep subjected to similar loads, we found that they increased when Pdi was decreasing (155). Coupled with our blood flow findings, these data suggest that oxygen consumption by the diaphragm decreased at that time despite the maintenance of oxygen delivery to the muscle, and that this may be secondary to failure of cellular mechanisms to utilize energy in the muscle itself.

Of note is the fact that there are fewer studies in the newborn examining the changes in blood flow to the respiratory muscles with loading. In a study by Mayock et al. in anesthetized piglets, no impairment of blood flow was found during resistive loading (156). This is contrary to what has been shown by Nichols et al. in the newborn lamb during electrical stimulation of the diaphragm (157). Further studies are needed to address this important issue during development.

In addition to the role of blood flow and circulating energy substrates, another source of energy to the muscle resides in the tissue itself, i.e., the muscle stores of glycogen. In adult limb muscle, glycogen depletion has been temporally associated with muscle fatigue or exhaustion; however, there is evidence that the two phenomena are not causally related (158). We and others have shown that the diaphragm in the newborn animal is rich in glycogen at birth (159–161), but it is unclear whether the newborn diaphragm is equipped with the metabolic machinery necessary to utilize the glycogen for energy production. In the rat, the level of activity of several glycolytic enzymes is lower than in the adult (160,162,163), suggesting that at least in this species glycogen cannot be utilized effectively. However, in a recent report, we have shown that in the newborn lamb glycogen depletion occurs in the diaphragm of these animals when subjected to inspiratory resistive loads, as occurs in the adult sheep (Fig. 13) (161). It is possible that these

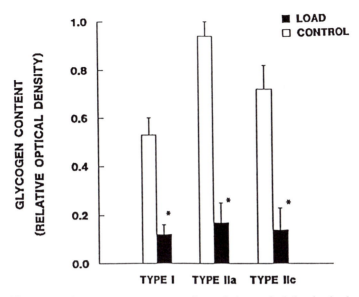

Figure 13 Mean glycogen content expressed as relative optical density in the costal diaphragm from control lambs and lambs subjected to severe inspiratory flow resistive loads. With these loads, glycogen content decreased in all fiber types, with the decrease being greatest in type IIa fibers, followed by type IIc and I fibers. *p, 0.005, loaded compared with control for each fiber type (161).

results can be explained by a greater degree of maturity of the newborn lamb as compared to the newborn rat.

B. Physiological Response to Loading

Diaphragmatic Endurance

As noted earlier, many reports in the literature support the belief that the adult diaphragm will fatigue when subjected to a high workload (129–133). In this context, diaphragmatic fatigue is defined as failure to generate the force required to meet ventilatory demands when the neuromuscular system is subjected to an increased load; upon removal of the load, functional recovery ensues. Using this definition, early studies have demonstrated that diaphragmatic fatigue occurs in the newborn human diaphragm as well (164,165). In these studies, diaphragmatic function was assessed by analyzing the change in the distribution of the frequency components of the diaphragm electromyogram (EMG) recorded with surface (skin) electrodes. This technique derives from studies of skeletal muscle that have shown that an increase in the low-frequency components of the EMG precedes the decrease in force generation (166,167). The shift in the spectral density to lower frequencies is expressed as a decrease in either the centroid frequency or the high (frequency)-to-low (frequency) ratio (H/L). In premature infants and infants being weaned from mechanical ventilation, electromyographic evidence of diaphragmatic fatigue was found (164,165). For example, Muller et al. found that the diaphragm EMG H/L decreased in infants who failed to be weaned from mechanical ventilation, but not in infants who could be weaned successfully. Evidence of diaphragmatic fatigue has been reported from neonatal animals such as the piglet, rabbit, and lamb (161, 168,169). In the animal studies Pdi was measured during loaded breathing as an index of force generated by the diaphragm. This measurement was lacking in the human studies. These experiments provide more conclusive evidence that diaphragmatic fatigue, as defined above, can occur in the newborn subjected to a respiratory load.

Factors Affecting Diaphragmatic Performance

Several properties of the respiratory system in the neonate differ from that of the adult and may affect the response of the diaphragm to load. The first of these factors is the neonatal thoracic cage. The newborn rib cage is highly compliant, providing little support of the chest wall for diaphragmatic action (170–172). Hence the rib cage may be distorted easily with increased respiratory effort (170–172). This propensity to distortion is compounded by the fact that the tonic intercostal muscle activity, which usually provides support for the rib cage, is inhibited during rapid eye movement (REM) sleep (165,173). As the diaphragm contracts during REM sleep, the rib cage moves inward and the abdominal wall outward, resulting in "paradoxical breathing" (174). In addition, phasic diaphragmatic activity may be increased during REM sleep, to compensate for the loss of intercostal activity (169,173). As a significant proportion of the work of the diaphragm is expended on chest wall distortion rather than effective ventilation, it has been suggested that increased diaphragmatic work during REM sleep in the newborn may result in diaphragmatic fatigue (164).

Other factors contribute to the effectiveness of diaphragmatic force output also. The ribs in the newborn thorax are oriented horizontally, in comparison to the oblique orientation of the adult ribs. Because of this, contraction of the intercostal muscles provides little additional increase in thoracic volume (173). In addition, the newborn infant spends most of the time supine, a position that has been shown to lead to up to a 15% decrease in functional residual capacity as compared to the upright position (171).

The mechanical disadvantage may not be limited to the rib cage and intercostal muscles, but may reside in the diaphragm as well. Recent data has confirmed the notion that the diaphragm is flattened in the newborn with a small area of apposition (172). Such a configuration, similar to that in lung hyperinflation, is thought to be mechanically disadvantageous, resulting in less shortening and less force production and airflow into the lungs (175). This speculation has been supported by data in the piglet showing that as lung volume decreased, the force response to electrical stimulation increased more in the older than in the newborn piglet (176,177). Because chest wall compliance was the same in these two groups of animals, the authors concluded that the difference in the response may be explained by a difference in diaphragmatic configuration (176).

C. Neuromuscular Interactions and Sites of Failure as a Function of Age

The various sites of respiratory muscle fatigue have been grouped in two broad categories: central and peripheral. Central failure refers to the central nervous system, and peripheral sites include the nerve fibers, the neuromuscular junction, or the muscle itself.

Central Fatigue

Central fatigue refers to two conditions. In the first condition, the excitatory drive diminishes without a concomitant decrease in force. In the second situation, a loss of force is also observed. In both conditions, there is an attempt by motoneurons to optimize their firing pattern to the needs and capability of the muscle. For instance, if the muscle is incapable of maintaining contraction because of failure of its contractile machinery, a drop in the firing discharge of the motoneurons may occur in an attempt to "protect" the muscle from depletion of high-energy phosphates or acetylcholine. This neural adaptation hypothesis postulates that there is a reflex decrease in firing discharge, possibly mediated by an effluent metabolite such as lactate or potassium ion (178). Although it has been suggested that central failure plays a role in the development of diaphragmatic fatigue in the adult (178,179), few studies have examined this directly in the newborn. In one study in anesthetized infant monkeys during prolonged inspiratory resistive loading (180), central output was assessed by measuring diaphragmatic minute EMG activity (respiratory frequency × peak EMG moving time average). This index was found to decrease during sustained loading, but the decrease was primarily due to bradypnea. These data, however, do not take into account alteration in neuromuscular transmission, which would not be appreciated if the EMG alone is examined.

Peripheral Fatigue

Peripheral mechanisms of muscle fatigue involve several potential sites. These sites include the nerve fibers along which axonal conduction failure may occur, failure of transmission across the neuromuscular junction, and failure of excitation-contraction coupling or of the contractile machinery.

In the in vitro nerve-muscle preparation from an adult animal, neuromuscular transmission failure can be easily elicited (181–184). In the intact subject, neuromuscular transmission failure has not been considered an important site of skeletal muscle fatigue (185). However, recent work by Aldrich (186) and from our laboratory (187) suggests that at least in animals subjected to inspiratory resistive loading, neuromuscular transmission failure may be an important mechanism that contributes to the development of diaphragmatic fatigue. Of interest also is the finding from our laboratory and others (188,189) that in the newborn rat diaphragm in vitro, force generation cannot be maintained during nerve stimulation for brief periods. This finding was not observed with direct muscle stimulation or with either stimulation route in the adult (Fig. 14). These data suggest that neuromuscular transmission failure may be more important as a site of fatigue in the newborn diaphragm than in the adult. These data do not, however, identify the mechanisms leading to this failure.

The neuromuscular axis is a dynamic system, undergoing major remodeling during early development. Innervation of muscle fibers is polyneuronal at birth, with synaptic elimination occurring during the first few weeks in rodents (190–192). The neuromuscular junctional folds increase in number and complexity (193), and the density of acetylcholine (ACh) receptors increases as well (194). Extrajunctional receptors found in early postnatal life disappear so that the receptors become concentrated in the junction (195,196). Structural and functional properties of the ACh receptor change as well; embryonic subunits are replaced by adult types (197). The opening time of the channel is slower in the neonate than in the mature muscle (198). Quantal content and release of ACh and safety factor have all shown to be less in the newborn than in the more mature muscle (199–201). Hence, with the tremendous change associated with maturation and development, it would not be surprising if neuromuscular transmission was found to be more susceptible to failure in the newborn. To investigate some of these possible mechanisms, we have begun to examine the electrophysiological changes in single muscle fibers during contraction in response to nerve stimulation (202). In this study, we found that in the newborn rat diaphragm muscle, action potentials failed to follow nerve stimulation at 50 Hz in about one-half of the fibers studied. The areas devoid of action potentials showed smaller deflections that were most likely end-plate potentials (epps) (Fig. 15). These data suggested that failure of adequate neurotransmitter release in the newborn led to generation of subthreshold epps and hence no action potentials. A more direct assessment of neurotransmitter release is needed to support this hypothesis. This might be performed by applying recently described optical techniques that utilize fluorescent dyes that bind to the membrane of neurotransmitter vesicles (203). Changes in the intensity of fluorescence can be correlated with vesicle release (203). However, this mechanism is only one of many possibilities. A recent report by Fournier et al. also analyzed epps in newborn rat diaphragms (188). Contractions were inhibited in this preparation by adding curare to the perfusate to partially block ACh receptors and render epp amplitude subthreshold. The results of this study suggest that axonal conduction block may be the mechanism underlying

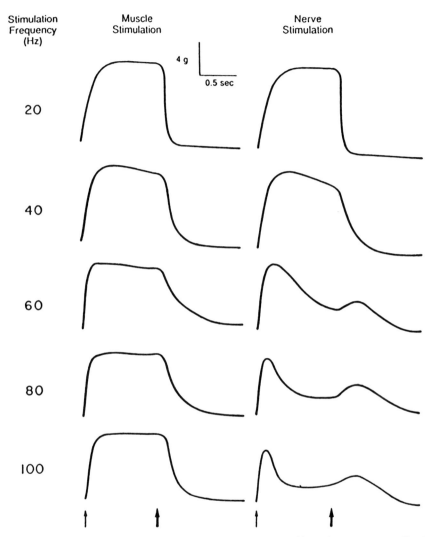

Figure 14 Force developed by diaphragm from a 7-day-old rat in response to direct muscle and nerve stimulation at 20, 40, 60, 80, and 100 Hz. Arrows mark the beginning (light arrow) and end (heavy arrow) of the 1-sec stimulus train. At nerve stimulation frequencies ≥ 40 Hz, peak force is not maintained during the stimulus (189).

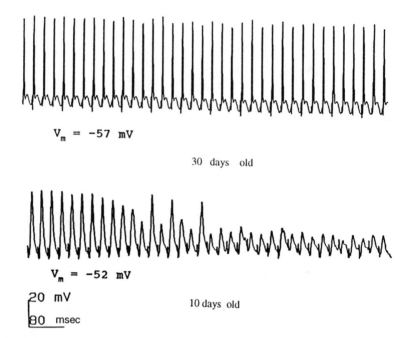

$V_m = -57$ mV

30 days old

$V_m = -52$ mV

20 mV

80 msec

10 days old

Figure 15 Intracellular recording from a 30-day-old (top) and 10-day-old (bottom) diaphragm muscle fiber during phrenic nerve stimulation at 50 Hz. Note that in the 10-day-old fiber, less than 50 action potentials are generated, and that the absent action potentials are replaced by smaller deflections, possibly epps (202).

neuromuscular transmission failure in the newborn diaphragm. Further studies are needed to explain these mechanisms more completely.

Clearly, a contraction cannot be produced if the muscle contractile machinery cannot respond to the preceding chain of events. As these events are electrical in nature and are expressed as a series of ionic currents, the process of excitation-contraction (EC) coupling is the link between these events. Studies of diaphragmatic function and fatigue in the newborn have suggested that EC coupling is an important site of failure at this age. For instance, the sarcoplasmic reticulum in the newborn baboon diaphragm is poorly developed (135), which results in delayed release and uptake of Ca^{2+}. The functional significance of this is reflected in the slow contraction and relaxation times in the newborn diaphragm (135). Although diaphragmatic fibers in the newborn baboon have high mitochondrial content, the prolonged relaxation time may impede blood flow and impair oxidative capacity.

The contractile proteins in the developing diaphragm have been the focus of attention in recent years. The previously applied histochemical categorization of developing diaphragmatic muscle fibers using adult criteria has not explained the observed fatigue resistance of the newborn diaphragm. As described above, oxidative capacity is uniformly low in the neonatal diaphragm and increases with age (142). Fatigue resistance follows the opposite trend and does not correlate with oxidative capacity (144). To better understand the basis for muscle contractile properties, immunohistochemical techniques have been used to identify isoforms of the myosin heavy chain (MHC) within the muscle fiber. In the newborn and adult muscle, four types of MHC have been reported: slow (type I), fast (type IIA), fast (type IIB). These MHC isoforms are usually found in the histochemically identified fiber types with the corresponding name (204–205). A fourth isoform, fast (type IIX), has also been recently identified (206). During development, two additional isoforms, MHC-embryonic and MHC-neonatal, are transiently expressed (207,208). In the neonatal rat diaphragm, recent studies have shown that MHC-neonatal and MHC slow are expressed initially, and that with maturation the adult fast isoforms appear while the neonatal form disappears (209,210). Of note is the fact that the rate of myofibrillar ATPase activity is lower in the developing muscle than in the adult (143). It has been speculated that the slow MHC isoforms present in early postnatal life with their slower cross-bridging have a lower energy requirement and hence may be more resistant to fatigue; the lower oxidative capacity of these fibers may reflect this balance (143).

The respiratory muscles play a major role in maintaining ventilation during loaded breathing in the neonate. Although information is available with respect to some of the factors that determine the response of respiratory muscles, many factors remain unknown. In addition, little is understood regarding the cellular and molecular processes that underlie proper and improper functioning of these muscles at a time when major development and remodeling occurs. Hence it is of utmost importance that we try to understand these mechanisms so that we may provide the therapies necessary in the newborn period, an age when respiratory problems remain a major cause of morbidity and mortality.

In summary, the understanding of the respiratory control system and its development is entering a new era. This is not unlike what is now being experienced in other systems, conditions, disease states, and disciplines. The exciting new approaches that are possible now, whether at the level of the integrated system, single cells, or gene, will no doubt revolutionize our thinking regarding how cells in the central nervous system divide, migrate, differentiate, and communicate with one another, to ultimately form, underlie, and refine intricate animal behavior, including respiration.

References

1. Rakic P, Bourgeois JP, Eckenhoff MF, Zecevic N, Goldman-Rakic PS. Concurrent overproduction of synapses in diverse regions of the primate cerebral cortex. Science 1986; 232(4747):232–235.

2. Donnelly DF, Haddad GG. Respiratory changes induced by prolonged laryngeal stimulation in unanesthetized piglets. J Appl Physiol 1986; 61:1018–1024.

3. Haddad GG, Lai TL, Mellins RB. Determination of the ventilatory pattern in REM sleep in normal infants. J Appl Physiol 1982; 53(1):52–56, 1982.

4. Haddad GG, Mellins RB. Hypoxia and respiratory control in early life. Annu Rev Physiol 1984; 46:629–643.

5. Rigatto H. A critical analysis of the development of peripheral and central respiratory chemosensitivity during the neonatal period. In: von Euler C, Lagercrantz H, eds. Central Nervous Control Mechanisms in Breathing. Oxford, UK: Pergamon, 1979: 137–148.

6. Bowes G, Townsend ER, Kozar LF, Bromley SM, Phillipson EA. Effect of carotid body denervation on arousal response to hypoxia in sleeping dogs. J Appl Physiol 1981; 51:40–45.

7. Bureau MA, Lamarche J, Foulon P, Dalle D. Postnatal maturation of respiration in intact and carotid body chemodenervated lambs. J Appl Physiol 1985; 59:869–874.

8. Bureau MA, Lamarche J, Foulon P, Dalle D. The ventilatory response to hypoxia in the newborn lamb after carotid body denervation. Respir Physiol 1985; 60:109–119.

9. Nakayama K. Surgical removal of the carotid body for bronchial asthma. Dis Chest 1961; 40:595–604.

10. Winter BJ. Carotid body resection in chronic obstructive pulmonary disease. Chest 1991; 100:883.

11. Blanco CE, Hanson MA, McCooke HB. Studies of chemoreceptor resetting after hyperoxic ventilation of the fetus in utero. In: Riberio JA, Pallot, DJ, eds. Chemoreceptors in Respiratory Control. London: Croom Helm, 1988:221–227.

12. Jansen AH, Purves MJ, Tan ED. The role of sympathetic nerves in the activation of the carotid body chemoreceptors at birth in the sheep. J Dev Physiol 1980; 2: 305–321.

13. Bureau MA, Begin R. Postnatal maturation of the respiratory response to O_2 in awake newborn lambs. J Appl Physiol 1982; 52:428–433.

14. Bureau MA, Cote A, Blanchard PW, Hobbs S, Foulon P, Dalle D. Exponential and diphasic ventilatory response to hypoxia in conscious lambs. J Appl Physiol 1986; 61:836–842.

15. Donnelly DF, Haddad GG. Prolonged apnea and impaired survival in piglets after sinus and aortic nerve section. J Appl Physiol 1990; 68:1048–1052.

16. Hofer MA. Lethal respiratory disturbance in neonatal rats after arterial chemoreceptor denervation. Life Sci 1984; 34:489–496.

17. Hofer MA. Sleep-wake state organization in infant rats with episodic respiratory disturbance following sinoaortic denervation. Sleep 1985; 8:40–48.

18. Haddad GG, Donnelly DF. The interaction of chemoreceptors and baroreceptors with the central nervous system. Ann NY Acad Sci 1988; 533:221–227.

19. Cole S, Lindenberg LB, Gallioto FM, Howe PE, DeGraff C, Davis JM, Lubka R, Gross EM. Ultrastructural abnormalities of the carotid body in sudden infant death syndrome. Pediatrics 1979; 63:13–17.

20. Naeye RL, Fisher R, Ryser M, Whalen P. Carotid body in sudden infant death syndrome. Science 1976; 191:567–569.

21. Perrin DG, Cutz E, Becker LE, Bryan AC, Madapallimatum A, Sole MJ. Sudden infant death syndrome: increased carotid body dopamine and noradrenaline content. Lancet 1984; 8:535–537.
22. Eden GJ, Hanson MA. Effects of chronic hypoxia from birth on the ventilatory response to acute hypoxia in the newborn rat. J Physiol (Lond) 1987; 392:11–19.
23. Hanson MA. Peripheral chemoreceptor function before and after birth. In: Johnston BM, Gluckman PD, eds. Respiratory Control and Lung Development in the Fetus and Newborn. Perinatology Reprod Series, 1986:311–330.
24. Hertzberg T, Hellstrom S, Lagercrantz H, Pequignot JM. Development of the arterial chemoreflex and turnover of carotid body catecholamines in the newborn rat. J Physiol (Lond) 1990; 425:211–225.
25. Carroll JL, Bureau MA. Decline in peripheral chemoreceptor excitatory stimulation during acute hypoxia in the lamb. J Appl Physiol 1987; 63:795–802.
26. Lawson EE, Long WW. Central origin of biphasic breathing pattern during hypoxia in newborns. J Appl Physiol 1983; 55:483–488.
27. Goiny M, Lagercrantz H, Srinivasan M, Ungerstedt U, Yamamoto Y. Hypoxia-mediated in vivo release of dopamine in nucleus tractus solitarii of rabbits. J Appl Physiol 1991; 70:2395–2400.
28. Biscoe TJ, Purves MJ, Sampson SR. Types of nervous activity which may be recorded from the carotid sinus nerve in the sheep fetus. J Physiol (Lond) 1969; 202:1–23.
29. Blanco CE, Dawes GS, Hanson MA, McCooke HB. The response to hypoxia of arterial chemoreceptors in fetal sheep and newborn lambs. J Physiol (Lond) 1984; 351:25–37.
30. Blanco CE, Hanson MA, Johnson P, Rigatto H. Breathing pattern of kittens during hypoxia. J Appl Physiol 1984; 56:12–17.
31. Hanson MA, Kumar P, McCooke HB. Post-natal resetting of carotid chemoreceptor sensitivity in the lamb. J Physiol (Lond) 1987; 382:57P.
32. Mulligan E, Bhide S. Non-sustained responses to hypoxia of carotid body chemoreceptor afferents in the piglet. FASEB J 1989; 3:A399.
33. Marchal F, Bairam A, Haouzi P, Crance JP, DiGiulio C, Vert P, Lahiri S. Carotid chemoreceptor response to natural stimuli in the newborn kitten. Respir Physiol 1992; 87:183–193.
34. Fitzgerald RS, Dehghani GA. Neural responses of the cat carotid and aortic bodies to hypercapnia and hypoxia. J Appl Physiol 1982; 52:596–601.
35. Kholwadwala D, Donnelly DF. Maturation of carotid chemoreceptor sensitivity to hypoxia: in vitro studies in the newborn rat. J Physiol (Lond) 1992; 453:461–473.
36. Eden GJ, Hanson MA. Maturation of the respiratory response to acute hypoxia in the newborn rat. J Physiol (Lond) 1987; 392:1–9.
37. Hanson MA, Kumar P, Williams BA. The effect of chronic hypoxia upon the development of respiratory chemoreflexes in the newborn kitten. J Physiol (Lond) 1989; 411:563–574.
38. Hertzberg T, Hellstrom S, Holgert H, Lagercrantz HM, Pequignot JM. Ventilatory response to hyperoxia in newborn rats born in hypoxia—possible relationship to carotid body dopamine. J Physiol (Lond) 1992; 456:645–654.

39. Mulligan E. Discharge properties of carotid bodies: developmental aspects. In: Haddad GG, Farber J, eds. Developmental Neurobiology of Breathing. New York: Marcel Dekker, 1991:321–349.

40. Schwieler GH. Respiratory regulation during postnatal development in cats and rabbits and some of its morphological substrate. Acta Physiol Scand 1968; 72: 1–123.

41. Acker H, Lubbers DW, Purves MJ, Tan ED. Measurement of the partial pressure of oxygen in the carotid body of foetal sheep and newborn lambs. J Dev Physiol 1980; 2:323–338.

42. Clarke JA, deBurgh Daly M, Ead HW. Comparison of the size of the vascular compartment of the carotid body of the fetal, neonatal and adult cat. Acta Anat 1990; 138:166–174.

43. Moore PJ, Clarke JA, Hanson MA, de B Daly M, Ead W. Quantitative studies of the vasculature of the carotid body in fetal and newborn sheep. J Dev Physiol 1991; 15:211–214.

44. McDonald DM. Peripheral chemoreceptors: structure-function relationships of the carotid body. In: Hornbein TF, ed. Regulation of Breathing. New York: Marcel Dekker, 1981:105–320.

45. Biscoe TJ, Purves MJ. Carotid body chemoreceptor activity in the new-born lamb. J Physiol (Lond) 1967; 190:443–454.

46. Neil E, O'Regan RG. The effects of electrical stimulation of the distal end of the cut sinus and aortic nerves on peripheral arterial chemoreceptor activity in the cat. J Physiol (Lond) 1971; 215:15–32.

47. Acker H. Measurements of potassium changes in the cat carotid body under hypoxia and hypercapnia. Pflüger's Arch 1978; 375:229–232.

48. Band DM, Linton RAF. Plasma potassium and the carotid body chemoreceptor in the cat. J Physiol (Lond) 1984; 345:33P.

49. Pokorski M, Lahiri S. Effects of naloxone on carotid body chemoreception and ventilation in the cat. J Appl Physiol 1981; 51:1533–1538.

50. Joels N, Neil E. The idea of a sensory transmitter. In: Torrance R, eds. Arterial Chemoreceptors. Oxford, UK, 1968:153–178.

51. Kondo H. An electron microscopic study on the development of synapses in the rat carotid body. Neurosci Lett 1976; 3:197–200.

52. Scheibner T, Read DJ, Sullivan CE. Distribution of substance P–immunoreactive structures in the developing cat carotid body. Brain Res 1988; 453:72–78.

53. Prabhakar N, Runold M, Yamamoto Y, Lagercrantz H, vonEuler C. Effect of substance P antagonist on hypoxia-induced carotid chemoreceptor activity. Acta Physiol Scand 1984; 121:301–303.

54. Donnelly DF, Smith EJ, Dutton RE. Neural response of carotid chemoreceptors following dopamine blockade. J Appl Physiol 1981; 50:172–177.

55. Lahiri S, Nishino T, Mokashi A, Mulligan E. Interaction of dopamine and halo-peridol with O_2 and CO_2 chemoreception in carotid body. J Appl Physiol 1980; 49: 45–51.

56. Gonzalez C, Almaraz L, Obeso A, Rigual R. Oxygen and acid chemoreception in the carotid body chemoreceptors. TINS 1992; 15:146–153.

57. Donnelly DF. Electrochemical detection of catecholamine release from rat carotid body, in vitro. J Appl Physiol 1993; 74(5):2330–2337.

58. Fidone S, Gonzalez C, Yoshizaki K. Effects of low oxygen on the release of dopamine from the rabbit carotid body in vitro. J Physiol (Lond) 1982;333: 93–110.

59. Gonzalez C, Fidone S. Increased release of 3H-dopamine during low O_2 stimulation of rabbit carotid body in vitro. Neurosci Lett 1977; 6:95–99.

60. Ganfornina MD, Lopez-Barneo J. Single K^+ channels in membrane patches of arterial chemoreceptor cells are modulated by O_2 tension. Proc Natl Acad Sci USA 1991; 88:2927–2930.

61. Peers C. Hypoxic suppression of K+ currents in type I carotid body cells: selective effect on the Ca^{2+}-activated K^+ current. Neurosci Lett 1990; 119:253–256.

62. Donnelly DF, Kholwadwala D. Hypoxia decreases intracellular calcium in adult rat carotid body glomus cells. J Neurophysiol 1992;67:1543–1551.

63. Ponte J, Sadler CL. Interactions between hypoxia, acetylcholine and dopamine in the carotid body of rabbit and cat. J Physiol (Lond) 1989; 410:395–410.

64. Biscoe TJ, Duchen MR. Responses of type I cells dissociated from the rabbit carotid body to hypoxia. J Physiol (Lond) 1990; 428:39–59.

65. Lopez-Barneo J, Lopez-Lopez JR, Urena J, Gonzalez C. Chemotransduction in the carotid body: K current modulated by Po_2 in type I chemoreceptor cells. Science 1988; 241:580–582.

66. Urena J, Lopez-Lopez J, Gonzalez C, Lopez-Barneo J. Ionic currents in dispersed chemoreceptor cells of the mammalian carotid body. J Gen Physiol 1989; 93: 979–999.

67. Peers C. Effect of lowered extracellular pH on Ca^{2+}-dependent K^+ currents in type I cells from the neonatal rat carotid body. J Physiol (Lond) 1990; 422:381–395.

68. Biscoe TJ, Duchen MR. Electrophysiological responses of disassociated type I cells of the rabbit carotid body to cyanide. J Physiol (Lond) 1989; 413:447–468.

69. Katz DM, Black IB. Expression and regulation of catecholaminergic traits in primary sensory neurons: relationship to target innervation in vivo. J Neurosci 1986; 6:983–989.

70. Dekin MS, Haddad GG. Membrane and cellular properties in oscillating networks: implications for respiration. J Appl Physiol 1990; 69:809–821.

71. Getting PA. Mechanisms of pattern generation underlying swimming in *Tritonia*. I. Neuronal network formed by monosynaptic connections. J. Neurophysiol 1981; 46:65–79.

72. Getting PA. Mechanisms of pattern generation underlying swimming in *Tritonia*. II. Network reconstruction. J Neurophysiol 1983; 49:1017–1035.

73. Getting PA. Mechanisms of pattern generation underlying swimming in *Tritonia*. III. Intrinsic and synaptic mechanisms for delayed excitation. J Neurophysiol 1983; 49:1036–1050.

74. Robertson RM, Pearson, KG. Neural circuits in the flight system of the locust. J. Neurophysiol 1985; 53:110–128.

75. Robertson RM, Pearson KG, Reichert H. Flight interneurons in the locust and the origin of insect wings. Science 1982; 217:177–179.

76. Selverston AI, Russell DF, Miller JP, King D. The stomatogastric nervous system: structure and function of a small neural network. Prog Neurobiol 1976; 7:215–290.

77. Calabrese RL. The roles of endogenous membrane properties and synaptic interaction in generating the heartbeat rhythm of the leech, *Hirudo medicinalis*. J Exp Biol 1979; 82:163–176.

78. Getting PA. Comparative analysis of invertebrate central pattern generators. In: Cohen AH, Rossignol S, Grillner S, eds. Neural Control of Rhythmic Movements in Vertebrates. New York: Wiley, 1988:101–127.

79. LeGallois JJC. Experiments on the principle of life. In: Comroe JH Jr, ed. Pulmonary and Respiratory Physiology, Part II. Pennsylvania: Dowden, Hutchinson & Ross, 1813:12–16.

80. Richter DW, Ballanyi K, Schwarzacher S. Mechanisms of respiratory rhythm generation. Curr Opin Neurobiol 1992; 2:788–793.

81. Smith JC, Ellenberger H, Ballanyi K, Richter DW, Feldman JL. Pre-Bötzinger complex: a brainstem region that may generate respiratory rhythm in mammals. Science 1991; 254:726–729.

82. Haddad GG, Mazza NM, Defendini RF, Blanc WA, Driscoll JM, Epstein RA, Mellins RB. Congenital failure of automatic control of ventilation, gastrointestinal motility and heart rate. Medicine 1978; 57:517–526.

83. Jiang C, Agulian S, Haddad GG. Cl$^-$ and Na$^+$ homeostasis during anoxia in hypoglossal neurons: intracellular and extracellular in-vitro studies. J Physiol (Lond) 1992; 448:697–708.

84. Feldman JL, Smith JC, Liu G. Respiratory pattern generation in mammals: in vitro en bloc analyses. Curr Opin Neurobiol 1991; 1:590–594.

85. Feldman JL, Smith JC, Ellenberger HH, Connelly CA, Greer JJ, Lindsay AD, Otto MR. Neurogenesis of respiratory rhythm and pattern: emerging concepts. Am J Physiol 1990; 259:879–886.

86. Farber JP. Medullary inspiratory activity during opossum development. Am J Physiol 1988; R578–R584.

87. Sica AL, Donnelly DF, Steele AM, Gandhi MR. Discharge properties of dorsal medullary inspiratory neurons in newborn pigs. Brain Res 1987; 408:222–226.

88. Richerson GB. The respiratory centers of the guinea pig: in vivo and perfused brain studies. Ph.D. dissertation, University of Iowa, 1987.

89. Farber JP. Motor responses to positive pressure breathing in the developing opossum. J Appl Physiol 1985; 58:1489–1495.

90. Farber JP. Medullary expiratory activity during opossum development. J Appl Physiol 1989; 66:1606–1612.

91. Millhorn DE, Bayliss DA, Erickson JT, Gallman EA, Szymeczek CL, Czyzyk-Kreska M, Dean JB. Cellular and molecular mechanisms of chemical synaptic transmission. Am J Physiol Lung Mol Cell Physiol 1989; 3:289–317.

92. Farber JP. Effects on breathing of rostral pons glutamate injection during opossum development. J Appl Physiol 1990; 69:189–195.

93. Lawson EE, Schwarzacher SW, Richter DW. Postnatal development of the medullary respiratory network in cat. In: Elsner N, Richter DW, eds. Rhythmogenesis in Neurons and Networks. Proceedings of the 20th Gottingen Neurobiology Conference, Stuttgart. New York: Thieme, 1992:69.

94. Jiang C, Cummins TR, Haddad GG. Membrane ionic currents and properties of freshly dissociated rat brainstem neurons. Exp Brain Res (in press).

95. Dekin MS, Getting PA. In vitro characterization of neurons in the ventral part of the nucleus tractus solitarius in guinea pigs. II. Ionic basis for repetitive firing properties. J Neurophysiol 1987; 58:215–229.

96. Dekin MS, Johnson S, Getting PA. In vitro characterization of neurons in the ventral part of the nucleus tractus solitarius in guinea pigs. I. Identification of neuronal types and repetitive firing properties. J Neurophysiol 1987; 58:195–214.

97. Haddad GG, Getting PA. Repetitive firing properties of neurons in the ventral region of the nucleus tractus soliarius. In-vitro studies in the adult and neonatal rat. J Neurophysiol 1989; 62:1213–1224.

98. Grillner S. Neurobiological bases of rhythmic motor acts in vertebrates. Science 1985; 228:143–149.

99. Grillner S, Buchanan JT, Wallen P, Brodin, L. Neural control of locomotion in lower vertebrates: from behavior to ionic mechanisms. In: Cohen AH, Rossignol S, Grillner S, eds. Neural Control of Rhythmic Movements in Vertebrates. New York: Wiley, 1988:1–41.

100. Haddad GG. Cellular and membrane properties of brainstem neurons in early life. In: Haddad GG, Farber, JP, eds. Developmental Neurobiology of Breathing. New York: Marcel Dekker, 1991:155–175.

101. Haddad GG, Donnelly DF, Getting PA. Biophysical membrane properties of hypoglossal neurons in-vitro: intracellular studies in adult and neonatal rats. J Appl Physiol 1990; 69:1509–1517.

102. Haddad GG, Donnelly DF. O_2 deprivation induces a major depolarization in brainstem neurons in the adult but not in the neonate. J Physiol (Lond) 1990; 429:411–428.

103. Jiang C, Haddad GG. The effect of anoxia on intracellular and extracellular K^+ in hypoglossal neurons in-vitro. J Neurophysiol 1991; 66:103–111.

104. Donnelly DF, Jiang C, Haddad GG. Comparative responses of brainstem and hippocampal neurons to O_2 deprivation: in vitro intracellular studies. Am J Physiol 1992; 262:L549–554.

105. Dean JB, Gallman EA, Zhu WH, Millhorn DE. Multiple effects of hypoxia on neurons in dorsal motor nucleus (X) and nucleus tractus solitarii (NTS). Soc Neurosci 1991; 17:465 (abstract).

106. Jiang C, Agulian S, Haddad GG. O_2 tension in adult and neonatal brain slices under several experimental conditions. Brain Res 1991; 568:159–164.

107. Haddad GG, Jiang C. Mechanisms of anoxia-induced depolarization in brainstem neurons: in-vitro current and voltage clamp studies in the adult rat. Brain Res 1993; 625:261–268.

108. Siesjo BK. Historical overview: calcium, ischemia, and death of brain cells. Ann NY Acad Sci 1988; 522:638–661.

109. Smith ML, Auer RN, Siesjo BK. The density and distribution of ischemic brain injury in the rat following 2–10 min of forebrain ischemia. Acta Neuropathol 1984; 64:319–332.

110. Kwei S, Jiang C, Haddad GG. Acute anoxia-induced alterations in MAP2 immunoreactivity and neuronal morphology in rat hippocampus. Brain Res 1993; 620:203–210.

111. Schmidt-Kastner R, Freund TF. Selective vulnerability of the hippocampus in brain ischemia. Neuroscience 1991; 40(3):599–636.

112. Fujiwara N, Hihashi H, Shimoji K, Yoshmura M. Effects of hypoxia on rat hippocampal neurons in vitro. J Physiol (Lond) 1987; 384:131–151.

113. Mourre C, Ben Ari Y, Bernardi H, Fosset M, Lazdunski M. Antidiabetic sulfonylurea: location of binding sites in the brain and effects on the hyperpolarization induced by anoxia in hippocampal slices. Brain Res 1989; 486:159–164.

114. Krnjevic K and Leblond J. Changes in membrane currents of hippocampal neurons evoked by brief anoxia. J Neurophysiol 1989; 62:15–30.

115. Leblond J, Krnjevic K. Hypoxic changes in hippocampal neurons. J Neurophysiol 1989; 62:1–14.

116. Kawasaki K, Traynelis SF, Dingledine R. Different responses of CA1 and CA3 regions to hypoxia in rat hippocampal slice. J Neurophysiol 1990; 63:385–394.

117. Cummins TS, Donnelly DF, Haddad GG. Effect of metabolic inhibition on the excitability of isolated hippocampal CA1 neurons: developmental aspects. J Neurophysiol 1991; 66:1471–1482.

118. Hansen AJ, Jounsgaard J, Hahnsen H. Anoxia increases potassium conductance in hippocampal nerve cells. Acta Physiol Scand 1982; 115:301–310.

119. Lipton P, Whittingham TS. The effect of hypoxia on evoked potentials in the in vitro hippocampus. J Physiol (Lond) 1979; 287:427–438.

120. Cherubini E, Ben-Ari Y, Krnjevic K. Anoxia produces smaller changes in synaptic transmission, membrane potential, and input resistance in immature rat hippocampus. J Neurophysiol 1989; 62:882–895.

121. Rosen AS, Morris ME. Anoxic depolarization of neocortical pyramidal neurons in vitro. Soc Neurosci 1990; 16:277 (abstract).

122. Doll CJ, Hochachka PW, Reiner PB. Effects of anoxia and metabolic arrest on turtle and rat cortical neurons. Am J Physiol 1991; 260(29):R747–755.

123. Jiang C, Haddad GG. Differential responses of neocortical neurons to glucose and/or O_2 deprivation in the human and rat. J Neurophysiol 1992; 68(6):2165–2173.

124. Cummins TR, Jiang C, Haddad GG. Human neocortical excitability during anoxia via sodium channel modulation. J Clin Invest 1993; 91:608–615.

125. Fazekas JF, Alexander FAD, Himwich HE. Tolerance of the newborn to anoxia. Am J Physiol 1941; 134:281–287.

126. Kabat H. The greater resistance of very young animals to arrest of the brain circulation. Am J Physiol 1940; 130:588–599.

127. Xia Y, Jiang C, Haddad GG. Oxidative and glycolytic pathways in rat (newborn, adult) and turtle brain: role during anoxia. Am J Physiol 1992; 262:R595–603.

128. Kass IS, Lipton P. Mechanisms involved in irreversible anoxic damage to the in vitro rat hippocampal slice. J Physiol (Lond) 1982; 332:459–472.

129. Roussos C, Macklem PT. Diaphragmatic fatigue in man. J Appl Physiol 1977; 43:189–197.

130. Bazzy AR, Haddad GG. Diaphragmatic fatigue in unanesthetized sheep. J Appl Physiol 1984; 57:182–190.

131. Aubier M, Trippenbach T, Roussos C. Respiratory muscle fatigue during cariogenic shock. J Appl Physiol 1981; 51:499–508.

132. Moxham J, Morris AJR, Spiro SG, Edwards RHT, Green M. Contractile properties and fatigue of the diaphragm in man. Thorax 1981; 36:164–168.

133. Aldrich TK, Appel D. Diaphragm fatigue induced by inspiratory resistive loading in spontaneously breathing rabbits. J Appl Physiol 1985; 59:1527–1532.

134. Keens TG, Bryan AC, Levison H, Ianuzzo CD. Developmental pattern of muscle fiber types in human ventilatory muscles. J Appl Physiol 1978; 44:909–913.

135. Maxwell LC, McCarter RJM, Kuehl TJ, Robotham JL. Development of histochemical and functional properties of baboon respiratory muscles. J Appl Physiol 1983; 54:551–561.

136. Mayock DE, Hall J, Watchko JF, Standaert TA, Woodrum DE. Diaphragmatic muscle fiber type development in swine. Pediatr Res 1987; 22:449–454.

137. Brooke MH, Kaiser KK. Muscle fiber types: how many and what kind? Arch Neurol 1970; 23:369–379.

138. Burke RE, Levine DN, Tsairis P, Zajac FE. Physiological types and histochemical profiles of motor units of cat gastrocnemius. J Physiol (Lond) 1973; 234:723–748.

139. Close RI. Dynamic properties of mammalian skeletal muscles. Physiol Rev 1972; 52:129–197.

140. Sieck GC, Sacks RD, Blanco CE, Edgerton VR. SDH activity and cross-sectional area of muscle fibers in cat diaphragm. J Appl Physiol 1986; 60:1284–1292.

141. Bazzy AR, Kim YJ. Effect of chronic respiratory load on cytochrome oxidase activity in diaphragmatic fibers. J Appl Physiol 1992; 72:266–271.

142. Sieck GC, Fournier M, Blanco CE. Diaphragm muscle fatigue resistance during postnatal development. J Appl Physiol 1991; 71:458–464.

143. Sieck GC, Fournier M. Developmental aspects of diaphragm muscle cells. In: Haddad GG, Farber JP, eds. Developmental Neurobiology of Breathing, Lung Biology in Health and Disease. New York: Marcel Dekker, 1991: 375–428.

144. Sieck GC, Blanco CE. Postnatal change in the distribution of succinate dehydrogenase activities among diaphragm muscle fibers. Pediatr Res 1991; 29:586–593.

145. Enad JG, Fournier M, Sieck GC. Oxidative capacity and capillary density of diaphragm motor units. J Appl Physiol 1989; 67:620–627.

146. Sieck GC, Cheung TS, Blanco CE. Diaphragm capillarity and oxidative capacity during postnatal development. J Appl Physiol 1991; 70:103–111.

147. Roussos C. The failing ventilatory pump. Lung 1982; 160:59–84.

148. Rochester DF, Bettini G. Diaphragmatic blood flow and energy expenditure in the dog. J Clin Invest 1976; 57:661–672.

149. Robertson CH, Foster GH, Johnson RL. The relationship of respiratory failure to the oxygen consumption of, lactate production by, and distribution of blood flow among respiratory muscles during increasing inspiratory resistance. J Clin Invest 1977; 59:31–42.

150. Bark H, Supinski G, LaManna JC, Kelsen SG. Relationship of changes in diaphragmatic muscle blood flow to muscle contractile activity. J Appl Physiol 1987; 62: 291–299.

151. Bellemare F, Grassino A. Effect of pressure and timing of contraction on human diaphragm fatigue. J Appl Physiol 1982; 53:1190–1193.

152. Bellemare F, Wright D, LaVigne CM, Grassino A. Effect of tension and timing of

contraction on the blood flow of the diaphragm. J Appl Physiol 1983; 54:1597–1606.

153. Buchler B, Magder S, Roussos C. Effects of contraction frequency and duty cycle on diaphragmatic blood flow. J Appl Physiol 1985; 58:265–273.

154. Pang LM, Kim YJ, Bazzy AR. Blood flow to the respiratory muscles and major organs during inspiratory flow resistive loads. J Appl Physiol 1993; 74:428–434.

155. Bazzy AR, Pang LM, Akabas SR, Haddad GG. O$_2$ metabolism of the sheep diaphragm during flow resistive loaded breathing. J Appl Physiol 1989; 66:2305–2311.

156. Mayock DE, Standaert TA, Murphy TD, Woodrum DE. Diaphragmatic force and substrate response to resistive loaded breathing in the piglet. J Appl Physiol 1991; 70:70–76.

157. Nichols DG, Howell S, Massik J, Koehler RC, Gleason CA, Buck JR, Fitzgerald RS, Traytsman RJ, Robotham JL. Relationship of diaphragmatic contractility to diaphragmatic blood flow in newborn lambs. J Appl Physiol 1989; 66:120–127.

158. Vollestad NK, Sejersted OM. Biochemical correlates of fatigue: a brief review. Eur J Appl Physiol 1988; 57:336–347.

159. Dawes GS, Shelley HJ. Physiological aspects of carbohydrate metabolism in the foetus and newborn. In: Dickens F, Randle PJ, Whelan WJ, eds. Carboyhdrate Metabolism and Disorders. London: Academic Press, 1968:87–121.

160. Smith PB. Postnatal development of glycogen- and cyclic AMP-metabolizing enzymes in mammalian skeletal muscle. Biochim Biophys Acta 1980; 628:19–25.

161. Kim YJ, Bazzy AR. Glycogen content in neonatal diaphragmatic fibers in response to inspiratory flow resistive loads. Pediatr Res 1992; 31:354–358.

162. Collin-Saltin AS. Some quantitative biochemical evaluations of developing skeletal muscle in the human foetus. J Neurol Sci 1978; 39:187–198.

163. Powers S, Lawler J, Criswell D, Dodd S, Silverman H. Age-related changes in enzyme activity in the rat diaphragm. Respir Physiol 1991; 83:1–10.

164. Muller NL, Gulston G, Cade D, Whitton J, Froese AB, Bryan MH, Bryan AC. Diaphragmatic fatigue in the newborn. J Appl Physiol 1976; 46:688–695.

165. Lopes JM, Muller NL, Bryan MH, Bryan AC. Synergistic behavior of respiratory muscles after diaphragmatic fatigue in the newborn. J Appl Physiol 1981; 51:547–551.

166. Lindstrom L, Kadefors B, Petersen I. An electromyographic index for localized muscle fatigue. J Appl Physiol 1977; 43:750–754.

167. Schweitzer TW, Fitzgerald JW, Bowden JA, Lynne-Davies P. Spectral analysis of human inspiratory diaphragmatic electromyograms. J Appl Physiol 1979; 46:152–165.

168. Mayock DE, Badura RJ, Watchko JF, Standaert TA, Woodrum DE. Response to resistive loading in the newborn piglet. Pediatr Res 1987; 21:121–125.

169. Le Souef PN, England SJ, Stogryn HAF, Bryan AC. Comparison of diaphragmatic fatigue in newborn and older rabbits. J Appl Physiol 1988; 65:1040–1044.

170. Gerhardt T, Bancalari E. Chest wall compliance in full term and preterm infants. Acta Pediatr Scand 1980; 69:359–364.

171. Bryan AC, Gaulthier C. Chest wall mechanics in the newborn. In: Roussos C, Macklem PT, eds. Lung Biology in Health and Disease. New York: Marcel Dekker, 1985:871–888.

172. Watchko JF, Mayock DE, Standaert TA, Woodrum DE. The ventilatory pump: neonatal and developmental issues. Adv Pediatr 1991; 38:109–134.

173. Muller NL, Bryan A.C. Chest wall mechanics and respiratory muscles in infants. Pediatr Clin North Am 1979; 26:503–516.

174. Eichenwald EC, Stark AR. Respiratory motor output: effect of state and maturation in early life. In: Haddad GG, Farber JP, eds. Developmental Neurobiology of Breathing. Lung Biology in Health and Disease. New York: Marcel Dekker, 1991:551–587.

175. Roussos C, Fixley M, Gross D, Macklem PT. Fatigue of inspiratory muscles and their synergistic behavior. J Appl Physiol 1979; 46:897–904.

176. Watchko JF, Mayock DE, Standaert TA, Woodrum DE. Diaphragmatic pressure in piglets: transvenous versus phrenic nerve stimulation. Pediatr Pulmonol 1986; 2:198–201.

177. Watchko JF, Standaert TA, Woodrum DE. Diaphragmatic function during hypercapnia: neonatal and developmental aspects. J Appl Physiol 1987; 62:768–775.

178. Bigland-Ritchie, B. Functional aspects of human muscles and their central nervous system interactions: implications for muscle failure. In: Haddad GG, Farber JP, eds. Developmental Neurobiology of Breathing. New York: Marcel Dekker, 1991:429–453.

179. Bellemare F, Bigland-Ritchie B. Central components of diaphragmatic fatigue assessed by phrenic nerve stimulation. J Appl Physiol 1987; 62:1307–1316.

180. Watchko JF, Standaert TA, Mayock DE, Twiggs G. Ventilatory failure during loaded breathing: the role of central neural drive. J Appl Physiol 1988; 65:249–255.

181. Krnjevic K, Miledi R. Failure of neuromuscular propagation in rats. J Physiol (Lond) 1958; 140:440–461.

182. Kelsen SG, Nochomovitz ML. Fatigue of the mammalian diaphragm in vitro. J Appl Physiol 1982; 53:440–447.

183. Aldrich TK, Shander A, Chaudhry I, Nagashima H. Fatigue of the isolated diaphragm: role of impaired neuromuscular transmission. J Appl Physiol 1986; 61:1077–1083.

184. Kuei JH, Shadmehr R, Sieck GC. Relative contribution of neuromuscular transmission failure to diaphragm fatigue. J Appl Physiol 1990; 68:174–180.

185. Bigland-Ritchie B, Kukulka CG, Lippold OCJ, Woods J. The absence of neuromuscular transmission failure in sustained maximal voluntary contractions. J Physiol (Lond) 1982; 330:265–278.

186. Aldrich TK. Transmission fatigue of the rabbit diaphragm. Respir Physiol 1987; 69:307–319.

187. Bazzy AR, Donnelly DF. Diaphragmatic failure during loaded breathing: role of neuromuscular transmission. J Appl Physiol 1993; 74:1679–1683.

188. Fournier M, Alula M, Sieck GC. Neuromuscular transmission failure during postnatal development. Neurosci Lett 1991; 125:34–36.

189. Feldman JD, Bazzy AR, Cummins TR, Haddad GG. Developmental changes in neuromuscular transmission in the rat diaphragm. J Appl Physiol 1991; 71:280–286.

190. Bennett MR, Pettigrew AG. The formation of synapses in striated muscle during development. J Physiol. (Lond) 1974; 241:515–545.

191. Bixby JL, Van Essen DC. Regional differences in the timing of synapse elimination in skeletal muscles of the neonatal rabbit. Brain Res 1979; 169:275–286.

192. Bixby JL. Ultrastructural observations on synapse elimination in neonatal rabbit skeletal muscles. J Neurocytol 1981; 10:81–100.

193. Ishikawa H, Sawada H, Yamada E. Surface and internal morphology of skeletal muscle. In: Peachey LD, Adrian RH, eds. Handbook of Physiology. Section 10, Skeletal Muscle. Bethesda, MD: American Physiological Society, 1983:1–21.

194. Bevan S, Steinbach JH. The distribution of α-bungarotoxin binding sites on mammalian skeletal muscle developing in vivo. J Physiol (Lond) 1977; 267:195–213.

195. Diamond J, Miledi R. A study of foetal and newborn rat muscle fibers. J Physiol 1962; 162:393–408.

196. Dennis, MJ, Ziskind-Conhaim L, Harris AJ. Development of neuromuscular junctions in rat embryos. Dev Biol 1981; 82:266–279.

197. Reiness CG, Hall ZW. The developmental change in immunological properties of the acetylcholine receptor in rat muscle. Dev Biol 1981; 81:324–331.

198. Fischbach GD, Schuetze SM. A post-natal decrease in acetylcholine channel open time at rat end-plates. J Physiol (Lond) 1980; 303:125–137.

199. Kelly SS, Roberts DV. The effect of age on the safety factor in neuromuscular transmission in the isolated diaphragm of the rat. Br J Anaesth 1977; 49:217–222.

200. Kelly SS. The effect of age on neuromuscular transmission. J Physiol (Lond) 1978; 274:51–62.

201. Wilson DF, Cardaman RC. Age-associated changes in neuromuscular transmission in the rat. Am J Physiol 1984; 247:C288–C292.

202. Bazzy AR, Donnelly DF. Failure to generate action potentials in newborn diaphragm following nerve stimulation. Brain Res 1993; 600:349–352.

203. Betz WJ, Bewick GS. Optical analysis of synaptic vesicle recycling at the frog neuromuscular junction. Science 1992; 255:200–203.

204. Gauthier GF, Lowey S, Hobbs AW. Fast and slow myosin in developing muscle fibers. Nature 1978, 274:25–29.

205. Kelly AM. Emergence of muscle specialization. In: Peachey LC, Adrian RH, eds. Handbook of Physiology. Bethesda, MD: American Physiological Society, 1983; 507–537.

206. Schiaffino S, Ausoni S, Gorza L, Saggin L, Gundersen K, Lomo T. Myosin heavy chain isoforms and velocity of shortening of type 2 skeletal muscle fibers. Acta Physiol Scand 1988; 134:575–576.

207. Whalen RG, Sell SM, Butler-Browne GS, Schwartz K, Bouveret P, Pinset-Harstrom I. Three myosin heavy chain isozymes appear sequentially in rat muscle development. Nature 1981; 292:805–809.

208. Butler-Browne GS, Whalen RG. Myosin isoenzyme transitions occurring during the postnatal development of the rat soleus muscle. Dev Biol 1984; 102:324–334.

209. LaFramboise WA, Daood MJ, Guthrie RD, Butler-Browne GS, Whalen RG, Ontell M. Myosin isoforms in neonatal rat extensor digitorum Longus, diaphragm, and soleus muscles. Am J Physiol 1990; 259:L116–L122.

210. LaFramboise WA, Daood MJ, Guthrie RD, Schiaffino S, Moretti P, Brozanski B, Ontell MP, Butler-Browne GS, Whalen RG, Ontell M. Emergence of the mature myosin phenotype in the rat diaphragm muscle. Dev Biol 1991; 144:1–15.

17

Unique Issues in Neonatal Respiratory Control

SANDRA J. ENGLAND

UMDNJ–Robert Wood Johnson Medical
  School
New Brunswick, New Jersey

MARTHA J. MILLER
and RICHARD J. MARTIN

Case Western Reserve University
Cleveland, Ohio

I. Introduction

Respiratory control mechanisms in the newborn infant have received considerable interest in the past several decades. The transition from placental gas exchange during intrauterine life to air breathing, coupled with the continued postnatal maturation of central neuronal processes, peripheral afferent mechanisms, the respiratory musculature, and the lungs and chest wall, presents the infant with unique challenges in the maintenance of metabolic homeostasis. This chapter will focus on these maturational challenges in relation to respiratory control in the healthy infant and in infants with respiratory disease. Topics related to respiratory control mechanisms in general are covered in greater detail in other chapters in this volume, and a comprehensive discourse on the developmental neurobiology of respiration is available in another volume of this series (Haddad and Farber, 1991).

II. Development of Respiratory Control

A. Central Respiratory Neurons

Neuronal development is incomplete at birth. Membrane input resistance decreases with age in central neurons and in spinal motoneurons (Cameron et al.,

1991; Haddad and Getting, 1989). Recent data suggest that the wider action potentials observed in respiratory neurons of the neonate in contrast to the adult are due to a greater dependence on calcium rather than sodium inward currents (Haddad et al., 1990). While the adult complement of neurons is present in the full-term infant, synaptic development continues postnatally with increased dendritic arborization in both medullary neurons and spinal motoneurons (Cameron et al., 1990). The neurotransmitter and neuromodulator content of neurons changes during fetal and neonatal development (Millhorn et al., 1991).

Neurons with inspiratory, postinspiratory, and expiratory firing patterns have been identified in the medulla of neonatal animals (Farber, 1988, 1989; Lawson et al., 1989; Sica et al., 1987). The firing rates of inspiratory units are low, and the phrenic neuronal and diaphragmatic electromyographic activity during inspiration is brief and does not exhibit the ramp-like activity observed in more mature animals. Expiratory neurons in the developing opossum do not fire consistently and often have low firing rates (Farber, 1989). This finding may account for the lack of expiratory muscle activation during positive pressure breathing in these immature animals.

Postnatal development of respiratory neurons affords plasticity in functional maturation of the respiratory system, the significance of which is unknown at the present time. Clearly, more complete data are needed to define the maturation of central respiratory control mechanisms in the full-term infant, particularly in the infant born prematurely.

B. Pulmonary Mechanoreceptors and C-Fiber Afferents

Afferent neurons from the respiratory peripheral feedback receptors in the lungs and airways undergo increasing myelination postnatally (Krous et al., 1985; Marlot and Duron, 1979; DeNeef et al., 1982). The firing rates of pulmonary stretch receptors in response to a given transpulmonary pressure increase postnatally (Farber et al., 1984), and a greater percentage of receptors are active at transpulmonary pressures below 4 cm H_2O in the adult than in the newborn animal (Fisher and Sant'Ambrogio, 1982). Thus there is a presumed paucity of afferent neuronal feedback to the medullary respiratory control center in the early postnatal period.

However, functionally, afferent feedback from pulmonary receptors has a profound effect on respiration in the neonate, with prolonged lengthening of the subsequent inspiration occurring with end-expiratory occlusion in full-term infants (Fisher et al., 1982; Kosch et al., 1986; Thach et al., 1978). However, in the premature infant inspiratory time is shortened (Gerhardt and Bancalari, 1981; Knill and Bryan, 1976; Thach et al., 1978), but this response is presumably mediated by chest wall receptors. Vagotomy in both neonatal and more mature rats results in a slow, deep breathing pattern, but in the neonate there is a profound depression of minute ventilation due to an extreme lengthening of expiratory time, while overall ventilation is maintained in the more mature rat (Fedorko et al., 1988).

Augmented breaths, presumably due to activation of rapidly adapting pulmonary receptors, are common in infants (Cross et al., 1960; Duron and Marlot, 1980; Thach and Taeusch, 1976) and can be elicited with lung inflation (Cross et al., 1960). The presence of spontaneous deep breaths in the young opossum (Farber et al., 1984) demonstrates that pulmonary reflexes can be elicited even in an extremely immature respiratory system. It has been suggested that spontaneous deep breaths in infants increase homogeneity of ventilation and assist in establishing surfactant activity in the transition to air breathing (Thach and Taeusch, 1976).

Mechanical irritation of the airways in term infants results in increased inspiratory efforts, a response that is believed to be mediated by rapidly adapting pulmonary ("irritant") mechanoreceptors (Fleming et al., 1978). Such stimulation in the preterm infant results in decreased respiratory frequency or apnea. In rabbit pups, stimulation of rapidly adapting receptors by intravenous injection of histamine had an increasing effectiveness in shortening inspiratory time and increasing breathing rate over the first week of life (Trippenbach and Kelly, 1988). These data suggest maturation of either the receptors and their afferents or the reflex response to their stimulation postnatally, a premise supported by the fact that fewer rapidly adapting receptors can be identified in the immature animal (Farber et al., 1984; Fisher and Sant'Ambrogio, 1982).

Thus despite a paucity of action potentials from pulmonary mechanoreceptors, the functional effect of these receptors is greater than that observed in the adults of most mammalian species. Processing of afferent feedback at the level of medullary respiratory premotor neurons is the most likely source for this enhancement of reflex effects in the newborn.

There is only sparse data on the maturation of pulmonary C-fiber receptors and the reflex responses to their activation in the newborn. The adult response to stimulation of C-fiber afferents with phenyldiguanide (apnea, bradycardia, and hypotension) has been reported to be reduced or absent in newborn kittens (Kalia, 1976). Capsaicin administered to neonatal animals results in a failure of development of afferents containing substance P (Lundberg and Saria, 1983).

C. Upper Airway Receptors

Receptors in the nose, pharynx, and larynx responding to both mechanical and chemical stimuli send afferent information to the medullary respiratory neurons. Afferents carried in the trigeminal, glossopharyngeal, and superior laryngeal nerves provide information on airflow and pressures as well as contributing to defense of the lungs. In the newborn, the laryngeal afferents have been most completely studied, with four types identified.

Receptors stimulated by water and other liquids can be subdivided into two categories, one with short-latency, short-duration responses dependent on the lack of chloride ions (Anderson et al., 1990; Boggs and Bartlett, 1982) and a second with long-latency, long-duration responses dependent on the hypoosmolality of the solution (Anderson et al., 1990). The latter subtype shows respiratory-modulated activity whereas the former does not. These receptors are found in adult and newborn animals, but the reflex apnea (Boggs and Bartlett, 1982) and laryngeal adduction (Sherry and Megirian, 1974) elicited with stimulation of the nerve endings is far more profound in the newborn and is assumed to represent a defense mechanism preventing aspiration. In human preterm infants, prolonged central apnea results from instillation of a small volume of fluid in the larynx (Davies et al., 1988). In lambs during the first week of life prolonged apnea resulting in collapse requiring resuscitation has been observed with stimulation of these afferents (Johnson et al., 1975).

The remaining three types of receptors are activated by transmural pressure, airflow (cooling), and phasic contraction or passive movement of intrinsic laryngeal muscles ("drive" receptors) (Sant'Ambrogio et al., 1983; Fisher et al., 1985). The pressure receptors show a greater response to negative than positive pressures. Some overlap in activation by discrete stimuli is evident between receptor types, and cooling of the larynx reduces the response of pressure and "drive" receptors in addition to activating the flow receptors. The newborn has a smaller population of flow receptors than the adult, and a reduced discharge frequency of pressure receptors has also been noted (Mortola and Fisher, 1988), but these findings could reflect difficulties in dissecting and recording from small, unmyelinated fibers in the newborn.

The reflex response to airflow through the upper airway is a reduced respiratory frequency and tidal volume sometimes to the point of apnea. This response is mediated by cooling of the flow receptors in the larynx (Fisher et al., 1985). Stimulation of these receptors also induces cardioinhibitory responses (Sant'Ambrogio et al., 1985). Pressure receptors show the greatest response to negative collapsing pressure (Fisher et al., 1985), and their stimulation also results in decreased respiration. Reduced activation of inspiratory muscles during upper airway narrowing would reduce the collapsing pressure on the airway. The respiratory response to negative airway pressure is greatest in newborn puppies, with an absence of response by 1 month of age in anesthetized puppies. The respiratory effects of activation of drive receptors are not profound but do appear to inhibit activity of the intrinsic laryngeal abductor, the posterior cricoarytenoid (Mathew et al., 1986).

It is unclear what role, if any, these receptors play in eupneic respiration since sectioning of the superior laryngeal nerve containing their afferents does not alter breathing pattern in chronic newborn animal studies (Mortola and Rezzonico, 1989). Their role may be much more important during airway collapse or hyperpnea.

D. Peripheral and Central Chemoreceptors

The peripheral chemoreceptors, predominantly the carotid body receptors, are responsible for the increase in ventilation that occurs in response to hypoxemia. The initial increase in ventilation in response to hypoxia is less in the newborn than the adult animal (Bureau et al., 1985, 1986), and continued hypoxia is accompanied by a substantial decrease in ventilation, sometimes below the normoxic level, in the newborn (Haddad and Mellins, 1984).

In utero, the Po_2 of fetal arterial blood is only about 25 mmHg, with values rising quickly to over 60 mmHg upon the establishment of air breathing and closure of the ductus arteriosus at birth. Carotid chemoreceptor activity increases in the fetus in response to decreasing Po_2 below 25 mmHg (Blanco et al., 1984a). However, the Pao_2 range over which the chemoreceptors responded is much lower than in the adult. Resetting of the receptor responsiveness to higher Po_2's appears to occur over the first several weeks of life in the lamb (Blanco et al., 1984a, 1988; Hanson et al., 1987) and may be dependent on a sustained increase in arterial Po_2 (Blanco et al., 1988; Hanson et al., 1989). Minimal multiplicative interaction of hypoxic and hypercapnic stimulation of carotid chemoreceptors is observed in the early postnatal period (Blanco et al., 1984a; Mulligan, 1988). Therefore, maturation of the chemoreceptor response to a given level of hypoxemia occurs postnatally and probably accounts for the less pronounced increase in ventilation during the initial stages of hypoxemia in the newborn compared to the adult animal. The cellular basis of this maturation is poorly understood, but recent studies indicate postnatal increases in the tyrosine hydroxylase and catecholamine content of carotid body afferent neurons (Katz, 1990; Katz and Erb, 1989).

The failure to sustain an increased ventilation with continued hypoxia could result from a number of factors. It should be noted that adult animals of many species also show a decrease in ventilation over time with hypoxia, albeit slower and of a lower degree than that observed in the neonate (Neubauer et al., 1990). Decreased activation of central chemoreceptors due to hypocapnia induced by increased brain blood flow during hypoxia cannot account for the failure to maintain an elevated ventilation (Lawson and Long, 1983). Adaptation of carotid chemoreceptor discharge, a reduced activity during sustained hypoxia, has been shown to occur in some receptors in neonatal piglets (Mulligan et al., 1989) but not in kittens (Blanco et al., 1984b; Schwieler, 1968). Hypoxic depression of central respiratory neurons occurs in anesthetized piglets under some circumstances (England, 1993) and has been well documented in anesthetized adult cats

(Neubauer et al., 1990). A decrease in metabolism has been shown to occur during hypoxia in the neonate (Haddad et al., 1982) and may indicate that the fall in ventilation is not inappropriate for the metabolic activity of the hypoxic neonate. Changes in pulmonary mechanics have also been implicated in the decreased ventilation during sustained hypoxia (LaFramboise et al., 1983).

Central chemoreceptors responding to increases in CO_2 are active in the fetal lamb (Hohimer, 1983, 1985) and result in increases in both the amplitude and frequency of fetal breathing movements (Bowes et al., 1981; Jansen et al., 1982). Ventilatory increases in response to increased CO_2 have been reported as lower in the newborn than the adult in some species (Nattie and Edwards, 1981; Guthrie et al., 1980) but not in the term human infant (Avery et al., 1963; Krauss et al., 1975). Preterm infants show a reduced response (Rigatto et al., 1975; Krauss et al., 1976), which may be attributed to central insensitivity as well as mechanical disadvantages (Moriette et al., 1985; Rigatto, 1984).

III. Maintenance of End-Expiratory Lung Volume

The ribs of the neonate are cartilaginous rather than bony and extend at almost right angles from the vertebral column, resulting in a more circular rib cage than in the adult (Devlieger et al., 1991; Openshaw et al., 1984; Takahashi and Atsumi, 1955). These structural characteristics result in a relative mechanical inefficiency and a passive end-expiratory lung volume that is only approximately 10% of total lung capacity in contrast to 50% in the adult (Agostoni, 1959). However, the neonate employs various mechanisms to actively elevate end-expiratory lung volume, including postinspiratory activity of the diaphragm and intercostals (Kosch et al., 1988; Muller et al., 1979b) and expiratory laryngeal adduction (England et al., 1985; Harding et al., 1979). End-expiratory tracheal airway pressure in the neonatal dog pup employing these mechanisms is approximately 5 cm H_2O, a substantial inherent or occult PEEP (England and Stogryn, 1986). The maintenance of an elevated end-expiratory lung volume and, therefore, elevated transpulmonary pressure during tidal breathing above the relaxation volume may contribute to enhanced pulmonary stretch receptor activity.

Kosch and Stark (1984) estimated that dynamic end-expiratory lung volume in the neonate is about 14 ml above the relaxation volume. Thus expiratory central output to the diaphragm, intercostals, and laryngeal muscles enhances the stability of terminal airways and alveoli and provides a more adequate lung volume for the maintenance of gas exchange (Zamel et al., 1989). The age at which end-expiratory lung volume is no longer dynamically elevated above the relaxation volume is not known. Colin et al. (1989), based on the shape of the expiratory flow-volume curve, estimated that the transition occurs at about 12 months of age.

IV. Sleep and Respiration

The full-term infant spends approximately 50% of sleep time in rapid eye movement (REM) sleep and the preterm infant even a larger percentage. Since infants sleep a good portion of the day and night, the changes in respiratory control that occur in REM sleep have profound effects (Table 1). REM sleep is accompanied by atonia of skeletal muscles other than the diaphragm. Decreased intercostal muscle activity contributes to increased paradoxical inward movement of the rib cage during inspiration and increased diaphragmatic work for moving a given tidal volume when compared with non-REM sleep (Guslits et al., 1987). The rate and depth of breathing in REM sleep are highly irregular (Hathorn, 1974; Stevenson and McGinty, 1978). Respiratory rate is higher in REM than non-REM sleep (Haddad et al., 1979; Curzi-Dascalova et al., 1983), with more frequent and prolonged apneas occurring in REM (Hoppenbrouwers et al., 1979).

Loss of phasic expiratory and inspiratory activity in upper airway muscles contributes to a greater risk of upper airway obstruction during inspiration and a potential for reduced end-expiratory lung volume. As described above, active mechanisms are required to maintain an adequate end-expiratory lung volume in the neonate, but the effect of sleep state on end-expiratory lung volume remains controversial. Henderson-Smart and Read (1979) demonstrated a large (30%) fall in end-expiratory lung volume during REM sleep by body plethysmography in full-term infants. Indirect evidence for a decrease in lung volume during REM sleep has also been presented (Lopes et al., 1981; Stark et al., 1987). However, several studies employing helium dilution measurements of lung volume have

Table 1 Physiological Changes in REM Sleep and Effects on Respiration

Physiological change	Potential consequences
Decreased intercostal and upper airway muscle tone and phasic respiratory activity	Increased inspiratory chest wall paradox
	Susceptibility to upper airway collapse
	Increased diaphragmatic work of breathing
	Decreased end-expiratory lung volume
Decreased response to pulmonary afferent mechanoreceptor feedback	Decreased recruitment of abdominal muscles
Decreased response to peripheral and central chemoreceptor stimulation	Decreased ventilatory and arousal responses to hypercapnia and hypoxia

failed to find significant changes in lung volume accompanying changes in sleep state (Beardsmore et al., 1989; Moriette et al., 1983; Stokes et al., 1989). Walti et al. (1986) observed small, but significant decreases in lung volume during REM sleep in the presence of gross paradoxical inward rib cage motion during inspiration, presumably a time when active mechanisms for maintaining lung volume are at a nadir due to skeletal muscle atonia.

As cited above, afferent feedback from pulmonary and upper airway receptors potentially modulates respiration in the neonate. However, during REM sleep, the responses to this afferent feedback are reduced or disabled (Phillipson and Bowes, 1986). This fact may account for the irregular breathing pattern observed in infants during REM sleep (Hathorn, 1974). Additionally, the recruitment of abdominal muscles during CO_2 inhalation in human infants is greater in quiet than REM sleep (Praud et al., 1989). Abdominal muscle recruitment has been shown to be dependent on vagal afferent feedback in some neonatal and adult species (Farber, 1983; Bishop and Bachofen, 1972) but not in others (Kelson et al., 1977; Watchko et al., 1990).

The ventilatory response to activation of peripheral and central chemoreceptors is reduced in REM sleep in both adults (Phillipson, 1978) and newborns (Henderson-Smart and Read, 1979b; Honma et al., 1984; Jeffrey and Read, 1980; Moriette et al., 1985). However, at least a portion of this decrease in ventilation may be explained by a failure to recruit intercostal inspiratory muscles during REM (Hershenson et al., 1989; Honma et al., 1984), resulting in an inability to generate large tidal volumes. Arousal responses to hypoxia are reduced in REM sleep (Henderson-Smart and Read, 1979b; Jeffrey and Read, 1980).

V. Influence of Neonatal Lung Disease

A. Acute Lung Disorders

Despite the high incidence of both acute respiratory distress syndrome (RDS), typically secondary to surfactant deficiency, and chronic neonatal lung disease (bronchopulmonary dysplasia; BPD), their impact on respiratory control mechanisms is poorly understood. RDS is typically an acute, transient disorder characterized by low compliance and FRC with resultant alveolar hypoventilation and right-to-left shunting of blood at both intrapulmonary and extrapulmonary sites. This disorder is typically treated with a combination of supplemental oxygen, assisted ventilation, and exogenous surfactant therapy (Carlo, 1992), allowing little opportunity for traditional studies of respiratory control in these preterm infants. When breathing spontaneously, these infants have a rapid respiratory rate (>60/min) and low tidal volume, even in the face of normal blood gas status (in supplemental O_2). Presumably their tachypnea is contributed to by stimulation of irritant receptors and other pulmonary afferent pathways from atelectatic alveolar structures. The combination of low lung and high chest wall compliance results in visible intercostal and subcostal retraction, flaring of the alae nasi, and an audible expiratory grunt, widely held to be a mechanism for maintaining adequate FRC via the laryngeal muscles.

Spontaneously breathing preterm infants with RDS were observed by Carlo et al. (1982) to exhibit less apnea than appropriately matched prematures without RDS, over the first days of life. The relatively comparable blood gas status between groups suggested that excitatory vagal afferents rather than chemoreceptors contributed to the enhanced respiratory muscle activity of the infants with RDS. In contrast, when neonatal respiratory distress is due to pneumonia, apnea frequently results in both preterm and term babies. Murphy and associates (1992) induced group B streptococcal sepsis in spontaneously breathing, 2-week-old piglets and documented a significant decline in transdiaphragmatic pressure not associated with acidosis, hypercapnea, or hypoxia, but presumably a direct effect of sepsis on diaphragmatic function. Thus the effect of acute neonatal lung disease on respiratory muscle activity will vary as a function of the infant's pathophysiology.

B. Chronic Neonatal Lung Disease

Unlike RDS, which is characterized by uniformly diminished FRC and lung compliance, lungs of infants with BPD exhibit nonhomogeneously impaired pulmonary function. Areas of atelectasis and hyperinflation may coexist, often associated with increased pulmonary resistance and clinical evidence of bronchospasm (Bancalari, 1992). Overall tidal volume is reduced and respiratory rate increased, resulting in a normal or increased minute ventilation. Much greater attention has been given to studying pulmonary function than respiratory control in infants with BPD. Characteristics of respiratory control in infants with BPD include:

Asynchronous (or paradoxical) chest wall motion

Limited adaptation to resistive loading

Episodes of desaturation during feeding

Hypoxia-induced airway constriction

Increased incidence of SIDS

Furthermore, the spectrum of disease may range all the way from a 1-month-old, spontaneously breathing, preterm infant with a minimal need for supplemental O_2 to a severely disabled survivor of neonatal intensive care with prolonged O_2 or ventilator requirements.

Durand and Rigatto (1981) examined respiratory patterns in BPD infants with and without CO_2 retention at rest. Their findings indicated that the hypercapnic infants (whose pulmonary mechanics were probably worse) had lower tidal volumes and more rapid respiratory rates. They speculated that changes in respiratory pattern are mediated through stretch or irritant reflexes originating in the lung, secondary to the underlying disease state. Not surprisingly, infants with BPD are less able to increase tidal volume in response to increasing concentrations of inspired CO_2. They are also less able to increase respiratory drive when given an additional resistive load, and they exhibit a greater fall in minute ventilation than seen in loaded healthy preterm infants (Greenspan et al., 1992). It is tempting to speculate that such relative inability to respond to chemical or mechanical respiratory loads may play a role in the higher incidence of sudden infant death syndrome (SIDS) reported for infants with BPD (Werthammer et al., 1982).

In healthy preterm infants, diaphragm contraction is associated with inward (asynchronous or paradoxical) motion of the rib cage, especially during active sleep. This has been proposed as a mechanism for decreasing both FRC and Pao_2 in infants during active sleep (Henderson-Smart and Read, 1979; Martin et al., 1979b). However, in infants with BPD such asynchrony of rib cage and abdomen typically predominates during all sleep states, presumably secondary to the infant's impaired respiratory mechanics (Rome et al., 1987; Allen et al., 1991). Failure of rib cage recruitment may act as a severe mechanical handicap and impair an infant's response to hypercapnia, as has been reported in healthy neonates during active sleep (Honma et al., 1984). The extra workload on the diaphragm associated with such inward excursion of the rib cage during all or part of inspiratory flow may contribute to respiratory failure (Heldt and McIlroy, 1987). With advancing maturation, this asynchronous chest wall motion gradually disappears in healthy infants; however, in infants with BPD, this process is undoubtedly slower (Gaultier et al., 1987).

In addition to low pulmonary compliance and high chest wall compliance, high pulmonary resistance also contributes to thoracoabdominal asynchrony in infants, which may be relieved by bronchodilator therapy (Allen et al., 1990). Bronchospasm is a very troublesome clinical problem in infants with BPD. It has been proposed that inhalation of 100% inspired O_2 may diminish airway constriction in infants with BPD (Teague et al., 1988; Tay-Uyboco et al., 1989), although this has not been universally observed (Carlo et al., 1990). Unlike extrinsic loading studies, there are no available data on the ventilatory strategies adopted by infants in response to bronchoconstriction.

VI. Effect of Body Position and Airway Obstruction

A. Supine Versus Prone

Infants exhibit some unique characteristics of respiratory function and its regulation, related to the supine versus prone position they occupy and further influenced by the degree of neck flexion or extension. When placed in either the supine or prone position, the head of spontaneously breathing neonates falls to the side and almost never occupies the midline position. Yet most studies of neonatal respiratory function have been made with the head midline. Preterm infants appear most comfortable when prone, exhibiting less time awake, more quiet sleep, less energy expenditure (Masterson et al., 1987), and a slightly higher transcutaneously measured P_{O_2} (Martin et al., 1979a). The latter may be related to improved thoracoabdominal synchrony (as discussed earlier) in the prone position secondary to a greater area of apposition of the diaphragm to the anterior rib cage (Wolfson et al., 1992). Heimler et al. (1992) reported an increase in apneic episodes in preterm infants when supine, which may be related to the above mechanisms.

In contrast to the apparent benefits of prone positioning in preterm infants, the prone position has recently been increasingly implicated as a risk factor for SIDS (Fleming et al., 1990; Dwyer et al., 1991; Ponsonby et al., 1992) especially in the United Kingdom, New Zealand, and Australia. These observations have resulted in recommendations in the United States that the prone sleeping position be avoided in healthy sleeping babies over the first 6 months of life (AAP Task Force, 1992; Guntheroth and Spiers, 1992). This recommendation may be premature and has been challenged, in the absence of data derived from studies in North America (Hunt and Shannon, 1992). Proposed mechanisms for vulnerability to SIDS in the prone position include oropharyngeal obstruction, hypoxia or hypercapnia secondary to rebreathing, decreased arousal, and overheating due to impaired heat dissipation, all of which might be compounded by excessive or inappropriate bedding (Fig. 1). The ability of infants beyond the neonatal period to place their head midline when prone may also be a variable in predisposing to SIDS.

B. Neck Position and Induced Airway Obstruction

Preterm infants, particularly supine, are quite susceptible to excessive neck flexion, resulting in partial or complete airway obstruction and an increased frequency of apnea (Thach and Stark, 1979). When studied beyond the neonatal period, former preterm infants also increase resistance in response to neck flexion (Carlo et al., 1989). Upper airway obstruction was found to accompany apnea in preterm infants even in the absence of neck flexion (see later). Nonetheless, induced airway occlusion has frequently been used in infants to assess their respiratory muscle response to spontaneous airway obstruction, as might occur during neck flexion or in micrognathic infants (Roberts et al., 1986). Gauda et al. (1987) documented that end-expiratory airway occlusion caused the immediate appearance of genioglossus electromyogram (EMG) in almost 50% of nonapneic infants, while only 13% of apneic infants exhibited genioglossus EMG on the first occluded inspiratory effort. Inability to recruit upper airway dilator muscles

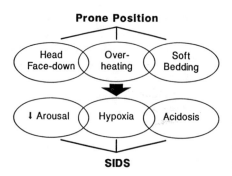

Figure 1 Series of proposed and potentially interrelated mechanisms whereby infants might be predisposed to SIDS when sleeping in the prone position.

during airway obstruction may be a source of vulnerability in some preterm infants. A proportion of preterm infants become apneic in response to external airway obstruction, although the mechanism by which apnea (rather than sustained inspiratory effort) occurs in response to obstruction is unclear (Upton et al., 1992b). Most preterm infants do, however, seem able to maintain upper airway patency in response to brief end-expiratory airway occlusions (Cohen and Henderson-Smart, 1986). Such induced airway occlusions do offer important physiological information, but do not appear to be a useful marker for vulnerability to spontaneous apnea (Gauda et al., 1989).

In the case of partial or complete obstruction of the nasal airway (as caused by excessive nasal secretions, nasal trauma, or choanal atresia), infants must resort to the oral route for maintenance of ventilation. Studies in term babies over the first days of life have revealed that 30% exhibit spontaneous periods of combined oral and nasal breathing and 40% respond to nasal obstruction with sustained oral breathing (Miller et al., 1985a). Thus, healthy term infants are best considered preferential rather than obligatory nasal breathers (Rodenstein et al., 1985). When trauma at the time of delivery leads to a high nasal resistance, nasal breathing may be supplemented or supplanted by the oral route (Fig. 2) (Miller et al., 1987). Preterm infants are more limited in their ability to initiate effective oral breathing during nasal occlusion, possibly secondary to immature coordination of the oral and pharyngeal musculature prior to 33–34 weeks postconceptional age (Miller et al., 1986).

VII. Interaction Between Breathing and Feeding

Feeding is a relatively complex activity that involves the coordination of neuromuscular activities involved in sucking, swallowing, and breathing. Durand et al. (1981) was the first to demonstrate that feeding can markedly influence respiratory

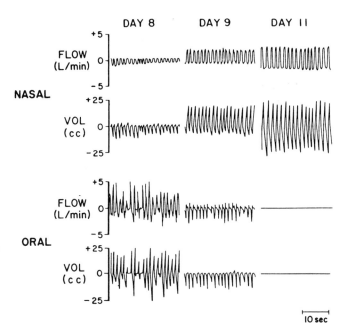

Figure 2 Transition from oral to nasal route of breathing over the second week of life in an infant who sustained nasal trauma at the time of delivery associated with a face presentation. On day 9 the infant exhibited combined oronasal breathing, inspiring predominantly through the nose and expiring through both routes. Inspiratory flow and volume are upward. (From Miller et al., 1987.)

control mechanisms in healthy term infants and depress their ventilatory response to CO_2. Subsequent studies confirmed that oral feeding significantly decreases minute ventilation, by declines in both respiratory frequency and tidal volume in preterm and term infants (Shivpuri et al., 1983; Mathew et al., 1985). Ventilation is most impaired during periods of continuous nutritive sucking of at least 30 sec duration, which typically occur at the onset of feeding.

In sharp contrast to the potentially adverse effect of oral feeding on ventilation and gas exchange, nonnutritive sucking appears to be associated with modest increases in both respiratory rate and transcutaneously measured Po_2 (Paludetto et al., 1984, 1986). These findings suggested that swallowing is the main mechanism for the decrease in ventilation during oral feeding. This was confirmed by Koenig et al. (1990), who documented that minute ventilation during bottle feeding was inversely related to swallow frequency. Swallows appeared to cause both inhibition of respiratory efforts for 0.5–1 sec and periods of airway closure. Swallows are more common during spontaneous apnea than nonapneic control periods, suggesting that both apnea and swallowing may be part of an airway protective response as might occur with accumulation of upper airway secretions (Menon et al., 1984; Pickens et al., 1988).

Linkage between ventilatory and feeding activities was recently demonstrated by Timms et al. (1993), who showed that hypercarbia (induced by CO_2 inhalation during feeding) significantly decreased sucking and swallowing frequencies and disrupted continuous sucking patterns in healthy preterm infants. Therefore, feeding can depress hypercapnic responses (Durand et al., 1981) and hypercapnia can disrupt feeding behavior (Timms et al., 1992). These observations strongly suggest competing drives for regulation of these activities in infants. This may present a particular problem in infants with BPD, who are known to exhibit dysfunctional feeding patterns. Such patients may manifest unsuspected hypoxemic episodes during feeding both prior to and after hospital discharge and must be closely monitored by pulse oximetry to determine any need for supplemental O_2 during feeding (Garg et al., 1988; Singer et al., 1992). It is possible that recurrent or prolonged periods of hypoxemia may contribute to the higher incidence of SIDS in this population of infants with BPD.

VIII. Apnea of Prematurity and SIDS

A. Pathophysiology of Neonatal Apnea

Definition

Idiopathic apnea is an extremely common disorder of prematurity that has the potential of severely compromising the well-being of infants unless it is promptly diagnosed and treated. Prolonged respiratory pauses of at least 10–15 sec duration associated with bradycardia (<100 beats/min) are generally referred to as apneic episodes, although the definition has varied widely (Daily et al., 1969; Kattwinkel et al., 1975; Miller and Martin, 1992). Infants may experience briefer respiratory pauses in conjunction with startles, movement, defecation, or swallowing during feeding (as already discussed). These short respiratory pauses are self-limiting and are usually not associated with significant bradycardia or hypoxemia, although this may not apply during oral feeding.

Apnea in premature infants is usually an isolated phenomenon, although clusters can occur. It is important to distinguish apnea from periodic breathing, during which the infant exhibits regular cycles of respiration 10–18 sec in length, interrupted by pauses at least 3 sec in duration, the pattern recurring for at least three cycles. Unlike apnea, periodic breathing has been considered a benign respiratory disorder in infancy because clinically significant hypercarbia or hypoxemia does not occur. Although periodic breathing in infants has been compared to periodic respiratory patterns (such as Cheyne-Stokes breathing) in later life, there is no clear evidence of a common pathophysiological basis between these disorders. The relationship between periodic breathing and apnea in infants is also unclear, although both decrease in frequency with advancing postconceptional age.

The reflex effects of apnea include sinus bradycardia, which may begin within 2 sec of the onset of apnea. A significant correlation has been found between the arterial desaturation and degree of bradycardia during apnea, and on this basis, it has been suggested that the decrease in heart rate might be due to hypoxic stimulation of the carotid chemoreceptors in the absence of respiratory efforts (Henderson-Smart et al., 1986). The reflex effects of apnea in infants have also been compared with the diving response of the seal. During reflex apnea in these animals, upper airway afferent input from superior laryngeal and trigeminal nerve stimulation may produce a greatly enhanced bradycardia. It is therefore possible that the rapid onset of bradycardia during apnea may be the consequence of multiple inhibitory reflex effects on the heart derived from upper airway receptors as well as the carotid bodies.

Central Neural Output

Immaturity of central respiratory control of the various ventilatory muscles has traditionally been accepted as a key factor in the pathogenesis of apnea of prematurity. Enhanced vulnerability of the bulbopontine respiratory areas to central or peripheral inhibitory mechanisms might explain why apneic episodes are precipitated in preterm infants by a wide diversity of metabolic, infectious, and cardiorespiratory events (Martin et al., 1986). Apnea may then reflect the final common response of incompletely organized and interconnected respiratory neurons to a multitude of inhibitory afferent stimuli. Because the maturation of central respiratory integrative mechanisms and their biochemical neurotransmitters is inaccessible to study in human infants, much current data are derived from studies performed in anesthetized newborn animal models. Endogenously released neuromodulators such as endorphins, prostaglandins, and adenosine have all been proposed as contributing to neonatal apnea, because they are known to depress central respiratory drive (Lagercrantz, 1987; Moss and Inman, 1989). The final respiratory output from the brainstem may be a complex function of many humoral and neural inhibitory and stimulatory inputs. The exact manner in which these are modulated during apnea of prematurity remains to be elucidated. Although idiopathic apnea of prematurity implies no underlying anatomical abnormality, occasionally underlying specific neuropathology such as brainstem infarction or a rare metabolic disorder can be identified.

Various physiological parameters have been employed to estimate central respiratory drive in human infants. These include mean inspiratory flow, inspiratory pressure generated during end-expiratory airway occlusion, and amplitude (or inspiratory slope) of the diaphragm EMG. Measurement of mean inspiratory flow is most influenced by the mechanics of the infant respiratory system, making it difficult to use this measurement as an index of respiratory center output. Respiratory muscle EMGs would appear to be optimal; technical difficulties, however, limit their use even as a research tool in human infants.

Sleep State and Arousal

It became apparent in the mid-1970s that respiratory control in infants is influenced by sleep state. It was observed that apnea occurs more commonly during active (REM) and indeterminate (transitional) sleep, when respiratory patterns are irregular in both timing and amplitude. The higher incidence of apnea during active sleep is probably secondary to the variability of respiratory rhythmicity that characterizes that state. Other factors may, however, enhance the infants' vulnerability to apnea during active sleep. As noted earlier, asynchronous chest wall movements during active sleep may predispose to apnea by decreasing lung volume and impairing oxygenation (Henderson-Smart and Read, 1979; Martin et al., 1986). The compensatory increase in diaphragm activity may predispose to diaphragmatic fatigue, suggesting that the enhanced vulnerability to apnea during active sleep may operate simultaneously at several levels of respiratory function (Muller et al., 1979a).

Arousal from sleep may play a role in the ability of an infant to quickly terminate an apnea. Furthermore, sleep state may determine whether arousal occurs in response to simultaneous development of hypercapnia and hypoxemia. In the lamb, repeated exposure to hypoxemia during sleep results in evidence of adaptation, i.e., increased time to arousal and decreased O_2 saturation at arousal (Fewell and Konduri, 1989). Miller et al. (1992) recently observed that repeated hypoxic exposure in the anesthetized piglet model causes a loss of hypercapnic sensitivity and aggravation of hypoxia-induced respiratory depression. Thus hypoxic respiratory depression, involving both arousal and nonarousal mechanisms, may increase the vulnerability of infants to apnea.

Spontaneous Upper Airway Obstruction

It is now well recognized that spontaneous airway obstruction, typically pharyngeal, commonly accompanies apnea in preterm infants (Milner et al., 1980; Mathew et al., 1982; Dransfield et al., 1983). Three classes of apneic events may be distinguished by the presence or absence of upper airway obstruction. Mixed apnea is probably the most common type observed in small premature infants and consists of obstructed inspiratory efforts as well as a central pause greater than or equal to 2 sec in duration (Fig. 3). In the relatively rare cases of purely obstructive apnea, obstructed breaths continue throughout the entire apnea. In purely central apnea, inspiratory efforts cease entirely and obstructed breaths are not observed. The presence of airway closure increases substantially with apneic episodes of

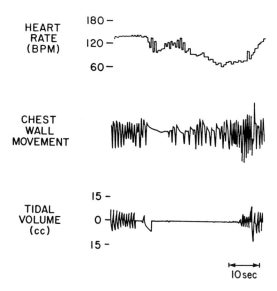

Figure 3 Representative mixed apnea in which cessation of airflow for approximately 10 sec is followed by a period with obstructed inspiratory efforts for at least 20 sec and accompanying bradycardia. Inspiratory volume is upward on the tidal volume tracing. (From Miller MJ, Martin RJ, Carlo WA: Diagnostic methods and clinical disorders in children. In: Edelman N, Santiago T, eds. Breathing Disorders of Sleep. New York: Churchill Livingstone, 1986:160.)

longer duration (Upton et al., 1992a). Thus it would appear that upper airway obstruction has the potential for prolonging short episodes of central apnea into clinically significant episodes of mixed apnea. While obstructed inspiratory efforts may occur at the onset of a mixed apnea, this sequence of events appear less commonly. Gauda et al. (1989) have documented a decrease in DIA EMG during the spontaneously obstructed inspiratory effects that characterize mixed apnea. Thus both central and mixed apneic episodes typically share an element of decreased respiratory center output to the respiratory muscles.

Because premature infants exhibit pharyngeal obstruction during spontaneous apnea, considerable interest has focused on the interaction between the various respiratory muscle groups in maintaining airway patency. A model was proposed for the pathogenesis of neonatal apnea by Thach (1983), whereby negative luminal pressures generated during inspiration may cause a compliant pharynx to collapse. Patency could be maintained by activation of upper airway muscles that would increase tone within the extrathoracic airway or elicit phasic contraction in synchrony with the chest wall muscles. The relative role played by active upper airway muscle contraction and passive rigidity of the anatomical framework of the upper airway in maintaining pharyngeal patency in preterm infants is as yet unknown.

Although many upper airway muscles, including the alae nasi and laryngeal abductor and adductor muscles, modulate patency of the extrathoracic airway, failure of genioglossus activation has been most widely implicated in mixed and obstructive apnea in both adults and infants (Remmers et al., 1978; Roberts et al., 1986). Carlo (1988) compared activity of the genioglossus muscle with that of the diaphragm in response to hypercapnic stimulation in infants. Consistent with data obtained in anesthetized and awake animal models, genioglossus activation was delayed after initiation of CO_2 rebreathing and occurred only after a CO_2 threshold of approximately 45 mmHg had been reached. In contrast, diaphragm EMG activity exhibited a more linear increase with progressive hypercapnia. In anesthetized newborn piglets, with central apnea induced by cooling of the ventral medullary surface, simultaneous development of hypercapnia and hypoxemia, as would occur during central apnea, was also associated with delayed recovery of neural output to the upper airway muscles versus the diaphragm (Martin et al., 1993).

Reflexes originating from the upper airway may directly alter the pattern of respiration in infants and play a crucial role in both the initiation and termination of apnea. Thach et al. (1989) have shown that, in tracheostomized human infants, negative pressure within the isolated upper airway depresses ventilation. These observations may also be relevant to the processes that initiate and resolve obstructive apnea. During such apnea, inspiratory efforts in the presence of an occluded upper airway would result in increased negative airway pressure below the site of the obstruction. Reflex inhibition of diaphragmatic contraction owing to increasing negative pressure in the airway lumen might then contribute to the subsequent development of a central pause characteristic of a mixed apnea. Resolution of the apnea could occur when chemoreceptor drive to phrenic and upper airway motoneurons overrides this inhibition, as already discussed.

B. Treatment of Apnea

Xanthines

Once precipitating factors have been excluded (most notably infectious and metabolic etiologies), the premature infant may be considered to have idiopathic apnea. The most widely used pharmacological agents for this disorder are the methylxanthines, theophylline and caffeine (Uauy et al., 1975; Aranda et al., 1983), which rapidly decrease the frequency of mixed, obstructive, and central apnea in premature infants. Therapeutic serum levels of theophylline (5–10 μg/ml) or caffeine (8–20 μg/ml) are usually free of toxicity. Indeed, the therapeutic effect of theophylline may include the additional effect of caffeine, for conversion of theophylline to caffeine does occur in premature infants. Central respiratory stimulation appears to be the major site of action of methylxanthines in premature infants with apnea. This is supported by the observation of Gerhardt et al. (1979) that respiratory center output increased and the threshold of the respiratory center to CO_2 decreased in human infants on aminophylline. These drugs may also increase strength of diaphragmatic contraction and decrease muscle fatigue (Aubier et al., 1983; Murciano et al., 1984) although this has not been confirmed in the piglet model (Mayock et al., 1990). Despite the multiple effects of the methylxanthines (Table 2), no serious consequences of treatment with theophylline or caffeine on growth or sleep/wake cycles have been reported in premature infants treated for apnea. Methylxanthine therapy is usually continued until the infant has reached 35–37 weeks' postconceptional age and apneic episodes have ceased. Maintenance of xanthine therapy beyond the neonatal period (and hospital discharge) is advocated by some (Hunt et al., 1983).

Continuous Positive Airway Pressure

Continuous positive airway pressure (CPAP) delivered by nasal prongs, nasal mask, or facemask at 2–5 cm water pressure has proved effective in the treatment of apnea in preterm infants (Kattwinkel et al., 1975). Initial studies suggested that the beneficial effects of CPAP are mediated by an alteration of the Hering-Breuer reflex (Martin et al., 1977), stabilization of the chest wall with reduction of the intercostal-phrenic inhibitory reflex (Hagan et al., 1977), or simply increase in oxygenation. Although such mechanisms may play a role in stabilization of ventilatory drive, nasal CPAP has been found to reduce predominantly mixed and obstructive apnea, with little or no effect on central apnea (Miller et al., 1985).

Table 2 Effects of Xanthines on Respiratory Control in Infants

Physiological effects
   Increased minute ventilation
   Shift of CO_2 response curve to left $\pm$ increased slope
   Improved pulmonary mechanics
   Decreased hypoxic ventilatory depression
   Altered sleep/wake cycles (?)
   Greater efficiency of diaphragmatic contraction (?)
Biochemical effects
   Inhibition of phosphodiesterase
   Central adenosine antagonism
   Increased metabolic rate
   Altered cellular calcium metabolism

Therefore, it appears likely that CPAP exerts its beneficial effect in infants by splinting the upper airway with positive pressure throughout the respiratory cycle. This is supported by the observation that CPAP in the therapeutic range (2–5 cm H_2O) reduces upper airway resistance in sleeping premature infants (Miller et al., 1990).

C. Potential Relationship of Neonatal Apnea to SIDS

Apnea of prematurity usually resolves by 36 weeks' postconceptional age; however, some premature infants do continue to have idiopathic apnea that requires prolonged monitoring as well as therapy. Epidemiological studies suggest at least a three- to fivefold increase of SIDS cases from low-birth-weight infants (Black et al., 1986), as indicated in Figure 4. A disorder of regulation of ventilation was first implicated in SIDS by Steinschneider (1972), and this observation has been expanded into the "apnea hypothesis" of SIDS, which may be stated as follows: Infants who are destined to die of SIDS manifest, at an early age, instability of ventilatory control that presents as recurrent apnea. Furthermore, it is this abnormality of ventilatory control that will ultimately result in the infant's demise.

Because the SIDS event occurs largely unanticipated, study of this disorder has been limited to retrospective evaluation of premature and term infants suffering an acute life-threatening event (ALTE) and to prospective analysis of heart rate and respiratory patterns in large cohorts of otherwise normal premature and term infants. In addition, detailed reports of families with more than one affected infant have prompted clinical studies of siblings of ALTE or SIDS infants.

A number of abnormalities of ventilatory control that resemble those found in apneic premature infants have been identified in ALTE infants. Among these are an increased frequency of apnea and periodic breathing during sleep (Guilleminault et al., 1975; Kelly and Shannon, 1981a). Some apneic events may have the

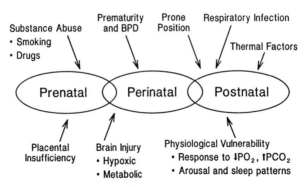

Figure 4   Model for pathogenesis of SIDS.

typical characteristics of mixed and obstructive apnea such as occurs in premature infants (Kelly and Shannon, 1981b; Kahn et al., 1988). Moreover, ALTE infants, like premature infants with apnea (Gerhardt and Bancalari, 1984), may exhibit impaired hypercapnic ventilatory responses (Shannon et al., 1977). The ventilatory response to hypoxia may also be abnormal, for Hunt et al. (1981) have reported that ALTE infants have a diminished ventilatory response to inhalation of 15% oxygen although there was moderate overlap with control infants. Hypoxic arousal also appears impaired in infants predisposed to apnea beyond the neonatal period (van der Hal et al., 1985). Despite these common features between neonatal apnea and SIDS, in the National Institute of Child Health and Human Development Cooperative Epidemiologic Study of SIDS Risk Factors, preterm infants subsequently dying of SIDS did not have a higher incidence of apnea of prematurity when matched with controls for birth weight and ethnicity (Hoffman et al., 1988). Furthermore, apnea of prematurity is more of a problem in supine infants (Heimler et al., 1992) whereas SIDS has been associated with the prone position. Thus it may not be apnea of prematurity, but prematurity itself, that is related to the underlying disorder in SIDS, and caution must be recommended in attributing the ventilatory responses exhibited by ALTE infants to any underlying disorder of respiratory control in SIDS.

To determine whether the abnormalities of cardiorespiratory control that have been described in small populations would apply to all infants at risk, large-scale prospective data have been collected in Great Britain. Southall et al. (1982) prospectively evaluated 24-hr recordings of respiratory and cardiac rhythms in low-birth-weight infants within 1 week of discharge from eight neonatal intensive care units. The resultant data failed to produce any evidence for an underlying disorder of respiratory pattern in SIDS. Specifically, the previously established markers for SIDS, such as excessive apneic pauses, periodic breathing, and abnormalities of heart rate spectra, failed to identify infants who would succumb.

It is certainly possible that a ventilatory control abnormality such as the one present in apnea of prematurity may underlie some cases of SIDS, and premature infants do remain at a higher risk for SIDS. It appears likely, however, that the apnea hypothesis in its current form cannot explain the majority of SIDS cases. Alternatively, it may be that the available techniques for measurement of ventilatory stability are inadequate to detect the disorder in future SIDS victims. The current development of new monitoring techniques, as well as their application to large-scale studies, may be required before the apnea hypothesis can be placed in its proper perspective in our overall understanding of SIDS.

References

AAP Task Force on Infant Positioning and SIDS. Positioning and SIDS. Pediatrics 1992; 89:1120–1126.

Agostoni E. Volume-pressure relationships to the thorax and lung in the newborn. J Appl Physiol 1959; 14:909–913.

Allen JL, Wolfson MR, McDowell K, Shaffer TH. Thoracoabdominal asynchrony in infants with airflow obstruction. Am Rev Respir Dis 1990; 141:337–341.

Allen JL, Greenspan JS, Deoras KS, Keklikian E, Wolfson MR, Shaffer TH. Interaction between chest wall motion and lung mechanics in normal infants and infants with bronchopulmonary dysplasia. Pediatr Pulmonol 1991; 11:37–43.

Anderson JW, Sant'Ambrogio FB, Mathew OP, Sant'Ambrogio G. Water-responsive laryngeal receptors in the dog are not specialized endings. Respir Physiol 1990; 79:33–44.

Aranda JV, Turmen T, Davis J, Trippenbach T, Grondin D, Zinman R, Watters G. Effect of caffeine on control of breathing in infantile apnea. J Pediatr 1983; 103:975–978.

Aubier M, Murciano D, Viires N, Lecocguic Y, Pariente R. Diaphragmatic contractility enhanced by aminophylline: role of extracellular calcium. J Appl Physiol 1983; 54: 460–464.

Avery ME, Chernick V, Dutton RE, Permutt S. Ventilatory response to inspired carbon dioxide in infants and adults. J Appl Physiol 1963; 18:895–903.

Bancalari E. Pathophysiology of chronic lung disease. In: Polin RA, Fox WW, eds. Fetal and Neonatal Physiology, 1st ed. Philadelphia: Saunders, 1992.

Beardsmore CS, MacFadyen UM, Moosavi SS, Wimpress SP, Thompson J, Simpson H. Measurement of lung volumes during active and quiet sleep in infants. Pediatr Pulmonol 1989; 7:71–77.

Bishop B, Bachofen H. Comparison of neural control of the diaphragm and abdominal muscle activated in the cat. J Appl Physiol 1972; 32:798–805.

Black L, David RJ, Brouillette RT, Hunt CE. Effects of birth weight and ethnicity on incidence of sudden infant death syndrome. J Pediatr 1986; 108:209–214.

Blanco CE, Dawes GS, Hanson MA, McCooke HB. The response to hypoxia of arterial chemoreceptors in fetal sheep and new-born lambs. J Physiol 1984a; 351:25–37.

Blanco CE, Hanson MA, Johnson P, Rigatto H. Breathing pattern of kittens during hypoxia. J Appl Physiol 1984b; 56:12–17.

Blanco CE, Hanson MA, McCooke HB. Effects on carotid chemoreceptor resetting of pulmonary ventilation in the fetal lamb in utero. J Dev Physiol 1988; 10:167–174.

Boggs DF, Bartlett D. Chemical specificity of a laryngeal apneic reflex in puppies. J Appl Physiol 1982; 53:455–462.

Bowes G, Wilkinson MH, Dowling H, Ritchie BC, Brodecky V, Maloney JE. Hypercapnic stimulation of respiratory activity in unanesthetized fetal sheep in utero. J Appl Physiol 1981; 50:701–708.

Bureau MA, Lamarche J, Foulon P, Dalle D. Postnatal maturation of respiration in intact and carotid body chemodenervated lambs. J Appl Physiol 1985; 59:869–874.

Bureau MA, Cote A, Blanchard PW, Hobbs S, Foulon P, Dalle D. Exponential and diphasic ventilatory response to hypoxia in conscious lambs. J Appl Physiol 1986; 61: 836–842.

Cameron WE, Brozanski BS, Guthrie RD. Postnatal development of phrenic motoneurons in the cat. Dev Brain Res 1990; 51:142–145.

Cameron WE, Jodkowski JS, Fang HE, Guthrie RD. Electrophysiological properties of developing phrenic motoneurons in the cat. J Neurophysiol 1991; 65:671–679.

Carlo WA, Martin RJ, Versteegh FGA, Goldman MD, Robertson SS, Fanaroff AA. The effect of respiratory distress syndrome on chest wall movements and respiratory pauses in preterm infants. Am Rev Respir Dis 1982; 126:103–107.

Carlo WA, Martin RJ, DiFiore JM. Differences in CO_2 threshold of respiratory muscles in preterm infants. J Appl Physiol 1988; 65:2434–2439.

Carlo WA, Beoglos A, Siner BS, Martin RJ. Neck and body position effects on pulmonary mechanics in infants. Pediatrics 1989; 84:670–674.

Carlo WA, Siner BS, DiFiore JM, Martin RJ. Oxygen saturation and pulmonary resistance in infants with bronchopulmonary dysplasia. Pediatr Res 1990; 27:201A (abstract).

Carlo WA. Assessment of pulmonary function. In: Fanaroff AA, Martin RJ, eds. Neonatal-Perinatal Medicine, 5th ed. St. Louis: Mosby-Year Book, 1992.

Cohen G, Henderson-Smart DJ. Upper airway stability and apnea during nasal occlusion in newborn infants. J Appl Physiol 1986; 60:1511–1517.

Colin AA, Wohl ME, Mead J, Ratken A, Glass G, Stark AR. Transition from dynamically maintained to relaxed end-expiratory volume in human infants. J Appl Physiol 1989; 67:2107–2111.

Cross KW, Klaus M, Tooley WH, Weisser K. The response of the newborn baby to inflation of the lungs. J Physiol (Lond) 1960; 151:551–565.

Curzi-Dascalova L, Lebrun F, Korn G. Respiratory frequency according to sleep states and age in normal premature infants: a comparison with full term infants. Pediatr Res 1983; 17:152–156.

Daily WJR, Klaus M, Meyer HBP. Apnea in premature infants: monitoring, incidence, heart rate changes, and an effect of environmental temperature. Pediatrics 1969; 43:510–517.

Davies AM, Koenig JS, Thach BT. Upper airway chemoreflex responses to saline and water in preterm infants. J Appl Physiol 1988; 64:1412–1420.

DeNeef KJ, Jansen JRC, Versprille A. Developmental morphometry and physiology of the rabbit vagus nerve. Dev Brain Res 1982; 4:265–274.

Devlieger H, Daniels H, Marchal G, Moerman PH, Casaer P, Eggermont E. The diaphragm of the newborn infant: anatomical and ultrasonographic studies. J Dev Physiol 1991; 16:321–329.

Dransfield DA, Spitzer AR, Fox WW. Episodic airway obstruction in premature infants. Am J Dis Child 1983; 137:441–443.

Durand M, Rigatto H. Tidal volume and respiratory frequency in infants with bronchopulmonary dysplasia (BPD). Early Hum Dev 1981; 5:55–62.

Durand M, Leahy FN, Maccallum M, Cates DB, Rigatto H, Chernick V. Effect of feeding on the chemical control of breathing in the newborn infant. Pediatr Res 1981; 15:1509–1512.

Duron B, Marlot D. Nervous control of breathing during postnatal development in the kitten. Sleep 1980; 3:323–330.

Dwyer T, Ponsonby ALB, Newman NM, Gibbons LE. Prospective cohort study of prone sleeping position and sudden infant death syndrome. Lancet 1991; 337:1244–47.

England SJ. Central Effect of hypoxia in the neonate. In: Speck DF, Dekin MS, Revelette WR, Frazier DT, eds. Respiratory Control: Central and Peripheral Mechanisms. Lexington: University of Kentucky Press, 1993:163–166.

England SJ, Stogryn HAF. Influence of the upper airway on breathing pattern and expiratory time constant in dog pups. Respir Physiol 1986; 66:181–192.

England SJ, Kent G, Stogryn HAF. Laryngeal muscle and diaphragm activities in conscious dog pups. Respir Physiol 1985; 60:95–108.

Farber JP. Expiratory motor responses in the suckling opossum. J Appl Physiol 1983; 54:919–925.

Farber JP. Medullary inspiratory activity during opossum development. Am J Physiol 1988; R578–R584.

Farber JP. Medullary expiratory activity during opossum development. J Appl Physiol 1989; 66:1606–1612.

Farber JP, Fisher JT, Sant'Ambrogio G. Airway receptor activity in the developing opossum. Am J Physiol 1984; 246:R752–R758.

Fedorko L, Kelly EN, England SJ. Importance of vagal afferents in determining ventilation in newborn rats. J Appl Physiol 1988; 65:1033–1039.

Fewell JE, Konduri GG. Influence of repeated exposure to rapidly developing hypoxemia on the arousal and cardiopulmonary response to rapidly developing hypoxemia in lambs. J Dev Physiol 1989; 11:77–82.

Fisher JT, Sant'Ambrogio G. Location and discharge properties of respiratory vagal afferents in the newborn dog. Respir Physiol 1982; 50:209–220.

Fisher JT, Mortola JP, Smith JB, Fox GS, Weeks S. Respiration in newborns. Development of the control of breathing. Am Rev Respir Dis 1982; 125:650–657.

Fisher JT, Mathew OP, Sant'Ambrogio FB, Sant'Ambrogio G. Reflex effects and receptor responses to upper airway pressure and flow stimuli in developing puppies. J Appl Physiol 1985; 58:258–264.

Fleming PJ, Bryan AC, Bryan MH. Functional immaturity of pulmonary irritant receptors and apnea in newborn preterm infants. Pediatrics 1978; 61:515–518.

Fleming PJ, Gilbert R, Azaz Y, Berry PJ, Rudd PT, Stewart A, Hall E. Interaction between bedding and sleeping position in the sudden infant death syndrome: a population based case-control study. Br Med J 1990; 301:85–89.

Garg M, Kurzner SI, Bautista DB, Keens TG. Clinically unsuspected hypoxia during sleep and feeding in infants with bronchopulmonary dysplasia. Pediatrics 1988; 81:635–642.

Gauda EB, Miller MJ, Carlo WA, DiFiore JM, Johnsen DC, Martin RJ. Genioglossus response to airway occlusion in apneic versus nonapneic infants. Pediatr Res 1987; 22:683–687.

Gauda EB, Miller MJ, Carlo WA, DiFiore JM, Martin RJ. Genioglossus and diaphragm activity during obstructive apnea and airway occlusion in infants. Pediatr Res 1989; 26:583–587.

Gaultier C, Praud JP, Canet E, Delaperche MF, D'Allest AM. Paradoxical inward rib cage motion during rapid eye movement sleep in infants and young children. J Dev Physiol 1987; 9:391–397.

Gerhardt T, Bancalari E. Maturational changes of reflexes influencing inspiratory timing in newborns. J Appl Physiol 1981; 50:1282–1285.

Gerhardt T, Bancalari E. Apnea of prematurity. I. Lung function and regulation of breathing. Pediatrics 1984; 74:58–62.

Gerhardt T, McCarthy J, Bancalari E. Effect of aminophylline on respiratory center activity and metabolic rate in premature infants with idiopathic apnea. Pediatrics 1979; 63:537–542.

Greenspan JS, Wolfson MR, Locke RG, Allen JL, Shaffer TH. Increased respiratory drive and limited adaptation to loaded breathing in bronchopulmonary dysplasia. Pediatr Res 1992; 32:356–359.

Guilleminault C, Peraita R, Souquet M, Dement WC. Apneas during sleep in infants: possible relationship with sudden infant death syndrome. Science 1975; 190:677–679.

Guntheroth WG, Spiers PS. Sleeping prone and the risk of sudden infant death syndrome. JAMA 1992; 267:2359–2362.

Guslits B, Gaston S, Bryan MH, England SJ, Bryan AC. Diaphragmatic work of breathing in premature human infants. J Appl Physiol 1987; 62:1410–1415.

Guthrie RD, Standaert TA, Hodson WA, Woodrum DE. Sleep and maturation of eucapnic ventilation and CO_2 sensitivity in the premature primate. J Appl Physiol 1980; 48:347–354.

Haddad GG, Farber JP. Developmental Neurobiology of Breathing. New York: Marcel Dekker, 1991.

Haddad GG, Getting PA. Repetitive firing properties of neurons in the ventral region of nucleus tractus solitatious: in vitro studies in adult and neonatal rat. J Neurophysiol 1989; 62:1213–1224.

Haddad GG, Mellins RB. Hypoxia and respiratory control in early life. Annu Rev Physiol 1984; 46:629–643.

Haddad GG, Epstein RA, Epstein MAF, Leistner HL, Marino PA, Mellins RB. Maturation of ventilation and ventilatory pattern in normal sleeping infants. J Appl Physiol 1979; 46:998–1002.

Haddad GG, Gandhi MR, Mellins RB. Maturation of ventilatory response to hypoxia in puppies during sleep. J Appl Physiol 1982; 52:309–314.

Haddad GG, Donnelly DF, Getting PA. Biophysical properties of hypoglossal motoneurons in vitro: intracellular studies in adult and neonatal rats. J Appl Physiol 1990; 69:1509–1517.

Hagan R, Bryan AC, Bryan MH, Gulston G. Neonatal chest wall afferents and regulation of respiration. J Appl Physiol 1977; 42:362–367.

Hanson MA, Kumar P, McCooke HB. Post-natal re-setting of carotid chemoreceptor sensitivity in the lamb. J Physiol 1987; 382:57P.

Hanson MA, Eden GJ, Nijhuis JG, Moore PJ. Peripheral chemoreceptors and other oxygen sensors in the fetus and newborn. In: Lahiri S, Forster RE II, Davies RO, Pack AI, eds. Chemoreceptors and Reflexes in Breathing: Cellular and Molecular Aspects. New York: Oxford University Press, 1989:113–120.

Harding R, Johnson P, McClelland ME. The expiratory role of the larynx during development and the influence of behavioral state. In: von Euler C, Lagercrantz H, eds. Central Nervous Control Mechanisms of Breathing. Oxford: Pergamon Press, 1979: 353–359.

Hathorn MKS. The rate and depth of breathing in newborn infants in different sleep states. J Physiol 1974; 243:101–113.

Heimler R, Langlois J, Hodel DJ, Nelin LD, Sasidharan P. Effect of positioning on the breathing pattern of preterm infants. Arch Dis Child 1992; 67:312–314.

Heldt GP, McIlroy MB. Distortion of chest wall and work of diaphragm in preterm infants. J Appl Physiol 1987; 62:164–169.

Henderson-Smart DJ, Read DJC. Reduced lung volume during behavioral active sleep in the newborn. J Appl Physiol 1979a; 46:1081–1085.

Henderson-Smart DJ, Read DJC. Ventilatory responses to hypoxaemia during sleep in the newborn. J Dev Physiol 1979b; 1:195–208.

Henderson-Smart DJ, Butcher-Peuch MC, Edwards DA. Incidence and mechanism of bradycardia during apnoea in preterm infants. Arch Dis Child 1986; 61:227–232.

Hershenson MB, Stark AR, Mead J. Action of the inspiratory muscles of the rib cage during breathing in newborns. Am Rev Respir Dis 1989; 139:1207–1212.

Hoffman HJ, Damus K, Hillman L. Risk factors for SIDS: results of the NICHHD SIDS Cooperative Epidemiologic Study. Ann NY Acad Sci 1988; 533:13–30.

Hohimer AR, Bissonnette JM, Richardson BS, Machida CM. Central chemical regulation of breathing movements on fetal lambs. Respir Physiol 1983; 52:99–111.

Hohimer AR, Bissonnette JM, Machida CM, Horowitz B. The effect of carbonic anhydrase inhibition on breathing movements and electrocortical activity in fetal sheep. Respir Physiol 1985; 61:327–334.

Honma Y, Wilkes D, Bryan MH, Bryan AC. Rib cage and abdominal contributions to ventilatory response to CO_2 in infants. J Appl Physiol 1984; 56:1211–1216.

Hoppenbrouwers T, Hodgman J, Harper RM, Hofmann E, Sterman MB, McGinty DJ. Polygraphic studies of normal infants during the first six months of life. III. Incidence of apnea and periodic breathing. Pediatrics 1977; 60:418–425.

Hunt, CE, Shannon DC. Sudden infant death syndrome and sleeping position. Pediatrics 1992; 90:115–118.

Hunt CE, McCulloch K, Brouiliette RT. Diminished hypoxic ventilatory responses in near miss sudden infant death syndrome. J Appl Physiol 1981; 50:1313–1317.

Hunt CE, Brouiliette RT, Hanson D. Theophylline improves pneumogram abnormalities in infants at risk for sudden infant death syndrome. J Pediatr 1983; 103:969–974.

Jansen AH, Ioffe S, Russell SJ, Chernick V. Influence of sleep state on the response to hypercaobia in fetal lambs. Respir Physiol 1982; 48:125–142.

Jeffrey HE, Read DJC. Ventilatory responses of newborn calves to progressive hypoxia in quiet and active sleep. J Appl Physiol 1980; 48:892–895.

Johnson P, Salisbury D, Storey AT. Apnea induced by stimulation of sensory receptors in the larynx. In: Bosma JF, Showacre J, eds. Development of Upper Respiratory Anatomy and Function: Implications for Sudden Infant Death. Washington, DC: U.S. Government Printing Office, 1975:160–178.

Kahn A, Blum D, Rebuffat E., Sottiaux M, Levitt J, Bochner A, Alexander M, Grosswasser J, Miller MF. Polysomnographic studies of infants who subsequently died of sudden infant death syndrome. Pediatrics 1988; 82:721–727.

Kalia M. Visceral and somatic reflexes produced by J pulmonary receptors in newborn kittens. J Appl Physiol 1976; 41:1–6.

Kattwinkel J, Nearman HS, Fanaroff AA, Katona PG, Klaus H. Apnea of prematurity. J Pediatr 1975; 86:588–592.

Katz DM. Molecular mechanisms of carotid body afferent neuron development. In: Lahiri S, Cherniack NS, Fitzgerald RS, eds. Biology of Oxygen Adaptation: Organ to Organelle. New York: Oxford University Press, 1990.

Katz DM, Erb MJ. Developmental regulation of tyrosine hydroxylase expression in primary sensory neurons of the rat. Dev Biol 1990; 137:233–242.

Kelly DH, Shannon DC. Treatment of apnea and excessive periodic breathing in the full-term infants. Pediatrics 1981a; 68:183–186.

Kelly DH, Shannon DC. Episodic complete airway obstruction in infants. Pediatrics 1981b; 67:823–827.

Kelson SG, Altose MD, Cherniack NS. Interaction of lung volume and chemical drive on respiratory muscle EMG and respiratory timing. J Appl Physiol 1977; 42:287–294.

Knill R, Bryan AC. An intercostal-phrenic inhibitory reflex in human newborn infants. J Appl Physiol 1976; 40:352–356.

Koenig JS, Davies AM, Thach BT. Coordination of breathing, sucking and swallowing during bottle feedings in human infants. J Appl Physiol 1990; 69:1623–1629.

Kosch PC, Stark AR. Dynamic maintenance of end-expiratory lung volume in full-term infants. J Appl Physiol Respir Environ Exercise Physiol 1984; 57:1126–1133.

Kosch PC, Davenport PW, Wozniak J, Stark A. Reflex control of inspiratory duration in newborn infants. J Appl Physiol 1986; 60:2007–2014.

Kosch PC, Hutchison AA, Wozniak JA, Carlo WA, Stark AR. Posterior cricoarytenoid and diaphragm activities during tidal breathing in neonates. J Appl Physiol 1988; 64: 1968–1978.

Krauss AN, Klain DB, Waldman S, Auld PAM. Ventilatory response to carbon dioxide in newborn infants. Pediatr Res 1975; 9:46–50.

Krauss AN, Waldman S, Auld PAM. Diminished response to carbon dioxide in premature infants. Biol Neonate 1976; 30:216–223.

Krous HF, Jordan J, Wen J, Farber JP. Developmental morphometry of the vagus nerve in the opossum. Dev Brain Res 1985; 20:155–159.

LaFramboise WA, Guthrie RD, Standaert TA, Woodrum DE. Pulmonary mechanics during the ventilatory response to hypoxemia in the newborn monkey. J Appl Physiol 1983; 55:1008–1014.

Lagercrantz H. Neuromodulators and respiratory control in the infant. In: Stern L, ed. The respiratory system in the newborn. Clin Perinatol 1987; 14:683.

Lawson EE, Long WA. Central origin of biphasic breathing pattern during hypoxia in newborns. J Appl Physiol 1983; 55:483–488.

Lawson EE, Richter DW, Bischoff A. Intracellular recordings of respiratory neurons in the lateral medulla of piglets. J Appl Physiol 1989; 66:983–988.

Lopes J, Muller NL, Bryan MH, Bryan AC. Importance of inspiratory muscle tone in the maintenance of the functional residual capacity in the newborn. J Appl Physiol 1981; 51:830–834.

Lundberg JM, Saria A. Capsaicin-induced desensitization of airway mucosa to cigarette smoke, mechanical and chemical irritants. Nature 1983; 302:251–253.

Marlot D, Duron B. Postnatal maturation of phrenic, vagus and intercostal nerves in the kitten. Biol Neonate 1979; 36:264–272.

Martin RJ, Nearman HS, Katona PG, Klaus MH. The effect of a low continuous positive airway pressure on the reflex control of respiration in the preterm infant. J Pediatr 1977; 90:976–981.

Martin RJ, Herrell N, Rubin D, Fanaroff A. Effect of supine and prone positions on arterial oxygen tension in the preterm infant. Pediatrics 1979a; 63:528–531.

Martin RJ, Okken A, Rubin D. Arterial oxygen tension during active and quiet sleep in the normal neonate. J Pediatr 1979b; 94:271–274.

Martin RJ, Miller MJ, Carlo WA. Pathogenesis of apnea in preterm infants. J Pediatr 1986; 109:733–741.

Martin RJ, Dreshaj IA, Miller MJ, Haxhiu MA. Differential recovery of respiratory neural output during central inhibition of respiratory drive in piglets. Pediatr Res 1993; 33:336A.

Masterson J, Zucker C, Schulze K. Prone and supine positioning effects on energy expenditure and behavior of low birth weight neonates. Pediatrics 1987; 80: 689–692.

Mathew OP, Roberts JL, Thach BT. Pharyngeal airway obstruction in preterm infants during mixed and obstructive apnea. J Pediatr 1982; 100:964–968.

Mathew OP, Clark ML, Pronske ML, Luna-Solarzano HG, Peterson MD. Breathing pattern and ventilation during oral feeding in term newborn infants. J Pediatr 1985; 106: 810–813.

Mathew OP, Sant'Ambrogio FB, Sant'Ambrogio G. Effects of cooling on laryngeal reflexes in the dog. Respir Physiol 1986; 66:61–70.

Mayock DE, Standaert TA, Watchko JF, Woodrum DE. Effect of aminophylline on diaphragmatic contractility in the piglet. Pediatr Res 1990; 28:196–198.

Menon AP, Schefft L, Thach BT. Frequency and significance of swallowing during prolonged apnea in infants. Am Rev Respir Dis 1984; 130:969–973.

Miller MJ, Martin RJ. Apnea of prematurity. In: Hunt CE, ed. Apnea and SIDS. Clin Perinatol 1992; 19(4):789–808.

Miller MJ, Carlo WA, Martin RJ. Continuous positive airway pressure selectively reduces obstructive apnea in preterm infants. J Pediatr 1985a; 106:91–94.

Miller MJ, Martin RJ, Carlo WA, Fouke JM, Strohl KP, Fanaroff AA. Oral breathing in newborn infants. J Pediatr 1985b; 107:465–469.

Miller MJ, Carlo WA, Strohl KP, Fanaroff AA, Martin RJ. Effect of maturation on oral breathing in sleeping premature infants. J Pediatr 1986; 109:515–519.

Miller MJ, Martin RJ, Carlo WA, Fanaroff AA. Oral breathing in response to nasal trauma in term infants. J Pediatr 1987; 111:899–901.

Miller MJ, DiFiore JM, Strohl KP, Martin RJ. The effects of nasal CPAP on supraglottic and total pulmonary resistance in preterm infants. J Appl Physiol 1990; 68:141–146.

Miller MJ, Haxhiu-Poskurica BA, Haxhiu MA, DiFiore JM, Martin RJ. Recurrent hypoxic exposure depresses the ventilatory response to hypoxia in the piglet. Pediatr Res 1992; 31:317A.

Millhorn DE, Szymeczek CL, Bayliss DA, Seroogy KB, Hökfelt T. Cellular, molecular, and developmental aspects of chemical synaptic transmission. In: Haddad GG, Farber JP, eds. Developmental Neurobiology of Breathing. New York: Marcel Dekker, 1991: 11–70.

Milner AD, Boon AW, Saunders RA, Hopkin IE. Upper airways obstruction and apnea in preterm babies. Arch Dis Child 1980; 55:22–25.

Moriette G, Chaussain M, Radvanyi-Bouvet MF, Walti H, Pajot N, Relier JP. Functional residual capacity and sleep states in the premature infant. Biol Neonate 1983; 43: 125–133.

Moriette G, Van Reempts P, Moore M, Cates D, Rigatto H. The effect of rebreathing CO_2 on ventilation and diaphragmatic electromyography in newborn infants. Respir Physiol 1985; 62:387–397.

Mortola JP, Fisher JT. Upper airway reflexes in newborns. In: Mathew OP, Sant'Ambrogio G, eds. Respiratory Function of the Upper Airway. New York: Marcel Dekker, 1988: 303–357.

Mortola JP, Rezzonico R. Ventilation in kittens with chronic section of the superior laryngeal nerves. Respir Physiol 1989; 76:369–382.

Moss IR, Inman JG. Neurochemicals and respiratory control during development. J Appl Physiol 1989; 67:1–13.

Muller N, Gulston C, Cade D, Whitton J, Froese AB, Bryan MH, Bryan AC. Diaphragmatic muscle fatigue in the newborn. J Appl Physiol 1979a; 46:688–695.

Muller NL, Volgyesi G, Becker L, Bryan MH, Bryan AC. Diaphragmatic muscle tone. J Appl Physiol 1979b; 47:279–284.

Mulligan E. Single fiber carotid body chemoreceptor responses in the piglet. FASEB J 1988; 2:A1293.

Mulligan E, Bhide S. Non-sustained responses to hypoxia of carotid body chemoreceptor afferents in the piglet. FASEB J 1989; 3:A399.

Murciano D, Aubier M, Lecocguic Y, Pariente R. Effects of theophylline on diaphragmatic strength and fatigue in patients with chronic obstructive pulmonary disease. N Engl J Med 1984; 311:349–353.

Murphy TD, Gibson RL, Standaert TA, Mayock DE, Woodrum DE. Effect of group B streptococcal sepsis on diaphragmatic function in young piglets. Pediatr Res 1993; 33:10–14.

Nattie EE, Edwards WH. CSF acid-base regulation and ventilation during acute hypercapnia in the newborn dog. J Appl Physiol 1981; 50:566–574.

Neubauer JA, Melton JE, Edelman NH. Modulation of respiration during brain hypoxia (review). J Appl Physiol 1990; 68:441–451.

Openshaw P, Edwards S, Helms P. Changes in rib cage geometry during childhood. Thorax 1984; 39:624–627.

Paludetto R, Robertson SS, Hack M, Shivpuri CR, Martin RJ. Transcutaneous oxygen tension during nonnutritive sucking in preterm infants. Pediatrics 1984; 74:539–542.

Paludetto R, Robertson SS, Martin RJ. Interaction between nonnutritive sucking and respiration in preterm infants. Biol Neonate 1986; 49:198–203.

Pickens DL, Schefft G, Thach BT. Prolonged apnea associated with upper airway protective reflexes in apnea of prematurity. Am Rev Respir Dis 1988; 137:113–118.

Phillipson EA. Respiratory adaptions in sleep. Annu Rev Physiol 1978; 40:133–156.

Phillipson EA, Bowes G. Control of breathing during sleep. In: Handbook of Physiology. Section 3. The Respiratory System. Vol. II. Control of Breathing, part 2. Washington, DC: American Physiological Society, 1986.

Ponsonby AL, Dwyer T, Gibbons LE, Cochrane JA, Jones ME, McCall MJ. Thermal environment and sudden infant death syndrome: case-control study. Br Med J 1992; 304:277–282.

Praud JP, Egreteau L, Benlabed M, Curzi L, Gaultier CL. The effect of rebreathing CO_2 on ventilation and respiratory muscle electromyography in infants. FASEB J 1989; 3:A1157.

Remmers JE, DeGroot WT, Sauerland EK, Anch AM. Pathogenesis of upper airway occlusion during sleep. J Appl Physiol 1978; 44:931–938.

Rigatto H. Control of ventilation in the newborn. Annu Rev Physiol 1984; 46:661–674.

Rigatto H, Brady JP, de la Torre Verduzco R. Chemoreceptor reflexes in preterm infants: the effect of gestational and postnatal age on the ventilatory response to inhalation of 100% and 15% oxygen. Pediatrics 1975; 55:604–613.

Roberts JL, Reed WR, Mathew OP, Thach BT. Control of respiratory activity of the genioglossus muscle in micrognathic infants. J Appl Physiol 1986; 61:1523–1533.

Rodenstein DO, Perlmutter N, Stanescu D. Infants are not obligatory nasal breathers. Am Rev Respir Dis 1985; 131:343–347.

Rome ES, Miller MJ, Goldthwait DA, Osorio IO, Fanaroff AA, Martin RJ. Effect of sleep state on chest wall movements and gas exchange in infants with resolving bronchopulmonary dysplasia. Pediatr Pulmonol 1987; 259–263.

Sant'Ambrogio G, Mathew OP, Fisher JT, Sant'Ambrogio FB. Laryngeal receptors responding to transmural pressure, airflow and local muscle activity. Respir Physiol 1983; 54:317–330.

Sant'Ambrogio G, Mathew OP, Sant'Ambrogio FB, Fisher JT. Laryngeal cold receptors. Respir Physiol 1985; 59:35–44.

Schwieler GH. Respiratory regulation during postnatal development in cats and rabbits and some of its morphological substrate. Acta Physiol Scand 1968; 72(Suppl 304): 1–123.

Shannon DC, Kelly DH, O'Connell K. Abnormal regulation of ventilation in infants at risk for sudden-infant death syndrome. N Engl J Med 1977; 297:747–750.

Sherry JH, Megirian D. Spontaneous and reflexly evoked activity in pharyngeal, laryngeal and phrenic motoneurons of cat. Exp Neurol 1974; 42:17–27.

Shivpuri CR, Martin RJ, Carlo WA, Fanaroff AA. Decreased ventilation in preterm infants during oral feeding. J Pediatr 1983; 103:285–289.

Sica AL, Donnelly DF, Steele AM, Gandhi MR. Discharge properties of dorsal medullary inspiratory neurons in newborn pigs. Brain Res 1987; 408:222–226.

Singer L, Martin RJ, Hawkins SW, Benson-Szekely LJ, Yamashita TS, Carlo WA. Oxygen desaturation complicates feeding in infants with bronchopulmonary dysplasia after discharge. Pediatrics 1992; 90:380–384.

Southall DP, Richards JM, Rhoden KJ, Alexander JR, Shinebourne EA, Arrowsmith WA, Cree JE, Fleming PJ, Goncalves A, Orme RLE. Prolonged apnea and cardiac arrhythmias in infants discharged from neonatal intensive care units: failure to predict an increased risk for sudden infant death syndrome. Pediatrics 1982; 70: 844–851.

Stark AR, Cohlan BA, Waggener TB, Frantz ID, Kosch PC. Regulation of end-expiratory lung volume during sleep in premature infants. J Appl Physiol 1987; 62:1117–1123.

Steinschneider A. Prolonged apnea and the sudden infant death syndrome: clinical and laboratory observations. Pediatrics 1972; 50:646–654.

Stevenson M, McGinty D. Polygraphic studies of kitten development: respiratory rate and variability during sleep-waking states. Dev Psychobiol 1978; 11:393–403.

Stokes GM, Milner AD, Newball EA, Smith NJ, Dunn C, Wilson AJ. Do lung volumes change with sleep state in the neonate? Eur J Pediatr 1989; 148:360–364.

Takahashi E, Atsumi H. Age differences in thoracic form as indicated by the Thoracic Index. Hum Biol 1955; 27:65–74.

Tay-Uyboco JS, Kwiatkowski K, Cates DD, Kavanagh L, Rigatto H. Hypoxic airway constriction in infants of very low birth weight recovering from moderate to severe bronchopulmonary dysplasia. J Pediatr 1989; 115:456–459.

Teague WG, Pian MS, Heldt GP, Tooley WH. An acute reduction in the fraction of inspired oxygen increased airway constriction in infants with chronic lung disease. Am Rev Respir Dis 1988; 137:861–865.

Thach BT. The role of pharyngeal airway obstruction in prolonging infantile apneic spells. In: Tilden JT, Roeder LM, Steinschneider A, eds. Sudden Infant Death Syndrome. New York: Academic Press, 1983.

Thach BT, Stark AR. Spontaneous neck flexion and airway obstruction during apneic spells in preterm infants. J Pediatr 1979; 94:275–281.

Thach BT, Taeusch HW Jr. Sighing in human newborn infants: role of inflation-augmenting reflex. J Appl Physiol 1976; 41:502–507.

Thach BT, Frantz ID III, Adler SM, Taeusch HW Jr. Maturation of reflexes influencing inspiratory duration in human infants. J Appl Physiol 1978; 45:203–211.

Thach BT, Menon AP, Schefft GL. Effects of negative upper airway pressure on the pattern of breathing in sleeping infants. J Appl Physiol 1989; 66:1599–1605.

Timms BJ, DiFiore JM, Martin RJ, Miller MJ. Increased respiratory drive inhibits oral feeding premature infants. J Pediatr 1993 (in press).

Trippenbach T, Kelly G. Respiratory effects of cigarette smoke, dust, and histamine in newborn rabbits. J Appl Physiol 1988; 64:837–845.

Uauy R, Shapiro DL, Smith B, Warshaw JB. Treatment of severe apnea in prematures with orally administered theophylline. Pediatrics 1975; 55:595–598.

Upton CJ, Milner AD, Stokes GM. Upper airway patency during apnoea of prematurity. Arch Dis Child 1992a; 67:419–424.

Upton CJ, Milner AD, Stokes GM. Response to external obstruction in preterm infants with apnea. Pediatr Pulmonol 1992b; 14:233–238.

van der Hal AL, Rodriguez AM, Sargent CW, Platzker ACG, Keens TG. Hypoxic and hypercapneic arousal responses and prediction of subsequent apnea in apnea of infancy. Pediatrics 1985; 75:848–854.

Walti H, Moriette G, Radvanyi-Bouvet MF, Chaussain M, Morel-Kahn F, Pajot N, Relier JP. Influence of breathing pattern on functional residual capacity in sleeping newborn infants. J Dev Physiol 1986; 8:167–172.

Watchko JF, O'Day TL, Brozanski BS, Guthrie RD. Expiratory abdominal muscle activity during ventilatory chemostimulation in piglets. J Appl Physiol 1990; 68:1343–1349.

Werthammer J, Brown ER, Neff RK, Taeusch HW. Sudden infant death syndrome in infants with bronchopulmonary dysplasia. Pediatrics 1982; 69:301–304.

Wolfson MR, Greenspan JS, Deoras EK, Allen JL, Shaffer TH. Effect of position on the mechanical interaction between the rib cage and abdomen in preterm infants. J Appl Physiol 1992; 72:1032–1038.

Zamel D, Revow M, England SJ. Expiratory airflow patterns and gas exchange in the newborn infant: results of model simulations. Respir Physiol 1989; 75:19–27.

18

Influences of Sex Steroids on Ventilation and Ventilatory Control

KOICHIRO TATSUMI

Chiba University
Chiba, Japan

BERNARD HANNHART

Laboratoire INSERM
Vandoeuvre-les-Nancy, France

LORNA G. MOORE

University of Colorado Health Sciences
  Center and University of Colorado at
  Denver
Denver, Colorado

I. Introduction

The purpose of this chapter is to review the influences of sex steroids on ventilation and ventilatory control. A previous, authoritative review (1) considered the influences of hormones and neurochemicals more generally; this review focuses on the ventilatory effects of endogenous and exogenous, female and male steroids.

Understanding the influences of sex steroids on ventilation and ventilatory control is important in view of the gender differences in susceptibility to hypoventilation disorders and the changes in ventilation occurring at various phases of the life cycle, including pregnancy, puberty, the menstrual cycle, and the menopause. Further, the detailed information acquired concerning the effects of sex steroids on ventilation and ventilatory control is important for understanding the sites and integrated modes of action by which ventilation is regulated in health and disease.

Our plan is first to summarize evidence concerning the importance of hormonal influences on ventilatory control in selected pathophysiological and physiological states. Second, we review, in detail, the effects of the female hormones, progestin and estrogen, on ventilation and ventilatory control. Third, we consider the ventilatory actions of the male hormone, testosterone. Fourth, we address the combined influences of gender, age, and sex steroids on ventilation and ventilatory control at different phases of the life cycle. Fifth, we conclude with our assessment of areas in which future research is needed for furthering our understanding of hormonal influences on ventilatory control in conditions of health and disease.

A. Importance of Hormonal Influences on Ventilatory Control

Female Protection from Hypoventilation Syndromes

Respiratory Disturbances During Sleep

These disturbances, including sleep apnea syndromes, dysrhythmic breathing, and snoring, are less common in women than men until after menopause (2–4). Particularly marked is the male predominance among persons with obesity hypoventilation syndrome (2–4). Further, while obesity increases the risk of developing sleep-disordered breathing in both sexes, women with sleep apnea syndromes are more massively obese than their male counterparts (5).

Several factors may contribute to the protection afforded premenopausal women, including the presence of female hormones, the absence of male hormones, and the effects of gender or age unrelated to sex hormones (2,3,6,7). These factors, in turn, appear to influence airway patency and ventilatory control.

Nasal breathing is important for maintaining ventilatory rhythmicity during sleep. Conversely, nasal obstruction is associated with apneic episodes (8,9). Nasal breathing accounts for a higher proportion of total nocturnal ventilation in women than men (95% vs. 71%, $p < 0.05$; Ref. 10). Pharyngeal resistance and hence the likelihood of pharyngeal collapse are greater in men than women (11). Further, nasal breathing declines and pharyngeal resistance increases with age in men but not in women. Differences in the effects of mass loading on respiratory compensation may be involved; obese women develop respiratory compensation with mass loading whereas obese men do not (12).

The effects of alcohol ingestion on breathing during sleep also differ in men and women. Whereas alcohol increased the number and severity of oxygen desaturation episodes in men, particularly with advancing age, women showed no effect of alcohol on breathing or oxygenation during sleep at any age (13,14). Alcohol ingestion produced selective blockade of genioglossal electromyogram (EMG) activity and an unfavorable balance between airway obstructing and dilating forces (15). The magnitude of the alcohol-associated decrease in genioglossal EMG activity was greater in men than women (16) and was reduced further in women during the luteal compared with the follicular phase of the menstrual cycle (17). Progesterone pretreatment also decreased the alcohol-induced mismatching of hypoglossal and phrenic activities in decerebrate cats (18).

The magnitude of the sleep-associated fall in hypoxic ventilatory response (HVR) and hypercapnic ventilatory response (HCVR) differs between the sexes.

Men reduce their HVR during sleep, but little change occurs in women (19) (Fig. 1). This may be attributable to gender differences in chemosensitivity and/or higher airway resistance in men during sleep. The lack of change in HVR among women was found in both the luteal and the follicular phase of the menstrual cycle although values were generally higher in the luteal phase.

Female as well as male hormones are likely to contribute to the gender differences in respiratory disturbances during sleep. Progestin administration has been shown to reduce the duration and severity of sleep-disordered breathing episodes in men with obesity hypoventilation syndrome but not in patients with obstructive sleep apnea syndromes without initial hypercapnia (20,21). The effects of female hormones are likely to involve estrogen as well as progesterone. We found that the number of sleep-disordered breathing episodes decreased after combined progestin and estrogen treatment in every postmenopausal woman studied even though the subjects were drawn from a group of healthy, nonobese volunteers with only modest numbers of sleep-disordered breathing episodes in the pretreatment state (Fig. 2) (22).

The apparent interaction between the effects of gender and obesity on the occurrence of sleep-disordered breathing may involve effects of sex steroids. Aromatization of estradiol occurs in adipose tissues and thus estradiol levels are likely to be augmented in obese persons (23). Since estrogen is required to induce progesterone receptors (24), the number of progesterone receptors and hence the response to normal circulating levels of progesterone may be enhanced in obese

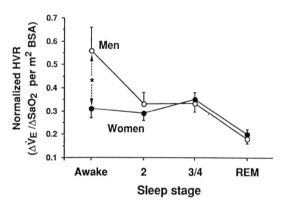

Figure 1   Hypoxic ventilatory response corrected for body surface area (BSA) in men and women. HVR is greater in men than women while awake but values decrease in men with NREM sleep and further with REM sleep. HVR values are preserved at awake values during NREM sleep and decrease slightly during REM sleep. V_E, expired ventilation; Sao_2, arterial O_2 saturation. (Reprinted from Ref. 19.)

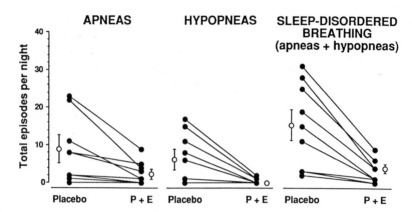

Figure 2 Number of apneas, hypopneas, and the total number of sleep-disordered breathing episodes per night decreased in every subject after 1 week of combined progestin and estrogen (P + E) treatment compared with numbers observed during placebo treatment. (Reprinted from Ref. 22.)

women. The presence of male sex hormones may also be involved in promoting sleep-disordered breathing in men as evidenced by the appearance of sleep apnea syndromes following testosterone treatment (7,25–27).

Syndromes of Altitude Sickness

High-altitude pulmonary edema (HAPE), subacute infantile, and chronic mountain sickness have been reported to be less common in females than males. Older reports suggesting female protection from acute mountain sickness (28,29,31) are not supported by more recent studies (30,32,33).

HAPE, a noncardiogenic form of pulmonary edema, is a rare occurrence in visitors who ascend rapidly to high altitude and in child or adolescent high-altitude residents after returning from brief sojourn at low altitude. The nonresident-ascent HAPE is more common in males than females (28,31,34–39). Interestingly, the sex difference appears in adulthood; girls and boys appear equally susceptible to the development of reascent HAPE (39,40).

It has been suggested that the male predominance in HAPE was simply due to a tendency for men to go to high altitude more frequently and/or exercise more vigorously (30). This is not supported by data derived form large numbers of tourists in Colorado (Honigman, personal communication). There also appears to be a different altitude threshold for HAPE in men and women; up to 11,000 ft, HAPE primarily affects men, whereas at higher altitudes, male and female visitors develop HAPE with equal frequency (30,34,37,39).

While the cause(s) of HAPE remain incompletely understood, hypoxic vasoconstriction, intravascular thromboses, and increased pulmonary capillary permeability are likely involved. Persons with a history of HAPE show a greater rise in pulmonary vascular resistance and impaired gas exchange during acute altitude exposure compared with normal subjects (41–44). A gender difference in the pulmonary vascular response to hypoxia has been observed; male rats, chickens, and pigs develop greater right ventricular hypertrophy than females after chronic exposure to high altitude (45–48). Hypoxic pulmonary vasoconstriction may have been attenuated by the presence of female hormones and/or the maintenance of higher alveolar and arterial oxygen tensions (49–51). While a low hypoxic ventilatory response has been implicated in the pathogenesis of HAPE (52–56), there does not appear to be a clear gender difference in hypoxic chemosensitivity (57–60). Females may be protected against hypoxic ventilatory depression (61,62), possibly owing to effects of progesterone (63). This may be important in the pathogenesis of HAPE since hypoxic ventilatory depression will manifest itself when the opposing peripheral chemoreceptor response to hypoxia is negligible or under conditions of severe hypoxemia (64,65).

A syndrome of subacute, infantile mountain sickness has been described among Han ("Chinese") infants born at low altitude and brought to reside in Lhasa, Tibet Autonomous Region, China at 3600 m (66). Symptoms of dyspnea, cough, cyanosis, sleeplessness, irritability, facile edema, and oliguria develop weeks to months after arrival at high altitude. Pathological findings indicate severe pulmonary hypertension and support the likelihood that death resulted from right heart failure. While only a small number of cases have been described, the majority (10/15) occurred in males ranging from 3 to 16 months of age (66). It is unknown whether gender differences in arterial O_2 saturation or pulmonary artery pressure exist in high-altitude infants. There is a generalized male susceptibility to other kinds of neonatal and infantile respiratory conditions. For example, worldwide boys succumb more frequently to sudden infant death than do girls (1.82 vs. 1.26 deaths per 1000 live births, respectively) (67).

Chronic mountain sickness is observed predominantly in men and is characterized by cyanosis, palpitations, headache, dizziness, and memory loss (68). First described in Andean highlanders (69), it has also been observed in Rocky Mountain and Himalayan high-altitude residents (68,70,71). The primary diagnostic symptom is excessive polycythemia. Compared with healthy residents of high altitude, chronic mountain sickness patients have lower arterial O_2 saturation particularly during sleep, elevated pulmonary arterial pressures, and right ventricular hypertrophy (72–76). Erythropoietin production is increased and may be exaggerated at a given level of arterial O_2 tension (148). Persons with chronic mountain sickness have a blunted hypoxic ventilatory drive (75,78,79). However, since long-term, healthy residents of high altitude also have blunted hypoxic ventilatory responses, a blunted drive may be permissive but is not likely to be the cause of chronic mountain sickness (71). The appearance of chronic mountain sickness is associated with advancing age (80,81) and often occurs in combination with some other pulmonary or cardiac abnormality, leading to the question of whether chronic mountain sickness is a discrete disease entity or is a complication of heart and lung diseases observed at high altitude.

Little attention has been paid to the factors responsible for the protection enjoyed by females in the development of chronic mountain sickness. This is surprising, particularly in light of studies showing that treatment with the synthetic progestin, medroxyprogesterone acetate, benefits men with the condition (82,83). While lower hemoglobin levels may be involved in protecting younger-aged women, there is little gender difference in hemoglobin in the over-50-year age group, who most commonly have chronic mountain sickness (84). The confounding effects of chronic obstructive lung disease are likely to be important. Women benefit from a reduced incidence of smoking and exposure to occupational conditions associated with the development of chronic lung disease. Further evaluation of the sources of this gender difference, with controls for the appropriate risk factors, is likely to be informative for identifying the etiological factor(s) responsible for the development of chronic mountain sickness.

Maternal and Fetal Well-Being During Pregnancy/ Gestation

Pregnancy is an important period during which female hormones influence ventilation and ventilatory control. As reviewed below, there is a pronounced early and progressive rise in ventilation during pregnancy accompanied by increased hypoxic and hypercapnic ventilatory sensitivity. Whereas the rise in ventilation has little effect on arterial O_2 saturation at sea level (since values are already nearly maximal), it raises arterial O_2 saturation and helps to maintain O_2 content at high altitude (85). The increase in ventilation, in turn, is correlated with an elevation in hypoxic ventilatory response (86).

The importance of the pregnancy-associated ventilatory changes is underscored by their relationship to fetal and maternal well-being. At high altitude, birth weight is reduced owing to retardation of intrauterine growth during the last trimester (87). In a series of studies, we have shown that the magnitude of rise in hypoxic ventilatory response and the resultant ventilation, arterial O_2 saturation, and arterial O_2 content correlate positively with infant birth weight at high altitude. In other words, women giving birth to lower-birth-weight infants hypoventilated and had lower levels of arterial oxygenation than women giving birth to normal-sized infants (86,88). The incidence of the maternal complication of pregnancy preeclampsia is also increased at high altitude (89; Zamudio, personal communication). Among preeclamptic as well as normal pregnant women at high altitude, arterial O_2 saturation correlates inversely with the level of blood pressure present; that is, the women with the lowest arterial O_2 saturation have the highest mean arterial pressure (89,90). While these observations indicate that the rise in maternal ventilation is likely to be important in relation to O_2 transport, the increased ventilation of pregnancy may also serve other functions such as facilitating CO_2 unloading from the fetal circulation.

II. Effects of Progestin and Estrogen on Ventilation and Ventilatory Control

Since the observations of Hasselbach in 1912, progestational hormones have been recognized to stimulate ventilation (91). Continuing studies have investigated the ventilatory effects of hormonal alterations during the menstrual cycle and pregnancy. Progestins have been administered to ameliorate hypoxemic episodes during sleep in persons with chronic obstructive lung disease and obesity hypoventilation syndromes. More recently, the steroid receptor-dependent mechanisms by which progestins influence ventilation and ventilatory control have begun to be investigated (92,93).

A. Alterations in Endogenous Hormone Levels: The Menstrual Cycle and Pregnancy

Ventilation

Arterial or alveolar P_{CO_2} falls in the luteal compared with the follicular phase of the menstrual cycle and progressively during pregnancy, implying an increase in alveolar ventilation per unit O_2 consumption (94–100). The increase in ventilation is due to an increase in tidal volume without a change in lung mechanics (101–103). Even though an upward shift of the diaphragm in late pregnancy reduces functional residual capacity, vital capacity remains unaltered (104). The increase in ventilation during the menstrual cycle is not due to increased metabolic rate since O_2 consumption does not change despite a rise in body temperature (95,100,105). Changes in ventilation begin before a detectable rise in metabolic rate during pregnancy (106). Nor are alterations in acid-base balance responsible since respiratory alkalosis is well compensated during the menstrual cycle and nearly fully compensated in pregnancy (85,99,105,107). The increase in resting ventilation is preserved during exercise (105). Neither maximum O_2 uptake nor aerobic power is changed in the luteal compared with the follicular phase or with pregnancy (102,108–110). That increased progesterone levels are involved is supported by a correlation between alveolar P_{CO_2} and the log of serum progesterone concentration during the menstrual cycle and pregnancy (Fig. 3) (100). Additionally, a reduction in ventilation is observed after the menopause (111,112) and in amenorrheic women (105).

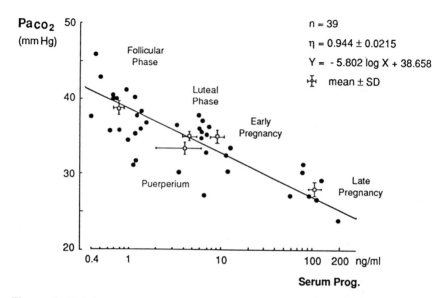

Figure 3 Relationship between Pa_{CO_2} and serum progesterone concentration during menstrual cycle, pregnancy, and puerperium. (Reprinted from Ref. 100.)

HVR, HCVR

An increase in HVR in the luteal compared with the follicular phase of the menstrual cycle has been observed in most, but not all, studies (57,101,105,110, 113). The augmentation is greater under conditions in which end-tidal P_{CO_2} is restored to follicular levels. HVR increases consistently with pregnancy in humans and other species (86,92,106,114–119). The rise in HVR begins before an elevation in metabolic rate, suggesting that hormonal or other pregnancy-specific factors are responsible. The magnitude of rise is not correlated with circulating progesterone levels among individual subjects (106,120). The increase in HVR after 20 weeks of pregnancy parallels the rise in metabolic rate (106).

The increase in HVR is an important contributor to the increase in resting ventilation during pregnancy at high altitude (86). Some effect on pregnancy ventilation occurs even at low altitude, due to steepening of the slope of the ventilatory response curve in the normoxic range (117).

HCVR has generally not been shown to change during the menstrual cycle (57,95,105,121). However, under conditions in which intersubject variability was carefully controlled, HCVR increased from the follicular to the luteal phase (122). During pregnancy there is a progressive rise in HCVR and shift to a lower CO_2 threshold (*x*-intercept) (96,106,117,123).

B. Separate and Combined Effects of Progestin and Estrogen

Progestin Alone

Döring et al. (96) first showed that progesterone administration increased alveolar ventilation in men. The rise in resting ventilation in males or females is qualitatively similar to that observed during the luteal phase of the menstrual cycle and pregnancy. End-tidal P_{CO_2} falls 2–6 mmHg owing to an increase in tidal volume (120,124–127). The ventilation rise is not dependent on an increase in body temperature or metabolic rate (57,114,128–130). No correlation has been observed between circulating progestin levels and the magnitude of fall in end-tidal P_{CO_2}.

The increase in ventilation observed at rest persists during exercise (114,131). Progestin administration in healthy persons does not modify arterial oxygenation, overall gas exchange, cardiac output, maximum O_2 uptake, or exercise performance (120,131,132).

The effect of progestin administration on HVR has been variable. Increases have been observed in most, but not all, studies and only when end-tidal P_{CO_2} was restored to pretreatment values (120,124,130,133–135) (Fig. 4). Progestin administration has not consistently raised HCVR in normal persons or patients with chronic obstructive pulmonary disease (20,57,105,120,124,130,134,136–139). Progesterone treatment enhanced the occlusion pressure ($P_{0.1}$) response to CO_2 (126).

There appears to be an interactive effect between progestin and metabolic rate on HVR such that elevated progestin levels potentiate the effect of mild exercise on HVR in women (113). It has been previously observed that women, unlike men, do not increase their HVR with mild exercise (140). Further, the correlation observed in men between normal variation in resting metabolic rate and HVR is not evident in women (141). However, in the presence of elevated progestin levels, mild exercise raises HVR in women, suggesting that progestin potentiates the effect of elevated metabolic rate on HVR in women (140). The source of the relationship between metabolic rate and HVR in men is not likely due to progesterone but could involve modulatory influences of testosterone.

Combined Progestin and Estrogen

In the natural settings of the menstrual cycle and pregnancy, elevations in progesterone are always preceded or accompanied by increases in estradiol. Estradiol alone does not raise ventilation in humans, rats, or cats (92,128,142, 143). Older reports suggested that the hyperventilatory effect of progesterone was prolonged when the two hormones were given together (128). More recently, we and others have demonstrated that estradiol is required for progesterone to raise effective alveolar ventilation and HVR. Rats or cats do not hyperventilate

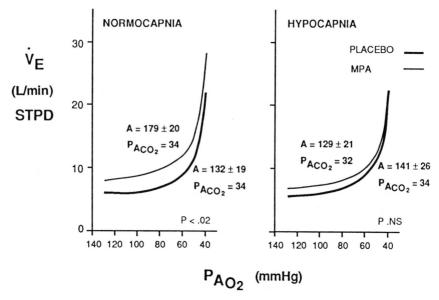

Figure 4   Hypoxic ventilatory response (HVR) during placebo and MPA administration. When measured at the pretreatment end-tidal P_{CO_2} levels (left), MPA raised HVR, but has no effect under the hypocapnic conditions present during room air breathing (right). (Reprinted from Ref. 130.)

in response to progestin alone, but when progestin is given in combination with estrogen, effective alveolar ventilation increases as indicated by a fall in arterial or end-tidal P_{CO_2} (92,143). Guinea pigs treated with combined progestin and estrogen have lower end-tidal P_{CO_2} levels than with either hormone alone although the change from pretreatment values did not differ among the various groups (144).

The two hormones combined have a greater and/or more consistent stimulatory effect on HVR than progestin alone. In awake cats, HVR rose after estrogen plus progestin treatment but did not change in response to either hormone alone (143). In women, the two hormones combined increased HVR more consistently than progestin alone, and the elevation in HVR was present both under the hypocapnic conditions observed during hormone treatment and when end-tidal P_{CO_2} was restored to pretreatment values (133). On the other hand, we did not find a greater effect of progestin on HVR when administered in the follicular than in the luteal phase of the menstrual cycle, despite the slightly higher estrogen values present (113). Combined progestin and estrogen administration in women also produced a greater rise in HCVR than progestin alone (133).

Estrogen does not appear to influence the interactive effect between progestin and metabolic rate on HVR. Mild exercise raised HVR only when progestin was administered during the luteal phase of the menstrual cycle, and the modulatory effect of progestin was not enhanced when given in the presence of elevated estrogen (113).

C. Central and/or Peripheral Sites of Action

Investigation of the sites at which progestin acts to increase ventilation and alters ventilatory control has been complicated in the past by the absence of a suitable experimental animal model. Progestin administration does not raise ventilation in ponies, cows, rabbits, goats, or rats (63,92,114–116); only the guinea pig hyperventilates in response to progestin (144,145). Other complicating factors have been a lack of control for the endocrine status of the animals studied and variation in the dosages employed. However, with the recognition that progestin stimulates ventilation in many of these same species in the presence of estrogen and the use of more physiological dosages in castrate or ovariectomized animals, the availability of animal models for investigating the site(s) of action has been enhanced.

Several lines of evidence support a central site of action for progestin in stimulating ventilation. Progesterone has clear central neural system effects; it crosses the blood-brain barrier (114), progesterone receptors have been found in the hypothalamus (especially in the ventromedial nucleus), and they are known to be important for progesterone-stimulated reproductive behaviors (146). In addition, progesterone has central neural system influences that are not dependent on traditional, steroid-receptor-mediated mechanisms. For example, progesterone at high doses has anesthetic effects (147) and, in a more physiological range, interacts with the A-type GABA receptor (32), interferes with adenosine uptake (33), and may be an endogenous ligand at the γ-opiate receptor (148). Progesterone also appears to have actions at the cell membrane not involving activation of intranuclear progesterone receptors that lead to a rise in intracellular calcium (77,149).

Progesterone has acute respiratory stimulant effects in carotid sinus nerve–denervated animals. In a series of studies in anesthetized, paralyzed cats with cut vagus and carotid sinus nerves, Bayliss and co-workers have shown that progesterone treatment acutely (within 45 min) raised integrated phrenic nerve activity (150). The increase in minute phrenic activity was not invoked by other steroid hormones (cortisol, estradiol, testosterone) and was prevented by the progesterone receptor blocker RU486. Other studies, described further in the next section, support the likelihood that these acute ventilatory effects of progesterone are receptor-dependent (151). Older reports also indicate that progesterone acts acutely at central sites; peripheral chemoreceptors were not required for acute stimulatory effects of progesterone in cross-circulated dogs (152), and progesterone applied directly to the medulla oblongata increased ventilatory sensitivity to hypercapnia (153). The acute nature of the preparations employed creates a difficulty for determining whether these central effects account for progesterone's stimulatory effects in the intact organism. In the intact organism, progesterone does not raise ventilation within the <1 hr time period over which these central neural effects of progesterone were examined (114). Thus, even though steroid-receptor-mediated, genomic effects of progesterone can take place within a <1 hr time period, the absence of acute ventilatory stimulation by progesterone in vivo raises the possibility that the central neural system sites operative acutely may not be the same as or include all those involved in chronic stimulation.

Progesterone may have peripheral sites of action operating in conjunction with or separately from central neural system effects. We have found increased ventilatory and carotid sinus neural output responses to hypoxia in pregnant compared with nonpregnant cats (117). That the increased carotid sinus neural output responsiveness was the major contributor to the increased hypoxic ventilatory response was supported by finding similar slopes of the ventilation versus carotid sinus neural output cross-plot in the pregnant and nonpregnant animals. In addition, there was no change in the carotid sinus neural output response to hypoxia after cutting the carotid sinus nerve and recording from the distal end. This implied that the responsible factors were intrinsic to the carotid body rather than due to decreased descending central neural inhibition or to increased descending central neural stimulation (117).

More direct evidence comes from carotid sinus nerve studies in cats treated with progesterone and/or estrogen (143). Progesterone increased the ventilatory and the carotid sinus neural output responses to hypoxia (Fig. 5). The increased

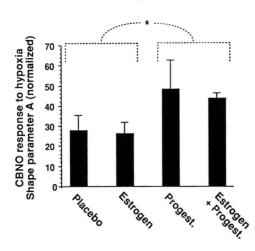

Figure 5   Carotid body neural output (CBNO) response to hypoxia shape parameter A was greater in the two groups of cats receiving progesterone (progesterone alone, estrogen + progesterone) than in the two groups not receiving progesterone (placebo, estrogen alone). $*p < 0.05$. (Reprinted from Ref. 143.)

carotid sinus neural response was not due to descending central stimulatory influences since the response recorded from the distal (carotid body) end remained elevated after the carotid sinus nerve was cut. Increased central nervous system translation of carotid body signal into ventilation was also not involved since progesterone treatment did not influence the slope of the ventilation versus carotid body neural output cross-plot (143). Whereas estrogen alone had no effect, estrogen in combination with progesterone raised the ventilatory and carotid sinus neural responsiveness to hypoxia. The effect of the combined hormones, however, was not greater than that of progesterone alone. Unexpectedly, estrogen increased the central nervous system translation of carotid sinus neural output into ventilation (143). Thus, in addition to the receptor-dependent mechanisms discussed below, estrogen may modify the effects of progesterone by acting centrally to modulate peripheral influences. The ventilatory response to hypercapnia was unaffected by acute progesterone treatment (154) but increased after chronic treatment with the two hormones combined (143).

D. Hormone Receptors and Receptor-Mediated Ventilatory Actions

Hormone Receptors

From studies in the breast and the endometrium, it is known that estradiol up-regulates the expression of estrogen and progesterone receptors and progesterone down-regulates both proteins (155–157). There are two progesterone receptors, A and B, with molecular weights of 79,000 daltons and 108,000 daltons, respectively (158), and a single estrogen receptor with a molecular weight of about 65,000 daltons. Recent gene-cloning data indicate that steroid receptors share three main regions (Fig. 6): the immunoreactive domain, the DNA-binding domain, and the steroid-binding domain (159,160). Once the receptor is activated by hormone, complex conformational changes occur that allow binding of the receptor to DNA (161).

Progesterone and estrogen are clearly defined activators of eukaryotic gene expression. Recent studies have revealed in detail the process by which progesterone and estrogen receptors bind as dimers to DNA regulatory enhancer sequences called steroid response elements (SREs) (162). The SREs are located in the 5′ flanking region of hormone-dependent genes and interact with other nuclear proteins in the activation of the transcriptional apparatus (Fig. 6). The resultant accumulation of new species of nuclear RNAs and their translation into specific proteins is characterized as a steroid hormone response (163,164).

In the breast, uterus, and brain, the effects of progesterone and estrogen on reproductive behaviors involve control over the expression of various genes and growth factors, as well as their own receptors (165). The mechanism whereby these hormones exert ventilatory or other effects (e.g., vascular) is unknown.

Steroid receptor domains:

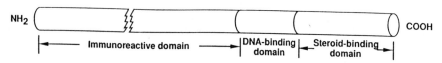

Steroid-regulated gene:

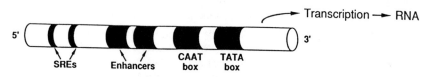

Figure 6 (Top) Three major domains of steroid receptors. The immunoreactive domain is of variable length, whereas the DNA-binding domain consists of approximately 70 amino acids and the steroid-binding domain consists of about 250 amino acids. (Bottom) Common organization of a steroid-regulated gene. (Adapted from Ref. 226.)

Progesterone and estrogen receptors have been found using immunocytochemistry, autoradiography, and radioactive ligand binding in a variety of vascular tissues, namely, endothelial and smooth muscle cells from human uterine artery and from baboon aorta, coronary artery, and myocardium (166,167). Progesterone receptors have also been found using immunocytochemistry in the infundibular and rostroventral periventricular nuclei of the hypothalamus and the preoptic area (93). Unknown is whether steroid hormone receptors exist in the carotid body.

The cellular mechanisms involved in ventilatory stimulation are unknown. That is, it is not clear whether estradiol and progesterone mediate a transcriptional response in central and/or peripheral tissues by acting through nuclear receptors to directly or indirectly regulate the expression of specific genes and, if so, what genes are up-regulated, and how they affect ventilation or ventilatory response. Further, not all actions of ovarian hormones necessarily involve activation of intranuclear receptors. For example, progesterone receptors have been identified on sperm cell membranes where they may act either as a calcium channel or be closely linked to a calcium channel to stimulate calcium influx (77,149).

Receptor-Mediated Ventilatory Actions

Several aspects of progesterone's ventilatory stimulant effects are consistent with a receptor-mediated mode of action. Progesterone has no immediate effect on ventilation in the intact organism; in men, a minimum of 48 hr is required to observe a ventilation rise, and maximal stimulation is seen after 1 week (114). Although there is a general relationship between the level of progesterone and the magnitude of hyperventilation (see Fig. 3), the stimulatory effect of progestin on ventilation does not depend closely on the level of circulating hormone, the dosage, or the luteinizing activity of the progestin employed. For example, while medroxyprogesterone acetate has a 15-fold greater and chlormadinone acetate has a 150-fold greater luteinizing activity than progesterone, their effects on end-tidal P_{CO_2} at a given dosage are similar (134,168,169). This time dependence and lack of clear dose effect suggest that characteristics of the target tissue are important determinants of hormone response.

Elevations in progesterone during the menstrual cycle or pregnancy are preceded or accompanied by increased estrogen levels. Thus, under natural circumstances, circulating levels of progesterone are raised in a setting in which estrogen levels are elevated and thus progesterone receptors are likely increased. The previously noted variability in ventilatory response to progestin may be attributable to differences in the levels of progesterone receptors present. In the rat, we showed that progestin administration failed to increase ventilation when given alone to animals whose progesterone receptor numbers were low (92). Elevation of progesterone receptor numbers with estradiol had no stimulatory effect on ventilation, but progestin administration did increase ventilation in animals whose progesterone receptor numbers had been elevated by estrogen pretreatment. Likewise in the cat, progestin alone did not affect resting ventilation but the combination of estradiol plus progesterone prompted a hyperventilatory response (143). In guinea pigs, the degree of hyperventilation (i.e., fall in arterial P_{CO_2}) was correlated with serum progestin levels when animals were treated with estrogen plus progestin but not with progestin alone (144,145). Finally, men with obesity-hypoventilation syndrome have a greater fall in arterial P_{CO_2} than normal men, perhaps as a result of their greater amounts of adipose tissue and higher estradiol levels (23) as well as their initial hypercapnia.

The acute, central neural stimulatory effects of progesterone have been shown to be receptor-mediated (93). Whereas progesterone alone had no effect, progesterone administration to ovariectomized, estradiol-pretreated cats produced an increase in minute phrenic activity. Pretreatment with either the estrogen receptor antagonist CI628, or the progesterone receptor antagonist RU486 decreased minute phrenic activity (Fig. 7) (151,170). That increased protein synthesis was involved was supported by the observation that pretreatment with the transcriptional inhibitor actinomycin D (ACTD) or the translational inhibitor anisomycin (ANI) attenuated the acute response to progesterone (171) (Fig. 7). Unknown is the extent to which progesterone's stimulatory effects on hypoxic ventilatory response are receptor-mediated.

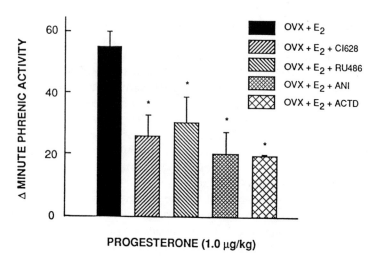

Figure 7 Effect of progesterone on minute phrenic activity (expressed as a percent of control) in ovariectomized (OVX), anesthetized, paralyzed cats after estradiol treatment (20 μg E_2/kg/day) and after pretreatment with estrogen and progesterone receptor antagonists (CI628 and RU486), the protein synthesis inhibitor (ANI, anisomycin), or the RNA synthesis inhibitor (ACTD, actinomycin-D). Samples sizes: OVX + E_2, $n = 8$; CI628, $n = 2$; RU486, $n = 3$; ANI, $n = 3$; ACTD, $n = 2$. *Significantly less than OVX + E_2. (Reprinted from Ref. 93.)

E. Therapeutic Uses of Progesterone and Estrogen

Two progestins, medroxyprogesterone acetate (MPA, 60 mg/day) and chlormadinone acetate (CMA, 5 mg/day), have been used as therapeutic agents for stimulating breathing in patients with a variety of hypoventilation disorders, including obesity-hypoventilation (Pickwickian) syndrome, chronic mountain sickness, and chronic obstructive pulmonary disease (137). No studies have evaluated the therapeutic efficacy of combined progestin and estrogen treatment for stimulating breathing although we observed that combined progestin and estrogen treatment decreased the number and duration of sleep-disordered breathing episodes in normal postmenopausal women (22).

For patients with sleep-disordered breathing, progestin treatment has been used as an alternative to tracheotomy (172) or nasal continuous positive pressure (173). In obese men with obstructive sleep apnea syndrome, MPA improved daytime ventilation, raised ventilatory responsiveness to hypoxia, and was protective during sleep in some, but not all, studies (127,174–178). Patients benefiting the most were those who were initially hypercapnic (179,180) and those able to decrease their end-tidal P_{CO_2} while awake (178,181) by increasing tidal volume and inspiratory effort (127).

For high-altitude residents with chronic mountain sickness at 3100 m, MPA administration for 10 weeks improved arterial blood gases, reduced hematocrit, and decreased the magnitude of O_2 desaturation during sleep (83,182). Among those without detectable lung disease, resting ventilation rose 20% and HVR was almost doubled but ventilatory response to hypercapnia was unchanged. There was no correlation between clinical improvement and the increase in ventilatory chemosensitivity.

Progestin treatment is of some benefit in patients with chronic obstructive pulmonary disease in situations where airway obstruction is not severe. Under circumstances of severe airway obstruction, an increase in ventilation is of limited benefit since the increased work of breathing produces more CO_2 than can be eliminated. Even among patients without mechanical restrictions, "responder" and "nonresponder" groups can be discerned; responders were defined as those who lowered Pa_{CO_2} by at lest 5 mmHg with voluntary hyperventilation or progestin treatment, whereas "nonresponders" did not (183). No other characteristics were able to clearly differentiate the two groups. CMA as well as MPA has been used to treat chronic obstructive pulmonary disease, particularly in patients who are elderly and/or initially hypercapnic (126,137). CMA treatment raised HVR and neuromuscular response to CO_2 in subjects who were able to decrease Pa_{CO_2} and enhanced the neuromechanical drive for load compensation as assessed by the ratio of the loaded to unloaded slope of the occlusion pressure response to CO_2.

Progestin treatment at the usual therapeutic dosage is well tolerated, and unwanted effects are rare. Decreased libido has been observed in a small number of subjects but was not accompanied by sexual impotence and was improved by a decrease in dosage (20,57,83,124). The other major side effect is dyspnea during exercise (124,131,184). However, dyspnea at rest has not been a problem even in subjects with marked rise in ventilation (57,124,183).

III. Effects of Testosterone on Ventilation and Ventilatory Control

A. Testosterone Effects on Ventilation During Wakefulness

Gender differences in ventilation and ventilatory control have frequently been attributed to actions of the female sex hormones, but male sex hormones or effects of gender unrelated to sex hormones may also be involved. In contrast with the large number of studies investigating the effects of the female sex hormones, there have been comparatively few studies of the male hormone, testosterone.

Administration of testosterone to hypogonadal or castrate males has resulted in an increase in ventilation and metabolic rate without a change in arterial or end-tidal P_{CO_2} (25,141,185). The increase in ventilation and metabolic rate has not been observed in all studies in hypogonadal men; White et al. (141) observed an increase, but Matsumoto et al. (25) found no change in ventilation or metabolic rate after testosterone treatment. Our results in neutered male cats were similar to those of White et al. (141). In awake animals, testosterone treatment raised resting ventilation and metabolic rate but did not alter end-tidal P_{CO_2} (185).

An increase in HVR with testosterone treatment has been observed in hypogonadal men or neutered male cats in whom a rise in metabolic rate was also present (25,141,185). The increase in HVR observed in neutered male cats occurred in both the awake and anesthetized conditions (185). The effect of testosterone on HCVR has been inconsistent; an increase (185), no change (25, 27,141), or a decrease (186) has been observed.

B. Testosterone Effects on Ventilation During Sleep

The greater frequency with which hypoventilation and sleep apnea disorders are observed in men than women (Section I.A) has prompted investigation of the influences of male hormones on ventilation during sleep. Testosterone replacement in hypogonadal men has been shown to increase the frequency of sleep-disordered breathing episodes (25,141). Several case studies report similar findings. Among a group of obese males, the only subject who experienced sleep-disordered breathing and arterial O_2 desaturation was hypogonadal (187). Testosterone administration was associated with the appearance of the obstructive sleep apnea syndrome in a male patient with primary hypogonadism and in a 54-year-old woman who was anemic owing to chronic renal failure (26,27). The sleep apnea symptoms improved with discontinuation and recurred with resumption of testosterone treatment. Among 13 women, four with obstructive sleep apnea had higher androgen levels than the others (146).

Several factors are likely to be involved in the increase in disordered breathing during sleep. Testosterone may facilitate the development of upper airway obstruction. Johnson et al. (26) observed an increase in supraglottal resistance following prolonged androgen treatment. In contrast, White et al. (141) found no change in upper airway dimensions as evaluated by computerized tomography or in upper airway resistance. However, the two subjects with an increased number of dysrhythmic episodes during sleep tended to have a higher supraglottic resistance and lower mean pharyngeal airway size than the other two subjects. Thus, anatomical differences in airway dimensions may contribute to interindividual variation in the effect of testosterone replacement on sleep-disordered breathing. White et al. (141) found no correlation between the effect of testosterone on HVR during wakefulness and the changes in breathing during sleep among individual subjects. However, both variables increased in most subjects, suggesting that interaction between an unstable ventilatory controller and decreased upper airway patency may also contribute to the development of sleep-disordered breathing (188,189).

C. Central and/or Peripheral Sites of Action

The increase in ventilation and HVR after testosterone treatment could be due to central and/or peripheral actions. One line of evidence suggesting that central sites are involved is the association between the increase in metabolic rate and the elevation in ventilation and HVR observed after testosterone treatment (57,133, 190). However, minute phrenic activity decreased after acute administration of testosterone in anesthetized, paralyzed cats with cut vagus and carotid sinus nerves (150).

We simultaneously measured the ventilatory and carotid sinus neural responses to hypoxia in castrate neutered male cats after testosterone or placebo treatment (185). Both the ventilatory and carotid sinus neural responses to hypoxia were increased in the testosterone-treated animals, but the central translation of the carotid sinus nerve activity into ventilation (i.e., slope of the ventilation–CSN activity cross-plot) was unaffected (Fig. 8). Thus, increased peripheral chemoreceptor responsiveness appeared responsible for the increase in HVR after

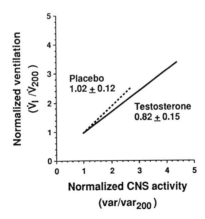

Figure 8 Simultaneously measured ventilatory and carotid sinus neural responses to hypoxia are computed using the normalized ventilation (V_I/V_{200}) and normalized carotid sinus nerve (CSN) activity expressed relative to the values obtained during hyperoxia. The slopes were similar in placebo and testosterone-treated cats, suggesting no difference between the two groups in the central nervous system translation of carotid sinus nerve activity into ventilation. (Reprinted from Ref. 185.)

testosterone treatment. The increase in peripheral chemoreceptor responsiveness may have been due, in part, to stimulatory central neural system influences since unilateral section of the carotid sinus nerve decreased the carotid sinus neural response to hypoxia in the testosterone-treated, but not the placebo, animals. An increase in metabolic rate is not likely to have raised carotid sinus neural response to hypoxia directly since several studies have shown that passive hindlimb stimulation fails to raise carotid body responsiveness to hypoxia (191,192).

D. Receptor-Mediated Actions

Testosterone acts through its specific steroid receptor in ways similar to those described above for progesterone and estrogen. Binding of the receptor-steroid complexes to DNA is accompanied by RNA synthesis (57), translation, and the formation of hormone-specific proteins that alter target cell functions (141).

Several factors are likely important for regulating androgenic actions in individual tissues: serum androgen concentration, the steroid-binding specificity of the androgen receptors, and the structure of the chromatin to which receptor-steroid complexes bind and activate gene transcription. The magnitude of change in ventilation, metabolic rate, HVR, or HCVR is not related to the absolute or relative change in serum testosterone in the normal to above-normal range (141,185). One factor that may be important is the length of time that the receptor-steroid complex is retained in the nucleus; the longer the complex is retained, the greater the degree of androgenic stimulation of responding genes (193). It is not known whether the ventilatory effects of testosterone are receptor-mediated and, if so, whether testosterone receptors are located in central and/or peripheral neural tissue.

The possible interaction among steroid hormones has been little explored. High dosages of progesterone suppress gonadal function and diminish serum testosterone levels (194). Testosterone and estrogen are capable of acting synergistically as well as antagonistically (195–198). Androgens also appear to interfere with the estrogen-dependent augmentation of progesterone receptors (199). The interactive effects of testosterone, progesterone, and estrogen on ventilation and ventilatory control remain to be investigated.

IV. Interactions of Gender, Age, and Sex Steroids

A. Circulating Hormones and/or Gender Effects

Sources of Gender Differences

Women have consistently been shown to have higher levels of effective alveolar ventilation (lower arterial or end-tidal P_{CO_2}) than men (49–51). As reviewed above, progesterone, particularly when combined with estrogen, increases ventilation (133,143). Testosterone also raises ventilation, but does not lower arterial or end-tidal P_{CO_2} (141,185). HVR and HCVR are increased by female as well as male hormones, but whether there are differences in HVR between men and women remains unclear (57–60). It is not clear whether the gender differences are due to the circulating levels of sex hormones present, effects of gender unrelated to levels of circulating sex steroids, or effects of prior sex-steroid exposure. Prior exposure to sex steroids is known to have organizational effects on the central neural system that influence the subsequent development of reproductive behavior (147), but its ventilatory consequences are unknown.

To explore the interaction between the effects of circulating hormones and those of gender, we studied intact versus castrate, male and female awake cats (200). We reasoned that comparison on intact versus castrate animals would be informative about the effects of normal circulating levels of sex hormones on ventilation and ventilatory responsiveness. The comparison of castrate males versus castrate females would provide information about the effects of gender. The intact females had a lower end-tidal P_{CO_2} than the awake, intact males, indicating an increased alveolar ventilation per unit CO_2 production, but castration did not change end-tidal P_{CO_2} in either sex (200). Comparison of the HVR values revealed that intact females had higher HVRs than intact males. HVR values were also higher in intact animals of both sexes compared with their neutered counterparts and higher in neutered female than in neutered male cats. These data suggested that normal circulating levels of sex hormones acted to raise HVR in both genders. Further, they implicated effects of gender unrelated to circulating sex hormones for raising HVR in intact females compared with intact males. However, since all the animals were castrate as adults, we were not able to separate effects of gender from those of prior hormonal exposure. Comparison of animals who had been castrate at birth with those who were castrate at adulthood would be useful for dissociating the effects of gender from those of prior hormonal exposure.

B. Gender Comparisons at Different Ages

Another approach toward exploring the interactions of gender and sex steroids is to consider ventilatory differences between males and females at different ages.

Developmental aspects of ventilatory control systems are further described in Chapter 16. Ventilatory control in newborns is distinctive in several respects. Newborns spend much of the time in REM sleep, which, unlike in adults, is marked by an increased respiratory center output (201) and unaltered peripheral and central chemoreceptor responsiveness (202). Newborns have a distinctive ventilatory response to hypoxia characterized by a transient hyperventilation followed by a progressive fall in ventilation (203–205). Ventilatory response to CO_2 increases with postnatal age (206,207).

Little is known about gender differences in maturational changes in ventilation and ventilatory control. In association with the menopause, ventilation falls and end-tidal or arterial P_{CO_2} rises toward but generally not to values observed in similarly aged men (208). With advancing age, changes occur in lung and chest wall mechanics, muscle mass, and strength that lead to a decline in maximal flow rate, vital capacity, and arterial O_2 saturation (209–212). A reduction in ventilatory as well as occlusion pressure response to hypercapnia and preservation of hypoxic ventilatory responsiveness have generally been observed in most, but not all, studies (213–218). The increment in tidal volume in response to hypercapnia appears reduced and inspiratory time prolonged in older subjects (218). Such a pattern may correspond to the normal response to a mechanically impeded respiratory pump. The effects of aging on ventilatory responses to chemical stimuli may be due to one or more of several factors: decreased peripheral and/or central chemoreceptor sensitivity to chemical stimuli, altered central nervous system processing of chemoreceptor input, decreased neural output to respiratory muscles, or changes in the mechanical properties of the respiratory system (209–211).

The rate of decline in pulmonary function with advancing age is greater in men than women (219). Compensation for increased mechanical loads is not complete, perhaps owing to a failure to detect small changes in respiratory resistance in older subjects. Compensation seems somewhat better preserved in women (220).

Sleep-disordered breathing increases with advancing age, especially among men (2,221–223). The types of sleep apnea do not differ in men and women, but men experience longer periods of maximum desaturation than women (222). Although sleep-disordered breathing can be predictive of increased mortality when especially severe, it does not seem to impair daytime functioning at sea level (224,225).

V. Summary and Future Research Directions

A. Summary

The importance of hormonal influences on ventilation and ventilatory control has been reviewed in relation to gender differences in the occurrence of respiratory disturbances during sleep, syndromes of altitude illness, and maintenance of maternal and fetal well-being during pregnancy and gestation.

Women appear to be protected against syndromes of sleep-disordered breathing through a combination of factors, including greater reliance on nasal breathing, decreased pharyngeal resistance, preservation of genioglossal EMG activity after alcohol ingestion, and maintenance of ventilatory chemosensitivity during sleep. Direct effects of female as well as male hormones and interactions with other factors affecting breathing disorders such as obesity are likely to be involved.

Female protection from HAPE, subacute infantile mountain sickness, and chronic mountain sickness may stem from gender differences in the pulmonary vascular response to hypoxia, alveolar ventilation, resistance to hypoxic ventilatory depression, and, possibly, erythropoietic sensitivity.

The influence of female hormones on raising ventilation during pregnancy has long been recognized. At high altitude, the level of maternal arterial oxygenation correlated positively with the birth weight of the offspring and negatively with maternal blood pressure. Thus, under circumstances of reduced maternal O_2 availability or fetal O_2 supply, the maternal hyperventilatory response to pregnancy appears to be important for preservation of maternal and fetal well-being.

Progesterone and estrogen exert ventilatory effects during the menstrual cycle and pregnancy phases of the female life cycle. In addition, increased progesterone levels appear to interact synergistically with metabolic rate to raise chemosensory response to hypoxia. Central (hypothalamic) actions of progesterone raise ventilation acutely via progesterone and estrogen receptor-dependent mechanisms. Chronic ventilatory stimulation by progestin is also likely to be progesterone and estrogen receptor-mediated; chronic progestin raises the carotid sinus neural response to hypoxia, and chronic estrogen treatment increases central neural translation of the carotid sinus signal into ventilation. However, the relative contribution of central and peripheral sites to the increase in resting ventilation with chronic elevations in progesterone and estrogen levels remains unclear. Progesterone has been of therapeutic benefit for raising ventilation under some clinical conditions. The therapeutic benefit of combined progestin and estrogen has not been evaluated.

Testosterone raises ventilation and ventilatory sensitivity to hypoxia when metabolic rate is elevated. The ventilatory consequences of variation in testosterone levels during the male life cycle have not been evaluated. Nor is it known whether the ventilatory effects of testosterone are receptor-dependent.

Gender differences in ventilation across the life cycle could be due to alterations in levels of circulating hormones, effects of gender independent of circulating hormones, or effects of prior sex steroid exposure. Only limited information is available to assess the relative contributions of these various factors.

B. Future Research Directions

In recent years, a beginning has been made for the linkage of knowledge concerning current concepts of steroid action based on their effects in reproductive tissues with information pertaining to the ventilatory effects of steroid hormones. Steroid receptors have been found in neurological tissues, but little is known concerning the specific cellular mechanisms whereby they affect ventilation and ventilatory response. Further research is required to determine whether steroid hormones act directly or indirectly on target genes and the specific genes involved. In addition, the possibility that the ventilatory effects are not receptor-mediated or not mediated through classic, intranuclear receptors requires investigation. Finally, whether the same mechanisms of action are operative at central and carotid body sites needs to be examined.

Studies designed to answer such questions will help to bridge the current gap between genetic, molecular, and physiological approaches to the understanding of hormonal actions. The benefits for such a line of investigation include the practical value of having improved therapeutic techniques available for the diagnosis and treatment of hypoventilation disorders. Scientific value will accrue from expanding our understanding of ventilatory control on a molecular level and from enabling an integration of molecular-based with physiological and evolutionary perspectives.

References

1. Dempsey JA, Olson EB Jr, Skatrud JB. Hormones and neurochemicals in the regulation of breathing. In: Fishman AP, Cherniack NS, eds. Handbook of Physiology. The Respiratory System. Control of Breathing. Section 3, vol II, part 1. Bethesda, MD: American Physiological Society, 1986:181–221.
2. Block AJ, Boysen PG, Wynne JW, Hunt LA. Sleep apnea, hypopnea and oxygen desaturation in normal subjects. A strong male predominance. N Engl J Med 1979; 300:513–517.
3. Block AJ, Wynne JW, Boysen PG. Sleep-disordered breathing and nocturnal oxygen desaturation in postmenopausal women. Am J Med 1980; 69:75–79.
4. Guilleminault C, van den Hoed J, Mitler MM. Clinical overview of the sleep apnea syndrome. In: Guilleminault C, Dement WC, eds. Sleep Apnea Syndrome. New York: Alan R Liss, 1978:1–12.
5. Guilleminault C, Quera-Salva MA, Partinen M, Jamieson A. Women and the obstructive sleep apnea syndrome. Chest 1988; 93:104–109.
6. Catterall JR, Calverley PM, Shapiro CM, Flenley DC, Douglas NJ. Breathing and oxygenation during sleep are similar in normal men and normal women. Am Rev Respir Dis 1985; 132:86–88.
7. Schneider BK, Pickett CK, Zwillich CW, et al. Influence of testosterone on breathing during sleep. J Appl Physiol 1986; 61:618–623.
8. Wynne JW. Obstruction of the nose and breathing during sleep (editorial). Chest 1982; 82:657–658.
9. Zwillich CW, Pickett C, Hanson FN, Weil JV. Disturbed sleep and prolonged apnea during nasal obstruction in normal men. Am Rev Respir Dis 1981; 124:158–160.
10. Gleeson K, Zwillich CW, Braier K, White DP. Breathing route during sleep. Am Rev Respir Dis 1986; 134:115–120.

11. White DP, Lombard RM, Cadieux RJ, Zwillich CW. Pharyngeal resistance in normal humans: influence of gender, age, and obesity. J Appl Physiol 1985; 58:365–371.

12. Kunitomo F, Kimura H, Tatsumi K, Kuriyama T, Watanabe S, Honda Y. Sex differences in awake ventilatory drive and abnormal breathing during sleep in eucapnic obesity. Chest 1988; 93:968–976.

13. Issa FG, Sullivan CE. Alcohol, snoring and sleep apnea. J Neurol Neurosurg Psychiatry 1982; 45:353–359.

14. Taasan VC, Block AJ, Boysen PG, Wynne JW. Alcohol increases sleep apnea and oxygen desaturation in asymptomatic men. Am J Med 1981; 71:240–245.

15. Bonora M, Shields GI, Knuth SL, Bartlett D Jr, St.John WM. Selective depression by ethanol of upper airway respiratory motor activity in cats. Am Rev Respir Dis 1984; 130:156–161.

16. Krol RC, Knuth SL, Bartlett D Jr. Selective reduction of genioglossal muscle activity by alcohol in normal human subjects. Am Rev Respir Dis 1984; 129: 247–250.

17. Leiter JC, Doble EA, Knuth SL, Bartlett D Jr. Respiratory activity of genioglossus. Interaction between alcohol and the menstrual cycle. Am Rev Respir Dis 1987; 135: 383–386.

18. St.John WM, Bartlett D Jr, Knuth KV, Knuth SL, Daubenspeck JA. Differential depression of hypoglossal nerve activity by alcohol. Protection by pretreatment with medroxyprogesterone acetate. Am Rev Respir Dis 1986; 133:46–48.

19. White DP, Douglas NJ, Pickett CK, Weil JV, Zwillich CW. Hypoxic ventilatory response during sleep in normal premenopausal women. Am Rev Respir Dis 1982; 126:530–533.

20. Sutton FD Jr, Zwillich CW, Creagh CE, Pierson DJ, Weil JV. Progesterone for outpatient treatment of Pickwickian syndrome. Ann Intern Med 1975; 83:476–479.

21. Lombard RM, Zwillich CW. Medical therapy of obstructive sleep apnea. Med Clin North Am 1985; 69:1317–1335.

22. Pickett CK, Regensteiner JG, Woodard WD, Hagerman DD, Weil JV, Moore LG. Progestin and estrogen reduce sleep-disordered breathing in postmenopausal women. J Appl Physiol 1989; 66:1656–1661.

23. Schneider G, Kirschner MA, Berkowitz R, Ertel N. Increased estrogen production in obese men. J Clin Endocrinol Metab 1979; 48:633–638.

24. Rao BR, Wiest WG, Allen WM. Progesterone "receptor" in rabbit uterus. I. Characterization and estradiol-17beta augmentation. Endocrinology 1973; 92:1229–1240.

25. Matsumoto AM, Sandblom RE, Schoene RB, et al. Testosterone replacement in hypogonadal men: effects on obstructive sleep apnoea, respiratory drives, and sleep. Clin Endocrinol (Oxf) 1985; 22:713–721.

26. Johnson MW, Anch AM, Remmers JE. Induction of the obstructive sleep apnea syndrome in a woman by exogenous androgen administration. Am Rev Respir Dis 1984; 129:1023–1025.

27. Sandblom RE, Matsumoto AM, Schoene RB, et al. Obstructive sleep apnea syndrome induced by testosterone administration. N Engl J Med 1983; 308: 508–510.

28. Ravenhill TH. Some experiences of mountain sickness in the Andes. J Trop Med Hyg 1913; 16:313–320.

29. Fitzmaurice FE. Mountain sickness in the Andies. Roy Naval Med Serv 1920; 6: 403–407.

30. Hackett PH, Rennie D. The incidence, importance, and prophylaxis of acute mountain sickness. Lancet 1976; 2:1149–1155.

31. Harris CW, Shields JL, Hannon JP. Acute altitude sickness in females. Aerosp Med 1966; 37:1163–1167.

32. Hackett PH, Rennie D. Rales, peripheral edema, retinal hemorrhage and acute mountain sickness. Am J Med 1979; 67:214–218.

33. Johnson TS, Rock PB. Acute mountain sickness. N Engl J Med 1988; 319:841–845.

34. Hultgren HN. High altitude medical problems. West J Med 1979; 131:8–23.

35. Ergueta J, Spielvogel H, Cudkowicz L. Cardio-respiratory studies in chronic mountain sickness (Monge's syndrome). Respiration 1971; 28:485–517.

36. Hultgren HN, Lopez C, Lundberge E, Miller H. Physiologic studies of pulmonary edema at high altitude. Circulation 1964; 29:393–408.

37. Hultgren HN, Spickard WB, Hellriegel K, Houston CS. High altitude pulmonary edema. Medicine (Baltimore) 1961; 40:289–313.

38. Hultgren HN. High altitude pulmonary edema. Adv Cardiol 1970; 5:24–31.

39. Sophocles AM Jr, Bachman J. High-altitude pulmonary edema among visitors to Summit County, Colorado. J Fam Pract 1983; 17:1015–1017.

40. Scoggin CH, Hyers TM, Reeves JT, Grover RF. High-altitude pulmonary edema in the children and young adults of Leadville, Colorado. N Engl J Med 1977; 297: 1269–1272.

41. Hultgren HN, Grover RF, Hartley LH. Abnormal circulatory responses to high altitude in subjects with a previous history of high-altitude pulmonary edema. Circulation 1971; 44:759–770.

42. Penaloza D, Sime F. Circulatory dynamics during high altitude pulmonary edema. Am J Cardiol 1969; 23:369–378.

43. Kleiner JP, Nelson WP. High altitude pulmonary edema. A rare disease? JAMA 1975; 234:491–495.

44. Houston CS, Dickinson J. Cerebral form of high-altitude illness. Lancet 1975; 2: 758–761.

45. Smith P, Moosavi H, Winson M, Heath D. The influence of age and sex on the response of the right ventricle, pulmonary vasculature and carotid bodies to hypoxia in rats. J Pathol 1974; 112:11–18.

46. Burton RR, Besch EL, Smith AH. Effect of chronic hypoxia on the pulmonary arterial blood pressure of the chicken. Am J Physiol 1968; 214:1438–1442.

47. Rabinovitch M, Gamble WJ, Miettinen OS, Reid L. Age and sex influence on pulmonary hypertension of chronic hypoxia. Am J Physiol 1981; 240:H62–H72.

48. McMurtry IF, Frith CH, Will DH. Cardiopulmonary responses of male and female swine to simulated high altitude. J Appl Physiol 1973; 35:459–462.

49. Fitzgerald MP, Haldane JS. The normal alveolar carbonic acid pressure in man. J Physiol (Lond) 1905; 32:486–494.

50. Fitzgerald MP. The changes in breathing and the blood at various high altitudes. Phil Trans R Soc Ser B 1913; 203:351–371.

51. Shock NW, Soley MH. Average values for basal respiratory functions in adolescents and adults. J Nutr 1939; 18:143–153.

52. Hackett PH, Rennie D, Hofmeister SE, Grover RF, Grover EB, Reeves JT. Fluid retention and relative hypoventilation in acute mountain sickness. Respiration 1982; 43:321–329.

53. Hackett PH, Roach RC, Schoene RB, Harrison GL, Mills WJ Jr. Abnormal control of ventilation in high-altitude pulmonary edema. J Appl Physiol 1988; 64:1268–1272.

54. Sutton JR, Bryan AC, Gray GW, et al. Pulmonary gas exchange in acute mountain sickness. Aviat Space Environ Med 1976; 47:1032–1037.

55. Moore LG, Harrison GL, McCullough RE, et al. Low acute hypoxic ventilatory response and hypoxic depression in acute altitude sickness. J Appl Physiol 1986; 60:1407–1412.

56. Lakshminarayan S, Pierson DJ. Recurrent high altitude pulmonary edema with blunted chemosensitivity. Am Rev Respir Dis 1975; 111:869–872.

57. White DP, Douglas NJ, Pickett CK, Weil JV, Zwillich CW. Sexual influence on the control of breathing. J Appl Physiol 1983; 54:874–879.

58. Hirshman CA, McCullough RE, Weil JV. Normal values for hypoxic and hypercapnic ventilatory drives in man. J Appl Physiol 1975; 38:1095–1098.

59. Aitken ML, Franklin JL, Pierson DJ, Schoene RB. Influence of body size and gender on control of ventilation. J Appl Physiol 1986; 60:1894–1899.

60. Rebuck AS, Kangalee M, Pengelly LD, Campbell EJM. Correlation of ventilatory responses to hypoxia and hypercapnia. J Appl Physiol 1973; 35:173–177.

61. Briton SW, Kline RF. Age, sex, carbohydrate, adrenal cortex, and other factors in anoxia. Am J Physiol 1945; 145:190–202.

62. Stupfel M, Demaria Pesce VH, Gourlet V, Bouley G, Elabed A, Lemercerre C. Sex-related factors in acute hypoxia survival in one strain of mice. Aviat Space Environ Med 1984; 55:136–140.

63. Kimura H, Mikami M, Kuriyama T, Fukuda Y. Effect of a synthetic progestin on ventilatory response to hypoxia in anesthetized rats. J Appl Physiol 1989; 67:1754–1758.

64. Cherniack NS, Edelman NJ, Lahiri S. Hypoxia and hypercapnia as respiratory stimulants and depressants. Respir Physiol 1970; 11:113–126.

65. Morrill CG, Meyer JR, Weil JV. Hypoxic ventilatory depression in dogs. J Appl Physiol 1975; 38:143–146.

66. Sui GJ, Liu YH, Cheng XS, Anand IS, Harris P, Heath D. Subacute infantile mountain sickness. J Pathol 1988; 155:161–170.

67. Kraus JF, Borhani NO. Post-neonatal sudden unexplained death in California: a cohort study. Am J Epidemiol 1972; 95:497–510.

68. Pei SX, Chen XJ, Si Ren BZ, et al. Chronic mountain sickness in Tibet. Q J Med 1989; 71:555–574.

69. Monge C. La enfermedad de los Andes (Sindromes eritremicos). An Fac Med Lima 1928; 11:314–318.

70. Hecht HH, McClement JH. A case of "chronic mountain sickness" in the United States. Am J Med 1958; 25:470–477.

71. Grover RF, Kryger MH. Polycythemia of chronic mountain sickness. In: Chamber-

layne EC, Condliffe PG, eds. Adjustment to High Altitude. Bethesda, MD: U.S. Department of Health and Human Services, 1983:37–41.

72. Cruz JC, Diaz C, Marticorena E, Hilario V. Phlebotomy improves pulmonary gas exchange in chronic mountain polycythemia. Respiration 1979; 38:305–313.

73. Winslow RM, Monge C, Brown EG, et al. Effects of hemodilution on O_2 transport in high-altitude polycythemia. J Appl Physiol 1985; 59:1495–1502.

74. Penaloza D, Sime F. Chronic cor pulmonale due to loss of altitude acclimatization (chronic mountain sickness). Am J Med 1971; 50:728–743.

75. Kryger MH, McCullough RG, Doekel RD, Collins D, Weil JV, Grover RF. Excessive polycythemia of high altitude: role of ventilatory drive and lung disease. Am Rev Respir Dis 1978; 118:373–390.

76. Kryger MH, Glas R, Jackson D, et al. Impaired oxygenation during sleep in excessive polycythemia of high altitude: improvement with respiratory stimulation. Sleep 1978; 1:3–17.

77. Blackmore PF, Neulen J, Lattanzio F, Beebe SJ. Cell surface-binding sites for progesterone mediate calcium uptake in human sperm. J Biol Chem 1991; 266: 18655–18659.

78. Severinghaus JW, Bainton CR, Carcelen A. Respiratory insensitivity to hypoxia in chronically hypoxic man. Respir Physiol 1966; 1:308–334.

79. Sun SF, Huang SY, Zhuang JG, et al. Decreased ventilation and hypoxic ventilatory responsiveness are not reversed by naloxone in Lhasa residents with chronic mountain sickness. Am Rev Respir Dis 1990; 142:1294–1300.

80. Monge C, Leon-Velarde F, Arregui A. Increasing prevalence of excessive erythrocytosis with age among healthy high-altitude miners (letter). N Engl J Med 1989; 321:1271.

81. Monge C, Leon-Velarde F. Physiological adaptation to high altitude: oxygen transport in mammals and birds. Physiol Rev 1991; 71:1135–1172.

82. Kryger MH, Glas R, Jackson D, et al. Impaired oxygenation during sleep in excessive polycythemia of high altitude: improvement with respiratory stimulation. Sleep 1978; 1:3–17.

83. Kryger MH, McCullough RE, Collins D, Scoggin CH, Weil JV, Grover RF. Treatment of excessive polycythemia of high altitude with respiratory stimulant drugs. Am Rev Respir Dis 1978; 117:455–464.

84. Zhuang JG, Zamudio S, Droma TS, Cai XF, Moore LG. Gender comparison of hemoglobin levels in Tibet. Am J Phys Anthropol 1992; 12(Suppl):192 (abstract).

85. Moore LG, Jahnigen D, Rounds SS, Reeves JT, Grover RF. Maternal hyperventilation helps preserve arterial oxygenation during high altitude pregnancy. J Appl Physiol 1982; 52:690–694.

86. Moore LG, Brodeur P, Chumbe O, D'Brot J, Hofmeister S, Monge C. Maternal hypoxic ventilatory response, ventilation and infant birth weight at 4300 m. J Appl Physiol 1986; 60:1401–1406.

87. Unger D, Weiser JK, McCullough RE, Keefer S, Moore LG. Altitude, low birth weight and infant mortality in Colorado. JAMA 1988; 259:3427–3432.

88. Moore LG, Maternal O_2 transport and fetal growth in Colorado, Peru and Tibet high altitude residents. Am J Hum Biol 1990; 2:627–638.

89. Moore LG, Hershey DW, Jahnigen D, Bowes W. The incidence of pregnancy-induced hypertension is increased among Colorado residents of high altitude. Am J Obstet Gynecol 1982; 144:423–429.
90. Zamudio S, Palmer SK, Dahms TE, et al. Blood volume expansion and pregnancy outcome at high and low altitude. J Appl Physiol 1993 (submitted).
91. Hasselbach KA. Ein Beitrag zur Respirationsphysiologie der Gravidität. Skand Arch Physiol 1912; 27:1–12.
92. Brodeur P, Mockus M, McCullough RE, Moore LG. Progesterone receptors and ventilatory stimulation by progestin. J Appl Physiol 1986; 60:590–595.
93. Bayliss DA, Millhorn DE. Central neural mechanisms of progesterone action: application to the respiratory system. J Appl Physiol 1992; 73:393–404.
94. Prowse CM, Gaensler EA. Respiratory and acid-base changes during pregnancy. Anesthesiology 1965; 26:381–392.
95. Takano N, Sakai A, Iida Y. Analysis of alveolar P_{CO_2} control during the menstrual cycle Pflüger's Arch 1981; 390:56–62.
96. Döring GK, Loeschke HH, Ochwadt B. Uber die Blutgase in der Schwangerschaft unter besonderer Berücksichtigung der arteriellen Sauerstoffsättigung. Arch Gynäkol 1949; 176:746–758.
97. Goodland RL, Pommerenke WT. Cyclic fluctuation of the alveolar carbon dioxide tension during the normal menstrual cycle. Fertil Steril 1952; 3:394–398.
98. Lyons HA. Respiratory effects of gonadal hormones. In: Salhanick HA, Kipnis DM, Van de Wiele RL, eds. Metabolic Effects of Gonadal Hormones and Contraceptive Steroids. New York: Plenum Press, 1969:394–402.
99. England SJ, Farhi LE. Fluctuations in alveolar CO_2 and in base excess during the menstrual cycle. Respir Physiol 1976; 26:157–161.
100. Machida H. Influence of progesterone on arterial blood and CSF acid-base balance in women. J Appl Physiol 1981; 51:1433–1436.
101. Takano N. Changes of ventilation and ventilatory response to hypoxia during the menstrual cycle. Pflüger's Arch 1984; 402:312–316.
102. Pernoll LM, Meltcalfe J, Kovach PA, Wachtel R, Dunham MJ. Ventilation during rest and exercise in pregnancy and postpartum. Respir Physiol 1975; 25:295–310.
103. Lotgering FK, Vandoorn MB, Struijk PC, Pool J, Wallenburg HC. Maximal aerobic exercise in pregnant women—heart rate, O_2 consumption, CO_2 production, and ventilation. J Appl Physiol 1991; 70:1016–1023.
104. Contreras G, Gutierrez M, Beroiza T, et al. Ventilatory drive and respiratory muscle function in pregnancy. Am Rev Respir Dis 1991; 144:837–841.
105. Schoene RB, Robertson HT, Pierson DJ, Peterson AP. Respiratory drives and exercise in menstrual cycles of athletic and nonathletic women. J Appl Physiol 1981; 50:1300–1305.
106. Moore LG, McCullough RE, Weil JV. Increased HVR in pregnancy: relationship to hormonal and metabolic changes. J Appl Physiol 1987; 62:158–163.
107. Milne JA, Pack AI, Coutts JR. Gas exchange and acid-base status during the normal human menstrual cycle and in subjects taking oral contraceptives. J Endocrinol 1977; 75:17P–18P.
108. Regensteiner JG, McCullough RG, McCullough RE, Pickett CK, Moore LG.

Combined effects of female hormones and exercise on hypoxic ventilatory response. Respir Physiol 1990; 82:107–114.

109. Eston RG. The regular menstrual cycle and athletic performance. Sports Med 1984; 1:431–445.

110. Dombovy ML, Bonekat HW, Williams TJ, Staats BA. Exercise performance and ventilatory response in the menstrual cycle. Med Sci Sports Exerc 1987; 19: 111–117.

111. Bokelmann O, Rother J. Zum Problem der extragenitalen Wellenbewegung im Leben des Weibes. Z Geburtschilfe Gynaekol 1924; 87:584–606.

112. Griffith FR Jr, Pucker GW, Brownell KA, Klein JD, Carmer ME. Studies in human physiology, alveolar air and blood gas capacity. Am J Physiol 1929; 89:449–470.

113. Regensteiner JG, McCullough RG, McCullough RE, Pickett CK, Moore LG. Combined effects of female hormones and exercise on hypoxic ventilatory response. Respir Physiol 1990; 82:107–114.

114. Skatrud JB, Dempsey JA, Kaiser DG. Ventilatory response to medroxyprogesterone acetate in normal subjects: time course and mechanism. J Appl Physiol 1978; 44: 939–944.

115. Keith IM, Bisgard GE, Manohar M, Klein J, Bullard VA. Respiratory effects of pregnancy and progesterone in Jersey cows. Respir Physiol 1982; 50:351–358.

116. Smith CA, Kellogg RH. Ventilatory response of rabbits and goats to chronic progesterone administration. Respir Physiol 1980; 39:383–391.

117. Hannhart B, Pickett CK, Weil JV, Moore LG. Influence of pregnancy on ventilatory and carotid body neural output responsiveness to hypoxia in cats. J Appl Physiol 1989; 67:797–803.

118. Gahlenbeck H, Frecking H, Rathschlag-Schaeffer AM, Bartels H. Oxygen and carbon dioxide exchange across the cow placenta during the second part of pregnancy. Respir Physiol 1968; 4:119–131.

119. Hoversland AS, Metcalfe J, Parer JT. Adjustments in maternal blood gases, acid-base balance, and oxygen consumption in the pregnant pygmy goat. Biol Reprod 1974; 10:589–595.

120. Bonekat HW, Dombovy ML, Staats BA. Progesterone-induced changes in exercise performance and ventilatory response. Med Sci Sports Exerc 1987; 19:118–123.

121. Damas-Mora J, Davies L, Taylor W, Jenner FA. Menstrual respiratory changes and symptoms. Br J Psychiatry 1980; 136:492–497.

122. Dutton K, Blanksby BA, Morton AR. CO_2 sensitivity changes during the menstrual cycle. J Appl Physiol 1989; 67:517–522.

123. Lyons HA, Antonio R. The sensitivity of the respiratory center in pregnancy and after the administration of progesterone. Trans Assoc Am Physicians 1959; 72: 173–181.

124. Schoene RB, Pierson DJ, Lakshaminarayan S, Shrader DL, Butler J. Effect of medroxyprogesterone acetate on respiratory drives and occlusion pressure. Bull Eur Physiopathol Respir 1980; 16:645–653.

125. Okita S, Kimura H, Kunitomo F, et al. Effect of chlormadinone acetate, a synthetic progesterone, on hypoxic ventilatory response in men. Jpn J Physiol 1987; 37: 137–147.

126. Kimura H, Hayashi F, Yoshida A, Watanabe S, Hashizume I, Honda Y. Augmentation of CO_2 drives by chlormadinone acetate, a synthetic progesterone. J Appl Physiol 1984; 56:1627–1632.

127. Skatrud JB, Dempsey JA, Iber C, Berssenbrugge AD. Correction of CO_2 retention during sleep in patients with chronic obstructive pulmonary disease. Am Rev Respir Dis 1981; 124:260–268.

128. Goodland RL, Reynolds JG, McCoord AB, Pommerenke WT. Respiratory and electrolyte effects induced by estrogen and progesterone. Fertil Steril 1953; 4:300–316.

129. Little BC, Matta RJ, Zahn TP. Physiological and psychological effects of progesterone in man. J Nerv Ment Dis 1974; 159:256–262.

130. Zwillich CW, Natalino MR, Sutton FD, Weil JV. Effects of progesterone on chemosensitivity in normal men. J Lab Clin Med 1978; 92:262–269.

131. Robertson HT, Schoene RB, Pierson DJ. Augmentation of exercise ventilation by medroxyprogesterone acetate. Clin Physiol 1982; 2:269–276.

132. Chiodi H. Aging and high-altitude polycythemia. J Appl Physiol 1978; 45:1019–1020.

133. Regensteiner JG, Woodard WD, Hagerman DD, et al. Combined effects of female hormones and metabolic rate on ventilatory drives in women. J Appl Physiol 1989; 66:808–813.

134. Morikawa T, Tanaka Y, Maruyama R, Nishibayashi Y, Honda Y. Comparison of two synthetic progesterones on ventilation in normal males: CMA vs. MPA J Appl Physiol 1987; 63:1610–1615.

135. Kimura H, Tatsumi K, Kunitomo F, et al. Progesterone therapy for sleep apnea syndrome evaluated by occlusion pressure responses to exogenous loading. Am Rev Respir Dis 1989; 139:1198–1206.

136. Lyons HA, Huang CT. Therapeutic use of progesterone in alveolar hypoventilation associated with obesity. Am J Med 1968; 44:881–888.

137. Tatsumi K, Kimura H, Kunitomo F, et al. Effect of chlormadinone acetate on ventilatory control in patients with chronic obstructive pulmonary disease. Am Rev Respir Dis 1986; 133:552–557.

138. Javaheri S, Guerra LF. Effects of domperidone and medroxyprogesterone acetate on ventilation in man. Respir Physiol 1990; 81:359–370.

139. Tyler JM. The effect of progesterone on the respiration of patients with emphysema and hypercapnia. J Clin Invest 1960; 39:34–41.

140. Regensteiner JG, Pickett CK, McCullough RE, Weil JV, Moore LG. Possible gender differences in the effect of exercise on hypoxic ventilatory response. Respiration 1988; 53:158–165.

141. White DP, Schneider BK, Santen RJ, et al. Influence of testosterone on ventilation and chemosensitivity in male subjects. J Appl Physiol 1985; 59:1452–1457.

142. Döring GK, Loeschke HH, Ochwadt B. Weitere Untersuchungen über die Wirkung der Sexualhormone auf die Atmung. Pflügers Arch 1950; 252:216–230.

143. Hannhart B, Pickett CK, Moore LG. Effects of estrogen and progesterone on carotid body neural output responsiveness to hypoxia. J Appl Physiol 1990; 68:1909–1916.

144. Hohimer AR, Hart MV, Resko JA. The effect of castration and sex steroids on ventilatory control in male guinea pigs. Respir Physiol 1985; 61:383–390.

145. Hosenpud JD, Hart MV, Morton MJ, Hohimer AR, Resko JA. Progesterone-induced hyperventilation in the guinea pig. Respir Physiol 1983; 52:259–264.
146. Mohamed G, Lopata M, Kukicia J, Schraufnagel D. Androgen levels in women with sleep apnea syndrome. Am Rev Respir Dis 1983; 127:237 (abstract).
147. McEwen BS. Basic Neurochemistry. Boston: Little, Brown, 1981.
148. Winslow RM, Chapman KW, Gibson CC, et al. Different hematologic responses to hypoxia in Sherpas and Quechua Indians. J Appl Physiol 1989; 66:1561–1569.
149. Tesarik J, Mendoza C, Moos J, Fenichel P, Fehlmann M. Progesterone action through aggregation of a receptor on the sperm plasma membrane. FEBS Lett 1992; 308:116–120.
150. Bayliss DA, Millhorn DE, Gallman EA, Cidlowski JA. Progesterone stimulates respiration through a central nervous system steroid receptor-mediated mechanism in cat. Proc Natl Acad Sci USA 1987; 84:7788–7792.
151. Bayliss DA, Cidlowski JA, Millhorn DE. The stimulation of respiration by progesterone in ovariectomized cat is mediated by an estrogen-dependent hypothalamic mechanism requiring gene expression. Endocrinology 1990; 126:519–527.
152. Mei SS, Cort D, Kao F. The investigation of respiratory effects of progesterone in cross-circulated dogs. Fed Proc 1977; 36:489 (abstract).
153. Tok G, Loeschke HH. Untersuchung über die zentrale Wirkung von Progesterone auf die Atmung and Vasomotorik bei Katzen. Z Atemweg Lungenkrankheiten 1981; 7:148–153.
154. Fitzgerald R, Johnson JWC. Progesterone and the carotid body. Physiologist 1975; 18:214 (abstract).
155. Kato J, Onouchi T, Okinaga S. Hypothalamic and hypophysial progesterone receptors: estrogen-priming effect, differential localization, 5-dihydroprogesterone binding, and nuclear receptors. J Steroid Biochem 1978; 9:419–427.
156. McLusky NJ, McEwen BS. Oestrogen modulates progestin receptor concentrations in some rat brain regions but not in others. Nature (Lond) 1978; 274:276–278.
157. Evans RM. The steroid and thyroid hormone receptor superfamily. Science 1988; 240:889–895.
158. Horwitz KB, Alexander PS. In situ photolinked nuclear progesterone receptors of human breast cancer cells: subunit molecular weights after transformation and translocation. Endocrinology 1983; 113:2195–2201.
159. Krust A, Green S, Argos P, et al. The chicken oestrogen receptor sequence: homology with V-erbA and the human oestrogen and glucocorticoid receptors. EMBO J 1986; 5:891–897.
160. Kumar V, Green S, Stack G, Berry M, Jin JR, Chambon P. Functional domains of the human estrogen receptor. Cell 1987; 51:941–951.
161. Kumar V, Green S, Staub A, Chambon P. Localisation of the oestrogen-binding and putative DNA-binding domains of the human oestrogen receptor. EMBO J 1986; 5: 2231–2236.
162. Gronemeyer H. Transcription activation by estrogen and progesterone receptors. Annu Rev Genetics 1991; 25:89–123.
163. O'Malley BW, Means AR. Female steroid hormones and target cell nuclei. Science 1974; 184:610–620.

164. Harlan RE. Regulation of neuropeptide gene expression by steroid hormones. Mol Neurobiol 1989; 2:183–200.

165. Vegeto E, Cocciolo MG, Raspagliesi F, Piffanelli A, Fontanelli R, Maggi A. Regulation of progesterone receptor gene expression. Cancer Res 1990; 50:5291–5295.

166. Sheridan PJ, McGill HC Jr. The nuclear uptake and retention of a synthetic progestin in the cardiovascular system of the baboon. Endocrinology 1984; 114:2015–2019.

167. Perrot-Applanat M, Groyer-Picard MT, Garcia E, Lorenzo F, Milgrom E. Immunocytochemical demonstration of estrogen and progesterone receptors in muscle cells of uterine arteries in rabbits and humans. Endocrinology 1988; 123:1511–1519.

168. Brennan DM, Kray RJ. Chlormadinone acetate, a new highly active gestation-supporting agent. Acta Endocrinol 1963; 44:367–379.

169. Tausk M. Pharmacology of orally active progestational compounds: animal studies. In: Tausk M, ed. Pharmacology of the Endocrine System and Related Drugs. Sect. 48, vol 2. Oxford, UK: Pergamon Press, 1972:35–216.

170. Baulieu EE. The progesterone receptor. In: Benagiano G, et al, eds. Progestogens in Therapy. New York: Raven Press, 1983:27–38.

171. Bayliss DA, Millhorn DE. Chronic estrogen exposure maintains elevated levels of progesterone receptor mRNA in guinea pig hypothalamus. Mol Brain Res 1991; 10:167–172.

172. Guilleminault C, Simmons FB, Motta J, et al. Obstructive sleep apnea syndrome and tracheostomy. Long-term follow-up experience. Arch Intern Med 1981; 141:985–988.

173. Sullivan CE, Issa FG, Berthon-Jones M, Eves L. Reversal of obstructive sleep apnoea by continuous positive airway pressure applied through the nares. Lancet 1981; 1:862–865.

174. Ingbar DH, Gee JB. Pathophysiology and treatment of sleep apnea. Annu Rev Med 1985; 36:369–395.

175. Dolly FR, Block AJ. Medroxyprogesterone acetate and COPD. Effect on breathing and oxygenation in sleeping and awake patients. Chest 1983; 84:394–398.

176. Cook WR, Benich JJ, Wooten SA. Indices of severity of obstructive sleep apnea syndrome do not change during medroxyprogesterone acetate therapy. Chest 1989; 96:262–266.

177. Hensley MJ, Saunders NA, Strohl KP. Medroxyprogesterone treatment of obstructive sleep apnea. Sleep 1980; 3:441–446.

178. Tatsumi K, Kimura H, Kunitomo F, Kuriyama T, Watanabe S, Honda Y. Effect of chlormadinone acetate on sleep arterial oxygen desaturation in patients with chronic obstructive pulmonary disease. Chest 1987; 91:688–692.

179. Orr WC, Imes NK, Martin RJ. Progesterone therapy in obese patients with sleep apnea. Arch Intern Med 1979; 139:109–111.

180. Strohl KP, Hensley MJ, Saunders NA, Scharf SM, Brown R, Ingram RH Jr. Progesterone administration and progressive sleep apneas. JAMA 1981; 245:1230–1232.

181. Daskalopoulou E, Patakas D, Tsara V, Zoglopitis F, Maniki E. Comparison of almitrine bismesylate and medroxyprogesterone acetate on oxygenation during

wakefulness and sleep in patients with chronic obstructive lung disease. Thorax 1990; 45:666–669.

182. Kryger MH, Weil JV, Grover R. Chronic mountain polycythemia: a disorder of the regulation of breathing during sleep? Chest 1978; 73:303–304.

183. Skatrud JB, Dempsey JA, Bhansali P, Irvin C. Determinants of chronic carbon dioxide retention and its correction in humans. J Clin Invest 1980; 65:813–821.

184. Lyons HA, Centrally acting hormones and respiration. Pharmacol Ther B 1976; 2: 743–751.

185. Tatsumi K, Hannhart B, Pickett CK, Weil JV, Moore LG. Effects of testosterone on hypoxic ventilatory and carotid body neural responsiveness. Am Rev Respir Dis 1993 (in press).

186. Strumpf IJ, Reynolds SF, Vash P, Tashkin DP. A possible relationship between testosterone central control of ventilation and the Pickwickian syndrome. Am Rev Respir Dis 1978; 117:A183 (abstract).

187. Harman E, Wynne JW, Block AJ, Malloy-Fisher. Sleep disordered breathing and oxygen desaturation in obese patients. Chest 1981; 79:256–260.

188. Cherniack NS. Sleep apnea and its causes. J Clin Invest 1984; 73:1501–1506.

189. Onal E, Lopata M, O'Connor T. Pathogenesis of apneas in hypersomnia-sleep apnea syndrome. Am Rev Respir Dis 1982; 125:167–174.

190. Weil JV, Byrne-Quinn E, Sodal IE, Kline JS, McCullough RE, Filley GF. Augmentation of chemosensitivity during mild exercise in normal man. J Appl Physiol 1972; 33:813–819.

191. Aggarwal D, Milhorn HTJ, Lee LY. Role of the carotid chemoreceptors in the hyperpnea of exercise in the cat. Respir Physiol 1976; 26:147–155.

192. Davies RO, Lahiri S. Absence of carotid chemoreceptor response during hypoxic exercise in the cat. Respir Physiol 1973; 18:92–100.

193. Janne OA, Bardin CW. Androgen and antiandrogen receptor binding. Annu Rev Physiol 1984; 46:107–118.

194. Southern AL, Gordon GG, Vittel J, Altman K. Effect of progestagens on androgen metabolism. In: Martini L, Motta M, eds. Androgens and Antiandrogens. New York: Raven Press, 1977:263–279.

195. Tokarz RR, Harrison RW, Seaver SS. The mechanism of androgen and estrogen synergism in the chick oviduct. Estrogen-modulated changes in cytoplasmic androgen receptor concentrations. J Biol Chem 1979; 254:9178–9184.

196. Huggins C, Hodges CV. Studies on prostatic cancer. I. The effects of castration, of estrogen and of androgen injection on serum phosphatases in metastatic carcinoma of the prostate. Cancer Res 1941; 1:293–297.

197. Roy AK, Milin BS, McMinn DM. Androgen receptor in rat liver: hormonal and developmental regulation of the cytoplasmic receptor and its correlation with the androgen-dependent synthesis of alpha2u-globulin. Biochim Biophys Acta 1974; 354:213–232.

198. MacIndoe JH, Etre LA. An antiestrogenic action of androgens in human breast cancer cells. J Clin Endocrinol Metab 1981; 53:836–842.

199. Horwitz KB, Costlow ME, McGuire WL. MCF-7; a human breast cancer cell line with estrogen, androgen, progesterone, and glucocorticoid receptors. Steroids 1975; 26:785–795.

200. Tatsumi K, Hannhart B, Pickett CK, Weil JV, Moore LG. Influences of gender and sex hormones on hypoxic ventilatory response in cats. J Appl Physiol 1991; 71: 1746–1750.

201. Finer NN, Abroms IF, Taeusch HW Jr. Ventilation and sleep states in newborn infants. J Pediatr 1976; 89:100–108.

202. Fagenholz SA, O'Connell K, Shannon DC. Chemoreceptor function and sleep state in apnea. Pediatrics 1976; 58:31–36.

203. Brady JP, Ceruti E. Chemoreceptor reflexes in the new-born infant: effects of varying degrees of hypoxia on heart rate and ventilation in a warm environment. J Physiol (Lond) 1966; 184:631–645.

204. Rigatto H, Brady JP, de la Torre Verduzco R. Chemoreceptor reflexes in preterm infants. I. The effect of gestational and postnatal age on the ventilatory response to inhalation of 100% and 15% oxygen. Pediatrics 1975; 55:604–613.

205. Albersheim S, Boychuk R, Seshia MMK, Cates D, Rigatto H. Effects of CO_2 on immediate ventilatory response to O2 in preterms infants. J Appl Physiol 1976; 41: 609–611.

206. Rigatto H, Brady JP, de la Torre Verduzco R. Chemoreceptor reflexes in preterm infants: II. The effect of gestational and postnatal age on the ventilatory response to inhaled carbon dioxide. Pediatrics 1975; 55:614–620.

207. Frantz ID, Adler SM, Thach BT, Taeusch HW Jr. Maturational effects on respiratory responses to carbon dioxide in premature infants. J Appl Physiol 1976; 41:41–45.

208. McPherson K, Healy KJ, Flynn FV, Piper KA, Garcia-Webb P. The effect of age, sex and other factors on blood chemistry in health. Clin Chim Acta 1978; 84:373–397.

209. Bode FR, Dosman J, Martin RR, Ghezzo H, Macklem PT. Age and sex differences in lung elasticity, and in closing capacity in nonsmokers. J Appl Physiol 1976; 41:129–135.

210. Mittman C, Edelman NJ, Norris AH, Shock NW. Relationship between chest wall and pulmonary compliance and age. J Appl Physiol 1965; 20:1211–1216.

211. Gibson GJ, Pride NB, O'cain C, Quagliato R. Sex and age differences in pulmonary mechanics in normal nonsmoking subjects. J Appl Physiol 1976; 41:20–25.

212. Kanber GJ, King FW, Eshchar YR, Sharp JT. The alveolar-arterial oxygen gradient in young and elderly men during air and oxygen breathing. Am Rev Respir Dis 1968; 97:376–381.

213. Kronenberg RS, Drage CW. Attenuation of the ventilatory and heart rate responses to hypoxia and hypercapnia with aging in normal men. J Clin Invest 1973; 52:1812–1819.

214. Altose MD, McCauley WC, Kelsen SG, Cherniack NS. Effects of hypercapnia and inspiratory flow resistive loading on respiratory activity in chronic airways obstruction. J Clin Invest 1977; 59:500–507.

215. Peterson DD, Pack AI, Silage DA, Fishman AP. Effects of aging on ventilatory and occlusion pressure responses to hypoxia and hypercapnia. Am Rev Respir Dis 1981; 124:387–391.

216. Patrick JM, Howard A. The influence of age, sex, body size and lung size on the control and pattern of breathing during CO_2 inhalation in Caucasians. Respir Physiol 1972; 16:337–350.

217. Rubin S, Tack M, Cherniack NS. Effect of aging on respiratory responses to CO_2 and inspiratory resistive loads. J Gerontol 1982; 37:306–312.

218. Chapman KR, Cherniack NS. Aging effects on the interaction of hypercapnia and hypoxia as ventilatory stimuli. J Gerontol 1987; 42:202–209.

219. Britt EJ, Shelhamer J, Menkes H, Cohen B, Meyer M, Permutt S. Sex differences in the decline of pulmonary function with age. Chest 1981; 80:79–80.

220. Kunitomo F, Kimura H, Tatsumi K, Kuriyama T, Watanabe S, Honda Y. Sex differences in awake ventilatory drive and abnormal breathing during sleep in eucapnic obesity. Chest 1988; 93:968–976.

221. Ancoli-Israel S, Kripke DF, Klauber MR, Mason WJ, Fell R, Kaplan O. Sleep-disordered breathing in community-dwelling elderly. Sleep 1991; 14:486–495.

222. Hoch CC, Reynolds CF, Monk TH, et al. Comparison of sleep-disordered breathing among healthy elderly in the seventh, eighth, and ninth decades of life. Sleep 1990; 13:502–511.

223. Bixler EO, Kales A, Cadieux RJ, Vela-Bueno A, Jacoby JA, Soldatos CR. Sleep apneic activity in older healthy subjects. J Appl Physiol 1985; 58:1597–1601.

224. Ancoli-Israel S, Klauber MR, Kripke DF, Parker L, Cobarrubias M. Sleep apnea in female patients in a nursing home. Increased risk of mortality. Chest 1989; 96:1054–1058.

225. Phillips BA, Berry DT, Schmitt FA, Magan LK, Gerhardstein DC, Cook YR. Sleep-disordered breathing in the healthy elderly. Clinically significant? Chest 1992; 101:345–349.

226. Harrison RW, Lippman SS. How steroid hormones work. Hosp Pract 1989; 24:63–76.

Part Five

LOADS, SENSATIONS, AND FAILURE

19

Mechanisms of Respiratory Load Compensation

MAGDY YOUNES

University of Manitoba
Winnipeg, Manitoba, Canada

I. Introduction

An added mechanical load may be defined as any mechanical change that makes it harder for the respiratory muscles to ventilate the lungs. Many respiratory disorders, particularly those in which ventilatory failure is a frequent outcome, are associated with an increase in the mechanical load. Thus, the system may be stiff (restrictive disorders), the airways may be narrowed (obstructive disorders), or the respiratory muscles may be placed at a mechanical disadvantage such as with hyperinflation and thoracic deformity

In disorders associated with increased mechanical load, arterial P_{CO_2} is usually normal until the very advanced stages of the disease. If ventilation is preserved despite a higher load, the muscles must be working harder. In other words, load compensation must have taken place. An important, and puzzling, aspect of these disorders is that the level of severity (i.e., mechanical disturbance) at which ventilatory failure ultimately develops varies greatly from one individual to another (1). Clinicians and investigators have been fascinated by this for decades. Although there are many possible explanations for this wide variability (2), the most plausible was felt to be that load compensation was more vigorous in some than in others. This accounts for the considerable interest in studying mechanisms of load compensation over the past several decades.

II. Methods of Study

Load compensation is usually studied through the use of external mechanical loads. The load is applied and the response is evaluated by measuring the changes in respiratory output. The responsible mechanisms are then dissected out by observing the time course of the response (e.g., immediate responses are likely mechanical or neural whereas delayed responses are likely nonneural) and by comparing the responses under various experimental conditions, which differ from one another in the potency of one or more of the putative mechanisms (e.g., selective deafferentation, application of loads to different anatomical regions, comparison of sleep vs. wakeful responses, etc.).

A. Types of External Loads

External loads may be resistive, elastic, pressure biasing, or threshold (3).

Resistive Loads

This is exemplified by breathing through narrow tubes or perforated discs. Here, the load is a function of flow. Extra pressure is required of the respiratory muscles only in the presence of flow. Thus, the load at the beginning and end of inspiration or expiration (zero flow) is not altered.

Elastic Loads

This is exemplified by breathing from rigid containers. Here, the opposing pressure (extra load) is a function of volume removed from, or added to, the container. Thus, with an inspiratory elastic load the pressure opposing the inspiratory muscles is greatest at end-inspiration, and so on. The severity of the load is determined by the volume of the rigid container, according to Boyle's law.

Pressure-Biasing Loads

Here, a constant pressure is applied to the respiratory system throughout inspiration and expiration. Examples include the use of continuous positive airway pressure (CPAP) and continuous negative airway pressure. The primary intent of these manipulations, as investigative tools, is to change the operating length of the respiratory muscles (and hence their mechanical advantage) by changing end-expiratory volume (however, see below).

Threshold Loads

Here, a valve is incorporated in the breathing circuit. The valve requires a certain pressure to remain open. Once open, it offers no resistive or elastic opposition to air movement. Once pressure decreases below the threshold level, the valve closes. These devices are intended to provide a constant load to either the inspiratory or expiratory muscles (depending on the phase in which they are applied).

B. Types of Load Application

With the exception of pressure biasing, which is always applied throughout the respiratory cycle, external loads can be applied during inspiration alone, expiration alone, or throughout. Application throughout the cycle approximates the disease state more closely; with few exceptions, the mechanical abnormality of disease exists during both phases (e.g., high resistance and greater stiffness in obstructive and restrictive diseases, respectively). Selective application to one or other phase is more useful in mechanistic studies, however. For example, one may be able to address the issue of whether the tachypnea occurring with elastic loading is related to the increasing load during inspiration or to the faster emptying during expiration. Likewise, continuous resistive load, while closer to the natural disease state, is more likely to result in dynamic hyperinflation, thereby confounding interpretation; the load on inspiratory muscles is no longer a simple resistive load but a combination of added resistance and a threshold load, and the muscles may function at a different operating length.

With the exception of threshold loads, external loads can be applied at the airway or to the body surface. The mechanical consequences of a given pressure are opposite at the two sites. Thus, continuous negative pressure to body surface is mechanically analogous to CPAP, and an elastic load applied to body surface should cause body surface pressure to increase in proportion to inspired volume.

Although the chest wall (including muscles) is affected similarly whether the load is applied to airway or body surface, other structures are not. This can be used to advantage to investigate site of afferent information producing a given loading response. Thus, with body surface loading, upper airway and intrathoracic pressures are not directly affected by the load and only the chest wall is loaded. Responses observed with this application can be attributed to chest wall mechanisms. An important advantage of this is the fact that the upper airway is not subjected to the abnormal pressure. Since the upper airway contains mechanoreceptors that can influence breathing (4), inclusion of the upper airway in the load (which does not happen naturally in diseases of the lung) compounds interpretation. On the other hand, body surface loading does not permit other mechanical consequences of natural loading, for example reduction in intrathoracic pressure, to take place. These changes may contribute to load responses through other mechanisms (5). When the load is applied simultaneously to airway and body surface (head out), the changes in airway and intrathoracic pressures are reproduced but the chest wall is not loaded (pressure is changed equally on both sides of the chest). When all three methods of application are compared (airway, body surface, and both together) insights can be obtained regarding site of origin of relevant afferent information (e.g., 5–7).

C. Appropriateness of External Loads as Disease Models

External loads are not analogous to natural disease for several reasons:

1.   Disease only rarely represents a simple change in mechanical load. There are virtually always compounding variables such as muscle weakness, pulmonary vascular disease, airway inflammation, parenchymal inflammation, obesity, hormonal and electrolyte disturbances, high ventilatory requirements (e.g., due to high dead space or metabolic rate), and so on (for review see Ref. 2). These are all variables that can affect the control of breathing. The breathing pattern observed in a given patient is the net result of load responses and the sum of effects of all these confounding variables.

2.   The naturally occurring mechanical load (in disease) generally develops over hours or years. This kind of development is difficult to reproduce experimentally. The long duration of the natural condition may be associated with receptor adaptation or central habituation that could profoundly affect the outcome. Two examples that can be cited in this regard are the resetting of CO_2 setpoint in the face of chronic hypercapnia and the habituation to the natural (normal) load. Thus, when the respiratory muscles of normal subjects are unloaded for a while and then the assist is removed, returning the load to its normal level, subjects experience a sense of loaded breathing. They are often surprised at how hard it is to breathe normally (personal observations; see also Chapter 20). Evidently some habituation to the normal load has occurred. There is evidence that this habituation takes place rather quickly (8). To the extent that load perception, and behavioral responses related to it, are important in acute load responses (see below), the long-term responses to load changes may be quite different from those observed in the usual brief laboratory experiment.

3.   The physical characteristics and mechanical consequences of the external loads commonly in use differ from the natural loads in several important respects. Only some of these will be discussed:

a.   *Resistive loads*: The most commonly studied load is an added inspiratory resistance with which flow increases monotonically with pressure (either linear or nonlinear). This type of load is virtually never encountered in real life. With the usual obstructive lung disease (COPD, asthma) the high resistance is present during both inspiration and expiration. The only time a predominantly inspiratory resistance is encountered is with dynamic upper airway narrowing (e.g., in snorers with or without obstructive sleep apnea, and with functional problems of the larynx and upper trachea). In all these cases, however, flow does not increase monotonically with effort but tends to reach a maximum level above which it is effort-independent (9–15). Since learning may be, or likely is, an important determinant of load responses in consciousness (see below), will the response to a flow limiting inspiratory resistance (no reward for extra effort) be the same as to one where flow increases with greater effort?

Again, the commonly used external expiratory resistance is not flow-limiting. The naturally occurring expiratory resistive load (e.g., COPD and asthma) is not only flow-limiting, but the maximum flow is volume-dependent (16). Will the two kinds of loads (volume-dependent, flow-limiting load and continuously effort-dependent resistive load) produce the same responses? Will expiratory muscles be recruited with the flow-limiting load even though this is futile? Or will the subjects, instead, tonically activate inspiratory muscles to take advantage of the greater maximum flow at higher volumes (as reportedly happens in acute asthma) (17,18)?

Even if one were to produce a volume-dependent, flow-limiting external expiratory resistor [e.g., as attempted by us (19)], the mechanical consequences are not the same as the internal load. With the latter, part of the airway, that downstream from the flow-limiting segment, will be compressed whereas with the external load the airway will be distended throughout. The effect of the two loads on airway mechanoreceptors, which reflexly or behaviorally affect breathing (20–22), will not be the same.

b. *Elastic loads*: Although the usually applied elastic loads may mimic the effect of increased lung stiffness on chest wall structures, they do not reproduce the effect of lung stiffness on lung and airway receptors. With naturally occurring lung stiffness, the change in transpulmonary pressure per unit volume (and hence the stimulus to pulmonary mechanoreceptors) is, by definition, increased. No manner of applying external elastic loads can reproduce that effect; the relation between volume and transpulmonary pressure is not altered whether the elastic load is applied at the airway or at body surface.

c. *Pressure biasing*: Although the primary intent of pressure biasing, as an investigative tool, is to change the operating length of the respiratory muscles (and hence their mechanical advantage) by changing end-expiratory volume, the change in load is actually quite varied and unpredictable and can in no way be equated to the hyperinflation of asthma or COPD. For example, the increase in end-expiratory volume intended to compromise the inspiratory muscles with CPAP may not materialize because of recruitment of expiratory muscles that oppose the applied pressure. Instead of being compromised, the inspiratory muscles may find their operating length unchanged (thanks to expiratory muscle recruitment) whereas their load may actually be markedly reduced since part of the inspiratory work is done passively (through relaxation of expiratory muscles), and upper airway resistance may become lower. Where end-expiratory volume actually increases, the load may be as much related to higher internal elastic load (volume cycling near total lung capacity where the pressure-volume curve is flatter) as to the decrease in mechanical advantage of the muscles. On the other hand, an obese subject who may be breathing near residual volume may find himself breathing in a more favorable region of the sigmoid pressure-volume curve during CPAP. The inspiratory muscles may, thus, become unloaded instead. Likewise, continuous negative airway pressure, intended to reduce operating volume and improve inspiratory muscle function, may inadvertently increase the internal load by causing volume to cycle in the stiff lower range of the *P-V* curve, or by resulting in higher upper airway resistance.

d. *Thresholds loads:* There is no natural counterpart to expiratory threshold loading. Inspiratory threshold load is the closest of any external load to simulate a natural load in that its impact is very similar to what happens with dynamic hyperinflation. In the latter case, inspiratory muscles must generate enough pressure to counteract the elastic recoil at end-expiration before flow can begin (23,24). Ironically, inspiratory threshold load is one of the least studied of external loads.

Notwithstanding their inadequacy as disease models, external loads have served as powerful tools to identify specific and nonspecific mechanisms available to the body. These will now be reviewed.

III. Ventilatory Response to Added External Loads

A. Inspiratory Loads

In anesthetized animals inspiratory loads invariably result in an immediate reduction in tidal volume and increase in inspiratory duration (25–30). Expiratory duration also increases so that the immediate reduction in ventilation is due to reduction in both V_T and F. With time both V_T and F gradually increase and ventilation is restored toward normal. Compensation, however, is not complete.

An important feature of the responses in anesthetized animals is that resistive and elastic loads elicit similar qualitative effects (i.e., T_i prolongation and reduction in frequency). Any quantitative difference in timing responses is explainable by mechanical factors [increased time constant with resistive loads and the opposite with elastic loads (30)].

The immediate response to added inspiratory loads in anesthetized humans differs from the response of animals in that there is little change in respiratory timing (31–35). The lack of timing responses may be related to the anesthetics used since Polacheck et al. (36) found significant prolongation of T_i in humans anesthetized with enflurane. As in anesthetized animals, V_T and V_E are depressed immediately in proportion to the added load, and there are no qualitative differences in response to elastic and resistive loads. Also as with anesthetized animals, the immediate depression in ventilation is followed by gradual return toward baseline (34). Whitelaw et al. (35) found that ventilatory output during sustained loading was no different from first breath responses when chemical factors (i.e., Po_2 and Pco_2) were matched.

The immediate response in conscious animals is also quite similar to that in anesthetized animals. Although comparisons between wakeful and anesthetized responses have not been done in the same animals, awake animals respond in the same fashion to elastic and resistive loads (e.g., 37–39), and in both cases T_i lengthens and tidal volume and ventilation decrease as a function of load severity. Hutt et al. (39) observed that the immediate increase in peak diaphragm activity was proportional to the increase in T_i. This suggests that the rate of rise in inspiratory activity was not immediately altered by the load (i.e., similar to anesthetized responses). The immediate reduction in ventilation is followed by a gradual return toward baseline values. Steady-state responses have been reported in conscious goats and sheep (40–43). Compensation is not complete and $Paco_2$ rises in proportion to the load. Conscious goats also appear to reduce their metabolic rate in response to sustained loads (40).

It therefore appears that conscious animals respond in a qualitatively similar manner to anesthetized responses. By contrast, the response of awake humans to inspiratory loads is substantially different from that of anesthetized humans and animals. The immediate responses to elastic and resistive loads are extremely variable (44), with V_T and timing changing in either direction with either load. The average responses, however, show a clear difference between elastic and resistive loads, with the former tending to result in shorter T_i and higher F and the latter producing opposite average responses.

With sustained load application the responses do not show as much variability. The steady-state response to inspiratory resistive loads is associated with an unchanged or slightly greater V_T, lengthened T_i, reduced respiratory rate, and a slightly decreased V_E (45–50). Sustained elastic loading is associated with a reduced V_T, a higher respiratory rate, and preserved ventilation (46,49–56). Thus, the qualitative differences between responses to elastic and resistive loads are preserved in the steady state.

B. Expiratory Loads

Expiratory loading in anesthetized animals invariably lengthens expiratory duration and slows breathing (57–61). This effect is more pronounced immediately after load application and wanes subsequently. The increase in T_e is not usually sufficient to return end-expiratory volume (EEV) to baseline. As a result, tidal volume tends to decrease immediately. With sustained loading, tidal volume tends to progressively increase, returning V_E toward normal. Compensation is never complete; V_E is invariably depressed in the steady state.

Awake humans also lengthen T_e and reduce frequency in response to expiratory resistive loading (47,62–66). Tidal volume generally increases to compensate for the decrease in frequency. In the steady state, ventilation is depressed only slightly (65).

C. Continuous Distending Pressure

In anesthetized animals continuous distending pressures result in prolongation of expiration with little or no change in T_i (67–69). Tidal volume is initially depressed but subsequently rises. Compensation is never complete and Pco_2 rises. Recruitment of expiratory muscles moderates the increase in end-expiratory volume, but this volume is always elevated relative to its baseline level.

In anesthetized humans, T_e lengthens slightly, T_i does not change, and end-expiratory volume rises to the level expected based on applied pressure and passive elastance, thereby indicating lack of expiratory muscle recruitment (70). Tidal volume and ventilation are depressed (70).

The response of awake humans to continuous positive pressure breathing has been extensively studied (71–76). The extent to which end-expiratory volume is defended varies greatly among subjects and is considerably influenced by training and prior instruction. In general, ventilation is well defended, and the steady-state changes in tidal volume and timing, while variable, are on average small.

IV. Effector Mechanisms

Load compensation is effected in part through muscular mechanisms (intrinsic properties of the muscles) and in part through changes in pattern of muscle activation.

A. Intrinsic Properties of Respiratory Muscles

As with other skeletal muscles, the force generated by respiratory muscles at a given level of activation is affected by the muscle's length and velocity of shortening (for reviews see 77–79). Respiratory muscle length is a function of respiratory volume, and the velocity of shortening is a function of flow rate. Since mechanical loads, by definition, reduce the volume change and flow rate attained at a given level of muscle activation, they alter the relation between muscle activity and pressure output. The direction of these effects is compensatory.

Effect of Volume on Pressure Output

1. When lung volume increases, inspiratory muscle length decreases. This affects the ability of inspiratory muscles to generate pressure in different ways:

a. According to the force-length relation (80,81), there is a length (L_O) at which tension developed (for a given activation) is maximal. Changes in length above and below this point are associated with a decrease in developed tension (80,81). For the diaphragm, L_O is at or below functional residual capacity (FRC) (81,82). Accordingly, the force-generating ability of the diaphragm decreases as the diaphragm descends during inspiration (81–84). There is evidence (85,86) that L_O of parasternal muscles is closer to total lung capacity (TLC). It follows that as lung volume increases from FRC, the mechanical advantage of the diaphragm deteriorates while that of the parasternals improves.

b. Effect of length on the frequency-force relation is as follows: When muscles shorten below L_O, the reduction in force output is relatively greater at low stimulation frequencies than at higher ones (79,87–89) (Fig. 1). It follows that

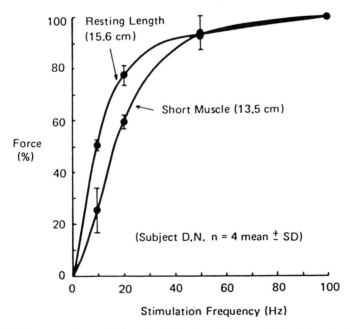

Figure 1 Frequency-force relation of a skeletal muscle at two different lengths. Force is normalized to the maximum obtained at each length. Note that force output is reduced relatively more at lower stimulation frequencies. (From Ref. 79.)

respiratory muscles are relatively more susceptible to the effects of shortening at submaximal levels of activation (as during spontaneous breathing) than during maximal stimulation.

2.   As lung volume increases, the shape, or more specifically the radii of curvature, of respiratory muscles may change. This alters the conversion of tension into pressure according to Laplace's relation (81,83,84,90).

3.   Composite effects of volume: It is clear from the above discussion that the effect of volume on the pressure-generating ability of respiratory muscles is complex and may depend on which muscles are active at the moment, the intensity of activation, and the variable and unpredictable effects on the shape of different muscles. Figure 2 shows some of the relationships observed in the past. With maximum voluntary activation in humans, the pressure generated by the combined action of all respiratory muscles decreases nonlinearly with volume, with the relation being concave to the volume axis (Fig. 2A). In anesthetized animals breathing spontaneously, the relation is linear and its slope increases with level of activation (Fig. 2B). When one looks at the diaphragm alone, the pressure (P_{di}) decreases nonlinearly as a function of volume but the line now is convex to the volume axis (Fig. 2C).

Although the various relations are quantitatively different, there is little doubt that the net effect of volume on pressure output is negative; at the same activity, respiratory muscles will generate less pressure at higher volume, and vice versa.

4.   Implication to load compensation: Figure 3 shows schematically the impact of this relation on load compensation. Assume that in a given state respiratory muscles are activated according to the pattern shown, and that this results in the pressure and volume patterns illustrated by the solid lines. The load is then increased. In the absence of the volume effect on the muscle's mechanical advantage, the pressure generated remains the same (dotted line in P_{mus} tracing). Because the load is higher, volume at any instant is lower (dotted line). However, since a lower volume increases the mechanical advantage of the muscles, P_{mus} at any instant should be higher even in the absence of neural compensation (dashed line). This extra pressure results in greater flow and volume than would otherwise be the case.

Clearly, compensation by this mechanism alone cannot be complete; if it were, volume would be unchanged and there would be no reason for P_{mus} to increase. The degree to which this mechanism succeeds depends on the slope of the active pressure-volume relation as represented in Figure 2. Available evidence indicates that this mechanism is quite potent. Thus, at the same activation, pressure output during occlusion at FRC appears to be about 50% greater than that developed at the usual end-inspiratory volume (83,92).

Effect of Flow on Pressure Output

As with other skeletal muscles (93–95), there is an inverse relation between pressure generated by the respiratory muscles and their velocity of shortening

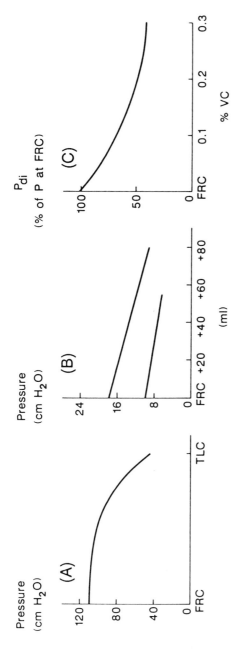

Figure 2 Effect of lung volume on pressure output. (A) Results obtained during maximal voluntary activation at different volumes in humans. FRC, functional residual capacity; TLC, total lung capacity. [From data of Agostoni and Mead (91).] (B) Results during occlusion at different volumes in spontaneously breathing cats. Pressure is airway pressure during occlusion and reflects the action of all muscles active at the time. The two lines depict different levels of activation. Level of activity is the same at all volumes in each line. Note that the relation here is linear and the slope increases with level of activity. [From data of Eldridge and Vaughn (92).] (C) Changes in pressure output of the diaphragm as a function of volume. VC, vital capacity. [Adapted from Younes and Riddle (77); originally redrawn from the data of Grassino et al. (84).]

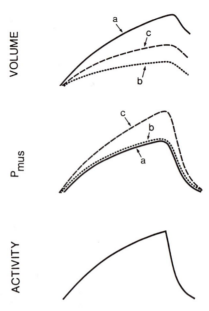

Figure 3 Schematic representation of the compensatory effect of the respiratory muscles' intrinsic properties. P_{mus} is pressure generated by inspiratory muscles. Solid lines: No added load. Dotted line: The load is increased but intrinsic properties are treated as nonexistent. In the absence of neural compensation (note no change in activity line), P_{mus} is unchanged. Total volume is depressed (line b). Dashed lines: P_{mus} increases as a result of the reduction in muscle shortening (less volume change). As a result, volume is not depressed as much (line C).

(96,97). The gain of this relation is such that pressure decreases by about 50% as flow increases from zero to maximum (nearly 8 l/sec in a normal subject) (96). In terms of load compensation, this effect operates in the same fashion as the effect of volume. Thus, an increase in load would tend to decrease flow. Pressure output would thus increase, thereby moderating the change in flow and volume that might otherwise occur.

At resting levels of ventilation, flow is not likely to have much effect on pressure output (77). This is because the average flow (ca. 0.4 l/sec) is a minuscule fraction of maximal inspiratory flow. It is, therefore, not likely that the force-velocity relation plays a significant role in load compensation at rest. Its role, however, may be expected to be greater in hyperpneic states.

B. Changes in Pattern of Muscle Activity

A variety of changes in pattern of respiratory muscle activation can be utilized to restore alveolar ventilation to, or toward, normal in the face of an increase in load.

In this section I will outline changes that have been noted and their significance. The neural mechanisms underlying these responses will be discussed in the following section.

The most obvious purpose of changes in motor output is the restoration of ventilation toward normal. These changes, however, may accomplish more subtle results such as minimization of discomfort or improvement in the efficiency of the lung as a gas exchanger. It has been found, for example, that in the face of an added inspiratory or expiratory resistance, end-tidal P_{CO_2} increases much less than is to be expected given the reduction in ventilation (45,65). This suggests that V_D/V_T has decreased, no doubt in part as a result of the altered pattern of breathing (slower deeper breathing). The reduction in V_D/V_T in turn reduces the need to increase muscle activation to restore P_{CO_2} to normal.

Respiratory motor output has many characteristics. There is the basic respiratory rate. Phasic respiratory muscle activity may be limited to inspiratory muscles or may also involve expiratory muscles (Fig. 4). Phasic activity in either muscle group is characterized by a rising phase and a declining phase (Fig. 4). Changes may involve the amplitude, duration, or shape of the rising phase or of the declining phase. Each of these variables can be, and has been noted to, change in response to added loads. In the next section, I will describe the functional significance of these changes.

Compensation for Inspiratory Loads

Changes in Respiratory Rate

Changes in respiratory rate have a reciprocal effect on the tidal volume required to maintain a given P_{CO_2}. Thus, an increase in rate would make it possible to attain a given ventilation with a smaller peak inspiratory effort. This may be useful in response to inspiratory loads where it is more difficult to attain a given V_T. On the other hand, such changes in pattern of breathing have implication to V_D/V_T. Otis (98) calculated the work of the respiratory muscles when different patterns of breathing are adopted under conditions of different mechanical loads, after allow-

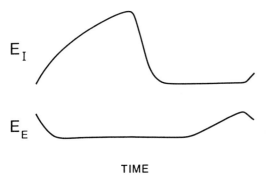

E_I

E_E

TIME

Figure 4   General pattern of inspiratory (E_I) and expiratory (E_E) muscle activation. One breathing cycle is represented (see text).

ing for changes in V_D/V_T. He found that for each set of respiratory mechanics there is an optimal respiratory rate associated with the least work. This optimal rate increased with increasing elastance and decreased with increasing resistance. Mead (99) carried out similar analysis but calculated the respiratory rate associated with the least mean inspiratory muscle pressure, an output variable akin to the more contemporary tension-time index (100). He came to similar conclusions. Both authors assumed that respiratory motor output is sinusoidal and that absolute V_D remained constant. Although these assumptions involve some simplification, conscious humans, by and large, follow these optimal patterns; they increase their rate with elastic loads and decrease it with resistive loads (see above). As indicated earlier, in anesthetized animals the rate response is similar with both loads.

Increase in Peak Amplitude of Inspiratory Activity

This is the most obvious way by which one can restore V_T in the face of an added inspiratory load and is a response that occurs with all types of loads under all experimental conditions. Because of the linear relation between inspiratory muscle activity and developed pressure at a given volume (101), the amount of increase in peak amplitude (all else remaining the same) required to restore V_T in the face of an added load is roughly the reciprocal of the fractional reduction in V_T that would result in the absence of neural compensation. Thus, a load that would reduce V_T to 50% of its baseline value would require roughly doubling of peak inspiratory activity to restore V_T, and so on (102).

The reduction in V_T that would result from inspiratory loads in the absence of neural compensation (but taking intrinsic muscle properties into account) varies greatly depending on the type of load, the baseline load, the duration of inspiration, and the shape of the rising phase of inspiratory activity (102). Figure 5 illustrates some of these relations. It can be seen that a given change in resistance has dramatically different effects on V_T depending on T_i. For example, an increase in resistance of 10 cmH$_2$O/L/sec (from 4 to 14) would decrease V_T to about 65% of its baseline value if T_i is 0.5 sec. This would necessitate a 50% increase in peak inspiratory activity to restore V_T. On the other hand, the same amount of added resistance would reduce V_T by less than 10% at a T_i of 2.5 sec, thereby necessitating a trivial increase in peak inspiratory activity to be offset. The same figure can be used to estimate the fractional reduction in V_T with elastic loads, with different baseline elastance and resistance values, and with different shapes of the rising phase.

Changes in Inspiratory Time

Figure 5 also shows that at the same peak amplitude (all points in this figure) and mechanics, V_T is larger the longer the T_i. This means that the effect of an added load on V_T can be partly or completely offset by simply increasing T_i (i.e., without

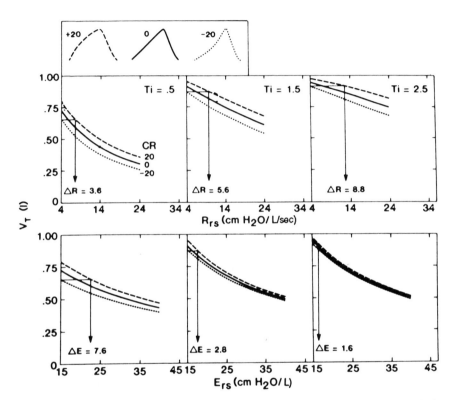

Figure 5 Effect of increasing resistance (R_{rs}) (top) and elastance (E_{rs}) (bottom) on tidal volume (V_T) at a constant level of peak inspiratory activity. Relation is given at different inspiratory durations (T_i) when rising phase is straight (CR = 0), concave to the time axis (CR = +20), or convex to time axis (CR = −20) (see inset at top). Straight lines and arrows indicate change in load ΔR and ΔE) that can be offset by indicated shape change. These data can also be used to compute the load compensatory potential of changes in T_i (see text). (From Ref. 102.)

any other neural changes). The load-compensating ability of T_i prolongation is greater if initial T_i is short, and with resistive loads.*

T_i prolongation makes it possible to restore V_T with a smaller change in peak amplitude. On the other hand, if respiratory rate is not altered, T_e will be shortened with the result that dynamic hyperinflation may occur particularly if expiratory resistance is also high. If rate slows down to maintain T_i/T_{tot}, then a greater V_T (and hence higher peak amplitude) is required. T_i prolongation is, therefore, not a universally beneficial response, and the net sparing effect (on increase in peak amplitude) will vary depending on a host of other variables.

It must be pointed out that mechanical T_i (onset of inspiratory flow to onset of expiratory flow) can change with added loads in the absence of changes in neural T_i (30,36,103). This is because inspiratory activity does not cease abruptly at the end of neural inspiration (Fig. 4), and this allows flow to continue beyond peak inspiratory activity. The delay between peak activity and flow reversal is affected by the mechanical properties of the respiratory system, being greater with long time constants (high R or compliance), and vice versa. Since added loads alter the time constant, inspiratory flow may continue for a longer (with added resistance) or shorter (with added elastance) time beyond peak neural activity. Accordingly, changes in mechanical T_i do not accurately reflect changes in neural T_i when the load is altered. Electromyography (EMG), or computation of driving pressure, is necessary to estimate the latter. Using these techniques, it has been found that neural T_i lengthens in intact anesthetized animals with both inspiratory elastic and resistive loads (30,104), whereas in conscious humans it lengthens with supraliminal (45) but not subliminal (105,106) resistive loads.

Changes in Curvature of the Rising Phase

Tidal volume can be increased by changing the curvature of the rising phase to one that is more concave to the time axis (compare the three lines in any panel in Fig. 5). Such a shape change can, therefore, be used to restore V_T in the face of added loads, and this response has been documented with inspiratory resistive loads in conscious humans (45,107). The arrows in Figure 5 indicate the load-compensating ability of shape changes. It can be seen that this response is more effective when T_i is long in the case of resistive loads, and when T_i is short in the case of added elastic loads.

In the case of resistive loads, compensation by shape changes is not without

---

*To obtain the load-compensating ability of an isolated change in T_i, begin at the Y intercept of any line in a panel (thereby indicating baseline V_T) and draw a horizontal line across panels to the right. Note the point at which the horizontal line intersects similar lines in the adjoining panels (e.g., solid, dashed, or dotted, indicating different shapes). The x value of the point of intersection is the load at which the same V_T will be obtained with the long T_i, all else (i.e., peak and shape) being the same (see 102 for additional details).

cost. Although the required increase in peak amplitude is less (45,107), the increase in mean inspiratory pressure [tension-time index (100)] is, in most cases, greater than if compensation is entirely effected by increases in peak amplitude (see Fig. 7 in 102). To the extent that mean inspiratory pressure is more relevant than peak pressure with respect to fatigue (100), a strategy that involves a shape change (more concave to time axis) is counterproductive with respect to potential for fatigue. Since this response does occur, however, some other benefit must be derived from it (? reduction in unpleasant sensation).

Recruitment of Expiratory Muscles

Expiratory muscle recruitment is potentially very effective in restoring V_T in the face of added inspiratory loads (102). In fact, it is rivaled in effectiveness only by changes in peak inspiratory amplitude. By forcing end-expiratory volume below passive FRC, elastic energy is stored. This can be utilized to restore tidal volume during inspiration, thereby moderating the necessary increase in inspiratory muscle activity. Figure 6 illustrates this potential. As can be seen, this response is effective with both elastic and resistive loads under all circumstances.

Although expiratory muscle recruitment was not observed with small resistive loads (45,107), it has been documented with larger loads (108–110).

Reduction in inspiratory muscle braking during expiration operates in the same direction as expiratory muscle recruitment in that it promotes faster emptying early in expiration, thereby enhancing the return to passive FRC and its further reduction by expiratory muscles. Such response has been documented with large inspiratory loads (109).

Expiratory Loads

Before discussing the various effector mechanisms used with expiratory loads, it is important to point out that not all expiratory loads need have a negative effect on ventilation. At rest, there is usually ample time for lung volume to return to passive FRC. Small to moderate increases in expiratory resistance will delay emptying. However, prevailing expiratory time may still permit volume to return to passive FRC with no additional responses. Normally, the time constant (resistance × compliance) of the passive respiratory system is about 0.3 sec (i.e., 3 × 0.1 = 0.3). This means that volume can passively return almost to FRC in less than 1 sec. Tripling the resistance would still be consistent with a passive return to FRC within a normal T_e. The fact that one or more of the compensatory responses described below is always observed, even with very small loads, suggests that preservation of ventilation is not the only objective of responses elicited by these loads.

Reduction in Postinspiratory Activity of Inspiratory Muscles

Inspiratory activity continues, albeit in a decrementing pattern, into the phase of mechanical expiration (45,64,65,103,107,111,112). This activity serves to brake

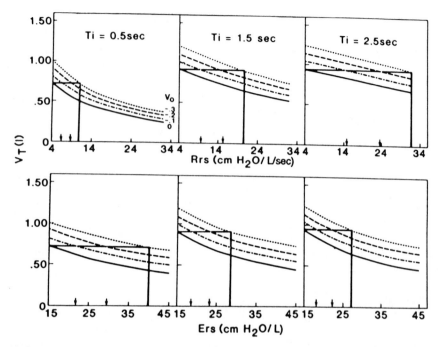

Figure 6 Effect of changes in R_{rs} (top) and E_{rs} (bottom) on V_T at different end-expiratory levels (V_0). V_0 is expressed in liters from passive functional residual capacity. Straight lines indicate load-compensating ability of a 0.3-liter reduction in V_0. Two arrows on abscissa indicate load-compensating ability of 0.1- and 0.2-liter reductions. See Figure 5 for abbreviations. (From Ref. 102.)

the process of lung emptying, which would otherwise be quite rapid. For example, without postinspiratory activity (PIA), the expiratory flow rate at the beginning of expiration following a tidal volume of 1 L (i.e., end-inspiratory elastic recoil = +10 cmH$_2$O) would be in excess of 3 L/sec ($10/R_{rs}$ = 10/3 = 3.3 L/sec). Reduction in the amount of PIA would be a highly efficient way of compensating for expiratory loads since extra pressure (elastic recoil) is released to facilitate flow with even a reduction in energy expenditure (less inspiratory muscle activity). This mechanism is not utilized in anesthetized animals (113) but has been reported in conscious cats (112). In conscious humans PIA also does not decrease when small loads are applied (64,65,114). However, it is likely that reduction in PIA is routinely utilized in conscious humans faced with higher resistive loads and expiratory threshold loads.

Prolongation of Expiration

Prolongation of T_e serves the obvious purpose of allowing more time for volume to return to passive FRC. The closer volume is to passive FRC at the beginning of inspiration, the less pressure inspiratory muscles must develop to attain the same V_T. Although this response makes intuitive sense, it is extremely inefficient, in fact counterproductive, in terms of protecting ventilation or sparing inspiratory muscle work. This is because expiratory flow is usually lowest toward the end of expiration. Prolonging T_e accomplishes relatively little further decrease in volume while respiratory rate decreases, making it necessary for inspiratory muscles to work harder to increase V_T. The balance of these two opposing consequences on inspiratory muscle function is such that inspiratory muscles would be better off if T_e prolongation did not take place. Yet, T_e prolongation is uniformly observed with all loads that impede expiration (Section III.B). T_e prolongation is clearly either a programmed response or subserves other functions (see later).

Recruitment of Expiratory Muscles

The functional significance of this response is quite obvious and will not be discussed further. Although expiratory recruitment may not be needed (see above) and often does not occur (64,65) with small expiratory loads, it is invariable with larger loads under all circumstances (47,62,63,66,115).

Inspiratory Muscle Recruitment

Increases in peak inspiratory activity result in an increase in end-inspiratory volume. This serves several purposes in the setting of added expiratory loads. First, it helps maintain tidal volume in the face of any increase in end-expiratory volume. Second, it can, by increasing V_T, offset the reduction in frequency produced by T_e prolongation. Third, the increase in elastic recoil at end-inspiration serves as an extra force promoting faster expiration.

Where it was looked for, augmentation in inspiratory activity was observed, or inferred, when expiratory loads, even small ones, were added (e.g., 62,65).

Continuous Distending Pressure

In the absence of any compensation, an increase in distending pressure (positive airway or negative chest wall pressure) increases end-expiratory volume (EEV) by an amount that equals applied pressure multiplied by respiratory compliance. Thus, with a compliance of 0.1 L/cmH$_2$O, an applied pressure of 10 cmH$_2$O should increase EEV by 1 L, and so on. The only predictable mechanical consequence of this would be to place the diaphragm at a mechanical disadvantage such that, all else being the same, it has to be activated more to attain the same V_T. Other variable consequences are concomitant changes in internal resistance (usually lower) or elastance (which may change in either direction, see above).

Two strategies can be adopted in response (116): First, an increase in inspiratory muscle activation would serve the obvious purpose of compensating for the adverse change in operating length of the diaphragm and any other increases in load. Such increases have been reported (73–76). The technical validity of these observations is, however, now in doubt (see below).

An alternate strategy is to resist the change in EEV through recruitment of expiratory muscles. In the event these muscles succeed in returning EEV to its original level, the inspiratory muscles will not only remain uncompromised but they are, in fact, considerably assisted. Thus, assume that EEV would increase by 1 L in the absence of any compensation (above example). If expiratory muscles reduce volume to its original EEV and then relax during inspiration, volume would passively increase by 1 L. In other words, a V_T of nearly 1 L would be obtained at no cost to the inspiratory muscles. In anesthetized animals expiratory muscles are routinely recruited (67–69) but compensation is not complete; EEV settles at an intermediate level between what it was and what it would have been without this recruitment. As indicated earlier, the change in EEV, and hence extent of expiratory recruitment, in humans is highly variable, with the responses ranging from total compensation (no change in EEV) to the total predictable change in EEV (i.e., no expiratory recruitment).

Slowing of respiratory rate, per se, serves no purpose and is counterproductive. The reduction in respiratory rate dictates an increase in V_T in order to maintain V_E, thereby adding to the stress imposed on the inspiratory muscles. Yet, respiratory slowing is the uniform response in anesthetized animals. A change in breathing to a faster and shallower pattern does help to reduce the elastic work of the inspiratory muscles. The breathing pattern response of conscious humans to this type of load is also highly variable (see Section III.C).

V. Afferent Mechanisms

The changes in respiratory neural output described earlier are necessarily mediated through perturbation, by the load, of afferent systems. In this section I will first outline some of the general features of these systems. This will be followed by a discussion of the specific mechanisms responsible for load compensation under anesthesia and in the conscious state.

A. General

The following systems have been identified as involved, or likely involved, in load compensation. Only those features relevant to load compensation will be outlined. The reader is referred to other chapters in this volume and other reviews (to be specified) for more detailed descriptions.

Chemical Feedback

These are responses mediated by changes in arterial and brain P_{O_2}, P_{CO_2}, and pH (for reviews see 117–119 and Chapters 9, 10, and 14). Because chemical responses are slow relative to neural responses, they are engaged only when compensation by the other systems is incomplete. Two features deserve mention at this point:

1. Although slower than other systems, chemical feedback is by no means slow. We have documented chemical responses within the second loaded breath (28). Furthermore, although complete (i.e., steady state) responses may take many minutes to be established, substantial chemical stimulation can be evident within 15–20 sec. For example, changes in P_{O_2} and P_{CO_2} produced by airway occlusion may result in tripling of the intensity of inspiratory activity within 20 sec, even in anesthetized animals (28). Thus, whereas responses within the first loaded breath can be reliably attributed to other mechanisms, the contribution of chemical feedback to subsequent breaths is difficult to exclude.

2. The load-compensating ability of chemical feedback in the steady state is enormous. Failure to appreciate this fact has led to unwarranted dismissal of its role. Thus, Figure 5 shows that, at a T_i of 1.5 sec, increasing resistance from 4 to 24 $cmH_2O/L/sec$ (a sixfold increase in respiratory resistance) or increasing elastance from 15 to 30 cmH_2O/L, results in a reduction in V_T to approximately 65% of its baseline value. As indicated earlier, a 50% increase in peak inspiratory activity would, singlehandedly, restore V_T. Assuming a ventilatory response to P_{CO_2} of 2.5 L/min/mmHg (or 30% of baseline ventilation/mmHg), this response can be mounted with a change of less that 2 mmHg in P_{CO_2}. An added resistance of 10 $cmH_2O/L/sec$ can be offset by a change in P_{CO_2} of less than 1 mmHg. Such changes are difficult to detect. It follows that, particularly with small and moderate loads, chemical feedback cannot be discounted on the grounds that P_{CO_2} and P_{O_2} did not change or changed only "very little."

Vagal Feedback

The vagus contains mechanoreceptors responsive to volume (i.e., transpulmonary pressure) and flow. Their various attributes and putative roles in the control of breathing have been reviewed extensively elsewhere (20,21,103). Their role in load responses is summarized below:

Responses Related to Volume

In the absence of load compensation, inspiratory loads would reduce tidal volume, expiratory loads would delay lung emptying, and continuous pressure loads would cause an increase in operating lung volume. These mechanical perturbations are sensed by volume-sensitive vagal receptors.

In the deeply anesthetized (barbiturate) animal, volume manipulations after vagotomy evoke no immediate respiratory responses (27,58,120). Responses to volume manipulations prior to vagotomy in this preparation can, thus, be reliably attributed to vagal volume-sensitive receptors. These responses are summarized in Figure 7.

1. Changes in tidal volume elicit reciprocal changes in the duration of inspiratory activity (T_i). As tidal volume is decreased, through an increase in mechanical load (27) or in ventilator gain (120), inspiratory duration increases and

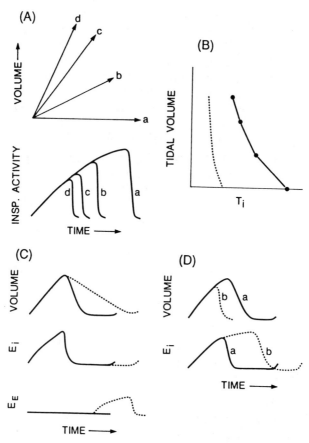

Figure 7 Relevant responses mediated by vagal volume-related feedback. T_i, durations of inspiratory activity; E_i, level of inspiratory activity; E_E, level of expiratory activity. See text for explanation. (From Ref. 193.)

inspiratory activity progresses to a higher level (Fig. 7A). In the face of an added inspiratory load, tidal volume would accordingly decrease less than it would otherwise.

A fundamental feature of this response in the deeply anesthetized animal is that the trajectory of inspiratory activity is not altered; the increase in peak activity is simply the result of T_i prolongation (27,104,120). This is quite relevant to load compensation. Thus, any compensation in V_T as a result of the increase in peak activity is at the expense of a longer T_i. Since changes in T_i evoke qualitatively similar changes in T_e (27,120), the V_T compensation is at the expense of a slower frequency. The net effect on ventilation is either neutral or, more commonly, negative (personal observations). It follows that although vagal volume feedback may contribute to observed responses, this contribution is, at least based on responses under deep anesthesia, not compensatory in the true sense.

The relation between V_T and T_i at a given respiratory drive is hyperbolic (27,120) (Fig. 7B). An important feature of this relation is that the dependence of T_i and peak inspiratory activity on V_T progressively decreases (line becoming progressively more vertical) as T_i without volume feedback (X intercept, Fig. 7B) decreases (36,121,122). This could happen, for example, with increases in body temperature, with some anesthetics, or in the presence of a tachypneic influence mediated by other vagal receptors (e.g., C-fibers) or by nonvagal mechanisms. This could lead to erroneous conclusions about the potency of vagal volume feedback (see below).

2. When lung emptying is delayed during expiration, as by increasing expiratory resistance, expiratory duration (T_e) is prolonged and there is usually recruitment of expiratory muscles (Fig. 7C) (57,112,123). Continuous elevation of lung volume, for example by CPAP, also elicits prolongation of T_e and recruitment of expiratory muscles (58,67,124). As indicated earlier, T_e prolongation in response to either load is, per se, not compensatory in terms of ventilation. By contrast, recruitment of expiratory muscles is a compensatory response. However, it is not clear that expiratory recruitment observed under these conditions is the direct result of vagal afferents. Although in the steady state expiratory muscle activity at any point in expiration is higher after than before the load, we (125) have found that the immediate response (i.e., before chemical feedback has had a chance to increase expiratory activity) is simply the result of T_e prolongation. In fact, when expiratory muscle activity was present prior to load application, the intensity of activity at corresponding times of expiration was lower when emptying was delayed (125).

It follows that vagal volume feedback, while able to exert powerful influences on breathing pattern under certain circumstances, is not necessarily a compensatory system.

It must be pointed out that the responses outlined above were observed under deep anesthesia. Vagal influence in consciousness may be different. At a minimum, it can serve as a source of information for behavioral responses (126) (see also Chapter 20).

3.   Withdrawal of lung volume prior to spontaneous termination of inspiratory activity results in prolongation of T_i (Fig. 7D) (127–129). To the extent that vagal volume feedback is inhibitory to T_i, this suggests that introduction of an inhibitory input and withdrawing it before it succeeded in terminating T_i results in a paradoxical response. Such paradoxical responses have also been observed with other inhibitory inputs, namely with stimuli to the rostal pons (130) and with electrical stimuli (inhibitory) to intercostal nerves (Younes, unpublished observations). Thus, it appears that this phenomenon is generalized and may serve to explain some load responses in conscious humans (see below).

4.   It has long been held that the effect of volume feedback on breathing is very weak in humans, conscious or anesthetized. The evidence for this belief, and a critique thereof, has been reviewed by Polacheck et al. (36) and will not be repeated. As concluded by these authors, the negative results observed in anesthetized humans are most likely related to the anesthetics used in humans, which either inhibit the relevant receptors or result in (are associated with) high baseline input to the inspiratory off-switch. Under the latter condition, even significant inspiratory inhibitory inputs have little effect on T_i (see Fig. 7B). In those individuals in whom baseline input was not so high under enflurane anesthesia (as indicated by a long T_i in the absence of volume feedback), there was a significant volume influence within the resting tidal volume range (36).

The techniques used to reliably quantitate the effect of volume feedback in anesthetized preparations (i.e., occlusion at end-inspiration to elicit T_e prolongation and occlusion at FRC to elicit T_i prolongation) are not suitable in conscious humans. For understandable reasons, the responses to such drastic interventions are dominated by behavioral reactions. The main evidence for the "weakness" of volume feedback in conscious humans is the failure of T_i to shorten during CO_2 inhalation until tidal volume exceeds two to three times the resting value; the change in frequency over this range is dominated by the reduction in T_e (112). A high volume threshold for the elicitation of volume feedback is thus postulated to exist in conscious humans (120). Polacheck et al. (36) outlined several reasons why this approach (i.e., V_T-T_i relation during CO_2 inhalation) may lead to false-negative results. These include a high level of off-switch inputs in the conscious state, independent effects of CO_2 on T_i control, and technical errors in measuring true T_i response. To these should be added the possible effect of consciousness on central adaptation. Thus, when conscious cats are tested in a similar manner, they also show little change in T_i as V_T increases with CO_2 inhalation (131).

We have recently had the opportunity to perform the appropriate tests (i.e., end-inspiratory and end-expiratory occlusions for single breaths) in two patients with the "locked-in" syndrome. In the full-blown syndrome, which these two patients had, all voluntary control over muscles supplied by spinal and lower cranial nerves is lost because of destruction of the motor pathways from the motor cortex to brainstem and spinal cord as they concentrate in the ventral pons (132). The patient, however, is left fully alert and with a full complement of sensory and reflex functions. End-inspiratory (two patients) and end-expiratory (one patient) occlusions produced highly reproducible prolongations in T_e (70–100%) and T_i (+20–30%), respectively, even though tidal volume was only in the 400- to 700-ml range (Fig. 8).

It follows that the notion that humans do not enjoy a significant lung volume influence on breathing pattern in the resting volume range must, at present, be viewed with suspicion.

Responses Related to Flow

In some studies on anesthetized animals an increase in inspiratory flow rate has been reported to result in an increase in inspiratory activity (133–135). This is observed in the same breath in which flow is increased and the response is abolished by vagotomy, thereby confirming that it is a vagally mediated reflex. This reflex has not been observed in all studies. The difference between studies is likely due to level of anesthesia; in those studies in which it was demonstrated, the response could be eliminated by supplemental doses of anesthesia (134).

We have recently studied the effect of inspiratory flow rate on spontaneous respiratory rate in ventilated normal subjects. Respiratory rate increased and P_{CO_2} decreased, sometimes dramatically, as inspiratory flow rate was increased at the same tidal volume (136).

Collectively, these two sets of observations indicate that inspiratory flow rate may appreciably affect the rate and intensity of inspiratory efforts in a positive feedback fashion. If so, then the reduction in flow rate engendered by added load would result in a reduction in respiratory motor output, a noncompensatory response.

Feedback from Chest Wall Including Muscles

This is discussed in detail in Chapter 12. Additional reviews are available (137–139). Only some general comments will be made here.

   1. Phrenic and intercostal nerves contain a variety of afferents that originate in the diaphragm and chest wall. These afferents respond to mechanical perturbations as well as to by-products of muscle contraction (see Chapter 12).

   2. Electrical stimulation of these nerves evokes highly varied and generally inconsistent responses. The observed responses indicate that afferents exist that can change respiratory timing and/or intensity of muscle activation in either direction. The potential is, therefore, there for these afferents to play a role in load responses although it is difficult to link responses observed with electrical stimulation to the mechanical and metabolic changes induced by loading.

   3. Muscle spindles, which normally mediate excitatory load responses at

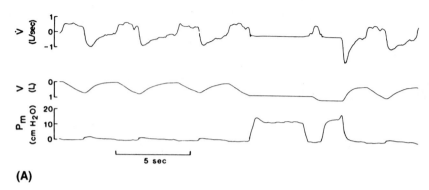

(A)

Figure 8 Results of end-inspiratory (A) and end-expiratory (B) occlusions in a patient with the "locked-in" syndrome. $\dot{V}$, flow, inspiratory flow up; V, volume, inspiration down; P_m, mouth pressure; DP, driving pressure computed according to the method of Im Hof et al. (45), reflecting inspiratory neural output. Following end-inspiratory occlusion (fourth breath in A), P_m increases reflecting elastic recoil. Onset of next inspiration is the time at which P_m begins declining from this elevated level. Note that expiratory duration of the occluded breath is longer than that of the preceding breaths. Following end-expiratory occlusion (fourth breath in B), driving pressure reaches a higher amplitude and inspiratory duration is increased. (Younes M, Sanii R, Daniels V, and Dubo H, unpublished observations.)

the spinal level in other muscles, are very sparse in the diaphragm and parasternal intercostals, the main muscles of breathing (138).

4. The only consistent response to mechanical loading that can be reliably attributed to chest wall afferents is reduction in T_i during inspiratory loading with no effect on inspiratory activity prior to termination; when the airway is occluded in vagotomized animals, T_i is shortened instead of the usual prolongation in animals with intact vagi (140–142). At a minimum, therefore, loading evokes inspiratory terminating activity from chest wall receptors. Although this response is rather weak, its intensity appears to depend on level of anesthesia. Thus, it is totally absent in deeply anesthetized animals and becomes noticeable as level of anesthesia lightens (140). This suggests that it may play a more important role in unanesthetized preparations.

The action of this reflex is similar to that of vagal volume feedback; T_i shortens without prior inhibition of inspiratory activity. Unlike its vagal counterpart, which responds to volume, this reflex responds to muscle tension. This may result in interesting composite responses. Thus, with natural increases in ventilation, both tidal volume and tidal increase in muscle tension are augmented. The two reflexes would thus operate in the same direction, helping to shorten T_i and increase respiratory rate. By contrast, the addition of load would reduce volume

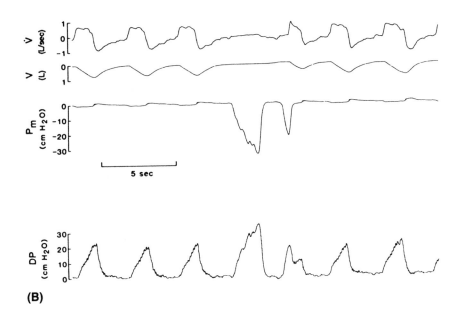

(B)

while increasing muscle tension. The two reflexes may thus counteract each other; the prolongation of T_i expected from reduced vagal volume feedback may be offset by the T_i shortening of increased muscle tension. It is thus evident that if the inhibitory chest wall reflex is operative in unanesthetized states, the net effect of inspiratory loading on T_i and respiratory rate will depend on the relative gains of the two reflexes. Thus, no change in T_i with loading may mean either that both reflexes are inactive or that the two gains are comparable.

Chest wall afferents project to the sensory cortex (see Chapters 12 and 20) and loads applied to the chest wall alone are sensed (5,6). Another likely contribution of these afferents is, therefore, via behavioral responses.

Behavioral Mechanisms

Changes in the mechanical load are readily sensed in awake subjects. Detection thresholds are in the range of $0.5-1.0$ cmH$_2$O/L/sec for added resistance and $1.0-2.5$ cmH$_2$O/L for added elastance (see 143 for review and references). Perception of the load may trigger behavioral responses that aim to minimize the unpleasant sensation or to compensate for perceived reduction in ventilation. Alternatively, the responses may simply be the result of anxiety. Behavioral responses are reviewed by Shea et al. (Chapter 20).

The very low threshold for detection makes it difficult to study reflex (i.e., automatic) control of breathing in awake subjects. A variety of paradigms have been utilized to bypass behavioral responses, including studies during sleep and with the use of special experimental designs. These will be reviewed later.

It may be argued that behavioral responses are an integral part of load compensation in the awake state and, as such, one should not attempt to avoid them. There is also the possibility that responses initiated in the awake state through conscious intervention may, in time, become automatic (see Chapter 20). Nonetheless, one can never be sure that the behavioral responses occurring during a short-term load application in a given subject necessarily reflect how this subject will respond to the load in the long run. This is because behavioral responses are necessarily modified by experience (see 144 for review), personality traits (144), adaptation (8), and probably a host of other factors. The relevance of responses observed during acute experiments to compensation in disease is, therefore, always dubious whereas automatic (reflex) responses are likely to be more robust.

Feedback from the Upper Airway

A variety of mechanoreceptors reside in the upper airway. Mechanical perturbations of the isolated upper airway have resulted in changes in respiratory output (for review see 4 and Chapter 11).

The upper airway is not involved in natural changes in respiratory load produced by lung and chest wall disease. They are, however, inadvertently subjected to the altered pressure and flow produced by experimental loads added at the mouth or nose. Receptors from the upper airway can, therefore, modify load responses either via the reflexes observed in anesthetized animals or by providing additional inputs relevant to behavioral control. This compounds interpretation of the results of external mechanical loading applied at the upper airway. The role of upper airway receptors in mediating responses to experimental loading has to be addressed before the relevance of these responses to disease states can be ascertained (see below).

Other Mechanisms

Vascular Mechanoreceptors

Loading alters intrathoracic pressure and blood volume as well as systemic arterial pressure. A variety of respiratory responses have been elicited during manipulations of vascular mechanoreceptors (145–150). The role of these reflexes in load responses is unknown.

Sympathetic Afferents

Some thoracic sympathetic afferents display respiratory modulation, and electrical stimulation of sympathetic nerves has resulted in apnea (see 151 for review). Sympathetic afferents do not contribute to load responses under anesthesia; as indicated earlier, no neural load responses are elicited after vagotomy in these preparations. A role for sympathetic afferents in consciousness cannot be ruled out, however.

Endogenous Opioids

Scardella et al. (40,41) found a progressive reduction in tidal volume in the course of resistive loading in conscious goats. This was partly reversed by administration of naloxone. These authors also demonstrated an increase in CSF B endorphin levels in these goats. Santiago et al. (152), from the same laboratory, had earlier found that some patients with COPD had an impaired response to added loads. Administration of naloxone restored a normal response in these patients. This finding was, however, not confirmed in a subsequent, controlled, study by Simon et al. (153). Although endogenous opioids clearly modulate load responses in conscious goats (41,42,152), their role in humans remains uncertain.

B. Mechanism of Load Compensation in Anesthetized Preparations

The specific responses observed with different loads have been outlined earlier. Their mechanisms will now be discussed.

Inspiratory Loads

First Breath

In anesthetized animals the increase in peak pressure output observed with the first loaded breath is due in part to the intrinsic properties of respiratory muscles (i.e., nonneural, see above) and in part to prolongation of inspiration allowing inspiratory output to progress to a higher level (25–27,30,104). There is no increase in diaphragmatic activity over the period corresponding to preloaded T_i (25–27,30, 104). Several investigators have observed small increases in external intercostal muscle activity over the same time period as control T_i (29,141,154,155). This response is eliminated by dorsal rhizotomy and is likely related to excitatory spindle reflexes; as indicated earlier, these receptors are abundant in intercostal muscles.

The prolongation of T_i during the first breath is exclusively related to the reduced vagal volume-related feedback (smaller V_T). This response is not observed in vagotomized animals (27,104,156).

Several studies have failed to show T_i prolongation during the first loaded breath in anesthetized humans (31,32,34,35,157). These studies, however, employed anesthetics that are known to attenuate vagal volume-related reflexes (see 36 for discussion). Polacheck et al. (36) found significant prolongation in several subjects under enflurane anesthesia.

It must also be reiterated that lack of T_i prolongation need not reflect an inactive vagal feedback but may be the result of opposing actions, during the first loaded breath, of vagal and chest wall reflexes (see above).

Subsequent to First Breath

In anesthetized animals the progressive increase in peak inspiratory activity and respiratory rate beyond the first breath is due to progressive deterioration in arterial Po_2 and Pco_2. We measured the breath-by-breath changes in blood gas tensions following applied loads in anesthetized cats and found that they could entirely account for the observed responses (28). This was subsequently confirmed in experiments where changes in blood gas tensions were minimized (158,159). Little or no further increases in respiratory output were observed beyond the first breath in these studies.

In anesthetized humans, the subsequent increase in respiratory output also appears to be mediated by chemical feedback. Margaria et al. (34) found that this recruitment was attenuated by O_2 breathing. That the remaining response was mediated by CO_2 was confirmed by Whitelaw et al. (35). These authors carried out CO_2 rebreathing tests with and without inspiratory load. In the loaded runs, the load was removed periodically for one to two breaths. These breaths were comparable to breaths obtained in the free (no load) runs at the same CO_2, indicating that sustained loading does not, per se, elicit any additional neural responses.

These results do not exclude a role for chest wall reflexes in mediating the progressive changes in respiratory output. As indicated earlier, a chest wall inhibitory reflex, likely responsive to tension in inspiratory muscles, may be operative under light anesthesia. Because the response to CO_2 is associated with increasing inspiratory muscle tension, this reflex may contribute to the progressive decrease in T_i and increase in respiratory rate that occur during sustained loading. This contribution, however, is part of the chemical response and not a primary response to the load.

Expiratory Loads and Continuous Pressure Application

In anesthetized animals, the prolongation of expiration and expiratory muscle recruitment observed during the first loaded breath are eliminated by vagotomy (57,58,60,61,67–69). Expiratory prolongation is part of the Hering-Breuer reflex and is related to increased pulmonary stretch receptor activity during expiration.

The subsequent responses to expiratory and continuous pressure loads (both of which tend to increase end-expiratory volume) have been studied by a large number of investigators (57,58,60,61,67–69,135,160–162). The results have been quite variable. The following is a rational explanation of the observed results:

The immediate response to these loads (T_e prolongation and increase in volume during expiration) has two inevitable consequences: a decrease in ventilation with consequent deterioration in blood gas tensions and an increase in expiratory activity of vagal slowly adapting receptors (SAR). Both changes have time-dependent effects on respiratory muscle activity and on respiratory timing. The effects of the two on any given variable may be concordant or discordant. The final result depends on the relative gains and the direction of action of these two influences.

Although SAR activity during inspiration tends to shorten T_i, sustained changes in SAR activity (i.e., tonic activity) have little or no effect on T_i (58,60,124,128,129). Sustained increases in end-expiratory volume, therefore, exert little influence, per se, on T_i. The T_e-prolonging effect of tonic SAR activity also adapts, but not completely (58,60,124,128,129). It follows that if all else remained the same (i.e., chemical drive, V_T) the response would be unchanged T_i, long T_e (but less than the first T_e), unchanged inspiratory muscle activity, and increased expiratory activity. The increase in expiratory activity would be less than that observed during the first expiration because of the relatively shorter T_e.

The changes in blood gas tensions that inevitably occur have the effect of producing time-dependent excitation of inspiratory and expiratory muscles. Increased chemical feedback may also cause T_i and T_e to shorten independent of vagal feedback (28,163).

In the course of sustained loads of this kind, expiratory muscles are subjected to two opposing influences: an inhibitory influence due to the decay in tonic vagal influence, and an excitatory influence due to increased chemical feedback. The net effect will essentially depend on the vigor of the chemical response. On the other hand, all factors tend to promote a progressive return of T_e toward preload T_e. Thus, expiratory activity of SAR will decrease due to receptor adaptation and, possibly, due to further reduction in end-expiratory volume on account of chemically induced expiratory muscle recruitment. There is also central adaptation to the residual tonic SAR activity, and increasing chemical feedback may independently shorten T_e. Steady-state T_e will thus always be intermediate between preload T_e and the first loaded T_e. The extent to which it remains longer than baseline T_e will depend on the potency of the various mechanisms affecting T_e as described above.

As indicated earlier, the residual effect of tonic SAR activity on T_i is minimal. T_i, however, remains subject to phasic SAR activity (a function of V_T), and to any independent effect of chemical feedback on T_i. Because V_T may be larger, smaller, or unchanged relative to baseline V_T (see below), the changes in phasic feedback may promote a longer or shorter T_i. The net effect on T_i will thus depend on what happens to V_T and on the potency of the independent effect of chemical feedback on T_i (usually quite weak in anesthetized animals).

The influences that determine steady-state V_T with these loads are most complex. The mechanical consequences may operate to decrease V_T. This is due to impaired mechanical advantage of inspiratory muscles and to the threshold load imposed by end-expiratory volume being higher than passive FRC (as in the case with pure expiratory load). On the other hand, and as indicated earlier, the inspiratory muscles may be better off if expiratory muscle recruitment succeeds in lowering end-expiratory level below the relaxation volume (as is the case with continuous positive pressure). The net mechanical effect on V_T will thus depend on the type of load (being less unfavorable with continuous than pure expiratory load), and on the extent of expiratory muscle recruitment. The net mechanical effect may be deleterious or salutary, as described before. Peak inspiratory activity will be subject to the excitatory effect of chemical feedback and the variable effect of phasic feedback of T_i. V_T is thus subject to many influences (mechanical, chemical, neural) that act in different directions, all of which are highly variable and interdependent. V_T may be larger than, smaller than, or similar to baseline V_T.

There has been very little in the way of exploring mechanisms in anesthetized humans. The study of Derenne et al. (70) in methoxyflurane-anesthetized humans indicated very little T_e prolongation or expiratory muscle recruitment during positive pressure breathing. This suggests that the vagal influence that normally mediates these responses is very weak. Whether this represents the actual situation in humans or is due to the anesthetic is unclear.

In summary, load responses in anesthetized preparations are mediated by chemical feedback and by vagal mechanoreceptor feedback with, at times, small contributions from chest wall reflexes. Because the vagal and chest wall reflexes observed under anesthesia are essentially not compensatory with respect to ventilation (see earlier), true load compensation under anesthesia is essentially mediated by chemical feedback (in addition to the automatic contributions by intrinsic properties of muscles). There has been no convincing evidence of the existence of any functionally significant neural load compensation under anesthesia.

C. Mechanisms of Load Responses in Unanesthetized Humans

By contrast to anesthetized preparations, where load compensation is essentially dependent on muscle properties and chemical feedback, in conscious preparations the entire spectrum of afferent mechanisms is potentially at play. The fact that humans retain a normal, or even subnormal, PCO_2 despite substantial mechanical problems imposed by disease indicates the existence of powerful nonchemical load compensatory mechanisms. Not only is the list of potential mechanisms extensive (see above), but because these mechanisms seem to be active only in unanesthetized preparations, our ability to dissect them apart is very limited. Nonetheless, a variety of approaches have resulted in useful insights. These will now be summarized.

Logical Approaches

These approaches are useful in excluding or including certain mechanisms based on well-established characteristics of these mechanisms. In this fashion the list of potential mechanisms is reduced. The following are examples:

1. Because the delay for chemical feedback is at least a few seconds, responses observed during the first loaded breath are necessarily neural in origin.

2. Responses during the first loaded breath are highly variable and bidirectional. In the studies by Axen and Haas (44), V_T and F were found to change in either direction, with either elastic and resistive loads, and the standard deviation of the change was substantially greater than the mean change. This is quite different from steady-state responses, which are qualitatively much more consistent and the coefficient of variation is usually less than one (e.g., 45,107). It is difficult to see how truly reflex responses can result in opposite changes in different individuals. One must, therefore, conclude that first-breath responses are dominated by behavioral mechanisms. Because much of this variability disappears later, first-breath responses in conscious humans are dominated by transitional behavioral reactions (startle responses) and likely have little relevance to load compensation.

3. Chemical feedback can also be excluded when subsequent (to first breath) responses are associated with unequivocal hypocapnia and no hypoxemia. Where P_{CO_2} is not significantly different from, or slightly higher than, baseline P_{CO_2}, chemical feedback cannot be excluded except where the load is severe. As indicated earlier, the acute increase in P_{CO_2} required to offset a small to moderate load is too small relative to measurement errors. Although in the occasional individual P_{CO_2} is lower than baseline during sustained loading, group averages invariably show P_{CO_2} in the steady state to be not different from (statistically) or slightly higher than control (e.g., 45,65,107). Chemical feedback, therefore, remains a distinct mediator of load responses in the steady state.

Axen et al. (50) quantitated average responses to inspiratory elastic and resistive loads in the first, fifth, and tenth loaded breaths in large numbers of individuals. They found a progressive increase in tidal volume and mean inspiratory flow rate with little progressive change in respiratory rate. These changes continued up to the tenth breath. Since the load was constant over the 10 breaths, these spirometric changes likely reflect a progressive increase in peak inspiratory output and in the mean rate of rise of inspiratory activity. In other words, both the time course and the nature of change in inspiratory output are highly consistent with chemical feedback. Furthermore, since V_E was, on average, decreased during the first breath [V_T decreased while F did not change or did not increase as much (44,50)], blood gas tensions must have deteriorated. It follows that not only was there a likely chemical stimulus, but the entire pattern beyond the first breath is consistent with chemical feedback. In fact, it is difficult to account for subsequent changes on the basis of other mechanisms.

Reflex responses are usually extremely fast. Slow reflex responses may be expected where the stimulus inciting them is increasing slowly. In the setting of added loads, inspiratory muscle fatigue and/or pulmonary congestion/edema could, theoretically, provide such slowly evolving reflex responses. The loads used in the studies by Axen et al. (up to 20 $cmH_2O/L/sec$ and 20 cmH_2O/L) are well below the range associated with either eventuality. Furthermore, with the development of either (fatigue or edema) the response should not be deeper efforts with no change in frequency; faster, shallower efforts would be expected.

It is possible that a hitherto unidentified neural mechanism exists that evolves over many seconds or minutes. Until this unlikely mechanism is discovered, the overwhelming likelihood is that chemical feedback is responsible for the compensatory changes observed in average responses beyond the first breath.

4.   The response of T_i to an inspiratory resistive load in conscious humans is similar to that of anesthetized animals (T_i lengthens). Since in anesthetized animals this response is mediated by vagal mechanoreceptors (see above), one is tempted to invoke the same mechanism for the human response. However, in humans V_T is not reduced and the reduction in V_T is responsible for the reduced vagal feedback in anesthetized animals. Furthermore, with elastic loads in humans T_i is not lengthened even though V_T is reduced. Despite superficial similarities, the actual responses are therefore opposite to what one might expect on the basis of vagal volume feedback. Im Hof et al. (45,107) used these arguments to conclude that T_i prolongation is not mediated by this mechanism.

5.   Likewise, the T_e prolongation with expiratory resistive loads in humans is qualitatively similar to what is observed in anesthetized animals with similar loads. The mechanism there is also vagal volume feedback. However, Poon et al. (65) argued that vagal feedback can only explain a small fraction of the response. Several reasons were cited, the principal one being that the extent of T_e prolongation is well in excess of what might be expected on the basis of established gain of vagal volume feedback even in animals where these reflexes are very prominent.

Studies in Patients with Selective Impairment of Putative Mechanisms

A variety of disorders interfere, naturally or through medical interventions, with certain potential mechanisms for load compensation. Patients with these disorders provide an opportunity for investigating mechanisms of load compensation in conscious humans. The following types of patients have been studied:

Patients with Tracheostomy

These patients provide an opportunity to examine the role of upper airway mechanoreceptors in load compensation.

Noble et al. (164) determined the detection threshold for resistive loads applied via tracheostomy in patients with minimal respiratory disease. These patients were able to detect loads as well as normals. There was also little improvement in detection threshold when the tracheostomy tube cuff was deflated, thereby also exposing upper airway receptors to the load (164). This study indicates that upper airway receptors are not critical for detection of externally applied loads. Behavioral load responses that depend on perception are, therefore, not likely to be accentuated as a result of the load being applied at the mouth.

O'Donnell et al. (49) studied the response to inspiratory and expiratory resistive loads and to elastic loads in patients with tracheostomy. When the loads were applied to the tracheostomy [i.e., upper airway (UA) receptors not included], the responses were qualitatively and quantitatively similar to the responses observed in normal subjects loaded at the mouth (i.e., where UA is also loaded). These authors also determined the response to the same loads selectively applied to the UA; with the cuff inflated, they used the flow and volume signals measured at the tracheostomy to generate pressure in proportion to flow and volume (analogous to resistive and elastic loads) that were applied to the UA. In 11 patients with total laryngectomy, pressure simulating inspiratory resistance produced a significant T_i prolongation. This is qualitatively similar to the general response to this type of load, but its magnitude was substantially smaller. Other types of loads had no effect when applied to UA. This observation indicates that involvement of nasopharyngeal and oropharyngeal receptors during experimental loading does not appreciably affect the response. The absence of the larynx was a problem in this study since the larynx is likely the most important site from which UA reflexes originate (4,165). Four additional subjects in the study by O'Donnell et al. (49) had a tracheostomy with an intact larynx. In one of these subjects elastic loading applied to UA alone produced rapid, shallow breathing. The other three showed no response. However, these three also had no response when the load was applied to the respiratory system via the tracheostomy (for discussion of possible reasons, see 49).

In summary, available results indicate that UA receptors do not alter the direction of responses to different loads but may contribute to their magnitude. The role of laryngeal receptors has, however, not been critically assessed yet.

Patients with Spinal Quadriplegia

Patients with complete transection of the lower cervical cord are devoid of afferent feedback from the rib cage and abdominal wall and from the sympathetic system. In fact, the only feedback available to them is via vagal, phrenic, and UA afferents. When loads are applied via a tracheostomy, these last afferents are also excluded. There is also a motor deficit. Although this deficit affects both inspiratory and expiratory muscles, it is more severe with expiratory muscles; with the most common lesions (C-5 to C-8) the diaphragm is generally intact, whereas virtually all expiratory muscles (including abdominals and internal intercostals) are paralyzed leaving only minor accessory muscles (notably the upper part of the pectoralis major muscle) to effect expiratory efforts (166). These patients, therefore, provide the opportunity of evaluating the role played by several afferent and effector mechanisms in various load responses. Several studies have been carried out (75,107,164,167–174). The following is a summary of their findings:

1. The threshold for load detection is not impaired in quadriplegics and remains very low (164,167,168,174). This is true also in quadriplegics loaded via tracheostomy (164).

2. Quadriplegic subjects do not decrease end-expiratory volume as much, if at all, in the face of large inspiratory loads (173). This is predictable given the severe deficit in expiratory muscles and does not provide any insights regarding afferent mechanisms.

3. With inspiratory resistive loads, quadriplegic subjects prolong T_i much less than normals (107,169,170,172). Quadriplegics also prolong T_e less than normals in response to expiratory resistive load (174). The increase in respiratory frequency with elastic loading is also depressed in this group (169,170). It, therefore, appears that afferents from the rib cage and/or abdomen play an important role in mediating the timing responses to added loads. On the other hand, Axen et al. (175) found similar effects on timing responses in patients with pure motor disorders, suggesting that the abnormalities in timing observed in quadriplegics may be somehow more linked to their motor deficit than to deafferentation. This last study by Axen et al. (175) examined only first-breath responses which are dominated by behavioral responses. It would be of considerable interest to see whether these deficits persist in the steady state. It must be pointed out that respiratory mechanics are often abnormal in patients with neuromuscular disorders (176), and that background resistance and elastance do influence the responses to added loads (177). Should it turn out that deficits in timing responses are common to all motor disorders, regardless of the state of integrity of afferents, then the results of quadriplegics might be explainable on nonspecific changes in background impedance and would cease to have mechanistic implications (in terms of responsible afferents).

4. The change in shape of the rising phase of inspiratory activity in response to inspiratory resistive loads is much depressed in quadriplegic subjects, suggesting that rib cage afferents (likely muscle spindles) mediate this response.

5. Notwithstanding the above deficits in load responses, quadriplegic subjects are as capable as normals of preserving ventilation, at least against small loads. Thus, the steady-state changes in end-tidal P_{CO_2} were not different from those of normal subjects (107,174). It must be reiterated that the timing and shape responses are basically noncompensatory in terms of ventilation (see above), and that very small (essentially unmeasurable) changes in P_{CO_2} are capable of offsetting inadequacies in neural response to small and moderate loads. The lack of significant difference in $\Delta P_{ET_{CO_2}}$ is, therefore, not surprising.

6. Banzett et al. (75) applied continuous negative pressure to the chest wall

in quadriplegics to evaluate the mechanism of increase in diaphragmatic activity with increases in lung volume [operating length compensation (73)]. They demonstrated a very rapid increase in diaphragm activity (within 5–10 sec) following application of negative pressure, despite a lower end-tidal P_{CO_2}. On the grounds that the only other (than phrenic afferents) potential feedback (vagal feedback) should work in the opposite direction, they suggested that the response is mediated by phrenic afferents. Unfortunately, behavioral responses could not be entirely eliminated, and considerable doubt has subsequently been cast regarding the comparability of diaphragm EMG at different lung volumes. Thus, supramaximal, and hence standardized, phrenic nerve stimuli produced substantially larger diaphragm EMG signals whenever diaphragm length decreased, and vice versa (178,179). Thus, the existence of operating length compensation mediated by phrenic afferents remains in doubt.

Patients with the Locked-in Syndrome (132)

These patients provide a unique opportunity for studying the role of mechanisms whose effector arm includes the motor cortex. The lesion is limited usually to the ventral pons in which corticospinal and corticobulbar tracts are concentrated. No other relevant tracts or nuclei (centers) exist in this area, so differences in responses between these patients and normals can be reliably attributed to loss of influence of the motor cortex on breathing.

We had the opportunity to study load responses in two patients with the complete syndrome. They were incapable of executing any voluntary respiratory acts (e.g., voluntary cough, breath hold, or any change in tidal volume) but coughed vigorously in response to tracheal irritation. Laughing and crying resulted in appropriate body and respiratory movements, indicating persistence of behavioral responses not mediated by the pyramidal tracts. All sensory modalities as well as auditory-evoked potentials were normal. CO_2 response measured in one patient was normal (4 L/min/mmHg). For all intents and purposes, these two patients lacked only voluntary control.

Figure 9 shows the average response to single-breath applications of an inspiratory resistive load (10 cmH$_2$O/L/sec) and a full elastic load (20 cmH$_2$O/L) in one subject. The other subject's responses were identical. Each load was applied on 8–10 occasions in each subject. The responses were highly consistent within each subject. The patients were fully awake when studied.

Tidal volume decreased with both loads, indicating incomplete compensation. The greater reduction in V_T with ΔE is due to its being a relatively larger load (see Fig. 5, ΔR of 10 vs. ΔE of 20). The most significant finding was the fact the T_i lengthened with both loads. This was true whether T_i was computed from the flow signal or driving pressure signal (akin to isometric P_{mus}; see 45 for technical details). This is in marked contrast to results observed in conscious subjects with intact pyramidal tracts where the average T_i responses are opposite in direction

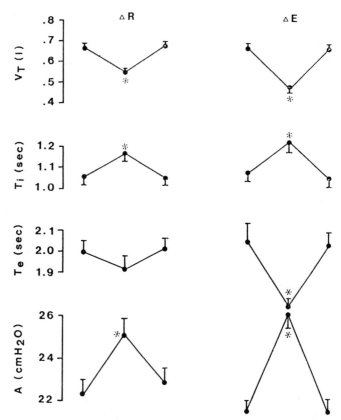

Figure 9 Average responses to single-breath applications of an added resistance (ΔR, 10 cmH$_2$O/L/sec, left) and an added elastance (ΔE, 20 cmH$_2$O/L) in a patient with the "locked-in" syndrome. $n = 8$ for ΔR and 10 for ΔE. V_T, tidal volume; T_i, inspiratory duration; T_e, expiratory duration. Both T_i and T_e were computed from driving pressure (see Fig. 8) and are, therefore, free of artifacts related to changes in respiratory system time constant due to added resistance and elastance. A, amplitude of driving pressure. The middle point in each case is the loaded breath, and the bracketing points reflect the values for the preceding and following unloaded breaths. Note that the responses to ΔR and ΔE are qualitatively similar. *Significant difference from control ($p < 0.01$ or better). (Younes M, Sanii R, Daniels V, and Dubo H, unpublished observation.)

with the two loads (44). The degree of T_i prolongation was commensurate with the expected reduction in vagal volume feedback, based on the reduction in V_T and the gain of this reflex (ΔT_i at end-expiratory occlusion, see Fig. 8). This T_i prolongation with resistive load (approximately 10%) was substantially less than what is observed in intact conscious humans with the same load [ca. 40% (44)].

Expiratory duration decreased with ΔE. This finding indicates that the reduction in T_e, which is usually observed with elastic loading in conscious intact humans, is clearly reflexic in origin, at least to a considerable extent. This may be related to faster emptying during expiration acting via vagal stretch receptors (less expiratory activity) or flow-sensitive receptors (e.g., rapidly adapting receptors). It may also be related to nonvagal reflexes that are more prominent in the unanesthetized state. It would be of interest to see whether T_e also shortens in these subjects when the elastic load is limited to inspiration and where expiratory flow is, therefore, not augmented.

Although peak inspiratory activity (A) increased, the increase was entirely due to T_i prolongation; there was no significant change in the rate of rise of inspiratory activity (A/T_i) (Fig. 9).

Expiratory resistive load for one breath resulted in slight (5%) prolongation of T_e, commensurate with the strength of the Hering-Breuer inflation reflex in these patients (Fig. 8). This is to be compared with the approximately 25% increase in normal subjects (65). End-expiratory volume did not return to the preload level prior to the next breath, indicating incomplete compensation.

With the exception of T_e shortening with added elastance, the responses observed in these two patients are identical to those observed in anesthetized animals; there are no qualitative differences between resistive and elastic loads, the increases in peak activity during the first breath are due to T_i prolongation, and the timing changes are related to differences in behavior of lung volume and are in the same direction as established vagal volume feedback. Although these results need to be confirmed in a larger sample, they suggest that, with one minor exception (T_e shortening with ΔE), any differences between awake intact humans and anesthetized animals are mediated by cortical mechanisms and conveyed via the pyramidal tracts.

The fact that T_i and T_e prolongation with inspiratory and expiratory resistive loads was substantially less than observed in intact subjects further supports earlier conclusions that the responses observed in intact subjects are largely not mediated by vagal feedback and likely represent the operation of higher mechanisms intended to reduce discomfort (44,65,107).

Other Patients with Impaired Feedback

Patients with lung, and heart-lung, transplantation offer an opportunity to study the role of vagal (and sympathetic) afferents in load responses. Inspiratory resistive load detection was reported to be normal in these patients (180). However, load responses have not yet been reported.

Likewise, the ventilatory response to CO_2 varies greatly among different normal subjects, and some patients have a nearly flat response despite normal mechanics (primary alveolar hypoventilation). It would be of considerable interest to compare steady-state responses to moderate loads in subjects with very different chemical sensitivity. This would shed light on the role of chemical feedback in subsequent (to first breath) compensation in awake humans. It should be kept in mind, however, that the difference in steady-steady P_{CO_2} between those with near-complete compensation and those with no subsequent compensation may be quite small (see earlier).

Studies During Sleep

The realization that upper airway resistance increases, often dramatically, during sleep has generated considerable interest in load responses in this state. Many studies have been carried out (for recent review see 10). The contrast between responses during sleep and wakefulness has provided considerable insight into mechanisms of load compensation in wakefulness.

One of the important features of load responses during sleep is their consistency (prior to arousal) within and between subjects. This contrasts sharply with awake responses (181,182) and indicates that interindividual differences in wakefulness are likely related to behavioral responses. However, the most significant feature is the apparent lack of neural compensation, with the defense of ventilation being left to chemical feedback.

The most frequently studied load is an added inspiratory resistance (181,183–185). Unlike the case in awake subjects, the immediate (first few breaths) response during sleep is characterized by reduction in V_T and V_E with a magnitude that is proportional to the load (Fig. 10). Not only is the compensation incomplete, but there does not appear to be any increase in peak diaphragmatic activity during the first few breaths, signifying no immediate compensatory neural response (183,184). The immediate prolongation of T_i, if any, is substantially less than during wakefulness (183–185) (Fig. 11). When the load is sustained, there is a progressive increase in respiratory output with a time course that is consistent with chemical feedback (181,183,185) (Fig. 10). Progressive recruitment of expiratory muscles was also observed (183) and this was also attributed to increased P_{CO_2}.

The comparison of time course of responses in wakefulness and sleep reported by Weigand et al. (Figs. 10 and 11) is instructive. The substantial differences observed immediately following load application gradually narrow, not only because of a chemically driven increase in the sleep values but also because of decline in awake values. The difference between awake and sleeping results becomes quite small at 4 min with all but the highest load, and one gets the impression that the differences would continue to narrow beyond 4 min. These

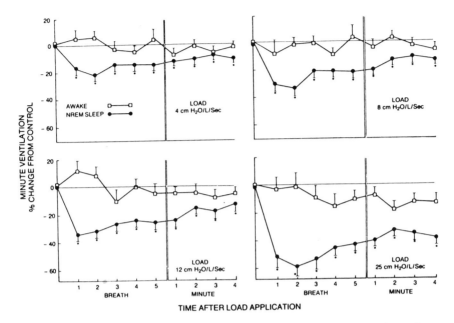

Figure 10   Mean (±SE) values for minute ventilation expressed as percent change from control over the first five consecutive breaths and 1–4 min after application of four different resistive loads during wakefulness and non-rapid-eye-movement (NREM) sleep. Note that minute ventilation was well maintained after resistive load application during wakefulness but decreased significantly from control values at all points after resistive load application during NREM sleep. □–□, awake subjects; ·——·, NREM subjects. *$p < 0.05$ different from control. (From Ref. 185.)

findings suggest that the apparently stronger defense in wakefulness is evanescent and that long-term responses may not be substantially different.

   The responses to inspiratory elastic loading and to complete occlusion at FRC were also reported (182,186,187). In general, they support the conclusions reached with resistive loading; there is very little immediate neural response and compensation takes place gradually with a time course that is consistent with chemical feedback (182,186,187). Interestingly, the reduction in T_e observed in conscious normal humans, as well as in locked-in patients (see above), was not observed during sleep. It is not clear whether this is related to the state of sleep or to the use of inspiratory (only) elastic load, as opposed to the continuous (I and E) load used in our locked-in patients, which tends to accelerate expiratory flow.

   Expiratory loads have not, to my knowledge, been tested in sleeping humans. However, the responses to continuous negative chest wall pressure (188) or to positive airway pressure (189) were reported. The responses in the steady

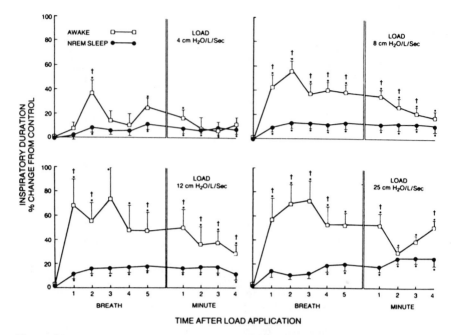

Figure 11   Mean (±SE) values for inspiratory duration (T_i) expressed as percent change from control over the first five consecutive breaths and 1–4 min after application of four different resistive loads during wakefulness and non-rapid-eye-movement (NREM) sleep. □–□, awake subjects; •——•, NREM sleep subjects. T_i increased dramatically after load application during wakefulness, with significantly smaller increments occurring during NREM sleep. *$p < 0.05$ different from control. †$p < 0.05$ different from NREM value. (From Ref. 185.)

state were generally small and consisted of a decrease in T_i, increase in T_e, and increase in diaphragm activity. There was no net change in ventilation or tidal volume (188). There was also no recruitment of expiratory muscles (189). Unfortunately, these results are confounded by the likely changes in upper airway resistance associated with the increase in lung volume and/or airway pressure and the uncertainty about the validity of EMG in the face of changing diaphragm position (178,179).

In summary, the responses to loading during sleep are much closer to those observed under anesthesia than to awake responses. This suggests that differences between wakefulness and anesthesia are simply due to lack of consciousness.

It may be argued that sleep is not a simple case of lack of consciousness but may involve specific suppression of reflex mechanisms. However, the similarity between the responses during sleep and in fully alert patients with the locked-in syndrome suggests that differences between awake and sleeping responses are related to mechanisms involving the motor cortex and executed by the pyramidal tracts.

Special Manipulations

A variety of experimental approaches have been utilized to circumvent the difficulties inherent in investigating conscious intact humans:

Role of Perception

As evident from the above discussion, timing responses to added loads are largely limited to the conscious state. An important issue is whether these responses represent automatic (reflex) mechanisms that are active only in the conscious state or are voluntary responses triggered by perception. This issue has been difficult to address because of the very low threshold for load detection (143). Thus, loads below the perceptual level are very small, and their consequences are expected to be too small relative to the noise of measurement (i.e., spontaneous breath-by-breath variability). Daubenspeck and associates (105,106,177) employed a highly sophisticated statistical approach (pseudorandom binary sequence, PRBS) that allowed them to detect, with confidence, very small changes in mechanical and neural responses to single-breath application of loads below the perceptual level. They found that inspiratory elastic and resistive loads elicit consistent reductions in neural T_e, thereby indicating that this response is reflexic. A similar conclusion was made from results of locked-in patients. These authors, however, did not find any changes in neural T_i in response to either load (105,106,177). One possible interpretation is that these responses require perception. On the other hand, because the loads were very small, it is possible that the mechanical perturbation was too weak to engage relevant reflexes.

Puddy and Younes (55) employed a different approach to permit assessment of responses to higher loads in the absence of perception. The magnitude of an elastic load was increased very slowly over a period of 18 min. They reasoned that since detection is related to the magnitude of step changes in load relative to background load [Weber's law (143)], this approach would increase the level of load at which perception occurs. This, in fact, is what happened, and they were able to evaluate responses up to a load of 6 cmH$_2$O/L in the absence of perception. There was a consistent and progressive reduction in both T_i and T_e as the load increased, indicating that both responses, although requiring consciousness, do not require perception. In five of the subjects, the load was suddenly increased at the end of the experiment to effect perception. Interestingly, whereas the preperceptual responses were consistent, the postperception responses were quite variable, with tidal volume and frequency changing in opposite directions in different subjects.

These two studies indicate that some of the differences between anesthetized and sleeping responses on one hand and conscious responses on the other are mediated by automatic mechanisms (i.e., do not require perception). These mechanisms, however, are operative only in the conscious state, and some (most notably T_i shortening with elastic loading) may even be effected by the cortico-spinal and corticobulbar tracts (cf. locked-in patients).

Why Do Inspiratory Resistive and Elastic Loads Elicit Opposite Effects on T_i?

As indicated earlier, the T_i prolongation with inspiratory resistive loads cannot be attributed to vagal feedback. The amount of prolongation in consciousness is also well in excess of that observed during sleep and anesthesia, or in patients with the locked-in syndrome, thereby indicating that it is largely due to higher mechanisms, requires consciousness, and is effected by the motor cortex. It is also clear that T_i shortening with inspiratory elastic loading is due to a higher-level mechanism and requires consciousness and intact efferent pathways from the motor cortex. The question arises as to how these higher mechanisms distinguish between the two loads even though both cause qualitatively similar perturbations to afferent mechanisms. Thus, in the absence of neural compensation, both loads would reduce volume-related vagal feedback and increase tension and decrease shortening of inspiratory muscles.

One possibility is that the subject recognizes an association between flow rate and the magnitude of an "abnormal" sensation related to the load (e.g., negative pressure or increased muscle tension) in the case of resistive loading (IRL) and a relation between volume and this "abnormal" sensation in the case of elastic loads (IEL). Strategies are then adopted to minimize these sensations, which would result in a reduction in flow rate in the case of IRL and in tidal volume in the case of IEL.

On the other hand, it is possible that the mechanism is much less sophisticated. Assume that the load, via increased tension or otherwise, results in an increase in activity of some afferent whose primary effect is to inhibit inspiration (e.g., tendon organs). In the case of IRL, this increase in inhibitory input will mirror flow, being maximal early in inspiration and declining later in that phase. With IEL, this inhibitory activity would progressively increase throughout inspiration. As indicated earlier, these two patterns of inhibitory inputs can result in opposite effects on T_i (129,130,190).

These possibilities were recently tested in two studies. In one (191), a sinusoidal negative-pressure load was applied during inspiration such that the load began declining within T_i. There was a significant prolongation of T_i even though there was no direct association between flow and pressure. However, the T_i prolongation was significantly less than that observed with an added resistance. This indicated that the association between flow and the abnormal pressure is also important. In a subsequent study, we (192) altered the phase relation between flow and the negative pressure. Negative pressure remained linked to flow, but the change in pressure was progressively delayed relative to flow. Phase shifts had little effect on the T_i response up to a point beyond which the T_i response abruptly decreased to an insignificant value. The results of these studies indicate that both the temporal pattern of pressure perturbation and an association between flow and pressure are important for the T_i responses observed in consciousness.

Role of Chest Wall Afferents in Mediating Load Responses in Consciousness

As indicated earlier, studies in anesthetized animals have suggested that chest wall reflexes may be sensitive to anesthesia. The possibility existed, therefore, that the differences between conscious and anesthetized responses were related to more active chest wall reflexes in the conscious state. Although studies in quadriplegic subjects do attempt to address this issue, it is not possible to completely isolate chest wall afferents from the load. Thus, in quadriplegia the diaphragm continues to be loaded.

We have developed a system whereby the chest wall alone can be loaded (i.e., no change in airway or intrathoracic pressure) or the opposite, where the load is applied at the airway but the chest wall (including diaphragm) is shielded from the load (5). We found that load detection deteriorates markedly when the chest wall alone is loaded whereas it is unaffected when the chest wall is protected from the load (5,6). This indicates that sources outside the respiratory muscles are more potent in signaling the load than chest wall afferents. More recently, we studied the steady-state response to elastic loading when the load was selectively applied to the chest wall and when the chest wall was shielded from the load (7). Tachypnea did not occur with either procedure although it developed when the load was applied in the usual way (i.e., at the mouth without protecting the chest wall). These studies indicate that higher centers likely utilize multiple inputs in the process of executing the timing responses to added loads.

VI. SUMMARY

Although some observations need to be confirmed and extended, there is sufficient information to allow the following tentative conclusions to be made about mechanisms of load compensation:

    1. Other than influences from the motor cortex, executed via the pyramidal tracts, there are only two major structural mechanisms for load compensation, the intrinsic properties of the respiratory muscles and chemical feedback. This applies across species and states (anesthesia, sleep, and wakefulness without cortical motor influences). The intrinsic properties temper the decrease in ventilation that might otherwise occur, and chemical feedback takes care of most of the rest to the

extent it is capable of. Vagal feedback makes a small contribution in defense of tidal volume (by lengthening T_i with inspiratory loading), but this is at the expense of frequency. Its influence on pattern also wanes as chemical feedback returns V_T toward control levels. Vagal feedback, therefore, plays a minor and temporary role. The role played by the vagus with expiratory loads (T_e prolongation) is essentially noncompensatory and very small over the range of loads to be reasonably expected in life (i.e., outside the laboratory).

2.   There are two minor compensatory responses that are also structural, a small increase in intercostal activity with inspiratory load (likely mediated by muscle spindles) and a reflex that shortens expiration during inspiratory loads. The latter appears to require consciousness but not perception.

3.   Cortical influences account for most of the differences between animals and between states. Cortical influences include timing responses and changes in intensity of muscle activity.

4.   Cortical influences account for the bulk of timing responses observed in conscious humans. These responses are, by and large, noncompensatory but serve to reduce abnormal sensation.

5.   The increase in intensity of respiratory muscle activation (i.e., rate of rise) in conscious preparations is almost entirely due either to chemical feedback or to cortical influences. There is no convincing evidence for the existence of any other neural reflexes capable of exciting respiratory neurons, to a functionally significant extent, in response to loads.

6.   Perception can clearly evoke cortically mediated changes in intensity of respiratory activation. It is not clear whether excitation via motor cortex can occur in the absence of perception.

7.   Subjective responses to perception account for the large interindividual differences in load responses. They also likely account for the different responses among different species while conscious. It is not clear whether the fundamental difference between reported conscious responses in some animals [e.g., dog (37,38) and goat (40–43) where conscious responses are hypercapnic and similar to sleeping responses] and human conscious responses (which are substantially different from sleeping responses) is related to differences in higher brain function among species or to extensive training, and hence adaptation, of these animals prior to formal testing.

8.   There is evidence that conscious responses to supraliminal loads wane with time, in addition to being influenced by experience. Virtually all experiments on conscious humans have not extended beyond a few minutes. It remains to be seen whether any nonchemical compensatory responses remain after longer-term load application. It is possible that with small and medium loads (i.e., those that can be readily compensated for by modest changes in blood gas tensions) responses after several hours of application may not be much different between consciousness and sleep or anesthesia. This information would clearly be relevant

to disease-related loading, which spans much longer periods than the usual laboratory experiments.

Acknowledgment

This work was supported by the Medical Research Council of Canada.

References

1. Anthonisen NR, Cherniack RM. Ventilatory control in lung disease. In: Hornbein TF, ed. Regulation of Breathing. New York: Marcel Dekker, 1981:965–987.
2. Younes M. Mechanisms of ventilatory failure. Curr Pulmonol 1993; 14:243–292.
3. Cherniack NS, Altose MD. Respiratory responses to ventilatory loading. In: Hornbein TF, ed. Regulation of Breathing. New York: Marcel Dekker, 1981:905–964.
4. Widdicombe JG. Reflexes from the upper respiratory tract. In: Cherniack NS, Widdicombe JG, eds. Handbook of Physiology: The Respiratory System, vol 2. Bethesda, MD: American Physiological Society, 1986:363–394.
5. Younes M, Jung D, Puddy A, Giesbrecht G, Sanii R. Role of the chest wall in detection of added elastic loads. J Appl Physiol 1990; 68(5):2241–2245.
6. Puddy A, Giesbrecht G, Sanii R, Younes M. Mechanism of detection of resistive loads in conscious humans. J Appl Physiol 1992; 72(6):2267–2270.
7. Giannouli E, Carlton T, Sanii R, Younes M. Mechanism of tachypnea with elastic loading in conscious humans. Am Rev Respir Dis 1993; 147:A166.
8. Killian KJ, Campbell EJM, Dyspnea. In: Roussos C, Macklem PT, eds. The Thorax. New York: Marcel Dekker, 1985:787–828.
9. Henke KG, Dempsey JA, Kowitz JM, Skatrud JB. Effects of sleep-induced increases in upper airway resistance on ventilation. J Appl Physiol 1990; 69:617–624.
10. Henke KG, Badr MS, Skatrud JB, Dempsey JA. Load compensation and respiratory muscle function during sleep. J Appl Physiol 1992; 72:1221–1234.
11. Hudgel DW, Hendricks C. Palate and hypopharynx sites of inspiratory narrowing of the upper airway during sleep. Am Rev Respir Dis 1988; 138:1542–1547.
12. Smith PL, Wise RA, Gold AR, Schwartz AR, Permutt S. Upper airway pressure-flow relationship in patients with obstructive sleep apnea. J Appl Physiol 1988; 64:789–795.
13. Schwartz AR, Smith PL, Wise RA, Gold AR, Permutt S. Induction of upper airway occlusion in sleeping individuals with subatmospheric nasal pressure. J Appl Physiol 1988; 64:789–795.
14. Miller RD, Hyatt RE. Obstructing lesions of the larynx and trachea: clinical and physiologic characteristics. Mayo Clin Proc 1969; 44:145–161.
15. Miller RD, Hyatt RE. Evaluation of obstructing lesions of the trachea and larynx by flow-volume loops. Am Rev Respir Dis 1973; 108:475–481.
16. Pride NB, Macklem PT. Lung mechanics in disease. In: Macklem PT, Mead J, eds. Handbook of Physiology: The Respiratory System, vol 3. Bethesda, MD: American Physiological Society, 1986:659–692.

17. Martin J, Powell E, Shore S, Emrich J, Engel LA. The role of respiratory muscles in the hyperinflation of bronchial asthma. Am Rev Respir Dis 1980; 121:441–447.

18. Muller N, Bryan AC, Zamel N. Tonic inspiratory muscle activity as a cause of hyperinflation in histamine-induced asthma. J Appl Physiol 1980; 49:869–874.

19. Sanii R, Younes M. Response of normal subjects to a flow-limiting expiratory resistance. Am Rev Respir Dis 1991; 143:A597.

20. Sant'Ambrogio G. Information arising from the tracheobronchial tree of mammals. Physiol Rev 1982; 62:531–569.

21. Coleridge HM, Coleridge JCG. Reflexes evoked from tracheobronchial tree and lungs. In: Cherniack NS, Widdicombe JG, eds. Handbook of Physiology: The Respiratory System, vol 2. Bethesda, MD: American Physiological Society, 1986: 394–430.

22. O'Donnell D, Anthonisen NR, Sanii R, Younes M. Effect of dynamic airway compression on breathing pattern and respiratory sensation in severe COPD. Am Rev Respir Dis 1987; 135:912–919.

23. Marini JJ. Lung mechanics determination at the bedside: Instrumentation and clinical application. Respir Care 1990; 35:669–696.

24. Smith TC, Marini JJ. Impact of PEEP on lung mechanics and work of breathing in severe airflow obstruction. The effect of PEEP on auto-PEEP. J Appl Physiol 1988; 65:1488–1499.

25. Lynne-Davies P, Couture J, Pengelly LD, Milic-Emili J. The immediate ventilatory response to added inspiratory elastic loads in cats. J Appl Physiol 1971; 30:512–516.

26. Lynne-Davies P, Couture J, Pengelly LD, West D, Bromage PR, Milic-Emili J. Partitioning of immediate ventilatory stability to added elastic loads in cats. J Appl Physiol 1971; 30:814–819.

27. Grunstein MM, Younes M, Milic-Emili J. Control of tidal volume and respiratory frequency in anesthetized cats. J Appl Physiol 1973; 35:463–476.

28. Younes M, Arkinstall W, Milic-Emili J. Mechanism of rapid ventilatory compensation to added elastic loads. J Appl Physiol 1973; 35:443–453.

29. Shannon R, Zechman FW. The reflex and mechanical response of the inspiratory muscles to an increased airflow resistance. Respir Physiol 1972; 16:51–69.

30. Miserocchi G, Milic-Emili J. Effect of mechanical factors on the relationship between rate and depth of breathing in cat. J Appl Physiol 1976; 41:277–285.

31. Read DJC, Freedman S, Kafer ER. Pressures developed by loaded inspiratory muscles in conscious and anesthetized man. J Appl Physiol 1974; 37:207–215.

32. Baydur A, Sassoon CS. Mechanisms of respiratory elastic load compensation in anesthetized humans. J Appl Physiol 1986; 60:613–617.

33. Zin WA, Behrakis PK, Luijendijk SC, Higgs BD, Baydur A, Boddener A, Milic-Emili J. Immediate response to resistive loading in anesthetized humans. J Appl Physiol 1986; 60:506–512.

34. Margaria CE, Iscoe S, Pengelly LP, Couture J, Don H, Milic-Emili J. Immediate ventilatory response to elastic loads and positive pressure in man. Respir Physiol 1973; 18:347–369.

35. Whitelaw WA, Derenne JP, Couture J, Milic-Emili J. Adaptation of anesthetized men to breathing through an inspiratory resistor. J Appl Physiol 1976; 41:285–291.

36. Polacheck J, Strong R, Arens J, Davies C, Metcalf I, Younes M. Phasic vagal influence on inspiratory motor output in anesthetized human subjects. J Appl Physiol 1980; 49:609–619.
37. Bowes G, Kozar LF, Andrey SM, Phillipson EA. Ventilatory responses to inspiratory flow-resistive loads in awake and sleeping dogs. J Appl Physiol 1983; 54(6):1550–1557.
38. Phillipson EA, Kozar LF, Murphy E. Respiratory load compensation in awake and sleeping dogs. J Appl Physiol 1976; 40:895–902.
39. Hutt DA, Parisi RA, Edelman NH, Santiago TV. Responses of diaphragm and external oblique muscles to flow-resistive loads during sleep. Am Rev Respir Dis 1991; 144:1107–1111.
40. Scardella AT, Santiago TV, Edelman NH. Naloxone alters the early response to an inspiratory flow-resistive load. J Appl Physiol 1989; 67:1747–1753.
41. Scardella AT, Parisi RA, Phair DK, Santiago TV, Edelman NH. The role of endogenous opioids in the ventilatory response to acute flow-resistive loads. Am Rev Respir Dis 1986; 133:26–31.
42. Petrozzino JJ, Scardella AT, Edelman NH, Santiago TV. Respiratory muscle acidosis stimulates endogenous opioids during inspiratory loading. Am Rev Respir Dis 1993; 147:607–615.
43. Bazzy AR, Haddad GG. Diaphragmatic fatigue in unanesthetized adult sheep. J Appl Physiol 1984; 57:182–190.
44. Axen K, Haas SS. Range of first-breath ventilatory responses to added mechanical loads in naive men. J Appl Physiol 1979; 46:743–751.
45. Im Hof V, West P, Younes M. Steady-state response of normal subjects to inspiratory resistive load. J Appl Physiol 1986; 60:1471–1481.
46. McIlroy MB, Eldridge FL, Thomas JP, Christie RV. The effect of added elastic and non-elastic resistances on the pattern of breathing in normal subjects. Clin Sci 1956; 15:337–344.
47. Zechman F, Hall FG, Hull WE. Effects of graded resistance to airflow in man. J Appl Physiol 1957; 10:356–362.
48. Daubenspeck JA. Influence of small mechanical loads on variability of breathing patterns. J Appl Physiol 1981; 50:299–306.
49. O'Donnell DE, Sanii R, Younes M. External mechanical loading in conscious humans: role of upper airway mechanoreceptors. J Appl Physiol 1988; 65:541–548.
50. Axen K, Haas SS, Haas F, Gaudino D, Haas A. Ventilatory adjustments during sustained mechanical loading in conscious humans. J Appl Physiol 1983; 55:1211–1218.
51. Freedman S, Weinstein SA. Effects of external elastic and threshold loading on breathing in man. J Appl Physiol 1965; 20:469–472.
52. Bland S, Lazerou L, Dyck G, Cherniack RM. The influence of the "chest wall" on respiratory rate and depth. Respir Physiol 1967; 3:47–54.
53. Pope H, Holloway R, Campbell EJM. The effects of elastic and resistive loading of inspiration on the breathing of conscious man. Respir Physiol 1968; 4:363–372.
54. Agostoni E, D'Angelo E, Piolini M. Breathing pattern in men during inspiratory elastic loads. Respir Physiol 1978; 34:279–393.

55. Puddy A, Younes M. Effect of slowly increasing elastic load on breathing in conscious humans. J Appl Physiol 1991; 70(3):1277–1283.

56. Lopata M, Pearle JL. Diaphragmatic EMG and occlusion pressure response to elastic loading during CO_2 rebreathing in humans. J Appl Physiol 1980; 49(4): 669–675.

57. Zechman FW, Frazier DP, Lally DA. Respiratory volume-time relationship during resistive loading in the cat. J Appl Physiol 1976; 40:177–183.

58. Grunstein MM, Wyszogrodski I, Milic-Emili J. Regulation of frequency and depth of breathing during expiratory loading in cats. J Appl Physiol 1975; 38:869–874.

59. Seaman RG, Zechman FW, Jr, Frazier DT. Responses of ventral respiratory group neurons to mechanical loading. J Appl Physiol 1983; 54:254–264.

60. D'Angelo E, Agostoni E. Immediate response to expiratory threshold loads. Respir Physiol 1975; 25:269–284.

61. Jammes Y, Bye PTP, Pardy RL, Katsardis C, Esau S, Roussos C. Expiratory threshold load under extracorporeal circulation: effects of vagal afferents. J Appl Physiol 1983; 55:307–315.

62. Gothe B, Cherniack NS. Effects of expiratory loading on respiration in humans. J Appl Physiol 1980; 49(4):601–608.

63. Daubenspeck JA, Bartlett DJ. Expiratory pattern and laryngeal responses to single-breath expiratory resistance loads. Respir Physiol 1983; 54:307–316.

64. Hill AR, Kaiser DL, Lu JY, Rochester DF. Steady-state response of conscious man to small expiratory resistance loads. Respir Physiol 1985; 61:369–381.

65. Poon CS, Younes M, Gallagher CG. Effects of expiratory resistive loads on respiratory motor output in conscious humans. J Appl Physiol 1987; 63(5):1837–1845.

66. Barnett TB, Rasmussen B. Separate resistive loading of the respiratory phases during mild hypercapnia in man. Acta Physiol Scand 1988; 133(3):355–364.

67. Bishop B, Bachofen H. Vagal control of ventilation and respiratory muscles during elevated pressures in the cat. J Appl Physiol 1972; 32:103–112.

68. D'Angelo E, Agostoni E. Tonic vagal influences on inspiratory duration. Respir Physiol 1975; 24:287–302.

69. Kelsen SG, Altose MD, Cherniack NS. The interaction of lung volume and chemical drive on respiratory muscle EMG and respiratory timing. J Appl Physiol 1977; 42: 287–294.

70. Derenne JP, Whitelaw WA, Couture J, Milic-Emili J. Load compensation during positive pressure breathing in anesthetized man. Respir Physiol 1986; 65:303–314.

71. Rahn H, Otis AB, Chadwick LE, Fenn WO. The pressure-volume diagram of the thorax and lung. Am J Physiol 1946; 146:161–178.

72. Agostoni E. Diaphragm activity and thoraco-abdominal mechanics during positive pressure breathing. J Appl Physiol 1962; 17:215–220.

73. Green M, Mead J, Sears TA. Muscle activity during chest wall restriction and positive pressure breathing in man. Respir Physiol 1978; 35:383–400.

74. Alex CA, Aronson, RM, Onal E, Lopata M. Effects of continuous positive airway pressure on upper airway and respiratory muscle activity. J Appl Physiol 1987; 62: 2026–2036.

75. Banzett RB, Inbar GF, Brown R, Goldman M, Rossier A, Mead J. Diaphragm electrical activity during negative lower torso pressure in quadriplegic men. J Appl Physiol 1981; 51:654–659.

76. Gillespie JR, Bruce E, Alexander J, Mead J. Breathing responses of unanesthetized man and guinea pigs to increased transrespiratory pressure. J Appl Physiol 1979; 47:119–125.

77. Younes M, Riddle W. A model for the relation between respiratory neural and mechanical outputs. I. Theory. J Appl Physiol 1981; 51:963–978.

78. Moxham J, Wiles CM, Newham D, Edwards RHT. Contractile function and fatigue of the respiratory muscles in man. In: Human Muscle Fatigue: Physiological Mechanisms. Ciba Found Symp 1981(82):197–206.

79. Edwards RHT, Faulkner JA. Structure and function of respiratory muscles. In: Roussos C, Macklem PT, eds. The Thorax. New York: Marcel Dekker, 1985:297–326.

80. Gordon AM, Huxley AF, Julian FJ. The variation in isometric tension with sarcomere length in vertebrate muscle fibres. J Physiol (Lond) 1966; 184:170–192.

81. Kim MJ, Druz WS, Danon J, Machnach W, Sharp JT. Mechanics of the canine diaphragm. J Appl Physiol 1976; 41:369–382.

82. Evanich MJ, Franco MJ, Lourenco RV. Force output of the diaphragm as a function of phrenic nerve firing rate and lung volume. J Appl Physiol 1973; 35:208–212.

83. Pengelly LD, Alderson A, Milic-Emili J. Mechanics of the diaphragm. J Appl Physiol 1971; 30:796–806.

84. Grassino A, Goldman MD, Mead J, Sears TA. Mechanics of the human diaphragm during voluntary contraction (statics). J Appl Physiol 1978; 44:829–837.

85. Farkas GA, Decramer M, Rochester DF, De Troyer A. Contractile properties of intercostal muscles and their functional significance. J Appl Physiol 1985; 59:528–535.

86. Jiang TX, Deschepper K, Demedts M, Decramer M. Effects of acute hyperinflation on the mechanical effectiveness of the parasternal intercostals. Am Rev Respir Dis 1989; 139:522–528.

87. Rack PMH, Westbury DR. The effects of length and stimulus rate on tension in the isometric cat soleus muscle. J Physiol (Lond) 1969; 204:443.

88. Edwards RHT. The diaphragm as a muscle: mechanisms underlying fatigue. Am Rev Respir Dis 1979; 119:81–84.

89. Farkas GA, Roussos C. Acute diaphragmatic shortening: in vitro mechanics and fatigue. Am Rev Respir Dis 1984; 130:434–438.

90. Marshall R. Relationships between stimulus and work of breathing at different lung volumes. J Appl Physiol 1962; 17:917–921.

91. Agostoni E, Mead J. Statics of the respiratory system. In: Handbook of Physiology. Respiration, sec 3, vol 1. Bethesda, MD: American Physiological Society, 1964: 387–409.

92. Eldridge FL, Vaughn KZ. Relationship of thoracic volume and airway occlusion pressure: muscular effects. J Appl Physiol 1977; 43:312–321.

93. Hill AV. The heat of shortening and the dynamic constants of muscle. Proc R Soc London Ser B 1938; 126:136–195.

94. Abbot BC, Wilkie DR. The relation between velocity of shortening and the tension-length curve of skeletal muscle. J Physiol (Lond) 1953; 120:214–223.

95. Ritchie JM. The relation between force and velocity of shortening in rat muscle. J Physiol (Lond) 1954; 123:633–639.
96. Agostoni E, Fenn WO. Velocity of muscle shortening as a limiting factor in respiratory airflow. J Appl Physiol 1960; 15:349–353.
97. Goldman MD, Grassino A, Mead J, Sears TA. Mechanics of the human diaphragm during voluntary contraction: dynamics. J Appl Physiol 1978; 44:840–848.
98. Otis AB. The work of breathing. In: Handbook of Physiology. Respiration, sec 3, vol 1. Bethesda, MD: American Physiological Society, 1964:463–476.
99. Mead J. Control of respiratory frequency. J Appl Physiol 1960; 15:325–336.
100. Bellemare F, Grassino. Effect of pressure and timing of contraction on human diaphragm fatigue. J Appl Physiol 1982; 53:1190–1195.
101. Eldridge FL. Relationship between respiratory nerve and muscle activity and muscle force output. J Appl Physiol 1975; 39:567–574.
102. Younes M, Riddle W. Relation between respiratory neural output and tidal volume. J Appl Physiol 1984; 56:1110–1119.
103. Younes M, Remmers J. Control of tidal volume and respiratory frequency. In: Hornbein TF, ed. Control of Breathing. New York: Marcel Dekker, 1981:617–667.
104. Younes M, Iscoe S, Milic-Emili J. A method for assessment of phasic vagal influence on tidal volume. J Appl Physiol 1975; 38:335–343.
105. Daubenspeck JA, Bennett FM. Immediate human breathing pattern responses to loads near the perceptual threshold. J Appl Physiol 1983; 55:1160–1166.
106. Kobylarz EJ, Daubenspeck JA. Immediate diaphragmatic electromyogram responses to imperceptible mechanical loads in conscious humans. J Appl Physiol 1992; 73:248–259.
107. Im Hof V, Dubo H, Daniels V, Younes M. Steady-state response of quadriplegic subjects to inspiratory resistive load. J Appl Physiol 1986; 60:1482–1492.
108. Martin J, Aubier M. Engel LA. Effects of inspiratory loading on respiratory muscle activity during expiration. Am Rev Respir Dis 1982; 125:352–358.
109. Martin JG, De Troyer A. The behaviour of the abdominal muscles during inspiratory mechanical loading. Respir Physiol 1982; 50:63–73.
110. Abbrecht PH, Rajagopal KR, Kyle RR. Expiratory muscle recruitment during inspiratory flow-resistive loading and exercise. Am Rev Respir Dis 1991; 144:113–120.
111. Citterio G, Agostoni E. Decay of inspiratory muscle activity and breath timing in man. Respir Physiol 1981; 43:117–132.
112. Remmers JE, Bartlett D Jr. Reflex control of expiratory airflow and duration. J Appl Physiol 1977; 42:80–87.
113. Zin WA, Pengelly LD, Milic-Emili J. Decay of inspiratory muscle pressure during expiration in anesthetized cats. J Appl Physiol 1983; 54:408–413.
114. Agostoni E, Citterio G, D'Angelo E. Decay rate of inspiratory muscle pressure during expiration in man. Respir Physiol 1979; 36:269–285.
115. Koehler RC, Bishop B. Expiratory duration and abdominal muscle responses to elastic and resistive loading. J Appl Physiol 1979; 46:730–737.
116. Banzett RB, Mead J. Reflex compensation for changes in operational length of inspiratory muscles. In: Roussos C, Macklem PT, eds. The Thorax. New York: Marcel Dekker, 1985:595–605.

117. Cunningham DJC, Robbins PA, Wolff CB. Integration of respiratory responses to changes in alveolar partial pressures of CO2 and O2 and in the arterial pH. In: Cherniack NS, Widdicombe JC, eds. Handbook of Physiology. The Respiratory System, vol 2. Bethesda, MD: American Physiological Society, 1986:475–528.

118. Fitzgerald RS, Lahiri S. Reflex responses to chemoreceptor stimulation. In: Cherniack NS, Widdicombe JG, eds. Handbook of Physiology: The Respiratory System, vol 2. Bethesda, MD: American Physiological Society, 1986:313–362.

119. Bledsoe SW, Hornbein TF. Central chemosensors and the regulation of their chemical environment. In: Hornbein TF, ed. Regulation of Breathing. New York: Marcel Dekker, 1981:347–428.

120. Clark FJ, von Euler C. On the regulation of depth and rate of breathing. J Physiol (Lond) 1972; 222:267–295.

121. Bradley GW, von Euler C, Marttila I, Roos B. Steady state effects of CO2 and temperature on the relationship between lung volume and inspiratory duration (Hering-Breuer threshold curve). Acta Physiol Scand 1974; 92:351–363.

122. Grunstein MM, Fisk WM, Leiter LA, Milic-Emili J. Effect of body temperature on respiratory frequency in anesthetized cats. J Appl Physiol 1973; 34:154–159.

123. Gautier H, Remmers JE, Bartlett D Jr. Control of the duration of expiration. Respir Physiol 1973; 18:205–221.

124. Bartoli A, Bystrzycak E, Guz A, Jain SK, Noble MIM, Trenchard D. Studies of the pulmonary vagal control of central respiratory rhythm in the absence of breathing movements. J Physiol (Lond) 1973; 230:449–465.

125. Younes M, Vaillancourt P, Milic-Emili J. Interaction between chemical factors and duration of apnea following lung inflation. J Appl Physiol 1974; 36:190–201.

126. Banzett RB, Lansing RW, Brown R. High-level quadriplegics perceive lung volume change. J Appl Physiol 1987; 62:567–573.

127. Younes M, Remmers JE, Baker J. Characteristics of inspiratory inhibition by phasic volume feedback in cats. J Appl Physiol 1978; 45:80–86.

128. Younes M, Polacheck J. Temporal changes in effectiveness of a constant inspiration terminating vagal stimulus. J Appl Physiol 1981; 50:1183–1192.

129. Younes M, Polacheck J. Central adaptation to inspiratory inhibitory, expiratory prolonging vagal input. J Appl Physiol 1985; 59:1072–1084.

130. Younes M, Baker J, Remmers JE. Temporal changes in effectiveness of an inspiratory inhibitory pontine stimulus. J Appl Physiol 1987; 62:1502–1512.

131. Gautier H. Pattern of breathing during hypoxia or hypercapnia of the awake or anesthetized cat. Respir Physiol 1976; 27:193–206.

132. Patterson JR, Grabois M. Locked-in syndrome: A review of 139 cases. Stroke 1986; 17:758–764.

133. Bartoli A, Cross BA, Guz A, Huszczuk A, Jefferies R. The effect of varying tidal volume on the associated phrenic motoneuron output: studies of vagal and chemical feedback. Respir Physiol 1975; 25:135–155.

134. Pack AI, Delaney RG, Fishman AP. Augmentation of phrenic neural activity by increased rates of lung inflation. J Appl Physiol 1981; 50:149–161.

135. Dimarco AF, von Euler C, Romaniuk JR, Yamamoto Y. Low threshold facilitation of inspiration by lung volume increments. Acta Physiol Scand 1980; 109:343–344.

136. Puddy A, Younes M. Effect of inspiratory flow rate on respiratory motor output in normal humans. Am Rev Respir Dis 1992; 146:787–789.
137. Shannon R. Reflexes from respiratory muscles and costovertebral joints. In: Fishman AP, ed. Handbook of Physiology. The Respiratory System, vol 2. Bethesda, MD: American Physiological Society, 1986:431–447.
138. Duron B. Intercostal and diaphragmatic muscle endings and afferents. In: Hornbein TF, ed. Regulation of Breathing. New York: Marcel Dekker, 1981:473–540.
139. Frazier DT, Revelette WR. Role of phrenic afferents in the control of breathing. J Appl Physiol 1991; 70:491–496.
140. Younes M, Youssef M. Effect of five human anesthetics on respiratory control in cats. J Appl Physiol 1978; 44:596–606.
141. Corda M, Eklund G, von Euler C. External intercostal and phrenic motor responses to changes in respiratory load. Acta Physiol Scand 1965; 63:391–400.
142. Remmers JE, Tsiaras WG. Effect of lateral cervical cord lesions on the respiratory rhythm of anesthetized, decerebrate cats after vagotomy. J Physiol (Lond) 1973; 233:63–74.
143. Zechman FW, Wiley RL. Afferent inputs to breathing: respiratory sensation. In: Cherniack NS, Widdicombe JG, eds. Handbook of Physiology. The Respiratory System. Control of Breathing, sec 3, vol 2, part 1. Bethesda, MD: American Physiological Society, 1986:449–474.
144. Cherniack NS, Milic-Emili J. Mechanical aspects of loaded breathing. In: Roussos C, Macklem PT, eds. The Thorax. New York: Marcel Dekker, 1985:751–786.
145. Aviado DM Jr, Li TH, Kalow W, Schmidt CF, Thurnbull GL, Peskin GW, Hess ME, Weiss AJ. Respiratory and circulatory reflexes from the perfused heart and pulmonary circulation of the dog. Am J Physiol 1951; 165:261–277.
146. Lloyd T Jr. Breathing response to lung congestion with and without left heart distension. J Appl Physiol 1988; 65:131–136.
147. Wead WB, Cassidy SS, Coast JR, Hagler HK, Reynolds RC. Reflex cardiorespiratory responses to pulmonary vascular congestion. J Appl Physiol 1987; 62:870–879.
148. Hatridge J, Haji A, Perex-Padilla JR, Remmers JE. Rapid shallow breathing caused by pulmonary vascular congestion in cats. J Appl Physiol 1989; 67:2257–2264.
149. Giesbrecht GG, Younes M. Respiratory response to pulmonary vascular congestion in conscious dogs. J Appl Physiol 1993; 74:345–353.
150. Grunstein MM, Derenne JP, Milic-Emili J. Control of depth and frequency of breathing during baroreceptor stimulation in cats. J Appl Physiol 1975; 39:395–404.
151. Kostreva DR, Hopp FA, Zuperku EJ, Igler FO, Coon RL, Kampine JP. Respiratory inhibition with sympathetic afferent stimulation in the canine and primate. J Appl Physiol 1978; 44:718–724.
152. Santiago TV, Remolina C, Scoles V III, Edelman NH. Endorphins and the control of breathing. N Engl J Med 1981; 304:1190–1195.
153. Simon PM, Pope A, Lahive K, et al. Naloxone does not alter response to hypercapnia or resistive loading in chronic obstructive pulmonary disease. Am Rev Respir Dis 1989; 139:134–138.
154. Bradley GW. The response of the respiratory system to elastic loading in cats. Respir Physiol 1972; 16:142–160.

155. Sant'Ambrogio G, Widdicombe JG. Respiratory reflexes acting on the diaphragm and inspiratory intercostal muscles of the rabbit. J Physiol (Lond) 1965; 180:766–779.

156. Jammes Y, Mathiot MJ, Delpierre S, Grimaud Ch. Role of vagal and spinal sensory pathways on eupneic diaphragmatic activity. J Appl Physiol 1986; 60:479–485.

157. Derenne J, Ph, Couture J, Iscoe S, Whitelaw, WA, Milic-Emili J. Regulation of breathing in anesthetized human subjects. J Appl Physiol 1976; 40:804–814.

158. Bruce EN, Smith JD, Grodins FS. Chemical and reflex drive to breathing during resistance loading in cats. J Appl Physiol 1974; 37:176–182.

159. Orthner FH, Yamamoto WS. Transient respiratory response to mechanical loads at fixed blood gas levels in cats. J Appl Physiol 1974; 36:280–287.

160. Iscoe S. Phrenic afferents and ventilatory control at increased end-expiratory lung volumes in cats. J Appl Physiol 1989; 66:1297–1303.

161. Fryman DL, Frazier DT. Diaphragm afferent modulation of phrenic motor drive. J Appl Physiol 1987; 62:2436–2441.

162. Finkler J, Iscoe S. Control of breathing at elevated lung volumes in anesthetized cats. J Appl Physiol 1984; 53:839–844.

163. Winning AJ, Widdicombe JG. The effect of lung reflexes on the pattern of breathing in cats. Respir Physiol 1976; 27:253–266.

164. Noble MIM, Frankel HL, Else W, Guz A. The sensation produced by threshold resistive loads to breathing. Eur J Clin Invest 1972; 2:72–77.

165. Sant'Ambrogio FB, Mathew OP, Clark WD, Sant'Ambrogio G. Laryngeal influences on breathing pattern and posterior cricoarytenoid muscle activity. J Appl Physiol 1985; 58:1298–1304.

166. De Troyer A, Estenne M, Heilporn A. Mechanisms of active expiration in tetraplegic subjects. N Engl J Med 1986; 314:740–744.

167. Noble MIM, Frankel HL, Else W, Guz A. The ability of man to detect added resistive loads to breathing. Clin Sci (Lond) 1971; 41:285–287.

168. Zechman FW, O'Neill R, Shannon R. Effect of low cervical spinal cord lesions on detection of increased airflow resistance in man. Physiologist 1967; 10:356. (abstract).

169. Axen K. Adaptations of quadriplegic men to consecutively loaded breaths. J Appl Physiol 1984; 56:1099–1103.

170. Axen K, Haas SS. Effect of thoracic deafferentation on load-compensating mechanisms in humans. J Appl Physiol 1982; 52:757–767.

171. Axen K. Ventilatory responses to mechanical loads in cervical cord-injured humans. J Appl Physiol 1982; 52:748–756.

172. Kelling JS, DiMarco AF, Gottfried SB, Altose MD. Respiratory responses to ventilatory loading following low cervical spinal cord injury. J Appl Physiol 1985; 59:1752–1756.

173. Manning H, McCool FD, Scharf SM, Garshick E, Brown R. Oxygen cost of resistive-loaded breathing in quadriplegia. J Appl Physiol 1992; 73:825–831.

174. O'Donnell DE, Sanii R, Dubo H, Loveridge B, Younes M. Steady-state ventilatory responses to expiratory resistive loading in quadriplegics. Am Rev Respir Dis 1993; 147:54–59.

175. Axen K, Bishop M, Haas F. Respiratory load compensation in neuromuscular disorders. J Appl Physiol 1988; 64:2659–2666.

176. De Troyer A, Pride NB. The respiratory system in neuromuscular disease. In: Roussos C, Macklem PD, eds. The Thorax. New York: Marcel Dekker, 1985:1089–1121.

177. Harver A, Daubenspeck JA. Human breathing pattern responses to loading with increased background impedance. J Appl Physiol 1989; 66:680–686.

178. McKenzie DK, Gandevia SC. Changes in human diaphragmatic electromyogram with positive pressure breathing. Neurol Sci Lett 1986; 7086–7090.

179. Brancatisano AS, Kelly SM, Tully A, Loring SH, Engel LA. Postural changes in spontaneous and evoked regional diaphragmatic activity in dogs. J Appl Physiol 1989; 66:1699–1705.

180. Tapper DP, Duncan SR, Kraft S, Kagawa FT, Marshall S, Theodore J. Detection of inspiratory resistive loads by heart-lung transplant recipients. Am Rev Respir Dis 1992; 145:458–460.

181. Iber C, Berssenbrugge A, Skatrud JB, Dempsey JA. Ventilatory adaptations to resistive loading during wakefulness and non-REM sleep. J Appl Physiol 1982; 52:607–614.

182. Wilson PA, Skatrud JB, Dempsey JA. Effects of slow wave sleep on ventilatory compensation to inspiratory elastic loading. Respir Physiol 1984; 55:103–120.

183. Badr MS, Skatrud JB, Dempsey JA, Begle RL. Effect of mechanical loading on inspiratory and expiratory muscle activity during NREM sleep. J Appl Physiol 1990; 68:1195–1201.

184. Hudgel DW, Hulholland M, Hendricks C. Neuromuscular and mechanical responses to inspiratory resistive loading during sleep. J Appl Physiol 1987; 63:601–608.

185. Wiegand L, Zwillich C, White D. Sleep and the ventilatory response to resistive loading in normal man. J Appl Physiol 1988; 64:1186–1195.

186. Kuna ST, Smickley JS. Response of genioglossus muscle activity to nasal airway occlusion in normal sleeping adults. J Appl Physiol 1988; 64:347–353.

187. Issa FG, Sullivan CE. Arousal and breathing responses to airway occlusion in healthy sleeping adults. J Appl Physiol 1983; 55:1113–1119.

188. Begle RL, Skatrud JB, Dempsey JA. Ventilatory compensation for changes in functional residual capacity during sleep. J Appl Physiol 1987; 62:1299–1306.

189. Begle RL, Skatrud JB. Hyperinflation and expiratory muscle recruitment during NREM sleep in humans. Respir Physiol 1990; 82:47–64.

190. Mathew OP, Farber JP. Effect of upper airway negative pressure on respiratory timing. Respir Physiol 1983; 54:252–268.

191. Sanii R, Younes M. Steady-state response of normal subjects to an inspiratory sinusoidal pressure load. J Appl Physiol 1988; 64(2):511–520.

192. Younes M, Sanii R. Effect of phase shifts in pressure-flow relationship on response to inspiratory resistance. J Appl Physiol 1989; 67(2):699–706.

193. Younes M. Patient-ventilator interaction with pressure-assisted modalities of ventilatory support. Semin Respir Med 1993; 14:299–322.

20

Respiratory Sensations and Their Role in the Control of Breathing

STEVEN A. SHEA
and ROBERT B. BANZETT

Harvard School of Public Health
Boston, Massachusetts

ROBERT W. LANSING

University of Arizona
Tucson, Arizona

I. Introduction

Humans (and presumably other animals) can perceive a wide range of respiratory sensations—perception of motion and position, localized irritation, and more generalized feelings including respiratory discomfort (e.g., an urge to breathe). Since we are able to voluntarily control breathing, we are able to alter breathing in response to these respiratory sensations.

This chapter considers techniques used to obtain reliable measurements of respiratory sensations, describes the different qualities of respiratory-related sensations and their afferent pathways, and discusses to what extent and under what circumstances respiratory sensations may influence breathing.

II. Measurement of Respiratory Sensations

A. Language

Most standard psychophysical experiments concern sensory responses to external stimuli (visual, auditory, or tactile) that are easily recognized and described by both the experimenter and the subject. Even these quantitative studies of perception assume a shared language between the experimenter and subject. In the usual psychophysical experiment, the subject has little difficulty in understanding what to do when asked to rate the intensity of a sound or light, but if asked to rate a respiratory sensation such as "breathlessness" or "breathing effort," different subjects may rate different aspects of their sensory experience. One reason is that respiratory sensations arise, in part, from visceral receptors (such as pulmonary receptors and chemoreceptors), and people seldom have the need or opportunity to learn to finely discriminate and describe visceral sensations. (It is no accident that the phrase "gut feeling" entered the vernacular as a synonym for knowledge that is very real, but is hard to describe.) The study of pain shares this apparent difficulty, yet studies of pain sensation in people of differing backgrounds have shown that common language can be developed to reliably communicate specific qualities of internal sensation (1). Similarly, recent studies have found that subjects can discriminate respiratory sensations produced by different clinical conditions or laboratory stimuli, and subjects can rate the intensity of respiratory sensations with precision and with a reliable relationship to the stimulus (2–5). Investigators have assessed respiratory sensations in many ways, which can create confusion when one attempts to compare results. For example, some studies examine "respiratory discomfort," others the detection of mechanical hindrances to breathing, and still others the scaling of sensations of spontaneous breathing. Investigators instruct subjects differently even in apparently similar experiments, and sometimes infer sensations without stating what subjects actually reported (for instance, many papers report that subjects experienced "dyspnea," but few subjects can be expected to use the word dyspnea). Some investigators have simply asked their subjects to describe their sensations, others have asked more specific questions, and others have systematically tested detection abilities or magnitude scaling without much reference to the character of the sensation. Subjective reports obtained in respiratory studies or clinical histories are limited by the verbal abilities and past experience of the subject and are easily influenced by the experimenter or physician. Descriptions given freely without guidance by the experimenter may differ from those given when the subject or patient is asked to accept or reject a descriptor. The number and kind of descriptors presented usually reflect the expectations of the experimenter. In designing or interpreting any respiratory psychophysical study, one must pay careful attention to language, both in defining the experimental task to the subject and in reporting the results.

B. Psychophysical Measures

Several measures of sensory performance have become fundamental to psychophysical studies since the inception of the field with the pioneering work of Fechner and Weber (reviewed in 6). "Detection" studies assess the smallest stimulus the subject can perceive ("absolute threshold") or the least perceptible stimulus change ("difference threshold"). "Magnitude" studies require the subject to judge the intensity of a range of stimuli, which may be done in several ways: (1) by asking the subject to rate the stimulus intensity on a numerical or verbal scale (magnitude scaling), requiring agreement on the meaning of points along the scale (this scale may have ordinal, interval, or, less frequently, ratio properties), (2) by asking the subject to reproduce the stimulus, say by turning a rheostat to match light intensity to the intensity of a stimulus light or moving a limb to copy a joint angle of the opposite limb (magnitude production), or (3) by asking the subject to produce another action of comparable intensity, say by gripping a hand dynamometer with different degrees of force to indicate the intensity of a sound (cross-modality matching). Another routine measurement is determination of the strongest level of noxious stimulus that a subject is willing to tolerate ("tolerance" or "upper threshold"). In all the above, the intensity of the physical stimulus is varied and subjects' responses are used to obtain a numerical estimate of discrimination or tolerance for stimulus change. The reader is referred to reviews on psychophysics (7,8). The literature on perception of pain and other sensations shows that absolute values for psychophysical measures vary with the testing procedures used and the subject studied. One can, however, discriminate changes in these measures in an individual subject with much greater resolution, enabling one to study the effects of various interventions.

Another category of sensory processing that must be considered in the detection of afferent signals is "perception without awareness" (9). This apparent contradiction in terms refers to the ability of subjects to consciously discriminate stimuli, even when they report that they are not "aware" of the stimulus. For instance, some subjects correctly identified tidal volume changes, even when they reported that they were only guessing (10). Sensory signals used to control voluntary movement include those the subject is aware of, those the subject is not aware of but can perceive, and those operating automatically at a completely unconscious level.

How Do Psychophysical Measures Relate to Sensory Performance Under More Natural Conditions?

In the laboratory the aim often is to test the limits of perceptual ability under optimal conditions; the type of stimulus and the time of presentation are known in advance, a single specific response is required, and attempts are made to control the levels of practice, attention, and motivation. Subjects in a respiratory psychophysical experiment are usually placed on a mouthpiece or other breathing device and instructed to attend to their respiratory sensations. Under such controlled conditions respiratory sensation can be quite sensitive; for instance, published reports show that people can discriminate 100-ml changes in tidal volume (see below). In natural circumstances conditions are not necessarily optimal: a single respiratory variable seldom changes in isolation, may change gradually, and changes occur when the subject is not attending to breathing so that discrimination is likely to be degraded. For instance, West and co-workers (11) showed that subjects did not report changes in tidal volume stimulated by exercise or hypercapnia until volume had doubled.

An additional caveat in translating laboratory results to real life is the difference in sensation that arises from different sources of motor control. Neural transmission in somatosensory pathways is modified by both the nature of the movement task and the source of the motor control. For example, when monkeys make preprogrammed rapid movements, there is less sensory input to the cortex than during slow and precisely guided movements (reviewed in 12). Similar effects are likely when breathing is measured in the laboratory, inasmuch as breathing is to some extent under voluntary control any time the subject thinks breathing is being studied. Respiratory sensations (e.g., sensitivity to volume change) may be different for spontaneous and voluntary breathing and may differ during different breathing tasks.

C. Behavioral measures

Behavioral changes in breathing can also be used to study sensitivity to respiratory stimuli, and circumvent the need for the experimenter and subject to agree on language. A subject's maximal breath-hold duration or the arterial gases at the "breakpoint" have frequently been used as behavioral measures of the tolerable limit of the sensation of an "urge to breathe" (e.g., 13–15). Similarly, the tolerance for stimuli such as external resistive loads or blood gas changes can be measured by the level at which the person elects to quit the procedure or signals for a change (e.g., 16). The natural response to a large external load is not to increase effort, but rather to pull the mouthpiece out (as often stated by Jere Mead). Procedures that do not depend on language have been used successfully to study sensory systems in animals (reviewed in 17). Such techniques recently have been applied to the study of respiratory load detection in dogs (which were trained to lift a paw when they detected a load; 18) and to sensitivity to hypoxia in rats (which were trained to withdraw from a chamber with low inspired Po_2 to avoid punishment; 19). Such behavioral measures permit the study of neural mechanisms of sensation in animals with various experimental interventions that are not possible in humans, including neural lesions.

D. Event-Related Potentials

Electrical potentials recorded from the scalp provide a direct measure of activity in sensory, cortical, and efferent pathways. These event-related potentials (ERPs) can be obtained noninvasively under reasonably natural conditions. Event related potentials can confirm the existence of a pathway to the cortex, can determine whether that pathway has been altered by experimental or clinical conditions, and can provide a nonverbal measure of signals reaching the cortex. They may be of particular advantage in comparing sensory physiology of humans with that of other animals. Sophisticated analysis of potentials recorded from many sites on the scalp may even allow three-dimensional mapping of sensory areas (20). An extensive literature is available on somatosensory potentials (21), but only recently have potentials associated with respiratory sensation and movement been investigated in humans (see Section III.B). Usually hundreds of responses that are triggered from the onset of the stimulus must be averaged to bring the sensory signal out of background noise. Respiratory stimuli can be presented only once per breath, requiring very long experimental sessions. In addition, many respiratory stimuli, such as blood gas changes, do not have the sharp stimulus onset needed to trigger evoked potential recordings. The very short-latency components (before 20 msec) appear to emanate from subcortical stations or projections, later components (20–80 msec) indicate the arrival of impulses in the primary sensory area, and still later components (80–400 msec) are associated with cognitive processes such as perception and recognition. These very late components are markedly influenced by memory, motivation, and state of expectancy, whereas the early potentials vary more directly with the physical properties of the stimulus. Neural afferent signals project to several brainstem and cortical areas, often along parallel paths (22). In some experiments the thresholds or intensity functions measured by somatosensory ERP waveforms closely match those obtained from psychophysical judgments, but in others they do not (21,23). Since ERP waveforms are composites of potentials originating from several cortical and subcortical sites and are unlikely to be identified with a single stage of sensory processing, even close correspondence between perception and potential cannot establish that they reflect the same neural events (24). These considerations argue against equating ERP waveforms with conscious perception of respiratory sensations; however, this technique has value for understanding the physiology of the sensory neural processing that precedes or underlies perceptions.

E. Individual Differences

Psychophysical studies show that people differ in their abilities to discriminate and report sensation. Since cognitive and decision processes intervene between afferent input and a subject's report of the sensation, some of this variability may represent differences in reporting, rather than differences in perception. Subject-to-subject differences in sensory threshold can reflect differences in each subject's criteria for deciding that a stimulus change has occurred. For instance, a subject may be reluctant to report feeling a sensation unless he or she is very certain; this "high decision criterion" will cause the experimenter to overestimate the stimulus strength necessary for detection. Decision criteria can be influenced by factors such as expectancy, motivation, and so forth. This problem with classical detection procedures has been addressed by signal detection approaches to psychophysics that systematically assess or eliminate the effect of decision criteria (25). These techniques have been used in a few respiratory studies (4,10,26–29). The relationship of perceptual judgments to stimulus intensity can also be influenced by the way the subject chooses to use numbers, verbal categories, or analog positions on a scale presented to him or her. As a result, the power law exponents that describe magnitude estimations can vary considerably among subjects for respiratory sensation as well as for other sensory modalities (30–32). Apart from the way in which subjects' decisions and experimental designs can systematically shape the results, a few subjects simply have difficulty in adjusting to experimental situations and in carrying out the sensory tasks given them. Their performance is inconsistent from trial to trial and does not improve with instruction or practice. It is common in many laboratories to exclude such "poor" subjects in favor of those who give reasonably reliable data over many successive trials (this is seldom, if ever, reported in print). This practice is valid when experiments are designed to test the limit of performance—but one must remember that such individuals exist and they may over-report or under-report symptoms in clinical situations.

F. Modulators of Respiratory Sensations

All measures of sensation can be influenced by a subject's motivation, state of fatigue, selective attention to available stimuli, and level of wakefulness or arousal. In the laboratory, these are usually controlled in such a way as to produce the best possible perceptual performance. Often, though, variation in one or more of these factors is intrinsic to the condition being studied; for example, changes in alertness accompany respiratory stimulation by hypoxia or hypercapnia; leg fatigue almost invariably accompanies respiratory stimulation during treadmill testing. Tolerance thresholds and intensity ratings of breathing discomfort (for example during hypercapnia) are also unquestionably influenced by the same personal characteristics that are known to influence response to pain: cultural differences, past experience, level of anxiety, perceived duration of the discomfort, perceived consequences of giving high or low ratings, and the ability to personally control the duration and intensity of the stimulus (e.g., 33–38).

III. Qualities of Respiratory Sensations and Afferent Pathways

Respiratory sensations can be divided into two broad (and not entirely separable) categories: respiratory proprioception and respiratory discomfort. These sensations arise from several afferent sources. Respiratory proprioception is the sense of the mechanical motion, displacements, position, and forces whether these sensations arise from somatic receptors or receptors in the lungs and other viscera, although all respiratory discomfort is often lumped under the single term "dyspnea." Comroe (39) recognized the difficulty this presented to understanding and suggested that "we must look for the sensory receptors, sensory pathways, and thalamic or cortical centers which are responsible for the perception of respiratory discomfort." Pain perception is a good analogy; studies of pain physiology and pain psychophysics have improved our understanding of the character of various kinds of pain and how to relate pain perception to the various pain pathways. However, we understand less about respiratory sensation than about pain and many other somatic perceptions. Our discussion here concentrates on identifiable respiratory sensations, largely neglecting the more complex constellations of sensation that comprise clinical reports of dyspnea.

Standard psychophysical procedures have been used to determine those respiratory variables that can be sensed, to quantify the resulting sensations, and to relate sensations to language used by subjects (e.g., 30,40,41). Subjects can accurately scale their perceptions of voluntarily produced respiratory muscle force (pressure) and movement (volume change) (42–44). For example, subjects can perceive and report changes of tidal volume as small as 50–100 ml (45–48). As one might expect, subjects describe changes in tidal volume as "smaller [or larger] breaths." The perception of external resistive and elastic loads has been well studied; the threshold for load detection is closely related to the airway opening pressure developed, and subjects are able to detect resistive or elastic loads that result in pressures of only about 1 cmH$_2$O (reviewed in 30). When large loads are applied, subjects speak of increased "effort" or "work" of breathing (2,44). Induced bronchoconstriction in asthmatics feels qualitatively different from external loading; subjects describe "chest tightness" in preference to "work" or "effort," and much greater external resistance is needed to evoke a similar degree of discomfort (49). Subjects can detect increases of 3–7 torr in end-tidal P$_{CO_2}$, reporting sensations such as "urge to breathe," "shortness of breath," and "starved for air" (4,28,50).

It is likely that one accommodates to continued respiratory stimuli—either centrally or at the receptor level. For instance, normal subjects whose ventilation is mechanically assisted for some period report that it feels "harder to breathe" when they resume normal breathing (51,52). This sensation disappears after a few breaths. It is plausible that gradual sensory accommodation to derangement in blood gases occurs in patients with lung disease, which would explain why some patients tolerate severe chronic hypercapnia and hypoxia.

A. Possible Afferent Origins of Perceived Sensations

Many afferent paths are available for the perception of breathing, and we know a great deal about the sensory receptors capable of transducing physical stimuli related to breathing and the reflex actions elicited by those receptors. These primary afferent pathways are well covered elsewhere in this book. Here we will briefly remind the reader of the receptors, their respective sensed variables, and discuss whether the afferent information reaches consciousness and what sensations are evoked. It took nearly 100 years to establish that limb muscle receptors give rise to perceived kinesthetic sensations (53), so it is not surprising that we know very little about the origin of breathing sensations. Natural sensations of respiratory movement undoubtedly result from combined afferent sources, even though one source may predominate, so introspection alone cannot be used to discover which receptors are contributing. To distinguish the contribution of each, the various possible afferent pathways must be selectively activated or selectively disrupted and the effects on perception studied. The many structures moved during a breath—the rib cage, spine, skin, airways, lungs, abdominal contents, and muscles of the head, neck, chest, and abdomen—are mechanically connected. It is, therefore, difficult to selectively stimulate respiratory mechanoreceptors. Changes in breathing usually produce changes in blood gases, and vice versa. If several alternate or parallel inputs to the brain exist, disruption of one may have little effect on the sensation detected.

Receptors in the Lungs and Lower Airways

A variety of visceral mechanoreceptors from the airways and lungs discharge in response to movement and pressures in the normal range of breathing (reviewed in 54,55). Short-latency responses have been evoked in the somatosensory cortex of cat and monkey following lung inflation or vagal stimulation (56,57). Sensations localized to the throat, chest, and abdomen have been elicited by stimulation of the human cortex (58). Subjects are certainly capable of perceiving a variety of mechanical stimuli in the thoracic and abdominal viscera and of localizing the region from which they arise. Mechanical or electrical stimulation of the large airways is perceived as irritating, tickling, uncomfortable, or painful, and in some cases can be localized on the left or right side or within a few inches longitudinally (59). Unpleasant "burning" sensations can be evoked by stimulating small fibers in the lungs with capsaicin (these sensations appear to be quite different from unpleasant sensations evoked by blood gas derangement) (60). Normal subjects can detect small changes in tidal volume, but this information could arise in the chest wall, upper airway, or pulmonary afferents.

Two strategies have been used to learn whether breathing movements can be perceived via intrathoracic afferents: their principal input to the brain (the vagus nerve) has been selectively blocked, or other possible sources have been eliminated leaving only the vagal input intact. Local anesthetic block of the vagus and glossopharyngeal nerves caused no change in the sensations of normal breathing or the detection of inspiratory loads in informed subjects; sensations during breath holding and hypercapnia were altered, presumably by the loss of peripheral chemoreceptors (61). Hence, disruption of pulmonary afferents has not yielded clear evidence of their normal contribution to perception, as might be expected because of the redundant pathways available from chest wall and upper airways. In the converse experiment, five quadriplegic subjects with C-1 to C-3 transections (mechanically ventilated through a tracheostomy, leaving only the vagus nerve as a sensory path for volume detection) detected 10% changes in ventilator-delivered tidal volume (10). (It is interesting to note that a given tidal volume is perceived as being smaller during hypercapnia; 4,28,62.) The ability of quadriplegics to detect volume changes was not substantially different from that of normal subjects ventilated through the mouth. These quadriplegic subjects were unaware of cues from the neck or head and were definite in localizing the source of their sensations within the chest. A further experiment in one of these subjects showed that volume detection could be abolished when pulmonary and lower airways' receptors were blocked with a high dose of lidocaine aerosol (63). These data suggest that pulmonary stretch receptors can provide conscious perception of volume.

Receptors in the Chest Wall

Muscle, tendon, and joint receptors are abundant in somatic respiratory structures (64), and their afferents terminate on motor centers throughout the nervous system: spine, brainstem, cerebellum, cortex (e.g., 65–68). Such afferents are important in the perception of limb motion (69) and can be expected to play a role in respiratory proprioception. Stimulation of intercostal and phrenic afferents has been shown to evoke potentials in the trunk area of the sensory cortex (68).

Lung volume is paralleled by chest wall volume; therefore, chest wall receptors could play a role in tidal volume perception. Spindle receptors in the intercostal muscles and joint receptors of the ribs are capable of reporting rib cage volume (reviewed in 70). Similarly, volume displacement of the diaphragm-abdomen pathway might be detected by the few spindles in the diaphragm and by spindles in the abdominal wall musculature. When inspiration is active, Golgi tendon organs could also contribute to volume perception, because lung inflation volume is strongly related to inspiratory muscle tension through respiratory system compliance. Accurate volume perception from the chest wall would necessitate a relatively complex integration of information—owing to the several degrees of freedom with which the chest wall can expand (71,72) and to the modulation of afferent information by both alpha and gamma motoneurons (73). Estimation of tidal volume is changed by interventions such as vibration, elastic loading, and fatigue, which are thought to alter respiratory muscle proprioception, demonstrating that in different situations chest wall afferents may improve accuracy or introduce error in volume perception (42,46,74). Volume perception has not yet been tested in subjects who lack afferent input from the lungs and upper airways (e.g., tracheostomized heart-lung transplant patients) to determine whether chest wall afferents alone can provide a good sense of tidal volume.

⅃

Perception of inspiratory loads is directly related to the pressure developed by inspiratory muscles (43,75). Therefore, it seems probable that respiratory muscle receptors play a role in detection of loads (e.g., 43,76), although in most experimental situations a corresponding pressure is developed across the extrathoracic airways thereby providing an alternative pathway for perception (see below). Force exerted by the respiratory muscles can be sensed by Golgi tendon organs or indirectly by the spindles. (Extrafusal and intrafusal fibers are coactivated; if muscle shortening is impeded, the intrafusal fibers will tend to stretch the spindle receptor, increasing its discharge.) Blockade of the vagus nerve with local anesthetic (61) or denervation of the lungs by transplantation (77) does not diminish the ability to detect external inspiratory loads, suggesting that pulmonary receptors are not needed for load perception. No single group of respiratory muscles has been found to be essential for load detection (78,79).

Nociceptive receptors innervated by small unmyelnated afferent fibers are also found in respiratory muscle (80–83). These receptors have been shown to have reflex effects and probably also give rise to sensation—perhaps the unpleasant sensations of respiratory muscle fatigue.

Upper Airway Receptors

The extrathoracic airways are endowed with temperature receptors excited by the flow of cool or dry air and mechanoreceptors sensitive to positive and negative transmural pressure swings (55). The "flow" receptors should be capable of providing information related to tidal volume, but this information will vary depending on ambient temperature and humidity. Activation of upper airway flow receptors, with substances such as menthol, can modify the perception of airflow (84). Upper airway mechanoreceptors can help to detect external loads applied by the physiologist or by more natural phenomena; they may help shape the behavioral response to problems such as obstruction of the nasal passages, turning one's face into the pillow at night, or breathing through a poorly designed industrial respirator. Aerosolized local anesthetic, sometimes used to eliminate upper airway receptor activation, does not degrade load detection (85), but the anesthetic may not penetrate below the mucosa to deeper mechanoreceptors. Bypass of the upper airways with tracheostomy diminished the ability to detect load (86). Younes and co-workers have shown that loads confined to the chest wall were not detected as well as loads applied to the extrathoracic airways, suggesting that upper airway mechanoreceptors are more sensitive than chest wall receptors (87,88). In direct contrast, Gandevia and co-workers (89) showed that pressure swings were not detected as well when confined to the oropharynx as when the glottis was open, suggesting that upper airway mechanoreceptors are less sensitive than chest wall receptors. Although the question of the relative sensitivity of these pathways is unsettled, the parallel pathways for load detection must be remembered in the design and interpretation of respiratory psychophysical experiments.

Corollary Discharge

Information related to respiratory muscle force generation is also available in the intensity of the motor signal dispatched to the muscles—it is thought that copies of motor signals (so-called corollary discharge) are sent to sensory areas of the cortex where they are perceived as a "sense of effort." Recently described rostral projections from brainstem respiratory motor neurons to the midbrain and thalamus in the cat provide a possible neural substrate for the conscious appreciation of respiratory corollary discharge (90,91). Similar projections may exist from the voluntary respiratory motor centers. The evidence that corollary discharge is perceived directly comes largely from perceptions reported during voluntary efforts of the limb motor system (69,92,93), but such perception has been questioned (94). The evidence concerning respiratory sense of effort comes from experiments in which subjects made voluntary inspiratory efforts after interventions that increase the motor command needed to develop a given force in the muscles: partial paralysis, fatigue, or shorter operational length. In these circumstances, subjects report making greater effort to overcome a given inspiratory load or to achieve a given inspiratory pressure (95–98). During total paralysis, then, one would expect subjects to report feeling great effort when attempting to produce maximal inspiratory pressure. Gandevia and co-workers (50) reported such a finding, but, in direct contrast, Lansing and Banzett (94) reported that such attempts were accompanied by no sense of effort. Therefore, it remains questionable whether corollary discharge alone can produce a sense of effort.

Although there has been no definitive experiment showing the role of medullary corollary discharge in sensation, patients with neurological lesions provide some tempting clues. Patients with congenital central hypoventilation syndrome have an absent ventilatory response and an absent perceptual response to hypercapnia (99). Similarly, spontaneously breathing quadriplegic subjects have abnormally low ventilatory responses and abnormally low respiratory discomfort during hypercapnia (100). These observations failed to demonstrate a divergence between the sensation response and the automatic ventilatory response. We await more conclusive experiments to *prove* that an urge to breathe accompanies automatic respiratory drive.

Since commands to respiratory muscles can originate either in the forebrain or in the automatic respiratory complex in the brainstem, both the existence and the quality of sensation arising from corollary discharge may well depend on the source of command; thus voluntary commands may result in a sense of effort, but automatic commands instead may give rise to sensations of an urge to breathe (e.g., air hunger or shortness of breath).

Arterial Chemoreceptors

Signals related to gas exchange status originate in chemoreceptors, both peripheral and central. In addition to the recognized respiratory chemoreceptors described elsewhere in this volume, there are other cerebral neurons that increase activity with high CO_2 (e.g., 101,102). Hypercapnia and hypoxia give rise to a sensation of an urge to breathe, or "air hunger." There is evidence from animal experiments that carotid chemoreceptor signals project directly to the cortex (103), although this does not prove that they are perceived. Other, less direct, routes to perception also are available; the reflex changes in ventilation evoked by changes in blood gases give rise to changes in breathing that can be sensed by the pathways noted above. Campbell and co-workers (104,105) showed that subjects paralyzed with curare did not perceive the discomfort of prolonged breath holding, giving rise to the opinion (which prevailed for over 20 years) that direct projections from chemoreceptors and medullary corollary discharge are not perceptible. However, the conclusions from those early studies have since been thoroughly refuted by experiments showing that subjects paralyzed by high spinal injury or complete neuromuscular block perceive the intense discomfort of hypercapnia or breath hold—indicating that direct projections of chemoreceptor afferents, corollary discharge from the medulla, or both, are important in perception (4,28,50).

Inputs Related to Exercise

Heavy exercise produces a sensation of shortness of breath, which is similar, but not identical, to the sensation of air hunger mentioned above: certainly they are both manifestations of an urge to breathe and are distinct from sensations such as the "tightness" of asthma, the "effort" associated with external loads, and so forth. In many individuals, shortness of breath is often the reason for quitting maximal exercise. This would be surprising if it were not so familiar, because it is generally believed that cardiac output, rather than ventilation, limits maximal exercise in healthy subjects (106,107); yet we perceive ourselves to be "out of breath," not "out of heart." Shortness of breath occurs at abnormally low exercise levels in some types of cardiopulmonary disease; thus it is both an important diagnostic symptom and a crippling effect (108).

The stimuli and afferent pathways giving rise to hyperpnea and to shortness of breath during exercise are not yet understood. Since Pa_{CO_2} falls and Pa_{O_2} rises during heavy exercise (109) at a time when the sensations are most marked, these blood gas stimuli cannot account for the sensation. Among the more popular current notions of stimuli that may cause exercise hyperpnea are chemoreceptors in the pulmonary circulation, metaboloreceptors and/or mechanoreceptors in the exercising limbs, and corollary discharge from limb motor centers that impinges on the medullary respiratory centers (reviewed in 110). The intensity of exercise that is associated with shortness of breath is also associated with lactic acidemia, which stimulates arterial chemoreceptors. Any or all of these stimuli could be directly and separately perceived as shortness of breath.

A unifying hypothesis that could explain the respiratory discomfort during exercise and during blood gas derangement is that there is a final common pathway: intense activity of the respiratory centers giving rise to corollary discharge that is perceived as air hunger or shortness of breath. The qualitative distinction between air hunger and shortness of breath may be due to the modifying effects of mechanoreceptive input related to exercise.

Miscellaneous Inputs

Several inputs not ordinarily considered as respiratory sensation deserve brief mention because they may be used to perceive breathing under special circumstances, and because they may form inadvertent cues during experiments. The chief among these is sound; during vocalization, airflow and sublaryngeal pressure information can be obtained from the acoustic signal; abnormal breath sounds often alert patients to respiratory problems; and apparatus or breath sounds can alert subjects to experimental interventions. Cutaneous receptors can detect respiratory movements, especially through contact with clothing or furniture. Mechanoreceptors in the vasculature or abdomen could also detect respiratory movement, although this has not been demonstrated.

B. Central Pathways and Processing of Afferent Information

In contrast to the vast amount of data on the cortical processing of visual, auditory, and limb proprioceptive input, there is little information about the cortical process of respiratory afferent signals. In considering aversive sensations like pain and dyspnea, it has been convenient to think of a "discriminable" component (information about location and intensity) and an "affective" component (motivational and distressing qualities). The cerebral systems that mediate discriminable responses to pain are different than those mediating affective responses (111,112). The structures mediating the affective component (medial thalamus, limbic system, prefrontal cortex) may also participate in perception of and response to respiratory discomfort. Pain itself cannot be identified with single localized sites in the forebrain, in contrast to sensations such as proprioception, touch, and sight. As stated by Campbell and Guz in the earlier edition of this volume (113), studies of direct cortical stimulation in conscious humans have failed to detect cerebral regions that subserve respiratory discomfort, and anencephalic humans exhibit signs of distress when breathing is obstructed. It is probably not possible to localize any single cortical area involved with respiratory discomfort, and it is likely that the neurons necessary for these perceptions are widely distributed throughout the cerebrum.

As expected from earlier psychophysical evidence, ERPs show that respiratory mechanoreceptor afferents reach the somatosensory regions of the cortex (e.g., 68, 114–116). The early potentials (less than 20 msec) elicited by respiratory stimuli have not yet been examined; however, the sequence of later waveforms elicited by respiratory stimuli is similar to those of other sensory modalities. Potentials evoked by external loads are systematically altered by the magnitude of the load—larger loads causing shorter latencies and greater amplitudes of certain waveforms. The later respiratory ERPs also vary systematically with age, suggesting changes in central processing of respiratory sensation, as seen in other sensory systems (117,118). It has been suggested that potentials evoked by loads are altered by respiratory disease, which may reflect altered central processing or altered afferent input (118–120).

IV. The Effect of Breathing on Respiratory Sensations

Before discussing the effect of respiratory sensation on breathing, we shall briefly review how breathing affects respiratory sensation. It is clear that the act of breathing diminishes the air hunger that is evoked by altered blood gases. The first demonstration of this phenomenon was the observation that the discomfort of breath hold could be relieved by rebreathing alveolar air, and the subject could immediately continue to perform another breath hold even though blood gases had worsened (13,14). A number of studies have shown that voluntarily reducing breathing below the spontaneous level at a given PET_{CO_2} produces discomfort (16,121–125). Several neural mechanisms, which are not mutually exclusive, could explain the relief of air hunger provided by breathing: (1) tidal expansion of the lungs and chest, sensed by mechanoreceptors of the lungs, respiratory muscles, and rib joints; (2) contraction of respiratory pump muscles, as sensed by spindle and tendon organ receptors; (3) release of the cortical effort needed to inhibit medullary respiratory centers (e.g., as at the end of breath holding); and (4) flow, sensed by receptors in the upper airways. Opie and co-workers (126) showed that mechanically ventilated polio patients could tolerate higher PET_{CO_2} when the ventilator tidal volume was higher, showing that at least part of the relief came from passively inflating the respiratory system. Experiments in ventilator-dependent quadriplegic patients have shown that vagal afferents alone can provide this relief (62). Eldridge and Chen (127) have shown that rostral projections from the brainstem respiratory centers are inhibited by lung inflation, and that this effect is mediated by the vagus.

Voluntarily overbreathing can cause some aspects of respiratory discomfort, but probably does not increase the urge to breathe. This remains unresolved because in different studies involving voluntary overbreathing, the subjects were asked to rate different aspects of respiratory discomfort: "breathlessness" (121, 124), "difficulty in breathing" (122,123), or "breathing discomfort" (125). Even in a given experiment a subject may have been rating different sensations when overbreathing (such as respiratory effort) versus when underbreathing (such as air hunger). In addition, when using volitional respiratory control to alter the relationship between breathing and sensation, we have to be aware that we may change their relationship because sensations may differ with different sources of motor command.

V. The Effect of Respiratory Sensations on Breathing

Skilled voluntary breathing maneuvers almost certainly are guided by respiratory sensation. In addition, respiratory discomfort can trigger a change from automatic to voluntary breathing or can alter breathing subconsciously. In most situations, our uncertainty of the source of the respiratory motor command and the fact that breathing and sensation are mutually interactive present difficulties in quantitatively assessing the effect of respiratory sensation on breathing.

A. Sources of Respiratory Motor Control

The respiratory muscles are unique in that they answer to different motor centers. The brain must solve complicated problems in the control of breathing muscles, particularly when ventilatory, postural, behavioral, and voluntary obligations must be met simultaneously (128). The automatic brainstem motor complex responds to homeostatic demands, mainly gas exchange, whereas the forebrain controls complex and precise conscious movements. Furthermore, breathing is affected by nonrespiratory behavioral drives associated with changes in the state of arousal or with pronounced changes in forebrain or midbrain neural activation. For example, breathing changes between wakefulness and sleep (129), with changes in posture, emotion, in association with mental imagery (130), in anticipation of exercise (131), and with visual and auditory stimulation (132,133). Such subconscious changes in breathing may be a by-product of arousal, with brainstem respiratory-related neurons being tonically stimulated from the cortex [as proposed by Fink (134)], from limbic structures (135,136), and/or via the reticular activating system (137,138).

Much is known about the discharge patterns and interconnections of respiratory-related neurons in the brainstem (reviewed elsewhere in this volume) but our understanding of their function is still far from complete. Many models of the brainstem respiratory controller have been proposed; the most attractive ones incorporate separate neural mechanisms for generating rhythm and for shaping the spatial and temporal pattern of muscle activation (e.g., 139). The automatic efferent rhythmic activity occurs in bulbospinal neurons having direct, monosynaptic connections to the phrenic spinal motoneurons (e.g., 140). Less is known about the manner in which voluntary drive from the cortex and behavioral drive from other forebrain structures interact with the medullary respiratory neurons. Emotions can still influence breathing (causing laughter or crying) when the voluntary respiratory pathways are totally ineffective (e.g., after a lesion in the pyramidal tracts), which provides evidence of respiratory pathways from limbic structures to the brainstem respiratory complex or directly to the respiratory neurons in the spinal cord (135,136). Humans can volitionally inspire via cortico-spinal pathways (141); alternatively, the cortex can inhibit or activate medullary neurons via corticobulbar fibers (e.g., 142–144). Some regions of cerebrum involved in the volitional control of breathing in humans have been identified. Maskill and co-workers (145) mapped those areas of the motor cortex where it was possible to activate diaphragm contraction with transcranial stimulation of motor command neurons; the diaphragm contraction was maximal (and predominantly contralateral) when the magnetic coil was placed just lateral to the vertex. This confirmed the pioneering work of Foerster (146), who had located the regions related to contraction of the diaphragm by electrical stimulation of exposed cortex. The cerebral regions activated during volitional inspiration and expiration have been located more precisely using positron emission tomography (147,148). With active inspiration (as opposed to passive inflation) regional cerebral blood flow increased in the primary motor cortex (dorsally and just lateral to the vertex), the supplementary motor area, and the ventrolateral thalamus. Similar areas were identified with active expiration, along with increased blood flow in the premotor cortex and the cerebellum.

Hence, there is opportunity for respiratory motor commands originating in the forebrain to bypass the medulla entirely, to utilize the medullary shaping apparatus to coordinate muscle action, or to alter the ongoing rhythm and shape of breaths originating in the medulla. It is possible that perceived respiratory sensation can invoke any of these pathways in order to guide breathing.

B. Determining the Effect of Respiratory Sensations on Breathing

Experimental Approaches

Measurement of Cortical Activation

It would be useful to be able to assess the cortical contribution to breaths that are ostensibly "automatic" since this could indicate that respiratory sensations may be affecting breathing via forebrain respiratory control centers.

Variation in the magnitude of the electromyographic response to submaximal stimulation of cortical motor command neurons can be used to assess the endogenous activity of the motor cortex. This cortical facilitation has been used to gauge the extent of voluntary input to various motor acts (e.g., 149,150) including breathing (151,152). This technique is rather imprecise; the sites of the activation of corticospinal pathways are not known (153–155) and the facilitatory effect may take place at least partly in the spinal cord (149).

Macefield and Gandevia (156) have proposed that we may be able to determine whether there is a cortical contribution to breathing in humans by recording electroencephalographic activity over the premotor and motor cortex, just as sensory cortical potentials can be recorded in response to respiratory-related afferent activity. They found that cerebral potentials just preceding inspiration could be detected close to the vertex during voluntary breathing maneuvers, and that these potentials were not detectable in relaxed subjects who were not thinking about their breathing (in electroencephalographic averages of up to 400 breaths). These authors suggested that during voluntary breathing these potentials represented efferent activity in the premotor and motor cortex, and that the cortex does not contribute consistently on a breath-by-breath basis to breathing during relaxed wakefulness in healthy subjects.

Recently, positron emission tomography has been used to localize respiratory-related cerebral activation during overt voluntary breathing acts (147,148), but such techniques have not yet been successfully applied to determine whether these cortical motor regions are involved in more natural breathing acts. Useful images require averaging data from many breaths in each of several subjects to limit radiation doses. The recently introduced "functional" magnetic resonance imaging, which gives better time resolution and does not use harmful radiation, also may be useful in determining whether breaths include cerebral components.

With the future development of these brain-mapping techniques, it is likely that it will soon be possible to study whether the respiratory motor cortex increases its activity in response to respiratory discomfort—for instance, during chemical stimulation, exercise, or in cardiopulmonary disease. These techniques may even prove useful in localizing specific respiratory sensations.

Comparison of Sleep and Wakefulness

Another way to measure the contribution of respiratory sensation to the control of breathing is to compare breathing during wakefulness to breathing during non–rapid eye movement (non-REM) sleep wherein sensations are unlikely to influence breathing. It is generally believed that during non-REM sleep the respiratory rhythm is governed exclusively by the automatic brainstem respiratory complex and is dependent on excitatory chemoreceptor input to the brainstem. Certainly, breathing is at its most regular during deep non-REM sleep (e.g., 136,157,158), and decreasing end-tidal PCO_2 by approximately 4 torr during non-REM sleep is enough to stop breathing (159,160), presumably because the brainstem respiratory complex is then below threshold. By contrast, reducing end-tidal PCO_2 by more than 4 torr has little effect on ventilation in waking subjects (52,134,159,160), and it has been assumed that during wakefulness the reticular activation system and/or varied forebrain activities influence the brainstem respiratory complex, keep it above threshold, and introduce variability. Further reasons to presume that forebrain influences on breathing are absent or minimal during non-REM sleep are that during this state: (1) phasic activity in respiratory-related neurons in the forebrain is reduced (e.g., 135); (2) the cortical facilitation of diaphragmatic activity induced by transcortical magnetic stimulation is reduced (152); (3) conditioned respiratory responses cannot be elicited (unless the stimulus arouses the subject) (e.g., 161); and (4) the late cortical components of respiratory ERPs, produced by airway occlusion and a resultant negative pressure in the airway, are profoundly altered (116).

To determine whether the abnormal breathing patterns associated with respiratory disease occur in response to discomfort, Shea and co-workers (158) studied eight patients with severe interstitial lung disease, who had the typical symptoms of breathlessness and a rapid shallow breathing pattern when awake at rest. These patients assumed a breathing pattern indistinguishable from age-matched controls during non-REM sleep—suggesting that the abnormal breathing pattern when awake may have been adopted in response to the respiratory discomfort, and that the sensation and the response disappear during sleep. In this study sleep hypoxemia was avoided by providing supplemental inspired oxygen. [In contrast, two other studies found that patients with interstitial lung disease still had a rapid, shallow breathing pattern when asleep, but in these studies hypoxemia also occurred, which could have stimulated breathing (162,163).]

The tolerance of severe hypoventilation during sleep in patients with chronic obstructive airways disease and sleep apnea (e.g., 164) could be explained by a lack of a sensation during sleep and therefore a reduced ventilatory response to disturbances in blood gases. If such hypoventilation occurred during wakefulness, it would cause severe discomfort, which would be overcome by voluntarily breathing. Arousal from sleep in response to blood gas derangements or airway irritants may be a measure of these stimuli reaching consciousness.

This approach of utilizing sleep to assess natural breathing in the absence of forebrain effects on breathing is useful, but we cannot be certain that the only change that affects breathing when we fall asleep is that respiratory sensation is absent.

Manipulation of the Relationship Between Breathing and Sensation

To study the effect of sensation on breathing one can manipulate their interrelationship, for example, by controlling the blood gases and thereby sensation while measuring the effect on breathing. A familiar example that illustrates that sensation affects a volitional breathing act is the voluntary breath hold paradigm: the limit (breakpoint) of breath hold is determined consciously by a contest between "will" and sensation (e.g., 13–15). If we assume that will is the same from trial to trial in a given subject, the time at which the maximum tolerable discomfort occurs can be altered by changing sensory stimuli such as blood gases or lung volume. Maximal breath hold duration is then a measure of the effect of sensory input on the volitional act of respiratory suppression. This approach, however, tells us little of what happens in more natural situations when rhythmic breathing does occur. As discussed in Section IV, several studies have utilized voluntary underbreathing or overbreathing to assess the effect of changing breathing level on the sensation of respiratory discomfort, but these studies do not tell us how sensation affects the level of breathing.

Since the volitional and reflex pathways can have the same effect on breathing, it is difficult to determine how much of the increase in ventilation is caused by sensation. Furthermore, it should be noted that directing a subject's attention to breathing can alter both of the variables of interest—breathing and sensation. No study has yet effectively determined whether increased sensations contribute to ventilatory responses when breathing is not controlled volitionally. Of primary interest are the time course and magnitude of the effect—it is possible that respiratory discomfort contributes to breathing only when the sensation reaches a certain threshold or if it is prolonged. A causal relationship between sensation and breathing is easiest to conceptualize if we assume that when severe discomfort does occur, then the voluntary respiratory pathway takes control completely from the automatic pathway. A more sophisticated approach is to envision a model in which the breathing pattern is determined at all times by parallel inputs to the respiratory controller from sensation and from automatic reflexes.

Mathematical Models Optimizing Breathing Sensation

There is a long-held notion that particular combinations of tidal volume and respiratory rate are adopted to minimize either respiratory work or the respiratory muscle force necessary to achieve the required alveolar ventilation (165–168), although the feedback mechanisms responsible were not explicitly considered. Poon (169) proposed a more elaborate model in which the level of ventilation is optimized on the basis of two conflicting demands: minimizing blood gas changes (modeled as a quadratic function of arterial P_{CO_2}) and minimizing "respiratory mechanical discomfort" (modeled as a logarithmic function of ventilation). The respiratory "discomfort" caused by increased breathing could be reflex and subconscious, but Poon acknowledges that conscious sensations of "respiratory effort" may be involved. Cherniack and co-workers (170), noting the capacity for humans to perceive sensations related to breathing and to voluntarily control breathing, have modified Poon's model with the notion that ventilation is determined to minimize perceived respiratory discomfort—based on inputs from the chemoreceptors and from a corollary discharge of the output of the ventilatory controller. The basis for this model is that discomfort increases above and below an optimum ventilation. This has been studied for voluntarily controlled breathing (discussed in Section IV) with the firm conclusion that the urge to breathe increases when breathing is constrained, but there remains disagreement on whether this sensation is increased when overbreathing (121–125).

Although models provide some basis for thinking about the problem, they are based on our scanty knowledge of the way in which subjects actually respond to respiratory sensations, and on as yet undemonstrated neurophysiological mechanisms. One serious problem is that the sensory transfer functions are based on magnitude scales with unknown properties (e.g., do they have ratio properties?). Another problem is the uncertainty, mentioned above, of the extent of cortical input to breathing. An example where these models fail to predict observed data is provided by subjects with congenital central hypoventilation syndrome (CCHS). These subjects do not increase ventilation or feel respiratory discomfort in the face of severe hypercapnia or hypoxia (99). Therefore, the optimum ventilation to minimize either respiratory work or discomfort ought to be zero—but it is not. Indeed, CCHS subjects have normal breathing patterns at rest, during mental activities, and these subjects even increase breathing in proportion of CO_2 production during aerobic exercise thereby maintaining their end-tidal P_{CO_2} (171–173).

C. Respiratory Sensations Guide Skilled Respiratory Movements

Voluntary respiratory movements can be controlled rapidly and precisely, as is demonstrated in singing and playing wind instruments. The afferent source of proprioceptive cues (chest wall, lung, and airways) may vary. Studies of human limb movements have shown that the particular set of cues a subject uses to guide a movement can change according to instructions given, the type of task performed (simple vs. complex, single vs. repetitive, or rapid vs. slow), and the movement phase (starting, in progress, or stopping) (174,175). Subjects can voluntarily respond to respiratory proprioceptive cues (as occurs with airway loading) within 100–150 msec—a reaction time comparable to that of hand movements (176, 177). With proprioceptive cues alone tidal volumes can be reproduced with an error of only about 100 ml of a target volume (45,46,74), and absolute lung volume, irrespective of the time required to reach that volume, is sensed to within 150 ml (178). With additional visual feedback on performance the accuracy of volume production is substantially improved to within 20 ml of a target volume (178). This suggests that respiratory precision, like manual precision (69), normally is limited by sensory input rather than by precision of efferent motor control. In untrained individuals the overall precision and dynamics of voluntary respiratory volume control during visual tracking tasks almost matches that observed for equivalent hand movements (179). Professional wind instrument players can more accurately reproduce tidal volumes than control subjects (180), suggesting that training can improve performance (although differences in inherent skill could have explained the results in this experiment).

Learning of Skilled Breathing Movements

There is little information about how sensory cues are used in the learning of skilled breathing movements. The cues a subject uses to guide limb movement change with the stage of learning (174,175). For example, in the early stages of learning visual cues predominate, but as learning progresses and the movement becomes more automatic proprioceptive cues are more important. Finally, with extended practice movement sequences can be executed with minimal or occasional feedback. It is probable that a subject's history of training may substantially affect how respiratory sensations are used. Highly learned movements may become less dependent on cortical motor planning, with subcortical structures becoming more involved (e.g., basal ganglia and cerebellum).

Such well-learned movement patterns proceed without awareness of the many sensory inputs guiding them; in fact, asking someone to attend to sensory inputs can seriously disrupt a well-programmed movement. Nevertheless, conscious sensations of movements are important in the initial stages of learning a motor act, providing feedback on the accuracy of the movement. These sensations can help to focus attention on only the most relevant proprioceptive cues, which themselves also can be associated with external events that can eventually trigger and/or guide the movement. There is growing evidence that the brain systems necessary for such conscious perception of stimuli are different from those used to acquire information without conscious recognition (181). The limited information available on learned respiratory movements or responses is discussed below.

D. Respiratory Discomfort May Trigger Change to Voluntary Breathing

We contend that it will be unusual for a subject not to modify either breathing or behavior when feeling marked respiratory discomfort, as may occur with blood gas derangements. Patients with severe cardiopulmonary disease often adopt volitional breathing strategies that minimize discomfort, such as breathing through pursed lips, bracing their arms to gain respiratory muscle advantage, or elevating functional residual capacity with tonic inspiratory muscle contraction (e.g., 182,183). Such patients also alter eating habits and speech patterns (and possibly language) in such a way as to minimize respiratory discomfort. For example, Lee and co-workers (184) found that patients with sarcoidosis, asthma, or emphysema adopted different patterns of breathing during conversational speech, and shortness of breath was avoided in each group, but when asked to count continuously they experienced shortness of breath.

Even in healthy subjects the uncomfortable perception of resistance to airflow during nasal congestion alerts the subject to increase respiratory muscle force or to switch to mouth breathing. Automatic mechanoreceptive reflexes are elicited when a breath is impeded by an external load (177,185), but these reflexes are too weak and brief to offer effective mechanical compensation, which can only be achieved by chemical feedback if the disturbance is prolonged or by voluntary intervention. Voluntary responses to such disturbances can be brought into play within the same breath (186). Indeed, voluntary breaths driven on the basis of sensation may provide more useful responses than automatic reflexes since voluntary reactions can be of widely varying strength and quality and can take into account both the prevailing situation and past experience. Upper airway receptors (including olfactory receptors) and intrapulmonary receptors provide sensations that can be used to protect against inhalation of foreign bodies, irritant agents, or very cold air—by voluntarily holding one's breath, altering breathing pattern, or leaving the area. Other examples where respiratory discomfort serves to alter behavior (so as to reduce the respiratory discomfort) include stopping exercise or terminating a prolonged breath hold.

It is noteworthy that respiratory sensations may not always fulfill a protective role or a role in optimizing breathing pattern on the basis of gas exchange or comfort. For example, chronic respiratory symptoms that accompany lung disease can become a debilitating facet of the disease itself. Furthermore, an inappropriate sensation of "breathlessness" or "air hunger" is a common symptom in hyperventilation syndrome (187,188). Indeed, it is possible that this sensation is itself the trigger for psychogenic hyperventilation.

E. Respiratory Sensations May Alter Spontaneous Breathing

Spontaneous breathing can be modulated by the action of the forebrain on medullary centers with or without the subject's awareness. We frequently think of respiratory stimuli as acting solely via the brainstem respiratory centers, but these stimuli are accompanied by an increased urge to breath or other respiratory discomfort (e.g., acidosis, hypoxia, exercise, and irritant stimuli) which can provoke forebrain action.

Using the ventilatory response to CO_2 as an example, it is believed that the response during sleep, which is less than that which occurs during wakefulness, reflects the pure automatic brainstem response (129). It seems possible that the greater response when awake is due, at least in part, to the perception of hypercapnia and a resultant cortical addition to the ventilatory response to CO_2— which may remain subconscious unless the sensation becomes overpowering. Murphy and co-workers (151) found a similar degree of cortical facilitation of the diaphragm (induced by transcranial magnetic stimulation of motor command neurons) during volitional breathing and CO_2-induced breathing. These authors inferred that an important part of the ventilatory response to hypercapnia originated in the cortex (and discuss why they do not favor the possible interpretation that spinal phrenic motoneurons driven from bulbospinal pathways were closer to threshold during hypercapnia). Although the sensations of an urge to breathe that accompany hypercapnia during wakefulness and the reduction in the ventilatory response to CO_2 during sleep suggest a facilitatory role for the cortex in the ventilatory response to CO_2, under some circumstances the cortex instead can inhibit the reflex brainstem output. The evidence includes an increased ventilatory response to CO_2 in decorticate animals (189) and in patients with bilateral cerebral infarction (190,191).

F. Learned Responses to Respiratory Sensations

Early studies of classical conditioning of respiratory responses to changes in blood gases are reviewed by Bykov (192). Interest has recently been revived in this area. The marked changes in breathing during the anticipation of exercise (131) probably represent a conditioned response. Martin and co-workers (193) demonstrated that goats repeatedly subjected to exercise in combination with added ventilatory dead space learned to increase their ventilation further; this response persisted for several trials during subsequent exercise after removal of the dead space. Adams and co-workers (194) have repeated this experiment in humans with similar results; both groups concluded that past experience can modify the ventilatory response to exercise. In a well-controlled study, Gallego and Perruchet (195) found, in humans, that following eight pairings of a sound and a brief hypoxic challenge, the sound alone produced an increase in breath duration. Orem and Netick (144) conditioned cats to hold their breath when presented with a tone by initially presenting the tone in combination with an inhalation of ammonia. Such adaptability of the ventilatory responses to, for example, exercise and hypoxia may be important in maintaining normal blood gases in the face of changes in physiological, mechanical, or environmental conditions.

Some of the nonautomatic breathing strategies mentioned previously, such as breathing when speaking or altering breathing in response to blood gas derangements, may be learned adaptations to respiratory sensations or behavioral situations. Learning could be based on the improvement in performance of a behavior, for example, taking a deep breath before a breath hold in order to prolong the breath hold, or learning to control subglottal pressure to produce a steady note. Alternatively, learning could be based on the minimization of respiratory discomfort, a possible example being the adoption of a rapid, shallow breathing pattern in patients with severe interstitial lung disease (158,196).

Several techniques in "breathing retraining" have been used in the rehabilitation of patients with lung disease, hyperventilation syndrome, or following thoracic surgery (e.g., 197–199). Gallego and co-workers (200) have found that the performance of a voluntarily altered breathing pattern can be improved with training, especially when there is feedback on performance. It has yet to be determined how long one can retain a voluntarily modified breathing behavior, and whether the learned pattern ever becomes completely automatic. In this respect, sleep may be a useful tool to distinguish automatic from subconsciously controlled breathing patterns.

With the possible exception of severe cardiopulmonary disease, we do not consciously attend to every breath while we are awake (in the same way that we do not attend to chronic tactile stimuli from our skin). But we do attend to our breathing when the afferent information is changed in an unexpected way (51): respiratory sensations are always available to the forebrain to direct motor activity. These sensations and the consequent conscious or subconscious forebrain influences on breathing may be important in shaping much of our breathing behavior while we are awake.

Acknowledgments

We thank Elizabeth Bloch-Salisbury for helpful comments on the manuscript, and Sarah Zurier and Christopher Kovacs for assistance with the references. This work was supported by NIH Grants HL 46690 and HL 19170.

References

1. Melzack R, Torgerson WS. On the language of pain. Anesthesiology 1971; 34: 50–59.
2. Simon PM, Schwartzstein RM, Weiss JW, Lahive K, Fencl V, Teghtsoonian M, Weinberger SE. Distinguishable sensations of breathlessness induced in normal volunteers. Am Rev Respir Dis 1989; 140:1021–1027.
3. Simon PM, Schwartzstein RM, Weiss JW, Fencl V, Teghtsoonian M, Weinberger SE. Distinguishable types of dyspnea in patients with shortness of breath. Am Rev Respir Dis 1990; 142:1009–1014.
4. Banzett RB, Lansing RW, Reid MB, Adams L, Brown R. "Air hunger" arising from increased P_{CO_2} in mechanically ventilated quadriplegics. Respir Physiol 1989; 76:53–67.
5. Elliott MW, Adams L, Cockcroft A, MacRae KD, Murphy K, Guz A. The language of breathlessness. Use of verbal descriptors by patients with cardiopulmonary disease. Am Rev Respir Dis 1991; 144:826–832.
6. Boring EG. A History of Experimental Psychology, 2nd ed. New York: Appleton-Century-Crofts, 1950.

7. Engen T. Psychophysics. I. Discrimination and detection. II. Scaling methods. In: Kling JW, Riggs LA, eds. Woodworth and Schlosberg's Experimental Psychology, 3rd ed. Vol. I: Sensation and Perception. New York: Holt, Rinehart and Winston, 1972:11–88.

8. Marks LE. Sensory Processes: The New Psychophysics. New York: Academic Press, 1974.

9. Dixon, NF. Preconscious Processing. Chichester: Wiley, 1987.

10. Banzett RB, Lansing RW, Brown R. High-level quadriplegics perceive lung volume change. J Appl Physiol 1987; 62:567–573.

11. West DW, Ellis CG, Campbell EJ. Ability of man to detect increases in his breathing. J Appl Physiol 1975; 39:372–376.

12. Prochazka A. Sensorimotor gain control: a basic strategy of motor systems? Prog Neurobiol 1989; 33:281–307.

13. Hill L, Flack M. The effect of excess of carbon dioxide and of want of oxygen upon the respiration and the circulation. J Physiol (Lond) 1908; 37:77–111.

14. Fowler WS. Breaking point of breath holding. J Appl Physiol 1954; 6:539–545.

15. Whitelaw WA, McBride B, Ford GT. Effect of lung volume on breath holding. J Appl Physiol 1987; 62:1962–1969.

16. Remmers JE, Brooks JE III, Tenney SM. Effect of controlled ventilation on the tolerable limit of hypercapnia. Respir Physiol 1968; 4:78–90.

17. Stebbins WC, Brown CH, Petersen MR. Sensory function in animals. In: Brookhart JM, Moutcastle VB, ed. Handbook of Physiology. Section 1. The Nervous System. Vol III. Sensory Processes. Bethesda, MD: American Physiological Society, 1984.

18. Davenport PW, Dalziel DJ, Webb B, Bellah JR, Vierck CJ. Inspiratory resistive load detection in conscious dogs. J Appl Physiol 1991; 70:1284–1289.

19. Arieli R. Can the rat detect hypoxia in inspired air? Respir Physiol 1990; 79: 243–253.

20. Homma I, Kanamaru A, Sibuya M. Mechanoreceptors and respiratory sensation. In: Takashima T, Cherniack NS, eds. Control of Breathing and Dyspnea. Oxford: Pergamon Press, 1991:229–234.

21. Regan D. Human Brain Electrophysiology. New York: Elsevier, 1989:289–292.

22. Merzenich MM, Kaas JH. Principles of Organization of sensory-perceptual systems. In: Sprague JM, Epstein AN, eds. Progress in Psychobiology and Physiological Psychology. Vol. 9. New York: Academic Press, 1980:1–42.

23. Hashimoto I, Gatayama T, Yoshikawa K, Sasaki M, Nomura M. Compound activity in sensory nerve fibers is related to intensity of sensation evoked by air-puff stimulation of the index finger in man. Electroenceph Clin Neurophysiol 1991; 81: 176–185.

24. Uttal WR. The Psychophysiology of Sensory Coding. New York: Harper & Row, 1973.

25. Green DM, Swets JA. Signal Detection Theory and Psychophysics. New York: Wiley, 1966.

26. Narbed PG, Marcer D, Howell JB, Spencer E. A signal detection theory analysis of the effect of chest cage restriction upon the detection of inspiratory resistive loads. Clin Sci 1983; 64:417–421.

27. Bonnel AM, Mathiot MJ, Grimaud C. Inspiratory and expiratory resistive load detection in normal and asthmatic subjects. A sensory decision theory analysis. Respiration 1985; 48:12–23.

28. Banzett RB, Lansing RW, Brown R, Topulos GP, Yager D, Steele SM, Londono B, Loring SH, Reid MB, Adams L, Nations CS. "Air hunger" from increased P_{CO_2} persists after complete neuromuscular block in humans. Respir Physiol 1990; 81: 1–17.

29. Harver A, Katkin ES, Bloch E. Signal-detection outcomes on heartbeat and respiratory resistance detection tasks in male and female subjects. Psychophysiology 1993; 30:223–230.

30. Zechman FWJ, Wiley RL. Afferent inputs to breathing: respiratory sensation. In: Cherniack NS, Widdicombe JG, eds. The Respiratory System. Section 3. Handbook of Physiology. Vol II. Bethesda, MD: American Physiological Society, 1986: 449–474.

31. Harver A, Tenney SM, Baird JC. A cautionary note on the interpretation of the power law for respiratory effort. Am Rev. Respir Dis 1986; 133:341–342.

32. Teghtsoonian R. The study of individuals in psychophysical procedures. In: Ljunggren G, Dornic S, eds. Psychophysics in Action. Berlin: Springer-Verlag, 1989: 95–102.

33. Sternbach R, Tursky B. Ethnic differences among housewives in psychophysical and skin potential responses to electric shock. Psychophysiology 1965; 1:241–246.

34. Kanfer FH, Goldfoot DA. Self-control and tolerance of noxious stimulation. Psychol Rep 1966; 18:79–85.

35. Johnson JE. Effects of accurate expectations about sensations on the sensory and distress components of pain. J Personal Soc Psychol 1973; 27:261–275.

36. Melzack R. The Puzzle of Pain. New York: Basic Books, 1973.

37. Evans FJ. The placebo response in pain reduction. In: Bonica JJ, ed. Advances in Neurology, vol 4. New York: Raven Press, 1974.

38. Hilgard ER. Pain perception in man. In: Held RN, Liebowitz HW, eds. Perception. Berlin: Springer-Verlag, 1975:849–875.

39. Comroe JH. Dyspnea. Mod Concepts Cardiovasc Dis 1956; 25:347–349.

40. Bakers JH, Tenney SM. The perception of some sensations associated with breathing. Respir Physiol 1970; 10:85–92.

41. Harver A, Mahler DA. The symptom of dyspnea. In: Mahler DA, ed. Dyspnea. Mount Kisko, NY: Futura, 1990:1–53.

42. Stubbing DG, Killian KJ, Campbell EJ. The quantification of respiratory sensations by normal subjects. Respir Physiol 1981; 44:251–260.

43. Altose MD, Dimarco AF, Gottfried SB, Strohl KP. The sensation of respiratory muscle force. Am Rev Respir Dis 1982; 126:807–811.

44. Stubbing DG, Ramsdale EH, Killian KJ, Campbell EJ. Psychophysics of inspiratory muscle force. J Appl Physiol 1983; 54:1216–1221.

45. Gliner JA, Folinsbee LJ, Horvath SM. Accuracy and precision of matching inspired lung volume. Percep Psychophys 1981; 29:511–515.

46. Wolkove N, Altose MD, Kelsen SG, Kondapalli PG, Cherniack NS. Perception of changes in breathing in normal human subjects. J Appl Physiol 1981; 50:78–83.

47. Katz-Salamon M. The ability of human subjects to detect small changes in breathing volume. Acta Physiol Scand 1984; 120:43–51.

48. Fox J, Kreisman H, Colacone A, Wolkove N. Respiratory volume perception through the nose and mouth determined noninvasively. J Appl Physiol 1986; 61: 436–439.

49. Schwartzstein R, Lilly J, Israel E, Basner R, Sparrow D, Weinberger S, Weiss JW. Breathlessness of asthma differs from that of external resistive loading. Am Rev Respir Dis 1991; 143:A596.

50. Gandevia SC, Killian K, McKenzie DK, Crawford M, Allen GM, Gorman RB, Hales JP. Respiratory sensations, cardiovascular control and kinaesthesia during complete paralysis in human subjects. J Physiol (Lond) 1993; 470:85–108.

51. Sears TA. Breathing: a sensori-motor act. Sci Basis Med Annu Rev 1971; 128–147.

52. Morrell MJ, Shea SA, Adams L, Guz A. Effects of inspiratory support upon breathing in humans during wakefulness and sleep. Respir Physiol 1993; 93:57–70.

53. Matthews PB. Muscle afferents and kinaesthesia. Br Med Bull 1977; 33:137–142.

54. Widdicombe JG. Nervous receptors in the respiratory tract and lungs. In: Hornbein TF, ed. Regulation of Breathing, Part I. New York: Marcel Dekker, 1981: 429–472.

55. Sant'Ambrogio G. Information arising from the tracheobronchial tree of mammals. Physiol Rev 1982; 62:531–569.

56. Kazakov VN. On the pulmonary receptor representation in cat brain cortex. [Russian]. Fiziol Z Sssr Imeni Sechenova 1966; 52:847–854.

57. O'Brien JH, Pimpaneau A, Albe-Fessard D. Evoked cortical responses to vagal, laryngeal and facial afferents in monkeys under chloralose anaesthesia. Electroencephal Clin Neurophysiol 1971; 31:7–20.

58. Penfield W, Jasper H. Epilepsy and the Functional Anatomy of the Human Brain. Boston: Little, Brown, 1954.

59. Morton DR. Klassen KP, Curtis GM. The clinical physiology of the human bronchi. I. Pain of tracheobronchial origin. Surgery 1950; 28:699–704.

60. Winning AJ, Hamilton RD, Shea SA, Guz A. Respiratory and cardiovascular effects of central and peripheral intravenous injections of capsaicin in man: evidence for pulmonary chemosensitivity. Clin Sci 1986; 71:519–526.

61. Guz A, Noble MI, Widdicombe JG, Trenchard D, Mushin WW. The effect of bilateral block of vagus and glossopharyngeal nerves on the ventilatory response to CO_2 of conscious man. Respir Physiol 1966; 1:206–210.

62. Manning HL, Shea SA, Schwartzstein RM, Lansing RW, Brown R, Banzett RB. Reduced tidal volume increases "air hunger" at fixed P_{CO_2} in ventilated quadriplegics. Respir Physiol 1992; 90:19–30.

63. Lansing RW, Banzett RB, Brown R, Reid M. Airway anesthesia diminished tidal volume perception in a C1–C2 quadriplegic. FASEB 1988; 2:A1298.

64. Duron B. Intercostal and diaphragmatic muscle endings and afferents. In: Hornbein TF, ed. Regulation of Breathing, Part I. New York: Marcel Dekker, 1981:473–540.

65. Bolser D, Remmers JE. Synaptic effects of intercostal tendon organs on membrane potentials of medullary respiratory neurons. J Neurophysiol 1989; 86:918–926.

66. Coffey GL, Godwin-Austen RB, MacGillivray BB, Sears TA. The form and

distribution of the surface evoked responses in cerebellar cortex from intercostal nerves in the cat. J Physiol (Lond) 1971; 212:129–145.

67. Davenport PW, Thompson FJ, Reep RL, Freed AN. Projection of phrenic nerve afferents to the cat sensorimotor cortex. Brain Res 1985; 328:150–153.

68. Gandevia SC, Macefield G. Projection of low-threshold afferents from human intercostal muscles to the cerebral cortex. Respir Physiol 1989; 77:203–214.

69. McCloskey DI. Kinesthetic sensibility. Physiol Rev 1978; 58:763–820.

70. Shannon R. Reflexes from respiratory muscles and costovertebral joints. In: Cherniack NS, Widdicombe JG, eds. Handbook of Physiology, Vol II. Section 3: The Respiratory System. Bethesda, MD: American Physiological Society, 1986: 431–447.

71. Agostoni E, Mognoni P, Torri G, Miserocchi G. Forces deforming the rib cage. Respir Physiol 1966; 2:105–117.

72. Konno K, Mead J. Measurement of the separate volume changes of rib cage and abdomen during breathing. J Appl Physiol 1967; 22:407–422.

73. Matthews PCB. Mammalian Muscle Receptors and Their Central Action. London: Arnold, 1972:243–246.

74. DiMarco AF, Wolfson DA, Gottfried SB, Altose MD. Sensation of inspired volume in normal subjects and quadriplegic patients. J Appl Physiol 1982; 53:1481–1486.

75. Muza SR, McDonald S, Zechman FW. Comparison of subjects' perception of inspiratory and expiratory resistance. J Appl Physiol 1984; 56:211–216.

76. Zechman FW, Muza SR, Davenport PW, Wiley RL, Shelton R. Relationship of transdiaphragmatic pressure and latencies for detecting added inspiratory loads. J Appl Physiol 1985; 58:236–243.

77. Peiffer C, Silbert D, Cerrina J, Le Roy Ladurie F, Dartevell P, Hervé P. Characteristics of respiratory sensation related to inspiratory resistive loads in lung transplant recipients. Am Rev Respir Dis 1993; 147:A169.

78. Eisele J, Trenchard D, Burki N, Guz A. The effect of chest wall block on respiratory sensation and control in man. Clin Sci 1968; 35:23–33.

79. Zechman FW, Wiley RL. Effect of chest cage restriction on perception of added airflow resistance. Respir Physiol 1977; 31:71–79.

80. Jammes Y, Buchler B, Delpierre S, Rasidakis A, Grimaud C, Roussos C. Phrenic afferents and their role in inspiratory control. J Appl Physiol 1986; 60:854–860.

81. Jammes Y, Mathiot MJ, Delpierre S, Grimaud C. Role of vagal and spinal sensory pathways on eupneic diaphragmatic activity. J Appl Physiol 1986; 60:479–485.

82. Revelette WR, Jewell LA, Frazier DT. Effect of diaphragm small-fiber afferent stimulation on ventilation in dogs. J Appl Physiol 1988; 65:2097–2106.

83. Frazier DT, Revelette WR. Role of phrenic nerve afferents in the control of breathing. J Appl Physiol 1991; 70:491–496.

84. Burrow AR, Eccles R, Jones AS. The effects of camphor, eucalyptus and menthol vapour on nasal resistance to airflow and nasal sensation of airflow. Acta Oto-Laryngol 1983; 96:157–161.

85. Chaudhary BA, Burki NK. The effects of airway anesthesia on detection of added inspiratory elastic loads. Am Rev Respir Dis 1980; 122:635–639.

86. Noble MIM, Eisele JH, Trenchard D, Guz A. Effect of selective peripheral nerve blocks on respiratory sensations. In: Porter R, ed. Breathing: Hering-Breuer Centenary Symposium. London: Churchill, Livingstone, 1970:233–251.

87. Younes M, Jung D, Puddy, A, Giesbrecht, G, Sanii R. Role of the chest wall in detection of added elastic loads. J Appl Physiol 1990; 68:2241–2245.

88. Puddy A, Giesbrecht G, Sanii R, Younes M. Mechanism of detection of resistive loads in conscious humans. J Appl Physiol 1992; 72:2267–2270.

89. Gandevia SC, Killian KJ, Campbell EJ. The contribution of upper airway and inspiratory muscle mechanisms to the detection of pressure changes at the mouth in normal subjects. Clin Sci 1981; 60:513–518.

90. Chen Z, Eldridge FL, Wagner PG. Respiratory-associated rhythmic firing of midbrain neurones in cats: relation to level of respiratory drive. J Physiol 1991; 437:305–325.

91. Chen Z, Eldridge FL, Wagner PG. Respiratory-associated thalamic activity is related to level of respiratory drive. Respir Physiol 1992; 90:99–113.

92. Hobbs SF, Gandevia SC. Cardiovascular responses and the sense of effort to contract paralysed muscles: role of the spinal cord. Neurosci Lett 1985; 57:85–90.

93. Gandevia SC. Roles for perceived voluntary commands in motor control. Trends Neurosci 1987; 10:81–85.

94. Lansing RW, Banzett RB. What do paralyzed awake humans feel when they attempt to move? J Motor Behav 1993; 25:309–313.

95. Campbell EJM, Gandevia SC, Killian KJ, Mahutte CK, Rigg JRA. Changes in the perception of inspiratory resistive loads during partial curarization. J Physiol (Lond) 1980; 309:93–100.

96. Gandevia SC, Killian KJ, Campbell EJ. The effect of respiratory muscle fatigue on respiratory sensations. Clin Sci 1981; 60:463–466.

97. Killian KJ, Gandevia SC, Summers E, Campbell EJ. Effect of increased lung volume on perception of breathlessness, effort, and tension. J Appl Physiol 1984; 57: 686–691.

98. Supinski GS, Clary SJ, Bark H, Kelsen SG. Effect of inspiratory muscle fatigue on perception of effort during loaded breathing. J Appl Physiol 1987; 62:300–307.

99. Shea SA, Andres LP, Shannon DC, Guz A, Banzett RB. Respiratory sensations in subjects who lack a ventilatory response to CO_2. Respir Physiol 1993 (in press).

100. Lieberman SL, Mourad I, Brown R, Schwartzstein RM. Spinal cord injury diminishes both the ventilatory response and air hunger due to steady state hypercapnia. Am Rev Respir Dis 1993; 147:A550.

101. Dell PC. Humoral effects on the brain stem reticular formations. In: Jasper HH, Proctor LD, Knighton RS, Noshay WC, Costello RT, eds. Reticular Formation of the Brain. Boston: Little, Brown, 1958:365–379.

102. Neubauer JA. Cellular mechanisms of central chemosensitivity. In: Speck DF, Dekin MS, Revelette WR, Frazier DT, eds. Respiratory Control: Central and Peripheral Mechanisms. Lexington: University Press of Kentucky, 1993:152–162.

103. Kukorelli T, Namenyi J, Adam G. Visceral afferent projection areas in the cortex. II. Representation of the carotid sinus receptor area. Acta Physiol Acad Sci Hungar 1969; 36:261–263.

104. Campbell EJ, Freedman S, Clark TJ, Robson JG, Norman J. The effect of muscular paralysis induced by tubocurarine on the duration and sensation of breath-holding. Clin Sci 1967; 32:425–432.

105. Campbell EJ, Godfrey S, Clark TJ, Freedman S, Norman J. The effect of muscular paralysis induced by tubocurarine on the duration and sensation of breath-holding during hypercapnia. Clin Sci 1969; 36:323–328.

106. Rowell LB. Human Circulation Regulation During Physical. New York: Oxford University Press, 1986.

107. Vanoverschelde JLJ, Essamri B, Vanbutsele R, D'Hondt AM, Cosyns JR, Detry JMR, Melin JA. Contribution of left ventricular diastolic function to exercise capacity in normal subjects. J Appl Physiol 1993; 74:2225–2233.

108. Adams L, Guz A. Dyspnea on exertion. In: Whipp BJ, Wasserman K, eds. Exercise, Pulmonary Physiology and Pathophysiology. New York: Marcel Dekker, 1991.

109. Wasserman K, Whipp BJ, Casaburi R. Respiratory control during exercise. In: Cherniack NS, Widdicombe JG, eds. Handbook of Physiology, vol II. Section 3: The Respiratory System. Bethesda, MD: American Physiological Society, 1986:595–619.

110. Eldridge FL, Waldrop TG. Neural control of breathing during exercise. In: Whipp BJ, Wasserman K, eds. Exercise, Pulmonary Physiology and Pathophysiology. New York: Marcel Dekker, 1991.

111. Fields HL. Pain. New York: McGraw-Hill, 1987:41–78.

112. Wall PD, Melzack R, ed. Textbook of Pain, 2nd ed. Edinburgh: Churchill Livingstone, 1989.

113. Campbell EJM, Guz E. Breathlessness. In: Hornbein TF, ed. Regulation of Breathing, Part II. New York: Marcel Dekker, 1981:1181–1196.

114. Davenport PW, Friedman WA, Thompson FJ, Franzen O. Respiratory-related cortical potentials evoked by inspiratory occlusion in humans. J Appl Physiol 1986; 60: 1843–1848.

115. Revelette WR, Davenport PW. Effects of timing of inspiratory occlusion on cerebral evoked potentials in humans. J Appl Physiol 1990; 68:282–288.

116. Wheatley JR, White DP. Influence of NREM sleep on respiratory-related cortical evoked potentials in normal humans. J Appl Physiol 1993; 74:1803–1810.

117. Pfefferbaum A, Ford JM, Wenegrat BG, Roth WT, Kopell BS. Clinical application of the P3 component of event-related potentials. I. Normal aging. Electroenceph Clin Neurophysiol 1984; 59:85–103.

118. Harver A, Bloch E. Correlation among age, lung function and event-related potentials. Psychophysiology 1992; 92(Suppl):537.

119. Harver A, Bloch E, Sampson M, Carter D. Respiratory-related evoked potentials in patients with obstructive sleep apnea and age-matched controls. FASEB J 1991; 5:A735.

120. Cruz M, Stecenko A, Davenport PW. Respiratory related evoked potentials in asthmatic children. Am Rev Respir Dis 1992; 145:A631.

121. Adams L, Lane R, Shea SA, Cockcroft A, Guz A. Breathlessness during different forms of ventilatory stimulation: a study of mechanisms in normal subjects and respiratory patients. Clin Sci 1985; 69:663–672.

122. Chonan T, Mulholland MB, Cherniack NS, Altose MD. Effects of voluntary

constraining of thoracic displacement during hypercapnia. J Appl Physiol 1987; 63: 1822–1828.

123. Chonan T, Mulholland MB, Altose MD, Cherniack NS. Effects of changes in level and pattern of breathing on the sensation of dyspnea. J Appl Physiol 1990; 69:1290–1295.

124. Schwartzstein RM, Simon PM, Weiss JW, Fencl V, Weinberger SE. Breathlessness induced by dissociation between ventilation and chemical drive. Am Rev Respir Dis 1989; 139:1231–1237.

125. Moosavi SH. Effect of volitionally induced "inappropriate" ventilation during exercise respiratory discomfort in man. J Physiol 1993; 459:351P.

126. Opie L, Smith A, Spalding J. Conscious appreciation of the effects produced by independent changes of ventilation volume and of end-tidal P_{CO_2} in paralysed patients. J Physiol 1959; 149:494–499.

127. Eldridge FL, Chen Z. Respiratory-associated rhythmic firing of midbrain neurons is modulated by a vagal input. Respir Physiol 1992; 90:31–46.

128. Loring SH, Banzett RB, Lansing RW. Activation of respiratory muscles. Semin Respir Med 1991; 12:270–276.

129. Phillipson EA, Bowes G. Control of breathing during sleep. In: Cherniack NS, Widdicombe JG, eds. Handbook of Physiology, vol II. Section 3: The Respiratory System. Bethesda, MD: American Physiological Society, 1986:649–689.

130. Golla FL, Antonovich S. The respiratory rhythm in its relation to the mechanism of thought. Brain 1929, 52:491–509.

131. Tobin MJ, Perez W, Guenther SM, D'Alonzo G, Dantzker DR. Breathing pattern and metabolic behavior during anticipation of exercise. J Appl Physiol 1986; 60:1306–1312.

132. Asmussen E. Regulation of respiration: "the black box." Acta Physiol Scand 1977; 99:85–90.

133. Shea SA, Walter J, Pelley C, Murphy K, Guz A. The effect of visual and auditory stimuli upon resting ventilation in man. Respir Physiol 1987; 68:345–357.

134. Fink BR. The influence of cerebral activity in wakefulness on regulation of breathing. J Appl Physiol 1961; 16:15–20.

135. Harper RM. State-dependent electrophysiological changes in central nervous system activity. In: Haddad GG, Farber JP, eds. Developmental Neurobiology of Breathing. New York: Marcel Dekker, 1991:521–549.

136. Munschauser FE, Mador MJ, Ahuka A, Jacobs L. Selective paralysis of voluntary but not limbically influenced automatic respiration. Arch Neurol 1991; 48:1190–1192.

137. Orem J, Osorio I, Brooks E, Dick T. Activity of respiratory neurons during NREM sleep. J Neurophysiol 1985; 54:1144–1156.

138. Hugelin A. Forebrain and midbrain influence on respiration. In: Cherniack NS, Widdicombe JG, eds. Handbook of Physiology. Section 3. The Respiratory System. Bethesda: American Physiological Society, 1986:69–91.

139. Feldman JL, Smith JC, Ellenberger HH, Connelly CA, Liu GS, Greer JJ, Lindsay AD, Otto MR. Neurogenesis of respiratory rhythm and pattern: emerging concepts. Am J Physiol 1990; 259:r879–886.

140. Ellenberger HH, Feldman JL, Goshgarian HG. Ventral respiratory group projections to phrenic motoneurons: electron microscopic evidence for monosynaptic connections. J Comp Neurol 1990; 302:707–714.

141. Aminoff MJ, Sears TA. Spinal integration of segmental, cortical and breathing inputs to thoracic respiratory motoneurons. J Physiol 1971; 215:557–575.

142. Planche D, Bianchi AL. Modification of bulbar respiratory neuron activity induced by cortical stimulation. [French]. J Physiol (Paris) 1972; 64:69–76.

143. Bassal M, Bianchi AL. Effects de la stimulation des structures nerveuses centrales sur l'activités respiratoires efferentes chez le chat. I. Responses a la stimulation corticale. J Physiol (Paris) 1981; 77:741–757.

144. Orem J, Netick A. Behavioral control of breathing in the cat. Brain Res 1986; 366:238–253.

145. Maskill D, Murphy K, Mier A, Owen M, Guz A. Motor cortical representation of the diaphragm in man. J Physiol 1991; 443:105–121.

146. Foerster O. Motorische Felden und Bahen, vol 6. In: Bumke O, Foerster O, eds. Handbook der Neurologie. Berlin: Springer, 1936:50–51.

147. Colebatch JG, Adams L, Murphy K, Martin AJ, Lammertsma AA, Tochon-Danguy HJ, Clark JC, Friston KJ, Guz A. Regional cerebral blood flow during volitional breathing in man. J Physiol (Lond) 1991; 443:91–103.

148. Ramsay SC, Adams L, Murphy K, Corfield DR, Grootoonk S, Bailey DL, Frackowiak RSJ, Guz A. Regional cerebral blood flow during volitional expiration in man: a comparison with volitional inspiration. J Physiol 1993; 461:85–101.

149. Berardelli A, Cowan JMA, Day BL, Dick J, Rothwell JC. The site of facilitation of the response to cortical stimulation during voluntary contraction in man. J Physiol (Lond) 1985; 360:52P.

150. Cullen JHS, Merton PA, Walker MC. Facilitation of the human long-latency thumb jerk by a cortical stimulus. J Physiol (Lond) 1986; 381:7P.

151. Murphy K, Mier A, Adams L, Guz A. Putative cerebral cortical involvement in the ventilatory response to inhaled CO_2 in conscious man. J Physiol 1990; 420:1–18.

152. Mier A, Murphy K, Shea SA, Guz A. Diaphragmatic EMG in response to cortical magnetic stimulation during sleep. Am Rev Respir Dis 1990; 141:A379.

153. Amassian VE, Quirk GJ, Stewart M. A comparison of corticospinal activation by magnetic coil and electrical stimulation of monkey motor cortex. Electroenceph Clin Neurophysiol 1990; 77:390–401.

154. Burke D, Hicks RG, Stephen JP. Corticospinal valleys evoked by anodal and cathodal stimulation of the human motor cortex. J Physiol 1990; 425:283–299.

155. Edgley SA, Eyre JA, Lemon RN, Miller S. Excitation of the corticospinal tract by electromagnetic and electrical stimulation of the scalp in the macaque monkey. J Physiol 1990; 425:301–320.

156. Macefield G, Gandevia SC. The cortical drive to human respiratory muscles in the awake state assessed by premotor cerebral potentials. J Physiol 1991; 439:545–558.

157. Shea SA, Horner RL, Banner NR, McKenzie E, Heaton R, Yacoub MH, Guz A. The effect of human heart-lung transplantation upon breathing at rest and during sleep. Respir Physiol 1988; 72:131–150.

158. Shea SA, Winning AJ, McKenzie E, Guz A. Does the abnormal pattern of breathing in patients with interstitial lung disease persist in deep, non-rapid eye movement sleep? Am Rev Respir Dis 1989; 139:653–658.

159. Skatrud JB, Dempsey JA. Interaction of sleep state and chemical stimuli in sustaining rhythmic ventilation. J Appl Physiol 1983; 55:813–822.

160. Datta AK, Shea SA, Horner RL, Guz A. The influence of induced hypocapnia and sleep on the endogenous respiratory rhythm in humans. J Physiol 1991; 440:17–33.

161. Badia P, Harsh J, Balkin T, Cantrell P, Klempert A, O'Rourke D, Schoen L. Behavioral control of respiration in sleep. Psychophysiology 1984; 21:494–500.

162. Bye PT, Issa F, Berthon JM, Sullivan CE. Studies of oxygenation during sleep in patients with interstitial lung disease. Am Rev Respir Dis 1984; 129:27–32.

163. Perez-Padilla R, West P, Lertzman M, Kryger MH. Breathing during sleep in patients with interstitial lung disease. Am Rev Respir Dis 1985; 132:224–229.

164. Weil JV, Cherniack NS, Dempsey JA, Edelman NH, Phillipson EA, Remmers JE, Kiley JP. NHLBI Workshop summary. Respiratory disorders of sleep. Pathophysiology, clinical implications, and therapeutic approaches. Am Rev Respir Dis 1987; 136:755–761.

165. Rohrer F. Physiologie der atembewegung. In: Bethe Aea, ed. Handbuch der Normalen und Pathologischen Physiologie, vol 2. Berlin: Springer, 1925:70–127.

166. Otis AB, Fenn WO, Rahn H. Mechanics of breathing in man. J Appl Physiol 1950; 15:592–607.

167. Mead J. Control of respiratory frequency. J Appl Physiol 1960; 15:325–336.

168. Yamashiro SM, Grodins FS. Respiratory cycle optimization in exercise. J Appl Physiol 1973; 35:522–525.

169. Poon CS. Ventilatory control in hypercapnia and exercise: optimization hypothesis. J Appl Physiol 1987; 62:2447–2459.

170. Cherniack NS, Oku Y, Saidel GM, Bruce EN, Altose MD. Optimization of breathing through perceptual mechanisms. In: Takishima T, Cherniack NS, eds. Control of Breathing and Dyspnea. Oxford: Pergamon Press, 1991:337–345.

171. Shea SA, Andres LP, Paydarfar D, Banzett RB, Shannon DC. Effect of mental activity on breathing in congenital central hypoventilation syndrome. Respir Physiol 1993; 94:251–263.

172. Shea SA, Andres LP, Shannon DC, Banzett RB. Ventilatory responses to exercise in humans lacking ventilatory chemosensitivity. J Physiol 1993; 468:623–640.

173. Paton JY, Swaminathan S, Sargent CW, Hawksworth A, Keens TG. Ventilatory response to exercise in children with congenital central hypoventilation syndrome. Am Rev Respir Dis 1993; 147:1185–1191.

174. Dickinson J. Proprioceptive Control of Movement. Princeton, NJ: Princeton University Press, 1976.

175. Keele SW. Movement control in skilled motor performance. Psych Bull 1968; 70:387–403.

176. Lansing RW, Meyerink L. Load compensating responses of human abdominal muscles. J Physiol 1981; 320:253–268.

177. Plassman BL, Lansing RW, Foti K. Inspiratory muscle responses to airway occlusion during learned breathing movements. J Neurophysiol 1987; 57:274–288.

178. Plassman BL, Lansing RW. Perceptual cues used to reproduce an inspired lung volume. J Appl Physiol 1990; 69:1123–1130.

179. Heywood P, Murphy K, Strong B, Belyavin A, Farmer E, Guz A. Is human cortico-spinal control of ventilation as precise as control of hand movement? J Physiol 1992; 452:30P.

180. Smith J, Kreisman H, Colacone A, Fox J, Wolkove N. Sensation of inspired volumes and pressures in professional wind instrument players. J Appl Physiol 1990; 68:2380–2383.

181. Squire L. Memory and Brain. New York: Oxford University Press, 1987.

182. Sharp JT, Druz WS, Moisan T, Foster J, Machnach W. Postural relief of dyspnea in severe chronic obstructive pulmonary disease. Am Rev Respir Dis 1980; 122: 201–211.

183. Martin JG, Shore SA, Engel LA. Mechanical load and inspiratory muscle action during induced asthma. Am Rev Respir Dis 1983; 128:455–460.

184. Lee L, Loudon RG, Jacobson BH, Stuebing R. Speech breathing in patients with lung disease. Am Rev Respir Dis 1993; 147:1199–1206.

185. Newsom Davis J, Sears TA. The proprioceptive reflex control of intercostal muscles during their voluntary activation. J Physiol 1970; 109:711–738.

186. Freedman S. The effects of added loads in man: Conscious and anaesthetized. In: Pengelly LD, Rebuck AS, Campbell EJM, eds. Loaded Breathing. Proceedings of an International Symposium on the Effects of Mechanical Loads on Breathing. Edinburgh: Churchill Livingstone, 1974:22–25.

187. Brashear RE. Hyperventilation syndrome. Lung 1983; 161:257–273.

188. Lewis RA, Howell JB. Definition of the hyperventilation syndrome. Bull Eur Physiopathol Respir 1986; 22:201–205.

189. Tenney SM, Ou LC. Ventilatory response of decoriticate and decerebrate cats to hypoxia and CO_2. Respir Physiol 1977; 29:81–92.

190. Heyman A, Birchfield RI, Sieker HO. Effects of bilateral cerebral infarction on respiratory center sensitivity. Neurology 1958; 8:694–700.

191. Brown HW, Plum F. The neurologic basis of Cheyne-Stokes respiration. Am J Med 1961; 30:849–860.

192. Bykov K. The Cerebral Cortex and the Internal Organs. New York: Chemical, 1957: 93–105.

193. Martin PA, Mitchell GS, Brown KL, Kaarakka P. Paired exercise and chemoreceptor stimulation alter subsequent ventilatory response to exercise. FASEB J 1990; 4:A540.

194. Adams L, Moosavi S, Guz A. Ventilatory response to exercise in man increases by prior conditioning of breathing with added dead space. Am Rev Respir Dis 1992; 145:A882.

195. Gallego J, Perruchet P. Classical conditioning of ventilatory responses in humans. J Appl Physiol 1991; 70:676–682.

196. Lourenço RV, Turino GM, Davidson LAG, Fishman AP. The regulation of ventilation in diffuse pulmonary fibrosis. Am J Med 1965; 38:199–216.

197. Johnston R, Lee K. Myofeedback: a new method of teaching breathing exercises in emphysematous patients. Phys Ther 1976; 56:826–831.

198. Van Doorn P, Folgering H, Colla P. Control of the end-tidal P_{CO_2} in the hyperventilation syndrome: effects of biofeedback and breathing instructions compared. Bull Eur Physiopathol Respir 1982; 18:829–836.

199. Blanc Gras N, Esteve F, Baconnier P, Benchetrit G. A new device for pulmonary rehabilitation based on visual feedback. IEEE, Proceedings of Meeting in Paris, 1992.

200. Gallego J, Ankaoua J, Lethielleux M, Chambille B, Vardon G, Jacquemin C. Retention of ventilatory pattern learning in normal subjects. J Appl Physiol 1986; 61:1–6.

21

Causes of Respiratory Failure

ROLF D. HUBMAYR and GARY C. SIECK

Mayo Clinic and Mayo Medical School
Rochester, Minnesota

I. Introduction

Respiratory failure refers to any condition in which the respiratory system fails to meet the gas exchange demands of the organism. External respiration, that is the exchange of O_2 and CO_2 between cell and atmosphere, proceeds along pathways containing diffusive and convective elements. Diffusion is the primary mode of gas transfer between alveolus and pulmonary capillary blood and between systemic capillary blood and the cell interior. The ventilatory pump and the cardiovascular system represent the convective elements of the gas transport chain. Since this book is devoted to the control of breathing, we will emphasize the role of the ventilatory pump and its neural control system in the pathophysiology of different respiratory failure syndromes. We find this perspective useful because insults to any one component of the cardiopulmonary system elicit control system responses of potential diagnostic and prognostic significance. In most instances, these responses are geared toward preserving alveolar ventilation. For this reason, acute hypercarbia is thought to reflect the overt failure of the ventilatory pump rather than a mere adaptive response compatible with steady-state load compensation.

System physiologists look at the ventilatory pump as a mechanism with a

959

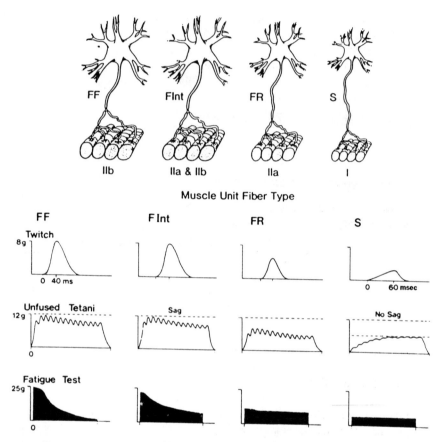

Figure 1 Diaphragm motor units are comprised of a phrenic motoneuron and the muscle fibers it innervates, i.e., the muscle unit. Muscle unit fibers have uniform histochemical staining profiles for myofibrillar ATPase after alkaline and acid preincubations such that they can be classified as type I, IIa, or IIb. Mechanical properties of muscle units also distinguish different motor unit types. Fast-twitch units are distinguished from slow-twitch units by the presence of "sag" in unfused tetani. Subclassification of fast-twitch units is based on fatigue resistance to repetitive stimulation. [Reprinted with permission from the publisher from Sieck GC. Organization and recruitment of diaphragm motor units. In: Roussos C, ed. The Thorax, 2nd ed. New York: Marcel Dekker (in press).]

control system composed of sensors (chemoreceptors and mechanoreceptors), an integrator/controller (brainstem rhythm and pattern generator), effector pathways (motor nerves), and a motor (the respiratory muscles), which moves a machinery (chest wall) and thereby provides ventilation to the lungs. A neurobiologist may look at the same system and see distinct populations of respiratory motor units composed of motor neurons and muscle fibers with specific structural, functional, and metabolic properties (Fig. 1). The motor units are excited or inhibited by premotor neurons and controlled by neuronal networks, which arguably interact with pacemaker cells. The system physiologist, who is often a physician, tries to attribute failure to a single or the "weakest" component of the ventilatory pump hoping to correlate integrated system responses such as respiratory rate, breathing patterns, and chest wall motion with specific mechanisms that may point to specific therapeutic approaches. The neurobiologist, who is often a basic scientist, may be more interested in motor unit plasticity, injury, and repair as the fundamental events that shape muscle output and is less concerned with whether and how such insults are expressed as altered breathing strategy. In the following sections, we discuss the pathobiology of respiratory failure syndromes from both perspectives.

II. Physiological Classification of Ventilatory Pump Failure Syndromes

Failure of the ventilatory pump may be attributed to disorders that affect the respiratory control system, the respiratory muscles, or the nerves that supply them. Failure may also result from excessive demands placed on these structures by inefficiencies in pulmonary gas exchange and by large mechanical loads. A classic example of primary control system failure is narcotics overdose, in which both rate and amplitude of the motor command to the respiratory muscles (and, thus, alveolar ventilation) are substantially reduced (1). Muscular dystrophy, myasthenia gravis, inflammatory polyneuroradiculopathy (Guillain-Barré syndrome), and amyotrophic lateral sclerosis (ALS) represent the most common causes of ventilatory pump failure from neuromuscular damage (2). However, these disorders are insignificant in number compared with lung diseases, which can stress the ventilatory pump to performance failure. Although it is conceptually useful to classify causes of respiratory failure according to the site of the primary insult, usually the problem is multifactorial. This is particularly true in elderly patients with chronic lung diseases who become ventilator dependent after surgical interventions. They represent at least half the patient population in chronic ventilator dependent units (3). Their respiratory muscles are uniformly weak, yet they face high inspiratory loads associated with increased ventilatory requirements from hypermetabolic states and abnormal respiratory system mechanics (4).

Because the respiratory muscles are the effector organs of the ventilatory control system and play such a pivotal role in compensating for pulmonary gas exchange problems, it has become popular to view most forms of acute hypercarbic respiratory failure as manifestations of respiratory muscle fatigue (5). The usefulness and inherent dangers of this oversimplified view are addressed in the following sections.

III. Respiratory Muscle Fatigue

Muscle fatigue has been defined as an inability to maintain an expected or required level of force (6). Applied to the study of the pathophysiology of hypercarbic respiratory failure, this definition has several shortcomings: (1) there is more than one respiratory muscle, (2) their separate or even combined force outputs cannot be measured directly, and (3) ventilatory control is sufficiently complex that defining *the expected or required level of respiratory muscle force*, i.e., *the muscle's load*, is possible only under highly specific experimental conditions. More recent attempts to define muscle fatigue have drawn attention to the reversibility of fatigue with rest and tried to distinguish between fatigue and weakness (7). This distinction lacks experimental support and it is unclear that separating weakness from fatigue has therapeutic consequences. The Respiratory Muscle Fatigue Workshop Group defined weakness as a condition in which the capacity of a *rested* muscle to produce force is impaired (7). The duration of inactivity (rest) required to separate weakness from fatigue was not specified. It is plausible that fatigued and injured (weak) motor units coexist within the same muscle and that both insults require rest for recovery and repair.

The maximal strength of a muscle and the load placed on it are important determinants of fatigue and endurance (8). Several investigators have tested and confirmed this hypothesis with respect to the respiratory system by studying ventilatory load responses in normal volunteers (5,9–14). In these studies, the ventilatory pump was loaded with an external resistance while subjects were instructed to generate a predetermined airway or transdiaphragmatic target pressure (P_{di}) during each breath. The inability to continue this task for prolonged periods of time was considered evidence for muscle fatigue. The validity of this assumption has been subsequently confirmed using bilateral phrenic nerve twitch stimulation (15).

Figure 2 shows the determinants of extrinsic-load-induced diaphragm fatigue as they have emerged from the above experiments (9,10). The quantity $P_{di}/P_{di}\text{MAX}$ on the abscissa is the target pressure or inspiratory load expressed as a fraction of the maximal force, or, more specifically, the pressure-generating capacity of the diaphragm. The quantity T_I/T_{TOT}, or duty cycle, on the ordinate is the inspiratory time expressed as a fraction of the total breath duration. Any

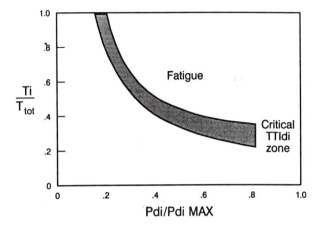

Figure 2 Determinants of the tension time index of the diaphragm (TTIdi) and its predictive value in experimental diaphragm fatigue. See text for further explanation. (Adapted with permission from the publisher from Ref. 10.)

combination of variables that defines a point to the right and upward of the shaded area identifies a load as nonsustainable or fatiguing, while a point to the left and down implies that the load will not induce fatigue and can be sustained "indefinitely." According to Figure 2, any load that is large relative to the maximal strength of the diaphragm and that has to be sustained over a large portion of the respiratory cycle is fatiguing. Because of the hyperbolic interface between the fatigue and nonfatigue zones (shaded area), fatiguing loads can be distinguished from nonfatiguing loads on the basis of a single variable, which is the product of $P_{di}/P_{di}\text{MAX}$ and T_I/T_{TOT}. This product is known as the tension time index of the diaphragm (*TTI*di). According to Figure 2, whenever *TTI*di is greater than 0.15, performance failure of the diaphragm is predicted (9).

Despite its scientific appeal, *TTI*di or related parameters have not proven useful in the clinical diagnosis of impending ventilatory pump failure (16–18). Possible reasons include (1) difficulties in measuring muscle strength in critically ill patients, and (2) the complexity of interactions between intrinsic load and the system's load response. Valid measurements of maximal respiratory muscle strength require the voluntary activation of all motor units. This is difficult to ascertain in highly motivated normal volunteers (19), let alone in patients. In contrast to laboratory-based experiments during which known, invariant loads (i.e., P_{di} targets) can be imposed to study ventilatory responses, patients with diseases of the respiratory system are not constrained to generate a unique P_{di}. Presumably, the respiratory pump's response to a load is designed to minimize the required force or power output of the respiratory muscles (12,20,21). The compensatory response of the respiratory pump to loading thus modifies the effective load on the respiratory muscles. A response that is out of proportion to the magnitude or type of mechanical load implies intrinsic respiratory muscle disease, impending muscle fatigue, or impending pump failure (22). This is distinct from overt failure, which is associated with hypoventilation and hypercarbia. What constitutes an appropriate load response requires a basic understanding of respiratory muscle dynamics and coordination. Defining impending pump failure on the basis of an abnormal load response is void of any mechanistic assumptions. Nevertheless, such an operational definition may be useful to the clinician, who must decide when to intervene and unload the ventilatory pump with mechanical ventilation.

Fatigue may occur at any one of numerous sites between the ventilatory controller and the muscle's contractile machinery (8). Fatigue is often classified as central or peripheral, depending on whether motoneurons generate action potentials. In other words, central fatigue implies reduced synaptic input to the motoneuron, while peripheral fatigue indicates the inability of muscle units to respond to adequate synaptic drive from the motoneuron. In turn, peripheral fatigue may occur at several potential sites, either presynaptic or postsynaptic. The site of fatigue appears to be highly task-specific and, thus, varies with the experimental setting. Electrical stimulation of motor axons using high stimulation rates predisposes them to neuromuscular transmission failure (Fig. 3) (23–27). Neuromuscular transmission failure may result from a failure of axonal action potential propagation (24), reduced quantal release of acetylcholine (ACh), increased hydrolysis of ACh or diffusion away from the motor end-plate, a desensitization of the ACh receptor, or a reduced excitability of the sarcolemmal membrane. The likelihood of neurotransmission failure varies with the rate of motoneuron excitation and with motor unit type; i.e., fast fatigable (F_f) and fast intermediate (F_{int}) motor units are most susceptible to this type of fatigue (25,28–30).

Muscle fatigue (postsynaptic) also depends on the rate of stimulation with a "low"- and "high"-frequency type of fatigue being commonly distinguished. High-frequency fatigue is generally attributed to alterations in t-tubule excitability such that forces generated at higher rates of stimulation are disproportionately affected. Accordingly, high-frequency fatigue recovers rapidly. Moreover, this type of muscle fatigue may influence certain types of muscle fibers with more extensive t-tubular systems and greater force-generating capacities (e.g., type IIb muscle fibers). Low-frequency fatigue is far more complex and may relate to any one of a number of mechanisms. For example, excitation-contraction coupling may fail because of inadequate calcium release from the sarcoplasmic reticulum. Calcium sensitivity of troponin may be altered. Cross-bridge cycling may be affected because of altered actomyosin adenosine triphosphatase (ATPase) activity on the accumulation of metabolites. Finally, there may be an inadequate energy supply through oxidative metabolism. A hallmark of low-frequency fatigue is slower recovery, which makes it difficult to distinguish from muscle weakness.

superimposed direct muscle stimulation

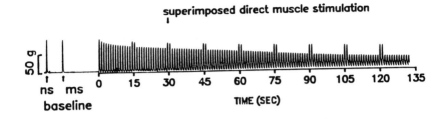

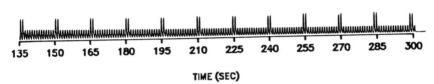

TIME (SEC)

Figure 3 Neuromuscular transmission failure in the rat diaphragm muscle was estimated by comparing forces generated by superimposed direct muscle stimulation with those generated by phrenic nerve stimulation. (Reprinted with permission from the publisher from Ref. 27.)

Muscle weakness can be distinguished from muscle fatigue by the presence of a structural defect or injury. In either case, the final common denominator is reduced force generation. Muscle injury has been observed following eccentric contractions and/or very forceful motor efforts (31). However, it is likely that muscle injury and repair are normal sequelae of muscle plasticity to a variety of conditions. Muscle weakness may result if the balance is tipped toward injury and repair mechanisms are swamped (e.g., with eccentric contractions) or inadequate (e.g., in aging). As with fatigue, muscle injury responds to rest, and thus, it would be difficult to distinguish muscle fatigue from muscle weakness solely on this basis.

Muscle fatigue or weakness need not involve the entire muscle. Indeed, abundant evidence indicates a wide range of susceptibility among muscle fiber types. Fatigability is a criteria for classifying different motor unit types (24,30,32), each comprising specific muscle fiber types (Fig. 1). Since ventilatory behaviors most likely require only limited motor unit recruitment, muscle fatigue and weakness may also be focal, depending on which motor units and muscle fibers are recruited. Indeed, the type of muscle fatigue may also vary depending on motor unit recruitment. For example, sustained low-level motor efforts may evoke predominantly low-frequency fatigue, whereas motor efforts involving short bursts of greater force may elicit high-frequency fatigue, neuromuscular transmission failure, or muscle injury.

Regardless, a key question is how the central nervous system responds to either the potential for or presence of fatigue. Clearly, one prophylactic mechanism adapted by the nervous system is an orderly recruitment of motor units, with less fatigable units recruited first. Thus, the central nervous system matches recruitment with the limitations of the motor units involved. But what if fatigue or weakness occurs among some motor units? The central nervous system may have the capability of alternating motor unit recruitment to allow recovery. Several investigators have reported motor unit rotation, that is, a redistribution of motor unit recruitment patterns within a muscle in the presence of fatiguing loads (33–36).

IV. Is Ventilatory Pump Failure a Manifestation of Respiratory Muscle Fatigue?

The relevance of peripheral fatigue, including neuromuscular transmission failure, as cause of reduced diaphragm muscle pressure output in ventilator-dependent patients is not known. Indeed, it has thus far not been possible to distinguish between diaphragm fatigue and weakness on clinical grounds. Virtually every study of respiratory muscle function in critically ill, ventilator-dependent patients has shown a profound reduction in diaphragm contractility. Although survivors tend to get stronger over time (37), the confounding influences of respiratory muscle inactivity and detraining during mechanical ventilation, intermittent fatigue related to weaning attempts, the resolution of disease and of hypermetabolic states, together with changes in nutritional status make it impossible to infer cause and effect from the time course of recovery in respiratory muscle function.

The clinical manifestations of ventilatory pump failure may provide clues about specific causes and the mechanisms underlying certain respiratory failure syndromes. In particular, observations made during weaning of patients from mechanical ventilation have been helpful because weaning offers an opportunity to prospectively evaluate the load response of a patient's ventilatory pump. In this respect, weaning is analogous to exercise testing in its goal to characterize the performance capacity and endurance of the cardiopulmonary systems and to identify weak links in these systems on the basis of physiological responses.

Although many weaning studies have been motivated by the desire to predict weaning outcome, they have also shed light on the sensitivity and specificity of certain physiological weaning response patterns. Physicians had become aware for some time that tachypnea frequently precedes overt gas exchange failure (38,39). A number of recent studies have drawn attention to reductions in tidal volume (V_T)

during unsuccessful weaning attempts (16,17,40). Table 1, adapted from Yang and Tobin (40), shows both threshold values and the accuracy of commonly used weaning indices. Results are based on a prospective-validation data set of 64 patients, 28 of whom failed weaning. Although the authors emphasized the value of the frequency/tidal volume ratio (a rapid shallow breathing index, f/V_T), it should be noted that a $V_T \geq 325$ ml was almost as good a predictor of weaning failure as a $f/V_T \leq 105$.

A system physiologist looks at V_T as the stroke volume of the ventilatory pump and makes comparisons with cardiac mechanics. This has proven useful insofar as it has drawn attention to some basic determinants of respiratory muscle

Table 1 Threshold Values and Accuracy of the Indices Used to Predict Weaning Outcome

Index	Value[a]	Positive predictive value[b]	Negative predictive value[b]
Minute ventilation (L/min)	≤ 15	0.55	0.38
Respiratory frequency (breaths/min)	≤ 38	0.65	0.77
Tidal volume (ml)	≥ 325	0.73	0.94
Tidal volume (ml)/patient's weight (kg)	≥ 4	0.67	0.85
Maximal inspiratory pressure (cmH$_2$O)[c]	≤ -15	0.59	1.00
Dynamic compliance (ml/cmH$_2$O)	≥ 22	0.65	0.58
Static compliance (ml/cmH$_2$O)	≥ 33	0.60	0.53
PaO$_2$/PA$_{O2}$ ratio	≥ 0.35	0.59	0.53
Frequency/tidal volume ratio (breaths/min/L)	≤ 105	0.78	0.95
CROP index (ml/breath/min)[d]	≥ 13	0.71	0.70

[a]Threshold values were those that discriminated best in the training data set between the patients who were successfully weaned and those in whom a weaning trial failed; $\geq$ and $\leq$ indicate whether the values above the threshold value or those below it are those that predicted a successful weaning outcome
[b]Values shown were derived from the complete prospective-validation data set, comprising 36 successfully weaned patients and 28 patients in whom weaning failed.
[c]To convert value to kilopascals, multiply by 0.09807.
[d]A weaning outcome index that integrates thoracic compliance, respiratory rate, arterial oxygenation, and P$_I$max.
Source: Adapted from Ref. 40 with permission from the publisher.

output, such as precontraction length (preload), contractility, and (after)load; these undoubtedly play a role in the regulation of V_T (41,42). Considering the number of conditions in which preload, contractility, and afterload of respiratory muscles are altered, (rapid) shallow breathing cannot be a specific manifestation of respiratory muscle fatigue. Rapid, shallow breathing caused by a reduced respiratory muscle preload is frequently seen in dynamically hyperinflated patients with airway obstruction; impaired contractility characterizes patients with either fatigue or weakness; and changes in lung or chest wall mechanics commonly increase the (after)load of respiratory muscles in disease. System physiologists often equate certain ventilatory parameters with parameters of muscle performance. For example, it is commonly assumed that in conditions during which respiratory rate or air flow is increased (e.g., exercise), the velocity of muscle shortening is also proportionately increased. This reasoning need not be correct, because it would imply a reduction in load on the muscle or the recruitment of muscle fibers with faster shortening velocities.

There are degrees of freedom in addition to rapid, shallow breathing with which the ventilatory pump can cope with a load. These include (1) a cyclic redistribution of motor outputs among different groups of respiratory muscles, the equivalent of motor unit rotation on a large scale (5,43), and (2) acceptance of a lower alveolar ventilation to minimize the respiratory muscles' overall force requirements.

The classic paper by Konno and Mead (44) introduced the idea that the careful inspection of chest wall shape and motion would provide information about respiratory muscle coordination. Several investigators have analyzed chest wall motion in disease, including during weaning from mechanical ventilation (38,45–50). In general, patients who fail weaning have more asynchronous chest wall movements between rib cage and abdomen than those who succeed. However, there is a great deal of overlap in asynchrony parameters between groups, such that none of them has sufficient predictive value to aid in clinical decision making. There is also a greater breath-to-breath variability of chest wall displacement patterns in failure patients. In Tobin's study, this was reflected in a greater standard deviation about the fraction of V_T, which was attributable to rib cage expansion ($\Delta V_{RC}/V_T$) (49). Individual $\Delta V_{RC}/V_T$ values were not clustered around two means as would be the case for true "respiratory alternans." Respiratory alternans describes an oscillation in chest wall displacement patterns between two distinct states, classically between rib cage and abdominal breathing. Such a strategy had been thought to provide alternating "rest" to different sets of respiratory muscles, i.e., diaphragm and inspiratory rib cage muscles.

To date it has not been possible to demonstrate a reversible change in the contractile properties of respiratory muscles, i.e., peripheral fatigue, in a clinical setting. Figure 4 shows a recording of gastric pressure (P_{ga}), flow ($\dot{V}$), and esophageal pressure (P_{es}) in a ventilator-dependent patient at the end of a 1-hr weaning trial that had to be aborted because of dyspnea. At that time, the

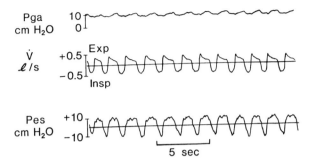

Figure 4 Recordings of gastric pressure (P_{ga}), gas flow ($\dot{V}$), and esophageal pressure (P_{es}) are shown from a ventilator-dependent patient at the end of a 1-hr weaning trial. For explanation see text. Exp, expiration; Insp, inspiration. (Reprinted with permission from the publisher from Hubmayr RD, Rehder K. Respiratory muscle failure in critically ill patients. Semin Respir Med 1992; 13:14–21.)

respiratory rate had risen to 40 breaths/minute. The shape of the expiratory flow wave tracing, with its convexity toward the time axis, demonstrates the presence of airway obstruction. Palpation of the abdomen revealed active expiration, which probably accounts for the increase in P_{es} to $+10$ cmH$_2$O at end-expiration. The inspiratory swings in P_{es} were relatively large (20 cmH$_2$O) and accompanied by a fall in P_{ga} as abdominal muscle activity decayed early during each breath. Figure 5 shows the result of two supramaximal bilateral phrenic nerve twitch stimulations, one performed before weaning (left) and one 5 min after the symptom-limited weaning trial (right). Even after prolonged respiratory muscle rest before weaning, intrathoracic (ΔP_{es} and ΔP_{ao}) and abdominal pressure swings (ΔP_{ga}) during supramaximal twitch stimulation of the phrenic nerves were significantly reduced. Normal volunteers generate a twitch $P_{di} \geq 20$ cmH$_2$O near relaxation volume (51) as opposed to the 6 cmH$_2$O in this patient who suffered from profound diaphragm weakness. After weaning, there was no further reduction in twitch P_{di}, suggesting that weaning had not induced peripheral diaphragm fatigue. These observations are consistent with the hypothesis that respiratory distress and compromise need not reflect contractile failure of the respiratory muscles themselves (peripheral fatigue) but may involve load perception and integrative responses on a central level. The example also points out that weakness and fatigue may share common load responses in terms of respiratory dynamics and muscle coordination.

V. The Control of Alveolar Ventilation in Acute Ventilatory Pump Failure

The inability to demonstrate peripheral diaphragm fatigue in the clinical setting has caused many to discard fatigue as an important mechanism in patients with

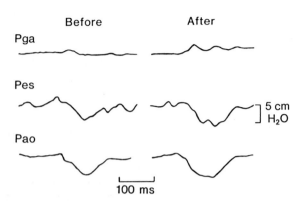

Figure 5 Gastric pressure (P_{ga}), esophageal pressure (P_{es}), and airway occlusion pressure (P_{ao}) were recorded during bilateral twitch stimulation of the phrenic nerves in the patient whose weaning response pattern is shown in Figure 4. The twitch pressure responses before and immediately after the symptom-limited weaning trial are identical. (Reprinted with permission from the publisher from Hubmayr RD, Rehder K. Respiratory muscle failure in critically ill patients. Semin Respir Med 1992; 13:14–21.)

acute hypercarbia. Such a view is not justified in light of the considerable methodological and conceptual difficulties inherent to all clinically feasible muscle function tests. It is, nevertheless, useful to ask whether and under what conditions the ventilatory control system sacrifices the maintenance of eucapneic CO_2 tensions in an attempt to reduce the work of breathing.

The arterial CO_2 tension reflects the CO_2 stores of the organism and is an important determinant of alveolar ventilation.

$$\text{Paco}_2 = \frac{\dot{V}CO_2\, k}{\dot{V}_E(1 - V_d/V_t)} \tag{1}$$

V_{CO_2} is the volume of CO_2 eliminated by the lungs, $\dot{V}_E$ the minute volume, and V_d/V_t the dead space to tidal volume ratio. In contrast to behavioral influences and mechanoreceptive feedback, CO_2 seems to have little effect on the regulation of breathing at partial pressures below 40 mmHg (52–56). On the other hand, it would be highly unusual to find Paco_2 in excess of 43 mmHg in an awake, spontaneously breathing normal human. This is because the normal ventilatory control system increases its output and, thus, ventilation in defense of normocarbia. There are some exceptions to this rule: Hypercarbia is not always a manifestation of ventilatory failure. The rise in Paco_2 during sleep reflects the reduced drive and chemoresponsiveness that accompany the loss of the wakefulness stimulus (52,57–60). Mechanically hyperventilated normal volunteers, in whom inspired gas is supplemented with CO_2, accept mild hypercarbia without a compensatory increase in respiratory muscle output (60). Sedatives and narcotics can blunt the ventilatory response to CO_2 without preventing the assumption of a new steady state, albeit at the expense of an increased CO_2 store.

How then is the physician to know whether mild acute hypercarbia represents an adaptive load response or impending pump failure? Normal volunteers seem unable (or unwilling) to sustain breathing against external resistive loads once end-tidal CO_2 starts to climb (61; Hubmayr RD, personal observation). To the extent to which this observation is relevant for the load response of patients with respiratory diseases, even mild load-induced (or weaning-induced) hypercarbia would be a sign of impending respiratory failure. Two recent studies in which unsuccessful weaning from mechanical ventilation was used as a human model of respiratory failure speak to this issue (16,17). Dunn et al. (16) measured the CO_2 responsiveness of the unloaded respiratory pump in difficult-to-wean patients with the recruitment threshold technique. Measurements of inspiratory muscle output were made during mechanical ventilation, and the machine settings were adjusted until phasic inspiratory muscle activity was completely suppressed. The CO_2 recruitment threshold (CO_2RT) was defined as the lowest Pa_{CO_2} at which the supplementation of CO_2 caused the reappearance of phasic inspiratory muscle activity (54). Since CO_2RT was determined during mechanical (hyper)ventilation, it was interpreted as a measure of the CO_2 "setpoint" of the unloaded respiratory pump. CO_2RT was then compared to the Pa_{CO_2} during unassisted spontaneous breathing (CO_2SB) in each patient (Fig. 6). Five patients who were successfully weaned maintained CO_2SB within 2 mmHg of CO_2RT. In contrast, seven of 10 patients who failed weaning because of dyspnea or sustained tachypnea (respiratory rate ≥ 30) retained CO_2SB compared with CO_2RT by more than 3 mmHg. Although patients who failed weaning tended to be weaker, there was a considerable overlap in parameters of mechanical load and inspiratory muscle strength between the groups. These findings underscore the interactions between load, load response, and CO_2 homeostasis. They suggest that load-induced reductions in tidal volume and alveolar ventilation often preclude the assumption of a new steady state.

The findings of Jabour et al., who evaluated a new weaning index based on ventilatory endurance and the efficiency of gas exchange, support the conclusion that the CO_2 gain of the ventilatory control system sets substantial limits to the load responses of the ventilatory pump (17). Jabour et al. applied the concepts illustrated in Figure 2 to the weaning assessment of ventilator-dependent patients. They defined a pressure time index (PTI) that was based on an estimate of the average inspiratory muscle pressure per breath (P_{breath}), the maximum voluntarily generated negative inspiratory pressure (NIP), and the inspiratory duty cycle, which is the inspiratory time (T_I) normalized by the total breath duration (T_{TOT})

$$PTI = (P_{breath}/NIP) \times (T_I/T_{TOT}) \tag{2}$$

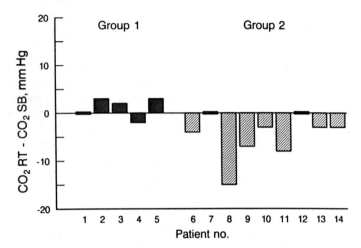

Figure 6 Differences between arterial CO_2 tensions (in mmHg) during recruitment testing (CO_2RT) and at the end of a weaning trial while breathing spontaneously (CO_2SB) are shown on the ordinate. Dark shaded bars (patients 1–5) represent observations in group 1 (success); light shaded bars (patients 6–14) represent observations in group 2 (failure). Note that three of the five patients in group 1 had lower arterial CO_2 tensions during spontaneous breathing than predicted from CO_2RT. Also note that seven of the nine patients in group 2 had arterial CO_2 tensions that exceeded CO_2RT by 3 mmHg or more. (Reprinted with permission from the publisher from Dunn WF, Nelson SB, Hubmayr RD. The control of breathing during weaning from mechanical ventilation. Chest 1991; 100:754–761.)

P_{breath} was calculated making the following assumptions: (1) the impedance of the respiratory system is independent of the mode of breathing, which means that the load on the inspiratory muscles during a spontaneous breath is the same as the load on a mechanical ventilator during a machine breath, (2) differences in inspiratory flow between the modes of breathing can be ignored, (3) there is no inadvertent positive end-expired pressure (PEEP), and (4) expiratory muscles do not contribute to the work of breathing. Therefore:

$$P_{breath} = (P_{pk} - PEEP) \times (V_Tsb/V_Tmv) \tag{3}$$

where P_{pk} is the peak airway pressure during mechanical ventilation, PEEP is the extrinsic positive end-expired airway pressure, and V_Tsb and V_Tmv the tidal volumes during spontaneous breathing and mechanical ventilation, respectively. Jabour et al. realized that PTI did not fully characterize the load on the inspiratory muscles and that the efficiency of the lungs as CO_2 eliminators also had to be taken into account (17). Their weaning index (WI), therefore, also contains an estimate

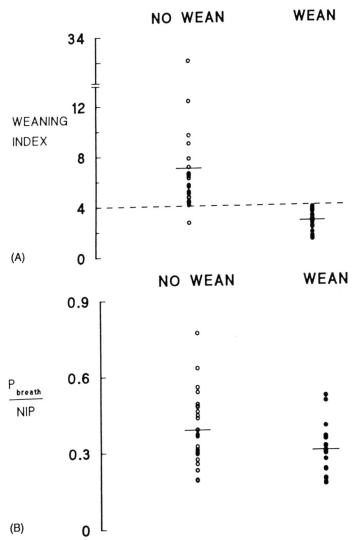

Figure 7 (A) Values of the weaning index (WI) in 44 weaning trials. Sensitivity, specificity, and predictive values of WI were ⩾0.95. (B) Values of inspiratory muscle pressure (P_{breath}) normalized by maximal negative inspiratory pressure (NIP) in 44 weaning trials. There is no difference between the weaning groups. (Reprinted with permission from the publisher from Ref. 17.)

of the minute volume ($V_E 40$, in ml/kg/min) that would have been required to achieve an arterial CO_2 tension (Pa_{CO_2}) of 40 mmHg.

$$WI = PTI \times V_E 40/V_T sb \tag{4}$$

$V_E 40$ was linearly interpolated from the actual V_E (in ml/kg BW) and Pa_{CO_2} during mechanical ventilation.

$$V_E 40 = (fmv \, V_T mv) \times (Pa_{CO_2} mv/40) \tag{5}$$

Although most of Jabour's assumptions are not strictly valid, the discriminative power of WI turned out to be very good (Fig. 7A). What is interesting about Jabour's approach is that patients are obviously not constrained to defend a Pa_{CO_2} of 40 mmHg during spontaneous breathing and their weaning index thus represents a hypothetical rather than an actual load. Indeed, PTI by itself did not distinguish very well between weaning success and weaning failure (Fig. 7B), which again suggests that under conditions of weaning-induced distress the power output of the respiratory muscles is insufficient to meet the target ventilation.

VI. The Control of Alveolar Ventilation in Chronic Respiratory Diseases

Although chronic hypercarbia and chronic respiratory acidosis are frequently referred to as *chronic respiratory failure*, it is better to view such abnormalities in alveolar ventilation as adaptive than to consider them manifestations of pump failure. In contrast to the constraints imposed by CO_2 sensitivity on acute load compensation, hypercarbia seems to be much better tolerated when insults and loads escalate gradually. Under these circumstances, reducing respiratory muscle work at the expense of alveolar ventilation seems to be a viable strategy for load compensation. Removal of an insult or load usually results in an augmentation of ventilation and a resetting of the Pa_{CO_2} toward normal. One example is the sustained improvement in pulmonary gas exchange in some patients with obstructive sleep apnea after CPAP therapy. Another example is the lowering of daytime Pa_{CO_2} in selected populations with intermittent nocturnal mechanical ventilation (INMV).

The efficacy of intermittent ventilatory assistance in patients with chronic hypercarbia secondary to neuromuscular diseases, chest wall deformities, and central hypoventilation syndromes has been shown in multiple studies (62–68). Although the majority of these studies were small and uncontrolled, their results were overwhelmingly positive. INMV restored daytime CO_2 tension and improved respiratory muscle strength. Whether nocturnal mechanical ventilation is efficacious in patients with severe chronic obstructive pulmonary disease (COPD) remains controversial (69–76). Our own preliminary experience with nocturnal

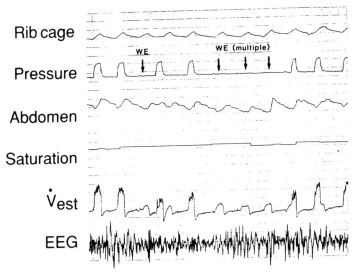

Figure 8 Strip chart recording of chest wall motion (rib cage, abdomen), airway pressure, oxygen saturation (pulse oximetry), flow ($\dot{V}$), and EEG in a sleeping nasally ventilated subject with COPD. The downward arrows indicate wasted efforts (WE), that is, breaths that failed to trigger a machine response. Also note that machine output and patient effort are out of phase following WE.

nasal positive pressure ventilation in COPD patients is very disappointing (Gay, PC, personal communication).

Benefit, defined as a reduction in daytime P_{CO_2} after several months of INMV, has been attributed to one of two possible mechanisms: (1) resting of respiratory muscles resulting in recovery from chronic fatigue and (2) prevention of nocturnal hypoventilation resulting in a lowering of the controller's setpoint for CO_2. There is no direct support for either hypothesis. Nevertheless, either mechanism requires optimal coupling between the respiratory muscle pump and the ventilator. Stroetz and Gay (77) used INMV on stable hypercarbic COPD patients and showed that even under research protocol conditions, up to 20% of spontaneous breathing efforts fail to elicit a machine response; they could not show that machine breaths are delivered in the absence of patient efforts (Fig. 8). In comparison, patients with neuromuscular diseases are easy to ventilate.

VII. Summary

Important insights into the mechanisms of ventilatory failure have resulted from collaborations between clinicians, system physiologists, and basic scientists interested in nerve and muscle biology. Significant challenges remain. The distinctions between normal adaptive responses, maladaptation, and failure continue to be blurry. Basic research on motor unit structure and function, together with clinical research using nocturnal mechanical ventilation to study patient-ventilator interactions and chronic unloading, should bring these distinctions into clearer focus.

Acknowledgment

This work was supported by Grants HL-45026 and HL-37680 from the National Institutes of Health.

References

1. Hickey RF, Severinghaus JW. Drug effects. In: Hornbein TF, ed. Regulation of Breathing, Part II. New York: Marcel Dekker, 1981:1251–1312.
2. Kaminski MJ, Young RR. Neuromuscular and neurological disorders affecting respiration. In: Roussos C, Macklem PT, eds. The Thorax, Part B. New York: Marcel Dekker, 1985:1023–1087.
3. Gracey DR, Viggiano RW, Naessens JM, Hubmayr RD, Silverstein MD, Koenig GE. Outcomes of patients admitted to a chronic ventilator-dependent unit in an acute-care hospital. Mayo Clin Proc 1992; 67:131–136.
4. Reinoso MA, Gracey DR, Hubmayr RD. Interrupter mechanics of patients admitted to a chronic ventilator dependency unit. Am Rev Respir Dis 1993; 148:127–131.
5. Roussos C, Macklem PT. The respiratory muscles. N Engl J Med 1982; 307:786–797.
6. Edwards RHT. Human muscle function and fatigue. In: Porter R, Whelan J, eds. Human Muscle Fatigue: Physiological Mechanisms. Ciba Foundation Symposium 82. London: Pitman Medical 1981:1–18.
7. NHLBI Workshop Summary. Respiratory muscle fatigue: report of the respiratory muscle fatigue workshop group. Am Rev Respir Dis 1990; 142:474–480.
8. Enoka RM, Stuart DG. Neurobiology of muscle fatigue. J Appl Physiol 1992; 72: 1631–1648.
9. Bellemare F, Grassino A. Effect of pressure and timing of contraction on human diaphragmatic fatigue. J Appl Physiol 1982; 53:1190–1195.
10. Bellemare F, Grassino A. Evaluation of human diaphragm fatigue. J Appl Physiol 1982; 53:1196–1206.
11. Gallagher CG, Im Hof V, Younes M. Effect of inspiratory muscle fatigue on breathing pattern. J Appl Physiol 1985; 59:1152–1158.
12. Jones GL, Killian KJ, Summers E, Jones NL. Inspiratory muscle forces and endurance in maximum resistive loading. J Appl Physiol 1985; 58:1608–1615.
13. McCool FD, McCann DR, Leith DE, Hoppin FG. Pressure-flow effects on endurance of inspiratory muscles. J Appl Physiol 1986; 60:299–303.
14. Roussos C, Macklem P. Diaphragmatic fatigue in man. J Appl Physiol 1977; 43: 189–197.

15. Aubier M, Murciano D, Lecocguic Y, Viires N, Pariente R. Bilateral phrenic stimulation: a simple technique to assess diaphragmatic fatigue in humans. J Appl Physiol 1985; 58:58–64.

16. Dunn WF, Nelson SB, Hubmayr RD. The control of breathing during weaning from mechanical ventilation. Chest 1991; 100:754–761.

17. Jabour ER, Rabil DM, Truwit JD, Rochester DF. Evaluation of a new weaning index based on ventilatory endurance and the efficiency of gas exchange. Am Rev Respir Dis 1991; 144:531–537.

18. Swartz M, Marino P. Diaphragmatic strength during weaning from mechanical ventilation. Chest 1985; 88:736–739.

19. Bellemare F, Bigland-Ritchie B. Assessment of human diaphragm strength and activation using phrenic nerve stimulation. Respir Physiol 1984; 58:263–277.

20. Mead J. Control of respiratory frequency. J Appl Physiol 1960; 15:325–336.

21. Yamashiro SM, Daubenspeck JA, Lauritsen TN, Grodins FS. Total work of breathing optimization in CO_2 inhalation and exercise. J Appl Physiol 1975; 38:702–709.

22. Rochester DF. Does respiratory muscle rest relieve fatigue or incipient fatigue. Am Rev Respir Dis 1988; 138:516–517.

23. Aldrich TK, Shander A, Chaudhry I, Nagashima H. Fatigue of isolated rat diaphragm: role of impaired neuromuscular transmission. J Appl Physiol 1986; 61:1077–1083.

24. Fournier M, Alula M, Sieck GC. Neuromuscular transmission failure during postnatal development. Neurosci Lett 1991; 125:34–36.

25. Johnson BD, Sieck GC. Differential susceptibility of diaphragm muscle fibers to neuromuscular transmission failure. J Appl Physiol 1993; 75:341–348.

26. Kelsen SG, Nochomivitz ML. Fatigue of the mammalian diaphragm in vitro. J Appl Physiol 1982; 53:440–447.

27. Kuei JH, Shadmehr R, Sieck GC. Relative contribution of neurotransmission failure to diaphragm fatigue. J Appl Physiol 1990; 68:174–180.

28. Clamman HP, Robinson AJ. A comparison of electromyographic and mechanical fatigue properties in motor units of the cat hindlimb. Brain Res 1985; 327:203–219.

29. Sandercock TG, Faulkner JA, Albers JW, Abbrecht PH. Single motor unit and fiber action potentials during fatigue. J Appl Physiol 1985; 58:1073–1079.

30. Sieck GC, Fournier M. Changes in diaphragm motor unit EMG during fatigue. J Appl Physiol 1990; 68:1917–1926.

31. Carlson BM, Faulkner JA. The regulation of skeletal muscle fibers following injury: a review. Med Sci Sports Exercise 1983; 15:187–198.

32. Burke RE, Levine DN, Zajac FE III, Tsairis P, Engel WK. Mammalian motor units: Physiological-histochemical correlation in three types of cat gastrocnemius. Science 1971; 174:709–712.

33. Forbes A. The interpretation of spinal reflexes in terms of present knowledge of nerve condition. Physiol Rev 1922; 2:361–414.

34. Enoka RM, Robinson GA, Kossev AR. Task and fatigue effects on low-threshold motor units in human hand muscle. J Neurophysiol 1989; 62:1344–1359.

35. Person RS. Rhythmic activity of a group of human motoneurones during voluntary contraction of a muscle. Electroenceph Clin Neurophysiol 1974; 36:585–595.

36. Seyffarth H. The behaviour of motor-units in voluntary contractions. Avhandlinger Utgitt Norske Videnskap-Akad Oslo. I. Matematisk-Naturvidenskapelig Klasse 1940; 4:1–63.

37. Criner GJ, Kreimer DT, Pidlaoan L. Patient outcome following prolonged mechanical ventilation (MV) via tracheostomy. Am Rev Respir Dis 1993; 147:A874.

38. Cohen CA, Zagelbaum G, Gross D, Roussos CH, Macklem PT. Clinical manifestations of inspiratory muscle fatigue. Am J Med 1982; 73:308–316.

39. Gilbert R, Auchincloss JH, Peppi D, Ashutosh K. The first few hours off a respirator. Chest 1974; 65:152–157.

40. Yang KL, Tobin MJ. A prospective study of indexes predicting the outcomes of trials of weaning from mechanical ventilation. N Engl J Med 1991; 324:1445–1450.

41. Hagan BM, Hubmayr RD. Respiratory failure: dynamics of breathing and coordination. In: Update in Intensive Care and Emergency Medicine. Vol 15: Ventilatory Failure. New York: Springer-Verlag 1991:75–96.

42. Hubmayr RD. Dynamics of breathing in ventilatory failure. In: Roussos C, ed. The Thorax, 2nd ed. New York: Marcel Dekker (in press).

43. Krieger BP, Ershowsky PF, Becker DA, Gazeroglu HB. Evaluation of conventional criteria for predicting successful weaning from mechanical ventilatory support in elderly patients. Crit Care Med 1989; 17:858–861.

44. Konno K, Mead J. Static volume-pressure characteristics of the rib cage and abdomen. J App Physiol 1968; 24:544–548.

45. Ashutosh K, Gilbert R, Auchincloss JH, Peppi D. Asynchronous breathing movements in patients with obstructive pulmonary disease. Chest 1975; 67:553–557.

46. Hoover CF. The diagnostic significance of inspiratory movements of the costal margins. Am J Med Sci 1920; 159:633–646.

47. Krieger BP, Ershowsky P. Noninvasive detection of respiratory failure in the intensive care unit. Chest 1988; 94:254–261.

48. Sharp JT, Goldberg NB, Druz WS, Fishman HC, Danon J. Thoracoabdominal motion in chronic obstructive pulmonary disease. Am Rev Respir Dis 1977; 115:47–56.

49. Tobin MJ, Guenther SM, Perez W, Lodato RF, Mador MJ, Allen SJ, Dantzker DR. Konno-Mead analysis of rib cage-abdominal motion during successful and unsuccessful trials of weaning from mechanical ventilation. Am Rev Respir Dis 1987; 135:1320–1328.

50. Tobin MJ, Perez W, Guenther SM, Lodato RF, Dantzker DR. Does rib cage-abdominal paradox signify respiratory muscle fatigue? J Appl Physiol 1987; 63:851–860.

51. Hubmayr RD, Litchy WJ, Gay PC, Nelson SB. Transdiaphragmatic twitch pressure: Effects of lung volume and chest wall shape. Am Rev Respir Dis 1989; 139:647–652.

52. Fink BR. Influence of cerebral activity in wakefulness on regulation of breathing. J Appl Physiol 1961; 16:15–20.

53. Hanks EC, Ngai SH, Fink BR. The respiratory threshold for carbon dioxide in anesthetized man: determination of carbon dioxide threshold during halothane anesthesia. Anesthesiology 1961; 22:393–397.

54. Prechter GC, Nelson SB, Hubmayr RD. The ventilatory recruitment threshold for carbon dioxide. Am Rev Respir Dis 1990; 141:758–764.

55. Simon PM, Leevers AM, Landry DM, Murty JL. Volume and frequency thresholds for inhibition of inspiratory motor output during mechanical ventilation. Am Rev Respir Dis 1993; 147:A166.

56. Simon PM, Skatrud JB, Landry DM, Dempsey JA. Level of chemical stimuli at initiation and termination of apnea in humans. Am Rev Respir Dis 1992; 145:A406.

57. Ingrassia TS III, Nelson SB, Harris CD, Hubmayr RD. Influence of sleep state on CO_2 responsiveness: a study of the unloaded respiratory pump in humans. Am Rev Respir Dis 1991; 144:1125–1129.

58. Lydic R, Orem J. Respiratory neurons of the pneumotaxic center during sleep and wakefulness. Neurosci Lett 1979; 15:187–192.

59. Orem J, Osorio I, Brooks E, Dick T. Activity of respiratory neurons during NREM sleep. J Neurophysiol 1985; 54:1144–1156.

60. Simon PM, Dempsey JA, Landry DM, Skatrud JB. Effect of sleep on respiratory muscle activity during mechanical ventilation. Am Rev Respir Dis 1993; 147:32–37.

61. Cherniack RM, Chodirker WB. Hypercapnia with relief of hypoxia in normal individuals with increased work of breathing. J Appl Physiol 1972; 33:189–192.

62. Curran FJ. Night ventilation by body respirators for patients in chronic respiratory failure due to late stage Duchenne muscular dystrophy. Arch Phys Med Rehabil 1981; 62:270–274.

63. Ellis ER, Bye PTP, Bruderer JW, Sullivan CE. Treatment of respiratory failure during sleep in patients with neuromuscular disease. Am Rev Respir Dis 1987; 135: 148–152.

64. Garay SM, Turino GM, Goldring RM. Sustained reversal of chronic hypercapnia in patients with alveolar hypoventilation syndromes: long-term maintenance with non-invasive nocturnal mechanical ventilation. Am J Med 1981; 70:269–274.

65. Gay PC, Patel AM, Viggiano RW, Hubmayr RD. Nocturnal nasal ventilation for treatment of patients with hypercapneic respiratory failure. Mayo Clin Proc 1991; 66:695–703.

66. Goldstein RS, Molotiu N, Skrastins R, Long S, De Rosie J, Contreras M, Pipkin J, Rutherford R, Phillipson EA. Reversal of sleep-induced hypoventilation and chronic respiratory failure by nocturnal negative pressure ventilation in patients with restrictive ventilatory impairment. Am Rev Respir Dis 1987; 135:1049–1955.

67. Kerby GR, Mayer LS, Pingleton SK. Nocturnal positive pressure ventilation via nasal mask. Am Rev Respir Dis 1987; 135:738–740.

68. Waldhorn RE. Nocturnal nasal intermittent positive pressure ventilation with bi-level positive airway pressure (BiPAP) in respiratory failure. Chest 1992; 101:516–521.

69. Braun NMT, Marino WD. Effect of daily intermittent rest of respiratory muscles in patients with severe chronic airflow limitation (CAL). Chest 1984; 84:59S–60S.

70. Celli B, Lee H, Criner G, Bermudez M, Rassulo J, Gilmartin M, Miller G, Make B. Controlled trial of external negative pressure ventilation in patients with severe chronic airflow obstruction. Am Rev Respir Dis 1989; 140:1251–1256.

71. Cropp A, Dimarco AF. Effects of intermittent negative pressure ventilation on respiratory muscle function in patients with severe chronic obstructive pulmonary disease. Am Rev Respir Dis 1987; 135:1056–1061.

72. Elliot M, Carroll M, Wedzicha J, Branthwaite M. Nasal positive pressure ventilation

can be used successfully at home to control nocturnal hypoventilation in COPD. Am Rev Respir Dis 1990; 141:322 (abstract).

73. Gutierrez M, Beroiza T, Contreras G, Diaz O, Cruz E, Moreno R, Lisboa C. Weekly Cuirass ventilation improves blood gases and inspiratory muscle strength in patients with chronic air-flow limitation and hypercarbia. Am Rev Respir Dis 1988; 138: 617–623.

74. Shapiro SH, Ernst P, Gray-Donald K, Martin JG, Wood-Dauphinee S, Beaupré A, Spitzer WO, Macklem PT. Effect of negative pressure ventilation in severe pulmonary disease. Lancet 1992; 340:1425–1429.

75. Strumpf DA, Millman RP, Carlisle CC, Grattan LM, Ryan SM, Erickson AD, Hill NS. Nocturnal positive-pressure ventilation via nasal mask in patients with severe chronic obstructive pulmonary disease. Am Rev Respir Dis 1991; 144:1234–1239.

76. Zibrak JD, Hill NS, Federman EC, Kwa SL, O'Donnell C. Evaluation of intermittent long-term negative-pressure ventilation in patients with severe chronic obstructive pulmonary disease. Am Rev Respir Dis 1988; 1515–1518.

77. Stroetz RW, Gay PC. Breath synchronization analysis criteria: a method to evaluate patient/ventilator interaction. Am Rev Respir Dis 1993; 147:A885.

Part Six

METABOLIC-STATE EFFECTS

22

Changes in Respiratory Motor Activity During Rapid Eye Movement Sleep

ALLAN I. PACK

University of Pennsylvania Medical Center
Philadelphia, Pennsylvania

I. Introduction

Sleep can be divided into a number of different stages. Broadly, it can be divided into non-rapid eye movement (NREM) sleep and rapid eye movement (REM), or active, sleep. REM sleep is a peculiar stage of our lives, first recognized in 1953 by Aserinsky and Kleitman (1). In this stage of sleep there are two major phenomena: atonia of postural muscles produced by active inhibition of motoneurons, and widespread flurries of activity (phasic events) throughout the brain and brainstem. Rapid eye movements, for which the state is named, are but one example of such phasic events. Phasic events are found not only in the brain, but also in peripheral outflows affecting such phenomena as heart rate, blood pressure, and coronary blood flow (for example, see 2).

These profound changes in REM sleep, not surprisingly, lead to changes in the neural systems controlling ventilation. This is of clinical import since apneas in the disease called obstructive sleep apnea are often longer in REM sleep than in other sleep states and are associated with greater oxygen desaturation (3). Thus, in this review, I concentrate on what we know about mechanisms leading to altered neural control of respiration in REM sleep.

The problem of understanding the neural basis of changes in ventilatory control in sleep is an order of magnitude more complex than the problem of respiratory rhythmogenesis discussed by Feldman and Smith in Chapter 2. Sleep is a rhythmic activity like respiration, but on a different time scale, and is inherently more complex since several different substates are involved. Moreover, understanding the changes in the neural control of ventilation during sleep involves investigation of the interaction between the neural circuitry controlling sleep and those generating breathing. Approaches to the problem involve techniques similar to those discussed by Feldman and Smith in Chapter 2, with some important differences. First, although investigators studying the neural mechanisms of sleep control have used in vitro approaches such as brain slices (for example, see 4–6), they have not utilized in vitro approaches in which a rhythm, e.g., REM sleep episodes, continues to be generated. On the one hand, a very extensive use has been made, however, of studies of sleep and also of breathing in chronic, normally behaving animals in which single unit activity has been recorded. It is interesting that one of the challenges to current concepts of respiratory rhythmogenesis comes from such studies (7,8). It seems important that insights gained from reduced or anesthetized preparations be more fully evaluated in the normally behaving animal.

II. Changes in Ventilation and Its Components During REM Sleep in Humans

Changes in ventilation and its components in REM sleep in humans have been assessed in several studies. Studies have shown that ventilation in REM sleep is reduced compared to that in wakefulness (9–14). In some studies respiratory frequency has been shown to be state-dependent (9,10), whereas others have shown the opposite, that it is state-independent (11). But REM sleep is a heterogeneous state where the intensity of phasic events varies from episode to episode. Since these phasic events influence respiration (16), the resultant average change may well be affected by how "phasic" the particular episode of REM sleep being studied is. Thus, as in all behaving subjects, ventilation during REM sleep cannot be interpreted simply in terms of chemical control of respiration. There are phasic influences that arise outside the traditional chemical control system for respiration that profoundly alter ventilatory output.

Ventilation in REM sleep, as compared to NREM sleep, is associated with a greater contribution of abdominal motion, compared with rib cage motion, to tidal volume (10,11,14,15,17). This is particularly so during the phasic events of REM sleep when the rib cage contribution to ventilation declines even further (14,15). These differences in the effect of REM sleep on rib cage and abdominal motion are likely to reflect differences in the output to the diaphragm and intercostal muscles (see further below).

Another change found during phasic events is asynchronous motion in the rib cage and abdomen (15). This asynchrony has been demonstrated in normal adults and is most marked during flurries of eye movements (15). It can at times be so extreme that paradoxical motion of the two compartments occurs.

Respiratory frequency also shows changes with phasic events. It increases in association with eye movements (14), primarily owing to decreases in expiratory duration, with alterations in inspiratory duration playing a much smaller role. Of the various variables that change in relationship to eye movements, increases in respiratory rate show the highest degree of statistical association (14). The variable with the second highest degree of association with the occurrence of phasic events is rib cage motion (14). This shows a progressive decrement with increases in eye movement density. Other variables, total ventilation and abdominal motion, show no association. There are both increases and decreases in these variables in association with eye movements, so there is no significant correlation for either with eye movement density.

Interestingly, for those variables (rib cage motion, respiratory frequency, and expiratory duration) that show the greatest association with eye movement density, the nature of the relationship is relatively consistent from episode to episode of REM sleep within one night in a single subject or across nights. However, there is significant intersubject variation. Some subjects (high responders) show larger changes in these variables with phasic events whereas other subjects have little variation (low responders).

These data suggest that the most major change in ventilation in REM sleep is the increased variability from breath to breath. A major source of this variability is the specific changes (reductions in expiratory duration with resultant increases in frequency and in rib cage motion) that occur in relationship to the phasic events of this sleep state. The magnitude of these changes varies from subject to subject, presumably reflecting differences in the impact of neural circuits activated during REM sleep on the respiratory neural control circuitry. A discussion of the basis of these changes observed in humans follows.

III. Changes in Electromyographic Activity During REM Sleep

At the next level of analysis, important changes are observed in electromyographic activity in REM sleep. A number of different patterns of change in respiratory muscle activity are found, which have different time courses (summarized in Table 1). First, atonia of limb and axial muscles occurs throughout REM sleep. Respiratory muscles are not completely spared from this effect; there are individual motor units even in the diaphragm that cease firing throughout REM sleep (18). Clearly, however, both the respiratory pump and upper airway muscles cannot

Table 1 Patterns of Alteration in Respiratory Motor Output in REM Sleep

Pattern	Time course	Comments
Atonia of muscle	Lasts duration of REM	Even single units in diaphragm can show this
Intermittent decrement	One to few breaths	Occurs in relation to phasic events
Intermittent augmentation	One to few breaths	Occurs in relation to phasic events
Fractionations (pauses in activity)	40–100 msec	Tends to occur in flurries in relation to phasic events
Asynchrony of activation	One to few breaths	Influences of REM sleep affect motoneuron pools in nonhomogeneous fashion

have as profound an atonia as limb muscles; otherwise respiration would not continue.

In addition to a tonic suppression, important changes in respiratory motor output occur in temporal association with the phasic events of REM sleep. In 1986, Kline et al. (19) analyzed the rate of rise of diaphragmatic electromyograms (EMGs) during sleep in cats. They found that in slow-wave sleep there is little variation from breath to breath. However, during REM sleep the variability of diaphragmatic activity increases. There are breaths in which the slope is depressed (intermittent decrement) and breaths in which it is increased (intermittent augmentation). The former are associated with lengthening of inspiratory duration and the latter with shortening. The occurrence of both intermittent decrements and augmentations of EMG is more common during periods with a high intensity of phasic events compared with periods when phasic events are less frequent. These phenomena are found in other respiratory motor outputs, although there may be some important quantitative differences. The influence of the neuronal mechanisms that lead on the one hand to a reduction and on the other hand to an increase in motor output may be different for different motor outputs. This has, however, not been directly addressed. There is some circumstantial evidence from the studies in humans described above (14). We found an increasing decline in rib cage motion with increasing phasic events (REM), while for abdominal motion there is essentially a balance between reductions and increases so that with increasing phasic events there is no net change in abdominal motion. These human studies also suggest that the duration of these phasic effects on different motor outputs may be different (14); abdominal motion might decline for a single breath during phasic events, rib cage motion is reduced for several breaths. In cats a reduction (or an increase) in diaphragmatic activity in association with phasic events is largely a single-breath phenomenon. While there has been no systematic study of the duration of intermittent decrements in various motor outputs, longer-lasting declines in the EMG of an upper airway dilator muscle (genioglossus) have been observed in humans (20) (see Fig. 1). Interestingly, in cats, electrical stimulation of one of the pathways that may be involved in these effects, the midpontine dorsal tegmentum, produces longer-lasting declines in activity of

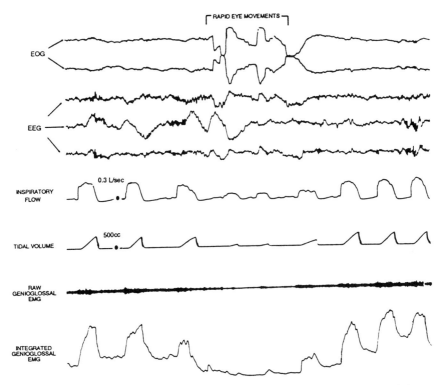

Figure 1 Intermittent decrement in upper airway muscle activity (genioglossus) in a human in association with phasic eye movements in REM sleep. From the top down: electro-oculograms (two traces); electroencephalogram (three traces); respiratory airflow; tidal volume; raw genioglossal EMG; integrated genioglossal EMG. In association with the eye movements (marked at top of record), there is reduction in airflow, tidal volume, and a loss of genioglossal EMG activity. (Reproduced from Ref. 20 by permission.)

hypoglossal nerve and soleus muscle than it does for diaphragmatic EMG activity (21,22). Diaphragm EMG activity returns to control levels even though the electrical stimulus is maintained. In contrast, the activity of hypoglossal and sciatic nerves is abolished throughout the period of stimulation and for a brief period thereafter.

Another type of change in respiratory muscle activity that is seen during the phasic events of REM sleep is what has been called by Orem "fractionations" (23) (see Fig. 2). These are brief pauses in activity of the muscle that last 40–100 msec and occur in clusters in association with the phasic events of REM sleep (see Fig. 2). Cross-correlation analysis shows that the reductions in diaphragmatic EMG are related temporally to the occurrence of ponto-geniculo-occipital (PGO) waves. PGO waves are an extremely sensitive marker of phasic events in REM sleep. They are large-voltage waves that can be recorded in the pons, lateral geniculate nucleus, and occipital cortex. PGO waves are normally found in REM sleep but can be induced in other states by sudden novel stimuli such as auditory tones (24–29). Associated with the induced PGO wave are changes in the activity of many peripheral muscles (29) and orienting behavior (28); the latter response habituates rapidly with repeated presentations of the stimulus (28). Fractionations in diaphragmatic activity also occur in association with PGO waves induced by auditory tones (30). They are particularly obvious when the auditory tone is applied in REM sleep. Decrements in the activity of the diaphragm can also be induced by auditory tones in NREM sleep, although there is sometimes an initial excitatory response that is not observed in REM sleep. Thus, there is evidence of a fairly tight

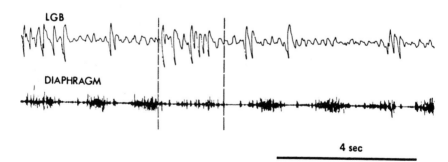

Figure 2 Fragmentations of diaphragm activity occurring in association with the phasic events of REM sleep. Recording of ponto-geniculo-occipital (PGO) waves from the lateral geniculate body (LGB) (top) and diaphragm EMG activity (bottom). PGO waves tend to occur in clusters. In association with these clusters, one observes that the normal diaphragm EMG burst is fragmented (area between dashed lines). This fragmentation is due to the presence of fractionations in activity (brief pauses of the order of 40–100 msec) that also tend to occur in clusters. (Reproduced from Ref. 23 by permission.)

connection between the neuronal mechanisms that produce PGO waves and descending drives to the diaphragm.

These phasic changes in motor output in REM sleep do not necessarily affect the entire motor output to a muscle simultaneously. This has been shown by Hendricks and Kline (31), who recorded simultaneously from two positions in the diaphragm, one in each hemidiaphragm or at two positions within one hemidiaphragm. During the phasic events of REM sleep, there is evidence of asynchronous activation of different portions of the muscle. Phasic changes in the motor output observed at one recording site may not be observed at the other. This suggests that the neural circuitry activated during phasic events in REM sleep does not project in a uniform manner to the relevant motoneuron pools.

During REM sleep, the neural mechanisms that are operative do not just affect motor output, but they may also change the magnitude of the relays of sensory afferent information. Studies of Ia pathways do not provide compelling evidence of the suppression of transmission during REM sleep (32). Evidence, however, exists for a REM sleep-related suppression in spinal ascending pathways (33). So far, there are no systematic studies of the state-related changes in the transmission in sensory pathways from respiratory afferents, e.g., from chemoreceptors or pulmonary receptors. Presynaptic inhibition of some respiratory afferents exist (see Chapter 5), yet it is not known whether this mechanism plays a role during REM sleep. There is a marked reduction of the Hering-Breuer reflex mediated by pulmonary stretch receptors during phasic REM sleep (34), yet the site and mechanism for this effect remain unknown.

IV. Relationship Between Phasic Events of REM Sleep and Occurrence of Apneas

The changes in respiratory motor output associated with phasic events are relevant to the occurrence of apnea during sleep, as shown by studies of an animal model of obstructive sleep apnea—the English bulldog. This animal, with obvious structural changes in its upper airway, has episodes of obstructive sleep apnea, particularly during REM sleep (35). Recordings of the EMG activity of the diaphragm and of an upper airway dilator muscle, the sternohyoid, reveal that obstructive apneas occur in relation to the phasic changes in respiratory motor output in REM sleep (36). Thus, tonic reduction in motor output is not sufficient, at least in this animal model, to lead to apnea. Rather, apneas occur when there is an additional phasic decrement in the activity of upper airway dilator muscles. Both periods of intermittent decrements in activity and periods with multiple fractionations can result in an apnea (36). Thus, understanding the basis of these phasic respiratory phenomena associated with REM sleep not only is intrinsically interesting, but also has great clinical relevance.

V. Neural Systems Involved in Generation of REM Sleep

Once we have described the changes that take place in muscle activity in REM sleep, particularly during phasic events, we must next try to understand the underlying neural mechanisms involved. Much has been learned about the neural mechanisms generating REM sleep since the original description of the state (1). It is necessary before discussing the neural mechanisms that might be responsible for the respiratory changes in REM sleep to briefly review what we know about these processes. [For excellent reviews on the neural mechanisms involved in REM sleep, the interested reader is referred to the reviews by Jones (37) and Siegel (38) and the monograph of Steriade and McCarley (39).]

The conventional wisdom is that REM sleep is generated in the brainstem. This conclusion comes from early studies in which transections of the brain were performed at various levels (40,41). The animals were allowed to recover and patterns of activity were subsequently studied. Animals with transections at the rostral end of the pons showed recurring periods that had many hallmarks of REM sleep—atonia, rapid eye movements, and so forth. In these preparations respiration during these REM-like periods was irregular (41). Although these studies do show that rhythmically occurring periods like REM sleep can be generated, this does not, of itself, prove that the brainstem is responsible for normal REM sleep. In other rhythmic systems, e.g., the heart, rhythm persists even though the normal rhythm generator (sinoatrial node) is removed. We do not know whether the normal control mechanism for REM sleep is maintained in these chronically decerebrate animals; i.e., should these REM-like episodes be interrupted, would there be evidence of increased pressure for REM sleep as in normal animals? Thus, in my view, the demonstration that cycles with features like that in REM sleep were maintained in the decerebrate preparation does not constitute sufficient proof that natural REM sleep is exclusively generated by brainstem mechanisms.

Nevertheless, the majority of work on the neural mechanisms of REM sleep has concentrated on the brainstem. Several groups of neurons have been identified whose firing changes with REM sleep. Cholinergic cells increase their firing in REM sleep; they have been called REM-on cells. In contrast, both serotonergic cells of the raphe and noradrenergic cells of locus coeruleus decrease their firing in REM sleep (REM-off cells). This has led to the reciprocal-interaction model for control of REM sleep. In brief, the reciprocal interaction model posits that there are mutually inhibitory connections between the cholinergic cells on the one hand and serotonergic and noradrenergic cells on the other. Thus the decline in the firing of raphe (42) and locus coeruleus (43,44) cells at the onset of REM sleep is thought to disinhibit cholinergic cells, allowing them to become active. (For a full, excellent description of the reciprocal interaction model, see 45.)

Much of the circuitry underlying this model has been elucidated, as have certain aspects of the cellular mechanisms involved. In the rostral pons, there are two groups of cholinergic cells—the pendunclo-pontine-tegmental muscles (PPT) and the laterodorsal tegmental nucleus (LDT). Lesions of the areas containing cholinergic cells markedly diminish or abolish the phasic events of REM sleep (PGO waves, eye movements) without affecting the amount of REM sleep (46). The number of PGO waves remaining after such lesions is correlated with the number of cholinergic cells remaining (46). Recent studies using more discrete lesions indicate that the PPT, rather than the LDT, is responsible for PGO waves in REM sleep (47). Within the PPT, there are cells that fire in association with PGO waves and are thought to be burst cells involved in the generation of these waves (48,49). The PPT is, however, unlikely to be a homogeneous system; rather, there is probably a distinct microorganization involved, but this has not been fully elucidated. We do know that there is an area toward the caudal end of PPT, close to the peribrachial region, where chemical stimulation produces profound, long-lasting increases in both REM sleep and the frequency of PGO waves (50). Cells in this region fire before the occurrence of PGO waves and before the firing of cells in the more rostral part of PPT (51). Thus, the burst generator may be situated here.

Cholinergic cells in the PPT are under the control of a number of different afferents. Important in this regard are serotonergic neurons presumably from the dorsal raphe since there is evidence of a projection from this region to LDT/PPT (52). Serotonergic cells from dorsal raphe are thought to inhibit cholinergic cells in PPT. There is considerable evidence to support this view: (1) depletion of serotonin (5-HT) by *p*-chlorophenylalanine (PCPA) results in the appearance of PGO waves in awake cats (53–55) [this does not occur in rats (56)]; (2) parasagittal lesions interrupting the presumed input from dorsal raphe release PGO waves in wakefulness (55); (3) the decline of firing of raphe cells during REM sleep (42) is temporally linked to the appearance of PGO waves (57–60); and (4) burst neurons in the LDT/PPT area are hyperpolarized by 5-HT (5,61), an effect that seems to be mediated by the 5-HT receptor of the 1A subtype (61).

But 5-HT may not be the only inhibitory neurotransmitter involved. An alternative view is that both noradrenaline and 5-HT are inhibitory and that the decline in both in REM sleep releases the PGO burst cells (62). The noradrenaline may come, at least in part, from neurons of the locus coeruleus (LC). In the rat, in which LC is a rather homogeneous noradrenergic group, the firing of these cells declines in REM sleep (43,44). In cats there is intermingling of noradrenergic cells with cholinergic neurons in the LDT/PPT area (63). The evidence for noradrenergic inhibition of burst cells is somewhat weaker than for 5-HT, since the effects of noradrenaline on cells in the LDT/PPT area are not as consistent as the effect of 5-HT (64). Thus, the neurochemical control of PGO wave generation (and consequently also the respiratory phasic events) is likely to be complex. This complexity is supported by there being a number of different neuron types in the PPT region that increase or decrease their firing in relation to PGO waves (65).

Neurons in the PPT have both ascending and descending projections. Cells in the PPT project to the thalamus (66–70) and produce facilitatory effects on their targets as revealed by a long-lasting muscarinic depolarization (71,72). In addition, PGO waves can be blocked in the lateral geniculate nucleus by nicotinic antagonists (73). Thus, respiratory phasic changes might involve the ascending pathways that lead to activation of cortical cells. As previously proposed (74), phasic changes in respiratory motor output may be a direct expression of dreams. Alternatively, phasic changes in respiratory motor output might be mediated by descending projections altering the activity of the relevant motoneurons and/or premotor cells. Recent anatomical studies reveal that cholinergic cells in the PPT also project caudally to the nucleus pontis oralis (PO) (75–77). Enhanced acetylcholine release in this region can be measured during state-dependent respiratory depression (78). Neurons from PO cells send axons that course both laterally (79) and along the dorsal midline to the medulla. Stimulation of this midline area results in a decrement in postural tone (80,81) and suppression of hypoglossal and diaphragmatic activity (21,22). There is, moreover, a projection from the LDT/PPT to the paramedian reticular nucleus of the caudal medulla (82), one of the medullary areas associated with the atonia of REM sleep (83).

One particularly important area in this descending pathway from the rostral cholinergic cells is located ventromedial to locus coeruleus in pontis oralis. It is called by some "subcoeruleus," a term used here. Small lesions of this area abolish, at least to some degree, the atonia that occurs in REM sleep (84,85), while larger lesions of pontis oralis allow more complex behaviors to be expressed in REM sleep (85). Lesions of subcoeruleus also alter respiratory motor output. Following such lesions, the rate of rise of diaphragmatic activity in REM sleep is increased compared with that in slow-wave sleep (86). Moreover, the fractionations of diaphragmatic activity in REM sleep (described above) are virtually abolished by such lesions (86). The region is cholinoceptive and can be activated by the muscarinic agonist carbachol.

VI. Changes in Respiratory Motor Output in the Carbachol Model of REM Sleep

The increase in cholinergic cell firing during REM sleep has prompted a number of studies to determine whether artificially simulating acetylcholine release can produce REM sleep or at least some components of the state. These studies usually involve the mixed nicotinic/muscarinic agonist carbachol. It was demonstrated as early as 1963 that local applications of carbachol into the pons produced a state like normal REM sleep (87). This technique has since been repeatedly applied and it has been found that microinjections of carbachol into the pontine reticular formation can lead to either a full-blown REM sleep-like state or dissociated states with, for example, increased phasic events without the other features of REM sleep or atonia without the other phenomena (88–90). The response obtained depends, at least to some extent, on the site of the microinjection (88–90). This is, however, not the sole explanation for different responses; injections at the same site in the same animal given at different times can produce different responses depending on the state of the animal at the time of injection (91). That the atonia produced resembles that in normal REM sleep is supported by the observation that the state-specific inhibitory postsynaptic potentials (IPSPs) produced following carbachol microinjection (92) are similar to those found in natural REM sleep (93–96).

Pontine carbachol injection thus presents a useful tool to study some of the changes in respiratory motor output that occur in REM sleep. For this purpose, the tool was first applied in studies in chronically instrumented animals (97–99). During episodes of REM sleep induced by carbachol, there is reduction in minute ventilation and respiratory rate that are similar, albeit more marked, than those occurring in natural REM sleep (97,98). The reductions in respiratory rate that accompany the depression of the respiratory motor output are positively correlated with the amount of endogenous acetylcholine released in the pontine tegmentum on the side opposite to that injected with carbachol (78). In these chronic animals, microinjections of carbachol also produced reductions in the activity of an upper airway muscle—the posterior cricoarytenoid (97,99). As in normal REM sleep, the percentage reduction in activity is much greater than the percentage reduction in ventilation. These observations both add support to the role of cholinergic mechanisms in REM sleep and demonstrate the usefulness of this approach to studying the changes in respiratory motor control in REM sleep.

Although the use of carbachol in chronically instrumented animals has the advantage of producing long-lasting episodes of REM sleep, one can study in chronic animals the respiratory changes in natural REM sleep itself. Even greater advantages are obtained by using carbachol in decerebrate animals. In such animals one can bring to bear a wide range of neurophysiological and pharmacological techniques, many of which cannot be used in the chronic animal. Thus our group has concentrated our studies using carbachol in decerebrate cats (100–105) and rats (106). Carbachol microinjections into the area ventromedial to the locus coeruleus (subcoeruleus), the same area that we lesioned in the studies reported in the previous section, produce profound changes in respiratory motor output (see Fig. 3). In the artificially ventilated, vagotomized, decerebrate cat with blood gases held constant, carbachol produces decrements in all respiratory motor outputs (see Fig. 3) and a reduction in respiratory rate. The degree of reduction in activity is different in the different motor outputs. The decrement in phrenic nerve activity is the least; there is a greater reduction in intercostal nerve activity, with the reduction in expiratory activity being much greater than that for inspiratory activity; and a marked suppression of hypoglossal nerve activity. The degree of suppression of hypoglossal nerve activity is comparable to the reduction in activity

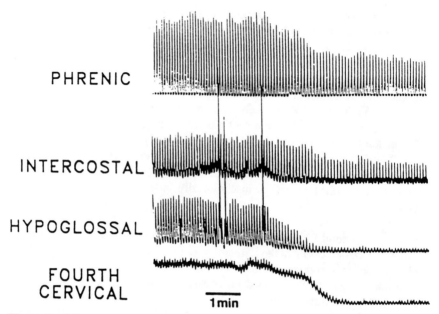

PHRENIC

INTERCOSTAL

HYPOGLOSSAL

FOURTH
CERVICAL

1 min

Figure 3 Effect of microinjection of carbachol into the pons on respiratory motor output. Moving average of activity recorded on four peripheral nerves: phrenic nerve, external intercostal nerve, hypoglossal nerve, and from a branch of C-4 to neck muscles. Carbachol was microinjected just before the beginning of these illustrated recordings. Carbachol produces decrements in the activity of all motor nerves although there are distinct differences in the magnitude of the effect on different motor outputs. For further details see text.

to postural neck muscles. Thus, there is a distinct hierarchy to the "state" dependence of the different respiratory motor outputs.

In this preparation the effects of activation of this cholinoceptive area on respiratory motor output are maximized. The microinjection of carbachol is likely to produce a simultaneous, powerful, and long-lasting activation of all cholinoceptive neurons. In natural REM sleep it seems unlikely that all such neurons are simultaneously activated. Furthermore, all feedback mechanisms that could compensate for the depression of motor output, e.g., changes in blood gas tensions sensed by peripheral and central chemoreceptors, are not operative in the decerebrate, paralyzed, artificially ventilated preparation. When such feedbacks are present, the effects are less marked; for example, in spontaneously breathing decerebrate cats, microinjection of carbachol produces only a transient reduction in phrenic nerve activity (105). The increase in carbon dioxide following carbachol results in phrenic nerve activity returning to baseline levels. However, intercostal and hypoglossal activity do not return to control levels until the effects of carbachol are reversed.

Thus, in the preparation that we employ, the effect of activation of this area on respiratory motor output is exaggerated. This exaggerated, reproducible, stable response is advantageous because it allows adequate time for experimental manipulation and data collection. The issue arises, however, whether results obtained from this approach are relevant to normal REM sleep. Our answer to this is yes. An important caveat, however, is that we are looking at only one component of the REM sleep mechanism, albeit an extremely important one. We know that in the area we are microinjecting carbachol, neuronal activity increases in REM sleep. Lesions of this area reduce the degree of atonia in REM sleep (84,85) and virtually abolish the fractionations of the diaphragm found in REM sleep (86). Species differences in the response to carbachol microinjections also support our assertion. In rats, inspiratory intercostal activity is little affected following carbachol injection (106). Similarly, inspiratory intercostal activity in rats is relatively preserved in natural REM sleep (107). Likewise, the duration of the reduction in motor activity following carbachol is relatively short in rats (106) compared with cats. Episodes of REM sleep in rats are also brief, of the order of 1 min (108).

These observations together suggest to us that activation of this area of the pontine reticular formation by acetylcholine during REM sleep is an important component of this process. Although our use of carbachol to mimic this activation leads to an exaggerated response in decerebrate animals, it points to the profound effect of this area on respiratory motor output, particularly to the upper airway (100), and also on cardiovascular variables (101). Thus, this approach provides a tool to begin to dissect the cellular and subcellular mechanisms of the reduction in respiratory motor activity that can occur in REM sleep.

VII. Insights from the Carbachol Model About Mechanisms of Depression of Respiratory Motor Output in REM Sleep

The use of carbachol microinjection provides a powerful approach to investigating changes at the cellular level. One logical question concerns whether there is a reduction in the activity of respiratory premotor cells. The answer to this question is yes. On average, the activity of cells in the ventral respiratory group (VRG) declines following carbachol microinjection (102). The magnitude of the decline in peak firing rate is similar for both inspiratory and expiratory neurons (about 12%) and is also similar to the decrement in phrenic nerve activity that is found (102). However, the magnitude of the decrement in peripheral expiratory motor output is much greater than the observed decline in the corresponding VRG expiratory premotor cells. This suggests that, for at least some respiratory motoneuron pools, there must be additional mechanisms that affect motoneuron activity through pathways other than alterations in the descending influence from the VRG.

At first sight, the effects of carbachol microinjection on the activity of VRG neurons might seem incompatible with the results of Orem (109), who studied the behavior of respiratory neurons in both the ventral and dorsal groups during natural REM sleep in chronically instrumented animals. He found that the discharge of both inspiratory and expiratory neurons increased in relationship to an increasing frequency of PGO waves. This increase in respiratory neuron activity involved an increase both in the frequency of respiratory bursts and in the cell's discharge frequency within a burst. When neuronal activity was extrapolated to a state where there is an absence of PGO waves (tonic REM sleep), neuronal activity in the ventral group was generally decreased compared to non-REM sleep, whereas in the dorsal group the responses were more variable.

In comparing these results one must remember that carbachol microinjection into subcoeruleus in decerebrate animals does not reproduce all the effects of REM sleep on respiration. Respiration is slowed following carbachol and not variable from breath to breath. In contrast, in natural REM sleep there is increased variability of respiration in relationship to phasic events, and respiration may accelerate at these times. Thus, carbachol microinjection activates only one component of a much more complex process that occurs in natural REM sleep, which involves both excitatory and inhibitory influences. However, the reduction in activity of VRG cells following carbachol that we observed (102) is compatible with the reduction that Orem found in the same cell group during "tonic" REM sleep (109).

Although our approach differs from that of Orem, the major conclusion of the two studies are identical. The marked suppression of respiratory motor activity, described previously, that can be observed during REM sleep, and can lead to apnea, cannot be explained solely by changes in activity of premotor respiratory neurons in the medulla. Rather, activation of inhibitory inputs to respiratory motoneurons or disfacilitation due to reductions in other so far unidentified excitatory inputs must occur. For postural motoneurons of the lumbar spinal cord, the most complete information about their behavior during REM sleep comes from the elegant studies of Chase and colleagues (93–95, 110–112, for review see 96) and from the studies of Glenn and Dement (113). Chase et al. have demonstrated that, in natural REM sleep, lumbar motoneurons are hyper-polarized, have decreases in membrane resistance, and have large inhibitory postsynaptic potentials that are characteristic of this state (93–95). As discussed previously, similar changes in the behavior of lumbar motoneurons are found following pontine microinjection of carbachol (92). These effects during natural REM sleep are likely to be mediated by glycine since they are abolished by iontophoresis of strychnine onto the motoneurons (110–112). Thus, the changes in respiratory motoneuronal activity following pontine microinjection of carbachol that we have described might similarly be related to postsynaptic inhibition of motoneurons by either glycine or gamma-aminobutyric acid (GABA). We have concentrated our investigation of this potential mechanism on the hypoglossal motor nucleus because of its great relevance to the clinical problem—obstructive sleep apnea.

In these studies, we have observed (somewhat to our surprise) that fast synaptic inhibition plays little, if any, role in the decrement of hypoglossal nerve activity produced by carbachol (103). Microinjections of strychnine, a glycine receptor antagonist, or bicuculline, a $GABA_A$ receptor antagonist, do not prevent the decrement in hypoglossal motor activity following carbachol. In these studies, we proved that the antagonists were operative by recording changes in the reflex motor response to lingual nerve stimulation. The latter produces a complex reflex response that has both a glycinergic and GABAergic component. Thus, for our negative result of the effects of the inhibitory amino acids antagonists on the carbachol response, there is a positive control. Further support for the lack of a major role of fast synaptic inhibition comes from studies with intracellular recording from hypoglossal motoneurons. There are, again, important differences between the results for lumbar motoneurons, discussed above, and the changes in hypoglossal motoneurons following carbachol. For hypoglossal motoneurons, the "state-specific" large IPSPs, found so uniformly in lumbar motoneurons (93–95), occur relatively infrequently. Moreover, for the hypoglossal pool, the motoneurons can still be activated antidromically after electrical stimulation of the hypoglossal nerve following carbachol. In contrast, antidromic invasion of lumbar motoneurons is often impossible particularly during bursts of rapid eye movements being blocked by the fast synaptic inhibition (94). Finally, in contrast to the profound decreases in the somatic membrane resistance characteristic of lumbar motoneurons during REM sleep (94,113), membrane resistance changes in hypoglossal motoneurons following pontine microinjections of carbachol are relatively small and inconsistent.

These results suggest that a different mechanism is operative at hypoglossal and potentially other orofacial motoneurons during REM sleep than in lumbar postural motoneurons. Since fast synaptic inhibition plays a minor role in the former, the focus must turn to disfacilitation. Two important premotor systems need to be considered—the raphe and locus coeruleus, since as discussed previously, the firing of both declines during REM sleep (42–44). A large component of the decline in raphe firing may be secondary to the atonia of REM sleep since lesions of the pontine tegmentum that lead to REM sleep without atonia also lead to a much lesser decline in raphe neuronal firing during REM (114). The midline raphe system of the brainstem consists of a number of distinct groups (for review, see 115). Cells in the caudal raphe—nucleus raphe pallidus and nucleus raphe obscurus—project to the hypoglossal motor nucleus (116–120,133) and their firing declines in REM sleep (115). These cells have as their major neuro-transmitter 5-HT, although neuropeptides such as thyrotropin-releasing hormone (TRH), substance P, met-enkephalin, somatostatin, and cholecystokinin are also colocalized in many of these cells (121–131). Serotonergic terminals are present in the hypoglossal nucleus (132) and the caudal raphe represents the primary source of serotonergic afferents (133).

Thus, the appropriate circuitry is present such that the decline in hypo-glossal motor activity following carbachol could be mediated, at least in part, by reductions in 5-HT input. For this to be the case, 5-HT would need to have a facilitatory effect on these motoneurons, as it does for facial motoneurons (134,135). In agreement with this prediction, microinjections of 5-HT into one hypoglossal motor nucleus produce a tonic long-lasting facilitation of motoneu-ronal activity without affecting the activity in the opposite, control, hypoglossal nerve (136) (see Fig. 4). A demonstration of the potential for 5-HT to facilitate

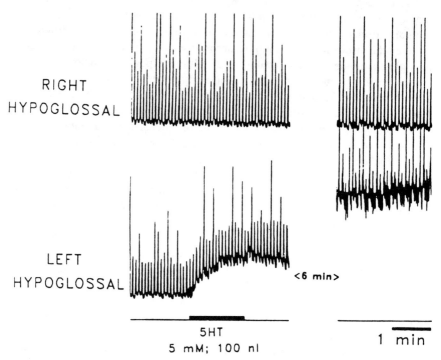

Figure 4   Effect of microinjection of serotonin (5 mM, 100 nl) into the left hypoglossal motor nucleus on hypoglossal nerve activity. The microinjection is followed by a relatively long-lasting tonic increase in activity on the injected side, while in the contralateral control side, activity is relatively unaffected. (Reproduced from Ref. 136 with permission.)

hypoglossal activity does not of itself prove that such facilitation is normally present. In the decerebrate cat, Kubin et al. (136) have shown that microinjections of methysergide, a broad-spectrum serotonin receptor antagonist, into the hypoglossal motor nucleus lead to long-lasting reductions in nerve activity to about half of its control level (see Fig. 5). Thus, at least in the decerebrate cat, there is evidence of a tonic, endogenous, serotonergic input into this pool of motoneurons. Based on the use of various antagonists and agonists of different specificities, we have concluded that the 5-HT receptors likely to be involved are type 1C or 2. The same receptors have been implicated in the excitation of facial motoneurons (135) and most consistently found to mediate excitatory effects (see 137–139). Serotonin type 2 receptors are found in the hypoglossal motor nucleus, as revealed by autoradiography (140).

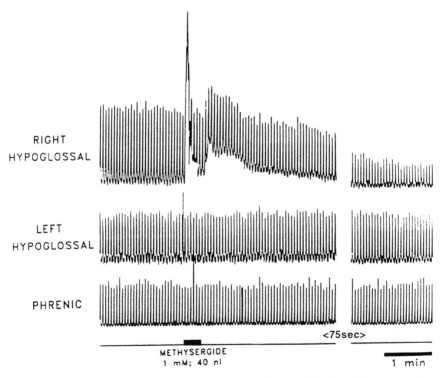

Figure 5 Effect of microinjection of methysergide (1 mM, 40 nl) into the right hypoglossal motor nucleus on hypoglossal nerve activity. The microinjection is followed by an initial excitation (methysergide is a partial agonist) and then by long-lasting suppression of activity. The activity on the contralateral, control side is unaffected. (Reproduced from Ref. 136 with permission.)

Evidence for the potential role of 5-HT in increasing the excitability of hypoglossal motoneurons is also supported by studies in brain slices (141). 5-HT produces a depolarization of motoneurons and increases the slope of the relationship between firing frequency and injected current (141). Brain slice studies also indicate that another transmitter from raphe neurons—the neuropeptide TRH— also produces depolarization of hypoglossal motoneurons (142,143). The effect of TRH is mediated by a G protein-coupled mechanism, although it does not involve either phospholipase or adenyl cyclase second-messenger systems (144). The potential interaction between TRH and serotonin has not yet been elucidated.

All of these studies point to the potential role of reductions in the serotonergic excitatory input from the caudal raphe in the suppression of hypoglossal motor activity following carbachol. More direct evidence comes from microdialysis studies. Reductions in the level of 5-HT in the hypoglossal motor nucleus are found following pontine microinjections of carbachol, and increases in 5-HT

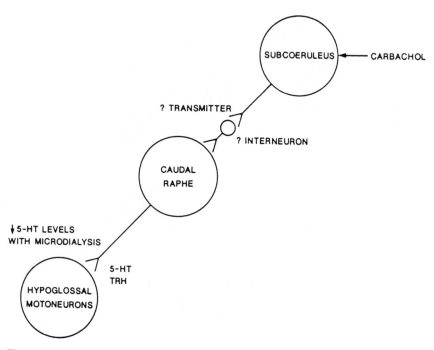

Figure 6 Proposed circuit that explains why the activity of hypoglossal motoneurons declines following carbachol microinjection in "subcoeruleus". Reduction in 5-HT levels at the motor nucleus have been demonstrated. The basis for the reduction in caudal raphe firing remains to be elucidated.

levels are observed when the carbachol effect is reversed by pontine microinjections of atropine (104). There is also evidence that the role of the medullary raphe system in state-dependent control of laryngeal motoneurons (145,146) may be similar to that discussed in more detail for hypoglossal motoneurons.

Thus, there seems little doubt that one component of the reduction in upper airway activity after carbachol is mediated by reductions in caudal raphe input to the relevant motoneurons (see Fig. 6). The evidence, in brief, is as follows: the relevant circuitry is present; caudal raphe firing declines during normal REM sleep and after carbachol microinjections; two of the neurotransmitters in raphe cells—5-HT and TRH—depolarize orofacial, including upper airway, motoneurons; and the level of 5-HT in the hypoglossal motor nucleus declines after carbachol microinjection. The mechanism of the reduction in caudal raphe firing itself remains to be determined; it may involve a local inhibitory interneuron, although this has not been studied.

While much information has been accumulated about the possible role of raphe cells in the carbachol response, the contribution of changes in the activity of cells in the locus coeruleus has not been studied.

VIII. Conclusions

The challenge of understanding how the neural control of respiration is altered during sleep is exciting. It involves bridging two disciplines—neural control of ventilation and neural control of sleep processes. The fundamental approach in both disciplines has been reductionist. The reductionist approach to sleep mechanisms has led to the identification of many of the important neuronal groups and neurotransmitters that are involved. While the role of these various groups in certain aspects of sleep, e.g., the postural atonia of REM sleep, has been elucidated, we know at present little about their role in mediating the characteristic changes in the neural control of respiration. The knowledge gained by basic investigators in sleep thus provides a powerful platform on which to build an approach to studies of changes in the neural control of ventilation in different states. The work of our group with carbachol in the decerebrate animal illustrates one such paradigm. By adapting a strategy that has been developed by those interested in fundamental questions about the generation and maintenance of REM sleep to a study of upper airway motor control, much has been learned. The future would seem to necessitate increasing interaction between the two disciplines. Those of us with a background in respiratory neural control should strive to convince our colleagues interested in sleep that studying the respiratory system as a model system for motor control is inherently interesting, and indeed more clinically relevant than the study of other motor systems.

Acknowledgments

I am extremely grateful to my colleagues (Dr. R. O. Davies, Dr. L. K. Kubin, Dr. A. R. Morrison, Dr. L. D. Sanford, and Dr. J. C. Hendricks) for helpful discussions and for the interesting science that we have done together. The original research was supported in part by NIH SCOR Grant HL-42236.

References

1. Aserinsky E, Kleitman N. Regularly occurring periods of eye motility, and concomitant phenomena during sleep. Science 1953; 118:273–274.
2. Kirby DA, Verrier RL. Differential effects of sleep stage on coronary hemodynamic function. Am J Physiol 1989; 256:H1378–H1383.
3. Findley LJ, Wilhoit SC, Suratt PM. Apnea duration and hypoxemia during REM sleep in patients with obstructive sleep apnea. Chest 1985; 87:432–436.
4. Leonard CS, Llinas RR. Electrophysiology of mammalian pedunculopontine and laterodorsal tegmental neurons in vitro: implications for the control of REM sleep. In: Steriade M, Biesold D, eds. Brain Cholinergic Systems. New York: Oxford University Press, 1990.
5. Leonard CS, Llinas RR. Serotonin (5-HT) inhibits mesopontine cholinergic neurons in vitro. Soc Neurosci Abstr 1990; 16:1233.
6. Kang Y, Kitai ST. Electrophysiological properties of pedunculopontine neurons and their postsynaptic responses following stimulation of substantia nigra reticulata. Brain Res 1990; 535:79–95.
7. Orem J, Trotter RH. Postinspiratory neuronal activities during behavioral control, sleep, and wakefulness. J Appl Physiol 1992; 72:2369–2377.
8. Orem J, Trotter RH. Medullary respiratory neuronal activity during augmented breaths in intact unanesthetized cats. J Appl Physiol 1993; 74:761–769.
9. Douglas NJ, White DP, Pickett CK, Weil JV, Zwillich CW. Respiration during sleep in normal man. Thorax 1982; 37:840–844.
10. Tabachnik E, Muller NL, Bryan AC, Levison H. Changes in ventilation and chest wall mechanics during sleep in normal adolescents. J Appl Physiol 1981; 51:557–564.
11. Stradling JR, Chadwick GA, Frew AJ. Changes in ventilation and its components in normal subjects during sleep. Thorax 1985; 40:364–370.
12. White DP, Weil JV, Zwillich CW. Metabolic rate and breathing during sleep. J Appl Physiol 1985; 59:384–391.
13. Gould GA, Gugger M, Molloy J, Tsara V, Shapiro CM, Douglas NJ. Breathing pattern and eye movement density during REM sleep in humans. Am Rev Respir Dis 1988; 138:874–877.
14. Neilly JB, Gaipa EA, Maislin G, Pack AI. Ventilation during early and late rapid-eye-movement sleep in normal humans. J Appl Physiol 1991; 71:1201–1205.
15. Millman RP, Knight H, Kline LR, Shore ET, Chung DC, Pack AI. Changes in compartmental ventilation in association with eye movements during REM sleep. J Appl Physiol 1988; 65:1196–1202.

16. Aserinsky E. Periodic respiratory pattern occurring in conjunction with eye movement during sleep. Science 1965; 150:763–776.

17. Tusiewicz K, Moldofsky H, Bryan AC, Bryan MH. Mechanisms of the rib cage and diaphragm during sleep. J Appl Physiol 1977; 43:600–602.

18. Sieck GC, Trelease RB, Harper RM. Sleep influences on diaphragmatic motor unit discharge. Exp Neurol 1984; 85:316–335.

19. Kline LR, Hendricks JC, Davies RO, Pack AI. Control of the activity of the diaphragm in rapid-eye-movement sleep. J Appl Physiol 1986; 61:1293–1300.

20. Wiegand L, Zwillich CW, Wiegand D, White DP. Changes in upper airway muscle activation and ventilation during phasic REM sleep in normal men. J Appl Physiol 1991; 71:488–497.

21. Kawahara K, Nakazono Y, Kumagai S, Yamauchi Y, Miyamoto Y. Neuronal origin of parallel suppression of postural tone and respiration elicited by stimulation of midpontine dorsal tegmentum in the decerebrate cat. Brain Res 1988; 474:403–406.

22. Kawahara K, Nakazono Y, Kumagai S, Yamauchi Y, Miyamoto Y. Inhibitory influences on hypoglossal neural activity by stimulation of midpontine dorsal tegmentum in decerebrate cat. Brain Res 1989; 479:185–189.

23. Orem J. Neuronal mechanisms of respiration in REM sleep. Sleep 1980; 3:251–267.

24. Bowker RM, Morrison AR. The startle reflex and PGO spikes. Brain Res 1976; 102:185–190.

25. Ball WA, Hunt WH, Sanford LD, Ross RJ, Morrison AR. Effects of stimulus intensity on elicited ponto-geniculo-occipital waves. Electroencephalogr Clin Neurophysiol 1991; 78:35–39.

26. Ball WA, Morrison AR, Ross RJ. The effects of tones on PGO waves in slow wave sleep and paradoxical sleep. Exp Neurol 1989; 104:251–256.

27. Ball WA, Sanford LD, Morrison AR, Ross RJ, Hunt WH, Mann GL. The effects of changing state on elicited ponto-geniculo-occipital (PGO) waves. Electroencephalogr Clin Neurophysiol 1991; 79:420–429.

28. Sanford LD, Ball WA, Morrison AR, Ross RJ, Mann G. Peripheral and central components of alerting: habituation of acoustic startle, orienting responses and elicited waveforms. Behav Neurosci 1992; 106:112–120.

29. Wu MF, Mallick BN, Siegel JM. Lateral geniculate spikes, muscle atonia and startle response elicited by auditory stimuli as a function of stimulus parameters and arousal state. Brain Res 1989; 499:7–17.

30. Kline LR, Hendricks JC, Silage DA, Morrison AR, Davies RO, Pack AI. Startle-evoked changes in diaphragmatic activity during wakefulness and sleep. J Appl Physiol 1990; 68:166–173.

31. Hendricks JC, Kline LR. Differential activation within costal diaphragm during rapid-eye-movement sleep in cats. J Appl Physiol 1991; 70:1194–1200.

32. Glenn LL, Dement WC. Group I excitatory and inhibitory potentials in hindlimb motoneurons during wakefulness and sleep. J Neurophysiol 1981; 46:1089–1101.

33. Soja PJ, Oka J-I, Fragoso M. Synaptic transmission through cat lumbar ascending sensory pathways is suppressed during active sleep. J Neurophysiol 1993; 70:1708–1712.

34. Sullivan CE, Murphy E, Kozar LF, Phillipson EA. Ventilatory response to CO_2 and

lung inflation in tonic versus phasic REM sleep. J Appl Physiol 1979; 47:1304–1310.

35. Hendricks JC, Kline LR, Kovalski RJ, O'Brien JA, Morrison AR, Pack AI. The English bulldog: a natural model of sleep-disordered breathing. J Appl Physiol 1987; 63:1344–1350.

36. Hendricks JC, Kovalski RJ, Kline LR. Phasic respiratory muscle patterns and sleep-disordered breathing during rapid eye movement sleep in the English bulldog. Am Rev Respir Dis 1991; 144:1112–1120.

37. Jones BE. Paradoxical sleep and its chemical/structural substrates in the brain. Neuroscience 1991; 40:637–656.

38. Siegel JM. Brainstem mechanisms generating REM sleep. In: Kryger MH, Roth T, Dement WC, eds. Principles and Practice of Sleep Medicine, 2nd ed. Philadelphia: Saunders, 1994:125–144.

39. Steriade M, McCarley RW. Brainstem Control of Wakefulness and Sleep. New York: Plenum Press, 1991:1–499.

40. Jouvet M. Recherches sur les structures nerveuses et les mécanismes responsables des différentes phases du someil physiologique. Arch Ital Biol 1962; 100:125–206.

41. Villablanca J. Behavioral and polygraphic study of "sleep" and "wakefulness" in chronic decerebrate cats. Electroencephalogr Clin Neurophysiol 1966; 21:562–577.

42. McGinty DJ, Harper RW. Dorsal raphe neurons: depression of firing during sleep in cats. Brain Res 1976; 101:569–575.

43. Aston-Jones G, Bloom FE. Activity of norepinephrine-containing locus coeruleus neurons in behaving rats anticipates fluctuations in the sleep-waking cycle. J Neurosci 1981; 1:876–886.

44. Foote SL, Bloom FE, Aston-Jones G. Nucleus locus coeruleus: new evidence of anatomical and physiological specificity. Physiol Rev 1983; 63:844–914.

45. Hobson JA, Lydic R, Baghdoyan HA. Evolving concepts of sleep cycle generation: from brain centers to neuronal populations. Behav Brain Sci 1986; 9:371–448.

46. Webster HH, Jones BE. Neurotoxic lesions of the dorsolateral pontomesencephalic tegmentum-cholinergic cell area in the cat. II. Effects upon sleep-waking states. Brain Res 1988; 458:285–302.

47. Shouse MN, Siegel JM. Pontine regulation of REM sleep components in cats: integrity of the pedunculopontine tegmentum (PPT) is important for phasic events but unnecessary for atonia during REM sleep. Brain Res 1992; 571:50–63.

48. McCarley RW, Nelson JP, Hobson JA. Ponto-geniculo-occipital (PGO) burst neurons: correlative evidence for neuronal generators of PGO waves. Science 1978; 201:269–272.

49. Nelson JP, McCarley RW, Hobson JA. REM sleep burst neurons, PGO waves, and eye movement information. J Neurophysiol 1983; 50:784–797.

50. Datta S, Calvo JM, Quattrochi JJ, Hobson JA. Long-term enhancement of REM sleep following cholinergic stimulation. Neuroreport 1991; 2:619–622.

51. Datta S, Hobson JA. Neuronal activity in the caudo-lateral peribrachial pons: relationship with PGO waves and REM. Soc Neurosci Abstr 1993; 19:567.

52. Cornwall J, Cooper JD, Phillipson OT. Afferent and efferent connections of the laterodorsal tegmental nucleus in the rat. Brain Res Bull 1990; 25:271–284.

53. Delorme F, Froment JL, Jouvet M. Suppression of sleep with *p*-chloromethamphetamine and *p*-chlorophenylalanine. C R Soc Seances Biol Fil 1966; 160: 2347–2351.

54. Pujol JF, Buguet A, Froment JL, Jones B, Jouvet M. The central metabolism of serotonin in the cat during insomnia. A neurophysiological and biochemical study after administration of *p*-chlorophenylanine or destruction of the raphe system. Brain Res 1971; 29:195–212.

55. Simon RP, Gershon MD, Brooks DC. The role of the raphe nuclei in the regulation of ponto-geniculo-occipital wave activity. Brain Res 1973; 58:313–330.

56. Kaufman LS. Parachlorophenylalanine does not affect pontine-geniculate-occipital waves in rats despite significant effects on other sleep-waking parameters. Exp Neurol 1983; 80:410–417.

57. Lydic R, McCarley RW, Hobson JA. Serotonin neurons and sleep. I. Long term recordings of dorsal raphe discharge frequency and PGO waves. Arch Ital Biol 1987; 125:317–343.

58. Lydic R, McCarley RW, Hobson JA. Serotonin neurons and sleep. II. Time course of dorsal raphe discharge, PGO waves, and behavioral states. Arch Ital Biol 1987; 126: 1–28.

59. Lydic R, McCarley RW, Hobson JA. Timing function of the dorsal raphe nucleus and the temporal organization of the ultradian sleep cycle. Exp Brain Res 1985; 12(suppl):125–144.

60. Lydic R, McCarley RW, Hobson JA. The time-course of dorsal raphe discharge, PGO waves, and muscle tone averaged across multiple sleep cycles. Brain Res 1983; 274:365–370.

61. Luebke JI, Greene RW, Semba K, Kamondi A, McCarley RW, Reiner PB. Serotonin hyperpolarizes cholinergic low-threshold burst neurons in the rat laterodorsal tegmental nucleus in vitro. Proc Natl Acad Sci USA 1992; 89:743–747.

62. Ruch-Monachon MA, Jalfre M, Haefely W. Drugs and PGO waves in the lateral geniculate body of the curarized cat. IV. The effects of acetylcholine, GABA and benzodiazepines on PGO wave activity. Arch Int Pharmacodyn Ther 1976; 219: 308–325.

63. Shiromani PJ, Malik MR, McCarley RW. Topographical distribution of noradrenergic, serotonergic and cholinergic perikaya in the feline pons: a 3D perspective. Sleep Res 1992; 21:77.

64. Muhlethaler M, Khatch A, Seralin M. Effects of monoamines and opiates on pedunculopontine neurons. In: Mancia M, Marini GI, eds. The Diencephalon and Sleep. New York: Raven Press, 1990:31–48.

65. Steriade M, Paré D, Datta S, Oakson G, Currò Dossi R. Different cellular types in mesopontine cholinergic nuclei related to ponto-geniculo-occipital waves. J Neurosci 1990; 10:2560–2579.

66. Hallanger AE, Levey AI, Lee HJ, Rye DB, Wainer BH. The origins of cholinergic and other subcortical afferents to the thalamus in the rat. J Comp Neurol 1987; 262:105–124.

67. Jones BE, Yang T-Z. The efferent projections from the reticular formation and the locus coeruleus studied by anterograde and retrograde axonal transport in the rat. J Comp Neurol 1985; 242:56–92.

68. Paré D, Smith Y, Parent A, Steriade M. Projections of brainstem core cholinergic and non-cholinergic neurons of cat to intralaminar and reticular thalamic nuclei. Neuroscience 1988; 25:69–86.

69. Steriade M. New vistas on the morphology, chemical transmitters and physiological actions of the ascending brainstem reticular system. Arch Ital Biol 1988; 126: 225–238.

70. Woolf NJ, Butcher LL. Cholinergic systems in the rat brain. III. Projections from the pontomesencephalic tegmentum to the thalamus, tectum, basal ganglia and basal forebrain. Brain Res Bull 1986; 16:603–637.

71. Curró Dossi R, Paré D, Steriade M. Short-lasting nicotinic and long-lasting muscarinic depolarizing responses of thalamocortical neurons to stimulation of mesopontine cholinergic nuclei. J Neurophysiol 1991; 65:393–406.

72. Steriade M, Curró Dossi R, Paré D, Oakson G. Fast oscillations (20–40 Hz) in thalamocortical systems and their potentiation by mesopontine cholinergic nuclei in the cat. Proc Natl Acad Sci USA 1991; 88:4369–4400.

73. Hu B, Bouhassira D, Steriade M, Deschenes M. The blockage of ponto-geniculo-occipital waves in the cat lateral geniculate nucleus by nicotinic antagonists. Brain Res 1988; 473:394–397.

74. Phillipson EA, Bowes G. Control of breathing during sleep. In: Cherniack NS, Widdicombe JG. Respiratory System's Control of Breathing, Vol III. Bethesda, MD: American Physiological Society, 1986:649–690.

75. Mitani A, Ito K, Hallanger AE, Wainer BH, Kataoka K, McCarley RW. Cholinergic projections from the laterodorsal and pedunculopontine tegmental nuclei to the pontine gigantocellular tegmental field in the cat. Brain Res 1988; 451:397–402.

76. Quattrochi JJ, Mamelak AN, Madison RD, Macklis JD, Hobson JA. Mapping neuronal inputs to REM sleep induction sites with carbachol-fluorescent microspheres. Science 1989; 245:984–986.

77. Shiromani PJ, Armstrong DM, Gillin JC. Cholinergic neurons from the dorsolateral pons project to the medial pons: a WGA-HRP and choline actyltransferase immunohistochemical study. Neurosci Lett 1988; 95:19–23.

78. Lydic R, Baghdoyan HA, Lorinc Z. Microdialysis of cat pons reveals enhanced acetylcholine release during state-dependent respiratory depression. Am J Physiol 1991; 261:R766–R770.

79. Sakai K, Sastre J-P, Salvert D, Touret M, Tohyama M, Jouvet M. Tegmentoreticular projections with special reference to the muscular atonia during paradoxical sleep in the cat: an HRP study. Brain Res 1979; 176:233–254.

80. Mori S, Kawahara K, Sakamoto T, Aoki M, Tomiyama T. Setting and resetting of level of postural muscle tone in decerebrate cats by stimulation of brain stem. J Neurophysiol 1982; 48:737–748.

81. Mori S, Sakomoto T, Ohta Y, Takakusaki K, Matsuyama K. Site-specific postural and locomotor changes evoked in awake, freely moving intact cats by stimulating the brainstem. Brain Res 1989; 505:66–74.

82. Shiromani PJ, Lai YY, Siegel JM. Descending projections from the dorsolateral pontine tegmentum to the paramedian reticular nucleus of the caudal medulla in the cat. Brain Res 1990; 517:224–228.

83. Lai YY, Siegel JM. Medullary regions mediating atonia. J Neurosci 1988; 8:4790–4796.
84. Henley K, Morrison AR. A re-evaluation of the effects of lesions on the pontine tegmentum and locus coeruleus on phenomena of paradoxical sleep in the cat. Acta Neurobiol Exp 1974; 34:215–232.
85. Hendricks JC, Morrison AR, Mann GL. Different behaviors during paradoxical sleep without atonia depend on pontine lesion site. Brain Res 1982; 239:81–105.
86. Hendricks JC, Kline LR, Davies RO, Pack AI. Effect of dorsolateral pontine lesions on diaphragmatic activity during REMS. J Appl Physiol 1990; 68:1435–1442.
87. Hernandez-Peon R, Chavez-Ibara G, Morgane PJ, Timo-Iaria C. Limbic cholinergic pathways involved in sleep and emotional behavior. Exp Neurol 1963; 8:93–111.
88. Baghdoyan HA, Rodrigo-Angulo ML, McCarley RW, Hobson JA. Site-specific enhancement and suppression of desynchronized sleep signs following cholinergic stimulation of three brainstem regions. Brain Res 1984; 306:39–52.
89. Baghdoyan HA, Rodrigo-Angulo ML, McCarley RW, Hobson JA. A neuroanatomical gradient in the pontine tegmentum for the cholinoceptive induction of desynchronized sleep signs. Brain Res 1987; 414:245–261.
90. Vanni-Mercier G, Sakai K, Lin JS, Jouvet M. Mapping of cholinoceptive brainstem structures responsible for the generation of paradoxical sleep in cat. Arch Ital Biol 1989; 127:133–164.
91. Lopez-Rodriguez F, Morales FR, Chase MH. Induction of muscle atonia by the microiontophoretic injection of cholinergic drugs into the brainstem reticular formation. Sleep Res 1992; 21:8.
92. Morales FR, Engelhardt JK, Soja PJ, Pereda AE, Chase MH. Motoneuron properties during motor inhibition produced by microinjection of carbachol into the pontine reticular formation of the decerebrate cat. J Neurophysiol 1987; 57:1118–1129.
93. Morales FR, Boxer P, Chase MH. Behavioral state-specific inhibitory postsynaptic potentials impinge on cat lumbar motoneurons during active sleep. Exp Neurol 1987; 98:418–435.
94. Morales F, Chase MH. Postsynaptic control of lumbar motoneuron excitability during active sleep in the chronic cat. Brain Res 1981; 225:279–295.
95. Morales FR, Chase MH. Repetitive synaptic potentials responsible for inhibition of spinal cord motoneurons during active sleep. Exp Neurol 1982; 78:471–476.
96. Chase MH, Morales FR. The atonia and myoclonia of active (REM) sleep. Annu Rev Psychol 1990; 41:557–584.
97. Lydic R, Baghdoyan HA. Cholinoceptive pontine reticular mechanisms cause state-dependent respiratory changes in the cat. Neurosci Lett 1989; 102:211–216.
98. Lydic R, Baghdoyan HA, Wertz R, White DP. Cholinergic reticular mechanisms influence state-dependent ventilatory response to hypercapnia. Am J Physiol 1991; 261:R738–R746.
99. Lydic R, Baghdoyan HA, Zwillich CW. State-dependent hypotonia in posterior cricoarytenoid muscles of the larynx caused by cholinoceptive reticular mechanisms. FASEB J 1989; 3:1625–1631.
100. Kimura H, Kubin L, Davies RO, Pack AI. Cholinergic stimulation of the pons depresses respiration in decerebrate cats. J Appl Physiol 1990; 69:2280–2289.

101. Kim A, Kubin L, Kimura H, Davies RO. Common origin of postural atonia and cardiorespiratory depression within the cholinoceptive pontine tegmentum (in preparation).

102. Kubin L, Kimura H, Tojima H, Pack AI, Davies RO. Behavior of VRG neurons during the atonia of REM sleep induced by pontine carbachol in decerebrate cats. Brain Res 1992; 592:91–100.

103. Kubin L, Kimura H, Tojima H, Davies RO, Pack AI. Suppression of hypoglossal motoneurons during carbachol-induced atonia of REM sleep is not caused by fast synaptic inhibition. Brain Res 1993; 611:300–312.

104. Kubin L, Tojima H, Taguchi O, Reignier C, Pack AI, Davies RO. Serotonin release in the hypoglossal (XII) nucleus region under conditions of suppressed raphe system activity. Soc Neurosci Abstr 1992; 18:1528.

105. Tojima H, Kubin L, Kimura H, Davies RO. Spontaneous ventilation and respiratory motor output during carbachol-induced atonia of REM sleep in the decerebrate cat. Sleep 1992; 15:404–414.

106. Taguchi O, Kubin L, Pack AI. Evocation of postural atonia and respiratory depression by pontine carbachol in the decerebrate rat. Brain Res 1992; 595:107–115.

107. Megirian D, Pollard MJ, Sherrey JH. The labile respiratory activity of ribcage muscles of the rat during sleep. J Physiol (Lond) 1987; 389:99–110.

108. Trachsel L, Tobler I, Achermann P, Borbely AA. Sleep continuity and REM–non-REM cycle in the rat under baseline conditions and after sleep deprivation. Physiol Behav 1991; 49:575–580.

109. Orem J. Medullary respiratory neuron activity: relationship to tonic and phasic REM sleep. J Appl Physiol 1980; 48:54–65.

110. Chase MH, Soja PJ, Morales FR. Evidence that glycine mediates the postsynaptic potentials that inhibit lumbar motoneurons during the atonia of active sleep. J Neurosci 1989; 9:743–751.

111. Soja PJ, Lopez-Rodriguez F, Morales FR, Chase MH. The postsynaptic inhibitory control of lumbar motoneurons during the atonia of active sleep: effect of strychnine on motoneuron properties. J Neurosci 1991; 11:2804–2811.

112. Soja PJ, Morales FR, Baranyi A, Chase MH. Effect of inhibitory amino acid antagonists on IPSPs induced in lumbar motoneurons upon stimulation of the nucleus reticularis gigantocellularis during active sleep. Brain Res 1987; 423:353–358.

113. Glenn LL, Dement WL. Membrane resistance and rheobase of hindlimb motoneurons during wakefulness and sleep. J Neurophysiol 1981; 46:1076–1088.

114. Trulson ME, Jacob BL, Morrison AR. Raphe unit activity during REM sleep in normal cats and in pontine lesioned cats displaying REM sleep without atonia. Brain Res 1981; 226:75–91.

115. Jacobs BL, Azmitia EC. Structure and function of the brain serotonin system. Physiol Rev 1992; 72:165–229.

116. Manaker S, Tischler LJ, Morrison AR. Raphespinal and reticulospinal axon collaterals to the hypoglossal nucleus in the rat. J Comp Neurol 1992; 322:68–78.

117. Borke RC, Nau ME, Ringer RL Jr. Brain stem afferents of hypoglossal neurons in the rat. Brain Res 1983; 269:47–55.

118. Holstege G. Descending motor pathways and the spinal motor system: limbic and non-limbic components. Prog Brain Res 1991; 84:307–421.

119. Takada M, Itoh K, Yasui Y, Mitani A, Nomura S, Mizuno N. Distribution of premotor neurons for the hypoglossal nucleus in the cat. Neurosci Lett 1984; 52: 141–146.

120. Ugolino G, Kuypers HGJM, Simmons A. Retrograde trans-neuronal transfer of Herpes simplex virus type I (HSVI) from motoneurons. Brain Res 1987; 422:242–256.

121. Bowker RM, Westlund KN, Sullivan MC, Wilber JF, Coulter JD. Transmitters of the raphe-spinal complex: immunocytochemical studies. Peptides 1982; 3:291–298.

122. Chiba T, Masuko S. Coexistence of varying combinations of neuropeptides with 5-hydroxytryptamine in neurons of the raphe pallidus et obscurus projecting to the spinal cord. Neurosci Res 1989; 7:13–23.

123. Conrath-Verrier M, Dietl M, Arluison M, Cesselin F, Bourgoin S, Hamon M. Localization of met-enkephalin-like immunoreactivity within pain-related nuclei of the cervical spinal cord, brainstem and midbrain in the cat. Brain Res Bull 1983; 11:587–604.

124. Hökfelt T, Elde R, Johansson O, Terenius L, Stein L. The distribution of enkephalin-immunoreactive cell bodies in the rat central nervous system. Neurosci Lett 1977; 6:25–31.

125. Hökfelt T, Ljungdahl A, Steinbusch H, Verhofstad A, Nilsson G, Brodin E, Pernow B, Goldstein M. Immunohistochemical evidence of substance P-like immunoreactivity in some 5-hydroxytryptamine-containing neurons in the rat central nervous system. Neuroscience 1978; 3:517–538.

126. Hökfelt T, Terenius L, Kuypers HGJM, Dann O. Evidence for enkephalin immunoreactive neurons in the medulla oblongata projecting to the spinal cord. Neurosci Lett 1979; 14:55–60.

127. Holets VR, Hökfelt T, Ude J, Eckert M, Penzlin H, Verhofstad AAJ, Visser TJ. A comparative study of the immunohistochemical localization of a presumptive proctolin-like peptide, thyrotropin-releasing hormone and 5-hydroxytryptamine in the rat central nervous system. Brain Res 1987; 408:141–153.

128. Hunt SP, Lovick TA. The distribution of serotonin, met-enkephalin and β-lipotropin-like immunoreactivity in neuronal perikarya of the cat brainstem. Neurosci Lett 1982; 30:139–145.

129. Johansson O, Hökfelt T, Pernow B, Jeffcoate SL, White N, Steinbusch HWM, Verhofstad AAJ, Emson PC, Spindel E. Immunohistochemical support for three putative transmitters in one neuron: coexistence of 5-hydroxytryptamine, substance P- and thyrotropin releasing hormone-like immunoreactivity in medullary neurons projecting to the spinal cord. Neuroscience 1981; 6:1857–1881.

130. Léger L, Charnay Y, Dubois PM, Louvet M. Distribution of enkephalin-immunoreactive cell bodies in relation to serotonin-containing neurons in the raphe nuclei of the cat: immunohistochemical evidence for the coexistence of enkaphalins and serotonin in certain cells. Brain Res 1986; 362:63–73.

131. Mantyh PW, Hunt SP. Evidence for cholecystokinin-like immunoreactive neurons in the rat medulla oblongata which project to the spinal cord. Brain Res 1984; 291:49–54.

132. Aldes LD, Marco LA, Chronister RB. Serotonin-containing axon terminals in the

hypoglossal nucleus of the rat. An immuno-electromicroscopic study. Brain Res Bull 1989; 23:249–256.

133. Manaker S, Tischler LJ. Origin of serotonergic afferents to the hypoglossal nucleus in the rat. J Comp Neurol 1993; 334:466–476.

134. McCall RB, Aghajanian GK. Serotonergic facilitation of facial motoneuron excitation. Brain Res 1979; 169:11–27.

135. Rasmussen K, Aghajanian GK. Serotonin excitation of facial motoneurons: receptor subtype characterization. Synapse 1990; 5:324–332.

136. Kubin L, Tojima H, Davies RO, Pack AI. Serotonergic excitatory drive to hypoglossal motoneurons in the decerebrate cat. Neurosci Lett 1992; 139:243–248.

137. Schmidt AW, Peroutka SJ. 5-Hydroxytryptamine receptor "families". FASEB J 1989; 3:2242–2249.

138. Bobker DH, Williams JT. Ion conductances affected by 5-HT receptor subtypes in mammalian neurons. Trends Neurosci 1990; 13:169–173.

139. Göthert M. Pharmacological, biochemical and molecular classification schemes of serotonin (5-HT) receptors with special reference to the 5-HT$_2$ class. Progr Pharmacol Clin Pharmacol 1990; 7:3–15.

140. Pazos A, Probst A, Palacios JM. Serotonin receptors in the human brain. IV. Autoradiographic mapping of serotonin-2 receptors. Neuroscience 1987; 21:123–139.

141. Berger AJ, Bayliss DA, Viana F. Modulation of neonatal rat hypoglossal motoneuron excitability by serotonin. Neurosci Lett 1992; 143:164–168.

142. Bayliss DA, Viana F, Berger AJ. Mechanisms underlying excitatory effects of thyrotropin-releasing hormone on rat hypoglossal motoneurons in vitro. J Neurophysiol 1992; 68:1733–1745.

143. Rekling JC. Excitatory effects of thyrotropin-releasing hormone (TRH) in hypoglossal motoneurons. Brain Res 1990; 510:175–179.

144. Bayliss DA, Viana F, Berger AJ. The mechanism mediating thyrotropin-releasing hormone (TRH) effects on motoneurons involves G-proteins but not protein kinase C, IP$_3$ or intracellular calcium. Soc Neurosci Abstr 1993; 19:988.

145. Arita H, Ochiishi M. Opposing effects of 5-hydroxytryptamine on two types of medullary inspiratory neurons with distinct firing patterns. J Neurophysiol 1991; 66:285–292.

146. Arita H, Sakamoto M, Hirokawa Y, Okado N. Serotonin innervation patterns differ among the various medullary motoneuronal groups involved in upper airway control. Exp Brain Res 1993; 95:100–110.

23

Interaction Between Metabolism and Ventilation: Effects of Respiratory Gases and Temperature

JACOPO P. MORTOLA

McGill University
Montreal, Quebec, Canada

HENRY GAUTIER

Faculty of Medicine St. Antoine
Paris, France

I. Introduction

Living organisms are biochemical machineries designed to extract, transform, store, and use energy. These functions can occur as long as an energy gradient is maintained, a process that is largely dependent on oxygen (O_2) and heat. O_2, acting as the final electron acceptor at the end of the electron-transport chain, effectively represents a sink for the proton gradient. By varying the degree of electron excitability, temperature (T), which is a measure of heat, influences the magnitude of the gradient and therefore the rate of the energy transfer. Cellular processes are very sensitive to variations of O_2 and T from the values selected for optimal function; the acceptable T range is much narrower than the variations of T observed on earth, and the toxic effects of O_2 have been known almost since its discovery.

Within the range compatible with the survival of the organism, the response to changes in T and O_2 span within two extremes. On the one end, cellular T and O_2 can conform to the prevailing environmental conditions; in such a case, metabolic rate and energy production vary as expected from the effects of T and O_2 on the energy flux. At the opposite extreme, cellular T and O_2 are protected and maintained constant by a variety of regulatory mechanisms. Mammals are thought

1011

to be among the optimal regulators, maintaining T and the O_2 supply to the vital organs within very narrow limits. In these regulations, lung ventilation plays a paramount role, not only for O_2 convection, but also for heat dispersion. In addition, metabolism itself, which is largely an aerobic process dependent on ventilation, since gas exchange other than via the lung is negligible, is a key aspect of thermoregulation; in fact, a substantial portion of the energy involved in the metabolic processes is dissipated as heat.*

The intricacies of the metabolism-ventilation coupling reflect numerous constraints. Since lung ventilation in mammals also represents the major route of CO_2 elimination and can be an important pathway of heat loss, the ventilatory contribution to the demands of the organism for homeothermy and adequate O_2 supply is confronted by the control of CO_2 and acid-base equilibrium and, in some cases, by that of heat and water balance. The structure itself of the ventilatory pump and the limits imposed by its mechanical characteristics are other obvious constraints to the ventilatory performance.

This chapter addresses the effects of changes in O_2 and T on body metabolism, ventilation, and their interrelation in mammals. The biochemical and neurophysiological bases of temperature and O_2 sensitivity at the cellular level are not discussed and can be found in separate articles and monographs (i.e., Poulos, 1981; Acker, 1988; Wilson and Rumsey, 1991). For clarity, the effects of changes in O_2 and T are reviewed separately, although their interaction will be repeatedly emphasized. The literature on the metabolic effects of changes in temperature and on the ventilatory response to changes in respiratory gases is voluminous; in keeping with the purpose of this review, attention is given to that portion of the literature which specifically addresses the interaction between metabolism, temperature, and respiratory gases, and to those studies which provide data and information pertinent to the discussion of this topic. Anesthesia can profoundly alter both metabolism and ventilation, as will be briefly discussed (Section IV.A); hence, almost exclusive priority is given to information obtained in humans or in conscious animal models.

II. Respiratory Gases

A. Acute Hypoxia

Metabolic Rate

Although the notion that hypoxia in mammals can decrease metabolic rate and body temperature (Tb) dates back more than a century, since the early observations

---

*Calorimetric measurements indicate that the total energy yield of 1 mole of glucose and 1 mole of ATP are, respectively, 2880 kJ and 30.6 kJ. Aerobic respiration of glucose yields 38 moles of ATP; hence, its efficiency is $(38 \times 30.6)/2880 = 40\%$, and 60% of the total energy is dissipated as heat.

of Legallois and Bert, it is only in the second half of this century that the phenomenon has been given more attention, with several studies attempting to elucidate its mechanisms and the interaction with $\dot{V}_E$. For the purpose of the present discussion, of particular interest are the studies performed by Cross et al. (1958) and Hill (1959). The former indicated that gaseous metabolism ($\dot{V}_{O_2}$ and $\dot{V}_{CO_2}$) decreased in human infants breathing 15% O_2, therefore demonstrating that hypometabolism could occur even with mild hypoxia. The latter study, on newborn kittens and adult guinea pigs, demonstrated that the metabolic drop was larger the lower the ambient temperature (Tamb), therefore emphasizing the importance of Tamb, and presumably of thermoregulatory mechanisms, in the hypoxic metabolic drop.

During the last 40 years the observations that in the newborn or young mammal $\dot{V}_{O_2}$ drops whenever the inspired O_2 decreases (hypoxic hypoxia, either normobaric or hypobaric) have been very numerous. Measurements were performed with different techniques in rats (Mourek 1959; Adolph and Hoy, 1960; Taylor, 1960; Saetta and Mortola, 1987; Mortola and Dotta, 1992), lambs (Acheson et al., 1957; Cross et al., 1959; Alexander and Williams, 1970; Sidi et al., 1983), kittens (Hill, 1959; Moore, 1959; Moore and Underwood, 1962; Mortola and Rezzonico, 1988; Frappell et al., 1991), puppies (Moore, 1956; Moore and Underwood, 1962), rabbits (Adamson, 1959; Blatteis, 1964; Dawkins and Hull, 1964; Várnai et al., 1971), monkeys (Dawes et al., 1960), and neonates of several other, less common, species (Mortola et al., 1989). During hypoxic hypoxia the drop in $\dot{V}_{O_2}$ is mostly due to a decrease in the arterial-venous O_2 difference, cardiac output remaining as in, or slightly above, the normoxic level (Alexander and Williams, 1970; Sidi et al., 1983). However, an experimental decrease in O_2 delivery by reduction of the cardiac output (stagnant hypoxia) also results in a drop of $\dot{V}_{O_2}$ (Fahey and Lister, 1989). The magnitude of the decrease in $\dot{V}_{O_2}$ depends on the age, being more marked in younger animals, the level of hypoxia, and the degree of development of the species at birth (Mourek, 1959; Taylor, 1960; Mortola et al., 1989; Frappell et al., 1991). In addition, the crucial parameter is the Tamb at which hypoxia occurs. At thermoneutrality, in some species, as in kittens (Hill, 1959), lambs (Cross et al., 1959; Sidi et al., 1983), newborn rabbits (Adamsons, 1959), and monkeys (Dawes et al., 1960), $\dot{V}_{O_2}$ decreases only if hypoxia is severe; in others, as the newborn rat, at thermoneutrality $\dot{V}_{O_2}$ drops even with moderate hypoxia (Taylor, 1960; Mortola and Dotta, 1992). At Tamb below thermoneutrality, the magnitude of the hypometabolic response varies mostly because the normoxic value is Tamb-dependent (Fig. 1). In human infants, presumably examined at the Tamb of the nursery, heat production and $\dot{V}_{O_2}$ decreased during 15% O_2 breathing (Brodie et al., 1957; Cross et al., 1958).

Among adult mammals, the drop in $\dot{V}_{O_2}$ during moderate hypoxia has been observed in cats (Gautier et al., 1989), squirrel monkeys (Horstman and Banderet, 1977), rats (Adolph and Hoy, 1960; Pappenheimer, 1977; Olson and Dempsey, 1978; Gautier and Bonora, 1992), guinea pigs (Hill, 1959), gophers (Lechner,

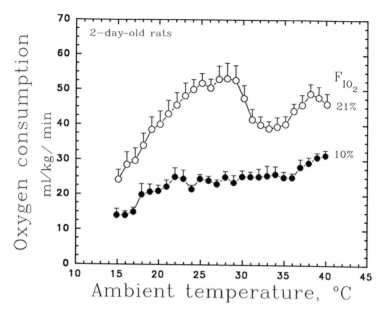

Figure 1 Oxygen consumption (means + 1 SEM) at different ambient temperatures in 2-days-old newborn rats, in normoxia (FI_{O_2} = 21%) and hypoxia (FI_{O_2} = 10%). Thermoneutrality in newborn rats is at Tamb = 32–34°C. (From Mortola, 1993, with permission; original data in Mortola and Dotta, 1992.)

1977), hamsters (Mortola, 1991), and many other rodents (Rosenmann and Morrison, 1975). In larger species, on the other hand, such as goats, ponies, and humans, the changes in $\dot{V}O_2$ during acute hypoxia were variable and inconsistent (reviewed by Dempsey and Forster, 1982). As in newborns, also in adults the metabolic response changed with Tamb (Lintzel, 1931; Blatteis, 1966; Dupre et al., 1988; Gautier et al., 1989, 1992), being small or absent at thermoneutrality, which is usually above the living range in Tamb of the species. In addition, both the magnitude and the threshold of the hypometabolic response to hypoxia can be conditioned by special habitats, such as for species living in burrows, at high altitude, or divers (Dejours, 1975; Tenney and Boggs, 1986). Recently (Frappell et al., 1992b), in a comparative study covering 27 mammalian species of six orders ranging in size from the 8-g broad-nosed bat to the 47-kg capybara, $\dot{V}O_2$, measured at Tamb of about 22°C, during 10% O_2 breathing decreased in almost all animals. The only exception was the armadillo, a mammal with an armored chest wall, which probably substantially raised the cost of breathing during the hypoxic hyperventilation. A proportionality emerged between the basal normoxic $\dot{V}O_2$ of the animal, expressed per unit of body weight ($\dot{V}O_2$/kg), and the magnitude of its drop during hypoxia, the decrease being larger in the smaller species, which have high $\dot{V}O_2$/kg. It is of interest that data previously obtained on newborn mammals studied at, or slightly below, thermoneutrality, overlapped with the adult relationship (Fig. 2). In other words, when normoxic $\dot{V}O_2$/kg was taken as the independent variable, age differences in the hypometabolic response to hypoxia were largely eliminated. This supports the argument, originally proposed by Hill (1959), that the more apparent hypometabolic response to hypoxia in the newborn may be due to the fact that, within each species, the $\dot{V}O_2$/kg of the young is higher than in the adult (Kleiber, 1932, 1961; Mortola, 1987), because of the small size, high anabolic requirements, and poor control of heat dissipation. In addition, the

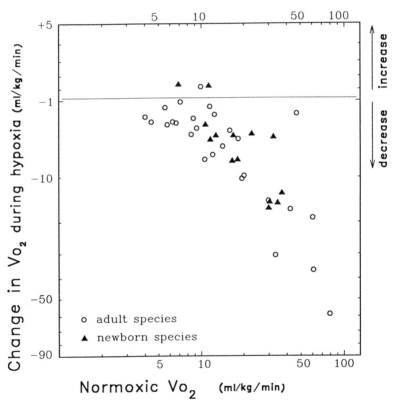

Figure 2 Double logarithmic representation of the drop in oxygen consumption ($\dot{V}O_2$/kg) during hypoxia versus the normoxic value for several newborn and adult mammals. Each data point refers to a different species. The magnitude of the $\dot{V}O_2$ drop seems to increase in the smaller animals, which have large resting values, whether newborns or adults. (From Mortola, 1993, with permission; original data in Frappell et al., 1992b.)

metabolic contribution of nonshivering thermogenesis, which is inhibited by hypoxia (Baum et al., 1970), is inversely proportional to body size (Heldmaier, 1971). A corollary of the above conclusion is that even in those large species with low resting $\dot{V}O_2$/kg the hypometabolic response to hypoxia should become apparent when normoxic $\dot{V}O_2$ is increased; some measurements in adult humans exposed to cold support this expectation (Kottke et al., 1948; Robinson and Haymes, 1990).

Mechanisms of Hypoxic Hypometabolism

A drop in Tb is often associated with the hypoxic decrease in metabolism and may be expected to lower metabolic rate via the Q_{10} effect.* Hence, the question has been raised of whether the decrease in Tb is an important contributor to, and perhaps the cause of, the hypometabolism (Moore, 1959). The answer to this question is negative for a number of reasons. First, the drop in $\dot{V}O_2$ occurs rapidly, often within 2 min from the onset of hypoxia, while the decrease in Tb is slow and gradual (Frappell et al., 1991; Mortola and Rezzonico, 1988). In fact, in some species, usually the largest, the drop in Tb can be apparent only after long exposures, presumably because of their long time constant for passive heat exchange. The drop in Tb is small compared to the metabolic drop; for example, in kittens after 15–30 min of 10% FI_{O_2}, $\dot{V}O_2$ can be 50% of control, while Tb decreases by 1–1.5°C (Mortola and Rezzonico, 1988), which would yield a Q_{10} several order of magnitudes higher than that expected from the passive effect of Tamb on biological reactions. Finally, in kittens exposed to hypoxia, Tb was artificially increased to the normoxic value by raising Tamb; this did not reverse the hypometabolic effect of hypoxia (Pedraz and Mortola, 1991).

In lambs during the first 2–3 months of life, breathing moderately hypoxic gases decreased $\dot{V}O_2$ with no increase in blood lactate or metabolic acidosis (Sidi et al., 1983; Moss et al., 1987). In kittens, blood lactate increased significantly during 10% O_2 breathing, when $\dot{V}O_2$ was 64% of control, but it was not changed during 15% O_2 breathing, with $\dot{V}O_2$ at 72% of control (Frappell et al., 1991). Hence, a drop in $\dot{V}O_2$ can occur without a parallel increase in lactate. Several objections have been raised about the interpretation of blood lactate levels as reflecting glycolytic rate, because of the various factors that can affect its concentration, including the rate of tissue release and washout, and the rate of hepatic and kidney removal. Nevertheless, the lactate data agree with results indicating that the O_2 debt during mild and moderate hypoxia is not, or is only minimally, paid back on restoration of normoxia; in fact, the immediate post-

---

*Q_{10} effect is the change in metabolic rate for 10°C change in T. In the physiological range of T, Q_{10} of enzymatic reactions is about 3. The Q_{10} of $\dot{V}O_2$ between two Tb (Tb′ and Tb″) is calculated as $Q_{10} = (\dot{V}O_2'/\dot{V}O_2'')^{[10/(Tb'-Tb'')]}$, where $\dot{V}O_2'$ and $\dot{V}O_2''$ are the $\dot{V}O_2$s at the corresponding Tb.

hypoxic $\dot{V}_{O_2}$ can be equal to, or even below, the prehypoxic level (Adolph and Hoy, 1960; Fahey and Lister, 1989; Frappell et al., 1991). These data on newborns are very similar to what is observed in adult dogs during stagnant hypoxia (Alpert, 1965) or hypoxic hypoxia (Alpert et al., 1958; Cain, 1977; Adams and Cain, 1983). In other words, the O_2 not used during hypoxia appears to correspond to a drop in energy utilization, with no compensatory increase in glycolysis*; therefore, on return to normoxia, no anaerobic debt needs to be paid back. This indicates that a portion of normoxic $\dot{V}_{O_2}$ represents "facultative" $\dot{V}_{O_2}$ and raises the question of what are the functions using facultative O_2.

Several energy-demanding functions could decline or be entirely suppressed during hypoxia: (1) tissue growth and differentiation, (2) tissue repair and maintenance, (3) muscle tone, and (4) thermoregulation. Function 1 applies mostly to newborn and young animals, but in some species, as in many rodents, body growth continues throughout the whole life. Functions 2, 3, and 4 are common to all mammals, irrespective of age, albeit to different degrees. The thermogenic component of thermoregulation varies substantially with age and size. In the early postnatal period, thermogenesis, present even in the least developed newborns, is often too modest for an effective protection of Tb against changes in Tamb and is therefore coupled to behavioral thermoregulation. Animal size is an important issue because the dispersion of heat, in first approximation, depends on body surface, which, relative to mass, is larger in smaller animals. Indeed, it is well known that small species have high specific metabolic rates ($\dot{V}_{O_2}$/kg) (Kleiber, 1932), possibly because of their large anabolic needs to maintain Tb, and nonshivering thermogenesis is inversely proportional to animal size (Heldmaier, 1971). Hence, the facts that, in hypoxia, the drop in $\dot{V}_{O_2}$ is minimal at thermoneutrality and it is larger in smaller species with high $\dot{V}_{O_2}$/kg (Fig. 2) are in favor of the argument that in mammals a large component of facultative $\dot{V}_{O_2}$ is determined by thermogenesis. However, the fact that in some species, and particularly in newborns, hypometabolism can be manifest even at thermoneutrality (Fig. 1) should not be overlooked. In addition, reptiles, amphibians, fish, and invertebrates have long been renowned for their capacity to conform to hypoxia, in some cases with extraordinarily long periods of hypometabolism (Hochachka, 1980; Robin, 1980; Wegener, 1988; Hicks and Wood, 1989; Burgreen and Roberts, 1991), and they are all ectothermic animals with little thermogenic control. Hence, unless one accepts the unlikely possibility of discontinuities in the phylogenetic scale, it seems reasonable to conclude that the decrease in thermogenesis in mammals represents an important mechanism, yet probably only one out of the many factors contributing to hypoxic hypometabolism.

---

*Pasteur described an increase in anaerobic glucose utilization as O_2 as acutely removed (Pasteur effect).

The involvement of the aortic and carotid bodies in the hypometabolic response to hypoxia has often been questioned; indeed, they are the main chemoreceptors sensing changes in arterial Po_2 (Pao_2), are known to project to the preoptic thermoregulatory regions, and, when stimulated, inhibit cold-induced shivering (Euler and Söderberg, 1958; Mott, 1963; Gautier et al., 1992). However, the results of several experiments, either on newborns or adults, provide a definite negative answer. The inhibition of cold-induced thermogenesis by hypoxia occurred even after chemodenervation, as well as during carbon monoxide hypoxia or anemia (Walters, 1927; Gautier et al., 1987a, 1989; Matsuoka et al., 1994a,b), which, by reducing the O_2 content without altering the Po_2, does not stimulate the carotid chemoreceptors (Lahiri et al., 1981). In addition, in newborn rabbits under ether anesthesia section of the carotid sinus nerves, vagus nerves, or both did not reverse the hypoxic drop of $\dot{V}o_2$ (Blatteis, 1964), and in conscious rats $\dot{V}o_2$ was reduced by hypoxia both before and after chemodenervation (Gautier and Bonora, 1992; Matsuoka et al., 1994a). Hence, the hypometabolic effect of hypoxia does not require the traditional chemosensory afferent information and must be searched for in the direct effects of O_2 on cellular function. In addition to the possible direct action of hypoxia on the hypothalamic thermosensory areas, O_2, by acting on smooth muscle cells (Duling, 1978), can influence the distribution of the microcirculation and, therefore, the relative contribution of tissues and organs to the $\dot{V}o_2$ of the whole body. The modulating effect of O_2 on the expression and regulation of genes is beginning to be recognized (Fanburg et al., 1992), but the molecular mechanisms of this regulation and the implications it could have on cellular function are largely unexplored.

In addition to the dominant role for substrate oxidation in the mitochondria, a less apparent and much less recognized function of O_2 is in a variety of biosynthetic reactions. In the cytosol, O_2 is used by several metabolic pathways either as electron acceptor, via oxidases, or as substrate, via O_2 transferases or oxygenases; this O_2, therefore, is not used by the mitochondrial cytochrome oxidase for oxidative phosphorylation (Bloch, 1962; Jöbsis, 1964; Hayaishii, 1974; Simon et al., 1978). Although the list of oxidases and oxygenases is long (Vanderkooi et al., 1991), it is difficult to calculate the magnitude of the non-respiratory fraction of $\dot{V}o_2$. Jöbsis (1964) estimated that the respiratory chain handles about 85–90% of $\dot{V}o_2$, and nonrespiratory $\dot{V}o_2$ is often evaluated at around 10–20% of the total (Duling, 1978; Robin, 1980; Cain, 1987). Irrespective of its actual magnitude, in the context of the present discussion, the nonrespiratory $\dot{V}o_2$ fraction is important for several reasons. First, the Km* for O_2 of many oxidases and oxygenases is very high, indicating a low O_2 affinity, quite differently from the cytochrome oxidase, which, with Km < 0.1 mmHg, has a very

---

*Michaelis constant, concentration that halves the maximal rate of the reaction.

high affinity for O_2 (Starlinger and Lübbers, 1973). This implies that a drop in O_2 supply can interfere with a number of nonrespiratory O_2-dependent metabolic functions before affecting oxidative phosphorylation. Because this metabolic component of $\dot{V}O_2$ does not participate to aerobic energy production, its reduction in hypoxia would not appear as an O_2 debt. Finally, it seems appropriate to note that any modification in the nonrespiratory O_2-dependent metabolic pathways offers the potential for the existence of O_2-sensing mechanisms activated before aerobic energy production is curtailed, as hypothesized for the control of the microvasculature (Duling, 1978). Whether nonrespiratory metabolites may contribute to the link between O_2 supply and cellular $\dot{V}O_2$, especially in those cases that seem to suggest a mismatch between changes in $\dot{V}O_2$ and any of the proposed regulators of tissue respiration (ATP, ADP, ATP/ADP, phosphocreatine, etc.) (Hogan et al., 1992a, b), is an attractive, but at present purely speculative, possibility.

Ventilation

Upon a sudden exposure to hypoxia, $\dot{V}E$ increases abruptly; then, it declines by a magnitude, and within a time, which vary greatly among species and with age. A few exceptions have been reported (Davis et al., 1988; Cao et al., 1992) but, rather than qualitative differences, they may only reflect a difference in the time scale of the phenomenon, which can be very long, as in ponies (Brown et al., 1992). In adult humans, $\dot{V}E$ after 10–30 min of hypoxia is about half of the initial increment (Weil and Zwillich, 1976; Kagawa et al., 1982; Easton et al., 1986). This time-dependent change in $\dot{V}E$ at the onset of hypoxia, often referred to as the "biphasic response," has attracted much attention, especially in newborns. The possibility that it is due to adaptation of the peripheral chemoreceptors is negated by numerous experimental studies; in fact, in both newborns and adults chemo-afferents had no or minimal (Biscoe and Purves, 1967; Schwieler, 1968; Blanco et al., 1984a, b; Marchal et al., 1992) adaptation to constant hypoxemia, even when $\dot{V}E$ was clearly changing (Blanco et al., 1984b; Vizek et al., 1987; Tatsumi et al., 1992). The hypothesis that a decrease in lung compliance was responsible for the time course of $\dot{V}E$ at the onset of hypoxia, based on findings in tracheotomized young monkeys (LaFramboise et al., 1983), did not agree with later measurements in intact animals (Côté et al., 1988). In anesthetized adult cats (Vizek et al., 1987) and kittens (Blanco et al., 1984b) temporal changes in V_T and phrenic or diaphragm electrical activities were closely related. A report suggesting that, in awake kittens, the hypoxic drop in V_T was not matched by a decrease in diaphragm electromyogram (Rigatto et al., 1988) could be explained by partitioning the diaphragm activity into its tonic and phasic components; the former increases in hypoxia, whereas the latter decreases along with V_T (Bonora et al., 1992).

The respiratory drive during hypoxia reflects a balance between the stimulation of the peripheral chemoreceptors and the central depression of hypoxia on respiration (see Chapter 6). Neither component is constant, because they express multiple events that change at different rates. The hypocapnia that accompanies the hyperventilation, blood pressure, metabolic rate, and temperature are only a few of the many variables known to influence the respiratory drive and changing during hypoxia, each according to its own dynamics. Hence, it may not be surprising that, following a squared drop in $F_{I_{O_2}}$, the ventilatory output does not immediately settle around a new steady value, but it responds first to the events with the shortest time constant, which are almost undoubtedly the peripheral chemostimuli. The existence of some relation between the steady $\dot{V}E$ value and that of the immediate increment at the onset of hypoxia (Bureau et al., 1985) and the findings that hypoxic $\dot{V}E$ can be increased either by pharmacological stimulation of the carotid bodies (McCooke and Hanson, 1985) or by decerebration (Martin-Body and Johnston, 1988) are some of the many observations that can be interpreted in light of such a dynamic balance.

In newborns, after a few minutes of hypoxia, $\dot{V}E$ can be close to, or even below, the normoxic value, but the degree of development at birth introduces important interspecies variations (Mortola et al., 1989); lambs and piglets, which are developmentally more mature at birth, during hypoxic breathing maintain $\dot{V}E$ much above the normoxic value (Davis et al., 1988, Bureau et al., 1984, 1986), differently from the majority of other laboratory species, including newborn cats, dogs, rabbits, and rodents (Haddad et al., 1982; Bonora et al., 1984; McCooke and Hanson, 1985; Saetta and Mortola, 1987; Bonora and Gautier, 1987; Mortola and Rezzonico, 1988; Rigatto et al., 1988; Mortola et al., 1989; Martin-Body and Johnston, 1988; Wangsnes and Koos, 1991). In infants, hypoxic $\dot{V}E$ can be similar to, or even below, the normoxic level (Cross and Oppé, 1952; Cross et al., 1954, 1959; Brady and Ceruti, 1966; Rigatto et al., 1975; De Boeck et al., 1984; Alvaro et al., 1992).

Breathing in hypoxia is usually rapid, although a slow pattern has been reported in premature infants and some adult species, reflecting a variability that may also depend on the degree of hypoxemia (Eden and Hanson, 1987; Mortola and Rezzonico, 1988). In most newborn animals, including infants at term (Bradi and Ceruti, 1966), tachypnea is associated with shallow breathing. In preterm infants, on the other hand, hypoxia more commonly decreases f (Cross and Oppé, 1952; Rigatto et al., 1975; Alvaro et al., 1992). Anesthesia can completely modify the response, slow respiration representing the most common pattern. The occurrence of a rapid, shallow pattern, particularly in those newborns with no or small hyperpnea, is of interest because it implies that alveolar ventilation, $\dot{V}A = f \times (V_T - V_D)$, is less than in normoxia.* Yet, the values of transcutaneous and arterial

---

*This would not be true if the dead space (V_D) was greatly reduced by hypoxia, but the available evidence suggests otherwise (Fisher et al., 1987; Wetzel et al., 1992).

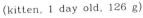

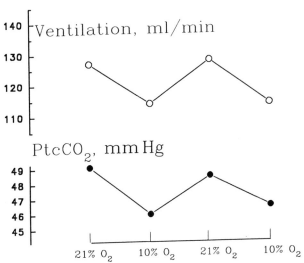

Figure 3   Minute ventilation (top) and transcutaneous P_{CO_2} (Ptc_{CO_2}, bottom) in a 1-day-old kitten during periods of normoxia ($F_{I_{O_2}}$ = 21%) and hypoxia ($F_{I_{O_2}}$ = 10%). During hypoxia, the drop in Ptc_{CO_2}, which reflects a similar decrease in arterial P_{CO_2}, despite the hypopnea is due to the large decrease in CO_2 production. (Modified from Mortola and Rezzonico, 1988.)

P_{CO_2} (Pa_{CO_2}) during hypoxia were 1–4 mmHg below the normoxic value (Haddad et al., 1982; Mortola and Rezzonico, 1988; Mortola and Matsuoka, 1993). In other words, in acute hypoxia the newborn can simultaneously present hyperventilation (i.e., drop in Pa_{CO_2}) and hypopnea (i.e., drop in $\dot{V}_A$) (Fig. 3). The few scattered data in human infants agree with the measurements on animals. For example, in term infants breathing 12% O_2 the end-tidal P_{CO_2} decreased even when $\dot{V}_E$ fell (Brady and Ceruti, 1966), and in preterm infants breathing 15% O_2 the end-tidal P_{CO_2} did not increase despite a 10–30% reduction in $\dot{V}_E$ (Rigatto and Brady, 1972b; Alvaro et al., 1992). Periodic breathing in hypoxic infants was also accompanied by a decrease in transcutaneous Pa_{CO_2} (Milerad et al., 1987). The combination of hypopnea and hyperventilation calls attention on the role played by the hypometabolism, specifically the decrease in $\dot{V}_{CO_2}$,* in the $\dot{V}_E$ response to hypoxia.

With growth, the hyperpneic response becomes progressively more appar-

---

*$\dot{V}_{CO_2}$ and alveolar (and arterial) P_{CO_2} are linked by the alveolar gas equation, $P_{A_{CO_2}}$ = Pb × $\dot{V}_{CO_2}/\dot{V}_A$, Pb being the dry barometric pressure.

ent (Sankaran et al., 1979; Bonora et al., 1984; Bonora and Gautier, 1987; Wangsnes and Koos, 1991), almost entirely because of the increase in V_T; for example, in kittens (Bonora et al., 1984) breathing $F_{I_{O_2}} = 11\%$ for 30–40 min, V_T and $\dot{V}_E$ were about 20–30% below normoxia until 2 weeks of age, just under normoxia at 4 weeks, and about 15–20% above normoxia by 2 months of age. In humans, no differences were seen between young adults and elderly subjects (Ahmed et al., 1991). Many adult species, in moderate hypoxia ($F_{I_{O_2}} = 10$–12%) maintain $\dot{V}_E$ at a level that is 30–50% above the normoxic value (Boggs and Tenney, 1984; Frappell et al., 1992b), but there are major interspecies variations, and in a few, as in newborns, $\dot{V}_E$ can be below normoxia (Frappell et al., 1992b).

In summary, the $\dot{V}_E$ response to acute hypoxia, within each animal, is time-dependent, probably reflecting the gradual adjustment of the balance among events with different dynamics. At equilibrium, the $\dot{V}_E$ response among individuals of the same species is consistently lower in younger animals.

Interaction Between Metabolism and Ventilation

The $\dot{V}_E$-$\dot{V}_{O_2}$ ratio (or "air convection requirement," Dejours et al., 1970) is relatively similar among species, whether newborns or adults, and in hypoxia it increases approximately by the same magnitude (Mortola et al., 1989; Frappell et al., 1992b). This implies that those species decreasing metabolic rate the most are also those with the smallest hyperpnea. Such reciprocal relation between the hypoxic changes in $\dot{V}_{O_2}$ and the magnitude of hyperpnea holds true also within the same species during development (Fig. 4): the youngest rats in hypoxia have a marked hypometabolism and little hyperpnea, while the opposite occurs in the oldest rats, which, in normoxia, have low $\dot{V}_{O_2}$/kg and $\dot{V}_E$/kg (Mortola et al., 1994).

A change in Tamb offers a convenient experimental opportunity to observe the strength of the metabolic-ventilatory interaction. Gautier and Bonora (1992) exposed adult rats to different Tamb, from 25°C to 5°C; $\dot{V}_{O_2}$ increased in the cold, and $\dot{V}_E$ followed closely, maintaining the $\dot{V}_E$-$\dot{V}_{O_2}$ ratio constant (see Section III.A). Upon exposure to hypoxia ($F_{I_{O_2}} = 12\%$), the $\dot{V}_E$-$\dot{V}_{O_2}$ ratio increased in all cases to approximately similar values, suggesting that at all Tamb the animals responded with a comparable hyperventilation. Indeed, in rats with chronic arterial catheters (Saiki et al., 1994) upon exposure to hypoxia ($F_{I_{O_2}} = 10\%$, $Pa_{O_2} = 33$–35 mmHg) the drop in Pa_{CO_2} (13–14 mmHg) was almost identical in warm (25°C) and cold (10°C) conditions (Fig. 5); in the warm condition, however, hypoxia had a minimal hypometabolic effect and almost doubled $\dot{V}_E$, whereas in the cold condition metabolism dropped by 29% and $\dot{V}_E$ increased by only 15%. Hence, exposure to the same degree of hypoxia resulted in the same hyperventilation, but with very different combinations of hyperpnea and hypometabolism. In adult rats in which core Tb was lowered, at constant Tamb, from 38°C to 35°C via a chronically implanted abdominal heat exchanger, the response to hypoxia was

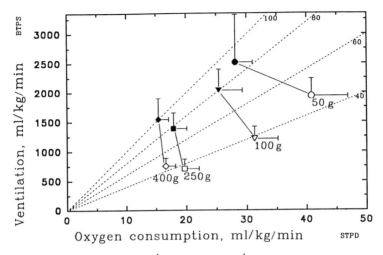

Figure 4 Oxygen consumption ($\dot{V}O_2$)-ventilation ($\dot{V}E$) relationship during normoxia (open symbols) or hypoxia (10% O_2, filled symbols) in rats of different body weights. Each data point is the average of 10 rats, five females and five males; bars are standard deviations. Oblique isopleths are $\dot{V}E$-$\dot{V}O_2$ ratios. (From Mortola et al., 1994.)

actually reversed, from hyperpnea (at 38°C) to hypopnea (at 35°C) (Maskrey, 1990). The opposite experiment, i.e., the increase in Tb, is known to increase the $\dot{V}E$ response to hypoxia in animals and humans (Petersen and Vejby-Christensen, 1977), but no measurements of metabolic rate during hyperthermic hypoxia are available.

In kittens (Mortola and Matsuoka, 1993), hypoxia ($F_{I_{O_2}}$ = 10%, Pa_{O_2} = 36 mmHg) in the cold condition (Tamb = 20°C) resulted in modest hyperventilation (Pa_{CO_2} decreased by 3 mmHg), and this was accompanied by hypopnea much more marked than in the warm condition (Tamb = 30°C), because of a larger decrease in V_T. These results, therefore, agree with the idea of an important metabolic contribution to the $\dot{V}E$ response to hypoxia. Because addition of 3–5% CO_2 to the hypoxic air resulted in sustained hyperpnea with large V_T, it was further hypothesized that the level of $\dot{V}E$ depends on the magnitude of CO_2 produced, possibly via the CO_2-mediated control of V_T (Mortola and Matsuoka, 1993).

In summary, despite the fact that changes in P_{O_2} and Tamb influence many variables, including the physicochemical relations determining the acid-base status of blood and brain tissue, the respiratory output seems to perfectly track the metabolic response. The response to hypoxia, therefore, can be listed as one more example, and an important extension, of the remarkable $\dot{V}E$-metabolism coupling well documented for conditions that increase metabolic rate, such as muscular

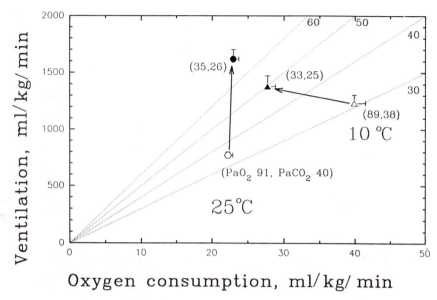

Figure 5 Oxygen consumption-ventilation relationship in adult rats during normoxia (open symbols) or hypoxia (10% O_2, filled symbols) at two ambient temperatures, 25 and 10°C. Symbols represent average values of 12 rats, bars indicate 1 SE. Oblique dotted isopleths indicate $\dot{V}E$-$\dot{V}O_2$ ratios. In parentheses, near each symbol, are the corresponding average values of arterial PO_2 and PCO_2. (From the data of Saiki et al., 1994).

exercise (Wasserman et al., 1986), pharmacological interventions (Huch et al., 1969; Levine and Huckabee, 1975), or cold exposure (see Section III.A), and for which no mechanism is as yet conclusively accepted (Dempsey and Forster, 1982; Wasserman et al., 1986). $\dot{V}CO_2$, more than $\dot{V}O_2$, closely relates to $\dot{V}E$ during exercise, and the proposal was made that the level of CO_2 returning to the lung sets the level of $\dot{V}E$ (Wasserman et al., 1977). This view is corroborated by a long series of experiments based on changes in venous CO_2 load (reviewed in Wasserman et al., 1986). The extension of these experiments to CO_2 unloading via an extracorporeal CO_2 membrane lung (Kolobow et al., 1977; Phillipson et al. 1981) is particularly relevant to the interpretation of the hypoxic hypometabolism-$\dot{V}E$ linkage; in fact, it showed a continuum $\dot{V}CO_2$-$\dot{V}E$ function not only above, but also below, the resting values (Phillipson et al., 1981). Hence, it seems appealing to view the hyperpneic response during hypoxia, and its interaction with hypometabolism, as an application of the concept that the CO_2 load governs the generation of the respiratory rhythm, although the precise nature of this linkage still needs to be understood.

B. Metabolism and Ventilation in Chronic Hypoxia

Acclimatization to Hypoxia

Many investigations have focused on the effect of high-altitude acclimatization on $\dot{V}O_2$; most of these studies examined the $\dot{V}O_2$ response to exercise, and particularly $\dot{V}O_2max$, since it offers an integrated view of the O_2 transport system. The study by Consolazio et al. (1966), with measurements on young healthy adults between 1 and 19 days upon ascent to 3465 m, can probably be quoted as typical of the conclusions of the majority of previous and following studies (Cerretelli and Di Prampero, 1987): $\dot{V}O_2$ during basal, sitting rest, and moderate exercise conditions was not markedly changed by altitude, whereas $\dot{V}O_2max$ was reduced. The reduction in $\dot{V}O_2max$ and the similarity in submaximal $\dot{V}O_2$ between high altitude and sea-level conditions find almost no exceptions in the literature; however, with respect to basal or resting $\dot{V}O_2$ during high-altitude acclimatization, all three possible results (no change, increase, or decrease at altitude) have been reported, with the weight of evidence perhaps in favor of an increase (Grover, 1963; Gill and Pugh, 1964; Phillips et al., 1969). The increase in basal $\dot{V}O_2$ could be attributed , at least partly, to the difficulties in reproducing basal conditions in the often unusual high-altitude environment, and some reports of its drop in the following days could reflect an habituation to the initially stressful conditions (Consolazio et al., 1966; Blatteis and Lutherer, 1976). Resting $\dot{V}O_2$ was reported to be increased (15–27%) during 6 days at high altitude (Huang et al., 1984), but the data of a later study by the same group (Moore et al., 1987) indicated that resting $\dot{V}O_2$ increased transiently during only the first day, with no significant changes from the low-altitude value during the following week. From the data of Reeves, Sutton, and colleagues in Operation Everest II (Reeves et al., 1987; Sutton et al., 1988) resting $\dot{V}O_2$ was below the sea-level value until the inspired PO_2 decreased to 63 mmHg, and it increased with more severe hypoxia. The facts that high altitude is a multienvironmental stressor of which hypoxia is the primary, but not the only, component (Monge and León-Velarde, 1991), and that chronic hypoxia triggers a number of hormonal responses known to influence metabolic rate (Heath and Williams, 1981), are among the most obvious explanations for the wide variability in the basal and resting metabolic data.

The metabolic response to cold exposure (10°C) during a 6-week sojourn at high altitude was found to be reduced, and immediately restored upon descent, despite a similar visible shivering intensity (Blatteis and Lutherer, 1976). This suggests some depression of nonshivering thermogenesis at high altitude, in agreement with the effect of acute hypoxia on the thermogenic response to cold (Section III.A).

As for the data on metabolism, measurements on resting $\dot{V}E$ of humans acclimatizing to high altitude are numerous, and the results are consistent, in both human and animal studies: with the persistence of the hypoxic stimulus $\dot{V}E$ progressively increases and Pa_{CO_2} decreases (Dempsey and Forster, 1982; Brown et al., 1992). Although the mechanisms of this gradual hyperventilation remain controversial, the two major theories seem to be an enhanced carotid body sensitivity to the hypoxic stimulus and a gradual compensation of the initial blood and spinal fluid alkalosis (Weil, 1986). To what extent resting metabolic rate contributes to the $\dot{V}E$ adjustments during high-altitude acclimatization is difficult to conclude in view of the uncertainties about the metabolic measurements. Nevertheless, some proportionality has been found between the changes in resting $\dot{V}O_2$ and the corresponding degree of hyperpnea, with no effect on the magnitude of the hyperventilation, evaluated from the drop in end-tidal P_{CO_2} (Huang et al., 1984; Moore et al., 1987). This underlines, once more, the importance of interpreting the mechanisms of the $\dot{V}E$ adjustments in the light of the corresponding metabolic condition. A clear example is provided by some measurements in rats acclimatizing at a simulated altitude of 4300m (Pb about 450 mmHg) (Olson and Dempsey, 1978): after the metabolic drop in the acute phase of hypoxia, $\dot{V}O_2$ gradually increased, with a parallel further increase in $\dot{V}E$, reaching the normoxic metabolic value between 1 and 4 days from the onset of hypoxia. A similar phenomenon of gradual recovery in $\dot{V}O_2$ and progressive increase in $\dot{V}E$ was also observed in newborn rats maintained in 10% FI_{O_2}, although the time course of the process seems to be longer (3–7 days) than in adults (Mortola et al., 1986; Piazza et al., 1988).

Living in Chronic Hypoxia

At high altitude, natives have lower resting $\dot{V}E$ and Pa_{O_2}, and higher Pa_{CO_2}, than newcomers (Severinghaus, 1972; Weil, 1986). Their $\dot{V}E$ response to acute hypoxia presents the typical hyperbolic shape as in lowlanders, but it is shifted to lower hypoxic values. In this respect, therefore, high-altitude natives behave like several other large native species, and differently from small mammals, which have a clearly reduced $\dot{V}E$ response after prolonged exposure to hypoxia (reviewed by Monge and León-Verlarde, 1991). An interpretation of these $\dot{V}E$ responses in light of the corresponding metabolic values would be appropriate, but information in this respect is scanty. Resting $\dot{V}O_2$ of high-altitude natives is similar or slightly higher than in lowlanders (Picón-Reátegui, 1961; Lefrancois et al., 1969; Nair et al., 1971), although the conclusion seems to depend on the type of normalization adopted (body weight, fat-free body weight, or body surface area). During exercise, $\dot{V}O_2$ was found to be similar to that of sea-level natives sojourning at high altitude; the increase in $\dot{V}E$, however, was less in the natives, indicating a greater ability to extract O_2 from the inspired gas (Lefrancois et al., 1969). Whether this ability is the expression of genetic traits or is a phenomenon acquired with prolonged exposure to hypoxia is unresolved, although some characteristics, such as the lower accumulation of lactic acid during exercise, persist on descent to sea level and have therefore been considered aspects of genetic adaptation (Hochachka et al., 1991).

Mammalian species resident at altitude, when exposed to hypoxia, have a lower hypometabolic response, and at a lower P_{O_2} threshold, than comparable lowland species (Bullard and Kollias, 1966; Rosenman and Morrison, 1975; Lechner, 1977). Their hyperpneic response to hypoxia is less than in sea-level controls (Monge and León-Verlarde, 1991). Animals living either permanently (fossorial) or intermittently (semifossorial) in burrows, where the gas composition can be substantially asphyxic (Kuhnen, 1985), also tend to have a diminished response to hypoxia, although the blunting of the $\dot{V}E$ response to hypercapnia has been more consistently documented (reviewed in Boggs et al., 1984; Tenney and Boggs, 1986). In the hamster, a semifossorial species, the $\dot{V}E$-$\dot{V}O_2$ ratio during FI_{O_2} = 10% increased about 30% less than in the white rat, a surface dweller, because of a lower hyperpnea and a slightly lower hypometabolism (Mortola, 1991).

In summary, adult mammals living in chronic hypoxia downplay the strategy adopted by lowlanders against acute hypoxia, which consists of variable combinations of hyperpnea and hypometabolism. Indeed, hypoxic hyperpnea is the obvious approach for the protection of homeothermy, but it is costly and can disturb the acid-base equilibrium. Hypometabolism, coupled to the redistribution of blood flow and hypothermia, permits long survival by sparing precious O_2 in favor of the life-supporting organs. However, it can have serious disadvantages especially in the developing organism, since the nonhomogeneous growth of tissues and organs may eventually become incompatible with survival (Mortola et al., 1993). The hyperpneic-hypometabolic response in mammals is likely to be an immediate, yet an emergency, type of response to hypoxia, not necessarily desirable in chronic conditions. Presumably, if the energy needs are not too stringent and the hypoxia not too severe, various mechanisms improving the extraction of O_2 from the inspired air and its delivery to the tissue have time to be implemented, gradually relieving the necessity of hyperpnea and hypometabolism. In this respect, it is of interest that infants born at high altitude have the same ventilatory and metabolic rates of lowland infants, whether of the same or different ethnic groups (Mortola et al., 1992b). In other words, the response of the high-altitude newborn to the low O_2 concentration of its environment is neither an increase in gas convection nor a reduction in O_2 use, but a more efficient extraction of O_2 from the total inspired quantity, a characteristic probably acquired via functional and structural alterations stimulated by fetal hypoxia.

C. Hyperoxia

Hyperoxia is a frequent occurrence in special aquatic environments, as in intertidal pools, because of the slow diffusion of gases and the cohabitation of plants and animals; in these conditions, Po_2 can oscillate from severe hypoxic levels to hyperoxic conditions of 300–400 mmHg (Truchot and Duhamel-Jouve, 1980). In air breathers, a rapid increase in Po_2 with respect to the predominant environmental level is experienced by some high-altitude animals and birds on descent at lower levels and by semifossorial species when they leave the hypoxic environment of the burrow. Birth and hatching are other common physiological conditions of a sudden increase in O_2 availability. In the human infant, Pao_2 rises from approximately 27 mmHg in utero to about 74 mmHg at 5 hr after birth (Polgar and Weng, 1979), an increase that is probably responsible for the transient silencing of the chemoreceptors (Cross and Malcom, 1952; Blanco et al., 1984a). Hyperoxia is a common event in the clinical setting, where concentrations of 40% or more can be administered for long periods of time, and its effects have also been investigated in the context of space physiology, diving, and hyperbaric medicine.

Metabolic Rate

Immediately after birth the newborn's $\dot{V}o_2$ is 2–3 times higher than in the fetus (Dawes and Mott, 1959; Dawes et al., 1960) and continues to rise in the following days (Mount, 1959; Baudinette et al., 1988; Cross et al., 1957, 1958). Several factors contribute to these changes, including the increase in muscle tone, the establishment of a steady ventilatory pattern, and the energy demands of rapid growth. In addition, thermogenic needs are probably of utmost importance (Dawes and Mott, 1959). In the marsupial tammar wallaby, where the first months of development are at the comfortable pouch temperature of 36°C, postnatal $\dot{V}o_2$/kg remains approximately constant (Baudinette et al., 1988). The question has been posed of whether the increasing energetic demands of the newborn are fully met by the availability of O_2. If not, one would expect that O_2 breathing would further increase $\dot{V}o_2$.

In newborn rats and mice breathing pure O_2 for 5–15 min at Tamb = 32–33°C, i.e., close to thermoneutrality, $\dot{V}o_2$ increased by about 10–25% (Mourek, 1959; Mortola and Tenney, 1986; Frappell et al., 1992a; Dotta and Mortola, 1992). Similar results were reported in human infants breathing 100% O_2 (Mortola et al, 1992a,b), while smaller increases in $\dot{V}o_2$ were observed in rat pups (Taylor, 1960) and lambs (Alexander and Williams, 1970) breathing lower hyperoxic concentrations ($Fi_{O_2} = 32$–54%). Measurements of $\dot{V}o_2$ in hyperoxia are often problematic, and the possibility of experimental errors, which usually lead to an overestimation of $\dot{V}o_2$, should be seriously considered (Hill et al., 1924–25; Welch and Pedersen, 1981; Cain, 1987). Somewhat reassuring is the fact that uniform results have been obtained with rather different experimental and analytical approaches, some of which, by assuming a respiratory quotient equal to unity, may have actually underestimated hyperoxic $\dot{V}o_2$ (Frappell et al., 1992a). In addition, the hyperoxic increase in $\dot{V}o_2$ has also been observed by direct measurements of cardiac output and arterial-venous O_2 difference (Alexander and Williams, 1970). Because of the damaging effects on tissues, hyperoxia was by necessity limited to brief exposures, especially in infants; however, the O_2 stores are so small that their potential contribution to an overestimate of the measurements of $\dot{V}_{O_2}$ seems unlikely even for exposures lasting only 5–10 min.

The phenomenon of increased $\dot{V}_{O_2}$ during O_2 breathing was interpreted as an indication that, in the normoxic newborn, $\dot{V}_{O_2}$ was limited by the concentration of available O_2 (Mortola and Tenney, 1986), as shown to occur in the avian embryo during the late phases of incubation and, possibly, in the mammalian fetus during late gestation (reviewed by Stock, 1988). However, in the newborn, it is not clear at which point of the O_2 cascade between alveoli and mitochondria such limitation would occur. One indication, in liver slices, that the critical P_{O_2}, i.e., the P_{O_2} below which $\dot{V}_{O_2}$ is supply dependent, is higher in younger kittens (Longmuir and Moore, 1958) may suggest that one place of O_2 resistance is at the cellular level, but more results are necessary for a persuasive conclusion. Alternatively, the nonrespiratory component of $\dot{V}_{O_2}$ may be involved in the hyperoxic increase of $\dot{V}_{O_2}$ (Section II.A), a possibility that has also been considered as explanation for the $\dot{V}_{O_2}$ dependence on O_2 supply in adult patients with sepsis or respiratory distress syndrome (Cain, 1984).

The neonatal increase in gaseous metabolism is more apparent with cold stimuli, when the O_2 demands are increased; it is accompanied by greater muscle activity and, in older animals, shivering, both contributing to a better protection of Tb (Mourek, 1959; Taylor, 1960; Alexander and Williams, 1970; Dotta and Mortola, 1992). In these conditions, anaerobic sources can participate in the energy needs, and hyperoxia, by favoring oxidative phosphorylation, may reduce lactate production; this, indeed, has been observed in lambs made hyperoxic during cold stimuli (Alexander and Williams, 1970). Hence, it is also possible that the increase in $\dot{V}_{O_2}$ during hyperoxia may reflect the stimulation of thermogenesis, by direct action on the hypothalamic centers or via inhibition of the chemoreceptors. Finally, it is of interest that in newborn rats at Tamb $= 25°C$, i.e., 7–8°C below thermoneutrality, breathing pure O_2 increased $\dot{V}_{O_2}$ to 64 ml/kg/min (Dotta and Mortola, 1992), a value that is substantially lower than the summit metabolic rates of normoxic adult rats or other adult mammals of small size (Thompson and Moore, 1968; Rosenmann and Morrison, 1974; Dawson and Olson, 1987) and not sufficient to protect their Tb. In other words, even with abundant O_2 supply, the newborn rat was unable to maintain Tb by reaching the $\dot{V}_{O_2}$ levels of the adult. This developmental difference in summit $\dot{V}_{O_2}$ indicates the existence of a limitation in the rate of maximal O_2 utilization which is independent of O_2 availability. A likely explanation is the absence of shivering, which deprives the newborn of an important mechanism of O_2 use and heat production; in addition, one cannot exclude the possibility that in these newborns the maximal speed of cellular respiration is lower than in adults.

Measurements in rats of different ages indicated that the hyperoxic effect on metabolism decreased with postnatal age, and by weaning age (about 21 days) the rise was only half of that observed in the first postnatal days (Mourek, 1959). In adult men, $\dot{V}O_2max$, but not resting $\dot{V}O_2$, was increased by hyperoxia (Wyndham et al., 1970; Welch, 1982; Cerretelli and Di Prampero, 1987; Powers et al., 1989), and lactate levels were generally reduced (Welch, 1982). In 20 healthy volunteers, breathing pure O_2 for about 15 min did not alter $\dot{V}O_2$; the arterial-venous O_2 difference and cardiac output were also unchanged (Barratt-Boyes and Wood, 1958). In conscious, instrumented dogs, hyperoxia has been shown to decrease whole body $\dot{V}O_2$ (Lodato, 1989), a result in agreement with a previous observation in adult dogs under anesthesia (Chapler et al., 1984). Although the latter findings are not consistent in the literature (Saunders et al., 1972), the reports of a drop in $\dot{V}O_2$ despite the increase in arterial O_2 content are of interest, also because of similar observations in critically ill patients, in whom $\dot{V}O_2$ decreased when the inspired O_2 concentration was raised (Reinhart et al., 1991). In these cases, cardiac output did not decrease, whereas heart rate did, but the probable decrease in cardiac $\dot{V}O_2$ would be too small to explain the drop in whole-body $\dot{V}O_2$ (Ganz et al., 1972). The observation that hyperoxia induced a reduction of $\dot{V}O_2$ in the in situ isolated canine hind-limb preparation despite the increase in O_2 delivery (Chapler et al., 1984) calls attention to phenomena occurring at the tissue or cellular level. The consistent finding in both the animal and human observations was the increase in mixed venous O_2 content and reduced O_2 extraction. This led to the hypothesis that hyperoxia may induce a phenomenon of overcompensation in the attempt to maintain tissue PO_2, with the paradoxical result of decreasing tissue oxygenation and $\dot{V}O_2$ (Chapler et al., 1984). Additional, or alternative, explanations may include systemic cellular O_2 toxicity and reduction in facultative, nonrespiratory, cellular O_2 use (Section II.A).

The observation that hyperoxia induced a modest drop in alveolar PCO_2 in the intact normothermic cat despite the absence of hyperpnea (Gautier et al., 1986) suggests some decrease in gaseous metabolism, which would be in agreement with the results in dogs mentioned above. On the other hand, under cold exposures, shivering was stimulated by hyperoxia in conscious cats (Gautier et al., 1989), and both shivering and $\dot{V}E$ were increased by hyperoxia in anesthetized cats (Euler and Söderberg, 1958; Gautier et al., 1992), with no changes in end-tidal PCO_2, which suggests a stimulatory effect of hyperoxia on thermogenesis, similarly to that seen in newborns under cold stimuli.

In summary, the effect of hyperoxia on resting gaseous metabolism seems to change during development, from stimulation in the neonatal period to modest depression in adulthood. Neither phenomenon is understood in its mechanisms. The fact that also in the adult, during cold, $\dot{V}O_2$ appears to be stimulated by hyperoxia suggests the involvement of thermoregulatory mechanisms.

Ventilation

During the first few breaths of hyperoxia $\dot{V}E$ decreases, in both newborns and adults. Because this does not occur after chemodenervation, the immediate drop is interpreted as due to the decrease in the chemoreceptor activity; indeed, the $\dot{V}E$ response to a few breaths of pure O_2 is often adopted as an indirect assessment of the chemoreceptor contribution to $\dot{V}E$ during normoxia (Dripps and Comroe, 1947; May, 1957; Dejours, 1957).

In infants, after the initial drop, $\dot{V}E$ rises to a steady value above the normoxic level (Graham et al., 1950; Cross and Warner, 1951; Cross and Oppé, 1952; Brady et al., 1964; Rigatto and Brady, 1972a; Davi et al., 1980; Mortola et al., 1992a), and breathing irregularities are reduced by even modest increases in inspired O_2 ($F_{I_{O_2}}$ = 25–40%; Weintraub et al., 1992). Because the increase in $\dot{V}E$ is mostly contributed by V_T, the rise in alveolar ventilation is actually greater than apparent from the $\dot{V}E$ measurements.

As in newborns, also in adults acute hyperoxia, after the brief hypoventilation, determines an increase in $\dot{V}E$ to, or even above, the control level (Dripps and Comroe, 1947; May, 1957; Lenfant, 1966; Miller and Tenney, 1975). In adult nonanesthetized cats O_2 breathing for 1 hr had no effects on $\dot{V}E$, whereas it induced a sustained hyperventilation after chemodenervation (Miller and Tenney, 1975; Gautier et al., 1986). Hence, hyperoxia appears to have a central stimulatory component that can be entirely masked by the decreased ventilatory drive of the chemoreceptors. In this light, in newborns, the more consistent hyperpneic response to hyperoxia may indicate that the balance between the central stimulatory action of hyperoxia and the decreased respiratory drive of the chemoreceptors is tilted in favor of the former. The increase in gaseous metabolism partly accounts for, but does not fully explain, the increase in $\dot{V}E$ (Mortola et al., 1992); the brain acidosis possibly accompanying cerebral vasoconstriction (discussed in Lambertsen et al., 1953), mild hypercapnia because of O_2-induced $\dot{V}E$-perfusion inequalities (Lenfant, 1986), or direct hyperoxic stimulation of the brainstem regions (Miller and Tenney, 1975) could represent the additional respiratory stimuli.

D. Carbon Dioxide

CO_2, like O_2, is a gas active on biological functions. Its effects on cellular properties and developmental processes have been known for many years (Nahas and Schaefer, 1974). The role on the metabolic rate of individual organs and of the whole body has also been the subject of several studies and seems to depend on the effects of two contrasting actions, the metabolic depression due to acidemia and the thermogenic action of catecholamines, the concentration of which is stimulated by CO_2 (Fenn and Asano, 1956; Tenney, 1956). In addition, CO_2 interferes with thermoregulation (Euler and Söderberg, 1958); hence, its net effect on metabolic rate is expected to reflect the balance among multiple factors.

At Tamb of 24–28°C, acutely inspired CO_2 in large concentrations ($F_{I_{CO_2}} >$ 8%) consistently reduced Tb, whereas the opposite seems to occur with lower $F_{I_{CO_2}}$ (reviewed by Schaefer et al., 1975), a difference that probably reflects the interplay of various factors on $\dot{V}O_2$ when $F_{I_{CO_2}}$ is increased (Karetzky and Cain, 1970; Stupfel, 1974; see also Sections III.A and III.B). In addition, the threshold for the thermogenic response to cold is shifted to lower values (see Kuhnen et al., 1987, for additional references). The acute metabolic effect of hypercapnia may change in chronic conditions, although very few data are available. Lechner et al. (1987) exposed weanling guinea pigs for 3 weeks either to hypercapnia ($F_{I_{CO_2}} = 5\% \ CO_2$) or air; $\dot{V}O_2$ measured at the end of the exposure during breathing the acclimation gas did not differ between the two groups.

Although the stimulatory effects of CO_2 on $\dot{V}E$ and its interaction with hypoxia have long been documented, the mechanisms mediating the short- and long-term adaptation to CO_2 are still controversial (Dempsey and Forster, 1982; Cunningham et al., 1986). In addition, the implications that metabolic changes may have on the CO_2-O_2 interaction have rarely been considered. In kittens (Mortola and Matsuoka, 1993), small concentrations of CO_2 added to the inspired air ($F_{I_{CO_2}} = 1\%$) did not have any measurable effect on metabolic rate, stimulated $\dot{V}E$, but did not modify the response to 10% O_2, which is characterized by rapid, shallow breathing with no hyperpnea (Section II.A); on the other hand, $F_{I_{CO_2}} = 3$ or 5% drastically changed the ventilatory response to hypoxia into a brisk, sustained hyperpnea. This could not be attributed to an increase in metabolic rate, because this level of hypercapnia, whether alone or added to the hypoxic gas, dropped $\dot{V}O_2$. These results could be interpreted as being in support of the view that the CO_2 drive dictates the ventilatory level (Section II.A); hence, the increased $F_{I_{CO_2}}$ would replace the drop in endogenously produced CO_2 during hypoxic hypometabolism. Along this view, it is of interest that the response of adult humans to low $F_{I_{CO_2}}$ (1–2%) is an *isocapnic* increase in $\dot{V}E$, a phenomenon interpreted as being in agreement with the idea that the magnitude of the oscillation in arterial CO_2, rather than the arterial P_{CO_2}, dictates the $\dot{V}E$ response to CO_2 (Anthonisen and Dhingra, 1978).

III. Temperature

Two major groups of animals may be distinguished with regard to their Tb: homeotherms and poikilotherms. In poikilotherms Tb conforms to the environmental temperature, approaching Tamb and following its oscillations. Homeotherms comprise a smaller group of animals, mammals and birds, which maintain an almost constant Tb over a wide range of Tamb, around a value (37–39°C) that is nearly the same for all eutherian endotherms. A third group of animals, hibernators and estivators, are endotherms (Prosser and Heath, 1991), which, under particular environmental conditions, permit Tb to fall to a value only slightly higher than Tamb.

Even in homeotherms, substantial T gradients exist between the inside, or "core" T (Tb), and body surface, or "shell," T, the surface being represented by the skin and underlying tissues. Only the former, usually estimated from colonic, abdominal, or esophageal measurements, is maintained within narrow limits, while the latter (Tskin) is subjected to wide variations. Tb may differ from the brain T (usually estimated from tympanic measurements) and, more precisely, from the T at the level of the thermoregulatory centers, because of the convective and evaporative heat exchange that may take place in the nasopharynx, especially during hyperthermia (Hunter and Adams, 1966). Although Tskin has wide regional variations, it is important to consider that (1) it determines to a great extent heat exchange with the environment, and (2) peripheral thermoreceptors located in the skin provide important input to the thermoregulatory centers (Prosser and Heath, 1991).

In steady-state conditions and for a large range of Tamb, the heat produced in the body (thermogenesis) is precisely balanced to the heat loss to the environment (thermolysis), so that Tb remains constant. The heat liberated during the metabolic conversion of chemical energy is dissipated into the environment by conduction, convection, radiation, and the evaporation of water from the skin and the respiratory tract.

During cold exposure, because of the increase in the gradient between Tskin and Tamb, thermolysis increases even though cutaneous vasoconstriction tends to decrease Tskin; thus, to maintain Tb, thermogenesis increases. This increase in metabolism is accompanied by a proportional augmentation in $\dot{V}E$. During heat exposure, thermolysis, represented by conduction, radiation, and convection, decreases because of the decrease in the gradient between Tskin and Tamb, even though cutaneous vasodilation tends to increase Tskin; eventually, when Tamb = Tskin, maintenance of Tb depends only on evaporation via the skin and the respiratory tract. In species with minimal or no sweating possibilities, the only way to evaporate water is through the respiratory tract; this is enhanced by increasing breathing rate, i.e., thermal polypnea or panting. It follows that $\dot{V}E$ is increased during both cold and heat exposures, in the former case because of the increased O_2 requirements for thermogenesis, in the latter to improve heat dissipation. Consequently, resting $\dot{V}E$ is expected to have a minimal value over a Tamb range close to thermoneutrality (Fig. 6).

The thermoregulatory system is unique among the major physiological functions in that it has, as effectors, no anatomically specialized structures, apart from the sweat glands. As a consequence, maintenance of a constant Tb requires the integration of many functions, including cardiorespiratory regulation and

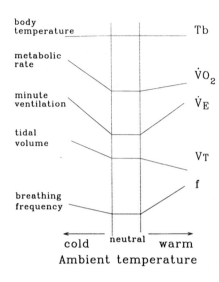

Figure 6 Schematic relationship between ambient temperature and body temperature (Tb), metabolic rate ($\dot{V}O_2$), minute ventilation ($\dot{V}E$), tidal volume (V_T), and breathing frequency (f). For modest drops or increases in Tamb (as assumed in this schema), Tb does not change. $\dot{V}O_2$ and $\dot{V}E$ have minimal values at thermoneutrality, and V_T increases and decreases, respectively, below and above thermoneutrality; f increases slightly with low Tamb, and markedly above thermoneutrality.

skeletal muscle control. The involvement of $\dot{V}E$ implies the existence of some constraints between thermoregulation and the regulation of the acid-base balance, particularly in conditions of hypoxia or hypercapnia.

A. Cold Exposure

Metabolic Rate

In endotherms exposed to cold, metabolism is increased. This increase is quite variable, from 2 to 5 times the minimal metabolic rate, and it depends on several factors such as the severity and duration of the cold exposure and the animal species, since smaller species, with larger body-surface-to-volume ratios, have relatively higher heat dispersion (Hemingway, 1963). This increase in metabolism is determined by combined nonshivering and shivering thermogenesis. Nonshivering thermogenesis can be defined as any heat-producing mechanism due to biochemical processes not involving muscular contractions (Jansky, 1973). Non-shivering thermogenesis is an effective means of heat production, particularly in neonates, including the human infant, and in adults after cold acclimation. Nonshivering thermogenesis is mostly based on the action of some mediators, particularly norepinephrine, on highly calorigenic tissues (brown fat tissues), and it is induced even by mild cold stimuli. Shivering thermogenesis, on the other hand, usually occurs with more severe cold stimuli, when Tb may begin to fall. In the rat, a very modest cold stress (Tamb = 20°C) increases $\dot{V}O_2$ by about 30% above the thermoneutral value, with no shivering. Shivering appears at lower Tamb, and at Tamb = 5°C metabolic rate is about 3 times greater than at 25°C

(Gautier et al., 1991). As a consequence, a significant relationship can be demonstrated between the intensity of shivering, as it can be quantified from electromyography, and heat production, calculated from $\dot{V}O_2$, in several animal species, such as rats (Gautier et al., 1991; Gautier and Bonora, 1992), cats (Gautier et al., 1989, 1992), and humans (Bell et al., 1992; Glickman et al., 1967). It should be remarked that, whereas in conscious animals exposed to cold the increase in thermogenesis matches the increase in thermolysis with no change in Tb, during anesthesia Tb decreases before thermogenesis is stimulated (Gautier et al., 1992), because the control of Tb is seriously impaired during anesthesia (Section IV.A).

Ventilatory Control

The great increase in metabolism observed during cold exposure is accompanied by an increase in $\dot{V}E$ in both humans (Glickman et al., 1967; Newstead, 1987) and animals (Gautier et al., 1992; Ingram and Legge, 1970; Kao and Schlig, 1956; Lim, 1960). This increase in $\dot{V}E$ results mainly from an increase in VT and to a lesser extent in f (Gautier et al., 1992; Horvath et al., 1956; Ingram and Legge, 1970; Lim, 1960). While in the pig $\dot{V}E$ increases less than the $\dot{V}O_2$ (Ingram and Legge, 1970), in other species such as rats (Gautier and Bonora, 1992; Saiki et al., 1994), cats (Gautier et al., 1992), dogs (Kao and Schlig, 1956; Lim, 1960), and humans (Glickman et al., 1967; Horvath et al., 1956; Newstead, 1987) $\dot{V}E$ increases approximately in proportion with metabolic rate. The same would occur in marsupial mammals (Hallam and Dawson, 1993). This indicates, as emphasized by Newstead (1987), that during cold exposure the regulation of breathing is precisely adjusted to the metabolic needs, not dissimilarly from what occurs during muscular exercise of moderate intensity.

It is well established that the control of thermoregulation results from an interaction between peripheral and central thermoreceptors with integration at the level of the hypothalamus (Simon et al., 1986). From recent studies, it appears that neural command signals from the hypothalamus are primarily responsible for the proportional driving of locomotion, respiration, and circulatory adjustments during exercise (Di Marco et al., 1983; Eldridge et al., 1985; Waldrop et al., 1986). Therefore, one could speculate the existence of some integrative mechanisms at the level of the hypothalamus, which, during cold exposure or muscular exercise, link the ventilatory and metabolic controls, with the result of no changes in arterial blood gases. This does not exclude the contribution to this regulation of peripheral inputs fine-tuning the ventilatory response, such as those from the muscles during exercise hyperventilation (Forster and Pan, 1991) or during cold-induced shivering (Euler, 1961).

Interaction with Hypoxia

It has been reported in many studies often carried out in young or small mammals (Gautier et al., 1989; Gautier and Bonora, 1992; Pedraz and Mortola, 1991; Wood,

1991) but also in humans (Blatteis and Lutherer, 1976) that hypoxia entails a decrease in the thermogenic response to cold exposure of even mild intensity (see also Section II.A). This is an inhibition of both shivering and nonshivering thermogenesis, accompanied by a lowering in Tb (Blatteis, 1972; Gautier et al., 1989, 1991, Pedraz and Mortola, 1991). Therefore, during cold exposure, hypoxia has two opposing effects on the control of $\dot{V}E$: a stimulatory effect via enhancement of the chemoreceptor input and a reduction in the respiratory drive linked to the decreased metabolic rate. In addition, the drop in Tb, not uncommon especially in newborns or small mammals, can have a direct effect on ventilatory control through the action on the respiratory centers (Section III.C).

Olson and Dempsey (1978) showed that, in adult rats studied at Tamb = 20–24°C, hypoxia ($F_{I_{O_2}}$ = 12–12.5%) induced a reduction of 25% in $\dot{V}_{O_2}$ and an increase in $\dot{V}E$ of only 12–20%. In a recent study also on adult rats, Gautier and Bonora (1992) have confirmed these results and extended the observations to various Tamb; at Tamb = 5°C, hypoxia ($F_{I_{O_2}}$ = 12%) induced a reduction of 25% in $\dot{V}_{O_2}$ and a 50% increase in $\dot{V}E$. If metabolic rate had not dropped, $\dot{V}E$ would have increased about 25% more, as was apparent from the $\dot{V}_{O_2}$-$\dot{V}E$ relationship constructed in normoxia at different Tamb.

The effects of hypoxia on the metabolic and ventilatory response to cold are not restricted to small or young mammals and have been observed in humans. For instance, in subjects exposed to a cold stress of 10°C for 3 hr, at high altitude the increase in $\dot{V}_{O_2}$ and $\dot{V}E$ was less than at sea-level (Blatteis and Lutherer, 1976).

The above results, globally considered, indicate the importance of metabolic adjustments in determining the $\dot{V}E$ response and fully support the remark by Olson and Dempsey (1978) that, during hypoxic exposure, the accompanying changes in metabolism introduce a potentially complex factor into the analysis of the ventilatory "drive."

It has been shown that many animal species including rodents, when exposed to hypoxia in a temperature gradient, select a cooler Tamb that accentuates the hypothermic effect of hypoxia (Wood, 1991; Gordon and Fogelson, 1991). This behavioral response suggests a lowering of the set point for thermoregulation during hypoxia, probably paralleled by a change in activity of the thermoregulatory neurons (Tamaki and Nakayama, 1987). A reduction in Tb during hypoxia may contribute to a reduction in the rate of enzymatic reaction and improves O_2 delivery by shifting to the left the hemoglobin dissociation curve.

Interaction with Hypercapnia

Several studies have dealt with the effects of CO_2 inhalation on Tb regulation, but very few have addressed the implications on $\dot{V}E$ control. In addition, there is no unanimous consensus about the effect of increased CO_2 on metabolic rate (Stupfel, 1974).

In small mammals exposed to cold, hypercapnia decreased $\dot{V}_{O_2}$ (for example, see Pepelko and Dixon, 1974). In larger mammals, such as dogs, ponies, and humans, hypercapnia ($F_{I_{CO_2}}$ up to 6%) at Tamb = 20–23°C resulted in a modest reduction in Tb and no changes or an increase in $\dot{V}_{O_2}$ (Jennings, 1979; Jennings and Laupacis, 1982; Kaminski et al., 1982). The increase in metabolism could represent a response to offset the increased respiratory heat loss of the hyperventilation. It could also be contributed by the cost of the hypercapnic hyperventilation; Pappenheimer (1977), however, argued that the increase in metabolism that he observed in rats during hypercapnia could not be caused by the increase in $\dot{V}_E$, because a similar hyperpnea during hypoxia was accompanied by a reduction in metabolic rate. In intubated dogs exposed to CO_2 at 2 or 18°C, it was shown that, whereas Tb was unchanged, metabolic rate increased more at 2°C than at 18°C, and in excess of the $\dot{V}_E$ response (Cain, 1971); it was suggested that the higher metabolic rate observed during hypercapnia in the cold was related to the increased shivering, whereas the hypoventilation in the cold presumably helped to conserve heat.

In humans in cold conditions (Tamb = 5°C) hypercapnia ($F_{I_{CO_2}}$ up to 6%) induced a decrease in Tb (Bullard and Crise, 1961; Wagner et al., 1983). In the study by Wagner et al. (1983) metabolism was found unchanged and hypothermia was attributed to the increase in respiratory evaporative heat loss of the hyperventilation. In contrast, in the study of Bullard and Crise (1961), the decrease in Tb was explained by a transient but marked decrease in metabolism and shivering. It was also found that CO_2 had a greater effect on $\dot{V}_E$ in the cold than at 30°C, in contrast to the above-mentioned results of Cain in dogs. Bullard and Crise (1961) have suggested that the effects of CO_2 on shivering and metabolism could result from a lowering of the threshold of the "cold-protection regulating centers" of the posterior hypothalamus. This seems supported by the finding that CO_2 increases the activity of warm-sensitive preoptic neurons, which decrease Tb (Tamaki and Nakayama, 1987).

In cats in a cold environment (Tamb = 5°C) hypercapnia ($F_{I_{CO_2}}$ = 3%) in normoxia had no effects on the thermoregulatory processes, while in hypoxia it counteracted the inhibitory effect of low O_2 on shivering and metabolism (Gautier et al., 1989).

In summary, the available information on the metabolic effect of CO_2 is much less abundant than that of hypoxia, and the results are rather mixed, especially with respect to the interaction with Tamb. Some of the data seem to suggest that in a warm environment CO_2 tends to increase $\dot{V}_{O_2}$, while the opposite may occur in cold conditions; across species, the smallest mammals may be more prone to a drop in $\dot{V}_{O_2}$ during hypercapnia. Hence, one may speculate that the effects of CO_2 on metabolic rate depend on the resting $\dot{V}_{O_2}$ of the animal, perhaps along a pattern similar to that discussed for hypoxia (Section II.A.). Despite the paucity of information, it seems appropriate to emphasize that a metabolic change during hypercapnia is a realistic possibility and must therefore be taken into account in the interpretation of the $\dot{V}E$ response to CO_2 (Pappenheimer, 1977).

Interaction with Muscle Exercise

The interaction between cold and muscular exercise upon metabolism and ventilatory control is of interest because both stimuli (thermal and exercise) influence $\dot{V}E$ markedly.

In humans studied between 5 and 28°C Tamb, at low level of exercise intensity metabolism was higher in the cold than in warm conditions (Lange Andersen et al., 1963). However, at high levels of work (above 300 kg × m/min), metabolic rate was not affected by Tamb, and the increase in Tb was similar by the end of the exercise. It was concluded that the heat generated during strenuous muscle exercise is sufficient to compensate for the heat loss in the cold. These results were confirmed in another study of the cost of muscle exercise in air at 25–27°C or in water at 18, 25, and 33°C (McArdle and al. 1976); during submaximal work, the metabolic rate was significantly greater in water at 18 and 25°C than in water at 33°C or in warm air, whereas, with heavier loads, the values of metabolic rate were the same. The increase in metabolic rate was accompanied by a proportional increase in $\dot{V}E$, along a relationship that was unaffected by Tamb. In addition, Newstead (1987) reported that the metabolism-$\dot{V}E$ relationship remained constant whether the increase in $\dot{V}O_2$ was due to shivering alone or to a combination of shivering and exercise.

It is of interest to examine the effect of hypoxia on the interaction between Tb regulation and gas exchange in exercise. In human subjects exercising at Tamb = 22°C, both $\dot{V}O_2$ and Tb attained similar values whether the exercise was performed at sea level or at simulated altitudes of 2000 and 4000 m, whereas, as expected, $\dot{V}E$ was greater at altitude (Greenleaf et al., 1969). Another recent study confirmed that, at Tamb = 25°C, Tb increased to the same level during an exercise performed in normoxia or in hypoxia ($FI_{O_2} = 12\%$) (Robinson and Haynes, 1990), although the metabolic rate was, perhaps surprisingly (see Section II.A), substantially lower in hypoxia than in normoxia; however, when the same exercise was performed at Tamb = 8°C, Tb was significantly lower in hypoxia than in normoxia.

In conclusion, it seems that the mechanisms integrating thermoregulation and exercise are not very sensitive to a drop in O_2 availability at thermoneutrality; on the other hand, during exercise in the cold, hypoxia appears to hinder thermoregulation, not dissimilarly from what was discussed above during resting conditions (Section III.A).

B. Heat Exposure

Most terrestrial vertebrates can lose heat by evaporating water (latent heat of vaporization, approximately 0.58 kcal/g at 35°C). Total evaporation heat loss can be expressed as the sum of the water losses from (1) the respiratory tract, influenced by $\dot{V}_E$, (2) transudation through the skin, and (3) active sweating. In birds and many mammals, which, differently from humans, do not have sweat glands, heat dissipation during exposure to high Tamb or exercise depends largely on evaporation from the respiratory tract. The evaporative loss from the respiratory tract is proportional to $\dot{V}_E$ and the difference in saturation density of expired and inspired gases.

Ventilatory Response

During heat exposure or during experimentally induced increase in Tb, the respiratory activity is markedly changed and the pattern of breathing consists generally in a large increase in f, while V_T is reduced. This particular pattern of breathing is often referred to as thermal polypnea or panting even though these terms are not clearly defined in the literature. Even in species that do not pant, but rely more on sweating than on respiratory evaporative heat loss (such as human or horse), $\dot{V}_E$ is in excess of metabolic needs.

During severe heat stress or when humidity in the ambient air is increased, thereby limiting heat loss from evaporation, the breathing pattern can eventually become slow and deep, i.e., opposite to the common response to modest heat stress (reviewed in Richards, 1970). Therefore, the relative changes in V_T, f, and $\dot{V}_E$ depend greatly on the severity and duration of heat stress; in addition, variability exists among species and can be introduced by the preparation under study. Anesthesia influences the $\dot{V}_E$ response to heat, and tracheostomy, often adopted in anesthetized preparations, deprives the animal of the upper airway control of heat and water balance.

Although a large component of the increased $\dot{V}_E$ during panting is almost entirely restricted to the dead space, an increase in $\dot{V}_A$ with consequent hypocapnia and respiratory alkalosis often occurs under conditions of heat stress. Then, a conflict may arise between the needs of maintaining an acceptable acid-base equilibrium and those of losing sufficient heat to preserve thermal homeostasis.

Several factors can contribute to the increase in $\dot{V}_{O_2}$ during heat exposure. Crawford (1962) has shown that, at least in the dog, panting frequency corresponds closely to the resonant frequency of the respiratory system, where the muscle force required for $\dot{V}_E$ is least, as discussed by Richards (1970). However, the increased respiratory work of the hyperventilation may eventually equal the heat dissipated during panting, possibly rendering panting ineffective in maintaining Tb constant. The increase in Tb can raise metabolic rate via the Q_{10} effect, approximately a 10% increase in metabolism for each 1°C increase in Tb. Other factors influencing metabolic rate during heat exposure have been proposed and are discussed by Richards (1970).

Panting

As for the control of the thermogenic response to cold, there is much evidence that panting is controlled by the activity of central thermoreceptors located in the hypothalamus and peripheral thermoreceptors in the skin (Simon et al., 1986). The former would be sensitive to blood temperature whereas the latter would respond to changes in Tamb and could activate panting before changes in blood T. The relative contribution of the central versus the peripheral components in the control of the respiratory response to heat has been the subject of many studies, with somewhat different results, partly because of differences in species and preparations used. For example, as already noticed in the last century, the conscious dog pants in the sun before any rise in Tb, whereas in the anesthetized animal, an appreciable increase in Tb is necessary to evoke panting because peripheral sensitivity has been reduced by anesthesia (Richards, 1970).

The genesis of the polypneic breathing has been investigated in many studies using unanesthetized animals. Pitts et al. (1939) produced polypnea in the cat by a high decerebration sparing the larger part of the hypothalamus. The same ventilatory pattern was also observed by Euler et al. (1970) and by Tenney and Ou (1977). Pitts et al. also noted that accessory movements of the tongue, nose, and jaws after high decerebration were similar to those observed during heat exposure. Polypnea after decortication could be reinforced by heating, but continued even at subnormal Tb. Furthermore, polypnea could not be obtained after transection of the midbrain, and Pitts et al. (1939), as well as Tenney and Ou (1977), concluded that some higher, hypothalamic structures must exert an accelerating influence on the brainstem respiratory centers. Finally, Tenney and Ou (1977) suggested that, normally, a tonic descending cortical inhibitory influence must operate on the diencephalon. The polypneic breathing of hypothalamic origin, in the absence of heat stress, has been observed in other situations. For example, Cohen (1964) has shown in the curarized and vagotomized cat that hyperventilation and the resulting hypocapnia induced a marked increase in the phrenic output (hypocapnic polypnea), which was enhanced after section through the anterior hypothalamus and eliminated by a midbrain section. Tachypneic breathing has been also observed in conscious carotid-body-denervated animals breathing hypoxic gases (Miller and Tenney, 1975), as well as in intact conscious cats during inhalation of small concentrations of CO, which does not significantly stimulate the carotid chemoreceptors (Gautier and Bonora, 1983). This hypoxic tachypnea was not observed after midcollicular decerebration. Therefore, it can be concluded that diencephalic or higher midbrain structures exert a tonic facilitatory influence on respiratory frequency, which is released from inhibition after removal of much of the forebrain or which can be evoked in the intact animal by central hypoxia, hypocapnia, or heat stress.

Interestingly, these different forms of rapid, shallow breathing have in common the fact that (1) they are almost exclusively observed in the un-anesthetized preparation, and (2) they can be markedly reduced by inhalation of moderate concentrations of CO_2, as will be discussed below.

Even though it is generally admitted that breathing is markedly controlled by the vagal activity, there are several observations showing that panting is largely unaffected by the section of the vagus nerves (Euler et al., 1970; Richards, 1970). This confirms the observations of Hammouda (1933) showing that, in the dog, the classical arrest of breathing during lung inflation (Breuer-Hering inspiratory inhibitory reflex) was absent during hyperthermic panting, indicating that, during hyperthermia, the central control of respiratory activity overrides the vagal peripheral control.

Interaction with Hypoxia

The effects of hypoxia on panting are less striking than the effects of hypercapnia. In anesthetized preparations, hypoxia seems to reduce f during thermal polypnea in dogs (Ruiz, 1973) and cats (Folgering, 1983). In agreement with these results, it has been found that pharmacological stimulation of arterial chemoreceptors with cyanide reduced panting in anesthetized dogs (Ruiz, 1975) and in conscious cats (Bonora and Gautier, 1990). However, in conscious noninstrumented cats, hypoxia clearly facilitated thermal panting; interestingly, this was also the case in carotid-denervated cats (Bonora and Gautier, 1989), which indicates that the facilitatory effects of hypoxia are centrally mediated. Furthermore, the comparison of the results obtained in intact and carotid-denervated cats in normoxia suggests that the latter were more sensitive to heat stress (Bonora and Gautier, 1989). This confirms the observations of Hales et al. (1975) in conscious sheep of a tendency for the maximal rapid, shallow breathing to occur sooner and at a lower degree of hyperthermia in the denervated than in the intact animal. Likewise, Folgering (1983) showed in anesthetized cats that severing of the carotid sinus nerves enhanced panting.

It follows that hypoxia seems to have two opposing effects on the control of thermal polypnea, a peripheral inhibitory component mediated by the arterial chemoreceptors, which can also operate during hypercapnia (Section III.B), and a central facilitatory component. The fact that the latter is very sensitive to anesthesia explains why the results concerning the effects of hypoxia on panting in intact conscious animals are different from those obtained in the anesthetized preparations.

Interaction with Hypercapnia

Thermal polypnea can be markedly reduced following inhalation of moderate concentrations of CO_2; this increases V_T and is accompanied by a marked reduction in f, with variable effects on $\dot{V}_E$ (Maskrey and Nicol, 1979; Maskrey et al., 1981). It may be suggested that this shift toward a greater V_T and lower f results from the removal of the "hypocapnic drive," which stimulates shallow and rapid breathing (Cohen, 1964; Miller and Tenney, 1975), as mentioned above (Section III.B).

Several nonexclusive hypotheses can be advanced as mechanisms mediating the changes in breathing pattern during CO_2 inhalation. For instance, the stimulating effect of CO_2 on the arterial chemoreceptors may be suggested, as it has been shown that pharmacological stimulation of these chemoreceptors is followed by a marked inhibition of panting in the cat (Bonora and Gautier, 1990). However, this mechanism cannot account for the reduction of hypoxic tachypnea, since it is observed in carotid denervated cats (Miller and Tenney, 1975). Apart from its action on the arterial chemoreceptors, it has been shown that CO_2 may also affect respiratory output during thermal panting through the stimulation of central chemoreceptors (See, 1984). The possible role of upper airways CO_2 sensory mechanism in the CO_2 attenuation of thermal tachypnea has been addressed, but it does not seem critical (Forster et al., 1985).

Another interesting hypothesis dealing with the inhibitory effects of CO_2 inhalation during heat or hypoxic tachypnea concerns the probable change in brain oxygenation. Indeed, it has been shown that, in the conscious sheep under heat stress, brain blood flow is reduced to about 70% of the control value (Hales, 1973). On the other hand, it is well known that cerebral blood flow is very dependent on the CO_2 level and the sensitivity to P_{CO_2} also increases with increasing T_b (Colton and Frankel, 1972). Therefore, administration of CO_2 during thermal tachypnea, by compensating the hypocapnia, is expected to increase cerebral perfusion and improve brain oxygenation. This mechanism may also apply to the CO_2 attenuation of the hypoxic tachypnea. The increased blood flow with CO_2 administration probably alters brain temperature (Hayward and Baker, 1968), which would by itself alter the activity of the central thermoreceptors. This effect, in addition to the sensitivity of the diencephalic thermoreceptors to CO_2 (Tamaki and Nakayama, 1987), may result in the decrease of panting during CO_2 inhalation.

Interaction with Muscular Exercise

During muscular exercise in a warm environment, $\dot{V}_E$ increases not only to satisfy the higher metabolic demands but also to increase the respiratory evaporative heat loss. Indeed, during a heavy or a prolonged exercise, even in a thermoneutral environment, T_b has been shown to increase, and the role of this rise as a contributing factor to the hyperventilation during prolonged exercise has been discussed (Forster and Pan, 1991).

In human subjects $\dot{V}_E$ increased more than metabolism in warm as compared to the thermoneutral environment and was accompanied by higher T_b

(Rowell et al., 1969; MacDougall et al., 1974). The increase in $\dot{V}E$ observed in hyperthermia can be attributed to several factors, such as the direct effect of higher Tb, the greater increase in blood lactate concentration, and, possibly, the thermally induced increased sensitivity to humoral stimuli (Section III.C). Finally, it should be noticed that, because during exercise, at any given $\dot{V}E$, VT was lower and f was higher in hyperthermia than in normothermia (Martin et al., 1979), the differences in $\dot{V}A$ between normothermia and hyperthermia may be less than apparent from the $\dot{V}E$ data.

C. Changes in Body Temperature

In the preceding sections (III.A and III.B), we have presented results about the ventilatory effects of changes in Tamb, with minimal or no changes in Tb; $\dot{V}E$ increased in both cold and warm environments, mostly because of, respectively, the increase in thermogenesis and the increase in thermolysis, and exposures to hypoxia or hypercapnia could significantly modify the ventilatory responses to changes in Tamb.

On the other hand, the study of the interaction between thermal and ventilatory control, and the effects upon it of the respiratory gases, can also be approached by artificial changes in Tb. This approach has most often been adopted on animal models under anesthesia, and extrapolation of the results to the conscious animal needs careful consideration.

Clark and von Euler (1972) have demonstrated in the anesthetized cat an inverse relationship between the duration of inspiration (TI) and VT during various respiratory stimulations. This dependency of TI on VT was referred to as the Breuer-Hering inspiratory threshold curve, since, after bilateral vagotomy, it was drastically changed, with TI being almost constant and independent of VT. Because TI was also found to be directly proportional to the expiratory time, any increase in VT had to be accompanied by an increase in f.

In anesthetized animals, increases in Tb well below the panting threshold shifted the TI-VT relationship toward lower values of TI, in such a way that a smaller VT was required to reach the Breuer-Hering inspiratory threshold and terminate inspiration (Grunstein et al., 1973; Bradley et al., 1974; Widdicombe and Winning, 1974). It was later suggested that mean inspiratory flow (VT/TI), presumably a reflection of the rate of buildup of central inspiratory activity, was increased during hyperthermia; hence, the combination of these two factors, the change in inhibitory threshold and the increase in VT/TI, would explain why TI was shortened by hyperthermia with only small effects on VT (Euler et al., 1976; Trippenbach and Milic-Emili, 1977). The expiratory duration was also markedly reduced during increases in Tb, hence contributing to the hyperthermic tachypnea (Euler and Trippenbach, 1976). Some effects of hyperthermia on pulmonary stretch receptors have been reported (Schoener and Frankel, 1972). However, because the changes in breathing pattern accompanying the increase in Tb persisted after vagotomy, they were attributed to inputs from the hypothalamic structures impinging on the brainstem mechanisms controlling ventilation.

In 1966, Hey et al., studying the effects of various respiratory stimuli on breathing in human subjects, described a linear relationship between $\dot{V}_E$ and V_T. The relationship was essentially unaltered by wide variations in PA_{CO_2}, PA_{O_2}, metabolic acidemia, and moderate muscular exercise; however, the effect of experimentally raising Tb was to increase the slope of the relationship; i.e., for a given $\dot{V}_E$, the pattern was more rapid and shallow during hyperthermia.

These results have been confirmed and extended by further measurements in humans. It has been shown that during induced hyperthermia, the $\dot{V}_E$ response to hypercapnia (Vejby-Christensen and Petersen, 1973) and to hypoxia (Petersen and Vejby-Christensen, 1977) was increased. In both studies, the increased responsiveness to these stimuli resulted from an increase in f.

In cats anesthetized with barbiturate or chloralose-urethan, the $\dot{V}_E$ response to CO_2 has been studied with Tb ranging between 33 and 41°C. Despite the large range in Tb explored, no shivering or panting was observed (Euler et al., 1970; Widdicombe and Winning, 1974), confirming that anesthesia seriously impairs the control of Tb. Two studies reported that, when Tb was raised, the $\dot{V}_E$ response to CO_2 was increased, mainly because of the augmentation in f (Euler et al., 1970; Widdicombe and Winning, 1974). However, another study showed no significant change in the responsiveness to CO_2 when Tb was changed (Olievier et al., 1982). It confirmed previous observations (Euler et al., 1970; Widdicombe and Winning, 1974) that Tb-induced changes in f persist after vagotomy, whereas they are abolished by midcollicular decerebration.

In conscious animals, experimental changes in Tb induce thermoregulatory responses reminiscent of those observed with changes in Tamb (Sections III.A and III.B). In conscious rats, Tb was changed by means of a heat exchange device implanted in the abdomen (Maskrey, 1990). It was found that the $\dot{V}_E$ response to hypoxia was not modified when Tb was raised from 38 to 41°C, while $\dot{V}_E$ was markedly reduced during hypoxia when Tb was decreased from 38 to 35°C. This was likely due to the inhibition of thermogenesis caused by hypoxia, as described in the previous sections. The $\dot{V}_E$ response to hypercapnia was slightly elevated in hyperthermia, whereas it was depressed by hypothermia, possibly because of the changes in thermogenesis caused by hypercapnia.

D. Fever

Fever may be defined as a controlled elevation of Tb above the normal range, resulting from an upward reset of the hypothalamic set point. It comprises several phases, often defined as febrile rise, flush, and defervescence, and the ventilatory control is expected to participate in several ways during these phases. For instance, during the febrile rise or chill, heat production increases and should be associated with an increase in $\dot{V}E$. During this phase, especially in a warm environment, a decrease in heat loss may also be expected. During the defervescence period, when thermolysis increases, $\dot{V}E$ is expected to participate, with sweating, to the evaporative heat loss.

To our knowledge, very little information is available on the $\dot{V}E$ response and its interaction with changes in metabolic rate during the various phases of fever, whether on humans or animal models (Dubois, 1948). In experimentally induced fever, the metabolic rate is increased by 25–40% over control, with a maximum observed during the chill or the flush period (Altschule et al., 1945; Cander and Hanowell, 1963; Moser et al., 1963; Malkinson et al., 1988; Cooper et al., 1992; Fewell, 1992; Suffredini et al., 1992). During the defervescence period, the metabolic rate seems to remain slightly elevated. From two studies in human subjects, it appears that $\dot{V}E$ was increased by about 30–40% during the chill phase and remained slightly elevated during the defervescence period. The increase in $\dot{V}E$ was mostly caused by an increase in VT during the chill phase whereas, during the defervescence period, f remained elevated (Cander and Hanowell, 1963; Moser et al., 1963). The data of a recent study in human subjects also suggested that $\dot{V}E$ increases markedly during fever induced by endotoxin administered intravenously. Three hours after the injection, metabolic rate increased by 30% and was accompanied by modest hypocapnia (Suffredini et al., 1992).

In anesthetized rats (Malkinson et al., 1988), f increased during centrally administered prostaglandin E1; on the other hand, in rabbits (Szelenyi and Szekely, 1979) the onset of pyrogen-induced fever was accompanied by a marked fall in f. It should be noticed that in the rabbit f was very high before the pyrogen injection, as it is often the case in this species. Hence, perhaps, the reduction in f with fever in the rabbit could be interpreted as a decrease in heat loss. In the lamb, Fewell (1992) has shown that PaO_2 was not significantly changed whereas the metabolic rate was increased by about 26% following injection of pyrogen. The study also demonstrated that carotid denervation eliminated the febrile and the metabolic response to the injection of the pyrogen.

IV. Special Cases

A. Anesthesia

Several excellent reviews have summarized the literature dealing with the effects of anesthesia on ventilatory control (Hickey and Severinghaus, 1981; Pavlin and Horbein, 1986). With respect to the present topics only a few aspects will be emphasized.

The effects of anesthesia on breathing can be quite variable. Apart from differences related to species, type of anesthesia, and dosage on neuronal activity, anesthesia induces many secondary effects, which, in turn, may impinge directly or indirectly on the generation of respiratory output. For example, (1) the loss of consciousness, which is the goal of the anesthetic procedure, is itself associated with changes in respiratory activity, not too dissimilarly from natural sleep. Hence, the changes in breathing pattern observed during anesthesia can reflect a balance between the withdrawal of the wakefulness stimulus and the specific effects of the drug on the brainstem and higher centers, but a quantitative separation between these two components is difficult to achieve. (2) Anesthesia can affect gas exchange by interfering with lung and chest wall mechanics, the coordinated activity of the respiratory muscles, and the ventilation-perfusion matching (Hedenstierna and Tokics, 1991); the consequent alterations in blood gases are expected to trigger compensatory reflexes. (3) Apart from the direct effect of the drug on the respiratory centers, anesthesia can markedly depress the peripheral and central chemosensitivity, with alteration of resting $\dot{V}E$ and its response to hypoxia and hypercapnia (Gautier, 1976). (4) Anesthesia introduces a significant decrease in metabolic rate and severely disrupts Tb regulation, as discussed in previous sections. For instance, during anesthesia the thresholds for vasoconstriction and shivering are decreased (Sessler, 1991); hence, thermogenesis is often depressed, and, depending on the effect on the control of the peripheral circulation, thermolysis is increased. Without external heating, the anesthetized animal in a moderate or cool environment usually presents severe hypothermia, with Tb possibly below 30°C. Under these circumstances, severe hypopnea can be observed, mostly because of a major decrease in f (Kiley et al., 1984; Gautier and Gaudy, 1986). Because the drop in $\dot{V}E$ often exceeds the drop in metabolic rate, it contributes to the hypoxemia and acidemia. Likewise, the sensitivity to CO_2 and hypoxia are markedly depressed (Natsui, 1969).

The changes on respiratory activity and its control introduced by anesthesia often appear to be even larger than expected on the basis of the factors listed above. Indeed, anesthesia is thought to have a direct effect also on the neurons involved in the generation of respiratory rhythmicity. Although there is an abundant literature describing the effects of anesthesia on the depth, rate, and pattern of each breath in various animal species, we have a very limited understanding of how each drug acts on the respiratory centers. Inhalational anaesthetics usually reduce $\dot{V}E$ and increase f. These changes in the pattern of breathing are probably mediated at a suprapontine level as they are markedly attenuated after midcollicular decerebration in the cat (Gautier et al., 1987b). Several agents administered intravenously, like barbiturates, in humans also reduce VT and increase f, whereas in the cat VT is only slightly depressed and f is markedly reduced (Gautier and Gaudy, 1978). Narcotics usually induce a marked depression of $\dot{V}E$ in humans mainly because of a decrease in f (Pavlin and Horbein, 1986).

In conclusion, although we are far from a complete understanding of the various mechanisms and their interplay, there is overwhelming evidence that anesthesia has profound effects on thermoregulation, ventilatory control, and their interaction. Because even the qualitative aspects of these effects are difficult to predict, extrapolation to the conscious intact animal of results on ventilatory control obtained in the anesthetized preparation is an exercise of optimism that can lead to erroneous conclusions.

B. Sleep

Three major physiological changes associated with sleep state have potential consequences on the regulation of breathing: (1) withdrawal of the wakefulness stimulus, (2) changes in metabolic rate, and (3) changes in Tb and thermoregulation, by a magnitude that depends on circadian influences. Interactions between metabolic rate, Tb, and $\dot{V}E$ are not easy to demonstrate during sleep because the changes observed in these functions are relatively small and sleep is not a unitary phenomenon (see Chapter 22).

At the onset of slow-wave sleep, a fall in Tb is observed. This is associated with a fall in metabolism of about 10% with respect to the relaxed wakefulness (Haskell et al., 1981; Palca et al., 1985; White et al., 1985). The drop in $\dot{V}A$ exceeds the drop in $\dot{V}CO_2$ with a modest rise in $Paco_2$. The major mechanism responsible for the hypoventilation during slow-wave sleep is the removal of the wakefulness stimulus, which emphasizes, therefore, the importance of state-dependent neural stimuli in driving breathing, in addition to the metabolic input (Phillipson and Bowes, 1986).

In human subjects metabolism is higher in rapid eye movement (REM) than in non-REM sleep (Haskell et al., 1981; Palca et al., 1986; Shapiro et al., 1984). In contrast to the human data, metabolism in animals tends to be lower during REM sleep than during non-REM sleep (Glotzbach and Heller, 1989). The most probable explanation for the difference between humans and animals in the direction of the metabolic change between REM and non-REM sleep is that in humans brain metabolism is a large contributor to whole-body metabolic rate, and cerebral blood flow and brain metabolism increase during REM sleep (Glotzbach and Heller, 1989).

Thermoregulatory responses are little affected during non-REM sleep, whereas they are markedly inhibited or absent during REM sleep. For example, during REM sleep shivering does not occur in a cool environment; heat loss mechanisms in warm conditions are also impaired, with a reduction of sweating or panting (Glotzbach and Heller, 1989; Parameggiani, 1990). Hence, non-REM sleep is a homeothermic state, whereas REM sleep tends to be a poikilothermic condition.

V. Conclusions

Probably the most general conclusion from the present overview is that metabolic rate in mammals is not a constant; on the contrary, it can substantially vary with temperature and respiratory gases. How metabolic rate is controlled and adjusted to the challenges is still unknown. In particular, the role of O_2 itself in controlling the speed of its own use is only beginning to be explored. Within this topic, the contribution of extramitochondrial O_2 and its potential implication in the regulation of metabolic rate deserve attention.

The notion that metabolism and ventilation participate together, both as dependent variables, in the control of thermogenesis, heat dissipation, tissue oxygenation, and acid-base control is of utmost importance for the understanding of the ventilatory pattern and its regulation; obviously, it implies that a correct interpretation of the ventilatory response is difficult without information about the metabolic condition.

The fact that $\dot{V}E$ accompanies the increase in metabolic rate during hypothermia is one more example of the coupling between these two variables in conditions of hypermetabolism, as it is well known to occur during exercise or with pharmacological stimulations of $\dot{V}O_2$. Hypoxia offers an interesting and less known example of this concept in the direction of hypometabolism and therefore represents an important extension of the relationship between metabolism and $\dot{V}E$. Hence, the metabolic-ventilatory response to hypoxia raises again the familiar question of the role of endogenously produced CO_2 in maintaining and regulating $\dot{V}E$. This is the same question that has long intrigued physiologists interested in the control of $\dot{V}E$ during muscle exercise, and its emergence from other areas of metabolic regulation suggests that it is probably the fundamental question at the core of respiratory control.

VI. Glossary of Terms and Units

a	arterial
A	alveolar
CO_2	carbon dioxide, mlSTPD
f	breathing frequency, breaths/min
FI_{O_2}	inspired fractional O_2 concentration
FI_{CO_2}	inspired fractional CO_2 concentration
O_2	oxygen, mlSTPD
Pb	barometric pressure, mmHg
PCO_2	partial pressure of CO_2, mmHg
PO_2	partial pressure of O_2, mmHg
Tamb	ambient temperature, °C
Tb	body temperature, °C
Tskin	skin temperature, °C
$\dot{V}A$	alveolar ventilation, mlBTPS/min
VD	dead space volume, mlBTPS

$\dot{V}_E$ minute ventilation, mlBTPS/min
$\dot{V}_{CO_2}$ carbon dioxide production, mlSTPD/min
$\dot{V}_{O_2}$ oxygen consumption, mlSTPD/min
V_T tidal volume, mlBTPS

Ectothermy: raise of Tb by external heat.
Endothermy: raise of Tb by internally produced heat.
Gaseous metabolism: $\dot{V}_{O_2}$ and $\dot{V}_{CO_2}$
Homeothermy: regulation of Tb around a constant value.
Hyper-, hypopnea: respectively, an increase and decrease of the absolute value of $\dot{V}_E$.
Hyper-, hypoventilation: respectively, an increase and decrease of $\dot{V}_E$ relative to $\dot{V}_{CO_2}$, irrespective of their absolute values.
Metabolism*:   cellular mechanisms consuming substrates and generating by-products in the process of creating chemically stored energy.
Poikilothermy: conformism of Tb to Tamb.
Respiration: processes governing transfer of respiratory gases between cells and environment in the process of creating chemically stored energy.
Thermoneutrality: range of Tamb over which Tb is maintained constant with minimal values of $\dot{V}_{O_2}$ during normoxia.

References

Acheson GH, Dawes GS, Mott JC. Oxygen consumption and the arterial oxygen saturation in foetal and new-born lambs. J Physiol (Lond) 1957; 135:623–642.

Acker H. Oxygen Sensing in Tissues. Berlin: Springer-Verlag, 1988.

Adams RP, Cain SM. Total and hindlimb oxygen deficit and "repayment" in hypoxic anesthetized dogs. J. Apppl Physiol 1983; 55:913–922.

Adamsons K Jr. Breathing and the thermal environment in young rabbits. J Physiol (Lond) 1959; 149:144–153.

Adolph EF, Hoy PA. Ventilation of lungs in infant and adult rats and its responses to hypoxia. J Appl Physiol 1960; 15:1075–1986.

Ahmed M, Giesbrecht GG, Serrette C, Georgopoulos D, Anthonisen NR. Ventilatory response to hypoxia in elderly humans. Respir Physiol 1991; 83:343–352.

Alexander G, Williams D. Summit metabolism and cardiovascular function in young lambs during hyperoxia and hypoxia. J Physiol (Lond) 1970; 208:85–97.

Alpert NR. Lactate production and removal and the regulation of metabolism. Ann NY Acad Sci 1965; 119:995–1011.

---

*Because energy production is generally an aerobic process, the terms *metabolic rate* and *gaseous metabolism* (or *oxygen consumption*) are used interchangeably in most of the chapter.

Alpert NR, Kayne H, Haslett W. Relationship among recovery oxygen, oxygen missed, lactate production and lactate removal during and following severe hypoxia in the unanesthetized dog. Am J Physiol 1958; 192:585–591.

Altschule MD, Freedberg AS, McManus MJ. Circulation and respiration during an episode of chill and fever in man. J Clin Invest 1945; 24:878–889.

Alvaro R, Alvarez J, Kwiatkowski K, Cates D, Rigatto H. Small preterm infants ($\leqslant$1500 g) have only a sustained decrease in ventilation in response to hypoxia. Pediatr Res 1992; 32:403–406.

Anthonisen NR, Dhingra S. Ventilatory response to low levels of CO_2. Respir Physiol 1978; 32:335–344.

Barratt-Boyes BG, Wood EH. Cardiac output and related measurements and pressure values in the right heart and associated vessels, together with an analysis of the hemodynamic response to the inhalation of high oxygen mixtures in healthy subjects. J Lab Clin Med 1958; 51:72–90.

Baudinette RV, Gannon BJ, Ryall RG, Frappell PB. Changes in metabolic rate and blood respiratory characteristics during pouch development of a marsupial, *Macropus eugenii*. Respir Physiol 1988; 72:219–228.

Baum D, Anthony CL, Stowers C. Impairment of cold stimulated lipolysis by acute hypoxia. Am J Dis Child 1971; 121: 115–119.

Bell DG, Tikuisis P, and Jacobs I. Relative intensity of muscular contraction during shivering. J Appl Physiol 1992 72:2336–2342.

Biscoe TJ, Purves MJ. Carotid body chemoreceptor activity in the new-born lamb. J Physiol (Lond) 1967; 190:443–454.

Blanco CE, Dawes GS, Hanson MA, McCooke HB. The response to hypoxia of arterial chemoreceptors in fetal sheep and new-born lambs. J Physiol (Lond) 1984a; 351: 25–37.

Blanco CE, Hanson MA, Johnson P, Rigatto H. Breathing pattern of kittens during hypoxia. J Appl Physiol 1984b; 56:12–17.

Blatteis CM. Hypoxia and the metabolic response to cold in new-born rabbits. J Physiol (Lond) 1964; 172:358–368.

Blatteis CM. Thermogenic processes during cold in hypoxia. Fed Proc 1966; 25:1271–1274.

Blatteis CM. Shivering and nonshivering thermogenesis during hypoxia. In: Smith RE, ed. Proc. Intern. Symp. Environ. Physiol., Bioenergetics. Bethesda, MD. Federation American Societies Experimental Biology, 1972:151–160.

Blatteis CM, Lutherer LO. Effect of altitude exposure on thermoregulatory response of man to cold. J Appl Physiol 1976; 41:848–858.

Bloch K. Oxygen and biosynthetic patterns. Fed Proc 1962; 21:1058–1063.

Boggs DF, Tenney SM. Scaling respiratory pattern and respiratory "drive." Respir Physiol 1984; 58:245–251.

Boggs DF, Kilgore DL, Birchard GF. Respiratory physiology of burrowing mammals and birds. Comp Biochem Physiol 1984; 77A:1–7.

Bonora M, Gautier H. Maturational changes in body temperature and ventilation during hypoxia in kittens. Respir Physiol 1987; 68:359–370.

Bonora M, Gautier H. Effects of hypoxia on thermal polypnea in intact and carotid body-denervated conscious cats. J Appl Physiol 1989; 67:578–583.

Bonora M, Gautier H. Role of dopamine and arterial chemoreceptors in thermal tachypnea in conscious cats. J Appl Physiol 1990; 69:1429–1434.

Bonora M, Marlot D, Gautier H, Duron B. Effects of hypoxia on ventilation during postnatal development in conscious kittens. J Appl Physiol 1984; 56:1464–1471.

Bonora M, Boule M, Gautier H. Diaphragmatic and ventilatory responses to alveolar hypoxia and hypercapnia in conscious kittens. J Appl Physiol 1992; 72:203–210.

Bradley GW, Euler C von, Martilla I, Roos B. Steady state effects of CO_2 and temperature on the relationship between lung volume and inspiratory duration (Hering-Breuer threshold curve). Acta Physiol Scand 1974; 92:351–363.

Brady JP, Ceruti E. Chemoreceptor reflexes in the newborn infant: effects of varying degrees of hypoxia on heart rate and ventilation in a warm environment. J Physiol (Lond) 1966; 184:631–645.

Brady JP, Cotton EC, Tooley WH. Chemoreflexes in the new-born infant: effects of 100% oxygen on heart rate and ventilation. J Physiol (Lond) 1964; 172:332–341.

Brodie HR, Cross KW, Lomer TR. Heat production in new-born infants under normal and hypoxic conditions. J Physiol (Lond) 1957; 138:156–163.

Brown DR, Forster HV, Lowry TF, Forster MA, Forster AL, Gutting SM, Erickson BK, Pan LG. Effect of chronic hypoxia on breathing and EMGs of respiratory muscles in awake ponies. J Appl Physiol 1992; 72:739–747.

Bullard RW, Crise JR. Effects of carbon dioxide on cold exposed human subjects. J Appl Physiol 1961; 16:663–638.

Bullard RW, Kollias J. Functional characteristics of two high-altitude mammals. Fed Proc 1966; 25:1288–1292.

Bureau MA, Zinman R, Foulon P, Begin R. Diphasic ventilatory response to hypoxia in newborn lambs. J Appl Physiol 1984; 56:84–90.

Bureau MA, Lamarche J, Foulon P, Dalle D. The ventilatory response to hypoxia in the newborn lamb after carotid body denervation. Respir Physiol 1985; 60:109–119.

Bureau MA, Côte A, Blanchard PW, Hobbs S, Foulon P, Dalle D. Exponential and diphasic ventilatory response to hypoxia in conscious lambs. J Appl Physiol 1986; 61:836–842.

Burggren W, Roberts J. Respiration and metabolism. In: Prosser CL, ed., Environmental and Metabolic Animal Physiology. New York: Wiley-Liss, 1991:353–435.

Cain SM. Ventilatory and metabolic responses of unanesthetized dogs to CO_2 at 2 and 18°C. J Appl Physiol 1971; 31:647–650.

Cain SM. Oxygen delivery and uptake in dogs during anemic and hypoxic hypoxia. J Appl Physiol 1977; 42:228–234.

Cain SM. Supply dependency of oxygen uptake in ARDS: myth or reality? Am J Med Sci 1984; 288:119–124.

Cain SM. Gas exchange in hypoxia, apnea, and hyperoxia. In: Farhi LE, Tenney SM, eds. Handbook of Physiology, vol 4, Gas Exchange, Bethesda, MD: American Physiological Society, 1987: 403–420.

Cander L, Hanowell EG. Effects of fever on pulmonary diffusing capacity and pulmonary mechanics in man. J Appl Physiol 1963; 18:1065–1070.

Cao K-J, Zwillich CW, Berthon-Jones M, Sullivan CE. Ventilatory response to sustained eucapnic hypoxia in the adult conscious dog. Respir Physiol 1992; 89:65–73.

Cerretelli P, Di Prampero PE. Gas exchange in exercise. In: Farhi LE, Tenney SM, eds. Handbook of Physiology, Section 3, Respiration, vol 4, Gas Exchange. Bethesda, MD: American Physiological Society, 1987: 297–339.

Chapler CK, Cain SM, Stainsby WN. The effects of hyeroxia on oxygen uptake during acute anemia. Can J Physiol Pharmacol 1984; 62:809–814.

Clark FJ, Euler C von. On the regulation of depth and rate of breathing . J Physiol (Lond) 1972; 222:267–295.

Cohen MI. Respiratory periodicity in the paralyzed, vagotomized cat: hypocapnic polypnea. Am J Physiol 1964; 206:845–854.

Colton JS, Frankel HM. Cerebrovascular response to CO_2 during hyperthermia. Am J Physiol 1972; 223:1041–1043.

Consolazio CF, Nelson RA, Matoush L-RO, Hansen JE. Energy metabolism at high altitude (3,475 m). J Appl Physiol 1966; 21:1732–1740.

Cooper AL, Horan MA, Little RA, Rothwell NJ. Metabolic and febrile responses to typhoid vaccine in humans: effect of β-adrenergic blockade. J Appl Physiol 1992; 72:2322–2328.

Côté A, Yunis K, Blanchard PW, Mortola JP, Bureau MA. Dynamics of breathing in the hypoxic awake lamb. J Appl Physiol 1988; 64:354–359.

Crawford EC Jr. Mechanical aspects of panting in dogs. J Appl Physiol 1962; 17:249–251.

Cross KW, Malcolm JL. Evidence of carotid body and sinus activity in new-born and foetal animals. J Physiol (Lond) 1952; 118:10P–11P.

Cross KW, Oppé TE. The effect of inhalation of high and low concentrations of oxygen on the respiration of the premature infant. J Physiol (Lond) 1952; 117:38–55.

Cross KW, Warner P. The effect of inhalation of high and low oxygen concentrations on the respiration of the newborn infant. J Physiol (Lond) 1951; 114:283–295.

Cross KW, Hooper JMD, Lord JM. Anoxic depression of the medulla in the new-born infant. J Physiol (Lond) 1954; 125:628–640.

Cross KW, Tizard, JPM, Trythall DAH. The gaseous metabolism of the newborn infant. Acta Paediatr 1957; 46:265–285.

Cross KW, Tizard JPM, Trythall DAH. The gaseous metabolism of the new-born infant breathing 15% oxygen. Acta Paediatr 1958; 47:217–237.

Cross KW, Dawes GS, Mott JC. Anoxia, oxygen consumption and cardiac output in newborn lambs and adult sheep. J Physiol (Lond) 1959; 146:316–343.

Cunningham DJC, Robbins PA, Wolff CB. Integration of respiratory responses to changes in alveolar partial pressures of CO_2 and O_2 and in arterial pH. In: Cherniack NS, Widdicombe JG, eds. Handbook of Physiology, section 3, Respiration. Bethesda, MD: American Physiological Society, 1986:475–528.

Davi M, Sankaran K, Rigatto H. Effect of inhaling 100% O_2 on ventilation and acid-base balance in cerebrospinal fluid of neonates. Biol Neonate 1980; 38:85–89.

Davis GM, Bureau MA, Gaultier C. The sustained ventilatory response to hypoxic challenge in the awake newborn piglet with an intact upper airway. Respir Physiol 1988; 71:307–314.

Dawes GS, Mott JC. The increase in oxygen consumption of the lamb after birth. J Physiol (Lond) 1959; 146:295–315.

Dawes GS, Jacobson HN, Mott JC, Shelley HJ. Some observations on foetal and new-born rhesus monkeys. J Physiol (Lond) 1960; 152:271–298.

Dawkins MJR, Hull D. Brown adipose tissue and the response of new-born rabbits to cold. J Physiol (Lond) 1964; 172:216–238.

Dawson TJ, Olson JM. The summit metabolism of the short-tailed shrew *Blarina brevicauda*: a high summit is further elevated by cold acclimation. Physiol Zool 1987; 60:631–639.

De Boeck C, Van Reempts P, Rigatto H, Chernick V. Naloxone reduces decrease in ventilation induced by hypoxia in newborn infants. J Appl Physiol 1984; 56:1507–1511.

Dempsey JA, Forster HV. Mediation of ventilatory adaptations. Physiol Rev 1982; 62: 262–346.

Dejours P. Intérêt méthodologique de l'étude d'un organisme vivant à la phase initiale de rupture d'un équilibre physiologique. C R Acad Sci (Paris) 1957; 245:1946–1948.

Dejours P. Principles of Comparative Respiratory Physiology. Amsterdam: North-Holland/American Elsevier, 1975.

Dejours P, Garey WF, Rahn H. Comparison of ventilatory and circulatory flow rates between animals in various physiological conditions. Respir Physiol 1970; 9:108–117.

Di Marco AF, Romaniuk JR, Euler C von, Yamamoto Y. Immediate changes in ventilation and respiratory pattern associated with onset and cessation of locomotion in the cat. J Physiol (Lond) 1983; 343:1–16.

Dotta A, Mortola JP. Effects of hyperoxia on the metabolic response to cold of the newborn rat. J Dev Physiol 1992; 17:247–250.

Dripps RD, Comroe JH Jr. The effect of the inhalation of high and low oxygen concentrations on respiration, pulse rate, ballistocardiogram and arterial oxygen saturation (oximeter) of normal individuals. Am J Physiol 1947; 149:277–291.

Dubois EF. Fever and the Regulation of Body Temperature. Springfield, IL: Charles C. Thomas, 1948:1–65.

Duling BR. Oxygen, metabolism, and microcirculatory control. In: Kaley G, Altura BM, eds. Microcirculation, vol. 2. Baltimore: University Park Press, 1978; 401–429.

Dupre RK, Romero AM, Wood SC. Thermoregulation and metabolism in hypoxic animals. In: Gonzales NC, Fedde MR, eds. Oxygen Transfer from Atmosphere to Tissues. New York: Plenum Press, 1988; 347–351.

Easton PA, Slykerman LJ, Anthonisen NR. Ventilatory response to sustained hypoxia in normal adults. J Appl Physiol 1986; 61:906–911.

Eden GJ, Hanson MA. Maturation of the respiratory response to acute hypoxia in the newborn rat. J Physiol (Lond) 1987; 392:1–9.

Eldridge FL, Milhorn DE, Kiley JP, Waldrop TG. Stimulation by central command of locomotion, respiration and circulation during exercise. Respir Physiol 1985; 59: 313–337.

Euler C von. Physiology and pharmacology of temperature regulation. Pharmacol Rev 1961; 13:361–398.

Euler C von, Söderberg U. Co-ordinated changes in temperature thresholds for thermoregulatory reflexes. Acta Physiol Scand 1958; 42:112–129.

Euler C von, Trippenbach T. Temperature effects on the inflation reflex during expiratory time in the cat. Acta Physiol Scand 1976; 96:338–350.

Euler C von, Herrero F, Wexler I. Control mechanisms determining rate and depth of respiratory movements. Respir Physiol 1970; 10:93–108.

Euler C von, Martilla I, Remmers JE, Trippenbach T. Effects of lesions in the parabrachial nucleus on the mechanisms for central and reflex termination of inspiration in the cat. Acta Physiol Scand 1976; 96:324–337.

Fahey JT, Lister G. Response to low cardiac output: developmental differences in metabolism during oxygen deficit and recovery in lambs. Pediatr Res 1989; 26:180–187.

Fanburg BL, Massaro DJ, Cerutti, PA, Gail DB, Berberich MA. Regulation of gene expression by O_2 tension (conference report). Am J Physiol 262 (Lung Cell Mol Physiol 6) 1992, L235–L241.

Fenn WO, Asano T. Effects of carbon dioxide inhalation on potassium liberation from the liver. Am J Physiol 1956; 185:567–576.

Fewell JE. Fever in young lambs: carotid denervation alters the febrile response to a small dose of bacterial pyrogen. Pediatr Res 1992; 31:107–111.

Fisher JT, Waldron MA, Armstrong CJ. Effects of hypoxia on lung mechanics in the newborn cat. Can J Physiol Pharmacol 1987; 65:1234–1238.

Folgering H. Adrenergic, cholinergic, and peripheral chemoreceptors effects on thermal panting in cats. In: Schläfke ME, Keopchen HP, See WR, eds. Central Neuron Environment. Berlin: Springer-Verlag, 1983; 82–87.

Forster HV, Pan LG. Exercise hyperpnea. Its characteristics and control. In: Crystal RG, West JB, eds. The Lung: Scientific Foundations. New York: Raven Press, 1991; 1553–1564.

Forster HV, Pan LG, Flynn C, Bisgard GE, Hoffer RE. Effect of upper airway CO_2 on breathing in awake ponies. J Appl Physiol 1985; 59:1222–1227.

Frappell P, Saiki C, Mortola JP. Metabolism during normoxia, hypoxia and recovery in the newborn kitten. Respir Physiol 1991; 86:115–124.

Frappell PB, Dotta A, Mortola JP. Metabolism during normoxia, hyperoxia, and recovery in newborn rats. Can J Physiol Pharmacol 1992a; 70: 408–411.

Frappell P, Lanthier C, Baudinette RV, Mortola JP. Metabolism and ventilation in acute hypoxia: a comparative analysis in small mammalian species. Am J Physiol 262 (Regul Integr Comp Physiol 31) 1992b, R1040–R1046.

Ganz W, Donoso R, Marcus H, Swan HJC. Coronary hemodynamics and myocardial oxygen metabolism during oxygen breathing in patients with and without coronary artery disease. Circulation 1972; 45:763–768.

Gautier H. Pattern of breathing during hypoxia or hypercapnia of the awake or anesthetized cat. Respir Physiol 1976; 27:193–206.

Gautier H, Bonora M. Ventilatory response of intact cats to carbon monoxide hypoxia. J Appl Physiol 1983; 55:1064–1071.

Gautier H, Bonora M. Ventilatory and metabolic responses to cold and hypoxia in intact and carotid body-denervated rats. J Appl Physiol 1992; 73:847–854.

Gautier H, Gaudy JH. Changes in ventilatory pattern induced by intravenous anesthetic agents in human subjects. J Appl Physiol 1978; 45:171–176.

Gautier H, Gaudy JH. Ventilatory recovery from hypothermia in anesthetized cats. Respir. Physiol. 1986; 64:329–337.

Gautier H, Bonora M, Gaudy JH. Ventilatory response of the conscious or anesthetized cat to oxygen breathing. Respir Physiol 1986; 65:181–196.

Gautier H, Bonora M, Schultz SA, Remmers JE. Hypoxia-induced changes in shivering and body temperature. J Appl Physiol 1987a; 62:2477–2484.

Gautier H, Bonora M, Zaoui D. Influence of halothane on control of breathing in intact and decerebrated cats. J Appl Physiol 1987b; 63:546–553.

Gautier H, Bonora M, Remmers JE. Effects of hypoxia on metabolic rate of conscious adult cats during cold exposure. J Appl Physiol 1989; 67:32–38.

Gautier H, Bonora M, Ben M'Barek S, Sinclair JD. Effects of hypoxia and cold acclimation on thermoregulation in the rat. J Appl Physiol 1991; 71:1355–1363.

Gautier H, Bonora M, Lahiri S. Control of metabolic and ventilatory responses to cold in anesthetized cats. Respir Physiol 1992; 87:309–324.

Gill MB, Pugh LGCE. Basal metabolism and respiration in men living at 5,800 m (19,000 ft). J Appl Physiol 1964; 19:949–954.

Glickman N, Mitchell HH, Keeton RW, Lambert EH. Shivering and heat production in men exposed to intense cold. J Appl Physiol 1967; 22:1–8.

Glotzbach SE, Heller HC. Thermoregulation. In: Kryger MH, Roth T, Dement WC, eds. Principles and Practice of Sleep Medicine. Philadelphia: Saunders, 1989; 300–305.

Gordon CJ, Fogelson L. Comparative effects of hypoxia on behavioural thermoregulation in rats, hamsters, and mice. Am J Physiol 260 (Regul Integr Comp Physiol 29) 1991; R120–R125.

Graham BD, Reardon HS, Wilson JL, Tsao MU, Baumann ML. Physiologic and chemical response of premature infants to oxygen-enriched atmosphere. Pediatrics 1950; 6:55–71.

Greenleaf JE, Greenleaf CJ, Card DH, Saltin B. Exercise-temperature regulation in man during acute exposure to simulated altitude. J Appl Physiol 1969; 26:290–296.

Grover RF. Basal oxygen uptake of man at high altitude. J Appl Physiol 1963; 18:909–912.

Grunstein MM, Younes M, Milic-Emili J. Control of tidal volume and respiratory frequency in anesthetized cats. J Appl Physiol 1973; 35:463–476.

Haddad GG, Gandhi MR, Mellins RB. Maturation of ventilatory response to hypoxia in puppies during sleep. J Appl Physiol 1982; 52:309–314.

Hales JRS. Effects of exposure to hot environments on the regional distribution of blood flow and on cardiopulmonary function in sheep. Pflügers Arch 1973; 344:133–148.

Hales JRS, Dampney RAL, Bennett JW. Influences of chronic denervation of the carotid bifurcation regions on panting in the sheep. Pflügers Arch 1975; 360:243–253.

Hallam JF, Dawson TJ. The pattern of respiration with increasing metabolism in a small dasyurid marsupial. Respir Physiol 1993; 93:305–314.

Hammouda M. The central and the reflex mechanism of panting. J Physiol (Lond) 1933; 77:319–336.

Haskell EH, Palca JW, Walker JM, Berger RJ, Heller HC. Metabolism and thermoregulation during stages of sleep in humans exposed to heat and cold. J Appl Physiol 1981; 51:948–954.

Hayaishii O, ed. Molecular Mechanisms of Oxygen Activation. New York: Academic Press, 1974: 678 pp.

Hayward JN, Baker MA. The role of the cerebral arterial blood in the regulation of brain temperature in the monkey. Am J Physiol 1968; 215:389–403.

Heath D, Williams DR. Man at High Altitude . Edinburgh: Churchill Livingstone, 1981: 247–258.

Heldmaier G. Relationship between non-shivering thermogenesis and body size. In: Jansky L, ed. Nonshivering Thermogenesis. Amsterdam: Swets and Zeitlinger, 1971: 73–80.

Hedenstierna G, Tokics L. Anesthesia. In: Crystal KG, West JB, eds. The Lung: Scientific Foundations. New York: Raven Press, 1991: 2175–2183.

Hemingway A. Shivering. Physiol Rev 1963; 43:397–422.

Hey EN, Lloyd BB, Cunningham DJC, Jukes MGM, Bolton DPG. Effects of various respiratory stimuli on the depth and frequency of breathing in man. Respir Physiol 1966; 1:193–205.

Hickey RF, Severinghaus JW. Regulation of breathing: drug effects. In: Hornbein TF, ed. Regulation of breathing, Part II. New York: Marcel Dekker, 1981; 1251–1312.

Hicks JW, Wood SC. Oxygen homeostasis in lower vertebrates. In: Wood SC, ed. Comparative Pulmonary Physiology, Current Concepts. New York: Marcel Dekker, 1989; 311–341.

Hill AV, Long CNH, Lupton H. Muscular exercise, lactic acid, and the supply and utilisation of oxygen. Parts IV–VI. Proc R Soc Lond Ser B 1924–25; 97:84–138.

Hill JR. The oxygen consumption of new-born and adult mammals. Its dependence on the oxygen tension in the inspired air and on the environmental temperature. J Physiol (Lond) 1959; 149:346–373.

Hochachka PW. Living Without Oxygen. Cambridge, MA: Harvard University Press, 1980; 1–237.

Hochachka PW, Matheson GO, Parkhouse WS, Sumar-Kalinowski J, Stanley C, Monge C, McKenzie DC, Merkt J, Man SFP, Jones R, Allen PS., Inborn resistance to hypoxia in high altitude adapted humans. In: Lahiri S, Cherniack NS, Fitzgerald RS, eds. Response and Adaptation to Hypoxia. Organ to Organelle. New York: Oxford University Press, 1991: 191–194.

Hogan MC, Arthur PG, Bebout DE, Hochachka PW, Wagner PD. Role of O_2 in regulating tissue respiration in dog muscle working in situ. J Appl Physiol 1992a; 73:728–736.

Hogan MC, Nioka S, Brechue WF, Chance B. A ^{31}P-NMR study of tissue respiration in working dog muscle during reduced O_2 delivery conditions. J Appl Physiol 1992b; 73:1662–1670.

Horstman DH, Banderet LE. Hypoxia-induced metabolic and core temperature changes in the squirrel monkey. J Appl Physiol 1977; 42:273–278.

Horvath SM, Spurr GR, Hutt BK, Hamilton LH. Metabolic cost of shivering. J Appl Physiol 1956; 8:595–602.

Huang SY, Alexander JK, Grover RF, Maher JT, McCullough RE, McCullough RG, Moore LG, Weil JV, Sampson JB, Reeves JT. Increased metabolism contributes to increased resting ventilation at high altitude. Respir Physiol 1984; 57:377–385.

Huch A, Kötter D, Loerbroks R, Piiper J. O_2 transport in anesthetized dogs in hypoxia, with O_2 uptake increased by 2:4-dinitrophenol. Respir Physiol 1969; 6:187–201.

Hunter WS, Adams T. Respiratory heat exchange influences on diencephalic temperature in the cat. J Appl Physiol 1966; 21:873–876.

Ingram DL, Legge KF. The effect of environmental temperature on respiratory ventilation in the pig. Respir Physiol 1969–70; 8:1–12.

Jansky L. Non-shivering thermogenesis and its thermoregulatory significance. Biol Rev 1973; 48:85–132.

Jennings DB. Body temperature and ventilatory response to CO_2 during chronic respiratory acidosis. J Appl Physiol 1979; 46:491–497.

Jennings DB, Laupacis A. The effect of body warming on the ventilatory response to CO_2 in the awake dog. Respir Physiol 1982; 49:355–369.

Jöbsis FF. Basic processes in cellular respiration. In: Fenn WO, Rahn H, eds. Handbook of Physiology, Section 3, Volume 1. Bethesda, MD: American Physiological Society, 1964: 63–124.

Kagawa S, Stafford MJ, Waggener TB, Severinghaus JW. No effect of naloxone on hypoxia-induced ventilatory depression in adults. J Appl Physiol 1982; 52:1030–1034.

Kaminsky RP, Forster HV, Klein JP, Pan LG, Bisgard GE, Hamilton LH. Effect of elevated PI_{CO_2} on metabolic rate in humans and ponies. J Appl Physiol. 1982; 52:1623–1628.

Kao FF, Schlig BB. Impairment of gas transport and gas exchange in dogs during acute hypothermia. J Appl Physiol 1956; 9:387–394.

Karetzky MS, Cain SM. Effect of carbon dioxide on oxygen uptake during hyperventilation in normal man. J Appl Physiol 1970; 28:8–12.

Kiley JP, Eldridge FL, Millhorn DE. The effect of hypothermia on central neural control of respiration. Respir Physiol 1984; 58:295–312.

Kleiber M. Body size and metabolism. Hilgardia 1932; 6:315–353.

Kleiber M. The Fire of Life. An Introduction to Animal Energetics. New York: Wiley, 1961.

Kolobow T, Gattinoni L, Tomlinson TA, Pierce JE. Control of breathing using an extracorporeal membrane lung. Anesthesiology 1977; 46:138–141.

Kottke FJ, Phalen JS, Taylor CB, Visscher MB, Evans GT. Effect of hypoxia upon temperature regulation of mice, dogs, and man. Am J Physiol 1948; 153:10–15.

Kuhnen G. O_2 and CO_2 concentrations in burrows of euthermic and hibernating golden hamsters. Comp Biochem Physiol 1986; 84A:517–522.

Kuhnen G, Wloch B, Wünnenberg W. Effects of acute hypoxia and/or hypercapnia on body temperatures and cold induced thermogenesis in the golden hamster. J Therm Biol 1987; 12:103–107.

Lahiri S, Mulligan E, Nishino T, Mokashi A, Davies RO. Relative responses of aortic body and carotid body chemoreceptors to carboxyhemoglobinemia. J Appl Physiol 1981; 50:580–586.

LaFramboise, WA, Guthrie RD, Standaert TA, Woodrum DE. Pulmonary mechanics during the ventilatory response to hypoxemia in the newborn monkey. J Appl Physiol 1983; 55:1008–1014.

Lambertsen CJ, Kough RH, Cooper DY, Emmel GL, Loeschcke HH, Schmidt CF. Oxygen toxicity. Effects in man of oxygen inhalation at 1 and 3.5 atmospheres upon blood gas transport, cerebral circulation and cerebral metabolism. J Appl Physiol 1953; 5: 471–494.

Lange Andersen K, Hart JS, Hammel HT, Sabean HB. Metabolic and thermal response of Eskimos during muscular exercise in the cold. J Appl Physiol 1963; 18:613–618.

Lechner AJ. Metabolic performance during hypoxia in native and acclimated pocket gophers. J Appl Physiol 1977; 43:965–970.

Lechner AJ, Blake CI, Banchero N. Pulmonary development in growing guinea pigs exposed to chronic hypercapnia. Respiration 1987; 52:108–114.

Lafrancois R, Gautier H, Pasquis P, Vargas E. Factors controlling respiration during muscular exercise at altitude. Fed Proc 1969; 28:1296–1299.

Lenfant C. Arterial-alveolar difference in P_{CO_2} during air and oxygen breathing. J Appl Physiol 1966; 21:1356–1362.

Levine S, Huckabee WE. Ventilatory response to drug-induced hypermetabolism. J Appl Physiol 1975; 38:827–833.

Lim TPK. Central and peripheral control mechanisms of shivering and its effects on respiration. J Appl Physiol 1960; 15:567–574.

Lintzel W. Über die Wirkung der Luftverdünnung auf Tiere. V. Mitteilung. Gaswechsel weisser Ratten. Pflügers Arch Ges Physiol 1931; 227:693–708.

Lodato RF. Decreased O_2 consumption and cardiac output during normobaric hyperoxia in conscious dogs. J Appl Physiol 1989; 67:1551–1559.

Longmuir IS, Moore RE. The change with age in the critical oxygen concentration of kitten liver slices. J Physiol (Lond) 1958; 138:44P (abstract).

MacDougall JD, Reddan WG, Layton CR, Dempsey JA. Effects of metabolic hyperthermia on performance during heavy prolonged exercise. J Appl Physiol 1974; 36: 538–544.

Malkinson TJ, Cooper KE, Veale WL. Physiological changes during thermoregulation and fever in urethan-anesthetized rats. Am J Physiol 255 (Regul Int Comp Physiol 24) 1988; R73–R81.

Marchal F, Bairam A, Haouzi P, Crance JP, Di Giulio C, Vert P, Lahiri S. Carotid chemoreceptor response to natural stimuli in the newborn kitten. Respir Physiol 1992; 87:183–193.

Martin BJ, Morgan EJ, Zwillich CW, Weil JV. Influence of exercise hyperthermia on exercise breathing pattern. J Appl Physiol 1979; 47:1039–1042.

Martin-Body RL, Johnston BM. Central origin of the hypoxic depression of breathing in the newborn. Respir Physiol 1988; 71:25–32.

Maskrey M. Body temperature effects on hypoxic and hypercapnic responses in awake rats. Am J Physiol 259 (Regul Int Comp Physiol 28) 1990; R492–R498.

Maskrey M, Nicol SC. Responses of conscious rabbits to CO_2 at ambient temperatures of 5, 20 and 25°C. J Appl Physiol 1979; 47:522–526.

Maskrey M, Hales JRS, Fawcett AA. Effect of a constant arterial CO_2 tension on respiratory pattern in heat-stressed sheep. J Appl Physiol 1981; 50:315–319.

Matsuoka T, Dotta A, Mortola JP. Metabolic response to ambient temperature and hypoxia in sinoaortic-denervated rats. Am J Physiol 266 (Regul Int Comp Physiol 35) 1994a, R387–R391.

Matsuoka T, Saiki C, Mortola JP. Metabolic and ventilatory responses to anemic hypoxia in conscious rats. J Appl Physiol 1994b (in press).

May P. L'action immédiate de l'oxygène sur la ventilation chez l'homme normal. Helv Physiol Acta 1957; 15:230–240.

McArdle WD, Magel JR, Lesmes GR, Pechar GS. Metabolic an cardiovascular adjustment to work in air and water at 18, 25, and 33°C. J Appl Physiol 1976; 40:85–90.

McCooke HB, Hanson MA. Respiration of conscious kittens in acute hypoxia and effect of almitrine bismesylate. J Appl Physiol 1985; 59:18–23.

Milerad J, Hertzberg T, Lagercrantz H. Ventilatory and metabolic responses to acute hypoxia in infants assessed by transcutaneous gas monitoring. J Dev Physiol 1987; 9:57–67.

Miller MJ, Tenney SM. Hyperoxic hyperventilation in carotid-deafferented cats. Respir Physiol 1975; 23:23–30.

Monge C, León-Velarde F. Physiological adaptation to high altitude: oxygen transport in mammals and birds. Physiol Rev 1991; 71:1135–1172.

Moore LG, Cymerman A, Huang S-Y, McCullough RE, McCullough RG, Rock PB, Young A, Young P, Weil JV, Reeves JT. Propranolol blocks metabolic rate increase but not ventilatory acclimatization to 4300 m. Respir Physiol 1987; 70:195–204.

Moore RE. The effect of hypoxia on the oxygen consumption of newborn dogs. J Physiol (Lond) 1956; 131:27P.

Moore RE. Oxygen consumption and body temperature in newborn kittens subjected to hypoxia and reoxygenation. J Physiol (Lond) 1959; 149:500–518.

Moore RE, Underwood MC. Hexamethonium, hypoxia and heat production in new-born and infant kittens and puppies. J Physiol (Lond) 1962; 161:30–53.

Mortola JP. Dynamics of breathing in newborn mammals. Physiol Rev 1987; 67:187–243.

Mortola JP. Hamsters versus rats: ventilatory responses in adults and newborns. Respir Physiol 1991; 85:305–317.

Mortola JP. Hypoxic hypometabolism in mammals. News Physiol Sci 1993; 8:79–82.

Mortola JP, Dotta A. Effects of hypoxia and ambient temperature on gaseous metabolism of newborn rats. Am J Physiol 263 (Regul Int Comp Physiol 32) 1992, R267–R272.

Mortola JP, Matsuoka T. Interaction between CO_2 production and ventilation in the hypoxic kitten. J Appl Physiol 1993; 74:905–910.

Mortola JP, Rezzonico R. Metabolic and ventilatory rates in newborn kittens during acute hypoxia. Respir Physiol 1988; 73:55–68.

Mortola JP, Tenney SM. Effects of hyperoxia on ventilatory and metabolic rats of newborn mice. Respir Physiol 1986; 63:267–274.

Mortola JP, Morgan CA, Virgona V. Respiratory adaptation to chronic hypoxia in newborn rats. J Appl Physiol 1986; 61:1329–1336.

Mortola JP, Rezzonico R, Lanthier C. Ventilation and oxygen consumption during acute hypoxia in newborn mammals: a comparative analysis. Respir Physiol 1989; 78:31–43.

Mortola JP, Frappell PB, Dotta A, Matsuoka T, Fox G, Weeks S, Mayer D. Ventilatory and metabolic responses to acute hyperoxia in newborns. Am Rev Respir Dis 1992a; 146:11–15.

Mortola JP, Frappell PB, Frappell DE, Villena-Cabrera N, Villena-Cabrera M, Peña F. Ventilation and gaseous metabolism in infants born at high altitude, and their responses to hyperoxia. Am Rev Respir Dis 1992b; 146:1206–1209.

Mortola JP, Gleed RD, Saiki C. Adaptation and acclimatization in the hypoxic newborn mammal. In: Speck DF, Dekin MS, Revelette WR, Frazier DT, eds. Respiratory Control: Central and Peripheral Mechanisms. Lexington: Kentucky University Press, 1993:176–180.

Mortola JP, Matsuoka T, Saiki C, Naso L. Metabolism and ventilation in hypoxic rats: effect of body mass. Respir Physiol 1994; 97:225–234.

Moser KM, Perry RB, Luchsinger PC. Cardiopulmonary consequences of pyrogen-induced hyperoxia in man. J Clin Invest 1983; 42:626–634.

Moss M, Moreau G, Lister G. Oxygen transport and metabolism in the conscious lamb: the effect of hypoxemia. Pediatr Res 1987; 22:177–183.

Mott JC. The effects of baroreceptor and chemoreceptor stimulation on shivering. J Physiol (Lond) 1963; 166:563–586.

Mount LE. The metabolic rate of the new-born pig in relation to environmental temperature and age. J Physiol (Lond) 1959; 147:333–345.

Mourek J. Oxygen consumption during ontogenesis in rats in environments with a high and low oxygen content. Physiol Bohemoslov 1959; 8:106–111.

Nahas G, Schaefer KE, eds. Carbon Dioxide and Metabolic Regulations. New York: Springer-Verlag, 1974; 353 pp.

Nair CS, Malhotra MS, Gopinath PM. Effect of altitude and cold acclimatization on the basal metabolism in man. Aerosp Med 1971; 42:1056–1059.

Natsui T. Respiratory response to hypoxia with hypocapnia or normocapnia and to CO_2 in hypothermic dogs. Respir Physiol 1969; 7:188–212.

Newstead CG. The relationship between ventilation and oxygen consumption in man is the same during both moderate exercise and shivering. J Physiol (Lond) 1987; 383: 455–459.

Olievier CN, Berkenbosch A, DeGoede J. Effect of temperature on the ventilatory response curve to carbon dioxide in anaesthetized cats. Respir Physiol 1982; 47:365–377.

Olson EB Jr, Dempsey JA. Rat as a model for humanlike ventilatory adaptation to chronic hypoxia. J Appl Physiol 1978; 44:763–769.

Palca JW, Walker JM, Berger RJ. Thermoregulation, metabolism, and stages of sleep in cold-exposed men. J Appl Physiol 1986; 61:940–947.

Pappenheimer JR. Sleep and respiration of rats during hypoxia. J Physiol (Lond) 1977; 266:191–207.

Parmeggiani P. Thermoregulation during sleep in mammals. News Physiol Sci 1990; 5: 208–212.

Pavlin EG, Hornbein TF. Anesthesia and the control of ventilation. In: Cherniack NS, Widdicombe JG, eds. Handbook of Physiology, The Respiratory System, vol II, Control of Breathing, part 2. Bethesda, MD: American Physiological Society, 1986; 793–813.

Pedraz, C, Mortola JP. CO_2 production, body temperature, and ventilation in hypoxic newborn cats and dogs before and after body warming. Pediatr Res 1991; 30:165–169.

Pepelko WE, Dixon GA. Elimination of cold-induced nonshivering thermogenesis by hypercapnia. Am J Physiol 1974; 227:264–267.

Petersen ES, Vejby-Christensen H. Effects of body temperature on ventilatory response to hypoxia and breathing pattern in man. J Appl Physiol 1977; 42:492–500.

Phillips RW, Knox KL, House WA, Jordan HN. Metabolic responses in sheep chronically exposed to 6,200 m. simulated altitude. Fed Proc 1969; 28:974–977.

Phillipson EA, Bowes G. Control of breathing during sleep. In: Cherniack NS, Widdicombe JG, eds. Handbook of Physiology: The Respiratory System, Vol 2, part 2. Bethesda, MD: American Physiological Society, 1986: 649–689.

Phillipson EA, Duffin J, Cooper JD. Critical dependence of respiratory rhythmicity on metabolic CO_2 load. J Appl Physiol 1981; 50:45–54.

Piazza T, Lauzon AM, Mortola JP. Time course of adaptation to hypoxia in newborn rats. Can J Physiol Pharmacol 1988; 66:152–158.

Picón-Reátegui E. Basal metabolic rate and body composition at high altitudes. J Appl Physiol 1961; 16:431–434.

Pitts RF, Magoun HW, Ranson SW. The origin of respiratory rhythmicity. Am J Physiol 1939; 127:654:670.

Polgar G, Weng TR. The functional development of the respiratory system. From the period of gestation to adulthood. Am Rev Respir Dis 1979; 120:625–695.

Poulos DA, chairman. Neurophysiology of temperature regulation (symposium). Fed Proc 1981; 40:2803–2850.

Powers SK, Lawler J, Demspey JA, Dodd S, Landry G. Effects of incomplete pulmonary gas exchange on $\dot{V}O_{2max}$. J Appl Physiol 1989; 66:2491–2495.

Prosser CL, Heath JE. Temperature. In: Prosser CL, ed. Environmental and Metabolic Animal Physiology. New York: Wiley-Liss, 1991: 109–165.

Reeves JT, Groves BM, Sutton JR, Wagner PD. Cymerman A, Malconian MK, Rock PB, Young PM, Houston CS. Operation Everest II: preservation of cardiac function at extreme altitude. J Appl Physiol 1987; 63:531–539.

Reinhart K, Bloos F, König F, Bredle D, Hannemann L. Reversible decrease of oxygen consumption by hyperoxia. Chest 1991; 99:690–694.

Richards SA. The biology and comparative physiology of thermal panting. Biol Rev 1970; 45:223–264.

Rigatto H, Brady JP. Periodic breathing and apnea in preterm infants. I. Evidence for hypoventilation possibly due to central respiratory depression. Pediatrics 1972a; 50:202–218.

Rigatto H, Brady JP. Periodic breathing and apnea in preterm infants. II. Hypoxia as a primary event. Pediatrics 1972b; 50:219–228.

Rigatto H, Brady JP, Verduzco de la Torre R. Chemoreceptor reflexes in preterm infants. 1. The effect of gestational and postnatal age on the ventilatory response to inhalation of 100% and 15% oxygen. Pediatrics 1975; 55:604–613.

Rigatto H, Wiebe C, Rigatto C, Lee DS, Cates D. Ventilatory response to hypoxia in unanesthetized newborn kittens. J Appl Physiol 1988; 64:2544–2551.

Robin ED. Of men and mitochondria: coping with hypoxic dysoxia. Am Rev Respir Dis 1980; 122:517–531.

Robinson KA, Haymes EM. Metabolic effects of exposure to hypoxia plus cold at rest and during exercise in humans. J Appl Physiol 1990; 68:720–725.

Rosenmann M, Morrison P. Maximum oxygen consumption and heat loss facilitation in small homeotherms by He-O$_2$. Am J Physiol 1974; 226:490–495.

Rosenmann M, Morrison PR. Metabolic response of highland and lowland rodents to simulated high altitudes and cold. Comp Biochem Physiol 1975; 51A:523–530.

Rowell LB, Brengelmann GL, Murray JA, Kraning KK II, Kusumi F. Human metabolic responses to hyperthermia during mild to maximal exercise. J Appl Physiol 1969; 26:395–402.

Ruiz AV. Ventilatory response of panting dog to hypoxia. Pflügers Arch 1973; 34: 89–99.

Ruiz AV. Effects of cyanide and doxapram during panting. Pflügers Arch 1975; 361:79–81.

Saetta M, Mortola JP. Interaction of hypoxic and hypercapnic stimuli on breathing pattern in the newborn rat. J Appl Physiol 1987; 62:506–512.

Saiki C, Matsuoka T, Mortola JP. Metabolic-ventilatory interaction in conscious rats: effect of hypoxia and ambient temperature. J Appl Physiol 1994; 76:1594–1599.

Sankaran K, Wiebe H, Seshia MMK, Boychuk RB, Cates D, Rigatto H. Immediate and late ventilatory response to high and low O_2 in preterm infants and adult subjects. Pediatr Res 1979; 13:875–878.

Saunders KB, Band DM, Ebden P, Van der Hoff JP, Maberley DJ, Semple SJG. Acid base status and gas exchange in the anaesthetized dog breathing pure oxygen. Respiration 1972; 29:305–316.

Schaefer KE, Messier AA, Morgan C, Baker GT III. Effect of chronic hypercapnia on body temperature regulation. J Appl Physiol 1975; 38:900–906.

Schoener EP, Frankel HM. Effects of hyperthermia and $PaCO_2$ on the slowly adapting stretch receptor. Am J Physiol 1972; 222:68–72.

Schwieler GH. Respiratory regulation during postnatal development in cats and rabbits and some of its morphological substrate. Acta Physiol Scand 1968; 304(Suppl): 8–123.

See WR. Interaction between chemical and thermal drives to respiration during heat stress. In: Hales JRS, ed. Thermal Physiology. New York: Raven Press, 1984: 353–358.

Sessler DI. Central thermoregulatory inhibition by general anesthesia. Anesthesiology 1991; 75:557–579.

Severinghaus JW. Hypoxic respiratory drive and its loss during chronic hypoxia. Clin Physiol 1972; 2:57–79.

Shapiro CM, Goll CC, Cohen GR, Oswald I. Heat production during sleep. J Appl Physiol 1981; 56:671–677.

Sidi D, Kuipers JRG, Heymann MA, Rudolph AM. Effects of ambient temperature on oxygen consumption and the circulation in newborn lambs at rest and during hypoxemia. Pediatr Res 1983; 17:254–258.

Simon E, Pierau F-K, Taylor DCM. Central and peripheral thermal control of effectors in homeothermic temperature regulation Physiol Rev 1986; 66:235–300.

Simon LM, Theodore J, Robin ED. Regulation of biosynthesis/biodegradation of oxygen-related enzymes by molecular oxygen. In: Robin ED, ed. Extrapulmonary Manifestations of Respiratory Disease. New York: Marcel Dekker, 1978: 151–169.

Starlinger H, Lübbers DW. Polarographic measurements of the oxygen pressure performed simultaneously with optical measurements of the redox state of the respiratory chain in suspensions of mitochondria under steady-state conditions at low oxygen tensions. Pflügers Arch 1973; 341:15–22.

Stock MK. The embryo—O_2 modulation of growth. In: Sutton JR, Houston CS, Coates G, eds. Hypoxia. The Tolerable Limits. Indianapolis, IN: Benchmark Press, 1988: 233–250.

Stupfel M. Carbon dioxide and temperature regulation in homeothermic mammals. In: Nahas G, Schaefer KE, eds. Carbon Dioxide and Metabolic Regulations. New York: Springer-Verlag, 1974: 163–186.

Suffredini AF, Shelhamer JH, Neumann RD, Brenner M, Baltharo RJ, Parrillo JE. Pulmonary and oxygen transport effects of intravenously administered endotoxin in normal humans. Am Rev Respir Dis 1992; 145:1398–1403.

Sutton JR, Reeves JT, Wagner PD, Groves BM, Cymerman A, Malconian MK, Rock PB, Young PM, Walter SD, Houston C. Operation Everest II: oxygen transport during exercise at extreme simulated altitude. J Appl Physiol 1988; 64:1309–1321.

Szelenyi Z, Szekely M. Comparison of the effector mechanisms during endotoxin fever in the adult rabbit. Acta Physiol Acad Sci Hung 1979; 54:33–41.

Tamaki Y, Nakayama T. Effects of air constituents on thermosensitivities of preoptic neurons: hypoxia versus hypercapnia. Pflügers Arch 1987; 409:1–6.

Tatsumi K, Pickett CK, Weil JV. Effects of haloperidol and domperidone on ventilatory roll off during sustained hypoxia in cats. J Appl Physiol 1992; 72:1945–1952.

Taylor PM. Oxygen consumption in new-born rats. J Physiol (Lond) 1960; 154:153–168.

Tenney SM. Sympatho-adrenal stimulation by carbon dioxide and the inhibitory effect of carbonic acid on epinephrine response. Am J Physiol 1956; 187:341–346.

Tenney SM, Boggs DF. Comparative mammalian respiratory control. In: Cherniack NS, Widdicombe JG, eds. Handbook of Physiology: The Respiratory System, vol 2, part 2. Bethesda, MD: American Physiological Society 1986: 833–855.

Tenney SM, Ou LC. Ventilatory response of decorticate and decerebrate cats to hypoxia and CO_2. Respir Physiol 1977; 29:81–92.

Thompson GE, Moore RE. A study of newborn rats exposed to the cold. Can J Physiol Pharmacol 1968; 46:865–871.

Trippenbach T, Milic-Emili J. Temperature and CO_2 effect on phrenic activity and tracheal occlusion pressure. J Appl Physiol 1977; 43:449–454.

Truchot J-P, Duhamel-Jouve A. Oxygen and carbon dioxide in the marine intertidal environment: diurnal and tidal changes in rockpools. Respir Physiol 1980; 39:241–254.

Vanderkooi JM, Erecinska M, Silver IA. Oxygen in mammalian tissue: methods of measurement and affinities of various reactions. Am J Physiol 260 (Cell Physiol 29) 1991, C1131–C1150.

Várnai I, Farkas M, Donhoffer S. The effect of hypoxia on heat production and body temperature in the new-born rabbit. Acta Physiol Acad Sci Hung 1971; 39:293–320.

Vejby-Christensen H, Petersen SE. Effect of body temperature and hypoxia on the ventilatory CO_2 response in man. Respir Physiol 1973; 19:322–332.

Vizek M, Pickett CK, Weil JV. Biphasic ventilatory response of adult cats to sustained hypoxia has central origin. J Appl Physiol 1987; 63:1658–1664.

Wagner JA, Matsushita K, Horvath SM. Effect of carbon dioxide inhalation on physiological responses to cold. Aviat Space Environ Med 1983; 54:1074–1079.

Waldrop TG, Mullins DC, Millhorn DE. Control of respiration by the hypothalamus and by feedback from contracting muscles in cats. Respir Physiol 1986; 64:317–328.

Walters FM. Effects of carbon monoxide inhalation upon metabolism. Am J Physiol 1927; 80:140–149.

Wangsnes KM, Koos BJ. Maturation of respiratory responses to graded hypoxia in rabbits. Biol Neonate 1991; 59:219–225.

Wasserman K, Whipp BJ, Casaburi R, Beaver WL. Carbon dioxide flow and exercise hyperpnea. Am Rev Respir Dis 1977; 115(Suppl):225–237.

Wasserman K, Whipp BJ, Casaburi R. Respiratory control during exercise. In: Cherniack NS, Widdicombe JG, eds. Handbook of Physiology: The Respiratory System, Vol 2, part 2. Bethesda, MD: American Physiological Society 1986: 595–619.

Wegener G. Oxygen availability, energy metabolism, and metabolic rate in invertebrates and vertebrates. In: Acker H, ed. Oxygen Sensing in Tissues. Berlin: Springer-Verlag, 1988: 13–35.

Weil JV. Ventilatory control at high altitude. In: Cherniack NS, Widdicombe JG, eds. Handbook of Physiology: the respiratory system, Vol 2, part 2. Bethesda, MD: American Physiological Society, 1986: 703–727.

Weil JV, Zwillich CW. Assessment of ventilatory response to hypoxia. Chest 1976; 70(Suppl):124–128.

Weintraub Z, Alvaro R, Kwiatkowski K, Cates D, Rigatto H. Effects of inhaled oxygen (up to 40%) on periodic breathing and apnea in preterm infants. J Appl Physiol 1992; 72:116–120.

Welch HG. Hyperoxia and human performance: a brief review. Med Sci Sport Exerc 1982; 14:253–262.

Welch HG, Pedersen PK. Measurement of metabolic rate in hyperoxia. J Appl Physiol 1981; 51:725–731.

Wetzel RC, Herold CJ, Zerhouni EA, Robotham JL. Hypoxic bronchodilation. J Appl Physiol 1992; 73:1202–1206.

White DP, Weil JV, Zwillich CW. Metabolic rate and breathing during sleep. J Appl Physiol 1985; 59:384–391.

Widdicombe JG, Winning A. Effects of hypoxia, hypercapnia, and change in body temperature on the pattern of breathing in cats. Respir Physiol 1974; 21:203–221.

Wilson DF, Rumsey WL. Factors affecting adaptation of the mitochondrial enzyme content to cellular needs. In: Lahiri S, Cherniack NS, Fitzgerald RS, eds. Response and Adaptation to Hypoxia. Organ to Organelle. Bethesda, MD: American Physiological Society, 1991: 14–24.

Wood SC. Interaction between hypoxia and hypothermia. Annu Rev Physiol 1991; 53: 71–85.

Wyndham CH, Strydom NB, van Rensburg AJ, Rogers GG. Effects on maximal oxygen intake of acute changes in altitude in a deep mine. J Appl Physiol 1970; 29:552–555.

24

Regulation of Hyperpnea, Hyperventilation, and Respiratory Muscle Recruitment During Exercise

JEROME A. DEMPSEY

University of Wisconsin
Madison, Wisconsin

HUBERT V. FORSTER

Medical College of Wisconsin
Milwaukee, Wisconsin

DOROTHY M. AINSWORTH

Cornell University
Ithaca, New York

I. Introduction

Muscular exercise makes unique and multifaceted demands on the ventilatory control system. The increase in CO_2 production by the locomotor muscles and therefore in CO_2 flow to the lung with increasing work rate means that there is little room for error in the magnitude and the proportionality of the ventilatory response. This gas exchange requirement becomes an especially demanding problem in heavy exercise as the buffering of metabolic acids produced by the locomotor muscles greatly augments the CO_2 load presented to the lung as well as the circulating hydrogen ion concentration, which must be compensated. In addition to this substantial requirement for gas exchange, feedback and feedforward mechanisms must be available and highly sensitive to protect against incurring excessively high levels of mechanical work and energy expenditures on the part of the chest wall muscles to meet ventilatory requirements. Finally, the ventilatory control system must also be designed to take into account that there are structural limits to the capability of the healthy lung to expand its volume and to increase flow rate and that the respiratory muscles in healthy humans and animals are indeed fatigable.

Our overview of the regulation of the ventilatory response to exercise is integrative and comprehensive. It includes a critical review of the abundant literature concerned with the continuing dilemma of the neurochemical regulation of exercise hyperpnea and an updated detailed consideration of the humoral mechanisms responsible for regulation of the hyperventilatory response to heavy exercise. This analysis is supplemented with recent data concerned with the regulation of respiratory muscle recruitment during exercise and a consideration of demand verses structural capacity as a determinant of the ventilatory response. We draw heavily on data obtained in the exercising human and in chronically instrumented, unanesthetized animal models—both intact and selectively denervated. We believe these models to be especially useful for addressing the question of ventilatory control during exercise, because a key aim and a major source of controversy in this research is to quantify the relative contributions of the various proposed mechanism to the total response. Thus it is important that the relative gains of the control system—and each of its elements—be as close to physiological as possible in the experimental models used. It is also crucial that the mode of "exercise" used to simulate the important metabolic and/or neurophysiological characteristics of exercise mimic actual locomotion as closely as possible. For our analysis of the mechanical limits to ventilation by the lung and chest wall, we include a variety of species and consider a broad range of fitness levels within a given species. This approach permits us to address the question of demand versus capacity in the ventilatory response to exercise across a broad continuum of demand.

II. Neurochemical Regulation of Exercise Hyperpnea and Hyperventilation

A description of an organ system's usual response to a stress is of value for many reasons, including the insights provided into the: (1) mechanism of the response, (2) importance of the response to health or survival, and (3) detection of abnormal responses. It therefore seems appropriate to begin this section with a description of the breathing responses to exercise.

A. Description of Breathing Responses to Exercise

Temporal Pattern of Breathing Response to Exercise

In humans, the temporal pattern of pulmonary ventilation ($\dot{V}_E$) during submaximal exercise has three rather distinct phases (1–10). The first phase is an increase that occurs immediately or within seconds after the onset of exercise. The second phase is a slow, gradual increase that occurs between about 5 sec and 2–3 min of exercise. The third phase is a stable $\dot{V}_E$ sustained for several minutes of exercise. Of the total increase in $\dot{V}_E$ from rest, the second phase is usually slightly larger than the first phase, and the magnitude of both the first and second phases increases as work intensity increases (1,3,4,8–10). The duration of the stable $\dot{V}_E$ is variable; by 5–10 min of exercise, the plateau in $\dot{V}_E$ is followed by a slow, gradual increase continues for the duration of exercise. In fact, during heavy exercise (>70% maximal), a steady state is rarely observed and the third phase consists continual increase usually at a rate slightly less than the phase 2 increase (3, Once exercise is terminated, $\dot{V}_E$ decreases within seconds to within 25–50% of and then it decreases to rest gradually over several minutes (1,2,5,7).

Mammals other than human also demonstrate fast and slow increases breathing during exercise (12–17). However, in some nonhuman mammals th phase 1 fast increase is followed by a plateau or an actual decrease in $\dot{V}_E$ toward control (13,15). Phase 2 follows as a gradual increase in $\dot{V}_E$, but different from human, a steady state is rarely reached. Phase 3 in nonhumans during submaximal exercise resembles phase 3 in humans during heavy exercise when there is a slow continual increase in $\dot{V}_E$.

Relationship of Ventilation to Metabolic Rate

In humans, $\dot{V}_E$ and alveolar ventilation ($\dot{V}_A$) are curvilinearly related to the increase in oxygen consumption ($\dot{V}O_2$) and carbon dioxide excretion ($\dot{V}O_2$) during dynamic muscular exercise (9,18–22). Specifically, between rest and 60–70% of maximal $\dot{V}O_2$, $\dot{V}_E$ and $\dot{V}_A$ increase in a nearly proportionate manner to the increase in $\dot{V}O_2$ and $\dot{V}CO_2$. This close relationship between breathing and metabolic rate during submaximal exercise is also evident in the temporal pattern of each, there is a highly significant correlation between the time constants of $\dot{V}_E$ and $\dot{V}O_2$ and an even higher correlation between $\dot{V}_E$ and $\dot{V}CO_2$ (21–23). At higher work rates $\dot{V}_E$ and $\dot{V}_A$ increase proportionately more than the increases in $\dot{V}O_2$ and $\dot{V}CO_2$.

The relationship between breathing and metabolic rate is influenced by several factors. For example, the $\dot{V}_E$-$\dot{V}O_2$ slope is greater during: (1) static than during dynamic muscular contractions (24,25), (2) upright treadmill walking than during sitting bicycle ergometry (24–27), (3) arm exercise than during leg exercise (24,28,29), (4) systemic metabolic acidosis than during normal acid-base conditions (30,31), (5) hypoxic than during normoxic levels of inspired O_2 (9,13, 24,32,33), and (6) conditions when certain hormones or neurotransmitters have been elevated above normal (34–36).

In nonhuman mammals, $\dot{V}_E$ and $\dot{V}_A$ increase during submaximal exercise proportionately more than the increase in metabolic rate (12,15–17, 37–44). Over the entire work range, the $\dot{V}_E/\dot{V}O_2$ relationship is probably curvilinear in nonhuman mammals. There is minimal published data to support this conclusion. However, $PaCO_2$ decreases progressively as exercise intensity increases (see below). For this to occur, $\dot{V}_A$ must increase more for a given increment in $\dot{V}O_2$ at high workloads than at low workloads (45).

Tidal Volume (V) and Breathing Frequency (f)
During Exercise

Usually, both V_T and f increase during exercise (9,19,37,44). The relationship in humans of f to metabolic rate appears to be linear while the V_T-$\dot{V}O_2$ relationship tends to be curvilinear. The change in f contributes relatively more to the increase in $\dot{V}_E$ than the change in V_T. In nonhumans, the f response to exercise tends to be more prominent than in humans; the V_T of most species changes minimally until 50% of maximal $\dot{V}O_2$ is achieved.

In both humans and nonhumans the magnitude of the $\dot{V}_T$ and f changes is affected by several factors. As the impedance of the respiratory system increases, there is a tendency for accentuation of the $\dot{V}_T$ response to exercise and attenuation of the f response (46–48). When the respiratory system makes a major contribution to eliminating heat, there is an accentuation of the f response to exercise (21,24,49–51). Finally, the type of exercise is an important determinant of the f and $\dot{V}_T$ responses; at equivalent $\dot{V}O_2$, f will be higher and V_T lower for treadmill running than for bicycle ergometry (17,25,40,52). This influence of limb movement frequency is a manifestation of entertainment whereby breathing and stride frequency are linked (see Section III).

Paco₂, Po₂, and Arterial pH During Exercise

In humans, $PaCO_2$, PaO_2, and arterial pH change minimally from rest during exercise up to approximately 60–70% of maximal $\dot{V}O_2$ (Fig. 1). In most healthy humans there is only a transient 1–3 mmHg hypocapnia at the onset of exercise and an even smaller change in $PaCO_2$ in the transition between mild and moderate exercise (Fig. 2) (26,53–55). In other apparently healthy humans, $PaCO_2$ transiently increases in rest-to-work and work-to-work transitions. The incidence and magnitude of transient hypercapnia are greater in asthmatic (Fig. 3) than in nonasthmatic humans, and hypercapnia is common with elevated impedance of the respiratory system (56–58). During steady-state conditions of submaximal exercise in healthy humans, $PaCO_2$ does not differ from rest or is at most 1–3 mmHg above rest (9,18–20,26,55). The tendency for a slight hypercapnia is greater for bicycle ergometry and treadmill walking than it is for treadmill running (26). Exceptional are individuals with above-normal respiratory impedance who consistently demonstrate a workload-dependent hypercapnia (56,57). Arterial pH and PaO_2 during steady-state submaximal exercise differ minimally from rest (Fig. 1) (18–20,26).

The relationship of $PaCO_2$ to submaximal exercise intensity is independent of the resting conditions. In other words, during such conditions as chronic metabolic acidosis and alkalosis or hormonal changes when $PaCO_2$ is altered from normal, $PaCO_2$ during exercise is regulated to near the altered resting level

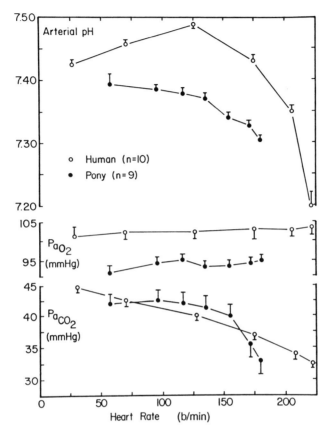

Figure 1 Arterial plasma pressure of CO_2 (Pa_{CO_2}) and O_2 (Pa_{O_2}) and arterial plasma pH of humans and ponies during treadmill exercise. Heart rate is used as an index of exercise intensity. (Data published in Refs. 15, 32, and 66.)

(30,31,36). Hypoxia is exceptional in that Pa_{CO_2} is lower during hypoxic exercise than during hypoxic rest (12,13,32,36).

Most healthy humans hyperventilate during exercise above 60–70% of maximal $\dot{V}_{O_2}$ (Fig. 1) (9,18–21,59). The hyperventilation is temporally associated and inversely related to plasma (lactate). A rise in PA_{CO_2} is observed before PA_{O_2} or Pa_{CO_2} decrease because of the extra CO_2 formed by the buffering of lactic acid by HCO_3 (21). Despite the increased PA_{O_2}, Pa_{O_2} is not increased above rest. Pa_{CO_2} is often decreased from rest by more than 10 mmHg during maximal exercise. Exceptional are superbly conditioned athletes who hyperventilate mini-

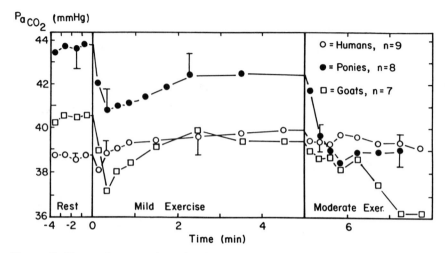

Figure 2 Temporal pattern of arterial plasma pressure of CO_2 ($Paco_2$) during mild and moderate exercise in humans, ponies, and goats. (Data published in Refs. 15, 26, and 43.)

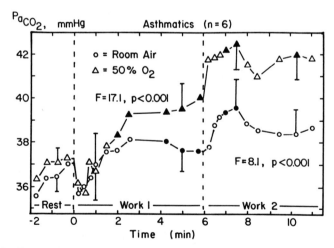

Figure 3 Temporal pattern of arterial plasma pressure of CO_2 ($Paco_2$) during mild and moderate bicycle ergometry in chemoreceptor intact asthmatics breathing room air or a 50% O_2–50% N_2 gas mixture. (Data published in Ref. 56.)

mally during heavy exercise and who experience a reduction in Pa_{O_2} that often is 30 mmHg below rest (60–62; see Section IV).

There are striking differences between humans and nonhumans in the effect of exercise on Pa_{CO_2} and arterial pH (Figs. 1 and 2) (12,13,15–17,38,40,41, 43,44,63–65). For example, it has been clearly shown that ponies and goats decrease Pa_{CO_2} in rest-to-work and work-to-work transitions (Fig. 2;15,40,43). Usually Pa_{CO_2} reaches a nadir during the first 30 sec of exercise with subsequently a slight, but definitely incomplete, return toward resting Pa_{CO_2}. The magnitude of the initial nadir in Pa_{CO_2} and the steady-state hypocapnia is related to the intensity of exercise (40). Nonhuman species also hyperventilate during heavy exercise, and in ponies at least, the magnitude of the hypocapnia is linearly related to work rate irrespective of arterial acid-base status (Fig. 1) (66). In other words, the onset of the acidosis is not associated, as in humans, with an accentuated reduction in Pa_{CO_2}. The hyperventilation causes a transient increase in Pa_{O_2} above rest, but during the steady state of mild, moderate, and heavy exercise Pa_{O_2} usually does not differ from rest (Fig. 1) (17,38,66). An exception are horses during heavy exercise (67,68). They do not hyperventilate; thus, Pa_{CO_2} is at or above normal and Pa_{O_2} is below normal. The reduced Pa_{O_2} is greater than expected from the change in Pa_{CO_2}; therefore, an alveolar-capillary diffusion limitation is probably a primary contributor to the hypoxemia (see Section III).

B. The Mechanism(s) Mediating the Exercise Hyperpnea

During the past century, there have been numerous studies attempting to gain insight into the mechanism(s) that mediates the exercise hyperpnea. As summarized, there is agreement that the stimulus or stimuli usually provide for a fast and slow increase in $\dot{V}_E$ to a steady state, that the stimulus is usually related to metabolic rate during submaximal exercise in humans in a manner that minimizes disruptions of arterial blood gases, and that several conditions can alter these basic relationships. Despite these common understandings, there are widely differing theories on the mechanisms of the hyperpnea (5,18,21,22,69,70). Most perplexing is that proponents of several theories provide data that seem to indicate that each can totally account for the hyperpnea.

A majority of theories have been historically classified as either "humoral" or "neural" (5,18). A theory is classified as humoral when it is proposed that exercise causes a change in some blood-borne agent that stimulates breathing at a receptor located outside the exercising muscle. On the other hand, a theory is classified as neural when it is proposed that the stimulus is not blood-borne but originates in the brain or in the exercising muscle and is transmitted to the medullary respiratory centers by either descending or ascending *neural* pathways. Some theories do not strictly fit into these classifications, and the case can be made that all proposed mechanisms have a neural component. Nevertheless, the distinction of blood-borne and non-blood-borne has utility as a conceptual framework; therefore, the following review of these theories will be organized in the traditional manner.

Humoral Theories

Geppert and Zuntz proposed in 1888 that an unknown blood substance produced by the exercising muscles provided the stimulus for the exercise hyperpnea (71). Subsequently, Haldane and Priestley demonstrated that breathing was increased by hypercapnia and hypoxia, and they proposed in 1905 that the increased CO_2 production during exercise could mediate the exercise hyperpnea (72). At this time, the existence of arterial and intracranial chemoreceptors was unknown; thus, it was assumed that CO_2 had a direct effect on the medullary respiratory control centers. However, Douglas and Haldane observed in 1909 that Pa_{CO_2} of humans did not change sufficiently during exercise to change medullary P_{CO_2} enough to account for the increased breathing (73). Eventually, in the 1930s, the arterial (74,75) and in the 1950s the intracranial (76,77) chemoreceptors were discovered. As a result, several theories have been formulated on carotid chemoreceptor mediation of the exercise hyperpnea, and studies have been completed in an attempt to determine whether intracranial chemoreceptor stimulus level might change during exercise. In addition, it has been proposed that sensory mechanisms in the great veins, heart, and/or lungs mediate the exercise hyperpnea.

Role of Carotid Chemoreceptors in Exercise Hyperpnea

Despite the nearly constant arterial blood gases and $[H^+]$ in humans during submaximal exercise, the carotid chemoreceptors could mediate the hyperpnea as a result of increased gain of these chemoreceptors. This hypothesis was supported by findings that carotid chemoreceptor firing rate was increased in anesthetized cats during passive hind-limb exercise (78). Section of the cervical sympathetic nerve or the postganglionic branch to the carotid body or section of the femoral and sciatic nerves eliminated this increased activity. In contrast, others (79) found that induced muscular contraction of hindlimb muscles of cats that stimulates breathing had no effect on afferent discharge from the carotid chemoreceptors. Moreover, others (80) studied humans during exercise before and after blocking carotid sympathetic innervation by injection of lidocaine into the stellate ganglia bilaterally. Lidocaine did not significantly alter $\dot{V}_E$ or blood gases during 9 min of submaximal exercise. The above data do not necessarily rule out increased chemoreceptor gain during exercise because factors unrelated to sympathetic innervation could increase carotid chemoreceptor activity and ventilatory responsiveness. In addition, the medullary controller and/or intracranial chemoreceptor gain could increase during exercise. If chemoreceptor gain is increased during exercise, the ventilatory response to P_{CO_2}, H^+, and P_{O_2} should be greater during exercise than at rest. From numerous studies, there is no clear indication that $\dot{V}_E$ responsiveness to CO_2-H^+ is increased during exercise (48,81–87). On the other hand, there is consensus that the $\dot{V}_E$ response to hypoxia is greater during exercise than at rest (18,82,87). However, there is no clear evidence that small (<5 mmHg) increases or decreases around the normal level of Pa_{O_2} during exercise has an effect on $\dot{V}_E$ (unpublished). Accordingly, it appears unlikely that potential changes in chemoreceptor sensitivity contribute to the hyperpnea of exercise.

Another hypothesized mechanism for carotid chemoreceptor mediation of the exercise hyperpnea is that a signal for breathing exists in the within-breath changes in P_{CO_2}, P_{O_2}, and H^+ (88,89). This postulate is based on findings that: (1) the within-breath changes are altered by exercise (90), (2) carotid chemoreceptor activity oscillates just like stimulus level at rest and during exercise (91,92), and (3) changes in these oscillations do influence breathing (93–96). However, the ventilatory changes secondary to changes in oscillation are small in magnitude (93–96). Moreover, from a recent study of ventilatory dynamics and oscillation during exercise by humans, it was concluded that oscillation in blood gases during exercise contributes minimally to the hyperpnea (97).

The carotid chemoreceptors could contribute to the exercise hyperpnea through the effect on chemoreceptor activity of exercise hyperkalemia. For both humans and ponies it has been shown that plasma $[K^+]$ during exercise is linearly related to CO_2 production and during submaximal exercise $\dot{V}_E$ is linearly related to plasma $[K^+]$ (97–102). In anesthetized cats it has been shown that intra-arterial injection of K^+ increases carotid chemoreceptor firing rate, and this increase is accompanied by an increase in $\dot{V}_E$, which is abolished by bilateral denervation of the carotid and aortic chemoreceptors (103–105). Supportive of a role for plasma $[K^+]$ in the exercise hyperpnea are data showing that in physically trained humans, both plasma $[K^+]$ and $\dot{V}_E$ are lower than in untrained subjects (98). Not supportive of a role for plasma K^+ are data showing that lowering of plasma $[K^+]$ in chronically hyperkalemic humans does not alter $\dot{V}_E$ (106,107). The potential contribution of elevated plasma $[K^+]$ has also been studied by intravenous infusion of K^+ in awake, exercising goats. Increases in plasma $[K^+]$ equivalent to moderate exercise had only a small affect on $\dot{V}_E$ (108). As a result, the evidence in support of K^+ at the carotid chemoreceptors contributing to the exercise hyperpnea remains largely circumstantial.

The evidence often cited in support of a carotid chemoreceptor contribution to the hyperpnea has been the findings of Wasserman et al. (58). They found, in carotid-chemoreceptor-resected (CCR) asthmatics, that the time constant of $\dot{V}_E$ during exercise was greater than in age-matched control subjects. As a result, there was a transient hypercapnia in the asthmatics but not the control subjects. These investigators subsequently found that any condition that increased carotid chemoreceptor activity (31,109) decreased the $\dot{V}_E$ time constant during exercise whereas conditions (110) that decreased chemoreceptor activity increased the time constant. As a result, Wasserman et al. concluded that the carotid chemoreceptors "are responsible, in part, for the rate of increase in $\dot{V}_E$ to steady state exercise." There are, however, two major concerns with these studies. First, changes in plasma [H$^+$] and Pao$_2$ affect breathing by mechanisms other than the carotid chemoreceptors (111); thus, control of breathing under these conditions is too complex to ascribe changes in ventilatory kinetics simply to the carotid chemoreceptors. Second, Wasserman's conclusion assumes that chemoreceptor resection rather than asthma was the cause of the abnormal response in the CCR asthmatics. However, it was not established whether the CCR asthmatics had normal pulmonary mechanics during exercise (58). Thus, it is conceivable that the exercise hypercapnia was due primarily to altered pulmonary mechanics or some other asthma-related factor. Increased airway resistance does indeed result in exercise hypercapnia accentuated by hyperoxia (which attenuates carotid chemoreceptor activity) (56,57). Moreover, recently it was found that carotid-chemoreceptor-intact asthmatics were hypercapnic during exercise and the hypercapnia was accentuated by hyperoxia (Fig. 3) (56). During hyperoxia, these chemoreceptor-intact asthmatics increased their Paco$_2$ by 5 mmHg between rest and moderate exercise. This increase is nearly identical to the increase in Paco$_2$ observed by Wasserman et al. in CCR asthmatics. It thus seems that the CCR asthmatics are not an appropriate model for assessing the role of the carotid chemoreceptors in the exercise hyperpnea. Their role in humans is suggested by the findings that during conditions when a significant hypercapnia occurs during exercise (ventilatory loading, asthma, chronic obstructive pulmonary disease), (56,57,112) this hypercapnia is accentuated by hyperoxia attenuation of carotid chemoreceptor activity. It appears that the role of the carotid chemoreceptors during exercise is to "fine-tune" alveolar ventilation to minimize disruptions in arterial blood gases and pH.

Data obtained on ponies (13,15,40), goats (12), and dogs (14) studied during exercise before and after CCR suggest that the normal role of the chemoreceptors in these species is to dampen an exercise hyperventilatory drive originating at another site. Specifically, the hyperventilation during the first 30 sec of a change in metabolic rate is greater in CCR animals than in normal animals. In ponies this effect is evident even when resting Paco$_2$ is the same in normal and CCR animals (Fig. 4), and the accentuated hyperventilation is also observed in normal ponies when chemoreceptor activity is attenuated through hyperoxia (40). In unusual situations when a pony hypoventilates during exercise (see below), the exercise hypoventilation is accentuated after CCR (113). In other words, these chemoreceptors minimize deviations in Paco$_2$ that occur in both directions from the normal Paco$_2$. Accordingly, as in humans, it appears that the role of the carotid chemoreceptors during exercise in nonhuman species is to "fine-tune" $\dot{V}_A$ to meet the metabolic needs for gas exchange.

In summary, it is clear that the within-breath changes in blood gases and the elevated plasma [K$^+$] during submaximal exercise potentially alter the input of the

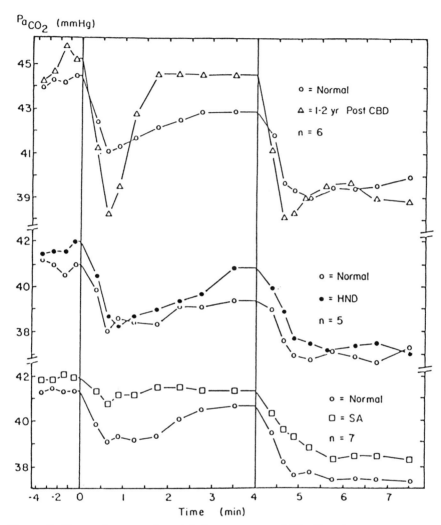

Figure 4 Temporal pattern of arterial plasma pressure of CO_2 (Pa_{CO_2}) at rest (top) and during mild (middle) and moderate (bottom) treadmill exercise in three groups of ponies studied before and after carotid body denervaration (CBD), pulmonary vagal denervation (HND), or partial spinal ablation (SA) at the 2nd lumbar level. (Data published in Ref. 113.)

carotid chemoreceptors to the medullary controllers. However, the magnitude of these potential effects and the results of studies in which chemoreceptor activity has been attenuated suggest that these chemoreceptors do not provide a "primary" drive for the exercise hyperpnea. Rather there is considerable data consistent with the concept of the chemoreceptors providing a fine-tuning function for $\dot{V}_A$ during exercise.

Role of Intracranial Chemoreceptors

Chemoreceptors are located within the brainstem which apparently respond to changes in $[H^+]$ or P_{CO_2} of cerebral interstitial fluid (76,77,114,115). The role of these chemoreceptors under any condition is unknown due to uncertainties in quantitating stimulus level (110,116). Nevertheless, it seems unlikely that mean stimulus level increases during exercise since P_{CO_2} and $[H^+]$ of both arterial and cerebral venous blood and cerebrospinal fluid (CSF) remain near normal or decrease during light and moderate exercise (37,117). In addition, manipulation of CSF $[H^+]$ does not alter the exercise hyperpnea (118). Furthermore, even though oscillations of pH in arterial blood can result in oscillation of brain extracellular fluid pH, these oscillations at rest are only 20% of the oscillations in blood, and it is unlikely that oscillations occur in brain pH at the breathing frequencies observed during exercise (70,119). Finally, because of their location and response kinetics, it is not intuitive for these chemoreceptors to be primary mediators or the major fine tuners of the exercise hyperpnea.

Great Vein, Cardiac, or Pulmonary Receptor Mediation of the Exercise Hyperpnea

Since mixed venous P_{CO_2} increases in humans during exercise (120,121), physiologists have been intrigued by the idea that receptors located in the great veins, the heart, or the lungs may mediate the exercise hyperpnea. This notion was proposed, tested, and rejected several years ago (122–128), but over the past 20 years there has been renewed and intense interest in this idea. This interest stemmed in large part from the close matching in humans of $\dot{V}_E$ to $\dot{V}_{CO_2}$ not only during steady-state exercise, but also during transitional conditions that, according to some investigators, provided for homeostasis of blood gases throughout exercise (22). These observations led to the hypothesis "that sensitive chemoreceptors on the arterial (high P_{O_2}) side of the pulmonary circulation function to change $\dot{V}_E$ pari passu to any change in CO_2 flow to the lungs" (22).

   The above hypothesis has been studied using extracorporeal gas exchangers, to either decrease (CO_2 scrubbing) or increase (CO_2 loading) venous P_{CO_2}. In some studies scrubbing and loading supposedly resulted in precise decreases or increases in $\dot{V}_E$ to maintain Pa_{CO_2} homeostasis (42,129–133). Others claim that owing to methodological deficiencies it was not possible to establish whether arterial isocapnia was maintained in many of these studies. Indeed, using more stringent protocols, it has been shown that $Paco_2$ changed during scrubbing and loading by an exact amount to account for the changes in $\dot{V}_E$ (134–139). Moreover, Orr et al. artificially ventilated cats to maintain $Paco_2$ homeostasis and found that phrenic output (as an index of ventilatory drive) was not altered with venous loading to a Pco_2 of 55 mmHg (140).

A limitation of these studies is the minimal amount that CO_2 is actually altered (~2–3 times normal). In this range of change in $\dot{V}co_2$, small departures of $\dot{V}_A$ to $\dot{V}co_2$ matching will cause significant changes in $Paco_2$, which easily could mediate the ventilatory changes through the carotid chemoreceptors (39,141). In other words, the "noise" of the system is too great for conventional measurement procedures to provide definitive resolution of the question.

A major concern with the CO_2 flow hypothesis has been that a receptor or signal has not been clearly identified to account for the exercise hyperpnea. In an attempt to elucidate a receptor, investigators have surgically isolated the pulmonary circulation from the systemic circulation. In support of pulmonary chemosensitivity, one study found that increasing pulmonary artery Pco_2 to 85 mmHg increased $\dot{V}_E$ but this response was much less than during systemic hypercapnia (142). A second study found that increasing pulmonary blood flow elicited a hyperpnea dependent on intact vagal nerves (143). Finally, it has been observed that these changes could be due to an effect of CO_2 on pulmonary stretch receptor activity (144–146). Even though these studies in total demonstrated that breathing could be altered by changing either pulmonary CO_2 or blood flow, they did not provide convincing evidence of a pulmonary receptor and signal with characteristics that would account for the exercise hyperpnea.

A third series of studies led to a theory known as "cardiodynamic" mediation of the exercise hyperpnea. In anesthetized animals, using bolus i.v. injections of isoproterenol (147) to increase cardiac output ($\dot{Q}_C$) or propanolol (148) to decrease $\dot{Q}_C$ it was found that $\dot{V}_E$ always changed in the same direction as $\dot{Q}_C$ and the magnitude of the $\dot{V}_E$ change maintained homeostasis of $Paco_2$. If the cardiac responses to the drugs were blocked, then there was no increase in $\dot{V}_E$. These changes in $\dot{V}_E$ were postulated due to a pulmonary mechanism that was activated by the change in $\dot{Q}_C$. However, other data supported the idea that cardiac mechanoreceptors might also influence $\dot{V}_E$. Passive distension of the right ventricle and increases in right ventricular, left ventricular, and pulmonary artery pressure have been shown to increase breathing (149–154). These studies in total demonstrate ventilatory changes secondary to cardiac events, but the role of these mechanisms in the hyperpnea of exercise is unclear.

The hypothesis of pulmonary receptor mediation of the exercise hyperpnea has been directly tested by studying the effect of attenuating or eliminating pulmonary vagal feedback. Humans were studied after lung transplant (155), dogs were studied after anesthetic block of the vagi (156), and dogs (157,158) and ponies (159,160) were studied before and after sectioning of the hilar branches of the vagus nerves bilaterally. All these preparations yielded similar results. Attenuation of vagal activity decreased breathing frequency and increased tidal volume at rest and during exercise. However, $\dot{V}_E$, $\dot{V}_A$, and P_{aCO_2} (Fig. 4), were not altered following vagi sectioning or anesthetic block. Moreover, in ponies lactic acid was infused intravenously before and after lung denervation (159). At rest and during mild and moderate exercise, the $\dot{V}_E$ and P_{aCO_2} response to pulmonary and systemic acidosis ($\Delta pH = 0.10$) was not altered by lung denervation. Also, in anesthetized cats (161), lactic acid was infused in the inferior vena cava while NaOH was infused into the left atrium resulting in a pulmonary acidosis ($\Delta pH = 0.1$) and a normal arterial pH. This level of pulmonary acidosis failed to increase ventilatory drive. These data warrant concluding that the exercise hyperpnea is not critically dependent on pulmonary afferents. Moreover, if a pulmonary CO_2-H^+ sensory mechanism exists, its gain is too low to provide the primary ventilatory drive during exercise.

The cardiodynamic theory of the exercise hyperpnea has also recently been directly tested. Goats (43) have been studied before and after complete denervation of the heart. Heart rate, cardiac output, and arterial blood pressure during exercise were lower after than before cardiac denervation. However, $\dot{V}_E$ and P_{aCO_2} during exercise were not altered by denervation. Similarly, in human cardiac transplant patients, the $\dot{V}_E$ response to exercise does not differ from normal (155,162,163). Finally, during exercise by awake animals with artificial hearts (164), $\dot{V}_E$ did not change directionally with changes in $\dot{Q}_C$. These findings do not support the concept of cardiodynamic mediation of the exercise hyperpnea.

In summary, it has been shown that sensory mechanisms in the heart and lungs influence breathing. These mechanisms appear suited to and probably are important in the ventilatory responses to small changes in lung CO_2 delivery. In addition, lung afferents influence the pattern of breathing and the recruitment of respiratory muscles (see below) during exercise. However, the data that supposedly suggest these mechanisms contribute to the exercise hyperpnea are circumstantial and/or controversial. On the other hand, direct tests of their potential contribution have uniformly shown that the exercise hyperpnea is not critically dependent on cardiac and lung sensory mechanisms.

Neural Theories

Central Command Mediation of the Exercise Hyperpnea

Late in the 19th century it was proposed by Zuntz and Geppert (127) and Johansson (165) that a signal originating above the pons was capable not only of driving locomotion, but also of providing the associated changes in ventilation and circulation. Subsequently, Krogh and Lindhard (8) postulated that these central command signals originated in the motor cortex. Their postulate was based primarily on the rapidity of the ventilatory and circulatory responses, which could not be accounted for by any humoral mechanism.

Strong support for the central command theory comes from studies on decorticate cats that ambulate on a treadmill spontaneously or during electrical or chemical stimulation of hypothalamic locomotor regions (166–170). At least three studies in the 1920s and 1930s using this model showed that the respiratory and cardiovascular responses actually preceded spontaneous locomotion (168–170). This temporal pattern suggested the responses were not dependent on feedback. These findings were confirmed by studies of DiMarco et al. (166) and Eldridge et al. (167) in the 1980s, who, in addition, found the ventilatory response was proportional to the walking speed. Furthermore, Eldridge et al. (167) found the ventilatory response to locomotion was the same whether locomotion was spontaneously or electrically or chemically (picrotoxin) induced; thus, neurons must be activated in the hypothalamus rather than by stimulation of fibers of passage as might occur with electrical stimulation. Eldridge et al. also found the response the same during spontaneous and fictive locomotion. In the latter studies paralyzed cats were studied while phrenic and muscle nerve activity were monitored; the identical responses under paralyzed and unparalyzed conditions are consistent with central command as opposed to feedback regulation. Finally, midcollicular decerebration eliminated all responses to hypothalamic stimulation, indicating that current or picrotoxin spread did not account for the respiratory and circulatory responses.

The data obtained on these decorticate cats have at least two limitations. First, as with many preparations, the decorticate cat may not duplicate physiological exercise. Second, metabolic rate was minimally increased in these cats during locomotion. As a result, until there are some further assurances regarding these limitations, definitive conclusions cannot be reached from these data.

Data obtained during spontaneous exercise appears to support central command mediation of the exercise hyperpnea (171–176). Ventilatory and circulatory responses to bicycle ergometry were obtained under normal conditions and a second time during partial neuromuscular blockade with tubocurarine. At the same $\dot{V}O_2$ or at the same absolute work intensity, ventilation and heart rate were greater than normal during neuromuscular blockade. Since muscle strength is reduced with blockade, the same amount of work can be achieved only by increasing the number of active motor units, which is achieved by increasing neural output from the motor cortex. The increased ventilation with blockade is thus purported to be due to the increased "central command."

Inconsistent with central command are data on humans comparing responses during spontaneous exercise with responses during electrically induced exercise (177–179). These data indicate that the ventilatory responses do not differ between voluntary and electrically induced exercise. The essential question is whether the voluntary or central command component is absent during electrically induced exercise. Several investigators have provided compelling arguments that central command was absent; thus, it seems that the exercise hyperpnea is not critically dependent on central command signals to the respiratory controller.

Short-Term Potentiation as a Component of the Exercise Hyperpnea

When in a paralyzed, vagotomized, artificially ventilated cat the carotid sinus nerve is stimulated at a constant level, phrenic nerve activity increases immediately and then gradually increases over several minutes of stimulation (180–183). Once the stimulus is removed, there is an abrupt decrease in phrenic nerve activity, but nerve activity remains above control and decreases exponentially to control over several minutes. This type of response has been observed with many different modes of stimulation (184–187). Moreover, the phenomenon occurs in other neuronal systems such as locomotion and shivering (188,189). Several mechanisms have been proposed to explain this phenomenon, including altered levels of neurotransmitters (190), altered transmembrane electrochemical differences (191), and basic properties of synaptic transmission (192). Relative to this review, the important point is that it is an accepted phenomenon, and certainly it must be considered as possibly contributing to phase II of the exercise hyperpnea. In other words, a primary drive (neural or humoral) mediates the phase I of the exercise hyperpnea and it activates short-term potentiation, which contributes to phase II. However, to our knowledge no evidence is available that permits a quantitation of the potential effect of this phenomenon.

Peripheral Neurogenic Mediation of the Exercise Hyperpnea

It seems intuitive that information regarding chemical and/or mechanical conditions in contracting muscles contributes to the exercise hyperpnea. Moreover, a neural signal from the muscles could account for the rapid onset of the hyperpnea and the signal could be proportional to metabolic rate, thereby accounting for the matching of $\dot{V}_E$ and $\dot{V}O_2$. In addition, passive movement of the legs increases $\dot{V}_E$ (193–196). Accordingly, numerous studies have induced muscle contractions in anesthetized animals (125,197–206) (electrical stimulation of spinal ventral roots, motor nerves, or the muscles directly) or awake humans (178,179,207,208) (muscle stimulation) to gain insight into the role of peripheral neurogenic afferents in the exercise hyperpnea.

A series of studies by Kao provide strong support for peripheral neurogenic mediation of the exercise hyperpnea (126,197). The key feature of these studies was the apparent isolation of muscle afferents from not only central command, but also humoral stimuli. Muscle contractions of the hindlimbs of a dog were electrically induced. The blood perfusing these muscles was provided by a second dog through anastomosis of the abdominal arteries and veins of the exercising and nonexercising dogs. At the onset of muscle contraction, $\dot{V}_E$ increased in the exercising dog, but in the nonexercising dog $\dot{V}_E$ did not increase until its Pa_{O_2} decreased and Pa_{CO_2} increased. The hyperpnea in the exercising dog was eliminated by ablation of the lateral spinal columns or by transection of the spinal cord. The hyperpnea in the nonexercising dog was quantitatively consistent with $\dot{V}_E$ responsiveness to the observed changes in arterial blood gases. Kao thus concluded, "there is certainly a peripheral neurogenic drive which must be considered as the, or one of the mechanisms of exercise hyperpnea."

Some (198–203) but not all (204–206) the other studies on anesthetized animals support the conclusion of Kao. In support are the studies of Mitchell et al., who stimulated the spinal ventral roots to elicit muscle contraction resulting in a hyperpnea that was abolished by sectioning of the corresponding dorsal roots. In contrast, other investigative groups have shown that spinal cord transection does not abolish the hyperpnea of electrically induced muscle contraction in anesthetized animals (204–206).

The role of peripheral neurogenic afferents in the exercise hyperpnea has been studied in humans. In paraplegics electrically induced contraction of the paralyzed muscles results in a hyperpnea that is indistinguishable from voluntary exercise in spinal-cord-intact humans (178,179,207,208). These findings suggest that the hyperpnea is mediated by a humoral mechanism. However, when, in paraplegics, cuffs around the contracting muscles were inflated to prevent venous return from the muscles, Pa_{CO_2} decreased and then there was a decrease in $\dot{V}_E$, which was predictable from the decrease in Pa_{CO_2} (208). In other words, these findings were inconsistent with humoral mediation of the hyperpnea in paraplegics during electrically induced exercise. The possibility therefore remains that an unknown neural pathway exists in the paraplegics, or indeed central command is somehow activated. The role of neurogenic afferents has also been studied in spinal-cord-intact humans using epidural anesthesia at L-3 to L-4 to block peripheral afferents. This procedure had no effect on the hyperpnea during bicycle exercise (209). A complication with the epidural block studies is that the block created a marked arterial hypotension, which per se may increase breathing (210). This increase potentially offsets the reduction in peripheral neurogenic stimuli resulting in a normal exercise hyperpnea. Accordingly, the paraplegic and epidural block data appear inconsistent with peripheral neurogenic mediation of the exercise, but complications render any conclusion tentative.

In many of the aforementioned studies, it is questionable whether the technique provides the exact type of contraction found during voluntary exercise. This consideration led to a recent study in which ponies were studied during exercise before and 3–4 weeks after attenuating spinal afferents through L-1 lesions of dorsal lateral spinal pathways (211). After lesioning, the exercise hyperpnea was less than normal, consistent with a contribution from peripheral neurogenic stimuli to the exercise hyperpnea (Fig. 4).

What is the possible source of peripheral neurogenic stimuli? Hornbein et al. found in humans that blockade of gamma-efferent fibers with lidocaine did not alter the hyperpnea during bicycle ergometry (212). These data indicate muscle spindles do not contribute to the hyperpnea. McCloskey and Mitchell (201) found that the hyperpnea during induced contractions in anesthetized animals was not altered by anodal block of large myelinated fibers, but it was abolished by anesthetic block of small myelinated and unmyelinated fibers. These group III and IV afferents could provide information relative to the mechanical or metabolic conditions in the muscles, and changes in extracellular $[K^+]$, $[H^+]$, or [lactate] might contribute to the latter (213,214,215).

As with each of the postulated mechanism for mediation of the exercise hyperpnea, there are data both supportive and not in support of a role for peripheral neurogenic stimuli. On balance, though, the evidence indicates muscle contractions do reflexly elicit an increase in breathing, but it is unclear to what extent these afferents contribute to the normal exercise hyperpnea.

Neural and Humoral Mediation of the Exercise Hyperpnea

It has been proposed that no single factor mediates the exercise hyperpnea. Dejours ascribes the initial, fast $\dot{V}_E$ response to a neural pathway and the phase II slow rise in $\dot{V}_E$ to humoral pathways (5). The exact nature of each component of this "neurohumoral" theory was not specified by Dejours, but it was emphasized that the combined effects of small changes in several blood-borne substances might constitute the humoral stimulus. In other words, for humans slight increases in plasma $[K^+]$, Pa_{CO_2}, catecholamines, pulmonary P_{CO_2}, and core temperature may provide sufficient stimulation to account for the phase II of the exercise hyperpnea, or phase II may result from short-term potentiation.

Yamamoto (216) proposed that there are "many sufficient mechanisms, each of which in a given, isolated circumstance, explains the whole phenomenon. When they act simultaneously, they mask each other." This reasoning attempts to reconcile the widely differing neural and humoral theories, many of which claim to be capable of explaining the entire exercise hyperpnea. There are two reported attempts to test this reasoning. Waldrop et al. (79) in anesthetized cats found that the summed $\dot{V}_E$ response to activation of central command and to neurogenic feedback when given separately exceeded the $\dot{V}_E$ response when the two mechanisms were activated simultaneously. Additional data suggest that the central command mechanism normally predominates. As stated previously, it is questionable whether this preparation represents physiological exercise.

Pan et al. (113) in awake ponies determined whether the breathing and Pa_{CO_2} response to exercise after three lesions [carotid body denervation (CBD), hilar nerve denervation (HND), and partial spinal lesion] was predictable from the individual effects of each lesion. Given their previous finding that at the onset of exercise CBD accentuates the exercise hypocapnia (15), HND does not affect the $Paco_2$ response (160), and partial spinal lesion attenuates the hypocapnia (211), they predicted the exercise hypocapnia would be less after all three lesions than it was with only CBD. They found, though, that the hypocapnia was greater after all three lesions than with CBD alone (Fig. 5). Moreover, they found that HND after CBD and spinal lesioning always accentuated the hypocapnia, which contrasts to absence of an effect on $Paco_2$ of HND alone or in combination with CBD or spinal lesioning. The accentuation after all three lesions was due to a markedly increased V_T during exercise. These data do not provide support for redundancy because the effect was actually opposite to expectations. However, these findings do not rule out redundancy because additional potential pathways for mediation of the hyperpnea were still intact. As a result, it is presently unclear whether indeed, as Yamamoto (216) proposed, there are redundant pathways for mediation of the exercise hyperpnea. Nevertheless, given the redundancy that exists in other aspects of ventilatory control (peripheral and central chemoreceptors, peripheral and central influences on termination of inspiration, etc.) and given the vital nature of the exercise hyperpnea to survival, the reasoning of Yamamoto seems intuitive.

Mechanism of Hyperventilation During Heavy Exercise

Increased H^+ stimulation of the carotid chemoreceptors is the most prevalent explanation for the hyperventilation in humans during heavy exercise (5,19,21, 217,218). This theory is suggested by the close correlation of the hyperventilation and plasma $[H^+]$. In other words, in humans hyperventilation is minimal and plasma pH is near normal at work intensities below about 60% of maximum, but between 60 and 70% of maximum $\dot{V}o_2$, hyperventilation is accentuated and a lactacidosis becomes apparent. Both hyperventilation and plasma lactacidosis progressively increase as work intensity is increased beyond 70% of maximum (19,21,32).

Carotid chemoreceptor mediation of the heavy exercise hyperventilation could result from factors in addition to increased $[H^+]$. Plasma K^+ (100,223) and catecholamine (224–229) concentrations are elevated during exercise, and each of these is known to increase chemoreceptor activity. Moreover, the exercise and hypoxic ventilatory stimuli are known to have a synergistic facilatory effect on ventilation (18,82,87,230). Finally, the synergism might also occur at the carotid chemoreceptors between H^+, Po_2, K^+, and catecholamines (100,111,230–232).

Carotid chemoreceptor mediation of the heavy exercise hyperventilation is supported by studies showing that increasing Pao_2 by increasing PI_{o_2} during heavy exercise results in a decrease in $\dot{V}_E$ and plasma (lactate) and an increase in $Paco_2$ and arterial pH (11,217,233). Hyperoxia presumably reduces both H^+ and Pao_2

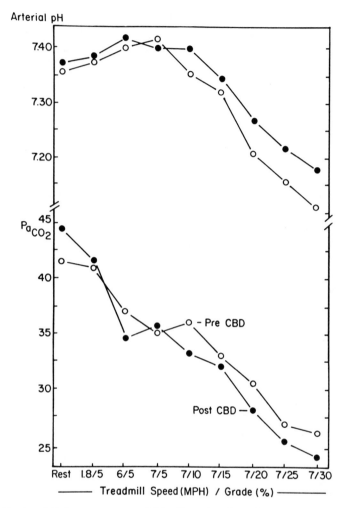

Figure 5 Arterial plasma pressure of CO_2 (Pa_{CO_2}) and arterial plasma pH in one pony during a progressive treadmill test to exhaustion before and two months after carotid body denervation. (Data obtained in laboratory of H. V. Forster.)

stimulation of carotid chemoreceptors. In addition, hyperoxia reduces the synergism between the P_{O_2} and the exercise stimuli and it likely also reduces the synergism among the humoral stimuli. There are thus several potential ways by which hyperoxia reduces chemoreceptor activity. Other evidence suggests, though, that the reduced $\dot{V}_E$ with hyperoxia might not be solely chemoreceptor-mediated. Specifically, increasing Pa_{O_2} from ~200 to 600 mmHg reduces $\dot{V}_E$ an amount similar to the decrease when Pa_{O_2} is increased from $\sim$90 to $\sim$200 mmHg (11,233). It seems unlikely that O_2-dependent chemoreceptor activity decreases further between a Pa_{O_2} of 200 and 600 mmHg. However, this change in P_{O_2} might reduce chemoreceptor responsiveness to H^+, K^+, and/or catecholamines. In addition, this increase in Pa_{O_2} might reduce plasma levels of the H^+, K^+, and/or catecholamines. Accordingly, uncertainty remains regarding the contribution of the carotid chemoreceptors to the reduction in $\dot{V}_E$ during heavy exercise when Pa_{O_2} is increased.

Often cited as support for carotid chemoreceptor mediation of the hyperventilation during heavy exercise are the findings that CCR asthmatics do not hyperventilate during heavy exercise (22,58). However, these CCR asthmatics were hypercapnic and acidotic even during mild exercise, and recent data (56) suggest that asthma and not CCR is the primary cause of their abnormal ventilatory response to exercise (Fig. 3). Moreover, the response of the asthmatics is comparable to the effect of ventilatory loading in nonasthmatic humans (56,57). Since it was not established that pulmonary mechanics were normal during exercise in the CCR asthmatics, it seems that the CCR asthmatics are not an appropriate model to gain insight into the role of the carotid chemoreceptors in the hyperventilation of heavy exercise.

Two different sets of data from human studies are inconsistent with H^+ mediation of heavy exercise hyperventilation. First through dietary manipulation, lactic acid production during heavy exercise can be attenuated, but this attenuation is not accompanied by attenuation of the hyperventilation (219–221). Second, humans with McArdle's syndrome are incapable of producing lactic acid, yet they hyperventilate in a normal manner during heavy exercise (222,223). Both series of studies provide evidence of a dissociation between hyperventilation and acidosis during heavy exercise. However, the appropriateness of McArdle's syndrome subjects as a model for these studies is questionable simply because these subjects hyperventilate even during submaximal exercise. In other words, some factor causes hyperventilation at all workloads in these subjects but this factor is probably not present in normal subjects. Thus, the data on these subjects, like the CCR asthmatics data, do not provide clear insights into the heavy-exercise hyperventilation mechanism.

Equines are the only nonhuman mammals that have been studied extensively during heavy exercise. In chemoreceptor intact ponies there is no accentuated hyperventilation during heavy exercise (Fig. 1) (66). Rather exercise hypocapnia is linearly related to work intensity irrespective of arterial pH, which is alkaline below about 60% of maximum $\dot{V}_{O_2}$ and then becomes progressively acidotic above 60% of maximum (Fig. 1). In thoroughbred horses during heavy exercise, Pa_{CO_2} is actually above normal despite a very severe lactacidosis (67,68). The reason for this hypoventilation might relate to a limitation on $\dot{V}_A$ imposed by the entrainment of breathing frequency and limb movement (see section IV). In any event, plasma acidosis during heavy exercise in equines is not associated with accentuated hyperventilation. Absence of a correlation between plasma H^+ and hyperventilation in ponies does not by itself indicate that H^+ has no influence on the hyperventilation. Indeed, it has been shown that ponies hyperventilate when lactic acid is infused intravenously at rest and during mild and moderate exercise (159).

One study in humans (234) where carotid chemoreceptor activity was attenuated by halothane and one study in carotid denervated dogs (235) support the concept of metabolic acidosis stimulation of $\dot{V}_E$ through the carotid chemoreceptors. However, studies in dogs (236), rabbits (237), goats (238), and ponies (159) have shown that CBD does not eliminate the hyperpnea induced by intravenous acid infusion. Moreover, lung denervation alone or in combination with CBD does not alter the ventilatory response to acid infusion at rest or during mild and moderate exercise (159). Finally, the hyperventilation during acid infusion can be accounted for on the basis of rapid changes in cerebral extracellular fluid $[H^+]$ (239). These data clearly show that the carotid chemoreceptors are not required for an exogenous lactacidosis-induced hyperventilation. However, exogenous lactacidosis does not replicate totally the conditions during exercise-induced lactacidosis; thus, these data do not establish the role of the carotid, lung, or intracranial chemoreceptors during the heavy-exercise hyperventilation.

Ponies are the only species known to have been studied during maximal exercise without airway disease before and after CBD (Fig. 5) (66,98). The absence of the chemoreceptors does not attenuate the hyperventilation at any workload, including maximal exercise. In fact, even though CBD ponies are mildly hypercapnic at rest, their $Paco_2$ decreases during maximal exercise often to a value 1–2 mmHg lower than before CBD. This 1–2 mmHg represents a large difference in $\dot{V}_A$ considering the absolute level of $Paco_2$ and rate of CO_2 production. Clearly, then, total stimulus level must be greater after CBD. Conceivably, at the carotid chemoreceptors in normal ponies the effect of hypocapnia outweighs the effect of the metabolic acids, hyperkalemia, and increased catecholamines, resulting in a net reduced level of chemoreceptor activity during maximal exercise. CBD thus removes an inhibitory influence on breathing during heavy exercise resulting in hyperventilation that is greater in CBD ponies than in normal ponies.

The powerful inhibitory effect of carotid chemoreceptor hypocapnia on breathing has recently been documented in studies on awake dogs and goats using an isolated carotid perfusion procedure (240,241). For example, reducing Pco_2 about 10 mmHg selectively at the level of the carotid chemoreceptor alone in the unanesthetized dog (240) resulted in an immediate reduction of 25–50% in V_T and $\dot{V}_E$. This inhibitory effect on ventilatory output persisted (although at a reduced level) throughout 2 min of perfusion despite significant increases in arterial Pco_2 (and presumably significant acidification of the medullary chemoreceptors). This substantial inhibitory effect of carotid body hypocapnia on V_T and $\dot{V}_E$ was also shown to be equivalent to that of hyperoxia also applied to the isolated, perfused carotid chemoreceptor.

In summary, there are considerable data inconsistent with the traditional theory that the hyperventilation in humans during heavy exercise without airway disease is mediated by increased H^+ stimulation of the carotid chemoreceptors. Alternate theories of hyperkalemia, catecholamines, and/or stimuli synergism contributing to the hyperventilation are also not supported by the studies on CBD ponies. Another possible explanation is suggested by the linear relationship in ponies between exercise hypocapnia and work intensity indicating that the "primary" exercise drive might be related curvilinearly to work rate resulting in the accentuated hyperventilation during heavy exercise. Possibly the crurae experiments support this view; that is, at high work intensities "central command" must increase out of proportion to work rate in order to complete the desired task. Conceivably, the marked effect of hyperoxia on breathing during heavy exercise is due primarily to increased O_2 delivery to the muscles, which increases aerobic metabolism and reduces central command. Clearly, the mechanisms responsible for the hyperventilation of heavy exercise remain controversial with seemingly strong evidence supportive of both a stimulatory and an inhibitory role for the carotid chemoreceptor.

C. Summary and Conclusions on Mechanisms of Exercise Hyperpnea

Although controversy remains regarding the exercise hyperpnea mechanism, certain conclusions are warranted, as depicted schematically in Figure 6.

We believe that several factors influence breathing during exercise. One factor is the primary stimulus. We believe, however, that there are exercise stimuli rather than an exercise stimulus. Blood pressure regulation, temperature regula-

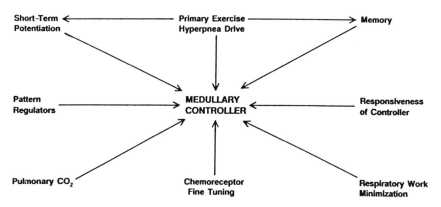

Figure 6 Schematic illustrating postulated role of various components of ventilatory control systems in hyperpnea of exercise.

tion, and other aspects of ventilatory regulation have redundant mechanisms, and therefore it is intuitive that redundancy exists in such a vital function as the exercise hyperpnea mechanism. There is no conclusive evidence for any of the postulated primary stimuli. However, there is rather convincing evidence that the known chemoreceptors and pulmonary afferents do not provide a primary drive. At rest or at low levels of CO_2 production, CO_2 delivery to the lungs or some factor related to it does appear to provide important information for breathing. However, this information or factor is normally superseded or overwhelmed by a distinct, non-CO_2 stimulus related to some other aspect of physiological exercise.

We feel that the primary exercise stimuli are feed-forward. Negative feedback as the primary mediator of the hyperpnea is not intuitive, and available evidence strongly suggests that during exercise the known feedback chemoreceptor mechanisms normally "fine-tune" breathing to the metabolic requirements.

We believe that short-term potentiation contributes to the hyperpnea. However, it cannot be considered "primary" because it requires activation by another stimulus.

We believe that chronic changes in $[H^+]$, chronic hypoxia, and/or neuromodulators influence the controller in a manner consistent with changes in its gain or responsiveness to the primary exercise drive.

We believe that spinal, lung, chest wall, respiratory muscle, and thermal afferents are important determinants of the pattern of breathing during exercise and that some of these afferents also are important in respiratory work minimization during exercise.

We believe that the exercise hyperpnea might be a learned response. Or, as Somjen (242) concludes, "the central nervous system (CNS) anticipates present and future needs on the basis of past experience." According to this theory negative feedback is of vital importance during infancy when "by having successfully corrected errors, the CNS learns how to prevent them." Learning by experience has been defined as "adaptive feed-forward control." Does such a system require central command, spinal afferents, and so forth to activate memory banks that evoke a ventilatory response that previously has been found successful, or do the brain's memory banks "employ principles different from all devices yet made by humans"? Conceivably, memory could account for inter- and intraspecies differences in the $\dot{V}_E$-$\dot{V}O_2$ relationship and differences or changes in the f and V_T responses to exercise.

III. Regulation of Respiratory Muscles During Exercise

Considerable emphasis has been placed on the regulation of exercise hyperpnea over the past 50 years. On the other hand, we know very little of how or by what mechanisms respiratory muscles are recruited during exercise to produce the appropriate hyperpnea. Only very recently have chronic animal models—especially the dog and pony—been utilized to study respiratory muscle recruitment during exercise. Considerable insight has been gained to date because of the use of a variety of quantitative techniques, such as chronically indwelling electromyographic (EMG) electrodes in a variety of primary accessory respiratory muscles, microsphere measurements of blood flow distribution among chest wall muscles, and sonomicrometry to measure dynamic changes in respiratory muscle length. We will concentrate on these data in the exercising quadruped. Unfortunately, in the human we must rely on more indirect techniques, such as body surface measurements of rib cage and abdominal compartments and of esophageal and gastric pressures to infer changes in respiratory muscle function during exercise. We will summarize both types of findings in this section, with emphasis on the more precise data obtained to date in the exercising quadruped.

A. Exercise-Induced Respiratory Muscle Activation in Quadrupeds

Numerous studies have shown that during quiet breathing in the standing awake quadruped (dog, pony, or horse), thoracic and abdominal expiratory muscle activity is normally present assisting the muscles of inspiration (243–247). In these three species, both inspiratory and expiratory muscle electrical activity is delayed relative to the onset of mechanical flow (Fig. 7), suggesting (1) that the initial generation of airflow during either phase of breathing is achieved by passive recoil of the antagonistic respiratory muscles and (2) that these species breathe *around* rather than from the relaxation volume (247). Ultimately, this delay in myoelectrical activation of respiratory muscles contributes, in part, to the biphasic airflow pattern normally seen during quiet breathing in the pony or horse.

However, during exercise the activation patterns of the major respiratory muscles change with respect to the *amplitude* and *onset* of myoelectrical activity. In addition, during exercise accessory muscles are recruited either tonically or phasically to assist the primary respiratory muscles, serving to stabilize the thoracic cage or to affect limb, head, or neck movements that may ultimately contribute to rib cage expansion.

Exercise-induced increases in inspiratory and expiratory muscles were first documented by DiMarco and colleagues (166), who examined phrenic nerve and intercostal muscle activity in decerebrate cats during spontaneously occurring or electrically induced walking. In either condition, they found *increases* in the peak phrenic neurogram and peak expiratory (internal) intercostal muscle activity. In contrast, peak inspiratory (external) intercostal muscle activity decreased. DiMarco et al. also found that during the onset of exercise, locomotory (quadriceps femoris) and respiratory muscles were simultaneously activated, suggesting that

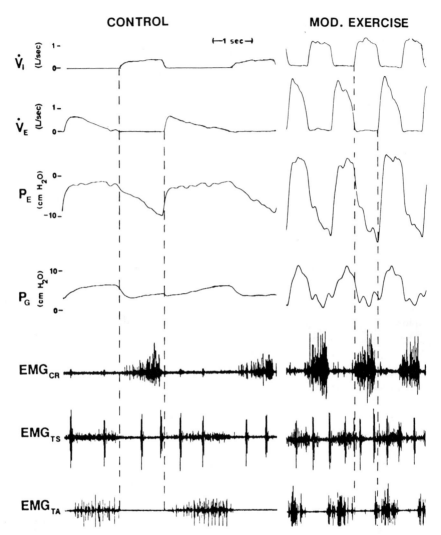

Figure 7 Inspiratory (V_I) and expiratory (V_E) flow rate, esophageal (P_E) and gastric (P_G) pressures, and EMG of the crural diaphragm (CR), triangularis sterni (TS), and transverse abdominal (TA) muscles during eupneic breathing and treadmill exercise (trotting) in a dog. The TS is contaminated by cardiogenic artifact. Note that during eupnea mechanical flow precedes electrical muscle activity and that gastric pressure decreases at the onset and throughout most of inspiration. During exercise, EMG activation is coincident with the mechanical flow, the qualitative features of gastric pressure signal are maintained, and end-expiratory esophageal pressure increases (248).

the primary input to respiratory muscle recruitment during exercise arose from descending inputs from the locomotory centers (see below). Yet, while an augmentation of respiratory muscle activity was clearly demonstrated in these studies, it remains uncertain to what extent the observed exercise bouts in this animal model (decerebrate cat) actually represented the coordinated natural walking activity of the intact cat. In addition, the severity of the exercise bouts remains uncertain as measurements of oxygen consumption or carbon dioxide production were not reported.

Using chronically instrumented dogs acclimated to treadmill exercise, Ainsworth and colleagues also examined exercise-induced alterations in both inspiratory and expiratory muscle electrical activity (248). In their study EMG activity was quantitated by dividing the area of the moving time averaged signal by the duration of electrical activity to yield the mean electrical activity (249). Using the mean electrical activity (MEA) as an index of activation, changes in the breathing pattern (decrements in inspiratory or expiratory times) or differences in the shape of the moving-time-averaged EMG signals (inspiratory vs. expiratory) were accounted for.

Ainsworth et al. (248) found that as $\dot{V}_{CO_2}$ and minute ventilation increased linearly with exercise intensity, phasic costal and crural electrical activity increased in a dose-dependent manner (Fig. 8). Such increases in electrical activity contributed to increases in phasic shortening of the diaphragm during exercise, as demonstrated in the sonomicrometry tracing from one chronically instrumented tracheostomized dog during treadmill exercise (Fig. 9). Such increases correlated well with the increase in both diaphragmatic EMG and tidal volume changes.

With regard to expiratory muscle activation during exercise, variable increases in abdominal or thoracic expiratory EMG occurred with low-intensity exercise (walking), but significant increases in phasic transverse abdominal or triangularis sterni (transverse thoracic) MEA were found only at the highest exercise intensity when the dogs were trotting—6.4 km/hr (Fig. 8). Furthermore, as ventilation increased, the onset of inspiratory and expiratory electrical activity occurred sooner and often coincided with the onset of mechanical flow (Fig. 7).

In this study, two additional but unique features of expiratory muscle activity during exercise were described. In some animals, phasic activation of *abdominal* muscles occurred during both inspiration and expiration and coincided with footplant. Such increases in EMG activity were clearly lacking in the thoracic expiratory muscles during exercise or in either abdominal or thoracic expiratory muscles during hypercapnic-induced hyperpneas at rest (250). This increased abdominal EMG activity in exercise supports a locomotory or a postural function for the transverse abdominal muscle. Second, exercise-induced increases in the *tonic* activity occurred in both the thoracic and abdominal expiratory muscles, as evidenced by positive shifts (1) in the mean gastric pressure signal and (2) in the baseline EMG activities of these muscles. Tonic alterations were not evident in the

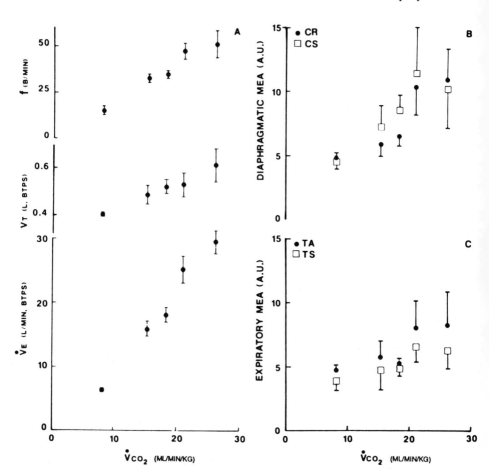

Figure 8 Mean (± standard deviation) ventilatory output (frequency, tidal volume, and minute ventilation) and respiratory muscle electrical activity (mean electrical activity) during eupnea and moderate treadmill exercise in chronically instrumented dogs. Crural (CR) and costal (CS) diaphragm EMG mean amplitude were significantly increased when V_{CO_2} exceeded 15.3 ml/min/kg. Triangularis sterni (TS) and transverse abdominal (TA) muscle activity were more variable and did not increase until $\dot{V}_{CO_2}$ exceeded 15.3 ml/min/kg (248).

diaphragmatic EMG. Thus increases in both *tonic* and *phasic* expiratory EMG activity contributed to decrements in end-expiratory lung volume (as inferred from increments in the end-expiratory esophageal pressure measurements) (251). Decrements in end-expiratory lung volume (EELV) due to expiratory muscle activation may have lengthened inspiratory muscles and improved their mechanical

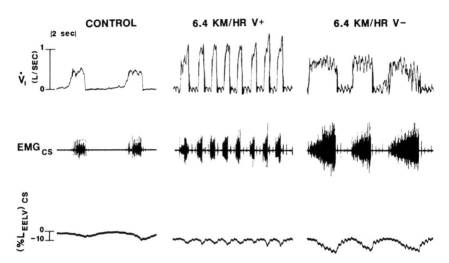

Figure 9 Inspiratory flow (V_I), costal diaphragmatic EMG, and sonomicrometry tracing from a chronically instrumented tracheotomized dog during eupnea and trotting with (V+) and without (V−) vagal blockade. Significant increases in diaphragmatic EMG occurred during exercise relative to the control. Removal of vagal afferent input from the lungs caused a further recruitment of the diaphragmatic EMG and increased tidal shortening. A significant lengthening of the diaphragm (end-expiratory length) was not found in this dog as a consequence of exercise-induced expiratory muscle recruitment.

efficiency. Such alterations in EELV were not noted during hypercapnic-induced hyperpneas where, despite comparable increases in phasic abdominal and thoracic expiratory muscle EMGs, tonic activation of the expiratory muscles was not evident (250).

Additional studies in equidae have further extended our understanding of respiratory muscle recruitment patterns during exercise. Gutting and co-workers (252) measured diaphragmatic and abdominal expiratory EMGs during graded treadmill walking in ponies (1.8 km/hr, 0%, 5%, and 10% grade). They found that as minute ventilation increased from 14 (eupnea) to 62 liters/min during exercise, significant linear increases in the rate of rise, peak, and MEA of the costal and crural EMG occurred during exercise. However, at this exercise intensity, significant increases in transverse abdominal MEA were not demonstrated. As a consequence, EELV failed to change with mild treadmill exercise. As the level of exercise and hyperpnea increased, Gutting et al. also found that (1) the delay between the onset of respiratory muscle electrical activity relative to the onset of mechanical flow was either eliminated or significantly reduced and (2) three of the four expiratory muscles (the rectus abdominous, the internal and external oblique muscles) exhibited phasic activity coincident with football.

In summary, the studies of Gutting and Ainsworth examining the muscle activation patterns of two types of quadrupeds during mild exercise have demonstrated (1) that abdominal expiratory muscle activity, normally present during eupneic breathing, is not significantly increased until a critical $\dot{V}_{CO_2}$ is exceeded, (2) that tonic activation of the expiratory muscles during exercise may serve a "shock absorber" function for the forces generated by footplant (253) and contribute to decrements in EELV, and (3) that abdominal expiratory muscles may assume functions that assist either locomotion or trunk stabilization.

While these studies have extended our knowledge of diaphragmatic and abdominal muscle recruitment patterns, the role of the "accessory" respiratory muscles—the interosseous intercostals, the sternocephalicus and scalenus— remains to be clearly defined. Do these muscles, which may not exhibit phasic activity during eupneic breathing, assume a role equal to that of primary respiratory muscles during exercise?

Additional studies provide *indirect* evidence for the activation of primary and accessory respiratory muscles during *high-intensity* exercise. Because muscle blood flow increases proportionately with muscle activity, Manohar's documentation of exercise-induced changes in equine respiratory muscle blood flow patterns has extended our understanding of muscle recruitment patterns during *maximal* exercise. Manohar studied galloping ponies that entrained their breathing frequency 1:1 with their stride frequency (254) (see below). Using radionuclide-labeled microspheres, he found that as oxygen consumption increased 38-fold during exercise to 126 ml/min/kg, there was a 22-fold increase in costal diaphragmatic blood flow (263 ml/min/100g tissue). On a per gram tissue basis, this increase in both costal diaphragmatic blood flow and oxygen delivery approximated the observed changes in blood flow to the hindlimb propulsive muscles, the gluteus medius and biceps femoris, or to the forelimb extensor muscle, the triceps brachii (254). Manohar concluded, based on the similarity of perfusion and oxygen delivery (per unit weight) to these two groups of muscles, that "diaphragmatic work and oxygen requirements during maximal exercise were not less than those of other vigorously working locomotory muscles of the pony."

In subsequent studies (255,256), exercise-induced increases in blood flow to other "inspiratory" muscles were documented. On a per gram tissue basis, crural flow more closely resembled that of the intercostal muscles. Furthermore, second to the diaphragm, the serratus ventralis showed the greatest percent increase in blood flow (Fig. 10). Lesser (but significant) increases in the blood flow to the external intercostals, serratus dorsalis, and scalenus muscles occurred (256). Among the "expiratory" muscles, the highest blood flows (on a per gram tissue basis) were found in the internal oblique and transverse thoracic (triangularis sterni) muscles. Blood flow to any expiratory muscle remained less than that to the

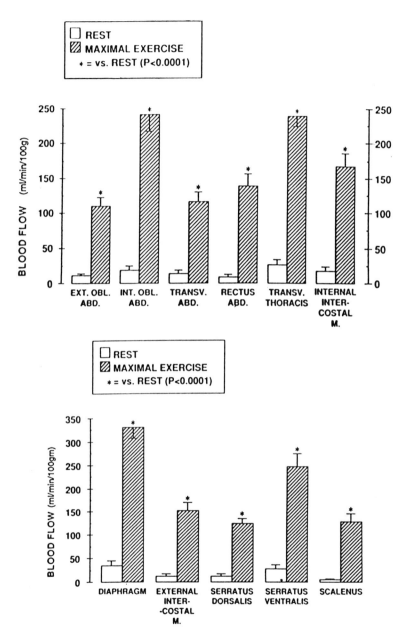

Figure 10 Blood flow to inspiratory (top) and expiratory (bottom) muscles during maximal treadmill exercise in ponies. Note the significant increases on a per tissue gram basis to all muscles examined (256).

diaphragm, which was surprising if, based on the studies of Gutting et al. (252), these muscles serve a locomotory role too. Collectively, the respiratory muscles received nearly 15% of the cardiac output during maximal exercise, with 8.4% of the cardiac output directed to the inspiratory muscles and 6.4% to the expiratory muscles (256).

As mentioned earlier, it is impossible to assess the *respiratory* role of these individual muscles based on perfusion values obtained during exercise. From these studies the locomotory or postural functions of these muscles cannot be partitioned out from the primary respiratory-related functions, especially given that respiration and locomotion were coupled 1:1 during exercise. Thus, it is uncertain whether these muscles function to primarily facilitate ventilation during exercise or whether their actions on the rib cage improve the mechanical efficiency of the diaphragm. However, based on the maximum or near-maximum blood flow rates observed by Manohar, there is no doubt that the metabolic requirements of these muscles increased markedly during maximal exercise.

B. Factors Regulating Respiratory Muscle Recruitment

Earlier we reviewed the theories on mechanisms of exercise hyperpnea. This section is devoted to the regulation and recruitment of respiratory muscle activity during exercise. Although our understanding of the specific input(s) remains limited, augmentation of inspiratory and expiratory muscle activities may be a consequence of (1) descending neural inputs from the locomotory centers (subthalamic and/or mesencephalic areas) activating respiratory centers in parallel, (2) proprioceptive inputs derived from pulmonary or chest wall mechanoreceptors modulating activity of medullary respiratory neurons, (3) peripheral or central chemoreceptor inputs responding to alterations in arterial gas tensions (hypoxia, hypercapnia) altering output of medullary respiratory neurons, and (4) non-respiratory-derived inputs (joint mechanoreceptors, muscle spindles) activating respiratory muscles recruited for the maintenance of posture or the movement of the limbs.

Proponents of the first hypothesis—that descending neural drives alter ventilation (and thus respiratory muscle recruitment)—advocate that motor pathways to both spinal locomotor pattern generators and respiratory neurons are simultaneously activated during exercise (8). The studies of DiMarco and colleagues (166), which demonstrated (1) synchronous changes in quadriceps and respiratory muscle EMG activity during the onset of exercise and (2) proportional increases between either integrated phrenic neurogram or expiratory intercostal EMG and the walking rate, have been cited as supportive evidence for this theory. However, one must remain cautious in concluding a causal relationship based on correlative data.

The facilitatory effects of pulmonary stretch receptor input on respiratory muscle activity during *eupneic* breathing have been investigated by several different groups using anesthetized or awake animal models (244,257–260). However, only recently have the modulating effects of pulmonary stretch receptors on respiratory muscle activity during exercise been defined in the canine species (261). Using the technique of reversible vagal cooling (156), Ainsworth studied respiratory muscle activation patterns in chronically instrumented tracheostomized dogs during moderate treadmill exercise (walking, trotting). Reversible cooling eliminated both phasic and tonic vagal inputs derived from slowly and rapidly adapting mechanoreceptors; inputs derived from nonmyelinated C-fibers, although attenuated, may have remained (262).

Ainsworth found that relative to the vagally intact exercise trials, at any given $\dot{V}CO_2$, vagal cooling was associated with further (significant) increases in the diaphragmatic, parasternal, and triangularis sterni EMG activity (Fig. 11). The increased EMG activity augmented tidal volume and diaphragmatic muscle tidal shortening (Fig. 9). This also suggested that during eupnea or during exercise, pulmonary mechanoreceptor inputs were normally *inhibitory* to the inspiratory and thoracic expiratory muscle activities. A comparable effect was not found with the transverse abdominal expiratory muscle (Fig. 11). During exercise with vagal blockade, transverse abdominal muscle EMG activity remained unchanged from the vagally intact exercise trials. That is, as tidal volume increased with vagal blockade during exercise, transverse abdominal muscle EMG activity did not increase *commensurate* with the tidal volume increases. Therefore, in the absence of pulmonary mechanoreceptor input, a greater percentage of the work of breathing during exercise was performed by the inspiratory and thoracic expiratory muscles. A similar finding was reported by Gutting et al., who studied diaphragmatic and transverse abdominal EMGs in hilar-denervated ponies during mild treadmill exercise (263). Thus vagal afferents influence respiratory muscle recruitment patterns and breathing patterns during exercise, even though these vagal influences are of little consequence to the overall hyperpnea (see above).

One additional important conclusion, pertinent to the underlying exercise-induced recruitment of respiratory muscle activity, became evident from the vagal blockade studies of Ainsworth. During these exercise trials, influences from pulmonary stretch receptor inputs were blocked and influences from chemoreceptors were unchanged or probably reduced because the dogs developed a mild hypocapnic-induced respiratory alkalosis during exercise. Nonetheless, large linear increases in inspiratory and expiratory EMG activity occurred as work rates increased. This must have been due to either feed-forward inputs from higher centers or from ascending inputs from the chest wall, diaphragm, or limb mechanoreceptors.

What evidence exists for ascending afferent modulation of respiratory muscle activity? Previous work in anesthetized or decerebrate cats has demonstrated the importance of intercostal muscles afferents on respiratory motoneuron

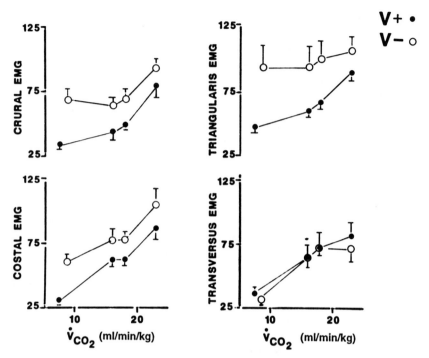

Figure 11   Mean electrical activity of the crural and costal diaphragm and two expiratory muscles, the triangularis sterni and transverse abdominal, during treadmill exercise in chronically instrumented tracheostomized dogs. Closed circles represent muscle activity (mean ± standard division, *n* = 5 dogs) during vagally intact exercise trials. Significant increases in inspiratory and thoracic expiratory activity occurred during vagal cooling (relative to vagally intact trials). No significant change in transverse abdominal activity occurred with vagal cooling, suggesting that locomotory-associated inputs assist in abdominal muscle recruitment during exercise (261).

activity. Decima et al. (264) demonstrated that proprioceptors in the lower thoracic intercostal and abdominal muscles exerted a facilitatory effect on phrenic motoneuron activity via spinal segmental pathways. In contrast, Remmers (265) found that afferent input from midthoracic segments exerted an inhibitory effect on phrenic output and that this effect was mediated via a supraspinal reflex. Furthermore, Shannon and colleagues found that selective stimulation of either external or internal intercostal tendon organs augmented only expiratory laryngeal motoneuron activity and either had no effect on or reduced the activity of the bulbospinal inspiratory or expiratory neurons (266,267). Although muscle spindles and tendon organs are relatively scarce within the diaphragm, group III and

IV thin-fiber afferents have been shown to stimulate inspiratory motor drive (268). However, whether these studies on muscle spindle afferents, tendon organs, or phrenic afferents, established in anesthetized or decerebrate animal models, can be extended to the awake exercising dog or horse is uncertain. Thus the effects of mechanoreceptor feedback from chest wall muscles or the diaphragm in the exercising quadruped remain to be established.

C. Entrainment of Breathing Frequency with Stride Frequency in the Quadruped

Locomotory-respiratory coupling (LRC) is a specialized breathing pattern adopted by many exercising mammals including the human (269). It has been observed in the trotting dog and pony (270,271) and in the cantering or galloping horse (272,273). A wide range of coupling ratios has been reported, but typically a 2:1 ratio is found in the trotting pony (271) and a 1:1 ratio in the galloping horse (272,273).

Although entrainment has been recognized in many cursorial mammals, little is presently known about the neural or biomechanical basis for it. In the model of the *cantering* horse proposed by Bramble and Jenkins (273) LRC is a consequence of biomechanical considerations. Inhalation begins as the horse becomes airborne and gathers all four limbs toward the trunk. Downward movement of the head and neck due to contraction of the sternocephalicus muscle simultaneously draws the rib cage forward. Forelimb extension prior to ground contact, enlarges the thoracic cage further, possibly through the action of the serratus ventralis muscle. Finally, in the last phase of inhalation, hip and hindlimb extension expands the abdominal cavity, decreases abdominal pressure, and causes a rearward displacement of the "visceral piston"—the liver and abdominal contents. These maneuvers aid the diaphragm in its caudal movement during inhalation. Accordingly, exhalation begins shortly after the impact of the nonleading forelimb. Concussive forces are transmitted to the thorax, thus externally loading and compressing the rib cage and decelerating the trunk. Expiration is further aided by contraction of the abdominal muscles, decreasing the abdominal volume and increasing the abdominal pressure.

Limited data support the plausibility of this biomechanical model. The required coordinated movements of the head-neck and hip-limb musculature, a biomechanical necessity, have been confirmed by kinematic analysis. While the role of the "visceral piston" has not been verified in the galloping horse, high-speed cineradiography of dogs running on a treadmill (273) suggests that there are substantial excursions of the liver and central diaphragm relative to the thoracic vertebral column during running.

Implicit in this biomechanical model is the importance of the accessory muscles (serratus ventralis, sternocephalicus) during locomotion. Specifically, their role may be to aid in either rib cage expansion or rib cage stabilization against longitudinal rotational forces incurred during forelimb ground contact. Furthermore, in this model, not only does the diaphragm serve as a primary muscle of respiration in the classical sense as a "pump," but this muscle, via its crural attachments, also provides a significant constraint on the inertial displacement of the visceral piston. Confirmation of this model awaits EMG and sonomicrometry studies demonstrating the tonic and phasic activities of primary and accessory respiratory muscles in exercising horses. Further modification of this biomechanical model is also required to describe the 2:1 entrainment ratios of the symmetrical gaits, the trot or pace, observed in either the horse or the dog.

What are the benefits of LRC? When one considers the substantial external loading forces that the thoracic cage is subjected to during locomotion and the subsequent shape and volume changes of the trunk produced with every stride, LRC would appear to be energetically beneficial to the exercising quadruped (273). That is, (1) muscles used for locomotion share in the task of airflow generation by expanding the rib cage, and (2) volume exchange is further aided either by externally applied concussive forces or by internal displacements of visceral tissue masses (liver, large intestine). However, such a beneficial role proposed for LRC is speculative, and such coordination may simply reflect evolution of the respiratory muscles from locomotory muscles rather than optimization of these two types of muscles (274,275).

However, consideration must also be given to the possible deleterious impact of entrainment on gas exchange. While stride frequency and respiratory frequency increase proportionately with exercise intensity during the canter or gallop, it is not known whether a proportionate increase in tidal volume occurs with changes in stride length. Can LRC limit further increases in tidal volume (and thus alveolar ventilation) relative to the changes in $\dot{V}CO_2$ or $\dot{V}O_2$ during maximal exercise in quadruped?

During mild exercise ($<60\%$ $\dot{V}O_{2max}$), the horse exhibits a ventilatory response analogous to that of other exercising quadrupeds with the development of a mild respiratory alkalosis. However, as oxygen consumption and carbon dioxide production increase to maximal levels of 142 ml/kg/min and 166 ml/kg/min, respectively, the horse fails to respond with an adequate hyperventilatory response (67). Severe respiratory and metabolic acidosis, arterial hypoxemia, and oxyhemoglobin desaturation in the face of isocapnia or hypercapnia ensue (67). The inability of the horse to achieve an appropriate compensatory hyperventilation theoretically could be the consequence of several factors, including (1) a mechanical limitation to the high ventilatory volumes required by the horse faced with an extraordinarily high CO_2 load, and (2) the imposition of a 1:1 LRC ratio restricting inspiratory and expiratory times available to achieve airflow rates sufficient to provide the needed alveolar ventilation. However, data from a recent study by Bayly and colleagues (276) suggested that LRC cannot explain CO_2 retention in heavy exercise. They attempted to determine the effects of increased stride frequency (and therefore increased breathing frequency) on exercise-induced CO_2 retention by comparing P_{aCO_2} between work rates that required the same $\dot{V}CO_2$ but had quite different breathing frequencies. This was accomplished by exercising the horses at different combinations of treadmill grade and speed (5, 7, 13 m/sec at grades 0–10%). Surprisingly, CO_2 retention still occurred to the same extent at a given exercise $\dot{V}CO_2$ independent of changes in the breathing frequency. Thus the rising CO_2 retention with increasing work rate could not be attributed to the accompanying increase in breathing frequency.

In summary, it would appear that at the exercise intensities examined in this study, entrainment did not contribute to the development of arterial hypercapnia. In fact, these investigators concluded that a 1:1 entrainment ratio, rather than a 2:1 ratio in which the tidal volume required for an adequate hyperventilatory response would have exceeded the vital capacity of the horse, appeared to be the best achievable ratio for the maximally exercising quadruped.

D. Exercise-Induced Respiratory Muscle Recruitment in the Human

In the healthy human knowledge of respiratory muscle recruitment depends primarily on indirect techniques. Measurements of diaphragmatic activity using gastric EMG electrodes placed near the gastroesophageal junction and transdiaphragmatic pressure show that the diaphragm is recruited roughly in proportion to the increasing exercise hyperpnea that occurs with increasing work rate (277). Estimating changes in body surface dimensions using respiratory inductive plethysmography suggests that the rib cage component contributes a greater proportion to the increasing tidal volume during exercise than at rest (278). The increased action of inspiratory accessory muscles is also suggested in humans (as it is in dogs) by the *reduction* in gastric pressure as rib cage volume expands during the initial phase of inspiration. This contrasts with the gastric pressure which increases throughout inspiration when the diaphragm is the sole inspiratory muscle, as is most likely the case under quiet resting conditions (278,279). The diaphragm muscle does not always recruit in proportion to increasing ventilation during exercise. For example, during exhaustive endurance exercise resulting eventually in diaphragmatic fatigue, the $\int P_{di}$ tends to plateau at a time when $\dot{V}_E$ and $\int P_e$ continue to increase markedly, suggesting that the diaphragm is contributing a smaller and smaller share to the total pressure generated by the inspiratory muscles as exercise proceeds (280). This finding in humans raises the intriguing possibility that the diaphragm might be "spared" from further fatigue during exhaustive endurance exercise by the recruitment of accessory inspiratory muscles—perhaps this inhibition occurs because the "beginnings" of fatigue-induced metabolic changes in the diaphragm might initiate inhibitory feedback via phrenic afferents (281).

The expiratory muscles in the abdominal wall become both tonically and phasically active even with very mild exercise such as loadless peddling on the bicycle ergometer at $\dot{V}_E \sim$ 15–20 L/min. This conclusion is based on many measurements of a progressive rise in gastric and esophageal pressure at end-expiration with increasing work rate and confirmed by a few measurements of abdominal muscle EMG using indwelling fine wire electrodes (282). The increasing abdominal muscle EMG phasic activity occurs in the transversus abdominus and rectus abdominus muscles in the human, although further analysis during the immediate recovery period suggests that much of the increased rectus abdominus activity is related more to locomotory activity such as hip flexion than to actual phasic expiration. During jogging or running marked tonic activation of the abdominal wall occurs—as is indicated by a sharp increase in the tonic level of gastric pressure in the transition from walk to jog (253,279). Grillner et al. (253) proposed that this increase in abdominal muscle tone is linked to the central locomotor "program" and may serve as a "shock absorber" for the vertebral column by dampening the force generated by the foot plant.

The phasic and tonic activation of expiratory abdominal muscles, together with the increased diameter and reduced resistance in the upper airway, results in an increase in expiratory flow rate that is sufficient to reduce end-expiratory lung volume progressively with increasing exercise despite a coincident progressive shortening of expiratory time with increasing work rate. Exercise appears to be unique in this respect because hyperpnea caused by only CO_2 rebreathing in upright subjects at rest rarely results in reduced EELV even when $\dot{V}_E$ is increased four to six times the air-breathing eupneic level (279). Advantages to be gained by abdominal muscle recruitment, increased gastric pressure, and reduced EELV during exercise are many. This recruitment is especially critical to ensuring a near-optimal length of the diaphragm and other inspiratory muscles at a time when the need for near-maximum generation of tension is required. A reduced EELV also protects against very high levels of end-inspiratory lung volume and therefore against incurring high elastic loads as tidal volume increases with increasing work rate.

Recruitment of pressure development by the expiratory muscles also appears to be quite efficient during exercise, as evidenced by the fact that pleural pressure during expiration does not exceed its maximum "effective" pressure. This "sparing" of expiratory pressure development by the expiratory muscles begins to become evident in the normal untrained subject in maximum exercise, but is more clearly demonstrated when extra CO_2 or hypoxia is superimposed at higher work rates (and higher $\dot{V}_E$ in the fitter subject) (also see section IV) (283). Additional (noneffective) expiratory pressures are not generated under these conditions—even though the superimposed chemoreceptor stimuli at these heavy workloads are very high ($Pa_{CO_2} > 50$ mmHg and $Pa_{O_2} < 40$–45 mmHg), and even though both locomotor-linked stimuli and hypercapnia normally do evoke strong expiratory muscle recruitment. Therefore, some very strong inhibitory overriding influences apparently prevail to prevent extensive, inefficient recruitment of expiratory muscles during maximum exercise. Alternatively, perhaps this is a "learned," feed-forward response from the higher central nervous system associated with the same descending neural pathways that produce limb locomotion and hyperpnea (284). In addition, we also know that there are strong inhibitory effects of afferent feedback from inspiratory muscles (diaphragm and intercostals) subjected to "fatiguing" loads or even excessive stretch (281). Perhaps these influences might also originate in expiratory muscles with a preponderance of spindle afferents. As discussed above, vagal feedback from lung stretch (i.e., pulmonary stretch receptors) has also been shown to be another important feedback mediator of rib cage and abdominal expiratory muscle activity, at least in the exercising dog (see Fig. 11).

IV. Mechanical Influences on Exercise Hyperpnea: Demand Versus Capacity

A. Lung and Chest Wall Mechanics in the Untrained

We are concerned in this final section with how mechanical properties of the lung and chest wall in a healthy person might impose significant constraints on flow rate, tidal volume, or respiratory muscle function during exercise. Certainly the bulk of the available evidence points to a near-ideally designed system in a healthy human to meet ventilatory requirements, as can be appreciated by examining the flow:volume and pressure:volume characteristics in healthy, young adults over a range of exercise intensities including the $\dot{V}_{O_{2max}}$ in the untrained (40–50 ml/kg/min) and that in the highly trained endurance athlete (65–82 ml/kg/min). In this first section we will concentrate on the response up to the normal untrained $\dot{V}_{O_{2max}}$.

As noted in Figure 12A and B, the tidal flow:volume and pressure:volume loop increases progressively with increasing exercise intensity, and end-expiratory lung volume is progressively reduced. At maximum exercise less than 10% of tidal volume is flow-limited and the expiratory pressure exerted barely reaches the lower limits of the maximum "effective" pressure, i.e., beyond which dynamic compression of airways occurs and further increases in expiratory pressure would not accomplish more flow rate. Finally, as noted in Figure 13, the dynamic capacity for pressure generation by the inspiratory muscles as determined at rest (283,285) is reduced with increasing exercise because inspiratory muscle length is reduced (with increasing tidal volume) and velocity of muscle shortening is increased (as flow rate increases). Nonetheless, the actual peak inspiratory muscle pressure

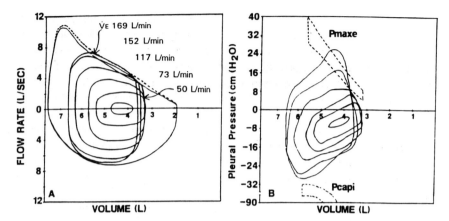

Figure 12 Mean flow:volume and pressure:volume loops in healthy young adult subjects shown across a continuum of work rates, including maximum $\dot{V}O_2$ in normally fit subjects ($\dot{V}_E$ = 117 L/min, $\dot{V}O_2$ = 40–50 ml/kg/min) and in highly fit subjects (maximum $\dot{V}O_2$ = 65–80 ml/kg/min; $\dot{V}_E$ = 169 L/min) (283).

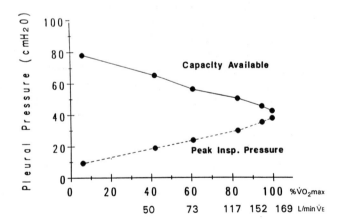

Figure 13 Capacity for inspiratory pleural pressure development (P_{cap_i}) versus the peak pleural pressure reached during tidal breathing, at increasing exercise intensities. The dynamic P_{cap_i} is determined at rest by volitionally varying the flow rate (velocity of shortening) and by performing maximum efforts against an occluded airway at varying lung volumes (i.e., varying inspiratory muscle length) (283).

developed with tidal breathing during maximum exercise is still only about 40% of the inspiratory muscle's capacity to generate pressure.

Despite the 10-fold increase in inspiratory-expiratory flow rates during exercise, airway resistance remains low and unchanged from rest primarily because of the regulation of the upper- and lower-airway caliber. First, the extrathoracic upper airway is both dilated and stiffened by increasing tonic motor activity—the latter being especially important because the extrathoracic airway is exposed to negative, collapsing transmural pressures during inspiration. Nasal airflow resistance is reduced in part owing to activation of the abductor alae nasae muscles and also because of vasoconstriction of the nares—the latter due to sympathetic activation (286). In addition, humans usually switch from a predominantly nasal route of ventilation to a much lower resistance oral route by means of the integrated action of the muscles controlling the oral pharynx and the position of the base of the tongue and soft palate (287). A key location in flow regulation occurs at the laryngeal aperture, whose diameter varies with the respiratory cycle, increasing during inspiration and narrowing during expiration. During all types of hyperpnea—including mild exercise—the expiratory narrowing of the laryngeal aperture is greatly attenuated—due primarily to the action of the posterior cricoarytenoid muscle (288). Finally, intrathoracic airway smooth muscle undergoes maximum relaxation and bronchodilation during exercise, causing a significant enlargement of the inspiratory and expiratory limbs of the maximum volitional flow:volume loop.

Just as with the regulation of the exercise hyperpnea, a complex variety of feedforward and feedback mechanisms are responsible for the regulation of intra- and extrathoracic airway caliber. One of these mechanisms is the stimulation of type III–IV nerve endings in contracting skeletal muscle, which has been shown to cause significant bronchodilation in anesthetized animals probably via inhibition at the medullary level of vagal efferent bronchoconstrictor activity (289). These are most likely the same muscle receptors (detailed in Section II) that have a significant effect on exercise hyperpnea. In addition, generation of negative pressure in the upper airway has been shown to produce a strong excitatory feedback effect via the superior laryngeal nerve to increase the stiffness and caliber of the upper airway (290). Although it has not yet been specifically demonstrated, we speculate that the feedforward, descending influences important in the activation of phrenic motor neurons and respiratory muscles of the chest wall during exercise also exert a strong effect on hypoglossal motor neurons and skeletal muscles controlling the stiffness and diameter of the upper airway.

These mechanisms cause maximum airway dilation, upper airway stiffness, and minimization of resistance to airflow during exercise, which in turn minimizes the pleural pressure required by the inspiratory muscles. A further benefit is that expiration can also be completed and hyperinflation avoided despite the greatly increased breathing frequency and reduced expiratory time that occur during heavy exercise.

Dynamic lung compliance is reduced by only 10–20% during exercise and only at maximum workloads. The likely major reason for this reduction is the encroachment of the tidal volume on the upper, alinear portion of the pressure:volume relationship as V_T exceeds 50% of vital capacity and 80% of total lung capacity. The fact that C_{dyn} is not markedly reduced (and therefore elastic loads greatly increased) is in part due to the careful regulation of frequency and tidal volume contributions to the ventilatory response. In turn, the activation of the inspiratory terminating "off switch" and therefore limitation of tidal volume in exercising humans is most likely due to inhibitory vagal feedback at tidal volumes greater than about 40–50% of inspiratory capacity—although the data concerning this mechanism in healthy humans are limited (291).

Why is it that inspiratory muscles generate only 40–50% of their capacity at maximum exercise in the untrained, healthy individual? Part of this answer is to be found simply in the low ventilatory requirements relative to the very large capacity of the diaphragm and other inspiratory muscles to generate pressure. An additional important factor that spares the relative intensity of inspiratory muscle pressure generation (for any given inspiratory flow rate) is the progressive reduction in end-expiratory lung volume with increasing exercise. This means that inspiratory muscles are operating at a longer and longer length and therefore at a much higher capacity for pressure development. Without this reduced end-expiratory lung volume, P_{cap_i} would have been reached during tidal breathing at heavy submaximal exercise in many normal subjects. As inferred from the foregoing discussion in Section III, several factors ensure a progressive decline in EELV with increasing exercise, including a lower airway resistance because of dilation of the intrathoracic airway and abduction and stiffening of the upper airway, as well as a reduced compliance of the abdominal compartment combined with a strong phasic activation of expiratory muscles of the abdomen and rib cage (279). Of course, none of this would be effective in reducing EELV in the face of an increasing breathing frequency and markedly reduced T_E if expiratory flow rate became significantly limited by dynamic compression of the airways during expiration. The fact that this does not occur speaks to the structural integrity of the intrathoracic airways, permitting them to remain patent over almost all of the tidal volume range at maximum exercise.

Up to this point we have emphasized the "overbuilt" structural capacity of the lung and chest wall in meeting the ventilatory requirements of exercise, but what does this mean in terms of the oxygen cost of hyperpnea and respiratory muscle fatigue? Furthermore, is the ventilatory output affected by the mechanical loads imposed?

While many and varied estimates of the cost of ventilation are available based on the $\dot{V}O_2$ that accompanies voluntary changes in ventilation in the resting subject, applying these estimates to heavy exercise is a major problem because the same level of hyperpnea accomplished during exercise will not usually require the same level of work or pattern of respiratory muscle recruitment as that accomplished voluntarily at rest (284). A recent study of Aaron et al. (292) has attempted to overcome this shortcoming by requiring the subjects to duplicate (via visual and audio feedback) their esophageal pressure:volume loop attained at submaximal and at maximal exercise—along with the breathing frequency and end-expiratory lung volume. The $\int P_{di}$ and $\int P_g$ experienced during exercise were also fairly closely duplicated by the voluntary "mimicking" trials. In nine normal subjects of varying fitness levels over a range of exercise $\dot{V}_E$ in the 75–120 L/min range with little or no expiratory flow limitation (as in Fig. 12), the oxygen cost *per liter* $\dot{V}_E$ increased about 10–15% (from 1.8 to 2.1 $mlO_2/min/L\dot{V}_E$) as $\dot{V}_E$ increased from 75 to 120 L/min. This amounted to an O_2 cost of ventilation that averaged 7–8% of $\dot{V}_{O_{2max}}$. This cost should not detract significantly from blood flow to locomotor muscles and is probably not sufficient to cause fatigue in the primary inspiratory muscles. Two types of evidence in humans speak against the possibility of inspiratory muscle fatigue under these short-term maximum exercise conditions. Levine and Henson (293) used the bilateral phrenic nerve stimulation technique to show objectively that short-term, progressive exercise to exhaustion did not result—with few exceptions—in significant decrements in the supramaximally stimulated P_{di}. Furthermore, when the pressure:volume (work) loop achieved doing maximum exercise was mimicked in the resting subject (as described above), the subject was able to maintain the $\int P_e$ for more than four times longer than the exercise period itself without evidence of task failure (292).

Finally, what role, if any, might be played by the mechanical loads incurred during exercise by the lung and chest wall on the regulation of exercise hyperpnea and/or respiratory motor output? The problem is controversial. On the one hand, some studies have used $He:O_2$ breathing to bring about a 35–40% reduction in airway resistance during exercise. At heavy workloads $He:O_2$ inhalation always caused an immediate and sustained increase in breathing frequency and $\dot{V}_I$. However, at more moderate workloads $He:O_2$ did not always result in significant increases in $\dot{V}_E$, but consistently caused immediate reductions in EMG activity of the diaphragm and transdiaphragmatic pressure coincident with the reduction in airway resistance, and these effects were immediately reversible upon return to air breathing and to normal airway resistance (294). These data point to the existence of a compensatory response during normal air-breathing exercise, which is sensitive to the mechanical load presented by the normal mechanical time constant of the respiratory system. This mechanoreceptor feedback-driven response should be considered an integral, although relatively small, portion of the total normal "drive" to breathe during exercise (see Section II). On the other hand, studies using a unique "proportional-assist" ventilator to provide even greater mechanical unloading during moderate exercise reported *no* compensatory ventilatory responses and claimed that the normal resistive load during exercise is without consequence to ventilation or respiratory motor output (295). Why there should be such marked differences between unloading studies is not clear, although the unloading techniques are certainly quite different, as are the means of measuring changes in respiratory motor output. This question of whether a normal mechanical impedance has any role in determining the normal respiratory motor output and exercise hyperpnea needs to be attacked comprehensively using various methods and degrees of "unloading" during varying levels of exercise intensity. Most important, measures of inspiratory and expiratory motor output in the form of EMG measurements of several primary and accessory respiratory muscles of the chest and abdominal wall need to be analyzed during the transitional and steady-state periods of unloading and loading.

Up to now we have considered several characteristics of the normal regulation of lung and chest wall mechanics during exercise, with the primary conclusion that exercise hyperpnea is carried out well within the structural reserves available to the healthy human. On the other hand, the metabolic cost of hyperpnea is indeed significant and the flow resistive load is probably "sensed" and at least partly compensated for by an augmented respiratory motor output. However, these costs and efforts are clearly not excessive, inspiratory and expiratory flow rates and volumes and inspiratory muscle pressure development are well below their respective capacities, and diaphragm fatigue does not occur. Accordingly, it is doubtful that the magnitude of exercise hyperpnea is constrained by mechanical limitation. On the other hand, this evidence does not permit us to conclude that substantial functional reserve is *always* present during exercise in *all* components of the healthy human pulmonary system or that exercise hyperpnea is *never* subjected to mechanical constraint or that the energy cost of hyperpnea is never excessive or may contribute to respiratory muscle fatigue. We now describe physiological conditions where this indeed may be the case.

B. Continuum of Demand Versus Capacity

A wide spectrum of maximum performance capacity exists among healthy humans as indicated by a more than twofold spread in $\dot{V}O_{2max}$ among normal healthy adults—even at any given age or gender. If homeostasis within the pulmonary system is to be maintained across this spectrum of demand, these changing metabolic requirements demand either of two circumstances:

1. That the existing capacities of the lungs, airways, and respiratory muscles have sufficient reserve (or are sufficiently "overbuilt") to meet the changing ventilatory demands as $\dot{V}O_{2max}$ increased, or

2. That these structures, like those of the locomotor and cardiac muscles, are adaptable and their respective capacities will increase proportionately.

Adaptability of the Pulmonary System Along the Fitness Continuum

The pulmonary system—lung and chest wall—shows only modest adaptability to chronic physical training when compared to other links in the gas transport chain. The lung gas exchange surface area undergoes virtually no structural adaptations—even when the maturing animal undergoes physical training (296). Furthermore, many athletic and nonathletic animals of similar body mass (e.g., cow vs. horse) may differ almost threefold in $\dot{V}o_{2max}$ (demand) and in mitochondrial volume of locomotor skeletal muscle, but will vary <50% in the area of their pulmonary diffusion surface (297). Lung volumes and flow rates also differ little between the highly fit and unfit human, as the maximum volitional flow:volume loops are virtually superimposable throughout inspiration and expiration (283). Structurally, then, one would expect lung elastic recoil and airway compressibility to be comparable among highly fit and normally fit subjects. Some exceptions to this rule may exist in the maturing competitive swimmer, who has exceptionally large lung volumes, or in the older fit subject (65–80 years), who has substantially increased MEF_{50} compared to his less fit contemporaries (298,299). Limited long-term data (300) suggest that swim training, per se, might actually cause 10–15% increases in vital capacity and total lung capacity, although in most studies it is difficult to distinguish between the effects of training and what the athlete has brought to the sport.

Respiratory muscles do tend to show significant, although somewhat limited, adaptability to physical training. Rats have been studied extensively in this regard. Consensus from a wide variety of studies is that aerobic enzymatic capacity does increase in respiratory muscles—but to a substantially lesser extent than in limb locomotor muscles of similar fiber type. The costal diaphragm is the most susceptible to change and the crural diaphragm the least susceptible. The relative intensity and duration of the training regimen does determine the degree of mitochondrial adaptability in some, but not all, respiratory muscles (301,302). Antioxidant enzymatic activity in the diaphragm also increases with physical training, thereby making this muscle better equipped to reduce the oxidative stress caused by the increased mitochondrial respiration. In humans, studies using running and swim training show increases in maximal sustainable ventilation, an indirect volitional test of respiratory muscle endurance (300,303). Maximum pressure development against the occluded airway, i.e., an estimate of inspiratory muscle strength, did not differ in the highly trained and untrained subjects.

So the adaptability of the healthy lung and chest wall to whole-body physical training is significant but limited. Accordingly, there are several examples of ventilatory demand either encroaching significantly on or sometimes even exceeding ventilatory capacity as metabolic and ventilatory requirements at maximum exercise increase with increasing fitness level. Examples are shown in the series of flow:volume loops in Figure 12A and B obtained during progressive exercise. As the fitter subject surpasses the normal $\dot{V}O_{2max}$, $\dot{V}_E$ rises and several signs of significant mechanical limitation begin to occur, all of which increase in severity as ventilatory demand increases and approaches closer and closer to the structural capacity of the airways, lung, and respiratory muscles.

First, more and more of the tidal volume experiences flow limitation during expiration with increasing exercise, starting with about 10% at 120 L/min and increasing progressively to 55–65% of the tidal volume at 160–170 L/min. End-expiratory lung volume rises back toward, but rarely ever above resting FRC. This relative hyperinflation is probably the *net* effect of some reduction in expiratory muscle pressure development in the face of greater and greater dynamic compression of the airways and flow limitation. Pressure generation by the expiratory muscles continues to increase but remains "effective" in terms of flow production and increasing $\dot{V}_E$. On the inspiratory side, peak pressure generated by the muscles increases with increasing ventilation whereas the dynamic *capacity* for generating inspiratory pressure is reduced because of decreasing muscle length (higher tidal volume and increasing EELV) and increasing velocity of muscle shortening (increased inspiratory flow rate) (see Fig. 13). So, the inspiratory muscles are working at a greater and greater fraction of their maximum capacity for pressure development, and as shown in Figure 13, in some really highly fit subjects the capacity is actually reached during tidal breathing at maximum exercise.

From rest through maximum exercise, inspiratory flow resistance remains constant but expiratory flow resistance eventually rises with increasing expiratory flow limitation. Thus during heavy exercise, ventilatory work rises markedly as inspiratory and expiratory flow rates continue to increase to >10 times resting levels. Elastic work also rises and C_{dyn} falls as an increasing tidal volume and a rise in EELV displace end-inspiratory lung volume to the upper, stiffer portions of the pressure:volume relationship. Accordingly the O_2 cost *per liter* ventilation begins to rise progressively with the onset of significant expiratory flow limitation, amounting to an increase of 30–50% as $\dot{V}_E$ increases from 120 to 160 L/min and inspiratory and expiratory work rises out of proportion to the rising $\dot{V}_E$. Thus, the O_2 cost of ventilation ($\dot{V}O_{2RM}$) requires more than 10% and as much as 15–17% of $\dot{V}O_{2Tot}$ at max exercise (292). Interestingly, despite these high costs per unit $\dot{V}_E$ and the fact that $\dot{V}_E$ is rising in a curvilinear fashion while the rate of increase in $\dot{V}O_{2Ttot}$ is falling at these high work rates, the increase in $\dot{V}_E$ remains "useful" as the O_2 cost of increasing $\dot{V}_E$ alone never exceeds the increase in total body $\dot{V}O_2$ (292).

Mechanical Constraints on the Hyperventilatory Response

What are the implications of these increasing demands along the normal continuum of increasing fitness levels to the regulation of exercise hyperpnea and hyperventilation? First it should be noted that absolute limitations to exercise ventilation are achievable in healthy subjects. This can be demonstrated in highly fit young adults (Figs. 12 and 14). Examination of the air-breathing flow:volume and pressure:volume loops at maximum exercise shows that the limits of flow and volume have indeed been nearly reached. This is suggested by the expiratory pressure development matching the effective maximum pressure and the peak inspiratory pressure development during a tidal breath matching P_{cap_i}. There are still small portions of the maximum volitional flow:volume loop at the initiation of inspiration and expiration that are not used. To test whether maximum "available" $\dot{V}_E$ was truly reached under these circumstances, hypercapnia up to >60 mmHg PET_{gO_2} or hypoxemia down to 75% Sao_2 was superimposed on maximum exercise. $\dot{V}_E$ and the flow:volume loops obtained during air breathing at maximum exercise remained unchanged despite these marked increases in chemoreceptor stimuli. Apparently, then, the maximum volitional breathing pattern is not chosen during maximum exercise regardless of the magnitude of the drive to breathe—probably because volitional breathing patterns commonly generate so much excessive, nonproductive pressure development, especially during early expiration.

Even at submaximal work loads and at more moderate levels of ventilatory requirement, there is indirect evidence of mechanical "constraint" on ventilatory output. For example, the slope of the ventilatory response to inhaled CO_2 remains unaltered with increasing levels of submaximal exercise until $\dot{V}_E$ is in the range of

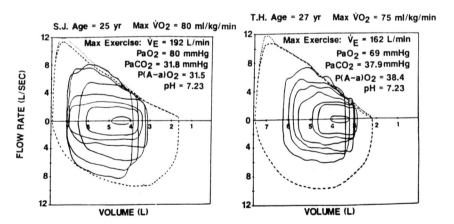

Figure 14 Flow:volume loops at varying exercise intensities including maximum and arterial blood gases at maximum exercise in two very fit runners. S.J. showed a substantial hyperventilation despite having reached complete (mechanical) limitation to flow and volume and having reached the capacity for pressure generation by the inspiratory muscles. On the other hand, T.H. was well short of his mechanical limits to ventilation, yet showed insignificant levels of hyperventilation and substantial arterial hypoxemia (283).

~120 L/min. Thereafter the response slope to inhaled CO_2 is reduced progressively (81). The hyperventilatory response to mechanical unloading via $He:O_2$ inhalation also becomes most consistent and prominent at these workloads (61). That this response to $He:O_2$ represents a true "unloading" effect at these high work rates may be appreciated by also noting that the hyperventilation caused by $He:O_2$ inhalation was substantially in excess of that caused by a superimposed hypoxia, even down to SaO_2 in the range of 70–75%. We could predict that this mechanical constraint effect on ventilatory output would begin to be manifested coincident with the occurrence of significant expiratory flow limitation, i.e., when >25% of the Vt is flow limited.

Mechanical limitation is certainly not the only factor determining the magnitude of the hyperventilatory response during heavy exercise. This hyperventilatory response is also determined to a significant extent by the available levels of feedforward and feedback stimuli and the degree of "responsiveness" to the combination of these stimuli at any given degree of mechanical limitation. This diversity among subjects' "responsiveness" is illustrated by contrasting two very fit subjects shown in Figure 14. Subject SJ showed a mild hyperventilation throughout exercise and a marked hyperventilatory response during his two final workloads, $PaCO_2$ was reduced to 31–32 mmHg with PaO_2 > 80 mmHg, and complete mechanical limitation of $\dot{V}_E$ was reached over the final two workloads. In contrast, subject TH showed moderate hyperventilation throughout exercise with significant but minimal hyperventilation (-2–3 mmHg $PaCO_2$) at very heavy and maximum work rates. This very minimal level of hyperventilation occurred *despite* an accompanying hypoxemia (PaO_2~65 mmHg) and acidosis and in the face of a significant mechanical reserve remaining for flow, volume, and inspiratory muscle pressure development. Clearly there is a marked difference between these subjects in their relative responsiveness to the many feedforward and feedback stimuli that accompany maximum exercise. We believe these individual differences in the degree of hyperventilation achieved during heavy exercise are attributable to inherent differences in responsiveness to the complex combination of mechanical loads placed on both the inspiratory and expiratory muscles and the available chemical stimuli.

Absence of CO_2 Retention in Health During Maximum Exercise

Do these mechanical constraints combined with sluggish ventilatory responses ever lead to a truly inadequate ventilation during heavy exercise? The clinical analogy here would be the patient with stable or reversible obstructed airway disease who commonly shows clear exercise-induced CO_2 retention. This ventilatory "failure" occurs very rarely in the healthy human or animal; i.e., ventilatory demand may equal but almost never exceeds mechanical capacity. Even in highly trained persons who reach mechanical limits of ventilation at maximum exercise (Fig. 12), absolute CO_2 retention never occurs. Rather, in these cases, reaching mechanical limitation coincided with their reaching maximal work capacity. Furthermore, the degree of mechanical limitation was *positively* correlated with and therefore *caused by* the magnitude of the ventilatory response rather than the maximum exercise being determined by the mechanical limitation of ventilation.

If these subjects had been capable of achieving even heavier work loads, it seems likely that Pa_{CO_2} would actually increase. We observed this to occur in some very rare instances in the highly trained in whom Pa_{CO_2} falls upon initiation of a heavy or maximum workload and then rises over time (61). The most extreme example we have observed to date in this regard is a 70-year-old, highly trained endurance athlete in whom the maximum flow:volume loop was reduced because of the normal aging-induced loss of lung elastic recoil and who reached the limits of his flow:volume loop at a workload slightly less than his maximum work rate. Thus, Pa_{CO_2} did rise slightly with further increasing work rate to maximum and over time during performance of the maximum work rate, despite marked increases in circulating humoral stimuli. In these extreme instances the subjects still remain normocapnic relative to rest or have Pa_{CO_2}'s in the range of 36–38 mmHg. Even though this is not CO_2 retention in the absolute sense, it is important to gas exchange at these high workloads because the A-aDo_2 is frequently widened to >35–45 mmHg, and it is important to have as much hyperventilation as possible to avoid severe exercise-induced arterial hypoxemia. Those athletes with the greatest arterial hypoxemia frequently also show either no or very minimal levels of hyperventilation during maximum exercise (61).

There are several other extreme examples in humans and quadrupeds in which CO_2 retention is also avoided even though the demands made on the ventilatory control system would appear to be extremely close to, if not in excess of, mechanical capacity. For example, the older athlete has a Vd:Vt ratio that is 25–35% greater than that in the young and significant flow limitation that is increased by 30–40% with an age-induced loss of lung elastic recoil; yet with very few exceptions the subjects complete maximum work rates, which are two times those of their sedentary contemporaries, and demonstrate highly significant hyperventilatory responses (298,299). The pony is capable of completing prolonged workloads requiring $\dot{V}_{CO_2}$'s that are 1.5 times those in the highly trained human athlete. Despite the fact that blood flow to the pony's diaphragm is at or very near maximum levels under these conditions and that blood flow to all respiratory muscles averages about 15% of cardiac output, the animal shows a substantial progressive hyperventilation (and arterial hypocapnia) throughout the duration of prolonged heavy exercise (255). Even the healthy human shows significant fatigue of the diaphragm as a result of very heavy endurance exercise to exhaustion, yet again shows a significant time-dependent hyperventilation throughout this exercise at 90–95% $\dot{V}_{O_{2max}}$ (280).

The most extreme and perplexing example of the balance struck between demand and capacity in the ventilatory control system is the thoroughbred horse, who, as mentioned earlier, begins to show graded CO_2 retention as exercise work rate increases beyond 60–70% of $\dot{V}O_{2max}$ (276). Arterial P_{CO_2} in the mid-50s or 10–15 mmHg greater than resting levels are not uncommon in the thoroughbred at maximum exercise. The likely implication is simply that the huge CO_2 production ($>$160–170 ml/kg/min, $P\bar{v}_{CO_2} > 120$ mmHg) outstrips the mechanical capability of the lung and chest wall to provide sufficient combinations of flow rate and Vt so that alveolar ventilation would match the increasing $\dot{V}_{CO_2}$. However, these data were obtained with work rates of only 2 min duration. If the maximum exercise load was continued for two times this period—with no further change in $\dot{V}_{CO_2}$ or in stride or in breathing frequency—the CO_2 retention did *not* persist. Rather P_{aCO_2} was returned to and even slightly below resting control levels. Although direct measurements of the ventilation are not available in these conditions, it seems clear the Vt and $\dot{V}_A$ must have increased substantially over the final few minutes of exercise—perhaps in response to the increasing arterial hypoxemia and metabolic acidosis, which worsened over this time period. Flow rate, volume, and pressure measurements are needed in this animal to confirm these estimates, and to solve this dilemma.

Collectively these findings speak to prioritization within the control system under conditions when ventilatory demand approximates capacity. Certainly there are many circumstances where mechanical considerations are very important in determining respiratory motor output, such as occurs during normal short-term heavy exercise where Vt is constrained to the lower, linear, and most mechanically efficient portion of the pressure-volume relationship and expiratory muscles exert just a sufficient amount of pressure to ensure achieving maximum flow rates without surpassing effective maximum pressures. Similarly, during endurance exercise the fatiguing diaphragm is spared as accessory inspiratory and expiratory muscles are recruited and play an ever increasing role in sustaining the ventilatory response. In some instances high levels of hyperventilation and ventilatory work are spared even though arterial hypoxemia is present and ventilatory responses would alleviate at least some of the hypoxemia (see Fig. 14). For example, the marked CO_2 retention experienced during very brief exercise in the thoroughbred horse is regarded by some as a "useful adaptation" because the increase in Vt and $\dot{V}_E$ required to maintain normocapnia will almost double the amount of ventilatory work (304,305).* On the other hand, significant CO_2 retention and asphyxia is

---

*These authors argued that the arterial hypoxemia caused by the hypoventilation would be offset by the increase in hemoglobin concentration in the exercising horse, which ensures that arterial O_2 content stays greater than resting levels (306). We agree that the increase in O_2-carrying capacity in the horse will prevent systemic O_2 transport and

simply not permitted by the normal control system—at least for any substantial period of time, even under the extreme work rates achieved in highly trained humans and some athletic animals. Accordingly, V_t and end-inspiratory lung volumes and flow rates and inspiratory and expiratory pressures are often increased markedly during heavy and maximum exercise with the goal of providing sufficient alveolar ventilation to prevent hypercapnia and hypoxemia with little apparent concern for mechanical efficiency or "minimization" of ventilatory work.

Physical Training Spares Exercise Hyperpnea

Finally, as an important footnote to the question of adaptability to the increase in maximum metabolic requirement along the fitness continuum, we wish to emphasize that despite the relative absence of structural adaptability in the lung and chest wall there is a substantial and important change in the regulation of exercise hyperpnea. This adaptation to training is manifested at work rates beyond moderate levels of exercise intensity, where—at any given external work rate of $\dot{V}O_2$— the trained person shows a significant reduction in ventilatory response. The training effect is often substantial, amounting to as much as 20–30% decrement in total $\dot{V}_E$ or 4–6 mmHg increase in Pa_{CO_2}, when comparisons are made pre- to posttraining at a fixed heavy, but submaximal work rate (300).

Precisely what mechanisms are responsible for this reduction in $\dot{V}_E$ is not known, although it is likely that this training/fitness effect is caused by a training-induced change in the aerobic capacity of the locomotor muscles. The reduction in $\dot{V}_E$ with training correlates positively with the decrease in circulating lactate (306). In turn, the reduced anaerobic metabolism is attributed to training effects on muscle mitochondrial volume and enzymes controlling glycolysis and fat oxidation. The decrease in circulating lactate may have two types of effects on $\dot{V}_E$. First, lactate produced in muscle is associated with increased $[H^+]$, which diffuses into plasma and reacts with bicarbonate in the red cell, which acts to buffer the increased $[H^+]$ and in so doing produces CO_2 (306,307). This effect of training may produce a 0.5 L/min decrease in $\dot{V}_{CO_2}$ at heavy work _tes and a smaller reduction in $\dot{V}O_2$ probably due to a reduced cost of metabolizing lactate. Second, at very heavy work rates, further increases in lactate causes progressive metabolic acidosis along with increasing levels of circulating K^+ and norepinephrine. Since

---

therefore $\dot{V}O_{2max}$ from falling as much as they would otherwise in the face of the exercise-induced arterial hypoxemia. However, we agree that the exercise-induced arterial hypoxemia, per se, would limit arterial O_2 content and therefore systemic O_2 transport below its maximum *achievable* level. Accordingly, we predict that the maximum arterial-to-venous O_2 content difference would also be reduced in the presence of arterial hypoxemia and thus $\dot{V}O_{2max}$ would be curtailed.

physical training results in reduced levels in all these potential circulating chemoreceptor stimuli, a cause:effect relationship with the reduced $\dot{V}_E$ is presumed (300). Similarly, over a broad range of work rates the reduction in $\dot{V}_{CO_2}$ with training is viewed appropriately as reduced ventilatory "requirement" and therefore a reduced ventilatory response "must" follow.

Certainly at first glance these explanations seem plausible—given the tight association of $\dot{V}_A$ to $\dot{V}_{CO_2}$ during exercise and the fact that circulating H^+, K^+, and norepinephrine all are known to stimulate carotid chemoreceptors. On the other hand, as explained in detail in Section II, we simply do not know precisely how $\Delta\dot{V}_{CO_2}$ during exercise translates into $\Delta\dot{V}_E$ because CO_2 flow to the lung lacks both a well-defined stimulus and a receptor site. Similarly, marked hyperventilation occurs in heavy exercise, even in the absence of carotid chemoreceptors, so we must question a key stimulatory role for *any* carotid chemoreceptor influence during heavy exercise in the trained or untrained (66,98).

Rather than a humoral-based cause of the training-induced decrease in ventilatory response, the mechanism might be purely "neural" in origin (see Section II for details). Suppose fatiguing locomotor muscles in heavy exercise would demand more input from the CNS to maintain tension development. This adaptation to increased motor output would also augment descending input ("central command") into the medullary respiratory pattern generator thereby causing heavy-exercise-induced hyperventilation. Accordingly, physical training might reduce this descending input—and therefore ventilatory output—by reducing the locomotor muscle fatigability at any given external work rate.

In summary, on the one hand, it seems clear that the substantial metabolic adaptability of locomotor muscles to physical training provides a critical means of ensuring a reduced hyperpnea in the trained state. This is an important adaptation in terms of sparing $\dot{V}_E$ and thereby ventilatory work, flow limitation, and so forth, at any given submaximal work rate in the trained—at least until eventually the higher maximum work rate and $\dot{V}_{CO_2}$ will demand much higher $\dot{V}_E$ in the trained than the untrained (see Fig. 12). However, in terms of mechanisms, we should not confuse associations of reduced $\dot{V}_E$ to reduced humoral stimuli with causation. This question of the mechanisms responsible for training-induced reductions in exercise hyperpnea must await the definitive elucidation of those mechanisms that are truly responsible for the hyperpnea and hyperventilation of exercise in all individuals.

C. Summary: Mechanical Limitations

Just as with exercise hyperpnea, the regulation of airway caliber, stretch of the lung parenchyma, and the tension developed by respiratory muscles is also near ideal during exercise. This results in a minimization of the effort and oxygen cost of breathing. While there is limited and controversial evidence that a portion of the drive to exercise hyperpnea may involve the "sensing" of and compensation for the mechanical impedance in a healthy subject, in general, the mechanical capacity to produce and sustain tidal volume, flow rate, and inspiratory muscle pressure far exceeds the ventilatory demands made during exercise. Nevertheless, because adaptations to fitness/training are limited at the level of the lung and chest wall—relative to other links in the gas transport chain—increasing fitness levels can produce sufficiently large ventilatory demands during maximum exercise, so demand will eventually seriously encroach on and sometimes even meet the mechanical capacity of the lung and chest wall. The earliest indication of this encroachment on the mechanical reserves is the occurrence of expiratory flow limitation, which in turn leads to increased end-expiratory lung volume shortening of inspiratory muscle length and eventually the generation of pressure by inspiratory muscles, which comes very close to their available dynamic capacity. In the very fit human, absolute mechanical limitations to volume, flow, and pressure are reached coincident with the achievement of maximum exercise. What are the consequences of this encroachment on mechanical reserve? First, the work and oxygen cost and circulatory cost of ventilation increase disproportionately at the very high workloads, and the diaphragm will fatigue if very high intensity exercise is sustained to exhaustion. However, the physiological ramifications of these "failures" and high physiological costs to exercise ventilation *or* to compromised blood flow to working locomotor muscles or to exercise performance itself remain unknown and for the most part untested. Mechanical constraint of the hyperventilatory response to very heavy or maximum exercise may occur to some extent, and this in turn will contribute to exercise-induced arterial hypoxemia in some cases. However, significant, sustained CO_2 retention is extremely rare in health, even under the most extreme conditions of exercise intensity and flow limitation.

Acknowledgments

The original work reported in this chapter was supported by grants from the National Heart, Lung, and Blood Institute, the Veterans Administration, and the American Lung Association. We are indebted to Paul Scherz and Gundula Birong for their assistance in the preparation of the manuscript.

References

1. Asmussen E. Ventilation at transition from rest to exercise. Acta Physiol Scand 1973; 89:68–78.
2. Beaver WL, Wasserman K. Transients in ventilation at start and end of exercise. J Appl Physiol 1968; 25:390–399.

3. Casaburi R, Barstow TJ, Robinson T, Wasserman K. Influence of work rate on ventilatory and gas exchange kinetics. J Appl Physiol 1989; 67:547–555.

4. D'Angelo E, Torelli G. Neural stimuli increasing respiration during different types of exercise. J Appl Physiol 1971; 30:116–121.

5. Dejours P. Control of respiration on muscular exercise. In: Handbook of Physiology, Respiration, Sect 3, Vol 1. Bethesda, MD: American Physiological Society, 1974: 631–648.

6. Diamond LB, Casaburi R, Wasserman K, Whipp BJ. Kinetics of gas exchange and ventilation in transitions from rest or prior exercise. J Appl Physiol 1977; 43: 704–708.

7. Hickman JB, Pryor WW, Page EB, Atwell RJ. Respiratory regulation during exercise in unconditioned subjects. J Clin Invest 1951; 30:503–516.

8. Krogh A, Lindhard J. The regulation of respiration and circulation during the initial stages of muscular work. J Physiol (Lond) 1913; 47:112–136.

9. Pearce DH, Milhorn HT Jr. Dynamic and steady-state respiratory responses to bicycle ergometer exercise. J Appl Physiol 1977; 42:959–967.

10. Torelli G, Brandi G. Regulation of ventilation at the beginning of muscular exercise. Intern Angew Physiol 1961; 19:134–139.

11. Asmussen E, Nielsen M. Pulmonary ventilation and effect of oxygen breathing in heavy exercise. Acta Physiol Scand 1958; 43:365–378.

12. Bisgard GE, Forster HV, Messina J, Sarazin RG. Role of the carotid body in hyperpnea of moderate exercise in goats. J Appl Physiol 1986; 52:1216–1222.

13. Forster HV, Pan LG, Bisgard GE, Kaminski RP, Dorsey SC, Busch MA. The hyperpnea of exercise at various P_{IO_2} in normal and carotid body denervated ponies. J Appl Physiol 1983; 54:1387–1393.

14. Flandrois R, Lacour JF, Eclache JP. Control of respiration in exercising dog: interaction of chemical and physical humoral stimuli. Respir Physiol 1974; 21: 169–181.

15. Pan LG, Forster HV, Bisgard GE, Kaminski RP, Dorsey SM, Busch MA. Hyperventilation in ponies at the onset of and during steady-state exercise. J Appl Physiol 1983; 54:1394–1402.

16. Powers SK, Beadle RE, Thompson D, Lawler J. Ventilatory and blood gas dynamics at onset and offset of exercise in the pony. J Appl Physiol 1987; 62:141–148.

17. Smith CA, Mitchell GS, Jameson LC, Musch TI, Dempsey JA. Ventilatory response of goats to treadmill exercise: grade effects. Respir Physiol 1983; 54:331–341.

18. Asmussen E. Exercise and the regulation of ventilation. In: Physiology of Muscular Exercise. American Heart Association 1967: 132–145.

19. Dempsey JA, Rankin J. Physiologic adaptations of gas transport systems to muscular work in health and disease. Am J Phys Med 1967; 46:582–647.

20. Dempsey JA, Reddan WG, Rankin J, Birnbaum ML, Forster HV, Thoden JS, Grover RF. Effects of acute through life-long hypoxic exposure on exercise pulmonary gas exchange. Respir Physiol 1971; 13:62–87.

21. Whipp B. Control of exercise hyperpnea. In: Hornbein TF, ed. Regulation of Breathing, Part II. New York: Marcel Dekker, 1981: 1069–1140.

22. Wasserman K, Whipp BJ, Casaburi R, Beaver WL, Brown HV. CO_2 flow to the lungs

and ventilatory control. In: Dempsey JA, Reed CE, eds. Muscular Exercise and the Lung. Madison: University of Wisconsin Press, 1977: 103–135.

23. Casaburi R, Whipp BJ, Koyal SN, Wasserman K. Coupling of ventilation to CO_2 production during constant load ergometry with sinusoidally varying pedal rate. J Appl Physiol 1978; 44:97–103.

24. Dempsey JA, Gledhill N, Reddan WG, Forster HV, Hanson PG, Claremont AD. Pulmonary adaptation to exercise: effect of exercise type, duration, chronic hypoxia, and physical training. In: The Marathon: Physiological, Medical, Epidemiological, and Psychological Studies. New York: New York Academy of Sciences 1977:243–261.

25. McMurray RG, Ahlborn SW. Respiratory responses to running and walking at the same metabolic rate. Respir Physiol 1982; 47:257–265.

26. Forster HV, Pan LG, Funahashi A. Temporal pattern of Pa_{CO_2} during exercise in humans. J Appl Physiol 1986; 60:653–660.

27. Kay JDS, Petersen ES, Vejby-Christensen H. Breathing in man during steady-state exercise on the bicycle at low pedaling frequencies and during treadmill walking. J Physiol (Lond) 1977; 272:553–561.

28. Jensen, JI. Neural ventilatory drive during arm and leg exercise. Scand J Clin Lab Invest 1972; 29:177–184.

29. Szal SE, Schoene RB. Ventilatory response to rowing and cycling in elite oarswomen. J Appl Physiol 1989; 67:264–269.

30. Forster HV, Klausen K. The effect of chronic metabolic acidoses and alkalosis on ventilation during exercise and hypoxia. Respir Physiol 1973; 17:336–346.

31. Oren A, Whipp BJ, Wasserman K. Effect of acid-base status on the kinetics of the ventilatory response to moderate exercise. J Appl Physiol 1982; 52:1013–1017.

32. Dempsey JA, Forster HV, Birnbaum ML, Reddan WG, Thoden J, Grover RF, Rankin J. Control of exercise hyperpnea under varying durations of exposure to moderate hypoxia. Respir Physiol 1972; 16:213–231.

33. Mitchell GS, Smith CA, Dempsey JA. Changes in the $V_I{:}V_{CO_2}$ relationship during exercise: role of carotid body. J Appl Physiol 1984; 57:1894–1900.

34. Knuttgen HG, Emersen K. Physiological response to pregnancy at rest and during exercise. J Appl Physiol 1974; 36:546–553.

35. Pernoll ML, Metcalfe J, Kovach PA, Wachtel R, Dunham M. Ventilation during rest and exercise in pregnancy and postpartum. Respir Physiol 1975; 25:295–310.

36. Schaefer SL, Mitchell GS. Ventilatory control during exercise with peripheral chemoreceptor stimulation: hypoxia versus domperidome. J Appl Physiol 1989; 67: 2438–2446.

37. Bisgard GE, Forster HV, Byrnes B, Stanek K, Klein J, Manohar M. Cerebrospinal fluid acid-base balance during muscular exercise. J Appl Physiol 1978; 45:94–101.

38. Clifford PS, Litzow JT, Coon, RL. Arterial hypocapnia during exercise in beagle dogs. J Appl Physiol 1986; 61:599–602.

39. Dempsey JA, Vidruk EH, Mitchell GA. Pulmonary control systems in exercise: update. Fed Proc 1985; 44:2260–2270.

40. Forster HV, Pan LG, Bisgard GE, Flynn C, Dorsey SM, Britton MS. Independence of exercise hypocapnia and limb movement frequency in ponies. J Appl Physiol 1984; 57:1885–1893.

41. Fregosi RF, Dempsey JA. Arterial blood acid-base regulation during exercise in rats. J Appl Physiol 1984; 57:396–402.
42. Phillipson EA, Bowes G, Townsend ER, Duffin J, Cooper JD. Role of metabolic CO_2 production in ventilatory response to steady-state exercise. J Clin Invest 1981; 68:768–774.
43. Brice AG, Forster HV, Pan LG, Brown DR, Forster AL, Lowry TF. Effect of cardiac denervation on cardiorespiratory responses to exercise in goats. J Appl Physiol 1991; 70:1113–1120.
44. Watken RL, Rostosfer HH, Robinson S, Newton JL, Baillie MD. Changes in blood gases and acid-base balance in the exercising dog. J Appl Physiol 1962; 17: 656–660.
45. Mines AH. Respiratory Physiology. New York: Raven Press, 1993: 50–51.
46. Mead J. Control of respiratory frequency. J Appl Physiol 1980; 49:528–532.
47. Otis AB, Fenn WO, Rahn H. Mechanics of breathing in man. J Appl Physiol 1950; 2:592–607.
48. Poon C-S. Ventilatory control in hypercapnia and exercise: optimization hypothesis. J Appl Physiol 1987; 62:2447–2459.
49. Barltrop D. The relationship between body temperature and respiration. J Physiol (Lond) 1954; 125:19–20P.
50. Dejours P, Teillac A, Girard F, Lacaisse A. Étude du rôle de l'hyperthermie centrale modérée dans la régulation de la ventilation de l'exercice musculaire chez l'homme. Rev Franç Études Clin Biol 1958; 3:755–761.
51. Whipp BJ, Wasserman K. Effect of body temperature on the ventilatory response to exercise. Respir Physiol 1970; 8:354–360.
52. Hanson P, Claremont A, Dempsey J, Reddan W. Determinants and consequences of ventilatory responses to competitive endurance running. Appl Physiol 1982; 52: 615–623.
53. Barr PO, Beckman M, Bjurstedt H, Brismar J, Hessler CM, Matell G. Time course of blood gas changes provoked by light and moderate exercise in man. Acta Physiol Scand 1964; 60:1–17.
54. Oldenburg FA, McCormack DO, Morse JLC, Jones NL. A comparison of exercise responses in stairclimbing and cycling. J Appl Physiol 1979; 46:510–516.
55. Young IH, Woolcock AJ. Changes in arterial blood gas tension during unsteady-state exercise. J Appl Physiol 1978; 44:93–96.
56. Forster HV, Dunning MB, Lowry TF, Erickson BK, Forster MA, Pan LG, Brice AG, Effros RM. Effect of asthma and ventilatory loading on $Paco_2$ of humans during submaximal exercise. J Appl Physiol 1993; 75:1385–1394.
57. Zechman F, Hull FG, Hull WE. Effects of graded resistance to tracheal air flow in man. J Appl Physiol 1967; 10:356–362.
58. Wasserman K, Whipp BJ, Koyal SN, Cleary MG. Effect of carotid body resection on ventilatory and acid-base control during exercise. J Appl Physiol 1975; 39:354–358.
59. Holmgren A, Linderholm H. Oxygen and carbon dioxide tension of arterial blood during heavy and exhaustive exercise. Acta Physiol Scand 1958; 44:203–215.
60. Powers SK, Lawler J, Dempsey JA, Dodd S, Landry G. Effects of incomplete pulmonary gas exchange on $\dot{V}o_2$ max. J Appl Physiol 1989; 66:2491–2495.

61. Dempsey JA, Hanson P, Henderson K. Exercise induced arterial hypoxemia in healthy humans at sea level. J Physiol (Lond) 1984; 355:161–175.

62. Rowell LB, Taylor HL, Wang Y, Carlson WB. Saturation of arterial blood with oxygen during maximal exercise. J Appl Physiol 1984; 19:284–286.

63. Kiley JP, Kuhlmann WD, Fedde MR. Arterial and mixed venous blood gas tensions in exercising ducks. Poultry Sci 1980; 59:914–917.

64. Kuhlmann WD, Hodgson DS, Fedde MR. Respiratory, cardiovascular and metabolic adjustments to exercise in the hereford calf. J Appl Physiol 1985; 58:1273–1280.

65. Mitchell GS, Gleason TT, Bennett AF. Ventilation and acid-base balance during activity in lizards. Am J Physiol 1981; 240:R29–R37.

66. Pan LG, Forster HV, Bisgard GE, Murphy CL, Lowry TF. Independence of exercise hyperpnea and acidosis during high intensity exercise in ponies. J Appl Physiol 1986; 60:1016–1024.

67. Bayly WM, Grant BD, Breeze RG, Kramer JW. The effects of maximal exercise on acid-base balance and arterial blood gas tensions in thoroughbred horses. In: Snow DH, Persson SG, Rose RJ, eds. Equine Exercise Physiology. Cambridge: Granta Editions, 1983: 400–404.

68. Hornicke H, Meixner R, Pollmann U. Respiration in exercising horses. In: Snow DH, Persson SG, Rose RJ, eds. Equine Exercise Physiology. Cambridge: Granta Editions, 1982: 7–16.

69. Forster HV, Pan LG. Exercise hyperpnea. In: Crystal RG, West JB, eds. The Lung: Scientific Foundations. New York: Raven Press, 1991: 1553–1564.

70. Eldridge FL, Waldrop TG. Neural control of breathing during exercise. In: Whipp BJ, Wasserman K, eds. Exercise: Pulmonary Physiology and Pathophysiology. New York: Marcel Dekker, 1991: 309–370.

71. Geppert J, Zuntz N. Ueber die Regulation der Atmung. Arch Ges Physiol 1888; 42: 189–245.

72. Haldane JS, Priestley JG. The regulation of the lung-ventilation. J Physiol (Lond) 1905; 32:225–266.

73. Douglas CG, Haldane JS. The regulation of normal breathing. J Physiol (Lond) 1909; 38:420–440.

74. Heymans C, Bouckaert JJ. Sinus Carotidiens et réflexes respiratoirés. C R Soc Biol 1930; 103:498–500.

75. Heymans JF, Heymans C. Sur les modifications directes et sur la regulation reflexes de l'activité du centre respiratoire de la tête isolié du chien. Arch Int Pharmacolodyn 1927; 33:273–372.

76. Leusen I. Chemosensitivity of the respiratory center. Influence of CO_2 in the cerebral ventricles in respiration. Am J Physiol 1954; 176:39–44.

77. Loeschcke HH, Koepchin HP. Ueber das Verhalten der Atmung und des arteriellen Drucks bei Einbringen von Veratridin, Lobelin und cyanid in den Liquor cerebrospinales. Pflüger's Arch Ges Physiol 1958; 266:586–610.

78. Biscoe TJ, Purves MJ. Factors affecting the cat carotid chemoreceptor and cervical sympathetic activity with special reference to passive hind-limb movements. J Physiol (Lond) 1967; 190:425–441.

79. Waldrop TG, Mullins DC, Millhorn DE. Control of respiration by the hypothalamus

and by feedback from contracting muscles in cats. Respir Physiol 1986; 64: 317–328.

80. Eisele JH, Ritchie BC, Severinghaus JW. Effect of stellate ganglion blockade on the hyperpnea of exercise. J Appl Physiol 1967; 22(5): 966–969.

81. Clark JM, Sinclair RD, Lenox JB. Chemical and nonchemical components of ventilation during hypercapnic exercise in man. J Appl Physiol 1980; 48:1065–1076.

82. Asmussen E, Nielsen M. Ventilatory responses to CO_2 during work at normal and at low oxygen tensions. Acta Physiol Scand 1957; 39:27–35.

83. Cunningham DJC, Lloyd BB, Patrick JM. The relation between ventilation and end-tidal P_{CO_2} in man during moderate exercise with and without CO_2 inhalation. J Physiol (Lond) 1963; 169:104–106.

84. Duffin J, Bechbache RR, Gorda RC, Chung SA. The ventilatory response to carbon dioxide in hyperoxic exercise. Respir Physiol 1980; 40:93–105.

85. Miyamura J, Yamishina T, Honda Y. Ventilatory response to CO_2 rebreathing at rest and during exercise in untrained subjects and athletes. Jpn J Physiol 1976; 26: 245–254.

86. Kelly MA, Owens GR, Fishman AP. Hypercapnic ventilation during exercise: effects of exercise methods and inhalation techniques. Respir Physiol 1982; 50: 75–85.

87. Weil JV, Byrne-Quinn E, Sodal IE, Kline JS, McCullough RE, Filley GF. Augmentation of chemosensitivity during mild exercise in normal man. J Appl Physiol 1972; 33:813–819.

88. Band DM, Cameron IR, Semple SJG. Oscillations in arterial pH with breathing in the cat. J Appl Physiol 1969; 26:261–267.

89. Goodman NW, Nail BS, Torrance RW. Oscillations in the discharge of single carotid chemoreceptor fibres of the cat. Respir Physiol 1974; 20:251–266.

90. Cross BA, Davey A, Guz A, Katona PG, Maclean M, Murphy K, Semple SJC, Stidwell R. The pH oscillations in arterial blood during exercise: a potential signal for the ventilatory response in the dog. J Physiol (Lond) 1982; 329:57–73.

91. Band DM, Willshaw P, Wolff CB. The speed of response of the carotid body chemoreceptor. In: Paintal AS, ed. Morphology and Mechanisms of Chemoreceptors. New Delhi, India: Navchetan Press, 1976: 197–207.

92. Black AMS, Torrance RW. Respiratory oscillations in chemoreceptor discharge in control of breathing. Respir Physiol 1971; 13:221–237.

93. Black AMS, Goodman NW, Nail BS, Rao, PS, Torrance RW. The significance of the timing of chemoreceptor impulses for their effect upon respiration. Acta Neurobiol Exp 1973; 33:139–147.

94. Grant B, Semple SJG. Mechanisms whereby oscillations in arterial carbon dioxide tension might affect pulmonary ventilation. In: Paintal AS, ed. Morphology and Mechanisms of Chemoreceptors. New Delhi, India: Navchetan Press, 1976.

95. Saunders KB. Oscillations of arterial CO_2 tension in a respiratory model: some implications for the control of breathing in exercise. J Theor Biol 1980; 84:163–179.

96. Yamamoto IH, Edwards MW. Homeostasis of CO_2 during intravenous infusion of CO_2. J Appl Physiol 1960; 15:807–818.

97. Ward SA, Whipp BJ. Phase-coupling of arterial blood-gas oscillations and ventilatory dynamics during exercise in humans. FASEB J 1993; 7:3664.

98. Forster HV, Lowry TF, Murphy CL, Pan LG. Role of elevated plasma [K⁺] and carotid chemoreceptors in hyperpnea of exercise in awake ponies. J Physiol (Lond) 1990; 417:112P.

99. McCoy M, Hargreaves M. Potassium and ventilation during incremental exercise in trained and untrained men. J Appl Physiol 1992; 73(4):1287–1290.

100. Paterson DJ. Potassium and ventilation in exercise. J Appl Physiol 1992; 72:811–820.

101. Linton RAF, Lim M, Wolff CB, Wilmshurst P, Band DM. Arterial potassium measured continuously during exercise in man. Clin Sci (Lond) 1984; 67:427–431.

102. Conway J, Paterson DJ, Petersen ES, Robbins PA. Changes in arterial potassium and ventilation in response to exercise in humans. J Physiol 1986; 374:26P.

103. Linton RAF, Band DM. The effect of potassium on carotid chemoreceptor activity and ventilation in the cat. Respir Physiol 1985; 59:65–70.

104. Band DM, Linton RAF, Kent R, Kurer FL. The effect of peripheral chemodenervation on the ventilatory response to potassium. Respir Physiol 1985; 60:217–225.

105. Jarisch AS, Londgren EN, Zotterman Y. Impulse activity in the carotid sinus nerve following intra-carotid injection of potassium chloride, veratrine sodium citrate, adenosenetriphosphate, and alpha dinitrophenol. Acta Physiol Scand 1952; 25:195–211.

106. Donaldson GC, Newstead CG. In man at rest undergoing haemodialysis, reduction in arterial potassium does not influence minute ventilation. J Physiol (Lond) 1988; 407:29P (abstract).

107. Paterson DJ, Friedland JS, Oliver DO, Robbins PA. The ventilatory response to lowering potassium with dextrose and insulin in subjects with hyperkalemia. Respir Physiol 1989; 76:393–398.

108. Warner MM, Mitchell GS. Ventilatory responses to hyperkalemia and exercise in normoxic and hypoxic goats. Respir Physiol 1990; 82:239–250.

109. Griffiths TL, Henson LC, Huntsman D, Wasserman K, Whipp BJ. The influence of inspired O₂ partial pressure on ventilatory and gas exchange kinetics during exercise. J Physiol (Lond) 1980; 306:34P (abstract).

110. Casaburi R, Stremal RW, Whipp BJ, Beaver WL, Wasserman K. Alteration by hyperoxia of ventilatory dynamics during sinusoidal work. J Appl Physiol 1980; 48:1083–1091.

111. Bisgard GE, Neubauer JA. Chapter 14, this volume.

112. Nery LE, Wasserman K, Andrews JD, Huntsman DJ, Hansen JE, Whipp BJ. Ventilatory and gas exchange kinetics during exercise in chronic airway obstruction. J Appl Physiol 1982; 53:1594–1602.

113. Pan LG, Forster HV, Brice AG, Lowry TF, Murphy CL, Wurster RD. Ventilatory response to exercise in ponies after elimination of 3 afferent pathways. J Appl Physiol (in press).

114. Fencl V, Miller TB, Pappenheimer JR. Studies on the respiratory response to disturbances of acid-base balance with deductions concerning the composition of cerebral interstitial fluids. Am J Physiol 1966; 210:459–472.

115. Pappenheimer JR, Fencl V, Heisey SR, Held D. Role of cerebral fluids in control of respiration as studied in unanesthetized goats. Am J Physiol 1965; 208:436–450.

116. Bledsoe SW, Hornbein TF. Central chemosensors and the regulation of their chemical environment. In: Hornbein TF, ed. Regulation of Breathing, Part I. New York: Marcel Dekker, 1981:347–428.

117. Dempsey JA, Pelligrino D, Aggarwal D, Olson EB. The brain's role in exercise hyperpnea. Med Sci Sports Exercise 1979; 11:213–220.

118. Smith CA, Jameson LC, Dempsey JA. Effects of altered CSF [H⁺] on ventilatory responses to exercise in the awake goat. J Appl Physiol 1988; 65:921–927.

119. Eldridge FL, Kiley JP, Paydarfar D. Dynamics of medullary hydrogen ion and respiratory responses to square-wave change of arterial carbon dioxide in cats. J Physiol (Lond) 1987; 385:627–642.

120. Casaburi R, Daly J, Hansen JE, Effros RM. Abrupt changes in mixed venous blood gas composition after the onset of exercise. J Appl Physiol 1989; 67:1106–1112.

121. Edwards RHT, Denison DM, Jones G, Davies CTM, Campbell EJM. Changes in mixed venous gas tensions at start of exercise in man. J Appl Physiol 1972; 32: 165–169.

122. Armstrong BW, Hurt HH, Blide RW, Workman JM. The humoral regulation of breathing. Science 1961; 133:1897–1906.

123. Aviado DM, Li TH, Kalow W, Schmidt CF, Turnbull GL, Peskin GW, Hess ME, Weiss AJ. Respiratory and circulatory reflexes from the perfused heart and pulmonary circulation of the dog. Am J Physiol 1951; 165:261–277.

124. Comroe JH. The location and function of the chemoreceptors of the aorta. Am J Physiol 1939; 127:176–191.

125. Dejours P, Methoefer JC, Teillac A. Essai de nise en evidence de chemorecepteurs veineux de ventilation. J Physiol (Paris) 1955; 47:160–163.

126. Kao FF. An experimental study of the pathways involved in exercise hyperpnea employing cross-circulation techniques. In: Cunningham DJC, Lloyd BB, eds. The Regulation of Human Respiration. Philadelphia: F. A. Davis, 1963:461–502.

127. Zuntz N, Geppert J. Ueber die Natur der normalen Atemreize und den Ort ihrer Wirkung. Arch Ges Physiol 1886; 38:337–338.

128. Cropp GJA, Comroe JH Jr. Role of mixed venous CO_2 in respiratory control. J Appl Physiol 1961; 16:1029–1033.

129. Wasserman K, Whipp BJ, Casaburi R, Huntsman DJ, Castagna J, Lugliani R. Regulation of arterial P_{CO_2} during intravenous CO_2 loading. J Appl Physiol 1975; 38:651–656.

130. Linton RAF, Miller R, Cameron R. Ventilatory response to CO_2 inhalation and intravenous infusion of hypercapnic blood. Respir Physiol 1976; 26:383–394.

131. Stremel RW, Whipp BJ, Casburi R, Huntsman DJ, Wasserman K. Hypopnea consequent to reduced pulmonary blood flow in the dog. J Appl Physiol 1979; 46: 1171–1177.

132. Phillipson EA, Duffin J, Cooper JD. Critical dependence of respiratory rhythmicity on metabolic CO_2 load. J Appl Physiol 1981; 50:45–54.

133. Lamb TW. Ventilatory responses to intravenous and inspired carbon dioxide in anesthetized cats. Respir Physiol 1966; 2:99–104.

134. Bennett FM, Tallman RD, Grodins FS. Role of V_{CO_2} in control of breathing of awake exercising dogs. J Appl Physiol 1984; 56:1335–1337.

135. Fordyce WE, Grodins FS. Ventilatory response to intravenous and airway CO_2 administration in anesthetized dogs. J Appl Physiol 1980; 48:337–346.

136. Grant BJB, Stidweill RP, Cross BA, Semple SJG. Ventilatory response to inhaled and infused CO_2: relationship to the oscillating signal. Respir Physiol 1981; 44: 365–380.

137. Greco EC, Fordyce WE, Gonzalez F, Reischl P, Grodins FS. Respiratory responses to intravenous and intrapulmonary CO_2 in awake dogs. J Appl Physiol 1978; 45: 109–114.

138. Lewis SM. Awake baboon's ventilatory response to venous and inhaled CO_2 loading. J Appl Physiol 1975; 39:417–422.

139. Ponte J, Purves MJ. Carbon dioxide and venous return and their interaction as stimuli to ventilation in the cat. J Physiol (Lond) 1977; 274:455–475.

140. Orr JA, Fedde MR, Shams H, Roskenbleck H, Scheid P. Absence of CO_2-sensitive venous chemoreceptors in the cat. Respir Physiol 1988; 73:211–224.

141. Bennett FM, Fordyce WE. Gain of the ventilatory exercise stimulus: definition and meaning. J Appl Physiol 1988; 65:2011–2017.

142. Sheldon JI, Green JF. Evidence for pulmonary CO_2 chemosensitivity: effects on ventilation. J Appl Physiol 1982; 52:1192–1197.

143. Green JF, Sheldon MI. Ventilatory changes associated with changes in pulmonary blood flow in dogs. J Appl Physiol 1983; 54:997–1002.

144. Coleridge HM, Coleridge JCG, Banzett RB. Effect of CO_2 on afferent vagal endings in the canine lung. Respir Physiol 1978; 34:135–151.

145. Green JF, Schertel ER, Coleridge HM, Coleridge JCG. Effect of pulmonary arterial P_{CO_2} on slowly adapting pulmonary stretch receptors. J Appl Physiol 1986; 60:2048–2055.

146. Mitchell GS, Cross BA, Hiramoto T, Scheid P. Effects of intrapulmonary stretch receptor discharge in dogs. Respir Physiol 1980; 40:29–48.

147. Wasserman K, Whipp BJ, Castagan J. Cardiodynamic hyperpnea: hyperpnea secondary to cardiac output increase. J Appl Physiol 1974; 36:457–464.

148. Brown HV, Wasserman K, Whipp BJ. Effect of beta-adrenergic blockade during exercise on ventilation and gas exchange. J Appl Physiol 1976; 41:886–892.

149. Crisp AJ, Hainsworth R, Tutt SM. The absence of cardiovascular and respiratory responses to changes in right ventricular pressure in anesthetized dogs. J Physiol (Lond) 1988; 407:1–13.

150. Kostreva DR, Hopp FA, Zuperku EJ, Ingler FO, Coon FL, Kampine JP. Respiratory inhibition with sympathetic afferent stimulation in the canine and primate. J Appl Physiol 1978; 44:718–724.

151. Kostreva DR, Hopp FA, Zuperku EJ, Kampine JP. Apnea, tachypnea, and hypotension elicited by cardiac vagal afferents. J Appl Physiol 1979; 47:312–318.

152. Lloyd TC. Effect on breathing of acute pressure rise in pulmonary artery and right ventricle. J Appl Physiol 1984; 57:110–116.

153. Uchida Y. Tachypnea after stimulation of afferent cardiac sympathetic nerve fibers. Am J Physiol 1976; 230:1003–1007.

154. Jones PW, Huszczuk A, Wasserman K. Cardiac output as a controller of ventilation through changes in right ventricular load. J Appl Physiol 1982; 53:218–224.
155. Banner N, Guz A, Heaton R, Innes JA, Murphy K, Yacoub M. Ventilatory and circulatory responses at the onset of exercise in man following heart or heart-lung transplantation. J Physiol 1988; 399:437–449.
156. Phillipson EA, Hickey RF, Bainton CR, Nadel JA. Effect of vagal blockade on regulation of breathing in conscious dogs. J Appl Physiol 1970; 29:475–479.
157. Clifford PS, Litzow JT, von Colditz JH, Coon RL. Effect of chronic pulmonary denervation on ventilatory response to exercise. J Appl Physiol 1986; 61:603–610.
158. Favier R, Kepenekian G, Desplanches D, Flandrois R. Effects of chronic lung denervation on breathing pattern and respiratory gas exchange during hypoxia, hypercapnia and exercise. Respir Physiol 1982; 47:107–119.
159. Erickson BK, Forster HV, Pan LG, Lowry TF, Brown DR, Forster MA, Forster AL. Ventilatory compensation for lactacidosis in ponies: role of carotid chemoreceptors and lung afferents. J Appl Physiol 1991; 70:2619–2626.
160. Flynn C, Forster HV, Pan LG, Bisgard GE. Role of hilar nerve afferents in hyperpnea of exercise. J Appl Physiol 1985; 59:798–806.
161. Orr JA, Carrithers JA, Liu F, Shirer HW. Failure of pulmonary acidosis to increase respiratory drive. J Appl Physiol 1992; 73:672–678.
162. Ehrman J, Keteyian S, Fedel F, Rhoads K, Levine TB, Shepard R. Cardiovascular responses of heart transplant recipients to graded exercise testing. J Appl Physiol 1992; 73(1):260–264.
163. Savin WM, Haskell WL, Schroeder JS, Stinson EB. Cardio-respiratory responses of cardiac transplant patients to graded, symptom-limited exercise. Circulation 1980; 45:1183–1194.
164. Huszczuk A, Whipp BJ, Adams TD, Fisher AG, Crapo RO, Elliot CG, Wasserman K, Olsen DB. Ventilatory control during exercise in calves with artificial hearts. J Appl Physiol 1990; 68:2604–2611.
165. Johansson JE. Ueber die Einwirkung der Muskeltaetigkeit auf die Atmung und die Herztaetigkeit. Skand Arch Physiol 1893; 5:20–66.
166. DiMarco AF, Romaniuk JR, von Euler C, Yamamoto Y. Immediate changes in ventilation and respiratory pattern associated with onset and cessation of locomotion in the cat. J Physiol (Lond) 1983; 343:1–16.
167. Eldridge FL, Milhorn DE, Kiley JP, Waldrop TG. Stimulation by central command of locomotion, respiration and circulation during exercise. Respir Physiol 1985; 59:313–337.
168. Hinsey JC, Ransom SW, McNattin RF. The role of the hypothalamus and mesencephalon in locomotion. Arch Neurol Psychiatry 1930; 23:1–43.
169. Ransom SW, Magoun HW. Respiratory and pupillary reactions induced by electrical stimulation of the hypothalamus. Arch Neurol Psychiatry 1933; 29:1179–1193.
170. Schaltenbrand G, Girndt O. Physiologische Beobachtungen Am Thalamuskatzen. Pflüger's Arch 1925; 209:333–361.
171. Asmussen E, Johansen SH, Jorgensen M, Nielsen M. On the nervous factors controlling respiration and circulation during exercise. Acta Physiol Scand 1965; 63:343–350.

172. Bonde-Petersen F, Gollnick PD, Hansen TI, Hulten N, Kristensen N, Secher JH, Secher N. Glycogen depletion pattern in human muscular fiber during work under curarization d-tubocuraine. In: Howard H, Poortmans JR, eds. Metabolic Adaptation to Prolonged Exercise. Basel: Berkhausen Verlag, 1975:422–430.

173. Galbo H, Kjaer M, Secher NH. Cardiovascular, ventilatory and catecholamine responses to maximal dynamic exercise in partially curarized man. J Physiol 1987; 389:557–568.

174. Goodwin GM, McCloskey DI, Mitchell JH. Cardiovascular and respiratory responses to changes in central command during isometric exercise at constant muscle tension. J Physiol (Lond) 1972; 226:173–190.

175. Hobbs SF. Central command during exercise: parallel activation of the cardiovascular and motor systems by descending command signals. In: Smith OA, Galosy RA, Weiss SM, eds. Circulation, Neurobiology and Behavior. Amsterdam: Elsevier Science Publishers, 1982:217–231.

176. Ochwadt B, Bucherl BE, Kreuger H, Loeschcke HH. Beeinflussung der Atemsteigerung bei Muskelarbeit durch partiellen neuromuskularen Block (Tuborcurarine). Pflüger's Arch 1959; 269:613–621.

177. Adams L, Frankel H, Garlick J, Guz A, Murphy K, Semple SJG. The role of spinal cord transmission in the ventilatory response to exercise in man. J Physiol 1984; 355:85–97.

178. Asmussen E, Nielsen M, Welth-Pedersen G. Cortical or reflex control of respiration during muscular work? Acta Physiol Scand 1943; 6:168–175.

179. Brice AG, Forster HV, Pan LG, Funahashi A, Lowry TF, Murphy CL, Hoffman MD. Ventilatory and $Paco_2$ response to voluntary and electrically-induced leg exercise. J Appl Physiol 1988; 64:218–225.

180. Viala D, Vidal C, Freton E. Coordinated rhythmic bursting in respiratory and locomotor muscle nerves. Neurosci Lett 1979; 11:155–159.

181. Gesell R, Brassfield CR, Hamilton MA. An acid-neuro-humoral mechanism of nerve cell activation. Am J Physiol 1942; 136:604–608.

182. Eldridge FL, Gill-Kumar P. Central neural respiratory drive and afterdischarge. Respir Physiol 1980; 40:49–63.

183. Eldridge FL. Maintenance of respiration by central neural feedback mechanisms. Fed Proc 1977; 36:2400–2404.

184. Budzinska K, Karczewski WA, Naslonska E, Romaniuk JR. Post-stimulus effects and their possible role for stabilizing respiratory output. In: von Euler C, Lagercrantz H, eds. Central Nervous Control Mechanism in Breathing. Oxford: Pergamon Press, 1980:115–127.

185. Eldridge FL. Central neural respiratory stimulatory effect of active respiration. J Appl Physiol 1974; 37:723–735.

186. Millhorn DE, Eldridge FL, Waldrop TG. Effects of medullary area I(s) cooling on respiratory response to chemoreceptor input. Respir Physiol 1982; 49:23–29.

187. Vis A, Folgering H. Phrenic nerve afterdischarge after electrical stimulation of the carotid sinus nerve in cats. Respir Physiol 1981; 45:217–227.

188. Binzis L, Hemingway A. Shivering as a result of brain stimulation. J Neurophysiol 1957; 20:91–99.

189. Larabee MG, Bronk DW. Prolonged facilitation of synaptic excitation in sympathetic ganglia. J Neurophysiol 1946; 10:139–154.

190. Millhorn DE, Eldridge FL, Waldrop TG. Pharmacologic study of respiratory afterdischarge. J Appl Physiol 1981; 50:239–244.

191. Sykova E. Activity-related fluctuations in extracellular ion concentration in the central nervous system. News Physiol Sci 1986; 1:57–61.

192. Magleby KL. Synaptic transmission, facilitation, augmentation, potentiation, depression. In: Edelman G, ed. Encyclopedia of Neuroscience. Boston: Brekhauser, 1987:1170–1174.

193. Comroe JH Jr, Schmidt CF. Reflexes from the limbs as a factor in the hyperpnea of muscular exercise. Am J Physiol 1943; 138:536–547.

194. Grandpiene R, Franck C, Violettie F, Arnould P. Effets reflexes respiratories declenches par les mouvements possifs. J Physiol Paris 1952; 44:253–255.

195. Harrison TR, Harrison WG, Calhoun JA, Marsh JP. Congestive heart failure. The mechanism of dyspnea on exertion. Arch Intern Med 1932; 50:690–720.

196. Honda Y, Menoguchi M. Studies on the alkalosis caused by passive movement. J Physiol Soc Jpn 1957; 19:465–467.

197. Kao FF. The peripheral neurogenic drive: an experimental study. In: Dempsey JA, Deed CE, eds. Muscular Exercise and the Lung. Madison: University of Wisconsin Press, 1977:71–85.

198. Bennett F. A role for neural pathways in exercise hyperpnea. J Appl Physiol 1984; 56:1559–1564.

199. Bessou P, Dejours P, Laporte Y. Action ventilatoire reflexe de fibers afferentes de grand diametre d'origine musculaire chez le chat. J Physiol (Paris) 1959; 51:400–401.

200. Lamb TW. Ventilatory responses to hind limb exercise in anesthetized cats and dogs. Respir Physiol 1968; 6:88–104.

201. McCloskey DI, Mitchell JH. Reflex cardiovascular and respiratory responses originating in exercising muscle. J Physiol (Lond) 1972; 224:173–186.

202. Mitchell JH, Reardon WC, McCloskey PI. Reflex effects on circulation and respiration from contracting skeletal muscle. Am J Physiol 1977; 233:H374–H378.

203. Senapati JM. Effect of stimulation of muscle afferents on ventilation of dogs. J Appl Physiol 1966; 21:242–246.

204. Cross BA, Davey A, Guz A, Katona PG, MacLean M, Murphy K, Semple SJG, Stidwell R. The role of spinal cord transmission in the ventilatory response to electrically induced exercise in the anesthetized dog. J Physiol (Lond) 1982; 329:37–55.

205. Weissman ML, Whipp BJ, Huntsman DJ, Wasserman K. Role of neural afferents from working limbs in exercise hyperpnea. J Appl Physiol 1980; 49:239–248.

206. Tibes U. Reflex inputs to the cardiovascular and respiratory centers from dynamically working canine muscles. Circ Res 1977; 42:332–341.

207. Brice G, Forster HV, Pan L, Funahashi A, Hoffman M, Lowry T, Murphy C. Is the hyperpnea of muscle contractions critically dependent on spinal afferents? J Appl Physiol 1988; 64:226–223.

208. Brown DR, Forster HV, Pan LG, Brice AG, Murphy CL, Lowry TF, Gutting SM, Funahashi A, Hoffman M, Powers S. Ventilatory response of spinal-cord lesioned subjects to electrically induced exercise. J Appl Physiol 1990; 68:2312–2321.

209. Fernandez A, Galbo H, Kjaer M, Mitchell JH, Secher NH, Thomas SN. Cardiovascular and ventilatory responses to dynamic exercise during epidural anesthesia in man. J Appl Physiol 1990; 420:281–293.

210. Ohtake PJ, Jennings DB. Ventilation is stimulated by small reduction in arterial pressure in the awake dog. J Appl Physiol 1992; 73:1549–1557.

211. Pan LG, Forster HV, Wurster RD, Murphy CL, Brice AG, Lowry TF. Effect of partial spinal cord ablation on exercise hyperpnea in ponies. J Appl Physiol 1990; 69:1821–1827.

212. Hornbein TF, Sorensen SC, Parks CR. Role of muscle spindles in lower extremities in breathing during bicycle exercise. J Appl Physiol 1969; 27:476–479.

213. Kaufman MP, Longhurst JC, Rybicki KJ, Wallach JH, Mitchell JH. Effects of muscular contraction on impulse activity of groups III and IV afferents in cats. J Appl Physiol 1983; 55:105–112.

214. Tibes U, Hemmer B, Boning D. Heart rate and ventilation in relation to venous K^+, osmolality, pH, P_{CO_2}, P_{O_2}, orthophosphate, and lactate at transition from rest to exercise in athletes and non-athletes. Eur J Appl Physiol 1977; 36:127–140.

215. Rybicki KJ, Waldrop TG, Kaufman MP. Increasing gracilis muscle interstitial potassium concentration stimulates group III and IV afferents. J Appl Physiol 1984; 58:936–941.

216. Yamamoto WS. Looking at the regulation of ventilation as a signalling process. In: Dempsey JA, Reid CE, eds. Muscular Exercise and the Lung. Madison: University of Wisconsin Press, 1977:137–149.

217. Asmussen E, Nielsen M. Studies on the regulation of respiration in heavy work. Acta Physiol Scand 1946; 12:171–188.

218. Nielson M, Asmussen E. Humoral and nervous control of breathing in exercise. In: Cunningham DJC, Lloyd BB, eds. The Regulation of Human Respiration. Philadelphia: Davis, 1963:504–513.

219. Green HJ, Hughson RL, Orr GW, Ranney DA. Anaerobic threshold, blood lactate and muscle metabolites in progressive exercise. J Appl Physiol 1983; 54:1032–1038.

220. Hagenhauser GJT, Sutton JR, Jones NL. Effect of glycogen depletion on the ventilatory response to exercise. J Appl Physiol 1983; 54:470–474.

221. Hughes EF, Turner SC, Brooks GA. Effect of glycogen depletion and pedaling speed on "anaerobic threshold." J Appl Physiol 1982; 52:1598–1607.

222. Hagberg JM, Coyle EF, Carrol JE, Miller JM, Martin WH, Brooke MH. Exercise hyperventilation in patients with McArdle's disease. J Appl Physiol 1982; 52: 991–994.

223. Paterson DJ, Friedland JS, Bascom DA, Clement ED, Cunningham DA, Painter R, Robbins PA. Changes in arterial K^+ and ventilation during exercise in normal subjects and subjects with McArdle's syndrome. J Physiol (Lond) 1990; 429: 339–348.

224. Coles DR, Duff F, Shepherd WHT, Whelan RF. The effect on respiration of infusions of adrenaline and noradrenaline into the carotid and vertebral arteries in man. Br J Pharmacol 1956; 11:346–350.

225. Cunningham DJC, Hey EN, Lloyd BB. The effect of intravenous infusion of noradrenaline on the respiratory response to carbon dioxide. Q J Exp Physiol 1958; 43:394–399.

226. Euler USV, Hellner S. Excretion of noradrenaline and adrenaline in muscular work. Acta Physiol Scand 1952; 26:183–191.

227. Flandrois R, Favien R, Pequignot JM. Role of adrenaline in gas exchanges and respiratory control in the dog at rest and exercise. Respir Physiol 1977; 30:291–303.

228. Haggendal J, Harley LH, Saltin B. Arterial noradrenaline concentration during exercise in relation to the relative work loads. Scand J Clin Lab Invest 1970; 26: 337–342.

229. Whelan RF, Young IM. The effect of adrenaline and noradrenaline infusions on respiration in man. Br J Pharmacol 1953; 8:98–102.

230. Cunningham DJC, Spurr D, Lloyd BB. The drive to ventilation from arterial chemoreceptors in hypoxic exercise. In: Torrance RW, ed. Arterial Chemoreceptors. Oxford: Blackwell, 1968:301–323.

231. Folgering H, Ponte J, Sadig T. Adrenergic mechanisms and chemoreception in the carotid body of the cat and rabbit. J Physiol 1982; 325:1–21.

232. Burger RE, Estavillo JA, Kumar P, Nye PLG, Patterson DJ. Effects of potassium, oxygen, and carbon dioxide on the steady state discharge of cat carotid body chemoreceptors. J Physiol 1988; 401:519–531.

233. Bannister RG, Cunningham DJC. The effects on the respiration and performance during exercise of the addition of oxygen to the inspired air. J Physiol 1954; 125: 118–137.

234. Knill RL, Clement JL. Ventilatory responses to acute metabolic acidemia in humans awake, sedated, and anesthetized with halothane. Anesthesiology 1985; 62: 733–745.

235. Bainton CR. Canine ventilation after acid-base infusions, exercise, and carotid body denervation. J Appl Physiol Respir Environ Exercise Physiol 1978; 44(1):28–35.

236. Kaehny WD, Jackson JT. Respiratory response to HCL acidosis in dogs after carotid body denervation. J Appl Physiol 1979; 46:1138–1142.

237. Nattie EE. Ventilation during acute HCL infusion in intact and chemodenervated conscious rabbits. Respir Physiol 1983; 54:97–107.

238. Steinbrook RA, Javaheri S, Gabel RA, Donovan JC, Leih DE, Fencl V. Regulation of chemodenervated goats in acute metabolic acidosis. Respir Physiol 1984; 56:51–60.

239. Teppema LJP, Barts WJA, Folgering HT, Evers JAM. Effects of respiratory and (isocapnic) metabolic arterial acid-base disturbances on medullary extracellular fluid pH and ventilation in cats. Respir Physiol 1983; 53:379–395.

240. Smith CA, Saupe KW, Henderson KS, Xi L, Chow CM, Dempsey JA. Contribution of carotid body hypocapnia to unstable breathing during sleep. Am Rev Respir Dis 1993; 147:A952.

241. Daristotle L, Bersssenbrugge AD, Engwall MJ, Bisgard GE. The effects of carotid body hypocapnia on ventilation in goats. Respir Physiol 1990; 79:123–136.

242. Somjen GG. The missing error signal—regulation beyond negative feedback. News Physiol Sci 1992; 7:184–185.

243. Smith CA, Ainsworth DM, Henderson KS, Dempsey JA. Differential responses of expiratory muscles to chemical stimuli in awake dogs. J Appl Physiol 1989; 66:384–391.

244. De Troyer A, Gilmartin JJ, Ninane V. Abdominal muscle use during breathing in unanesthetized dogs. J Appl Physiol 1989; 66:20–27.

245. Brice AG, Forster HV, Pan LG, Lowry RF, Murphy CL. Respiratory muscle electromyogram responses to acute hypoxia in awake ponies. J Appl Physiol 1990; 68:1024–1032.

246. Koterba AM, Kosch PC, Beech J, Whitlock T. Breathing strategy of the adult horse (*Equus caballus*) at rest. J Appl Physiol 1988; 64:337–346.

247. Hall LW, Aziz HA, Groenendyk J, Keates H, Rex MAE. Electromyography of some respiratory muscles in the horse. Res Vet Sci 1991; 50:328–333.

248. Ainsworth DM, Smith CA, Eicker SW, Henderson KS, Dempsey JA. The effects of locomotion on respiratory muscle activity in the awake dog. Respir Physiol 1989; 78:145–162.

249. Ledlie JF, Pack A, Fishman AP. Effects of hypercapnia and hypoxia on abdominal expiratory nerve activity. J Appl Physiol 1983; 55:1614–1622.

250. Ainsworth DM, Smith CA, Eicker SW, Henderson KS, Dempsey JA. The effects of chemical versus locomotory stimuli on respiratory muscle activity in the awake dog. Respir Physiol 1989; 78:163–176.

251. Sharratt MT, Henke KG, Pegelow DF, Aaron E, Dempsey J. Exercise-induced changes in functional residual capacity. Respir Physiol 1988; 70:313–326.

252. Gutting SM, Forster HV, Lowry TF, Brice AG, Pan LG. Respiratory muscle recruitment in awake ponies during exercise and CO_2 inhalation. Respir Physiol 1991; 86:315–332.

253. Grillner S, Nillson J, Thorstensson A. Intra-abdominal pressure changes during natural movements in man. Acta Physiol Scand 1978; 103:275–283.

254. Manohar M. Blood flow to the respiratory and limb muscles and to abdominal organs during maximal exertion in ponies. J Physiol 1986; 377:25–35.

255. Manohar M. Costal vs. crural diaphragmatic blood flow during submaximal and near-maximal exercise in ponies. J Appl Physiol 1988; 65:1514–1519.

256. Manohar M. Inspiratory and expiratory muscle perfusion in maximally exercised ponies. J Appl Physiol 1990; 68:544–548.

257. Bishop B. Reflex control of abdominal muscles during positive-pressure breathing. J Appl Physiol 1962; 19:224–232.

258. De Troyer A, Ninane V. Effect of posture on expiratory muscle use during breathing in the dog. Respir Physiol 1987; 67:311–322.

259. Farkas GS, Baer RE, Estenne M, De Troyer A. Mechanical role of expiratory muscles during breathing in upright dogs. J Appl Physiol 1988; 64:1060–1067.

260. Ainsworth DM, Smith CA, Johnson BD, Eicker SW, Henderson KS, Dempsey JA. Vagal contributions to respiratory muscle activity during eupnea in the awake dog. J Appl Physiol 1992; 72:1355–1361.

261. Ainsworth DM, Smith CA, Johnson BD, Eicker SW, Henderson KS, Dempsey JA. Vagal modulation of respiratory muscle activity in awake dogs during exercise and hypercapnia. J Appl Physiol 1992; 72:1362–1367.

262. Pisarri TE, Yu J, Coleridge HM, Coleridge JCG. Background activity in pulmonary vagal C-fibres and its effects on breathing. Respir Physiol 1986; 64:29–43.

263. Gutting SM, Forster HV, Brice AG, Lowry TF, Pan LG, Murphy CL. The pattern of respiratory muscle activity during exercise in normal and hilar nerve denervated ponies. FASEB J 1988; 2:A1297 (abstract).

264. Decima EE, Euler C von, Thoden U. Intercostal-to-phrenic reflexes in the spinal cat. Acta Physiol Scand 1969; 75:568–579.

265. Remmers JE. Extra-segmental reflexes derived from intercostal afferents: phrenic and laryngeal responses. J Physiol 1973; 233:45–62.

266. Shannon R, Bolser DC, Lindsey BG. Medullary expiratory activity: influence of intercostal tendon organs and muscle spindle endings. J Appl Physiol 1987; 62: 1057–1062.

267. Bolser DC, Lindsey BG, Shannon R. Medullary inspiratory activity: influence of intercostal tendon organs and muscle spindle endings. J Appl Physiol 1987; 62: 1046–1056.

268. Hussain SNA, Magder S, Chatillon A, Roussos C. Chemical activation of thin-fiber phrenic afferents: respiratory responses. J Appl Physiol 1990; 69:1002–1011.

269. Bechbache RR, Duffin J. The entrainment of breathing frequency by exercise rhythm. J Physiol (Lond) 1977; 272:553–561.

270. Bramble DM, Carrier DR. Running and breathing in mammals. Science 1983; 219: 251–256.

271. Art T, Desmecht D, Armory H, Lekeux P. Synchronization of locomotion and respiration in trotting ponies. J Vet Med Assoc 1990; 37:95–103.

272. Attenburrow DP. Time relationships between the respiratory cycle and the limb cycle in the horse. Eq Vet J 1982; 14:69–72.

273. Bramble DM, Jenkins FA. Mammalian thoracic kinematics during locomotor-respiratory integration. Am Zool 1990; 30:74A (abstract).

274. Dumont JPC, Robertson RM. Neuronal circuits: an evolutionary perspective. Science 1986; 233:849–852.

275. Tenney SM, Leiter JC. The control of breathing: an uninhibited survey from the perspective of comparative physiology. Chapter 1, this volume.

276. Bayly WM, Hodgson DR, Schulz DA, Dempsey JA, Gollnick PD. Exercise-induced hypercapnia in the horse. J Appl Physiol 1989; 67:1958–1966.

277. Bye PT, Esau SA, Walley KR, Macklem PT, Pardy RL. Ventilatory muscles during exercise in air and oxygen in normal men. J Appl Physiol 1984; 56:464–471.

278. Grimby G, Goldman M, Mead J. Respiratory muscle action inferred from ribcage and abdominal V-P partitioning. J Appl Physiol 1976; 41:739–751.

279. Henke KG, Sharratt M, Pegelow D, Dempsey JA. Regulation of end-expiratory lung volume during exercise. J Appl Physiol 1988; 64:135–146.

280. Johnson BD, Babcock MA, Suman OE, Dempsey JA. Exercise induced diaphragmatic fatigue in healthy humans. J Physiol (Lond) 1993; 460:385–405.

281. Jammes Y, Buchler B, Delpierre S, Rasidakis A, Grimaud C, Roussos C. Phrenic afferents and their role in inspiratory control. J Appl Physiol 1986; 60:854–860.

282. Dempsey JA, Johnson BD, Saupe KW. Adaptations and limitations in the pulmonary system during exercise. Chest 1990; 97:815–875.

283. Johnson BD, Saupe KW, Dempsey JA. Mechanical constraints on exercise hyperpnea in endurance athletes. J Appl Physiol 1992; 73:874–886.

284. Klas JV, Dempsey JA. Voluntary versus reflex regulation of maximal exercise flow:volume loops. Am Rev Respir Dis 1983; 127:725–734.

285. Leblanc P, Summers MD, Inman NL, Jones EJ, Campbell M, Killian KJ. Inspiratory muscles during exercise: a problem of supply and demand. J Appl Physiol 1988; 65: 2482–2489.

286. Ohki M, Hasegawa M, Kurita N, Wantanbe I. Effects of exercise on nasal resistance and nasal blood flow. Acta Otolaryngol (Stockh) 1987; 104:328–333.

287. Wheatley JR, Amis TC, Engel LA. Oro-nasal partitioning of ventilation during exercise in man. J Appl Physiol 1991; 71:546–551.

288. England SJ, Bartlett D. Changes in respiratory movements of the human vocal chords during hyperpnea. J Appl Physiol 1982; 52:780–785.

289. Kaufman MP. Afferents from limb skeletal muscle. Chapter 13, this volume.

290. Mathew OP. Control of upper airway muscle activity in regulation of breathing. Chapter 11, this volume.

291. Winning AJ, Hamilton RD, Shea S, Knott C, Guz JA. The effect of airway anesthesia on the control of breathing and the sensation of breathlessness in man. Clin Sci 1985; 68:215–225.

292. Aaron EA, Johnson BD, Pegelow D, Dempsey JA. The oxygen cost of exercise hyperpnea: implications for performance. J Appl Physiol 1992; 72:1818–1825.

293. Levine S, Henson D. Low-frequency diaphragmatic fatigue in spontaneously breathing humans. J Appl Physiol 1988; 64:672–680.

294. Hussain SNA, Pardy RL, Dempsey JA. Mechanical impedance as determinant of inspiratory neural drive during exercise in humans. J Appl Physiol 1985; 59(2): 365–375.

295. Gallagher CG, Younes M. Effect of pressure assist on ventilation and respiratory mechanics in heavy exercise. J Appl Physiol 1989; 66:1824–1837.

296. Ross KA, Thurlbeck WM. Lung growth in newborn guinea pigs: Effects of endurance exercise. Respir Physiol 1992; 89:353–364.

297. Hoppeler H, Kayar SR, Claassen H, Uhlmann E, Karas RH. Adaptive variation in the mammalian respiratory system in relation to energetic demand. III. Skeletal muscles: setting the demand for oxyge. Respir Physiol 1987; 69:27–46.

298. Johnson BD, Reddan WG, Seow KC, Dempsey JA. Mechanical constraints on exercise hyperpnea in an aging population. Am Rev Respir Dis 1991; 143:968–977.

299. Johnson B, Dempsey J. Demand vs. capacity in the aging pulmonary system. In: Holloszy J, ed. Exercise and Sport Science Review. Philadelphia: Williams & Wilkins, 1991: 171–210.

300. Clanton TL, Dixon GF, Drake J, Gadek JE. Effects of swim training on lung volumes and inspiratory muscle conditioning. J Appl Physiol 1987; 62(1):39–46.

301. Powers SK, Criswell D, Lawler J, Martin D, Ji LL, Herb R, Dudley G. Regional differences in training-induced alterations in diaphragmatic oxidative and anti-oxidant enzyme activity. Respir Physiol 1994; 95:227–237.

302. Powers S, Criswell D, Lieu F-K, Dodd S, Silverman H. Diaphragmatic fiber type specific adaptation to endurance exercise. Respir Physiol 1992; 89:195–207.

303. Robinson EP, Kjeldgaard JM. Improvement in ventilatory muscle function with running. J Appl Physiol Respir Environ Exercise Physiol 1982; 52(6):1400–1406.

304. Art T, Anderson L, Woakes AJ, Roberts C, Butler PJ, Snow DH, Lekeux P.

Mechanics of breathing during strenuous exercise in thoroughbred horses. Respir Physiol 1990; 82:270–294.

305. Butler PJ, Woakes AJ, Anderson LS, Roberts CA, Martin DJ. Stride length and respiratory tidal volume in exercising thoroughbred horses. Respir Physiol 1993; 93:51–56.

306. Casaburi R, Storer TW, Wasserman K. Mediation of reduced ventilatory response to exercise after endurance training. J Appl Physiol 1987; 63:1533–1538.

307. Taylor R, Jones NL. The reduction by training of CO_2 output during exercise. Eur J Cardiol 1979; 9:53–62.

AUTHOR INDEX

Italic numbers give the page on which the complete reference is listed.

SUBJECT INDEX

A

Abdominal motion, 984–987
Abdominal motoneurons (see
  Motoneurons)
Acclimatization, 1025
  to hypoxia, 636–649
  to long-term hypoxia, 646–649
  to short-term hypoxia, 636–646
    central chemoreceptor mechanisms,
      637–639
    CNS mechanisms, 639–640
    peripheral chemoreceptor
      mechanisms, 640–645
    time course, 636
Acetazolamide, 478–480, 493, 496
Acetylcholine (cholinergic cells), 702,
  990–993
Acetylcholinesterase, 489–490
Acidosis, 473, 486, 544, 548, 1016,
  1031
Adaptation, 556–557, 563–568, 570–
  573
  to airway occlusion, 556–558, 564–
    565, 571
  to bronchospasm, 567–568
  to dense gas breathing, 566–567

[Adaptation]
  to loaded breathing, 563–568, 570–
    573
Adenosine, 622–623, 634
β-Adrenergic pathways, 587
Afferent connections, 325, 330
Afferent fibers, 544–571, 573
  in abdominal nerve, 549, 555, 558,
    561, 570
  activation procedures, 544–555, 559–
    565, 567–568, 571
  blocking agents, 558–559, 565–567
  in intercostal nerve, 549, 553–554,
    556, 561, 570
  in limb muscle nerve, 544–546, 553,
    561, 569
  in phrenic nerve, 547, 550, 555, 573
  in vagus nerve, 556, 559–561, 563–
    568, 569
Afferent nerves
  intercostal, 930
  phrenic, 930
  vagal, 930–932, 936
Age effects, 834, 849
Airway smooth muscle, 585
Airway tone, 556–558
Alcohol ingestion, 830

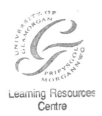
Learning Resources
Centre